Clinical Manual of Contact Lenses
FOURTH EDITION

Clinical Manual of Contact Lenses

FOURTH EDITION

Edward S. Bennett, OD, MSEd, FAAO
Professor of Optometry
Assistant Dean for Student Services
and Alumni Relations
Co-Chief, Contact Lens Service
Director of Student Services
College of Optometry
University of Missouri–St. Louis
St. Louis, Missouri

Vinita Allee Henry, OD, FAAO
Clinical Professor of Optometry
Co-Chief, Contact Lens Service
Director of Clinical Operations & Residencies
College of Optometry
University of Missouri–St. Louis
St. Louis, Missouri

Wolters Kluwer | Lippincott Williams & Wilkins
Health
Philadelphia • Baltimore • New York • London
Buenos Aires • Hong Kong • Sydney • Tokyo

Acquisition Editor: Ryan Shaw
Product Manager: Kate Marshall
Vendor Manager: Bridgett Dougherty
Senior Manufacturing Coordinator: Beth Welsh
Marketing Manager: Alexander Burns
Designer: Teresa Mallon
Production Service: S4Carlisle Publishing Services

© 2014 by LIPPINCOTT WILLIAMS & WILKINS, a WOLTERS KLUWER business
Two Commerce Square
2001 Market Street
Philadelphia, PA 19103 USA
LWW.com

Third Edition © 2009 by Lippincott Williams & Wilkins
Second Edition © 2000 by Lippincott Williams & Wilkins
First Edition © 1994 by Lippincott Williams & Wilkins

All rights reserved. This book is protected by copyright. No part of this book may be reproduced in any form by any means, including photocopying, or utilized by any information storage and retrieval system without written permission from the copyright owner, except for brief quotations embodied in critical articles and reviews. Materials appearing in this book prepared by individuals as part of their official duties as U.S. government employees are not covered by the above-mentioned copyright.

Printed in China

Library of Congress Cataloging-in-Publication Data

Clinical manual of contact lenses / [edited by] Edward S. Bennett, Vinita Allee Henry.—4th ed.
   p. ; cm.
Includes bibliographical references and index.
ISBN 978-1-4511-7532-5 (alk. paper)
I. Bennett, Edward S. II. Henry, Vinita Allee.
[DNLM: 1. Contact Lenses. WW 355]
RE977.C6
617.7'523—dc23

2013010440

Care has been taken to confirm the accuracy of the information presented and to describe generally accepted practices. However, the authors, editors, and publisher are not responsible for errors or omissions or for any consequences from application of the information in this book and make no warranty, expressed or implied, with respect to the currency, completeness, or accuracy of the contents of the publication. Application of the information in a particular situation remains the professional responsibility of the practitioner.

   The authors, editors, and publisher have exerted every effort to ensure that drug selection and dosage set forth in this text are in accordance with current recommendations and practice at the time of publication. However, in view of ongoing research, changes in government regulations, and the constant flow of information relating to drug therapy and drug reactions, the reader is urged to check the package insert for each drug for any change in indications and dosage and for added warnings and precautions. This is particularly important when the recommended agent is a new or infrequently employed drug.

   Some drugs and medical devices presented in the publication have Food and Drug Administration (FDA) clearance for limited use in restricted research settings. It is the responsibility of the health care provider to ascertain the FDA status of each drug or device planned for use in their clinical practice.

To purchase additional copies of this book, call our customer service department at (800) 638-3030 or fax orders to (301) 223-2320. International customers should call (301) 223-2300.

Visit Lippincott Williams & Wilkins on the Internet: at LWW.com. Lippincott Williams & Wilkins customer service representatives are available from 8:30 am to 6 pm, EST.

10 9 8 7 6 5 4 3 2

To our families for their devotion and encouragement:

Jean Bennett OD, Matt, Josh, and Emily

ESB

Sam, Amanda, Emily, Elizabeth, and my parents,
Vincel and Anita Allee

VAH

Contributing Authors

Joseph T. Barr, OD, MS, FAAO
Professor of Optometry Emeritus
College of Optometry
The Ohio State University
Columbus, Ohio
Vice President, Global Clinical and
 Medical Affairs and Professional
 Services Vision Care
Private Practice
Rochester, New York

Carolyn G. Begley, OD, MS, FAAO
Professor
School of Optometry
Indiana University
Bloomington, Indiana

William J. Benjamin, OD, MS, PhD, FAAO
Professor
University of Alabama at Birmingham
 School of Optometry
Birmingham, Alabama

Edward S. Bennett, OD, MSEd, FAAO
Assistant Dean for Student Services
 and Alumni Relations
Co-Chief, Contact Lens Service
Director of Student Services
College of Optometry
University of Missouri–St. Louis
St. Louis, Missouri

Dennis Burger, OD, FAAO
Clinical Professor
School of Optometry
University of California
Berkeley, California

J. Bart Campbell, OD, FAAO
Chair, Department of Optometric Education
Southern College of Optometry
Memphis, Tennessee

Carmen Castellano, OD, FAAO
Adjunct Assistant Professor
College of Optometry
University of Missouri-St. Louis
The Koetting Associates
St. Louis, Missouri

Larry J. Davis, OD, FAAO
Dean and Associate Professor
College of Optometry
University of Missouri–St. Louis
St. Louis, Missouri

John de Brabander, PhD
University Eye Clinic Maastricht
The Netherlands

Julie Ott DeKinder, OD, FAAO
Associate Clinical Professor of
 Optometry
College of Optometry
University of Missouri–St. Louis
St. Louis, Missouri

Gregory W. DeNaeyer, OD, FAAO, FSCS
Arena Eye Surgeons
Columbus, Ohio

Olivia K. Do, OD, FAAO
Assistant Professor of Optometry
Southern California College of Optometry
Fullerton, California

Contributing Authors

Kathryn Dumbleton, BSc (Hons), MSc, MCOptom, FAAO, FBLA
Head of Clinical Logistics
Centre for Contact Lens Research
Adjunct Associate Professor
School of Optometry
University of Waterloo
Waterloo, Ontario

S. Barry Eiden, OD, FAAO
President and Medical Director
North Suburban Vision Consultants, Ltd.
Deerfield, Illinois
President and Co-Founder
EyeVis Eye and Vision Research Institute
Assistant Clinical Professor
Department of Ophthalmology Cornea and Contact Lens Service
University of Illinois Medical Center
Chicago, Illinois

Arthur B. Epstein, OD, FAAO, FABCO, FBCLA
Phoenix Eye Care, PLLC
Phoenix, Arizona
Adjunct Clinical Associate Professor
Midwestern University
Arizona College of Optometry Eye Institute
Glendale, Arizona

Vinita Allee Henry, OD, FAAO
Clinical Professor of Optometry
Co-Chief, Contact Lens Service
Director of Clinical Operations & Residencies
College of Optometry
University of Missouri–St. Louis
St. Louis, Missouri

Cary M. Herzberg, OD, FAIO
President, International Academy of Orthokeratology
President, Orthokeratology Academy of America
Aurora, Illinois

John Mark Jackson, OD, FAAO
Associate Professor of Optometry
Southern College of Optometry
Memphis, Tennessee

Jason Jedlicka, OD, FAAO, FSLS
Cornea and Contact Lens Institute of Minnesota
Edina, Minnesota

Lyndon Jones, PhD, FCOptom, DipCLP, DipOrth, FAAO, FIACLE
Centre for Contact Lens Research
School of Optometry
University of Waterloo
Waterloo, Ontario

Frans H. M. Jongsma
University Eye Clinic Maastricht
Maastricht, the Netherlands

Matthew Kauffman, OD
Private Practice
Family Vision Solutions and Specialty Contact Lens Center
Houston, Texas

Eric Kawulok, OD
Casey Eye Institute–Waterfront
Portland, Oregon

Beth T. Kinoshita, OD, FAAO
Assistant Professor
Pacific University College of Optometry
Forest Grove, Oregon

Randy Kojima, FAAO, FOAA
Research Scientist and Clinical Instructor
Pacific University College of Optometry
Forest Grove, Oregon

Nicky Lai, OD, MS, FAAO
Associate Professor of Clinical Optometry
Chief, Contact Lens Service
College of Optometry
The Ohio State University
Columbus, Ohio

Dawn Y. Lam, MS, OD, FAAO
Assistant Professor
Southern California College of Optometry
Fullerton, California

Matthew Lampa, OD, FAAO
Assistant Professor
Pacific University College of Optometry
Forest Grove, Oregon

Kimberly A. Layfield, OD
Private Practice
St. Louis, Missouri

Derek J. Louie, MSc, OD, FAAO
Assistant Professor, Ophthalmology
Casey Eye Institute
Oregon Health & Sciences University
Portland, Oregon

Ron Melton, OD, FAAO
Private Practice
Charlotte, North Carolina
Adjunct Faculty
Salus University, Pennsylvania College
  of Optometry
Elkins Park, Pennsylvania
Adjunct Faculty
Indiana University School of Optometry
Bloomington, Indiana

Chandra V. Mickles, OD, MS
Clinical Assistant Professor, Optometry
University of the Incarnate Word
Rosenberg School of Optometry
San Antonio, Texas

Bruce W. Morgan, OD, FAAO
Chief of Cornea and Contact
  Lens Service
Director of Residencies
Michigan College of Optometry,
  Ferris State University
Big Rapids, Michigan

Clarke D. Newman, OD, FAAO
Adjunct Assistant Professor
University of Houston
College of Optometry
Plaza Vision Center
Dallas, Texas

Keith Parker
President
Advanced Vision Technologies
Golden, Colorado

Judyith W. Perrigin, MT (ASCP), OD, FAAO
Professor
University of Houston
College of Optometry
Houston, Texas

Thomas G. Quinn, OD, MS, FAAO
Partner
Drs. Quinn, Quinn and Associates
Clinical Assistant Professor
Ohio University College of Medicine
Athens, Ohio

Marjorie J. Rah, OD, PhD, FAAO
Manager
Global Medical Affairs, Vision Care
Bausch + Lomb Inc.
Rochester, New York

Terry Scheid, OD, FAAO
Associate Clinical Professor
Diplomate AAO Cornea, CL, and Refractive
  Surgery Section
State University of New York
New York, New York

Muriel M. Schornack, OD, FAAO, FSLS
Consultant
Department of Ophthalmology
Mayo Clinic
Assistant Professor of Ophthalmology
Mayo College of Medicine
Rochester, Minnesota

Glenda Secor, OD, FAAO, Dip CCLRT
Huntington Beach, California

Christine W. Sindt, OD, FAAO
Director, Contact Lens Service
Associate Professor, Clinical Ophthalmology
University of Iowa Hospitals & Clinics
Iowa City, Iowa

**Luigina Sorbara, MSc, FAAO, FBCLA,
  Dip CCLRT**
Associate Professor
Head, Contact Lens Clinic
Researcher, CCLR
School of Optometry and Vision Science
University of Waterloo
Waterloo, Ontario

Loretta Szczotka-Flynn, OD, PhD, FAAO
Associate Professor of Ophthalmology
Department of Ophthalmology
Case Western Reserve University
Cleveland, Ohio

Randall Thomas, OD, MPH, FAAO
Private Practice
Concord, North Carolina

Eef C. J. van der Worp, PhD
University Eye Clinic Maastricht
Maastricht, the Netherlands

Heidi Wagner, OD, MPH, FAAO
Professor of Optometry
Nova Southeastern University
Health Professions Division
College of Optometry
Fort Lauderdale, Florida

Jeffrey J. Walline, OD, PhD, FAAO
Associate Professor
College of Optometry
The Ohio State University
Columbus, Ohio

Ronald K. Watanabe, OD, FAAO
Associate Professor of Optometry
Department of Specialty
  and Advanced Care
The New England College
  of Optometry
Boston, Massachusetts

Stephanie L. Woo, OD, FAAO
Havasu Eye Center
Lake Havasu, Arizona

Preface

Clinical Manual of Contact Lenses addresses a wide variety of clinical topics, including rigid gas-permeable lens design and fitting, soft lens problem solving, astigmatic management, and bifocal correction. It is written so the practitioner can easily locate a topic and information about that topic without having to read an entire chapter. Each chapter concludes with sample cases that reinforce and demonstrate the practical nature of the chapter's topic. Nomograms and proficiency checklists also summarize and emphasize the important points in the chapters.

The purpose of this book is to help students and practitioners fit, evaluate, and troubleshoot contact lenses, especially specialty contact lens designs. We hope this strictly clinical text will aid in everyday fitting situations and be an easy reference source to answer questions that might arise during the evaluation of a contact lens patient. It is written generically to be current for many years to come.

In this fourth edition of the *Clinical Manual of Contact Lenses*, we have sought to not only update and revise this manual, but also introduce new chapters on exciting new development in the field of contact lenses. To this extent, the chapter on scleral lenses by renowned experts Drs. Greg DeNaeyer, Jason Jedlicka, and Muriel Schornack is a must-read. Likewise, a new chapter on the contact lens fitting of young people addresses an important area that is certainly expanding, and we are fortunate to have Drs. Jeff Walline, Christine Sindt, and Marjorie Rah authoring it. A much-needed optics chapter with important clinical background information has been added to complement Dr. Joe Benjamin's other chapter pertaining to optics formulas and problems. Of course, the information pertaining to clinical management in such areas as keratoconus, postsurgical, orthokeratology, presbyopia, extended wear, and correction of astigmatism has been greatly revised and updated —as much as possible—to be current for the next several years. A very popular chapter in the third edition that was updated for this edition is the one pertaining to the management of contact lens complications by two foremost experts in the field, Drs. Ron Melton and Randall Thomas.

Both of us have been active in the Association of Contact Lens Educators (AOCLE), and we are honored that many educators involved with this organization have assisted with chapters in this text.

Edward S. Bennett, OD, MSEd
Vinita Allee Henry, OD

Acknowledgements

It is not possible to author a clinical text without it being a collaborative effort. We would like to first acknowledge our contributors, without whom this text would not have been possible. They include Joe Barr, Carolyn Begley, Denny Burger, Joe Benjamin, Bart Campbell, Carmen Castellano, Larry Davis, John de Brabender, Julie DeKinder, Greg DeNaeyer, Olivia Do, Kathy Dumbleton, Barry Eiden, Art Epstein, Cary Herzberg, John Mark Jackson, Jason Jedlicka, Frans Jongsma, Lyndon Jones, Eric Kawulok, Matt Kauffman, Beth Kinoshita, Randy Kojima, Dawn Lam, Matt Lampa, Nicky Lai, Kim Layfield, Derek Louie, Ron Melton, Chandra Micklas, Bruce Morgan, Clarke Newman, Keith Parker, Judy Perrigin, Tom Quinn, Marjie Rah, Terry Scheid, Muriel Schornack, Glenda Secor, Christine Sindt, Gina, Loretta Szczotka-Flynn, Randall Thomas, Stephanie Woo, Eef van der Worp, Heidi Wagner, Jeff Walline, and Ron Watanabe.

We appreciate the assistance of our graphical artist, Janice White for her contributions to this text. We would also like to acknowledge cases submitted by the 2012–2013 class of Cornea and Contact Lens residents. The support of Lippincott Williams & Wilkins is greatly appreciated.

The support of our families, and especially our spouses Jean and Sam, made it possible for us to devote the time necessary to make this text as timely and clinically applicable as humanly possible.

This year marks the 30th year of our working together. It has been a privilege and a blessing to work as a team. Only the most fortunate have the opportunity to have a professor become a mentor, colleague, and close friend and—conversely—have a student become a resident, co-worker, exceptional role model, and close friend. This book is a celebration of that friendship.

Finally, we would like to acknowledge all practitioners who believe that contact lenses, and, in particular, specialty lens designs, have an important application in their respective practices. We hope this text serves as a beneficial guide in helping you build your contact lens practice as well as for our students who will be the future of our profession.

Contents

Contributing Authors vi
Preface x
Acknowledgements xi

SECTION I. Introduction 1
1 Preliminary Evaluation 2
2 Optical Considerations in Contact Lens Practice 30

SECTION II. Gas-Permeable Lenses 53
3 Corneal Topography 54
4 Gas-Permeable Material Selection 89
5 Gas-Permeable Lens Design, Fitting, and Evaluation 112
6 Gas-Permeable Lens Care and Patient Education 157
7 Verification of Gas-Permeable Lenses 187
8 Gas-Permeable Lens Problem Solving 203
9 Modification of Gas-Permeable Lenses 229

SECTION III. Soft Lenses 251
10 Soft Lens Material Selection 252
11 Soft Lens Fitting and Evaluation 270
12 Soft Lens Care and Patient Education 287
13 Soft Lens Problem Solving 313

SECTION IV. Challenging Cases 343
14 Correction of Astigmatism 344
15 Bifocal Contact Lenses 395

16 Overnight Contact Lens Wear 435

17 Aphakia 473

18 Children and Contact Lenses 497

19 Keratoconus 518

20 Postsurgical Contact Lens Fitting 578

21 Scleral Lenses 609

22 Orthokeratology 648

23 Management of Contact Lens-Associated
    or Lens-Induced Pathology 670

24 Contact Lens Practice Management 691

Appendices 702
Index 707

Section I

Introduction

Chapter 1

Preliminary Evaluation

Edward S. Bennett, Judith M. Perrigin, Ronald K. Watanabe, and Carolyn G. Begley

PURPOSE

A comprehensive preliminary evaluation is the essential first step in the contact-lens-fitting process. It is extremely important for the practitioner to evaluate every potential contact lens wearer to determine whether the patient is suitable for contact lens wear. This will minimize the risk of future failures or problems because of poor patient selection. If the patient is deemed a good candidate, the information obtained during the prefitting examination will help determine the most appropriate lens material, lens design, wearing time, and care regimen. It also serves as baseline data with which changes caused by contact lens wear can be compared.

HISTORY

A good history includes the patient's reasons for wanting to wear contact lenses, ocular and medical histories, and any previous contact lens history. The history should guide the clinician in determining which tests to perform and the expected results for those tests. It should also contribute to the fitter's recommendations on contact lens types, care regimens, and wearing schedules.

Reasons for Contact Lens Wear

1. Cosmesis. Many patients do not like their appearance in glasses. Others may have corneal scars or other disfigurements that can be masked by standard or custom-tinted lenses.
2. Inconvenience of glasses. They may be uncomfortable, get misplaced or broken, and have to be cleaned.
3. Improved vision. Patients with high ametropias, anisometropia, high astigmatism, keratoconus, corneal trauma, corneal distortion, and poor refractive surgery outcomes benefit visually from contact lenses.
4. Sports and recreation. Most athletes, both professional and recreational, benefit from the wider field of vision provided by contact lenses. Tints may be customized for specific sports to improve contrast and tracking. Scleral and hybrid lenses are available for crisp optics and low risk of loss or decentration during sports activities.
5. Occupation. In addition to athletes, individuals in the performing arts benefit greatly from contact lens wear. Celebrities, politicians, and others in the public eye may prefer their cosmetic appearance in contact lenses. However, contact lenses are contraindicated for patients who work in dusty or dirty environments (e.g., coal miners, sanitation workers) where debris and particulate matter may become trapped under the lens. In addition, individuals such as laboratory workers and hairdressers who work around noxious fumes are borderline contact lens candidates because of the possibility of a chemical keratitis and lens surface contamination. Some workers such as plumbers and automobile mechanics may experience difficulty cleaning all of the dirt and oils off their hands and may therefore be poor candidates. Other individuals, such as pilots, flight attendants, and video display

terminal operators, may work in low-humidity environments and perform tasks during which blinking is inhibited. These individuals are not contraindicated for contact lens wear, but should be managed as potential dry-eye patients.
6. Vision therapy. Patients may be more accepting of and more compliant in wearing occluder contact lenses than eye patches. These can either be lenses with opaque pupils or very high plus powers.
7. Color vision defects. Patients with color vision defects, particularly red–green, may be able to better discriminate between colors by wearing a red- or magenta-tinted lens in one eye. This may enable them to qualify for certain jobs or activities that were not an option without the lens.

Ocular History

1. Previous correction. Glasses or contact lenses?
2. Strabismus and amblyopia. Significantly reduced acuity? Diplopia? Past treatment?
3. Vision therapy. Binocular vision problems or symptoms?
4. Eye trauma or infections.
5. Eye surgery.
6. Glaucoma or other ocular diseases.

Medical History

The following symptoms and conditions may contraindicate or restrict contact lens wear:

1. Itching, burning, or tearing.
2. Seasonal or chronic allergies.
3. Recurrent ocular infection or inflammation.
4. Sinusitis.
5. Dryness of mouth, eyes, or mucous membranes.
6. Nocturnal lagophthalmos.
7. Convulsions, epilepsy, or fainting spells. Such an individual should be identified as a contact lens wearer.
8. Diabetes. Type 1 diabetics, in particular, may have varying degrees of corneal anesthesia, poor corneal epithelial healing, and the potential to develop neurotrophic keratitis.
9. Collagen vascular disorders. Patients with rheumatoid arthritis and related collagen vascular disorders may have Sjögren's syndrome with keratoconjunctivitis sicca and associated tear film abnormalities. They may chronically use systemic medications, which adversely affect corneal healing and tear film. In addition, handling difficulties may be present.
10. Pregnancy. During pregnancy, particularly the third trimester, the tear film and corneal curvature may change significantly. This usually stabilizes shortly after childbirth. Many patients successfully wear their contact lenses throughout their pregnancy.
11. Psychiatric treatment. Patients on medications to control anxiety, depression, or manic–depressive states should be screened but not necessarily discouraged from contact lens wear, especially if contact lenses would benefit them visually.
12. Thyroid imbalance. Hyperthyroidism, for example, may result in exophthalmos and lack of blinking, which can make contact lens wear difficult because of insufficient tear flow to the cornea.
13. Systemic medications. Certain medications can affect contact lens wear by reducing production of the aqueous phase of the tear film. Patients currently taking any of these medications should either be contraindicated as a contact lens wearer until the medication is discontinued or placed on a limited wearing schedule and carefully monitored. These medications include antihistamines, anticholinergics, some β-adrenergic blockers, tricyclic antidepressants, and oral contraceptives.[1]

14. Topical ocular medications. Patients using topical ocular medications may have restricted wearing times during contact lens wear. Soft lenses absorb the medication and alter drug delivery to the cornea, while gas-permeable (GP) lenses may block access to the cornea or increase contact time for any medication that collects under the lens.[2] In general, topical medications should be instilled 15 to 20 minutes before application of contact lenses or after they are removed.
15. Smokers. Individuals who smoke have been shown to be at greater risk for serious ocular complications and should not be recommended for overnight wear.[3,4]

Contact Lens History

If the patient is currently wearing lenses or has worn them in the past, it is important to determine why the person desires a refit, since this will likely affect what lens material and design will be used. The following questions should be asked:

1. What type of contact lens does (or did) the patient wear? Satisfaction? Symptoms?
2. What is (are) the reason(s) for discontinuing wear or desiring a change?
3. What is the patient's current wearing and lens replacement schedule?
4. What is the patient's care regimen (if appropriate)? Satisfaction? Symptoms? Compliance?
5. Is there a history of a contact lens-related problems or complications in the past?
6. Is there a frequent history of changing lens materials (i.e., "shopper")?

ANATOMIC MEASUREMENTS

Ocular and eyelid dimensions influence the selection of lens type, initial lens parameters, and fitting technique to be used (i.e., lid attachment vs. interpalpebral).

Horizontal Visible Iris Diameter

1. Horizontal visible iris diameter (HVID) provides an approximation of the corneal diameter, and ranges from 10 to 13 mm.
2. HVID is measured with a pupillary distance (PD) ruler tilted inward and read using the horizontal scale (Fig. 1.1).
3. This measurement will help determine overall diameter of the contact lens.

Pupil Diameter

1. Measurement of pupil diameter is similar to that for HVID (Fig. 1.2).
2. Perform this measurement under both normal and dim illumination. The latter will help in determining the optical zone diameter of a GP lens, which should be 1 to 2 mm larger

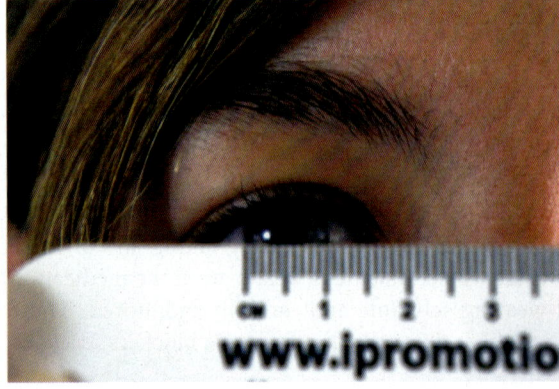

FIGURE 1.1 Proper measurement of corneal diameter.

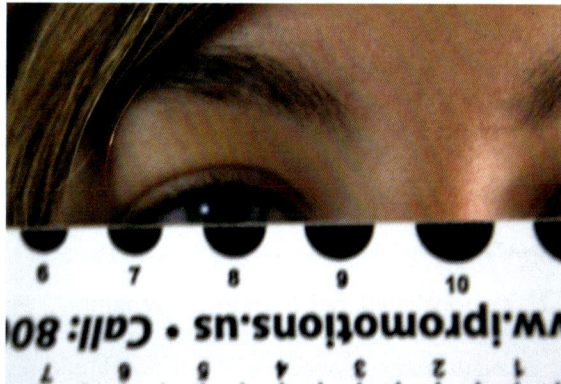

FIGURE 1.2 Measurement of pupil diameter.

than the pupil to minimize flare with vertical blink movement and pupil dilation in dim lighting conditions (e.g., driving at night).
3. Pupil sizes (dim illumination) are categorized as follows:
Small pupil: <5 mm.
Medium pupil: 5 to 7 mm.
Large pupil: >7 mm.
4. For large pupil sizes, select a large optical zone (e.g., >8 mm) or a soft lens with a large optical zone. (Do not assume all soft lenses have large optical zones!)

Palpebral Aperture Height/Lid Position

1. Palpebral aperture height is equal to the vertical measurement of the opening between the upper and lower lids, with the patient gazing straight ahead.
2. Perform this measurement with the patient relaxed and looking straight ahead (Fig. 1.3); also note and record the lid-to-cornea relationship.
3. This procedure will help determine type of lens and lens diameter for optimum patient comfort. A patient with an abnormally large palpebral fissure (e.g., ≥12 mm) will need a large-diameter lens for stability and comfort; likewise, a patient with an abnormally small palpebral fissure (e.g., ≤9 mm) will require a small-diameter lens.
4. Similarly, the position of the lower and upper lid to the limbus should be determined. A patient with a low upper lid that overlaps a large portion of the superior cornea is more likely to have superior lid attachment. Likewise, a patient with a high upper lid that does not overlap much of the superior cornea is more likely to result in an inferior lens position.[5] Lid position may also influence the type of rigid multifocal selected for presbyopic patients.

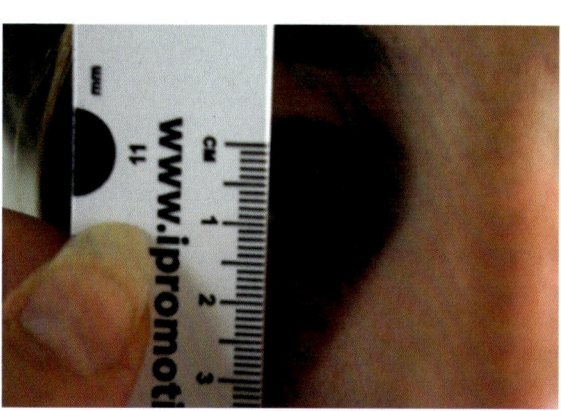

FIGURE 1.3 Measurement of palpebral aperture height.

Lid Tension

1. Lid tension is determined by lid eversion. Grasping the upper lid between the thumb and forefinger and gently pulling outward will give the practitioner an estimation of the lid tension over the globe.
2. Tight lids will pull a lens upward or may squeeze it downward (watermelon seed effect). Loose (heavy, fatty) lids will displace a lens downward.

Blink Rate

1. A normal blink rate is 10 to 15 per minute.
2. Blink rate should be measured without the patient's knowledge; note the amplitude, length, and completeness of a typical blink.
3. If the patient presents with only 10% to 50% completeness of the blink, GP lenses are contraindicated unless a lid attachment or superior fitting relationship exists after the blink.[6] If the patient is a very infrequent blinker, daily disposable soft lenses for social/occasional wear are recommended. On follow-up of patients with incomplete blinks, interpalpebral corneal and conjunctival desiccation should be monitored.

REFRACTIVE INFORMATION

An evaluation of corneal topography and refractive status, with subsequent determination of predicted residual astigmatism, is imperative for proper contact lens design and parameter selection so that the likelihood of future success is maximized.

Corneal Topography

An evaluation of the patient's corneal topography is important in determining the appropriate lens parameters to be diagnostically fit. The base curve radius (BCR) and diameter for both GP and soft lens materials are selected based on corneal curvature measurements.

Corneal Contour

The cornea is an aspheric surface with greatest curvature at the apex and progressively flatter curvature toward the periphery. It is classically visualized as consisting of an essentially spherical central corneal cap (apical zone/apical cap) and a surrounding peripheral zone that gradually flattens. The corneal cap is defined as the area within which the corneal power does not change more than 1 D and is approximately 4 mm in diameter. A more accurate description of the corneal contour is an ellipsoid centrally, with progressively increasing radius of curvature and eccentricity toward the periphery.[7] It is important to understand this corneal shape so that a contact lens can be optimally fit. For example, two patients having identical central corneal curvatures but different peripheral corneal curvatures and eccentricities are likely to be optimally fit with different contact lens parameters.

Evaluation

Methods for evaluating corneal topography include keratometry, autokeratometry, photokeratoscopy, and videokeratography (computer-assisted corneal topographic modeling).

Keratometer: The most common instrument for measuring corneal topography, the keratometer averages the curvature values of a few points on the cornea separated by approximately 3 mm in both the vertical and horizontal meridians. This instrument has the advantages of both ease of use and low cost. However, there are disadvantages:

- Only the central 3 mm of the cornea (approximately 8% of the corneal area) is evaluated.
- The apex is not directly measured.

- The central 3 mm of the cornea is assumed to be spherical, which may not be true. The magnitude of error is related to the rate of peripheral corneal flattening.
- A decentered corneal apex may cause inaccuracy.
- Examiner error is possible.
- Keratometric change may not correspond with refractive change.

Despite its drawbacks, many practitioners still use keratometry for the initial selection of lens parameters because of its accessibility and ease of use. In fact, for initial base curve selection and prediction of residual cylinder, it has proven to be quite reliable. However, fluorescein pattern evaluation is still the most important assessment in GP contact lens fitting, while centration and lens lag are most important for soft lens fit assessments.

Autokeratometer: Currently available automated keratometers provide accurate and consistent measurements of the central corneal curvature. Many simultaneously perform autorefraction as well as autokeratometry. These combination autorefractor autokeratometers have become increasingly common. The Humphrey Autokeratometer also assesses a larger area of the cornea (6.4 mm in the vertical meridian; 2.6 mm in the horizontal meridian), calculates the corneal curvature at the apex, provides the location of the apex, and calculates the shape factor. The disadvantages of automated keratometers include a much higher cost to the practitioner and, in some, a limited area of evaluation.

Photokeratoscope: A photokeratoscope presents a hemispherical, lighted Placido disk image to the cornea. The observer focuses on a virtual image (plus sign) reflected from the corneal apex. A Polaroid photo is taken and analyzed to determine corneal curvature. Since the camera magnification is fixed and known, the amount of separation between rings can be used to determine curvature.[8] The advantages of these instruments are their ability to provide a topographic analysis of at least 55% of the corneal surface, their ability to detect subtle topographic shifts, and the availability of data. The disadvantages include the more complicated data analysis and presentation, the limited availability of the instrument (it is no longer in production), and the expense.

Videokeratography: The videokeratograph (computer-assisted corneal topography system) is a state-of-the-art instrument that measures and analyzes thousands of points on the corneal surface to provide information on corneal curvature and contour. Today it is generally referred to as simply a corneal topographer. It produces a color-coded corneal topographic map that provides the examiner with an easy-to-read representation of the curvature of virtually the entire corneal surface. Most systems use a combination of computer technology and a photokeratoscopic (Placido disk) image (Fig. 1.4) to produce a comprehensive topographic map of the cornea. Alternative methods utilizing projected grids (raster photogrammetry),[9] pachymetry,[10]

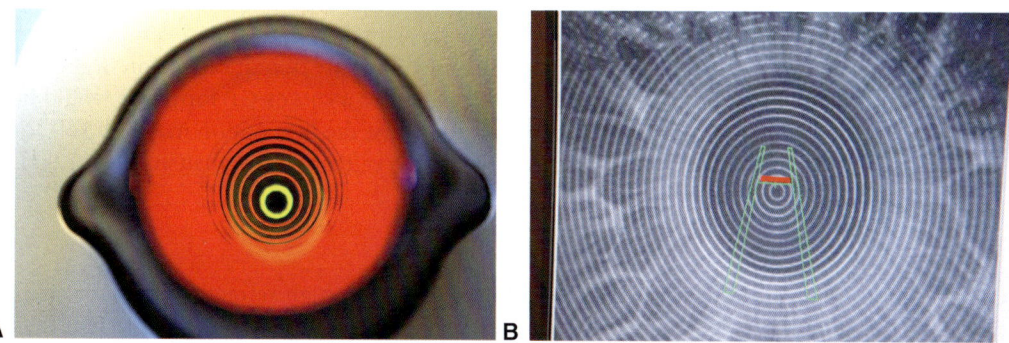

FIGURE 1.4 (A) Photokeratoscopic cone used in Placido disk-based videokeratographers. (B) Image projected on the cornea.

and Fourier analysis of sine waves[11] have also been developed. Topographers may also be used to determine noninvasive tear breakup time (NIBUT).

In addition to calculating corneal curvature, videokeratography software is able to determine corneal eccentricity, surface regularity, and elevation. With this information, the practitioner can detect corneal irregularities that may be causing reduced visual acuity and more effectively manage corneal distortion induced by contact lens wear, trauma, or surgery. Also, all videokeratographers have software that can design GP contact lenses based on the topographic information it has obtained. These software programs can design GP contact lenses successfully, but for most normal corneas, it may still be more efficient and just as accurate for the practitioner to use keratometry values for initial lens selection.[12,13] For irregular corneas, videokeratography more extensively describes the corneal contour, which may allow the practitioner to make contact-lens-fitting decisions with greater confidence.[14]

The advantages of videokeratography include the availability of significantly more information, the ease of use and analysis, and the most accurate method of monitoring topographic changes over time. The primary disadvantage is cost, although most systems are becoming very affordable for most practitioners.

Final Analysis

Despite the vast amount of information that videokeratography provides, most still consider keratometry the method of choice for diagnostic lens selection for normal corneas; however, it is important to remember that it represents only a starting point. As more accurate and accessible contact-lens-fitting software becomes available for videokeratography, it may replace keratometry. Currently, it is more valuable for qualitative evaluations of the overall shape of the cornea, particularly for distorted and highly astigmatic corneas, for which both initial fitting and long-term management are enhanced.

Refraction

It is important to perform a careful binocular refraction to help calculate the contact lens power and expected residual astigmatism. Residual astigmatism for spherical soft lenses is simply equal to the refractive astigmatism. For GP contact lenses, calculated residual astigmatism is determined by the following formula:

$$\text{CRA (calculated residual astigmatism)} = \text{Refractive astigmatism} - \text{Keratometric astigmatism}$$

Example:

$$\text{Keratometry} = 42.00 \ @ \ 180; \ 42.25 \ @ \ 090$$

$$\text{Refraction} = -2.00 - 1.00 \times 180$$

$$\text{CRA} = (-1.00 \times 180) - (-0.25 \times 180) = -0.75 \times 180$$

Typically, if the actual residual astigmatism (ARA) measured by refracting over a GP contact lens is >0.75 D, a spherical GP lens is not recommended because of reduced vision. Depending on the amount of keratometric (corneal) astigmatism, either a soft or GP toric lens would be a better option. In the above case, if the ARA equals the CRA, the best option may be a soft toric lens since the ARA with a spherical soft lens will equal the refractive astigmatism (or −1.00 D).

BINOCULAR VISION STATUS

Contact lenses may alter the binocular status of patients with high refractive errors or significant binocular anomalies. It is therefore important to test binocular function prior to lens fitting and make the necessary recommendations for lens wear.

Accommodation and Convergence

Pre-presbyopic moderate to high myopes may experience accommodative problems when switching from spectacles to contact lenses. In addition, they should be advised that a bifocal correction will probably be required at an earlier age. Convergence is similarly affected. A spectacle-corrected myope has a base-in prism effect when viewing at near, while a spectacle-corrected hyperope has a base-out prism effect. When contact lenses are worn, the myope loses the base-in prism effect at near and must converge more. Likewise, the contact lens-corrected hyperope loses the base-out prism effect at near and must converge less. Exophoric myopes and esophoric hyperopes may therefore experience more nearpoint symptoms with contact lenses than with spectacles.

Prismatic Correction

If base-in or base-out prism is necessary to provide binocularity and relieve asthenopic stress, it must be prescribed in spectacles. Although contact lenses can be worn together with spectacles, most patients would not appreciate the benefits of contact lens wear if glasses must also be worn. A small amount of base-down prism can be corrected in a contact lens, but base-up prism must be placed in spectacles.

SLIT-LAMP EVALUATION

A comprehensive slit-lamp examination plays a vital role in determining whether the patient is a good contact lens candidate. The following should be evaluated on all prospective contact lens wearers:

External Observation

It is important to evaluate the eyelashes and external eyelids for the following conditions:

Blepharitis

Swollen, inflamed lid margins reduce prognosis for successful contact lens wear. Debris from the lids may act as an irritant, and abnormal meibomian gland secretions will create an oily film on the lens surface. Staphylococcal blepharitis is also a potential cause of corneal infiltrates and may predispose the wearer to peripheral corneal ulcers. Acute and chronic forms of blepharitis should be treated before the patient is fit with contact lenses.

Meibomian Glands

Capped or inspissated glands may indicate poor tear film quality, an increased tendency for tear film evaporation, and a shortened tear breakup time (TBUT). Meibomian gland disease (MGD) or dysfunction should be treated prior to fitting with lenses. Treatment may include warm compresses, lid hygiene, gland expression, and oral omega-3 supplements.

Entropion/Trichiasis

In-turned or disorganized lash patterns are not a contraindication for contact lens wear. In fact, a soft lens would protect the cornea from irritation caused by in-turned lashes.

Conjunctiva

The bulbar and tarsal conjunctiva should be evaluated biomicroscopically with white light. Rose bengal and lissamine green dye can be used to stain damaged or dead conjunctival cells, thus visualizing defects. Upper eyelid eversion is also required.

Bulbar Conjunctiva

Moderate injection of the bulbar conjunctiva, especially if persistent, may be caused by infection, dry eye, blepharitis, an allergic reaction, or other inflammatory process, and may contraindicate contact lens wear. Interpalpebral conjunctival staining is also suggestive of dry eye and should be investigated further with a tear film evaluation prior to contact lens fitting. Dense or coalesced rose bengal or lissamine green staining of the interpalpebral conjunctiva is often associated with the symptoms of dry eye. The presence of a pinguecula could necessitate a low modulus soft lens material or GP lens if the edge of a higher modulus silicone hydrogel lens irritates this condition. The presence of a pterygium should contraindicate contact lens wear; however, if only a small region of the peripheral cornea is affected, contact lenses can be considered.

Tarsal Conjunctiva

After upper eyelid eversion, the superior tarsal conjunctiva should be evaluated with and without fluorescein using the following scale[15]:

0 = satin. No papillae are observable.
1 = mildly elevated papillae, 0.1 to 0.2 mm in diameter, with uniform distribution (several papillae per millimeter of lid area).
2 = papillae are 0.5 to 1.0 mm in diameter, with nonuniform distribution.
3 = papillae 1 mm in diameter or greater are present on all regions of the upper lid.

Seasonal allergies result in mild papillary hypertrophy of the upper lid, usually of grade 1. A patient with giant papillary conjunctivitis (GPC, also known as contact lens papillary conjunctivitis [CLPC]) will exhibit large, irregularly sized papillae of grade 2 or 3 on the superior tarsal plate, which may be flattened and scarred if the condition is chronic (Fig. 1.5). GPC improves when a new contact lens is worn or with cessation of contact lenses. Thus, a new patient with GPC may be fitted in a daily disposable soft lens or a 2-week disposable lens, in combination with a decreased lens wearing time until the condition resolves. A combination mast cell inhibitor–antihistamine topical solution or a corticosteroid may be used initially to decrease the inflammation.

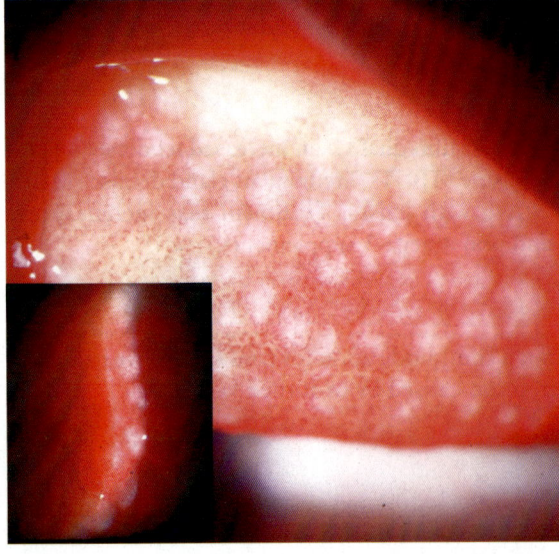

FIGURE 1.5 A reverted upper lid from a patient with giant papillary conjunctivitis (GPC), showing grade 3 papillae on the upper tarsal plate.

Cornea

It is critical to carefully evaluate all aspects of the cornea prior to fitting. The presence of any significant corneal defect or disease process contraindicates contact lens wear until the condition has resolved. Many corneal defects are best visualized using the technique of indirect illumination. Chronic conditions, such as corneal dystrophies, may alter the type of contact lens, wearing schedule, and care regimen prescribed.

Limbal Vasculature

A 360-degree evaluation of the limbal vessels should be performed. Documentation of limbal vessel encroachment onto the cornea should be made. It is important to differentiate normal limbal vasculature from contact lens-induced vascularization. Encroachment of 1 to 2 mm suggests chronic hypoxia and may indicate the need for refitting with a silicone hydrogel, even on a daily wear (DW) basis, or refitting with GP lenses. Encroachment of >2 mm requires refitting to increase oxygen to the cornea, a decreased wearing time, and careful monitoring to prevent further advance of the neovascularization.

Epithelial Staining

Fluorescein application using a fluorescein strip moistened with preservative-free saline is essential when evaluating a new patient. A yellow, Wratten number 12 filter should be used in addition to the cobalt filter; if not, subtle staining may not be detected. Sequential staining with liquid fluorescein has also been recommended.[16] Any areas of punctate epithelial staining should be noted. The presence of dense, coalesced staining may contraindicate fitting at that time and require treatment. Always perform this procedure even if it is likely that the patient desires soft lenses. The eye can be thoroughly irrigated to rinse out the dye before lens application. TBUT can be performed at this time as well.

Edema

The presence of deep stromal striae or folds, epithelial microcysts and vacuoles, or epithelial and stromal clouding indicates corneal edema and may contraindicate contact lens wear. The cause of the edema should be determined and treated, if possible. Occasionally, corneal dystrophies may cause edema; contact lenses are sometimes used in the management of these conditions. Epithelial microcysts are commonly found in extended-wear patients, and indicate that a period of oxygen deprivation has occurred.

Opacities: Scars versus Infiltrates

Carefully scan the cornea to differentiate an active from an inactive condition. Any active corneal infection or inflammation (e.g., corneal infiltrates, microbial keratitis) contraindicates contact lens wear at that time and requires the appropriate treatment.[17] Corneal scars and other inactive opacities are not contraindications to contact lens wear.

Endothelium

Evaluate the endothelial layer for the presence of guttata and polymegethism. The presence of an endothelial dystrophy may contraindicate contact lens wear.

TEAR FILM EVALUATION

The preocular tear film plays an important role in contact lens wear. It maintains hydration of soft contact lenses, determines lens surface wettability, acts as the primary anterior refracting surface, and deposits protein, lipids, and mucin onto the lens surface. Poor tear quality or quantity will reduce the patient's prognosis for successful contact lens wear. There are several tear evaluations that should be performed to determine whether a patient is a good contact lens candidate.

Tear Meniscus Evaluation

The height and quality of the lower tear prism (lacrimal lake) are evaluated during the slit-lamp examination. This is a good test for detecting the borderline dry-eye patient. If the tear prism is not sufficient, an aqueous deficiency is present. The anterior border of the tear meniscus is just behind the meibomian gland orifices. Where the meniscus meets the cornea, a black line exists that represents localized thinning. To evaluate the tear meniscus, fluorescein should be applied over the inferior bulbar conjunctiva about 1 to 2 minutes before evaluation[4] and then observed with cobalt blue and Wratten number 12 filters. When the meniscus is so thin that it appears as a fine line, it is a significantly insufficient tear meniscus (Fig. 1.6).

Tear Breakup Time

TBUT is the most widely used test of tear film quality and a good predictor of contact lens success. It is equal to the postblink time for dry spots to form in the tear film, and it is theoretically caused by contamination of the mucin layer by lipids. Fluorescein is instilled, and the cornea is evaluated with a wide slit-lamp beam (i.e., 2–4 mm) under low magnification (i.e., 10× to 20×) with the

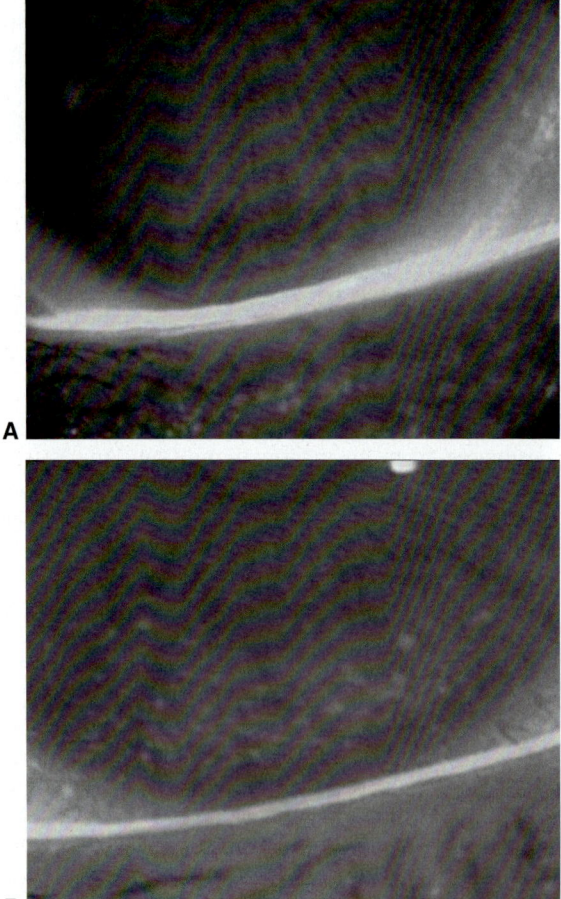

FIGURE 1.6 The inferior meniscus of a normal **(A)** and a dry-eye patient **(B)**. Note the inferior corneal staining in the dry-eye patient. (Courtesy of Wendy Harrison.)

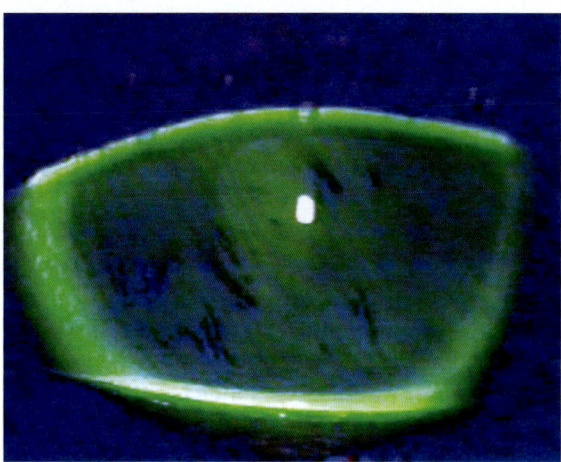

FIGURE 1.7 The formation of dry spots in the precorneal tear film observed when measuring tear breakup time (TBUT).

cobalt blue and yellow Wratten number 12 filters. When wetting the fluorescein strip with saline, it is important to use unpreserved saline and shake excess moisture from the strip to avoid artificially destabilizing the tear film. The number of seconds until a dry spot forms is recorded. These dry spots appear as dark regions in the green-dyed tear film (Fig. 1.7). The patient is instructed to refrain from blinking during this period. An average, normal value is 15 to 20 seconds. Less than 8 to 10 seconds indicates the patient may have dry eye, although many asymptomatic patients show TBUT in this range.[18] However, a low TBUT indicates that the patient is best suited for DW, may suffer from end-of-the-day dryness, and may not be able to obtain a comfortable all-day wearing schedule. Several important considerations could affect results:

- Do not manipulate the lids immediately prior to testing.
- Avoid forced blinks as this may cause eye make up to contaminate the tear film and shorten the breakup time.
- It is best to use unpreserved saline to wet the fluorescein strip.
- No applanation tonometry should be performed before the test.
- Repeat the test several times, especially if low values are being obtained.
- Fluorescence of the tear film is enhanced if a Wratten number 12 or similar yellow filter is placed over the observation system.
- Do not perform this test immediately after contact lens removal. Wearing contact lenses decreases TBUT, possibly for several hours after lens removal.

Two NIBUT tests have been developed to minimize any disruption to the tear film.[19] In one technique, a grid pattern is projected onto the anterior ocular surface, which is observed using a biomicroscope under low magnification.[20] When the grid pattern is disrupted, the tear film is breaking up. A second NIBUT technique involves using the keratometer or topographer mire image to observe tear film rupture.[21] In both techniques, a value of 8 to 10 is the cutoff for dry eye.

Interference Phenomena Evaluation

The lipid layer can be evaluated by specular reflection or interferometry of the tear film. Clinically, the slit lamp can be used, but the viewable area is very limited. The Keeler Tearscope is a commercially available instrument that provides a larger area of specular reflection, which allows the majority of the precorneal tear lipid layer to be visualized at once. With either technique, colored interference patterns of the lipid layer will be observed. A good lipid layer will have an amorphous pattern that appears gray to brown in color. Thinner lipid layers have a marble-like pattern, and if the lipid layer is absent, no interference patterns will be observed.[22,23]

Schirmer Tear Test

The Schirmer tear test evaluates basal tear secretion and part of the reflex secretion and has been used to screen contact lens candidates for suitability for lens wear. Although this is a simple test to administer, it has several problems including discomfort, inconsistency, and unreliability.[24–26] Nevertheless, it can be useful in detecting the aqueous-deficient dry-eye patient.

With the patient viewing superiorly, place a Schirmer test strip over the lower lid such that the 5-mm notched portion of the strip is approximately one-third of the way from the outer canthus. Several techniques are used to perform the test. In one technique, the patient continuously looks upward with the room illumination lowered to reduce reflex tearing from light sensitivity (Fig. 1.8). After 5 minutes, the strip is removed, and the amount of wetting is measured in millimeters. Another technique is to ask the patient to keep the eyes closed after placement of the strip. A cutoff value of 5 mm in 5 minutes is considered normal.[27] The Schirmer tear test is most useful when a very low volume of tears is detected. A very high volume of tears, noted by the wetting of the complete strip or most of the strip, may not be repeatable, whereas an extremely low volume, noted by a very small area of strip coverage (0–4 mm), usually indicates aqueous deficiency. This test can be performed with or without anesthetic. If anesthetic is used, it is best to perform the test several minutes after the anesthetic is instilled. However, performing the test without anesthetic is more useful for evaluating the success of contact lens wear because it demonstrates the more natural response of the ocular surface response to irritation. If the patient's tear volume is low and little or no tearing results from instillation of the irritating Schirmer's strip, then the volume of tears is likely to remain low with contact lens wear. Thus, a low Schirmer's value indicates that the patient will be likely to suffer from dry-eye symptoms with contact lens wear.

Important considerations when performing the Schirmer tear test include the following:

- Use low room illumination.
- The strip should rest in a slightly temporal position so that when the lower lid kicks inward during blinking, contact with the cornea, which may cause excess ocular irritation and reflex tearing, is avoided.

Phenol Red Thread Test

The phenol red thread test, developed by Hamano et al.,[28] consists of a high-quality 70-mm cotton thread soaked in phenol red dye. It is performed similar to the Schirmer test: the end of the thread is inserted over the lower lid onto the temporal palpebral conjunctiva while the patient views superiorly. The test is performed for 15 seconds, and the amount of the test strip that has turned to red color is measured (Fig. 1.9). The average value in the United States has

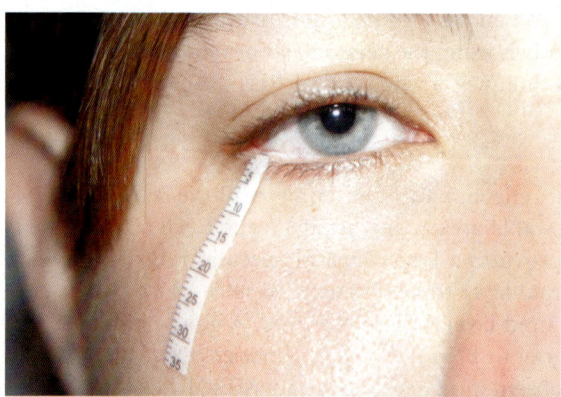

FIGURE 1.8 Proper Schirmer strip placement at the outer one-third of the lower eyelids.

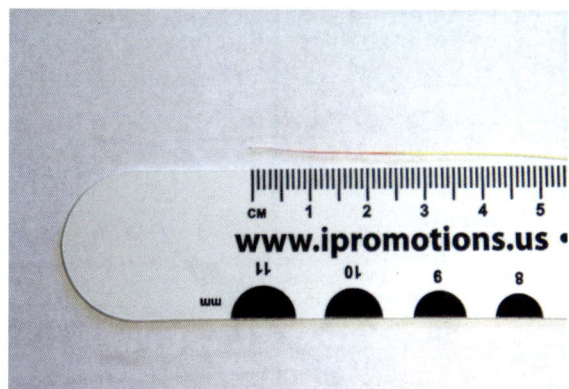

FIGURE 1.9 The phenol red thread test.

been found to be 24.3 mm.[29] A value below 9 mm has been diagnostic of dry eye. The benefits of this test include the following:

1. No anesthesia necessary; minimal discomfort.
2. A 15-second test time.
3. Little reflex secretion.
4. More valid than the Schirmer tear test.[30]
5. Minimal environmental effects such as humidity because of the short testing time.

Criticisms of this test include the following:

1. Relatively low absorption capacity; individuals may secrete tears at a higher rate than can be absorbed by the thread.[31]
2. This test may only measure residual tears in the cul-de-sac, not tear volume.

Rose Bengal

Rose bengal stains damaged ocular surface cells that are not protected by an intact mucin layer. Therefore, the dye stains cells on the ocular surface of dry-eye patients, whose conjunctival cells become keratinized and lose their mucins.[32–34] For that reason, it has traditionally been used as a conjunctival stain for the dry-eye patient, although it is noticeably painful for those patients because it shows cellular toxicity if the mucin layer is breached.[35] A drop of 1% rose bengal (or use of an impregnated strip moistened with unpreserved saline) is instilled into the conjunctival sac; this is followed by irrigation of the external eye with an isotonic saline solution. The amount and location of the red stain will dictate the severity of the condition. Typically in keratoconjunctivitis sicca, the inferior cornea and conjunctiva will exhibit a large amount of staining. It particularly stains dead cells an intense red color, while it stains cells that are devitalized a weaker color. In marginally dry eyes, the conjunctival surface may stain in a discrete punctate fashion (Fig. 1.10), whereas in pathologic dry eye, it is more coalesced. Typically, the adjacent triangular sections of the exposed bulbar conjunctiva, both nasally and temporally, will stain. After the patient has blinked three to six times and the excess dye has been washed away by the tears, the eye is examined with white light. The following grading sequence has been recommended for evaluating this condition[36]:

0 = absence of staining.
1 = staining of <1/3 of the cornea.
2 = staining of between 1/3 and 2/3 of the cornea.
3 = staining of between 2/3 and the entire cornea.
4 = staining over the entire cornea.
5 = inferior conjunctival staining.

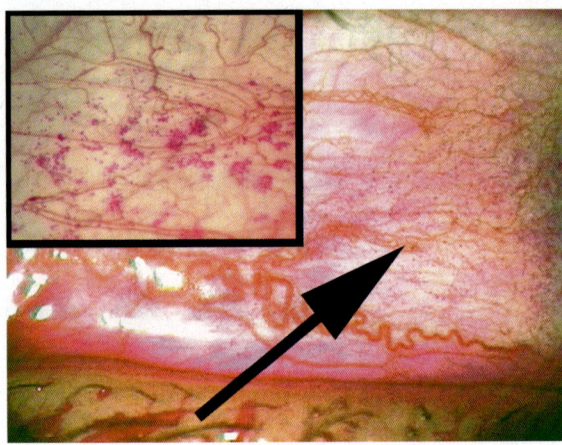

FIGURE 1.10 Rose bengal staining of the conjunctiva in a dry-eye patient (*arrow*). Staining is magnified in the inset showing the typical punctate pattern.

Lissamine Green

Lissamine green is a dye that provides information similar to the more traditional rose bengal dye, but without pain or discomfort for the patient. It is available in both strips and liquid form. It works by diffusing into damaged or keratinized cells,[37,38] similar to sodium fluorescein. One drop of 1% lissamine green is instilled in the lower cul-de-sac, and the ocular surface is then examined with the slit lamp in white light. It has been shown that this dye yields staining scores that are not significantly different from those obtained with rose bengal. In addition, lissamine green produces noticeably less irritation than rose bengal, and the irritation is of shorter duration.[38] Therefore, lissamine green can be used interchangeably with rose bengal when evaluating the eye for keratitis sicca. The grading scale is the same as for rose bengal.

Lid Wiper Epitheliopathy

The lid wiper is the area of the upper lid at the junction of the cutaneous and conjunctival tissue. The wiper is the "windshield wiper" of the ocular surface and contact lens during blinking. If the tissue is rough, trauma due to friction to the corneal epithelium and sensitivity can occur and the contact lens may not wet well. As described by Korb,[39,40] lid wiper epitheliopathy (LWE) is a diagnostic sign of dry-eye disease. Often, when all other tests are normal on symptomatic patients, LWE will be positive.[41] Contact lens wearers with dryness symptoms exhibit significant degrees of LWE even in the absence of corneal staining and bulbar injection. Fluorescein staining of the lid wiper area is graded on a scale of 0 (no staining) to grade 3. It is graded separately on linearity and severity, and then the two scores are averaged. Rose bengal or lissamine green dye is then applied to the wiper area and scored in the same manner as for fluorescein, but using white and red-free light. Scores are averaged for the two dyes for the final result:

0.5 to 1.0 = Grade 1 (mild LWE)
1.25 to 2.0 = Grade 2 (moderate)
2.25 to 3.0 = Grade 3 (severe)

Tear Osmolarity

Aqueous deficient and evaporative dry-eye conditions result in increased concentration/osmolarity of the tear film. This in turn can interfere with homeostasis and lead to inflammation and ocular surface disease. Thus, elevated tear osmolarity values (>308 mOsms/L) can be indicative of dry eye.[42] Previously, osmolarity measurements were available primarily in research settings. However, with the recent reclassification of the TearLab Osmolarity System as a waived instrument under the federal Clinical Laboratory Improvement Amendments (CLIA), tear osmolarity testing will likely become more common in private and group practice settings which manage dry-eye patients.[43] The TearLab Osmolarity System by TearLab Corp (San Diego, California) is designed to be an in-office instrument for in vitro diagnostic tear testing. The procedure is rapid, noninvasive and requires only 50 nL of tears. Practitioners must obtain a CLIA Certificate of Waiver in order to perform the testing in their offices. This is required whether or not they are charging for the procedure. Filing for the Certificate of Waiver, in most cases, simply involves completing and submitting CMS form 116 and paying a registration fee. Certain states may require a state form.

Dry-Eye Questionnaire

The use of a dry-eye questionnaire can be beneficial in determining if the patient has some dryness characteristics or is in an environment that could be prone to inducing dryness. One such questionnaire, adapted from McMonnies et al.,[30,44] is given in Box 1.1. It can also be useful to ask about end-of-the-day dryness because that is a common complaint among contact lens wearers.[45]

BOX 1.1. DRY-EYE QUESTIONNAIRE*

1. Age_____
2. Gender   Male   Female
3. Currently wearing (circle one) no contact lenses, rigid contact lenses, soft contact lenses.
4. If you wear contact lenses, do you have a modified wearing schedule because of dryness?
5. Are your eyes usually sensitive to cigarette smoke, smog, air conditioning, or central heating?
   Yes (2)   No (0)   Sometimes (1)
6. Do you take (please underline) antihistamine tablets (1); antihistamine eyedrops (1); diuretics (1); sleeping tablets (1); tranquilizers (1); oral contraceptives (1); medication for duodenal ulcer (1) or digestive problems (1), high blood pressure (1), hormone replacement pills (1), or other (write)?
7. Do you have arthritis?
   Yes (2)   No (0)   Uncertain (1)
8. Do you have a connective tissues disorder?
   Yes (2)   No (0)
9. Do you have a thyroid abnormality?
   Yes (2)   No (0)   Uncertain (1)
10. Do you experience dryness of the nose, mouth, throat, chest, or vagina?
    Never (0)   Sometimes (1)   Often (2)   Constantly (3)
11. Are you known to sleep with your eyes open?
    Yes (2)   No (0)   Sometimes (1)
12. Do you have eye irritation upon waking from sleep?
    Yes (2)   No (0)   Sometimes (1)
13. Have you ever had drops prescribed or other treatment for dry eyes?
    Yes (2)   No (0)

*Numbers in parentheses represent score for each answer.

What Series of Tests Should Be Used?

1. TBUT reveals tear quality and should be performed on all prospective contact lens wearers. However, contact lens wear decreases the TBUT, so the test is not accurate just after lens removal.
2. Biomicroscopic evaluation of the tear prism would indicate whether an aqueous tear deficiency is present. The presence of inferior corneal and conjunctival fluorescein staining also indicates a dry-eye condition. Staining of the lid wiper area with fluorescein and rose bengal or lissamine green is important for detection of LWE.
3. A tear volume test can also be performed.
4. Tear osmolarity can also be evaluated.
5. Lissamine green is preferred over rose bengal when evaluating a dry-eye suspect for conjunctival staining because of the increased comfort with that dye.

FINAL CONSULTATION

Evaluation of Motivation

Motivation may be the most important factor in determining success versus failure of a contact lens wearer. A highly motivated patient can often tolerate discomfort and other problems that would be difficult for the patient who has only a superficial motivation.[46] Motivation can be tested by explaining that contact lenses are a healthcare device and must be cared for constantly and without error. The patient's motivation to wear them is twofold: the desire to see well and the desire to improve his or her appearance. The greater a patient's need for contact lenses, either visual or psychological, the more likely that motivation will be high.[47] Other factors to consider include the following:

1. Satisfaction with spectacles: is the patient exhibiting only a casual interest in contact lenses ("shopping")?
2. With a younger child, is it the child who really desires the contact lenses or is a vanity-conscious parent the only one who desires them? If the latter is true, the child is not ready for lens wear.
3. Limited wearing time (e.g., because of borderline dry eye) may decrease the patient's motivation to wear contact lenses.
4. If the patient has excessive concerns (e.g., high fees, discomfort, or possible complications), success is unlikely.
5. If the patient exhibits hypochondriac-like concerns about minor ailments, he or she may not be willing to tolerate the initial discomfort and adaptation associated with contact lens wear. Likewise, if the patient is quite timid, successful contact lens wear is much less probable than for patients who are independent and confident.[48]
6. If the patient does not agree with the practitioner's recommendations (e.g., GPs not soft, hydrogen peroxide not chemical disinfection, DW only not extended wear), lenses should not be ordered and careful documentation in the patient's record is required.

Benefits of Contact Lenses versus Spectacles

The benefits of contact lenses versus spectacles can also be explained to a new prospective contact lens candidate. Several studies have demonstrated that contact lens wearers are more outgoing, optimistic, athletic, and less self-conscious than their spectacle-wearing counterparts.[48] Myopic children fitted in rigid contact lenses may progress in myopia more slowly than their spectacle-wearing counterparts.[49] Additionally, children and teens wearing contact lenses of any type may show greater confidence and self-esteem than their peers wearing spectacles.[50] The following benefits can also be mentioned:

1. Contact lenses increase magnification of the retinal image for moderate to high myopes.
2. The contact lens wearer is free from obstruction by the spectacle frame.

3. A slight increase in light transmission is present. (This is also why some new contact lens wearers complain that they experience more photophobia in daylight conditions.)
4. Fewer optical aberrations are present because the patient views through the optical center of the lens at all times.

Comparison of Gas-Permeable and Soft Lenses

A discussion of which lens material is best for a given patient is important. The factors that can be considered when discussing this decision with a patient are presented in Tables 1.1 and 1.2.

Comfort

Comfort is an important factor in the eventual decision. Discomfort is the number one reason for discontinuation of contact lens wear.[45,51] If the patient is very concerned about discomfort, soft lenses should be considered (assuming the patient is even motivated for contact lens wear in general). Always tell the patient what to expect before the diagnostic fitting process. The initial comfort can also be judged at this time. If the patient is a high reactor (e.g., if the patient is still tearing and has little desire to gaze straight ahead even after a 15- to 30-minute period), soft lenses should be considered. Likewise, if the patient demonstrates greater than average sensitivity during the examination (e.g., during drop instillation, lid eversion, tonometry), soft lenses are often preferable. Due to their large size, scleral GP lenses are typically more comfortable than standard GPs as are hybrid lenses.

Myths

This is the perfect time to dispel any myths the patient may believe in about contact lenses. Some of these include the following:
1. "The contact lens will get behind my eye."
2. "The contact lenses will break on my eye."
3. "I can't be fit because I have 'stigmatism.'"
4. "Contact lenses damage the eye."
5. "Shouldn't you be at least 16 years old to wear contact lenses?"
6. "Contact lenses HURT!"
7. "They don't make contacts for bifocal wearers."
8. I have trouble getting lenses in and out, so I should wear the kind I can sleep in for a month at a time.

TABLE 1.1 Advantages of Gas-Permeable and Soft Lenses

GP ADVANTAGES	SOFT LENS ADVANTAGES
Vision	Initial comfort
Ocular health	Oxygen transmission (silicone hydrogels)
High oxygen transmission	Variable wear
Wettability	Disposability = convenience
High astigmatic correction	No foreign body sensation
Ease of care/easier compliance	Athletes (see Table 1.2)
Long-term comfort	Ability to change eye color
Stability/durability	Residual cylinder with GPs
Benefit irregular cornea patient	Reduced initial chair time
Eye protection	

TABLE 1.2 Preferred Contact Lens Correction in Sports

SPORT	SOFT	SOFT OR GP	HYBRID OR SCLERAL
Baseball	•	•	•
Contact sports			
Basketball	•		•
Boxing	•		•
Football	•		•
Hockey	•		•
Soccer	•		•
Wrestling	•		•
Golf	•		•
Hunting		•	•
Jogging		•	•
Mounting climbing		•	•
Racquet sports/handball			
Handball	•		•
Racquetball	•		•
Squash	•		•
Tennis	•		•
Scuba diving	•		
Snow skiing		•	•
Swimming	•		

Another myth to consider with employed patients is that contact lenses offer no protection to the eye. It is very likely that contact lenses can help protect the cornea from injury by various flying objects. One study reported on 125 cases that included sports, automobile, workshop, and chemical accidents in which eyes were protected by contact lens wear.[52] However, because of the trauma that can occur from a hard object in addition to substances that can result in toxicity reactions, contact lenses should never be substituted for the appropriate safety eyewear. Likewise, protective goggles should be worn in most sports, especially racquetball and squash.

OTHER CONSIDERATIONS

What about the −0.50 D Myope?

It is not uncommon for low ametropic patients to be told they are not good contact lens candidates. Often this results from the practitioner's preconception that the patient really does not need to wear any lenses and/or lacks motivation because of the low refractive error. In most cases, these patients are good contact lens candidates. If they appear to be motivated or have an occupational need for contact lenses, they should be fit with lenses. As a result of the low ametropia, soft lenses are often recommended, especially if occasional wear is desired.

How to Approach the Borderline Dry-Eye Patient

Dry eye is the most common problem associated with contact lens wear, and is one of the most common reasons that patients discontinue contact lens wear. As many as 50% of contact lens wearers report dry-eye symptoms, often worse later in the day.[53,54] Some borderline dry-eye patients present at the initial fitting visit with occasional dry-eye symptoms, whereas others are asymptomatic. In either case, contact lens wear usually aggravates dry-eye symptoms. It is often difficult to decide how to fit the borderline dry-eye patient (e.g., a patient with a low TBUT, reduced tear prism, or antihistamine use). There are several considerations that can help maximize the borderline dry-eye patient's likelihood for comfortable contact lens wear.[55]

Gas-Permeable versus Soft

Hydrogel and silicone hydrogel lenses have the advantages of initial comfort and ability to rehydrate with application of rewetting drops. GP lenses often present a healthier alternative, in terms of oxygen availability to the corneal epithelium. The final decision may be determined by the case history and the prefitting evaluation. Would the patient benefit visually from GP lenses? Is the patient interested only in occasional wear? Is there a history of corneal infection or GPC? If the patient appears to be a candidate for either GP or soft lenses, he or she may achieve a longer wearing time with soft lenses because of the ability to rehydrate the lenses, either by applying rewetting drops frequently or performing a 10-minute saline soak in the middle of the wearing period.

Soft Lens Selection

Among traditional hydrogel lenses, water content, lens thickness, and surface deposit resistance are the hydrogel material properties that help minimize dryness. Most agree that low-water-content lenses dehydrate less because there is less water to lose and that thicker lenses maintain a greater "reservoir" of water whose dehydration is lower than that in thinner lenses.[56] In one study, more borderline dry-eye patients preferred a low-water-content thick hydrogel lens (8) than low-water thin (5), GP (5), high-water thick (4), and high-water thin (4) lenses. Lens surface treatments can also increase the on-eye wettability of soft lenses. Silicone hydrogel materials typically use surface treatments or internal wetting agents to improve wettability, thus providing another option for fitting the dry-eye patient. Several studies have shown that fitting dry-eye patients with silicone hydrogels improved dryness symptoms.[57,58]

Gas-Permeable Lens Selection

GP lenses have the advantage of not dehydrating and obtaining water from the postlens tear film. However, they may induce peripheral corneal desiccation in patients with dry eye. If a GP lens is desired, a highly wettable material, such as a medium-oxygen-permeability (Dk) fluorosilicone acrylate, is recommended. Scleral GP lenses may be used as a means of maintaining a tear reservoir for those with moderately to severely dry eyes.

Care

Many care systems are available to patients, mostly chemical disinfection with preservatives. A patient who has been successfully using a particular care system should be kept with the same system. However, the care system of any patient who has shown a possible allergic reaction to a preservative or who has dry eye should be evaluated. It is important to be aware of the preservative in each care system to avoid giving that patient a similar system with the same preservative. Preservative-free care systems are an option for patients with possible allergies or dry eye. Daily cleaning with a good surfactant cleaner is recommended for dry eye because the patients tend to show more lens deposits. Cleaners with abrasive components may benefit patients who develop protein deposits rapidly. Patients who experience rapid protein deposition despite diligent cleaning may require a refit to weekly or daily disposable lenses.

Wearing Schedule

A reduced wearing schedule may be necessary for dry-eye patients. Daily wear is mandatory. These recommendations should be made the first visit after tear film testing has been completed. Proactive education will prepare the patient for limited but successful lens wear.

Adjunct Therapy

The use of rewetting drops during lens wear is essential in maintaining good comfort and ocular surface health for dry-eye patients. Midday lens cleaning and saline soaks will allow the patient to prolong lens wear in the latter half of the day when dry-eye symptoms typically increase. This is particularly important for those wearing scleral GPs as it replenishes the tear reservoir behind the lens. If rewetting drops and saline soaks are not sufficient, punctal occlusion may be a good option. Initial diagnostic evaluation with dissolvable collagen plugs, followed by permanent occlusion with nondissolvable silicone plugs or cautery can significantly increase tear retention and decrease dry-eye symptoms. Before applying punctal plugs, care must be taken to be sure the etiology of the problem has truly decreased tear production, but not inflammation, infection, or blepharitis. Restasis can be used to increase tear production when appropriate. If there is an allergic component to the dry eye, topical medications such as mast cell stabilizer–antihistamine combinations can be considered as long as the patient does not instill the drops while soft lenses are on the eyes. Oral omega-3 supplements may also be helpful in improving tear quality and resolving symptoms of dryness.

FINAL ANALYSIS

The goal of the preliminary evaluation is to be able to answer the question, "Is the patient a suitable candidate for contact lens wear?" In this final assessment, you must consider the patient's goals, history, refractive status, and ocular health. In addition to answering this question, you must determine the most appropriate contact lens option that will meet the patient's needs without creating clinical problems. Table 1.3 provides an overview of good, borderline, and poor candidates for contact lens wear.

TABLE 1.3 Good, Borderline, and Poor Contact Lens Candidates

GOOD	BORDERLINE	POOR
• Motivated	• Borderline dry eye	• Unmotivated
• High ametropia	• Allergies/occasional antihistamine use	• Dusty, dirty environment
• Children/adolescents (if motivated/mature)	• Excessive fear about foreign body on eye	• Poor hygiene
• Aphakia	• Lab workers and hairdressers	• Diabetes
• Refractive anisometropia	• Mild (1–1.5 mm) limbal vessel encroachment	• Pathologic dry eye
• Irregular cornea	• Pinguecula	• Active corneal infection (e.g., neovascularization, infiltrates, coalesced staining)
• Good ocular/systemic health	• Preexisting corneal scars	• Pterygium
• Normal binocular vision	• Entropion, ectropion, trichiasis	• Chronic blepharitis
• Good manual dexterity	• Patient under psychiatric care	• Endothelial dystrophy
	• Hypochondriasis	• Immunosuppressed patients
		• Lateral prism in correction
		• Poor manual dexterity
		• Chronic alcoholism

SUMMARY

Careful patient selection is paramount to successful contact lens wear. If a comprehensive history, refractive and ocular evaluation, and assessment of suitability are performed, it is likely that the patient will be a successful contact lens wearer. Whether or not the patient is ultimately fit with contact lenses, providing an honest appraisal of the probability of successful contact lens wear will eventually benefit both doctor and patient.

CLINICAL CASES

CASE 1

A 38-year-old automobile mechanic visits the office for a complete eye examination. During the course of your examination, he casually asks if you think he could wear contact lenses. His motivation results from having to clean his spectacles frequently because of oil, grease, and dirt coming in contact with them from a car or his hands. Otherwise he is quite pleased with the vision and wearing of spectacles. You observe that his hands appear to be quite dirty.

Should this patient be fitted with contact lenses?

SOLUTION: If this patient's dissatisfaction with his spectacles was greater and his hygiene was better, he may have been a good contact lens candidate. But his dirty hands and work environment would increase the risk of serious eye infection from lens contamination as compared to the general population. Therefore, it would be preferable to advise this patient that he is not a good contact lens candidate.

CASE 2

A 16-year-old woman visits the office for a complete eye examination and contact lens fitting. She has never worn contact lenses before but strongly dislikes wearing spectacles, which she needs to wear constantly because of her nearsightedness. During the case history she indicates to you that she has seasonal allergy problems, necessitating occasional antihistamine use. You also observe that her palpebral conjunctiva has a grade 1 papillary hypertrophy. All other ocular health findings are normal. Her refraction is as follows:

$$OD\ -3.25 - 1.00 \times 170$$
$$OS\ -2.75 - 1.25 \times 005$$

Should this patient be fitted with contact lenses?

SOLUTION: Because this patient is very motivated and uses antihistamines only on an occasional basis, she is a good contact lens candidate. However, her allergies that have resulted in papillary hypertrophy may lead to dryness symptoms and lens deposits, especially during an allergy season. For this reason, a DW schedule is highly advisable. In addition, the patient should be warned that reduction in wearing time and possible temporary discontinuation of lens wear may be required during the allergy season. Some patients can also be fitted with a daily disposable lens during the allergy season, or all year, to avoid the excessive lens deposits often associated with allergies. For the same reason, a GP lens material which can be easily cleaned may also be recommended. Some patients are able to continue lens wear during allergy season by using newer topical medications such as combination mast cell stabilizer–antihistamine drops. These are available both in prescription and over-the-counter form.

CASE 3

A 21-year-old woman visits the office with a desire to be fitted with contact lenses. She wore GP lenses intermittently for 2 years, but could never wear them for long periods of time because of dryness. When she last visited her doctor 1 year ago, he mentioned to her that she is not a good candidate for contact lenses because she has dry eyes. Nevertheless, she is very motivated for contact lens wear and is receptive to any recommendations on lens material and wearing time. She finds her spectacles to be unacceptable cosmetically while also inconvenient during the many athletic activities in which she participates during her spare time. Her refraction is the following:

$$OD\ -4.00-1.25\times 010$$
$$OS\ -3.50-1.00\times 180$$

Slit-lamp evaluation shows an absence of staining and papillary hypertrophy. However, the TBUT is only 6 seconds.

Should this patient be fitted with contact lenses?

SOLUTION: Yes, this patient should become a satisfied contact lens wearer. Based on her motivation and past contact lens-wearing history, the best choice is to fit her into a 1-day disposable toric soft lens. She should also be warned not to expect all-day wear and to be careful about not overwearing the lenses. For patients whose prescription is not available in a daily disposable toric, a 2-week disposable hydrogel or silicone hydrogel soft toric lens can be fitted, but it may be desirable to add a cleaner to the care system to help keep the lenses clean. Preservative-free or transient preservative rewetting drops may also help with dryness symptoms later in the day. For some patients, removing the lenses midday and cleaning or soaking them briefly in saline may also help. For those not using daily disposables, a nonpreserved lens care system helps relieve dryness symptoms for some patients.

CASE 4

A 24-year-old patient enters the office inquiring about contact lenses. He is a professional musician who has never worn contact lenses before and wears spectacles only for reading music and night driving. He feels the spectacles are a hindrance while performing in the orchestra because he frequently has to shift fixation and they tend to obstruct his view. However, as excellent vision is critical for viewing both his music and the conductor, he feels a vision correction is necessary. The refraction results in the following:

$$OD\ -0.50-0.25\times 180$$
$$OS\ -0.50\ DS$$

Should this patient be fitted with contact lenses?

SOLUTION: Because of the critical vision demand required in his occupation, in combination with his dissatisfaction with spectacles, this patient would make a good contact lens candidate. However, as a result of his low refractive error, soft lenses would be recommended to accommodate a probable occasional lens-wearing schedule. Daily disposable lenses would be the best choice if he does wear them occasionally.

CASE 5

A 33-year-old woman inquires about contact lenses during her routine eye examination. She states that she has to wear her glasses constantly and would like to be able to see without having to wear them. She reports that she has never tried contact lenses before because she was afraid that they would damage her eyes. She asks many questions about the potential hazards of contact lens wear and seems overly concerned about discomfort during the adaptation process. She also appears very timid and nervous during your testing, particularly during tonometry and ophthalmoscopy. Her keratometry and refraction are as follows:

OD 41.00 @ 090; 41.75 @ 180 $-0.50-0.75\times 090$
OS 41.50 @ 090; 42.00 @ 180 $-0.75-0.50\times 095$

Should this patient be fitted with contact lenses?

SOLUTION: Although this patient seems motivated to wear contact lenses, her exaggerated concerns about potential risks reduce the likelihood that she will be a satisfied wearer. In addition, her apprehension during ocular testing may indicate that she will have difficulty learning application of contact lenses, which may further discourage her. Because of her concerns about initial comfort, a soft lens would be advisable; however, her refraction suggests that a spherical lens may not provide her with sharp acuity. A soft toric may provide better acuity but could be less comfortable initially. This patient is not a good candidate. However, if after a comprehensive discussion on the risks and benefits of contact lens wear she still desires to be fitted, proceed with caution.

CASE 6

A 54-year-old patient presents for his routine eye examination. During the examination, he expresses a desire to be fitted with contact lenses for his outdoor activities, which include golf, jogging, and working in his garden. His main complaint is that his glasses get dirty and fog up during these activities. He has never worn contact lenses before. His ocular history includes primary open-angle glaucoma, for which he takes timolol 0.5% b.i.d. in both eyes. His refraction is the following:

$$OD\ -3.00 - 0.25 \times 180$$
$$OS\ -2.50 - 0.50 \times 170$$
$$Add\ +1.75$$

Slit-lamp evaluation reveals normal ocular structures with no corneal staining or papillary hypertrophy. His TBUT is 10 seconds.

Should this patient be fitted with contact lenses?

SOLUTION: This patient is a good part-time contact lens candidate. Aside from his glaucoma, his ocular and systemic health are good, and he is motivated to eliminate spectacle wear during sports and other outdoor activities. The main concern is his use of topical medications. First, the contact lenses may alter the delivery of the medication to the eye, which may cause undue fluctuations in his intraocular pressure. Second, preservatives in the drops may discolor or damage the contact lenses. To address these concerns, a disposable soft lens (daily disposable being an excellent option) should be prescribed. This will allow the patient to replace his lenses frequently so that the drops do not adversely affect them. In addition, the patient should be instructed to wait 15 to 20 minutes after drop instillation before applying his lenses in the morning, and to wait until after removal to instill his drops in the evening. A soft lens also allows him to wear contact lenses on a part-time basis. Finally, the issue of single-vision versus multifocal options should be discussed (see Chapter 15).

CASE 7

A 14-year-old boy presents for his annual eye examination. During the examination he reports that, although he wears sports goggles, they become dirty and limit his field of view during his junior high school football games. He has been told in the past that he can't wear contact lenses because of his astigmatism, but inquires if he can wear them during practice and in games. Your keratometry and refraction reveal the following:

$$OD\quad 43.25\ @\ 175;\ 45.50\ @\ 85\quad -0.50 - 2.50 \times 175$$
$$OS\quad 43.75\ @\ 010;\ 45.50\ @\ 100\quad -1.00 - 1.75 \times 010$$

Slit-lamp examination reveals no corneal staining or tarsal abnormalities. His tear meniscus appears normal, and his TBUT is 15 seconds.

Should this patient be fitted with contact lenses?

SOLUTION: Yes, this patient is a great contact lens candidate. Most teenagers are mature enough to handle the responsibilities of contact lens wear and care, but it is important to individually assess each patient's maturity level. This patient has significant astigmatism and was told that he could not wear contact lenses. However, soft and GP lens designs are available that will be able to correct his vision quite well (see Chapter 14). Because of the physical nature of football, soft lenses should be fitted to avoid lens loss during games. In addition, a disposable or frequent replacement lens should be considered so that he can dispose of his lenses when they become soiled. This may occur as often as every game, which is possible with a disposable toric lens. Another option which would provide excellent vision and not dislodge during football is hybrid lenses. These are becoming increasingly popular for those needing the crispness and stability of vision offered by a GP lens while participating in sports. He may even discover that his vision with contact lenses is good enough to consider full-time wear.

CASE 8

A 24-year-old architect presents for a contact lens fitting. He is currently earning his recreational pilot's license and is concerned that if he were to lose his glasses during turbulence, he would be unable to land his plane. Otherwise, he has no other complaints with his glasses. He reports that he had tried soft contact lenses in the past but did not continue with them because his work demands the sharpest vision possible. His keratometry and refraction are as follows:

$$OD \quad 43.50 @ 175; 44.25 @ 085 \quad -1.50 - 0.75 - 175$$
$$OS \quad 43.75 @ 180; 44.25 @ 090 \quad -2.00 - 0.50 \times 180$$

Should this patient be fitted with contact lenses?

SOLUTION: This patient is a good candidate for part-time soft lens wear. A spherical design should provide enough clarity for most visual tasks, including flying. If sharper vision is desired, a soft toric can be fitted in the right eye. A GP contact lens would provide sharper acuity, but they are not as suitable for part-time wear. In addition, the patient may experience dry eyes while flying, which can be minimized with proper soft lens selection.

CASE 9

A 38-year-old woman presents for a contact lens fitting. She reports that she would like the cosmetic benefit of not having to wear her glasses, which she wears full time. She reports that she has prism in her glasses, and without them she sees double. Lensometry reveals 2 prism diopters of base-out OD and OS. Your refraction is as follows:

$$OD \quad -3.50 \, DS \quad\quad\quad 20/20$$
$$OS \quad -1.75 - 1.50 \times 170 \quad 20/20$$

Binocular testing reveals an intermittent alternating esotropia of 10 prism diopters with 2 prism diopters of base-out prism over each eye, she is able to fuse. Slit-lamp evaluation reveals good ocular health.

Should this patient be fitted with contact lenses?

SOLUTION: Because this patient requires lateral prism to prevent diplopia, contact lenses are not a good option. Even if her vision is correctable to 20/20 in each eye with contact lenses, she would require plano spectacles with the lateral prism to wear over her contact lenses. If the patient is mainly concerned about the poor cosmesis with thick myopic lenses with base-out prism, contact lens wear can significantly reduce the edge thickness of the glasses. A smaller frame size will further decrease edge thickness. However, the patient may decide over time that she is not appreciating much benefit from the contact lenses and discontinue wear. If the patient desires contact lens wear without spectacles, she should be advised that she is a poor candidate.

CASE 10

A 28-year-old man presents for a comprehensive eye examination and contact lens fitting. He is a salesman who feels that his glasses prevent him from making eye contact with his clients. He has never worn contact lenses in the past. He has no ocular complaints other than periodic redness and irritation. His general health is good. His refraction reveals the following:

$$OD \quad -5.50\ DS$$
$$OS \quad -5.75 - 0.25 \times 180$$

Slit-lamp examination reveals flakes and crusts on his eyelashes, clogged meibomian gland orifices, mild conjunctival injection, and grade 1 inferior corneal staining. TBUT is 3 seconds.

Should this patient be fitted with contact lenses?

SOLUTION: This patient has a classic case of chronic blepharitis and meibomitis with mild conjunctival and corneal involvement. He should not be fitted with contact lenses at this time, although he may eventually become a good candidate once this condition is resolved. However, chronic blepharitis is very difficult to eradicate completely and will likely require continued maintenance treatment. The patient should be advised at this visit to begin a course of hot compresses and lid scrubs twice a day. The patient should then be re-evaluated in 2 weeks. If the condition has cleared sufficiently such that no injection or corneal staining is present, the patient can then be fitted with contact lenses. Either disposable soft or GP lenses can be fitted, and diligent cleaning and disinfection are crucial. This patient may suffer from dry-eye symptoms in contact lenses, even with treatment, so silicone hydrogels or daily disposables may be a good choice. Continued lid hygiene is also important in preventing future complications.

CLINICAL PROFICIENCY CHECKLIST

- Primary reasons for patient interest in contact lenses include cosmesis, inconvenience of spectacles, better vision, sports, and occupational considerations.
- Among the contraindications to contact lens wear are chronic allergies necessitating antihistamine use, dryness, juvenile diabetes, cardiovascular disorders, and pregnancy.
- If the patient is a current contact lens wearer, it is important to obtain a comprehensive contact lens history, including his or her satisfaction with current lenses and lens parameter verification.
- It is important to perform keratometry or videokeratography on all potential contact lens wearers. The use of videokeratography is especially beneficial for all high astigmatic and irregular cornea patients.
- A careful binocular refraction should be performed to predict the final lens power and determine residual astigmatism.
- The patient's binocular vision status should be evaluated; if lateral prism is necessary, the patient may not be a good contact lens candidate.
- Anatomic measurements such as corneal diameter, pupil diameter, and palpebral aperture height, in addition to determination of lid tension and blink rate, will help determine both the material to be used and the specific lens parameters.
- A comprehensive slit-lamp examination to evaluate eyelashes, tarsal and bulbar conjunctiva, and corneal integrity is important; a 360-degree evaluation of the limbus and fluorescein evaluation of the cornea are also important.
- Preocular tear film quality and volume should be evaluated by a combination of tests such as TBUT, tear prism evaluation, corneal and conjunctival staining, and phenol red thread test.

(continued)

- During the final consultation, the patient's motivation should be evaluated. In addition, it may be necessary to discuss the benefits of spectacles versus contact lenses and GP versus soft lens materials.
- The very low ametrope is a good contact lens candidate. Part-time DW is usually recommended for these patients.
- The borderline dry-eye patient may be an acceptable contact lens candidate; careful contact lens selection and patient education are keys to creating a successful contact lens wearer.

REFERENCES

1. Jaanus SD, Bartlett JD, Hiett JA. Ocular effects of systemic drugs. In: Bartlett JD, Jaanus SD, eds. *Clinical Ocular Pharmacology*. 3rd ed. Boston, MA: Butterworth Heinemann; 1995:970–972.
2. Bartlett JD. Medications and contact lens wear. In: Silbert JA, ed. *Anterior Segment Complications of Contact Lens Wear*. New York, NA: Churchill Livingstone Inc; 1994:474–482.
3. Stapleton F, Keay L, Jalbert I, et al. The epidemiology of contact lens related infiltrates. *Optom Vis Sci*. 2007; 84:257–272.
4. Morgan PB, Efron N, Brennan NA, et al. Risk factors for the development of corneal infiltrative events associated with contact lens wear. *Invest Ophthalmol Vis Sci*. 2005;46:3136–3143.
5. Carney LG, Mainstone JC, Carkeet A, et al. Rigid lens dynamics: lid effects. *CLAO J*. 1997;23(1):69–77.
6. Josephson JE. Examination of the anterior ocular surface and tear film. In: Stein H, Slatt B, Stein R, eds. *Fitting Guide for Rigid and Soft Contact Lenses*. 3rd ed. St. Louis, MO: CV Mosby; 1990:39–50.
7. Mandell RB. The enigma of the corneal contour. *CLAO J*. 1992;18(4):267–273.
8. Rowsey JJ, Reynolds AE, Brown R. Corneal topography: corneascope. *Arch Ophthalmol*. 1981;99:1093–1100.
9. Belin M, Litoff D, Strods S, et al. The PAR Technology Corneal Topography System. *Refract Corneal Surg*. 1992;8:88–96.
10. Snook RK. Pachymetry and true topography using the ORBSCAN System. In: Gills JP, Sanders DR, Thornton SP, et al., eds. *Corneal Topography: The State of the Art*. Thorofare, NJ: SLACK Inc; 1995:89–103.
11. Mejia-Barbosa Y, Malacara-Hernandez D. A review of methods for measuring corneal topography. *Optom Vis Sci*. 2011;78(4):240–253.
12. Chan JS, Mandell RB, Johnson L, et al. Contact lens base curve prediction from videokeratography. *Optom Vis Sci*. 1998;75(6):445–449.
13. Jeandervin M. Computer-aided contact lens fitting with the corneal topographer. *Contact Lens Spectrum*. 1998;13(3):21–24.
14. Szczotka L. Contact lenses for the irregular cornea. *Contact Lens Spectrum*. 1998;13(6):21–27.
15. Allansmith MR, Korb DR, Greiner JV, et al. Giant papillary conjunctivitis in contact lens wearers. *Am J Ophthalmol*. 1977;83(5):697–708.
16. Korb DR, Herman JP. Corneal staining subsequent to sequential fluorescein instillations. *J Am Optom Assoc*. 1979;50(3):361–367.
17. Snyder C. Infiltrative keratitis with contact lens wear—a review. *J Am Optom Assoc*. 1995;66(3):160–177.
18. Andres S, Henriques A, Garcia ML, et al. Factors of the precorneal fluid break-up time (BUT) and tolerance of contact lenses. *Int Cont Lens Clin*. 1987;14(3):81–120.
19. Tomlinson A. Cont lens-induced dry eye. In Tomlinson A, ed. *Complications of Contact Lens Wear*. London: Mosby Year Book; 1992:195–218.
20. Mengher LS, et al. Noninvasive assessment of tear film stability in Holly FJ, ed. *Preocular Tear Film in Health, Disease, and Contact Lens Wear*. Lubbock, TX: Dry Eye Institute; 1986:64.
21. Patel S, Murray D, McKenzie A, et al. Effects of fluorescein on tear breakup time and on tear thinning time. *Am J Optom Physiol Opt*. 1985;62:188–190.
22. Guillon JP, Guillon M. Tear film examination of the contact lens patient. *Optician*. 1993;206(5421):21–29.
23. Doane MG, Lee ME. Tear film interferometry as a diagnostic tool for evaluating normal and dry-eye tear film. *Advances Exper Med Biol*. 1998;438:297–303.
24. Cho P, Yap M. Schirmer test. I. A review. *Optom Vis Sci*. 1993;70(2):152–156.
25. Bennett ES, Gordon JM. The borderline dry-eye patient and contact lens wear. *Contact Lens Forum*. 1989;14(7):52–74
26. Nichols, KK, Mitchell GL, Zadnik K. The repeatability of clinical measurements of dry eye. *Cornea*. 2004;23(3):272–285.
27. Methodologies to diagnose and monitor dry eye disease: Report of the Diagnostic Methodology Subcommittee of the International Dry eye Workshop (2007). *Ocul Surf*. 2007;5(2):108–152.

28. Hamano T, Mitsunaga S, Kotani S, et al. Tear volume in relation to contact lens wear and age. *CLAO J.* 1990; 16(1):57–61.
29. Sakamoto R, Bennett ES, Henry VA, et al. The phenol red thread tear test: A cross-cultural study. *Inv Ophthalmol Vis Sci.* 1993;34(13):3510–3514.
30. Elliott L, Henderson B, Bennett ES, et al. Comparison of overall performance of hydrogel and rigid gas permeable lens materials in the contact lens management of the borderline dry eye patient. Presented at: Annual Meeting of the American Academy of Optometry; 1996; Orlando, FL, December.
31. Lupelli L. A review of lacrimal function tests in relation to contact lens practice: I. *Contact Lens J.* 1988;16(7):4–17.
32. Feenstra RP, Tseng SC. What is actually stained by rose bengal? *Arch Ophthalmol.* 1992;110(7):984–993.
33. Tseng SC, Zhang SH. Interaction between rose bengal and different protein components. *Cornea.* 1995;14(4):427–435.
34. Danjo Y, Watanabe H, Tisdale AS, et al. Alteration of mucin in human conjunctival epithelia in dry eye. *Invest Ophthalmol Vis Sci.* 1998;39(13):2602–2609.
35. Argüeso P, Tisdale A, Spurr-Michaud S, et al. Mucin characteristics of human corneal-limbal epithelial cells that exclude the rose bengal anionic dye. *Invest Ophthalmol Vis Sci.* 2006;47(1):113–119.
36. Zuccaro VS. Rose bengal: a vital stain. *Contact Lens Forum.* 1981;6:39–43.
37. Chodosh J, Dix RD, Howell RC, et al. Staining characteristics and antiviral activity of sulforhodamine B and lissamine green B. *Invest Ophthalmol Vis Sci.* 1994;35(3):1046–1058.
38. Manning F J, Wehrly SR, Foulks G, et al. Patient tolerance and ocular surface staining characteristics of lissamine green versus rose bengal. *Ophthalmology.* 1995;102(12):1953–1957.
39. Korb DR, Greiner JV, Herman JP, et al. Lid-wiper epitheliopathy and dry-eye symptoms in contact lens wearers. *CLAO J.* 2002;28(4):211–216.
40. Korb DR, Herman JP, Blackie CA, et al. Prevalence of lid wiper epitheliopathy in subjects with dry eye signs and symptoms. *Cornea.* 2010;29(4):377–383.
41. Pult H, Purslow C, Berry M, et al. Clinical tests for successful contact lens wear: relationship and predictive potential. *Optom Vis Sci.* 2008;85(10):E924–E929.
42. TearLab Corp www.tearlab.com. Accessed June 2012.
43. Foulks GN, Lemp MA, Berg M. TearLab™ Osmolarity as a Biomarker for disease severity in mild to moderate dry eye disease. *Am Acad Ophthalmol.* PO382, 2009
44. McMonnies CA, Ho A. Patient history in screening for dry eye patients. *J Am Optom Assoc.* 1987;58(4):296–301.
45. Begley CG, Caffery B, Nichols KK, et al. Responses of contact lens wearers to a dry eye survey. *Optom Vis Sci.* 2000;77(1):40–46.
46. Harris MG, Gilman EL. Consultation, examination and prognosis. In: Mandell RB, ed. *Contact Lens Practice.* 4th ed. Springfield, IL: Charles C. Thomas; 1988:136–172.
47. White PF, Gilman EL. Preliminary evaluation. In: Bennett ES, Weissman BA, eds. *Clinical Contact Lens Practice.* Philadelphia, PA: Lippincott; 1992:chap. 17.
48. Terry R. The effect of glasses on personality perception. *Contact Lens Spectrum.* 1989;4(7):58.
49. Walline JJ, Jones LA, Mutti DO, et al. A Randomized trial of the effects of rigid contact lenses on myopia progression. *Arch Ophthalmol.* 2004;122(12):1760–1766.
50. Walline JJ, Sinnott L, Ticak A, et al. Children's attitudes about kids in eyeglasses (CAKE) Study [abstract]. *Invest Ophthalmol Vis Sci.* 2006:1149.
51. Hewett TT. A survey of contact lens wearers. II. Behaviors, experiences, attitudes, and expectations. *Am J Optom Physiol Opt.* 1984;61(2):73–79.
52. Rengstorff RH, Black CJ. Eye protection from contact lenses. *J Am Optom Assoc.* 1974;45(3):270–275.
53. Doughty MJ, Fonn D, Richter D, et al. A patient questionnaire approach to estimating the prevalence of dry eye symptoms in patients presenting to optometric practices across Canada. *Optom Vis Sci.* 1997;74(8):624–631.
54. Begley CG, Chalmers RL, Mitchell L, et al. Characterization of ocular surface symptoms from optometric practices in North America. *Cornea.* 2001;20(6):610–618.
55. Snyder C. Alleviating dryness in contact lens wear. *Contact Lens Spectrum.* 1998;13(8):35–40.
56. Sorbara L, Talsky C. Contact lens wear in the dry eye patient: predicting success and achieving it. *Can J Optom.* 1988;50(4):234–241.
57. Dillehay, SM, Miller MB. Performance of Lotrafilcon B silicone hydrogel contact lenses in experienced low-Dk/t daily lens wearers. *Eye Contact Lens.* 2007;33(6 Pt 1):272–277.
58. Schafer J, Mitchell GL, Chalmers RL, et al. The stability of dryness symptoms after refitting with silicone hydrogel contact lenses over 3 years. *Eye Contact Lens.* 2007;33(5):247–252.

Chapter 2

Optical Considerations in Contact Lens Practice

Chandra V. Mickles and William J. Benjamin

Practitioners who are cognizant of the optical effects of contact lenses are in a better position to optimize outcomes and prevent disappointments with this mode of refractive correction. Hence, knowledge of optical principles surrounding the wear of contact lenses is critical for achieving success in their prescription.

The purpose of this chapter is to review the optics of contact lens practice as a quick reference source for the clinician. It is intended to be a practical companion to Chapters 26 and 27 of *Borish's Clinical Refraction,* which discuss the optics of contact lenses in greater detail.[1,2] The reader can refer to these chapters for a more extensive analysis of the optical considerations in contact lens practice.

In the first half of this chapter, clinically relevant topics will be presented. The second half will offer the practitioner a practical guide to key formulae, clinical guidelines, and a worksheet for computing refractive powers of rigid contact lenses. A set of optical problems is also included at the end of the chapter, so that the busy practitioner or student can relatively quickly prove his or her knowledge in this area.

REFRACTIVE CORRECTION

As technological advancements continue to expand contact lens practice, it is easy to forget the fundamental reason for their existence. Simply put, contact lenses provide patients with excellent vision through refractive correction.

As an optical device, contact lenses have the ability to bend parallel light rays into focus to fulfill the optical correction of ametropia. In other words, contact lenses have refractive power, which is the magnitude that a lens diverges or converges light. Although thin in appearance, contact lenses are treated in geometrical optics as a *thick* lens. Unlike thin lenses, the refraction of light as it passes through the thickness of the lens must be taken into consideration. Hence, the refractive power of contact lenses is not simply equivalent to the sum of refractive powers of the anterior and posterior surfaces. The refractive power of a contact lens results from the power of the anterior and posterior surfaces, the refractive index of the material, and the center thickness (CT) of the contact lens material.

The refractive power that is most used for contact lenses is the back vertex power, or BVP. The point of reference for the BVP is the back vertex of the lens, and this point is easily localized during measurement using a lensometer. The thick lens formula for computing the BVP of a typical contact lens of meniscus design (Fig. 2.1) is

$$BVP = \frac{F_1}{1-(t/n')F_1} + F_2$$

where

$\quad\quad$ BVP = the back vertex power, in diopters

$\quad\quad$ $F_1 = (n' - n)/r_1$ = the refractive power of the anterior lens surface

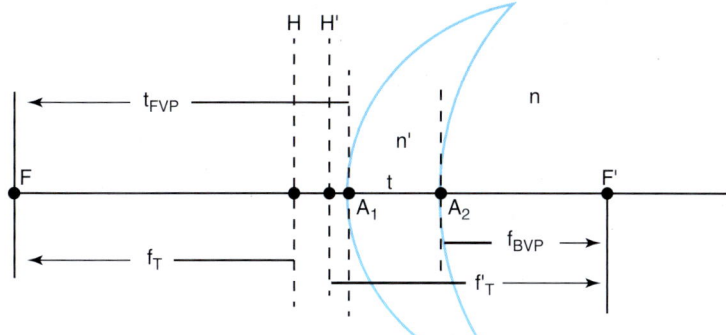

FIGURE 2.1 A typical contact lens is a thick lens, optically speaking. It has a meniscus design such that the principal planes (H, H') lie anterior to a plus lens, as shown, but posterior to a minus lens. Made of material having a refractive index (n') greater than air (n), the front (convex) lens surface has a plus power (F1), and the back (concave) lens surface a minus power (F2). The front surface vertex (A1) and the back surface vertex (A2) are separated by center thickness (t). The refractive power of the lens is a function of F1, F2, t, and n', but it depends on the reference points from which focal lengths are measured. The diagram indicates three possible reference points from which focal length can be measured (f_T, f_{FVP}, and f_{BVP}, respectively): (1) principal planes (f_T); (2) front vertex (FVP); and (3) back vertex (BVP). (Modified from Benjamin W. Visual optics of contact lens wear. In: Bennett ES, Weissman BE, eds. Clinical Contact Lens Practice. Philadelphia, PA: JB Lippincott; 1991:9.)

$F_2 = (n - n')/r_2$ = the refractive power of the posterior lens surface
t = the CT of the lens, in meters
n' = the refractive index of the lens material
r_1 = the radius of curvature of the anterior surface, in meters
r_2 = the radius of curvature of the posterior surface, in meters

Clinical Measurement of Refractive Power

When measuring the BVP, the concave (back) surface of the contact lens is placed against the lens stop such that the back vertex is located at the lens stop. Although most contact lenses are specified by BVP by convention, the relatively steep curvatures of contact lenses make correct positioning of the concave surface of the contact lens on the lens stop more difficult than on the convex (front) surface. Thus, many clinicians routinely measure the front vertex power (FVP) of contact lenses, as correct positioning of the contact lens on the lens stop is easier with this measurement. Measuring from the front vertex instead of the back vertex is inconsequential when measuring thin contact lenses because the two powers are comparable. However, as lens thickness increases, the difference between the FVP and BVP becomes clinically significant (Table 2.1). Practitioners must be mindful of this disparity, particularly with high plus powers that have large CT. For correct positioning of the back vertex of contact lenses in the measurement of BVP, a contact lens stop that is smaller than the conventional lens stop can be fitted on most lensometers.

Vertexing the Power

Lenses are said to have equivalent effective power if their focal points are at the same axial position. When correcting ametropia, this is at the far point, the point conjugate to the retina of a patient. Ametropia is corrected when the correcting lens's focal point is placed at the far point of the eye. The focal length required to form a focus at the far point varies with the distance of the correcting lens from the anterior corneal surface known as the vertex distance. For example, as a minus lens is brought closer to the corneal plane (decreasing vertex distance), a

TABLE 2.1 Differences between Front and Back Vertex Powers for Rigid Lenses

BACK VERTEX POWER (D)	FRONT VERTEX POWER (D)	CENTER THICKNESS (mm)	POWER DISPARITY (D)
−10	−9.92	0.10	−0.08
−5	−4.95	0.12	−0.05
0	0.0	0.15	0.00
+5	+4.90	0.23	+0.10
+10	+9.71	0.32	+0.29
+15	+14.44	0.41	+0.56
+20	+19.06	0.50	+0.94

longer focal length (lower power) is required to form an image at the same far point. Therefore, if compensation is not made, lenses of the same refractive power yet different vertex distances will have different effective powers. The foci will not be placed on the same point, and the patient will not have clear vision at distance.

This is the case when comparing spectacle lenses to contact lenses. While spectacles are worn at vertex distances of typically 8 to 18 mm in front of the corneal apex, contact lenses are worn at a vertex distance of zero (Fig. 2.2).[1] Therefore, clinicians must convert the refractive power of a spectacle lens at its vertex distance to the equivalent effective power of the contact lens at the vertex distance of zero. Consequently, the focus will remain on the far point of the eye and the patient will see properly.

The change in focal length (1/BVP) to keep the lens focus on the far point of the eye is equal to the change in vertex distance. In other words, the difference in power between the spectacle plane and the corneal plane is related to the difference in focal lengths required by altering the

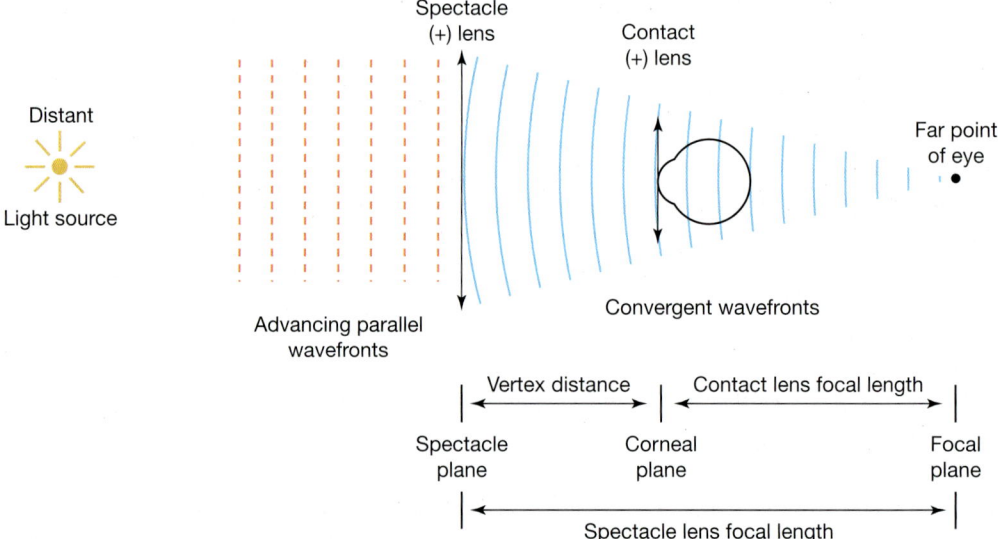

FIGURE 2.2 Refractive power with vertex distance. The refractive power of the correcting lens depends on the vertex distance. For a plus lens correction at the corneal plane will require a shorter focal distance than at the spectacle plane by an amount equal to the vertex distance. (Modified from Benjamin W. Visual optics of contact lens wear. In: Bennett ES, Weissman BE, eds. *Clinical Contact Lens Practice*. Philadelphia, PA: JB Lippincott; 1991:9.)

vertex distance. The effective power difference between corrections at the spectacle plane and cornea becomes clinically significant at lens powers greater than about ± 4.00 D.

Example 1: Minus Lens

An eye's spectacle refraction is −5.00 D at a vertex distance of 12 mm. One first calculates the focal length of this lens:

$$\text{Focal length} = \frac{1}{-5.00\,\text{D}} = -0.200\,\text{m}$$

The contact lens refractive power to keep the focal point on the eye's far point is then calculated by adjusting the prior focal length by the amount of the vertex distance:

$$\frac{1}{(-0.200\,\text{m} - 0.012\,\text{m})} = -4.72\,\text{D}$$

Example 2: Plus Lens

An eye's spectacle refraction is +5.00 D at a vertex distance of 12 mm. The focal length of this lens is

$$\text{Focal length} = \frac{1}{+5.00\,\text{D}} = +0.200\,\text{m}$$

The contact lens refractive power to keep the focal point on the eye's far point using a contact lens is then

$$\frac{1}{(+0.200\,\text{m} - 0.012\,\text{m})} = +5.32\,\text{D}$$

For those who might better use an equation to vertex powers from the spectacle plane to the corneal plane, the following equation can be used:

$$\text{BVP}_{\text{contact lens}} = \frac{\text{BVP}_{\text{spectacles}}}{(1 - d\text{BVP}_{\text{spectacles}})}$$

where
  BVP = back vertex power, in diopters
  d = vertex distance

For an astigmatic correction, this calculation must be performed for each primary meridian.

It can be observed above that, as a minus lens is brought closer to the eye, its effective power increases such that its refractive power must be decreased to keep the focus on the far point.[1] As a plus lens is brought closer to the eye, its effective power decreases such that its refractive power must be increased to maintain a constant amount of power relative to the eye.

Rather than resort to calculation, clinicians often use what is called a Vertex Distance Table (see Appendix 2) to determine the required BVP of a contact lens from the refractive correction found at the spectacle plane. Vertexing the BVP to the corneal plane is often one of the initial steps of fitting a contact lens.

Flexure of Contact Lenses on the Eye

Soft contact lenses are much flatter than the cornea and drape to the corneal surface. As a result, they flex a large amount when placed on the eye. This induces a clinically significant change in BVP for thick contact lenses, such as those having a plus power, predicted by the following equation:

$$F_{ch} = -300(t)\left[\left(1/r_k^2\right)-\left(1/r_2^2\right)\right]$$

where

F_{ch} = change in BVP induced by flexure, in diopters
t = CT of contact lens, in millimeters
r_k = the radius of curvature of the cornea, determined by keratometry, in millimeters
r_2 = radius of curvature of the posterior contact lens surface, in millimeters.

The power alterations result in a net reduction of plus power and can account for up to 0.75 D less plus power than that indicated on the packaging of lenses of large plus power, such as might be prescribed for an eye with aphakia. The power of minus lenses does not change sufficiently to be of clinical significance because they are so thin. Thus, clinicians do not have to be concerned about power changes of soft lenses due to flexure in cases of myopia, low hyperopia, or even usually medium hyperopia.

Rigid lenses do not conform to the corneal surface. Compared to soft lenses, then, flexure of spherical rigid lenses is generally small (≤1.50 D) and does not result in clinically significant changes of lens refractive power. However, rigid lens flexure creates astigmatic back-surface toricity that alters the power of the lacrimal lens. Flexure and its impact on the lacrimal lens will be reviewed further in Chapter 5 of this text and in many of the optics problems found in the Formulae for Optics section of this chapter.

The amount of flexure depends on the flexural strength of the rigid lens material. Lenses made of materials having greater oxygen permeability generally flex more than materials of low permeability, and thin lenses flex more than thick lenses. Flexure of the optical zones of spherical rigid lenses is not induced when the cornea is nontoric and is clinically insignificant when worn on corneas of low toricity. When the cornea is toric by a diopter or greater, the practitioner should consider the effects of flexure of spherical rigid lenses.

Many rigid lenses prescribed today are made of the more flexible oxygen-permeable materials and are designed as thin as possible to meet corneal oxygen demands and provide better comfort. Thus, flexure of rigid materials can become problematic for contact lens practitioners. Flexure can be minimized by increasing lens thickness, selection of a stiffer material, or by prescription of a bitoric lens for which the back curvatures better match a highly toric cornea.

Lacrimal Lens Power

The back surface of a rigid lens, unlike a soft contact lens, does not conform to the cornea. Thus, the space between the lens and the cornea is filled in with tear fluid. The reservoir of tear fluid behind the lens is referred to as a "lacrimal lens," "fluid lens," or "tear lens." The lacrimal lens has a power determined by its front surface, back surface, and thickness just like any other lens. Indeed, when an eye wears a rigid lens, it is wearing in actuality two lenses: the rigid lens and the lacrimal lens.

When the lacrimal lens is very thin, as is the case in most contact lens wearers, the power of the lacrimal lens is taken to be the difference between the back curve of the contact lens and the front curve of the corneal surface. The thickness of the lacrimal lens is in these cases insignificant from a refractive power point of view. The lacrimal lens power (LLP) is therefore defined as the base curve (D) − keratometry reading (D), both defined in keratometric diopters ($n' = 1.3375$) applied to the two primary meridians.

A "minus" lacrimal lens is created when the base curve is flatter than the corneal surface meridian and a "plus" lacrimal lens is created when the lens is steeper than the cornea (Fig. 2.3). In order to compensate for a minus-powered lacrimal lens, plus power can be incorporated into the contact lens prescription in compensation. Minus power can be incorporated into the

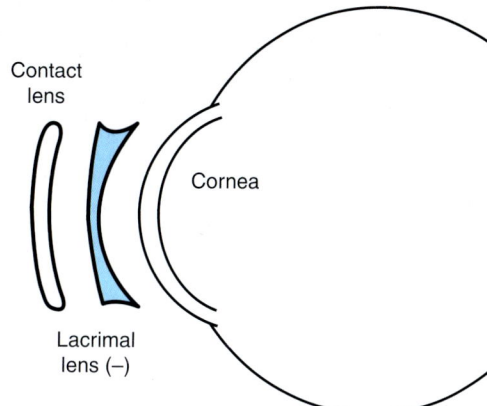

FIGURE 2.3 Lacrimal lens. (Modified from Benjamin W. Visual optics of contact lens wear. In: Bennett ES, Weissman BE, eds. *Clinical Contact Lens Practice*. Philadelphia, PA: JB Lippincott; 1991:9.)

contact lens prescription in compensation for a plus-powered lacrimal lens. Allowing for the LLP is illustrated in the following examples.

Lacrimal Lens Power Example

An eye's refraction is -1.00 D and it has a keratometry reading of 44.50 D. The plan is to fit the patient with a lens having a base curve of 45.50 D (7.42 mm). Note, in this case, the lens is steeper than the cornea.

LLP = 45.50 − 44.50 = +1.00 D. This is a "plus" lacrimal lens trapped between the cornea and the lens that is steeper than the cornea.

The power of -1.00 D is required to compensate for the lacrimal lens. Thus, the power of the contact lens needed to correct for the eye's myopia is predicted to be -2.00 D.

Frequently, in clinical practice, a diagnostic rigid contact lens is placed on the eye to assess the fitting of the lens and to ascertain the final contact lens power that will be ordered for a patient. Typically, the desirable diagnostic contact lens which matches exactly the base curve and refractive power needed is not available. A refraction over the best-fitting diagnostic lens is used to determine the final contact lens power (FCLP). This FCLP can be calculated with the following equation:

$$FCLP = DCLP + OR - \Delta LLP$$

where
    DCLP = Diagnostic CLP (D)
    OR = Overrefraction (D)
    ΔLLP = change in LLP in diopters, when altering from the diagnostic contact lens to the final contact lens.

The use of this equation is illustrated further in Chapter 5 of this text and in many of the optics problems found in the Formulae for Optics section of this chapter.

BINOCULAR VISION AND PERCEPTION

The minification or magnification of vision through contact lenses is different from spectacles, and it is important that practitioners are cognizant of the subsequent clinical ramifications.

Spectacle Magnification

Spectacle magnification (SM), or magnification of correction, indicates how much a corrective lens magnifies or minifies the retinal image compared to the same eye uncorrected.

A positive correcting lens will magnify and a negative correction lens will minify the retinal image.[3] The effect decreases with vertex distance. Placing a lens closer to the cornea, such as a contact lens, will result in less magnification for a positive lens and less minification for a negative lens. The equation for SM is

$$SM = \underbrace{\frac{1}{1 - h(BVP)}}_{\text{(power factor)}} \times \underbrace{\frac{1}{1 - (t/n')F_1}}_{\text{(shape factor)}}$$

where

SM = Spectacle magnification

BVP = the back vertex power of the correcting lens, in diopters

h = stop distance from the plane of the correction lens to the ocular entrance pupil, in meters = vertex distance + 3 mm

t = CT of the correcting lens (m)

n' = the refractive index of the correcting lens

F_1 = the front surface power of the correcting lens, in diopters

Technically speaking, SM will be affected in contact lens wear by the front surface curvature (F_1). However, contact lenses are so thin that thickness (t) offsets front surface curvature, making the shape factor clinically insignificant. The lacrimal lens could be included in this analysis, but its impact on magnification is usually considered clinically insignificant. Hence, the shape factor and lacrimal lens are omitted from most considerations of magnification in cases of contact lens wear.

The major factor that produces a difference in magnification of a contact lens compared to a spectacle lens is the stop distance (h). It is 3 mm (0.003 m) for contact lenses because the vertex distance is zero. If the vertex distance for a spectacle lens is 15 mm, the stop distance is 18 mm (0.018 m). Overall, SM will generally be greater than unity in hyperopia (indicating magnification) and less than unity in myopia (indicating minification), but will be much less with contact lenses than with spectacles.

Clinical Implications of Spectacle Magnification

Clinicians should consider the effects of changing retinal image size from the uncorrected to corrected state when fitting contact lenses. This is influenced by the type of correction. For high myopes, the minification of retinal image size in spectacles is much reduced with contact lenses. As a result, highly myopic patients often have enhanced visual acuity with contact lenses in comparison to spectacles. Hyperopes encounter the opposing effect, whereby a reduction in visual acuity can occur with contact lenses.

The equation below can be used by the clinician to estimate the change in magnification of correction when going from spectacle correction to a contact lens:

$$\frac{\text{Contact lens power factor}}{\text{Spectacle lens power factor}} = 1 - hBVP$$

where

h = the stop distance of the spectacle lens, in meters = vertex distance + 3 mm

BVP = the back vertex power of the spectacle lens, in diopters.

Let us assume a patient's spectacle Rx is +15 D at a 15-mm vertex distance. A contact lens will result in approximately 27% less magnification as shown below.

$$\text{Approximate SM} = 1 - (0.018 \times 15)$$
$$= 0.73 \text{ or } 27\% \text{ less magnification with the contact lens.}$$

The reduction of SM is important in unilateral aphakia. Spectacle correction can result in 25% to 30% magnification for the aphakic eye and create refractive and prismatic diplopia. In fact, 5% to 8% magnification can occur with contact lens correction. This causes a reduction of binocularity and, in a few unilateral cases, diplopia, even without the prismatic component. As a result, intraocular lenses, with h = 0, theoretically contribute little or no magnification of the retinal image, and are the correction of choice in unilateral aphakia.[1]

The clinical implications of the magnification of contact lenses extend to aniseikonia, unequal image size between eyes. This will be discussed later in this chapter.

Relative Spectacle Magnification

Relative spectacle magnification (RSM) compares the corrected ametropic retinal image size to that of the standard emmetropic schematic eye. There are two equations for RSM. One equation describes RSM in cases of axial ametropia and the other equation describes RSM in cases of refractive ametropia. However, the theoretical optical implications are confusing because ametropia is seldom purely axial or purely refractive, and because retinal stretching exists in axial myopia. Many clinicians therefore rely on SM for individual cases because the application of RSM has so many confounding factors.

Anisometropia and Aniseikonia

Aniseikonia is a binocular vision anomaly in which retinal image sizes are unequal between eyes, primarily due to the correction of anisometropia. As the stop distance is less for contact lenses than for spectacles, the difference in magnification or minification between the eyes is usually less with contact lenses. Thus, contact lenses are often the correction of choice in anisometropia.

There is the theoretical case of axial anisometropia in which the analysis of RSM would suggest that spectacle correction would be better. However, as mentioned, anisometropia is seldom purely axial and the retinal stretching of the more myopic eye may reduce or eliminate the theoretical advantage. Thus, contact lenses should be attempted even in cases of suspected axial anisometropia to see if binocularity will be better accomplished.

Prismatic Effects of Contact Lenses

Prism

Prism causes image displacement. The amount of the displacement varies with the distance from the optical center of lens and the lens power at that distance. Image displacement does not occur at the lens's optical center. The amount of prism present at a given point on a lens can be deduced using Prentice's Rule:

$$P = hBVP$$

where, in this case,

- h = the distance from the lens optical center to the point on the lens pierced by the line of sight, in meters
- BVP = back vertex power of the lens, in diopters

A lens will induce increasing amounts of image displacement when viewed through points farther from the optical center.

Prismatic Effects and Vergence with Contact Lenses

Contact lenses substantially reduce the prismatic effects common with spectacle wear.[1] This is because contact lenses follow the eye as it rotates into different gaze positions, whereas spectacle lenses do not (Fig. 2.4). Contact lenses, for instance, virtually eliminate the base-in effect of minus spectacle lenses upon convergence in near gaze and the base-out effect of plus spectacle lenses (Fig. 2.4). They eliminate the vertical imbalances created by spectacle lenses in cases of anisometropia. The prismatic effects of spectacle wear minimized in contact lens wear are presented in Table 2.2.

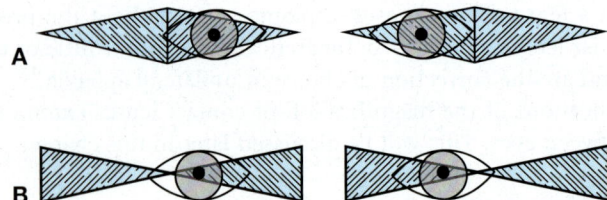

FIGURE 2.4 Prismatic effect of lens correction. Base-out effect of plus spectacle correction **(A)** and base-in effect of minus spectacle correction **(B)**. When a person converges to a near object, the eyes deviate from the optic axes of his or her spectacle lenses and generate prism according to Prentice's rule (Equation 26–30). (Modified from Benjamin W. Visual optics of contact lens wear. In: Bennett ES, Weissman BE, eds. *Clinical Contact Lens Practice.* Philadelphia, PA: JB Lippincott; 1991:9.)

There are some prismatic effects of significant contact lens movement on the blink and decantation, especially in cases of high ametropia or high anisometropia. In these cases, the displacement of the optical center of the contact lens from the patient's line of sight can result in prismatic fluctuations that are unsettling for some patients. Furthermore, although contact lenses reduce the undesirable prismatic effects of spectacles, beneficial prismatic effects of spectacles, such as the beneficial effect of minus lenses for exophoria at near and of plus lenses for esophoria at near, may also be reduced or eliminated.

Accommodative Demand

It is well-known that myopic corrections in spectacles reduce the amount of accommodative demand necessary to focus at near and that hyperopic spectacle corrections increase the demand at near. The wear of contact lenses brings the accommodative demand back to almost that of emmetropia. Therefore, clinicians should be wary of prescribing contact lenses to pre-presbyopic myopes and other myopes that have reduced accommodative amplitudes. Conversely, hyperopes receive a beneficial boost to their accommodative ability with contact lenses and anisometropes may obtain a more equal accommodative demand between the two eyes.

Contact Lens Optical Aberrations

Vision is affected by optical aberrations. Fortunately, contact lenses, unlike spectacles, follow the line of sight with eye rotation. As a result, the off-axis aberrations that influence central vision of patients wearing spectacles are minimized with contact lenses. Still, optical aberrations

TABLE 2.2 Prismatic Effects of Contact lenses

NEGATIVE EFFECTS	EFFECTS[a] MINIMIZED WITH CONTACTS

Prismatic fluctuations secondary to:
    Excessive lens movement
    Lens decentration
	"Base-out" effect for bilateral hyperopes, "base-in" effect for bilateral myopes

Prism imbalances with:
    Unilateral prism-ballasted torics
    Prism-ballasted bifocals for anisometropes
	Vertical prismatic effects and imbalances in down gaze resulting from anisometropia

Inability to correct significant prismatic deviations	Vergence demand alterations in anisometropia or antimetropia, required for right and left gaze
Increased near convergence demand for bilateral myopes	Increased near convergence demand for bilateral hyperopes

[a]The prismatic effects common to spectacle wear.

TABLE 2.3 Optical Aberrations of Correcting Lenses and Visual Deficits Produced During Lens Wear

ABERRATION	OBJECT POSITION	VISUAL DEFICIT	
		SPECTACLES	CONTACT LENSES
Spherical aberration	On axis	Central	Central
Coma	Off axis	Central and peripheral	Peripheral
Radial astigmatism	Off axis	Central and peripheral	Peripheral
Curvature of field	Off axis	Central and peripheral	Peripheral
Distortion	Off axis	Central and peripheral	Peripheral
Chromatic aberration	On and off axis	Central and peripheral	Central and peripheral
Prismatic dispersion	Off axis	Central and peripheral	Peripheral

of contact lenses do exist. Table 2.3 lists the various optical aberrations of contact lenses and spectacles. Several contact lens manufacturers have attempted to reduce optical aberrations of their contact lens designs with varying degrees of success. However, the future is promising for effectively correcting for optical aberrations or using them to the contact lens wearer's advantage.

Residual and High Astigmatism

Residual astigmatism, the refractive astigmatism left uncorrected when a contact lens is placed on the eye, and other calculations related to correction of astigmatism are thoroughly discussed in Chapter 14 of this text. Clinical optics guidelines and formulae useful for clinical practice in this area are also located at the end of this chapter. Additionally, there is a set of back-toric optics problems to assist the reader in gaining mastery of this topic.

FORMULAE FOR CONTACT LENS OPTICS

Refractive Correction

Reflection for rays at near-normal incidence:

$$R = [(n' - n)/(n' + n)]^2$$

Back vertex power:

$$BVP = \frac{F_1}{1 - (t/n')F_1} + F_2$$

Front vertex power:

$$FVP = F_1 + \frac{F_2}{1 - (t/n')F_2}$$

where

R = reflectance from 0 to 1.0
n = refractive index of medium surrounding surface
n' = refractive index of medium within lens
t = CT of contact lens (m)

BVP = back vertex power (D)
FVP = front vertex power (D)
F_1 = front surface power (D)
F_2 = back surface power (D)

Vertex Equation

$$F_{contact\ lens} = F_{spectacles}/1 - dF_{spec}$$

where

F = refractive power
d = vertex distance

Surface power:*

$$F = \frac{n' - n}{r}$$

Law of Gladstone and Dale:

$$n_{hydrated} = n_p V_p + n_s V_s$$

Water content:

$$WC = \frac{n_{dehydrated} - n_{hydrated}}{n_{dehydrated} - n_{saline}} \times 100$$

where

r = radius of curvature of contact lens surface (m)
F = refractive power of surface
V_p, V_s = fraction of material volume devoted to polymer, saline
n_p, n_s = refractive indices for the polymer, saline in a hydrogel
WC = water content, in %

Empirical effect of flexure on soft contact lens power:

$$\Delta F = -300(t)\left[\left(1/r_k^2\right) - \left(1/r_2^2\right)\right]$$

where

t = CT of lens
r_k = radius of curvature of cornea
r_2 = base curve radius of lens
ΔF = change of refractive power (D)

Lacrimal Lens

Lacrimal lens power:

LLP = BC − K

Fitting Formulae:**

CPR = CLP + OR + LLP
and
FCLP = CPR − LLP

Diagnostic lens formula:

FCLP = DCLP + OR − ΔLLP

Astigmatism Addition:

CPA = CA + IA

where

CPA = astigmatism at corneal plane (DC)
CA = corneal astigmatism (DC)
IA = internal astigmatism (DC)
BC = base curve (D)
K = keratometry reading (D)
LLP = lacrimal lens power (D)

ΔLLP = change in LLP (D)
CPR = corneal plane refraction (D)
CLP = contact lens power (D)
FCLP = final CLP (D)
DCLP = diagnostic CLP (D)
OR = overrefraction (D)

Binocular Vision and Perception

Spectacle magnification:

$$SM = \underbrace{\frac{1}{1 - d(BVP)}}_{\text{(power factor)}} \times \underbrace{\frac{1}{1 - (t/n')F_1}}_{\text{(shape factor)}}$$

Comparison of contact lens to spectacle lens power factors:***

$$\frac{\text{Contact Lens Power Factor}}{\text{Spectacle Lens Power Factor}} = 1 - d(BVP)$$

---

*In *keratometric* diopters, n' = 1.3375 and n = 1.0000.
**When an OR of zero is intended for the final lens order, these two equations are equivalent.
***BVP here is that of the spectacle lens.

where

> BVP = back vertex power (D)
> d = stop distance, from back vertex of correcting lens to entrance pupil of eye (m)*
> t = CT of correcting lens (m)
> SM = spectacle magnification relative to 1.0

Magnification of Spectacle–contact lens telescope:**

$$M_t = \frac{-F_e}{F_o} \times \frac{F_{acd}}{4}$$

where

> M_t = magnification of telescope relative to 1.0
> F_o = power of objective, spectacle lens (D)
> F_e = power of eyepiece, contact lens (D)
> F_{add} = power of add in spectacle lens (D)

Prentice's rule:*

$$P = h(BVP)$$

Prism thickness formula:

$$P = \frac{100(n'-1)(BT-AT)}{BAL}$$

where

> P = prismatic power in prism diopters ($^\Delta$)
> h = half of the chord diameter, 2h
> BVP = back vertex power (D)
> BT = thickness of prism base
> AT = thickness of prism apex
> BAL = length of the base-apex line

Other Optical Considerations

Sagittal depth equations:

$$s = r - \sqrt{r^2 - h^2}$$

$$s_p = \left(\frac{r_{a-p}}{1-e^2}\right) - \sqrt{\left(\frac{r_{a-p}}{1-e^2}\right)^2 - \left(\frac{h^2}{1-e^2}\right)}$$

$$s_o = r_{a-o}(1-e^2) - \sqrt{[r_{a-o}(1-e^2)]^2 - h^2(1-e^2)}$$

$$s_p = \frac{h^2}{2r_{a-p}}$$

$$s_p = \left(\frac{r_{a-p}}{1-e^2}\right) + \sqrt{\left(\frac{r_{a-p}}{1-e^2}\right)^2 - \left(\frac{h^2}{1-e^2}\right)}$$

where

> e = eccentricity
> r_a = apical radius of curvature
> r_{a-p} = prolate apical radius of curvature
> r_{a-o} = oblate apical radius of curvature
> s_p, s_o = prolate, oblate sagittal depths

---

*Stop distance = vertex distance + 3 mm.
**When no add is in the spectacle lens, ($F_{add}/4$) is omitted from this equation.
***Note that here h is in centimeters

CLINICAL GUIDELINES FROM CONTACT LENS OPTICS

Differences between Front and Back Vertex Powers for Rigid Lenses

BACK VERTEX POWER (D)	FRONT VERTEX POWER (D)	CENTER THICKNESS (mm)	POWER DISPARITY (D)
−10	−9.92	0.10	−0.08
−5	−4.95	0.12	−0.05
0	0.0	0.15	0.00
+5	+4.90	0.23	+0.10
+10	+9.71	0.32	+0.29
+15	+14.44	0.41	+0.56
+20	+19.06	0.50	+0.94

Effect of Vertex Distance at 15 mm

HYPEROPIC (+) CORRECTION AT SPECTACLE PLANE	AMOUNT OF EFFECTIVE CHANGE WHEN REFERRED TO CORNEA (D)	MYOPIC (−) CORRECTION AT SPECTACLE PLANE
+4.00	±0.25	−4.25
+5.50	±0.50	−6.00
+6.75	±0.75	−7.50
+7.75	±1.00	−8.75
+9.25	±1.50	−10.75
+10.50	±2.00	−12.50
+12.75	±3.00	−15.75
+14.50	±4.00	−18.50
+16.00	±5.00	−21.00

Contact Lens Correction of Astigmatism*

CONDITION	CONTACT LENS OPTIONS
REFRACTIVE CYLINDER ≤0.75 DC	
Corneal toricity = Refractive cylinder	Spherical rigid lens* Spherical or aspheric soft lens
Corneal toricity ≠ Refractive cylinder	Spherical or aspheric soft lens* Spherical rigid lens
REFRACTIVE CYLINDER = CORNEAL TORICITY (WITHIN ±0.50 DC)	
Low astigmatism (0.75–2.00 DC)	Spherical rigid lens* Toric soft lens
High astigmatism (>2.00 DC)	Bitoric "SPE" rigid lens* Spherical rigid lens Custom toric soft lens
REFRACTIVE CYLINDER ≠ CORNEAL TORICITY (DIFFERENCE >0.50 DC)	
Low corneal toricity (≤2.00 DC)	Toric soft lens* Front toric rigid lens
High corneal toricity (>2.00 DC)	Bitoric "CPE" rigid lens* Custom toric soft lens

*Optimal option, on average, considering optical quality of correction, comfort, and fit of contact lenses.

Approximate Accommodative Demand at the Corneal Plane, Relative to Emmetropia for Near (40 cm) Object

DIFFERENCE IN CORNEAL PLANE ACCOMMODATIVE DEMAND COMPARED WITH EMMETROPIA (D)	BACK VERTEX POWER OF HYPEROPIC SPECTACLE LENS (D)	BACK VERTEX POWER OF MYOPIC SPECTACLE LENS (D)
±0.25	+3.25	−.87
±0.50	+6.00	−8.37
±0.75	+8.62	−13.75
±1.00	+10.87	−20.87

Figure 2.5 is rigid lens form 1040.

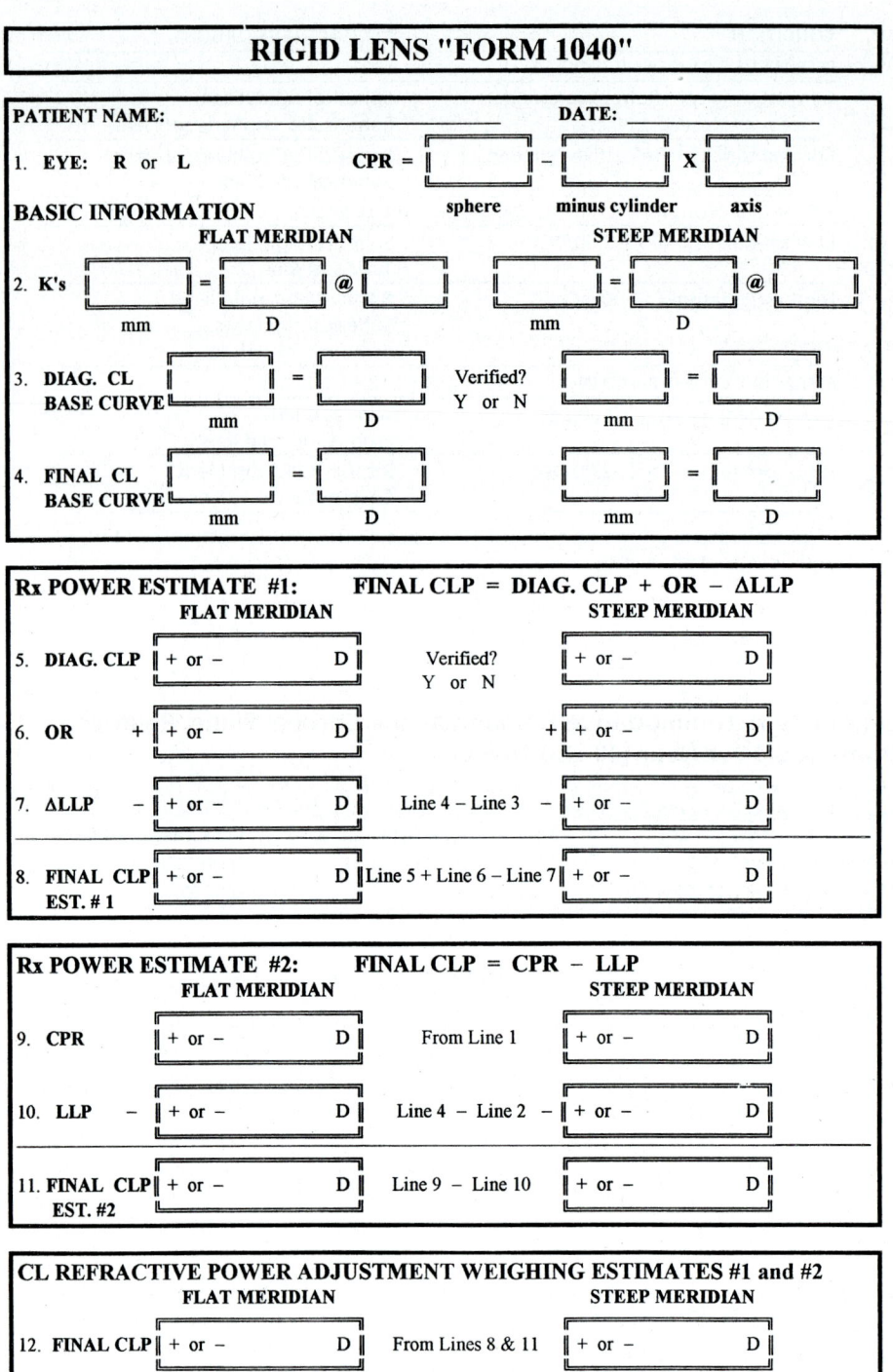

FIGURE 2.5 Rigid lens form 1040. CPR, corneal plane refraction; Diag. CL, diagnostic contact lens; Diag. CLP, diagnostic contact lens (refractive) power; Final CL, the contact lens that will be ordered; Final CLP, final contact lens (refractive) power; LLP, lacrimal lens (refractive) power; ΔLLP, change of LLP to that of the final contact lens base curve from that of the diagnostic contact lens base curve; OR, overrefraction at the corneal plane.

Chapter 2 • Optical Considerations in Contact Lens Practice

NOTES FOR USE:
- Generally fit approximately two-thirds or three-quarters of the corneal toricity.
- Judge credibility of estimate no. 1 versus credibility of estimate no. 2 before adjusting power to that which will be ordered (final CLP).
- Bias toward the "spherical power effect" when appropriate, where back-surface toricity in keratometric diopters (line 4) is equal to CLP refractive cylinder (line 12).

CLINICAL CASES

General Optical Concepts

1. Patient has a spectacle Rx of -11.00 DS at a vertex distance of 11 mm. What is the refractive error referred to the cornea?

    Answer: -9.81 DS

2. If the spectacle correction is $+15.00 - 5.00 \times 180$ at a vertex distance of 12 mm, what correction is required at the cornea?

    Answer: $+18.29 - 6.93 \times 180$

3. The following spectacle prescriptions for two ametropic eyes were obtained at a vertex distance of 12 mm: (A) $-5.25 - 3.50 \times 010$; (B) $+15.50 - 2.25 \times 165$. What are the powers referred to the cornea and rounded to the nearest eighth of a diopter?

    Answer: (A) $-5.00 - 3.00 \times 010$ (B) $+19.00 - 3.25 \times 165$

4. A contact lens has a back surface radius of 7.80 mm. (A) What is the refractive power of the surface in air if its refractive index is 1.49? (B) What would be the refractive power of the front surface of the tear film in air if it had the same radius of curvature as did the back surface of the contact lens (7.80 mm)? (C) How do these two values compare to the power of the posterior lens/tear film interface formed at the back surface of this lens?

    Answer: (A) -62.82 D   (B) $+43.08$ D
    (C) -19.74 D. Their sum is same as actual power calculated for the interface.

5. A polymethylmethacrylate (PMMA) contact lens has a BVP of -3.00 DS, a back surface radius of 8.00 mm, and a CT of 0.15 mm. What is the front surface radius of this lens?

    Answer: 8.46 mm

6. A contact lens has a back surface radius of 7.50 mm, a CT of 0.18 mm, a front optic radius of 7.95 mm, and a refractive index of 1.47. What are the vertex powers of this lens?

    Answer: BVP = -3.12 D   FVP = -3.07 D

7. A back surface concentric bifocal contact lens is to have a $+2.25$ DS peripheral addition. What posterior peripheral radius is required if the base curve is 7.60 mm, CT is 0.21 mm, refractive index is 1.49, and central power is -1.00 DS?

    Answer: 8.55 mm

8. If a front surface concentric bifocal contact lens is to have a $+2.25$ D peripheral add, what anterior peripheral radius is required if the base curve is 7.60 mm, CT is 0.21 mm, refractive index is 1.49, and central power is -1.00 DS?

    Answer: 7.55 mm if "add" is generated by FTP, 7.59 mm if "add" is generated by BVP

9. A patient has a −9.00 DS spectacle correction at a vertex distance of 13 mm. (A) When fitted with contact lenses, will the patient require more or less accommodation for a 40-cm viewing distance than with spectacles? What dioptric amount of accommodation would this patient require with spectacles (B) and with contact lenses (C) when viewing a target 40 cm in front of the spectacle plane?

Answer: (A) More accommodation required with contact lens
(B) Corneal plane accommodation = +1.95 D
C) Corneal plane accommodation = +2.42 D

10. A patient being fitted with a gel contact lens has the following Rx: −6.00 − 0.62 × 165 at a vertex distance of 15 mm. What is (A) the corneal plane refraction and (B) the expected equivalent sphere power required for the contact lens?

Answer: (A) −5.50 − 0.50 × 165   (B) −5.75 DS

11. In the problem above, the spectacle Rx was made of resin (n = 1.50), +3.75 base curve, and 2.0-mm CT. The contact lens has a 0.08-mm CT, n = 1.45, and the base curve is 8.60 mm on the eye. Using equivalent spherical correction, calculate the SM (A) when wearing spectacles and (B) when wearing contact lenses. (C) What is the net change in magnification when this eye switches from spectacles to contact lenses? (D) What is the net change in magnification attributable only to the power factors when switching from spectacles to contact lenses?

Answer: (A) 0.902, or −9.8% (minification)   (B) 0.986, or −1.4% (minification)
Note: Use power factor only.
(C) +8.4% (magnification)   (D) 1.1035, or +10.35% (magnification)

12. Keratometry readings for an eye are 41.50/46.75 @ 180. (A) What is the actual refractive astigmatism at the cornea that is a result of the difference between primary meridians? (B) What is the estimated refractive astigmatism encountered at the *posterior* corneal surface?

Answer: (A) −5.85 DC × 090   (B) +0.60 DC × 090

Hint: n = 1.3375 was used for the keratometer instead of n = 1.376 to account for the power of the posterior cornea.

13. A rigid gas-permeable contact lens has a base curve of 7.90 mm, CT of 0.15 mm, BVP of −4.00 D, and refractive index of 1.47. (A) What are the vertex focal lengths of this lens? (B) What would the front surface radius have to be for the lens to be of zero BVP?

Answer: (A) f_{BVP} = −250 mm; f_{FVP} = +253 mm   (B) 7.95 mm

14. The refractive index of a dry button of gel material is 1.49. It is to be made into a finished hydrophilic contact lens, which, when hydrated, will have a CT of 0.07 mm, BVP of −8.50 D, and base curve of 8.80 mm. (A) If the water content of hydrated material is 38.6%, what is the refractive index of the hydrated lens? (B) What is the radius of curvature of the front surface (hydrated)? (C) What is the FVP of the hydrated lens? (D) What would be the BVP of the lens (as if in air) when placed on the same cornea?

Answer: (A) n = 1.43   (B) 10.67 mm   (C) −8.45 D
(D) −8.57 D. This is a small change, into the minus, that is clinically insignificant.

15. An emmetropic low-vision patient requires the use of a spectacle–contact lens telescope. You feel that 1.5× is an excellent magnification to obtain for this patient and have the availability of prescribing up to a −40 D contact lens. (A) The patient's spectacle frame allows only a 15-mm vertex distance. What is the maximum magnification that you can obtain, and with what power of spectacle lens? (B) If you fit the patient with a frame that has adjustable pads, in which a vertex distance of 20 mm is attainable, what is the lowest power of spectacle lens that you can use and still obtain 1.5× magnification?

Answer: (A) 1×, with +25.00 D spectacle lens and −40.00 D contact lens
(B) +16.67 D, with contact lens of −25.00 D

Chapter 2 • Optical Considerations in Contact Lens Practice

Lacrimal Lens Problems

16. A patient who wears a rigid lens on one eye has come in for a checkup after 7 years without otherwise visiting your office. The lens was fitted over a central corneal graft, which originally had an average keratometry reading of 47.00 DS and now has a Keratometry reading of 43.00 DS. Yet the patient still wears the same lens. For smaller amounts of corneal shape alteration, the lacrimal lens should "mask" nearly all refractive changes as long as the rigid lens is worn. But for very large K changes, the lacrimal lens theory may not completely predict changes in the OR and the optimum rigid lens Rx. In this case, what OR could have resulted from the K change noted?

Answer: +0.47 DS

17. If a patient has keratometry readings of 43.00 @ 180, 43.00 @ 090; has a spectacle Rx of −3.00 DS; and is fitted with a lens with a base curve of 7.60 mm, what power is needed in the contact lens?

Answer: −4.37 DS

18. If a patient has keratometry readings of 44.00 @ 180, 44.00 @ 090; has a spectacle Rx of −4.00 DS; and is fitted with a lens with a base curve of 7.60 mm, what power is needed in the contact lens?

Answer: −4.37 DS

19. A patient has on his eye a diagnostic lens with a 7.50-mm base curve and power of −1.50 DS. A refraction over the lens indicates the need for an additional −1.25 DS and the practitioner's analysis of the fit indicates that a base curve of 7.40 mm would be better. (A) What refractive power is required if the 7.40-mm base curve is ordered? (B) If the patient required a lens with a base curve of 7.55 mm, what refractive power would be needed?

Answer: (A) −3.36 DS   (B) −2.47 DS

20. If a patient has keratometry readings of 45.00 @ 180, 47.00 @ 090; has a spectacle Rx of −1.00 − 2.00 × 180; and is fitted with a lens with a base curve of 7.50 mm, (A) what power is needed in the contact lens? (B) Did corneal toricity match refractive cylinder in this case?

Answer: (A) −1.00 DS   (B) Yes

21. If a patient has keratometry readings of 46.00 @ 180, 47.50 @ 090; has a spectacle Rx of −2.00 − 1.50 × 180; and is fitted with a lens with a base curve of 7.18 mm, what power is needed in the contact lens?

Answer: −3.00 DS

22. If a patient has keratometry readings of 44.00 @ 180, 45.50 @ 090; has a spectacle Rx of +2.00 − 2.00 × 180; and is fitted with a base curve of 7.50 mm, (A) what spherical power is needed in the contact lens and (B) what is the amount of residual astigmatism? (C) Did corneal toricity match refractive cylinder in this case?

Answer: (A) +0.75 DS, equivalent sphere   (B) −0.50 DC × 180   (C) No

23. A patient has keratometry readings of 45.00 DS and a spectacle prescription of −2.00 DS, and is to be fitted with a rigid lens (n = 1.49) with a base curve of 7.40 mm. What power would be required in the contact lens?

Answer: −2.61 DS

24. A patient has a spectacle prescription of −2.25 − 0.50 × 180 and keratometry readings of 45.00 @ 180, 45.50 @ 090. If a 7.40-mm base curve contact lens is fitted to this eye, (A) what power should be ordered and (B) how much residual astigmatism is expected? (C) Did corneal toricity match refractive cylinder?

Answer: (A) −2.86 DS   (B) None   (C) Yes

25. The spectacle prescription of a patient is +12.00 DS measured at a vertex distance of 14 mm, and his keratometry readings are 42.00 DS. He is to be fitted with a contact lens with a base curve of 7.89 mm. What power should be ordered in the contact lens?

    Answer: +13.65 DS

26. If a patient is wearing a 7.85-mm base curve and −4.00 DS corneal lens, and the OR is −1.25 DS, what power should be ordered in a new lens that has a 7.71-mm base curve?

    Answer: −6.03 DS

27. If a patient is wearing a 7.42-mm base curve and −2.50 DS lens, and the refraction over the lens is −0.75 DS, what power should be ordered in the new lens with a 7.50-mm base curve?

    Answer: −2.75 DS

28. A patient's Keratometry readings are 42.00 @ 180, 44.00 @ 090 and the spectacle Rx is −2.00 − 1.00 × 180. What is the predicted residual astigmatism with a spherical (A) rigid contact lens and with a spherical (B) soft contact lens?

    Answer: (A) −1.00 DC × 090   (B) −1.00 DC × 180

29. Find the predicted OR when a diagnostic rigid contact lens having a base curve of 42.00 D and power of −2.00 D is used on a patient with a spectacle Rx of −3.00 − 0.50 × 175 and keratometry readings of 41.75 @ 180, 43.00 @ 090.

    Answer: −0.50 − 0.75 × 095 or 090

30. A patient's eye has keratometry readings of 43.00 @ 180, 45.00 @ 090; has a spectacle Rx of −1.00 − 2.00 × 180, and is being fitted with a lens with a base curve of 7.76 mm. Your overkeratometry readings are 42.50 @ 180, 43.50 @ 090. (A) What is your expected refraction over a −1.50 DS diagnostic lens? (B) Did corneal toricity match refractive cylinder in this case?

    Answer: (A) pl − 1.00 × 180   (B) Yes

31. An eye has been fitted with a rigid contact lens having a base curve of 7.94 mm and a power of −3.00 DS. The keratometry readings are 42.50 @ 180, 44.00 @ 090 and the spectacle Rx is −2.00 − 0.75 × 180. (A) Assuming that this lens is inflexible, what is the expected OR for the lens? (B) What would be your recommended refractive power if you were to correct the ametropia with (B) a front toric rigid lens or (C) a toric soft lens, ignoring rotational and orientational effects on the eye?

    Answer: (A) +1.75 − 0.75 × 090   (B) −1.25 − 0.75 × 090   (C) −2.00 − 0.75 × 180

32. Surprise! You ordered a spherical rigid lens for the patient above with a power of −1.62 DS according to the spherical equivalent of your OR at the fitting session, and your overkeratometry readings now show at dispensing that the lens is flexing on the eye with-the-rule by 0.75 D! (A) What is your expected OR? (B) Given that you could order a lens of similar parameters that would flex in an identical manner, what spherical refractive power would you now order?

    Answer: (A) −0.37 DS   (B) −2.00 DS

33. A patient has a spectacle prescription of −3.50 − 1.00 × 180. While wearing a rigid contact lens with a base curve of 7.70 mm and a power of −2.00 DS, the obtained OR was −2.00 DS. What are this person's keratometry readings?

    Answer: 43.33 @ 180, 44.33 @ 090

34. A soft contact lens is fitted to a patient with keratometry readings of 43.00 @ 180, 44.25 @ 090 and a spectacle Rx of −3.00 − 0.75 × 180. What residual astigmatism would be expected with the soft lens on the eye?

    Answer: −0.75 DC × 180

35. A 1.00 DS myope with a Keratometry reading of 45.00 DS is fit with a plano powered rigid contact lens. What base curve must be used to optimally correct this person's ametropia?

    Answer: 7.67 mm

36. A patient was initially fit with a rigid contact lens having a base curve of 44.00 D and a power of −3.50 D. It was later necessary to change the base curve to 43.00 D. What power must now be ordered?

    Answer: −2.50 DS

37. Calculate the corneal curvatures using the following:

    Spectacle Rx: −2.50 − 0.75 × 180
    Diagnostic rigid lens: 43.00 BC, −3.00 power
    OR: +0.50 − 1.75 × 090

    Answer: 41.25 @ 180, 43.75 @ 090

38. Find the predicted OR when a rigid contact lens with a 42.25 BC and −3.00 D power is fitted on an eye having the following parameters:

    Spectacle Rx: −4.50 − 1.00 × 172
    Vertex distance: 13 mm
    Keratometry readings: 44.50 @ 180, 46.25 @ 090

    Answer: +1.87 − 0.87 × 090

39. Suppose that for the eye in the previous question, the OR was −1.25 − 1.50 × 180. What are the calculated Keratometry readings?

    Answer: 42.25 @ 180, 41.63 @ 090

40. You have placed an inflexible rigid lens on a 43.50/44.00 @ 090 cornea from your fitting set of −3.00 DS lenses. You meant to place a lens with a 7.90-mm base curve on the eye, but found out just after the lens was on the patient that your set of trial lenses had been mixed up. (A) If the spectacle Rx was −2.00 − 1.25 × 180 and the OR was +1.75 × 0.75 × 180, what was the base curve of the lens that you placed on the eye? (B) Suppose that you thought that the lens looked too "flat," and upon subsequent testing you found that a lens with a 7.70-mm base curve fitted the best. What should be your expected OR with your 7.70-mm base curve trial lens, rounded to the nearest eighth of a diopter? (C) You could prescribe the "equivalent sphere" Rx and forget about the cylinder in the OR, but you have the ability to increase flexure of the lens by making it thinner. If you could place a lens of the appropriate thickness on the eye such that it would flex to correct for the residual cylinder found with your inflexible trial lens, what amount of cylinder in the overkeratometry readings would be ideal? Is this realistically achievable?

    Answer: (A) 7.90 mm

    > Hint: Use lacrimal lens theory applied to both meridians.
    >
    > Note: Lucky! The correct lens was on the cornea.

    (B) +0.62 − 0.75 × 180

    (C) 0.75 DC, steeper in the horizontal meridian. No. This cannot be reasonably expected.

    > Hint: Flexure is attributed to the meridian of steepest corneal curvature. Lens power does not alter. Flexure can only correct for refractive astigmatism that is not the result of corneal toricity. Had the OR been +0.62 − 0.75 × 090 and corneal curvature remained the same, flexure could correct for the refractive cylinder.

41. A patient's eye is +8.50 −4.50 × 010 at a vertex distance of 14 mm, and has Keratometry readings of 43.50/48.00 @ 100. (A) A +5.00 D diagnostic rigid lens with 7.50-mm base curve seems to fit in a reasonable manner, for a spherical lens. What amount of residual astigmatism should show through the OR? (B) The lens flexes on the eye such that 0.50 D of flexure is revealed in the overkeratometry readings. What is the expected OR? (C) To obtain a better fit, you desire to order a bitoric rigid lens. Not having a bitoric diagnostic lens available, you estimate that about 2.50 D of back-surface toricity should be correct,

and order a lens with back surface radii of 7.60 mm and 7.20 mm. What refractive power should you order, assuming that this lens will not flex?

Answer: (A) −0.90 DC × 010

　　Hint: Refer power to cornea before using lacrimal lens theory.

　　Note: Although it appears that corneal toricity and refractive astigmatism are equal, once referred to the cornea they are not; therefore, astigmatism is not completely masked.

(B) +3.14 − 1.40 × 010

　　Hint: Flexure increases power of lacrimal lens into the plus/less minus in the steeper corneal meridian. Flexure in this case, as in most cases, worsens residual astigmatism.

(C) +8.75 − 3.37 × 010. Note that in most bitoric fits, increasing back toricity necessitates an increase of refractive astigmatic correction in the lens.

Back Toric Contact Lens Problems

42. A patient has a spectacle prescription of −0.50 − 3.50 × 180 and keratometry readings of 42.00 @ 180, 45.00 @ 090. If fitted with a toric base curve of 7.94/7.58 mm, what power must be ordered in the contact lens?

Answer: −1.00 − 2.50 × 180, or −1.00 D @ 180/−3.50 D @ 090

43. A refraction over a 7.70-mm base curve rigid diagnostic lens of −3.00 DS power is −1.75 −1.00 × 090. The lens ordered has a toric back surface with radii of 7.50/7.90 mm (on a with-the-rule cornea). What lens power should be specified for this lens to correct the patient's refractive error?

Answer: −4.64 − 1.27 × 180, or −4.64 D @ 180/−5.91 D @ 090

44. A patient has keratometry readings of 42.00 @ 180, 46.00 @ 090; has a spectacle Rx of −2.00 − 5.00 × 180 at a vertex distance of 12 mm; and is fitted with a contact lens with base curve radii of 7.95/7.50 mm. What power is needed in the contact lens?

Answer: −2.45 − 3.00 × 180, or −2.45 D @ 180/−5.45 D @ 090

45. A diagnostic lens with a base curve of 7.50 mm and −3.00 DS is placed on a patient's eye and a refraction over the lens indicates a need for the following additional power: −0.50 − 0.75 × 090. The lens to be ordered for this patient is to have a base curve of 7.35/7.70 mm (toric). What power is needed in the contact lens, assuming with-the-rule corneal toricity?

Answer: −3.08 − 1.34 × 180, or −3.08 D @ 180/−4.42 D @ 090

46. A patient has keratometry readings of 43.00 @ 180, 46.25 @ 090; has a spectacle Rx of −8.00 − 3.50 × 180 at a vertex distance of 12 mm; and is fitted with a lens with base curve radii of 7.45/7.85 mm. The lens has a diameter of 9.50 mm, optic zone of 7.50 mm, secondary curve radii of 8.45/8.85 mm, and CT of 0.12 mm. The refractive index of the rigid lens is 1.52. (A) What power should be ordered in the lens and (B) what front radii are needed?

Answer: (A) −7.30 − 1.86 × 180, or −7.30 D @ 180/−9.16 D @ 090
　　　　(B) 8.86 mm @ 180 and 8.62 mm @ 090

47. A patient has a spectacle prescription of −10.00 − 5.00 × 180 at a vertex distance of 12 mm, and keratometry readings of 44.00 @ 180, 49.00 @ 090. If the patient is fitted with a spherical rigid lens with a radius of 7.30 mm, (A) what spherical power would be required in the contact lens? (B) What residual astigmatism would be expected? (C) Does corneal toricity match refractive cylinder in this case? (D) Would lens flexure help or hinder in this case?

Answer: (A) −10.55 DS, equivalent sphere　　(B) −1.22 DC × 090
　　　　(C) Actually, it does not. Once the refractive cylinder is referred to the cornea, it amounts to −3.78 DC × 180, which is less than corneal toricity
　　　　(D) Up to 1.25 DC of flexure would help correct the refractive astigmatism.

48. If the above eye is fitted with a toric base curve lens with radii of 7.55/6.96 mm, (A) what power would be required in each meridian to correct the patient's refractive error? (B) This lens is representative of what optical fitting effect? (C) How much cylinder rotates with this lens on the eye?

   Answer: (A) −9.63 D @ 180, −12.20 D @ 090
   (B) Cylindrical power effect (CPE)
   (C) Approximately 1.25 DC

49. A patient's corneal toricity matches that of the refractive cylinder, yet the toricity does not allow a rigid contact lens with a spherical base curve to fit correctly. Keratometry readings are 40.00 @ 180, 44.50 @ 090 and the spectacle refraction is +1.00 − 4.50 × 180. With your office fitting set, you estimate that a bitoric lens having base curves of 8.33/7.76 would provide the best fit. (A) What would be the refractive power of the ordered lens (n = 1.47) in air? (B) What would be the power of the lens on the eye, its posterior surface immersed in tear fluid? (C) This lens is an example of what type of optical fitting effect? (D) How much cylinder rotates with this lens on the eye?

   Answer: (A) +0.50 − 3.00 × 180, or +0.50 D @ 180/−2.50 D @ 090
   (B) +40.79 @ 180, +40.83 @ 090 (essentially spherical)
   (C) Spherical power effect (SPE)
   (D) Almost none; zero

50. A bitoric rigid contact lens has base curve radii of 8.03 mm and 7.67 mm and has BVPs of −1.00 D and −4.00 D in those meridians, respectively. What amount of cylinder power rotates with this lens as it varies rotational orientation on the eye?

   Answer: 1.00 DC

CLINICAL PROFICIENCY CHECKLIST

- The true refractive power of a contact lens is calculated with the *thick* lens formula.
- FVP or BVP are measured clinically. The disparity between these powers becomes clinically significant with high plus powers (>+8) that have large CT.
- Effective power differences are clinically significant at ±4.00 D.
- Flexure of soft contact lenses when placed on the eye induces changes in BVP that are significant in the high plus powers.
- Highly oxygen-permeable rigid materials and thin lenses flex more. Manage flexure by increasing the lens thickness, using a stiffer material, or by designing a bitoric lens for the highly toric cornea.
- High myopes often have enhanced visual acuity with contact lenses as a result of the larger retinal image provided by the contact lens as compared to spectacles.
- Contact lenses are often the preferred correction in anisometropia and especially for refractive anisometropes in terms of retinal image size. Even in axial anisometropia, contact lenses can often provide excellent binocular vision.
- Contact lenses minimize the lateral and vertical prismatic effects that are common to spectacle lens wear.
- Myopes have increased accommodative demand with contact lenses than with spectacles. Hyperopes require less accommodative demand with spectacles compared to contact lenses. Thus, the clinician should be careful when contemplating contact lenses for pre-presbyopic myopes or myopes with low accommodative amplitudes.
- Myopes have increased convergence demand at near with contact lenses than with spectacles. Hyperopes require less vergence demand at near with spectacles than with contact lenses. Thus, the clinician should be careful when contemplating contact lenses for myopes with borderline near convergence ability.
- The impact of off-axis optical aberrations is minimized with contact lenses compared to spectacles.

ACKNOWLEDGMENTS

Portions of this chapter were modified from previous works of the coauthor, including Benjamin WJ. Optical phenomena of contact lenses. In Bennett ES, Weissman B, eds. *Clinical Contact Lens Practice*. Philadelphia, PA: Lippincott Williams & Wilkins; 2004:111–163.

REFERENCES

1. Benjamin WJ. Contact lenses: applied optics of contact lens correction. In: Benjamin WJ, ed. *Borish's Clinical Refraction*. 2nd ed. St. Louis, MO: Elsevier Medical Publications; 2006:1188–1245.
2. Benjamin WJ. Clinical optics of contact lens prescription. In: Benjamin WJ, ed. *Borish's Clinical Refraction*. 2nd ed. St. Louis, MO: Elsevier Medical Publications; 2006:1246–1273.
3. Douthwaite, WA. *Contact Lens Optics and Lens Design*. 3rd ed. Philadelphia, PA: Elsevier Butterworth-Heinemann; 2006:12, 21–22.

Section II

Gas-Permeable Lenses

Chapter 3

Corneal Topography

Eef van der Worp, John de Brabander, and Frans Jongsma

INTRODUCTION

Contact lens practitioners have a high interest in the shape of the cornea. When this shape is known, a contact lens that will optimize the cornea–lens relationship can be selected, fitted, or designed. Generally, mimicking the shape of the cornea promotes comfort of lens wear and reduces mechanical effects of the lens on the cornea.

The standard procedure in contact lens practice is to measure the cornea with a keratometer. But what exactly does keratometry tell us? It typically measures the average curve of the central 3 mm of the cornea in two meridians. This includes, at minimum, three limitations. First, a keratometer measures curves and curves are not the equivalent of shape. Second, it estimates, rather than measures, the average central curves. This means it does not provide information about the exact central point (not to mention the top) of the cornea. Third, and most important: 3 mm is a very small area of a cornea. A typical cornea is 11 to 12 mm in diameter. Contact lenses, in general, cover a much larger part of the cornea than 3 mm (Fig. 3.1), and a keratometer does not provide information about the periphery of the cornea.

Corneal topography also has its limitations, all of which will be discussed in this chapter. However, when compared to the keratometer, it provides the practitioner with much more information about the geometry of the cornea and therefore can aid in optimizing the lens-to-cornea fitting relationship.

Interestingly, the principle of corneal topography is as old as that of keratometry, dating back to the late 19th century. Is it impossible to measure corneal shape with a keratometer? Theoretically, peripheral corneal curve radii can be measured by performing keratometry and having the subject view at an angle of 25 or 30 degrees nasally, temporally, superiorly, and inferiorly. If this information about the peripheral corneal curves is related to the central curves of the cornea, some idea about the amount of flattening toward the periphery can be obtained. Apart from the fact that with a keratometer it is often challenging to obtain reliable peripheral curve data from the periphery of the cornea, computation of corneal shape from this data is difficult.

Overall, keratometry is not the best method to measure corneal shape, apart from being time consuming. Corneal topographers can provide information about thousands of data points on the cornea, which will result in a better understanding about corneal shape. More and more, practitioners will have to rely on corneal shape data rather than corneal curves. This is crucial when managing refractive surgery, orthokeratology (ortho-k), and keratoconus patients, but also, for the design and manufacturing of any type of contact lens, information about the shape of the cornea is essential.

In this chapter, history, principles, and recently developed devices to measure the shape of the eye's front surface are discussed. The primary goal is to explain how corneal topographers work, and how these devices can be used optimally in the contact lens practice.

HISTORY

For centuries, ophthalmologists, optometrists, and others involved in eye care have been using the reflection capacity of the first refractive surface of the eye to obtain a qualitative impression of the integrity of the cornea. Historically, it has been described to diagnose the integrity of the

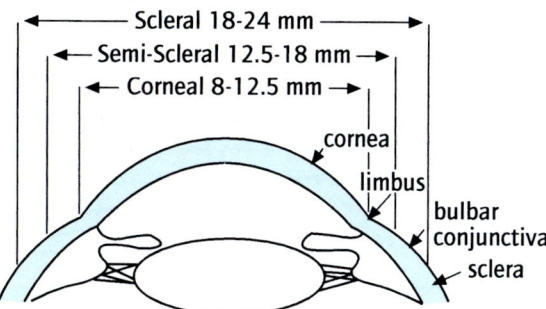

FIGURE 3.1 Contact lenses with various diameters in relationship to the eye dimensions.

cornea by viewing the reflected image of a rectangle window (Fig. 3.2). This simple diagnostic tool is based on the fact that the boundary air-tear film acts as a mirror.

From this, the basis for quantitative corneal topography was described by Von Helmholtz, Placido, and Gullstrand in the late 19th century. Von Helmholtz[1] measured the local slope of the cornea by observing the reflection of a pair of objects positioned at a known place with respect to the subject's eye (Fig. 3.3). The virtual image obtained this way is called the *first Purkinje image*. On the basis that the cornea can be considered as an optical equivalent to a spherical mirror, Javal[2] designed an instrument in which the objects could be rotated around the optical axis. In this way, it became possible to find the orientation of the flattest and steepest radius of curvature, so-called "principle meridians" of the cornea. With his device, more precise measurements of the cornea were introduced. Although Javal called it *ophthalmometry*, this technique is known today as *keratometry* (from *keratos*, Greek for *cornea*).

Instead of pairs of objects, Placido[3] used a disk with concentric rings with a central hole, through which he observed the image reflected by the subject's eye (Fig. 3.4).

This extended the observation to more meridians, and it evaluates an entire region rather than two or more points on the cornea. With this simple but ingenious invention (also called keratoscopy), the practitioner is able to make a qualitative diagnosis of corneal irregularities and, very importantly, to estimate the amount and direction of corneal astigmatism.

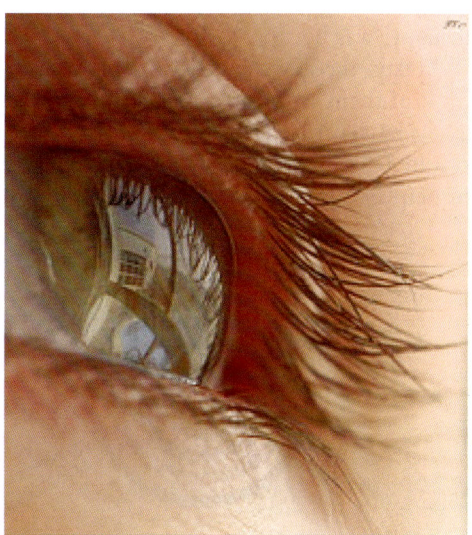

FIGURE 3.2 Image of a rectangle window as reflected by the cornea.

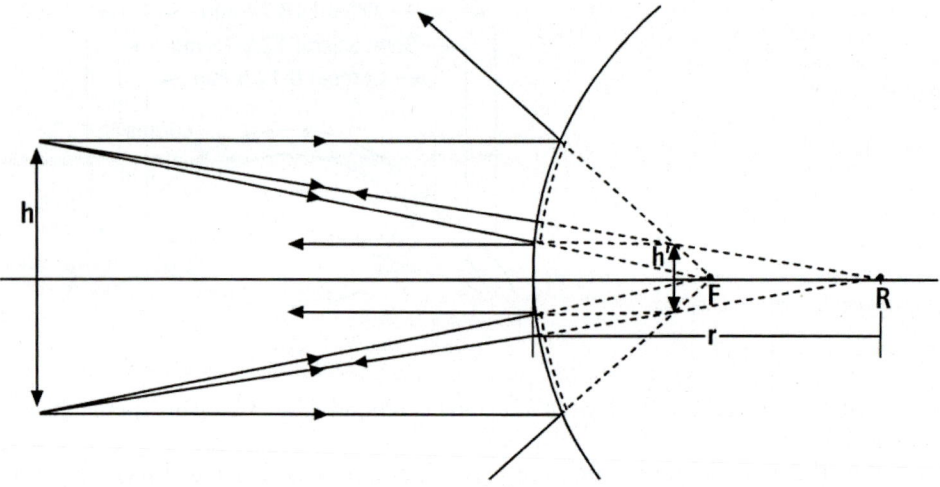

FIGURE 3.3 The principle of keratometry is based on image formation as with a convex mirror. The radius of curvature of the cornea (r) determines the difference in distance between the object mires (h) and the same at the reflected image side (h'). Note that only two small and separated areas of the cornea actually contribute to the measurement. Note also that the longer the distance between the object mires (h) and the cornea is, the closer the h' is located to the focal plane of the cornea.

Gullstrand[4] took a major step in quantification of corneal topography by placing a photographic camera in the central hole of the Placido disk (Fig. 3.5). Measuring the size of the rings on the photographs enabled Gullstrand to estimate the corneal radius of curvature quantitatively. The technique, no longer in use today, was referred to as photokeratoscopy.

Placido disk photographs from an irregular cornea (Fig. 3.6A) and a cornea with a very steep apex, a flat superior area, and a steep inferior area, all associated with keratoconus (Fig. 3.6B), are shown. It can be observed that only a very small area of the cornea can be imaged and other areas cannot typically be interpreted or only with severe error.

A century after the invention of photography, the first television was developed, leading to the small and inexpensive charge coupled device (CCD) television systems that are common today. The modern personal computer has had a comparable history. Coupling these two devices has made it possible to collect and process a quarter of a million data points in a very brief time. After the development of algorithms for surface reconstruction, a translation of the acquired image into clinically relevant data in the 1980s, called computer-assisted video keratoscopy, was born.[5]

Today, these systems are simply called corneal topographers and many devices exist, but most of them are still based on the old Placido disk principle. The inherent limitations of imaging by specular reflection (see section Using a Corneal Topographer later in this chapter) resulted in the development of alternatives. These topographic devices, based on different principles, opened new possibilities, but also introduced other limitations. This has resulted

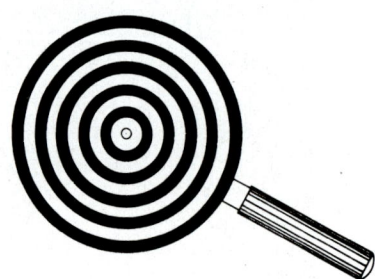

FIGURE 3.4 Hand-held Placido disk.

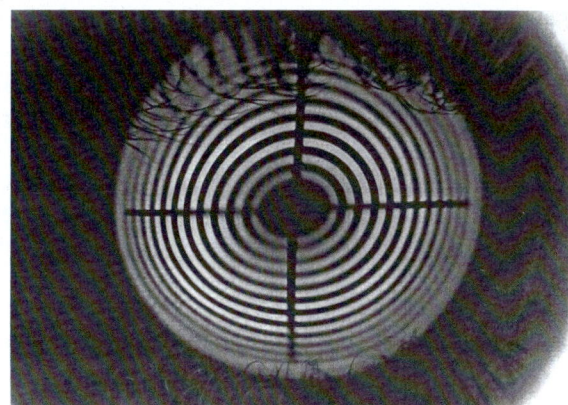

FIGURE 3.5 Photographic image of a Placido disk reflected on an astigmatic cornea.

in a somewhat confusing situation, where it is not always possible for the practitioner to link modalities of a given device to what is desired and/or practical. This also accounts for the way image data are transformed into data of eye shape and even more how this is presented in numbers, indices, or color-coded maps.

Corneal topography has led to the publication of a vast number of papers and patents. In a study at the University of Maastricht by Jongsma et al.,[6] information was found on 24 devices that were based on essentially different principles. Analyzing the principles of these devices revealed that all devices would fit into a system that discriminates between the combinations of used light sources and the way they interact with the eye's front surface (light–matter interaction). The literature descriptions yielded 12 modalities. The light source may be a

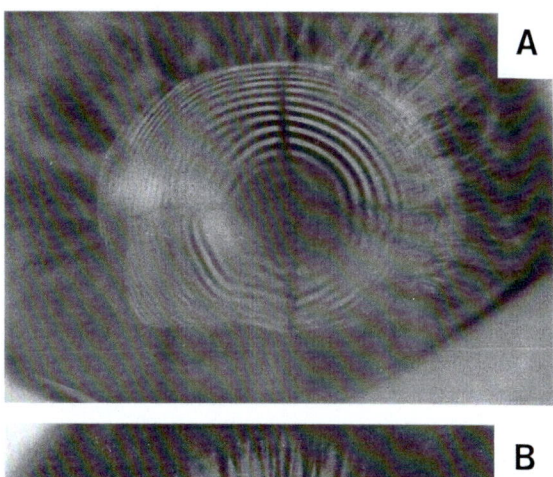

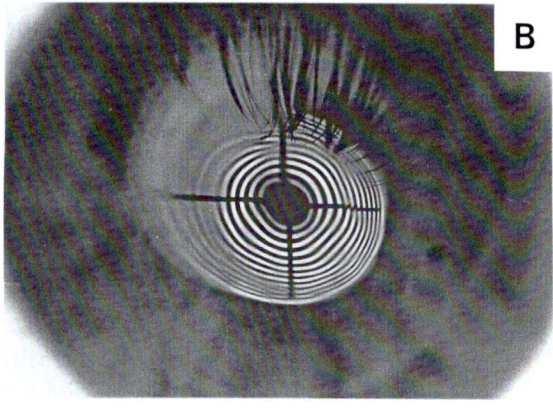

FIGURE 3.6 Placido disk photographs from an irregular cornea (**A**) and a cornea with a very steep apex, a flat superior part, and a steep inferior part (**B**; keratoconus).

light-emitting object (e.g., a Placido disk) or a projected image (e.g., a slit, lines, or a grid). The light used can be incoherent or coherent. The light–matter interaction can be specular reflection, scattering, diffuse reflection, total reflection, or a combination. Not all combinations of these are technically feasible. Some are possible but rather expensive, or very difficult to use in clinical settings. Most widely used are devices based on reflection from a light-emitting object, such as the keratometer and the keratoscopes. Devices based on projection (e.g., a scanning slit or optical coherence tomography [OCT]) have entered the market recently. Generally, these devices are found to be most prevalent in ophthalmology clinics.

There are numerous new developments in the field of reflection corneal topographers, which will improve the accuracy and usefulness of the procedure. Collins et al.[7,8] in Brisbane, Australia, for example, researched dynamic corneal topography, via which multiple topography maps can be made within seconds, creating an almost live movie of the corneal topography, showing its dynamic rather than static nature. Researchers in Amsterdam, the Netherlands, developed a modified Placido disk system using different colors.[9] They claim this system gives a more accurate representation about the periphery of the cornea, by preventing skew ray errors. This instrument has recently become commercially available.

In addition to this, corneal topographers are now integrated with wavefront aberrometers, which can be a major advantage in contact lens practice. Subtracting the anterior surface aberrations from the total aberrations will reveal the rest aberrations of the eye. Corneal topography then can be useful (see later section in this chapter) to aid in fitting contact lenses, and it is technically possible to add rest aberrations on the front surface of the lens.[10]

KERATOMETRY

In keratometry, the reflected image of small light-emitting targets, usually called *mires*, formed by the anterior surface of the cornea, is used to determine the outer radius for one meridian (see Fig. 3.3). By rotating the instrument about its optical axis, the principal meridians of the cornea (flattest and steepest) can be found. Actually, in keratometry, it is not the size of an object that is compared with a formed image—the separation between the two mires at the object plane is compared with the measured separation in the image. To exactly measure the latter separation, keratometers have a built-in doubling system. As can be observed from Figure 3.3, only a very small area of the cornea is used to reflect the two mires. The angle between the incoming ray from the mires and the reflected ray from the cornea, called the *collimator angle*, is normally about 17 degrees. However, some autokeratometers work with different collimator angles to measure the asphericity along meridians. The keratometer actually presents an average measurement using two small areas that are separated from each other (depending on the device and the radius of curvature of the cornea, from 2.0 to 3.5 mm). So, the apex is not measured but estimated to be spherical between the measured areas. In irregular corneal surfaces and/or a decentered corneal apex (as in keratoconus), this may cause clinically relevant inaccuracies. Also, the range of corneal curvatures that ensure proper images for measurements is limited (usually from 6 to 9 mm). Furthermore, the periphery of the cornea is not measured using standard keratometric methods. A problem in keratometry is also that the measurement is observer dependent. Errors by the observer are misalignment, improper positioning of the mires, ambiguity by distorted mires, focusing, and, most important, accommodation by the observer. In most keratometers, errors in focusing are restricted by using a Scheiner disk (double image if out of focus) or collimated mires and telecentric viewing systems (accommodation-independent systems).

Although strictly qualitative, the keratometer can still give the experienced user some information by judging the distortion of the imaged mires on corneal irregularities, tear film quality, and, indirectly, the fit and front surface quality of soft contact lenses. To decrease inaccuracies and also to reduce the inherent problem that the object is not placed in infinity and thus the image is not formed exactly at the focal plane of the cornea, Mandell[11] developed keratometers with a long working distance and small objects (small mire keratometry). With these devices, he performed measurements of the peripheral corneal curvature by having the patient fixate on a movable off-axis light source. The need for extra information on the corneal periphery can be easily deducted from Figure 3.1, if one realizes that the smallest contact lens has a diameter of 8.0 mm and classic keratometry only provides information on an area of around 3.0 mm (around 8% of the corneal surface).

Using the principle of off-axis fixation devices, Wilms[12] developed a method that can be used with most ordinary keratometers and delivers an estimation of *e*-values at 30 or 25 degrees from the central axis (Fig. 3.7). Apart from the fact that it is often difficult to obtain reliable peripheral curve data from the periphery of the cornea, it also should be considered that two different methods are being postulated—tangential and sagittal curves—which are difficult to compare.[13]

In summary, the (auto-) keratometer is a relatively easy-to-use device that, in normal corneas, provides average information on corneal curvature, including amount and axis of astigmatism. In contact lens practice, it is successfully used as an initial step to find parameters for a trial lens prior to evaluation by an experienced practitioner. More experienced users can also gain information on the quality of the central part of the corneal surface, the tear film, and the front surface of a soft contact lens.

KERATOSCOPY AND CORNEAL TOPOGRAPHY

Strictly, the name *keratoscopy* means viewing the cornea; therefore, the original Placido disk is a true keratoscope in the hands of the practitioner looking at the formed image. With photographing the image, the name of the device has historically been changed to *photokeratoscopy*. Examples of photokeratoscopic images are given in Figures 3.5 and 3.6.

When viewing these images, the qualitative information that can be gained is very evident for a trained clinician. Compared to the keratometer, the photokeratoscopic images give information on a relatively small area, but definitely a larger area than just two points.

With the replacement of the photo camera by a CCD camera, the name of the device was changed to a *videokeratoscope*. Over time, the name was changed to *videokeratograph* or, more common and most widely used, *corneal topographer* after the implementation of computer-assisted software algorithms to analyze the picture.

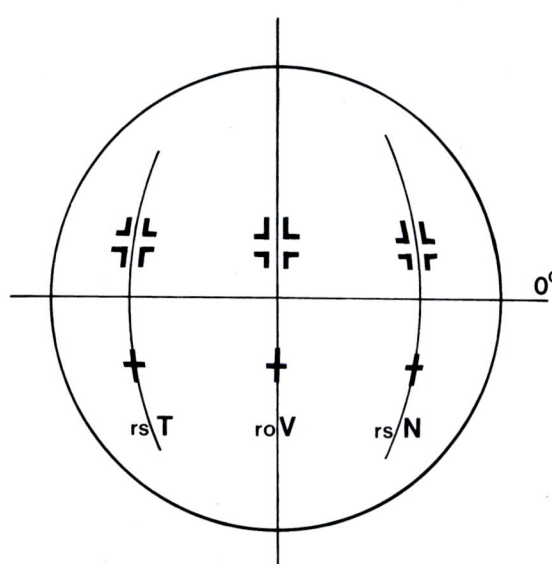

FIGURE 3.7 The areas measured using sagittal topography as proposed by Wilms. Note that the horizontal meridian is measured in the periphery with the keratometer mires in a vertical position.

The name *corneal topography* implies that the topography of the cornea is exactly measured. Is this true? Is the picture that is displayed as a color-coded map the true shape (topography) of the entire cornea? The answer could be no or sometimes yes, but important for clinical applications, the correct answer is "we don't know." The reason for this lies in the inherent problem of using a reflected image of an unknown surface that, in itself, is the object of the measurement. Without discussing complicated optical mathematics, some understanding of these inherent problems is useful for practitioners to understand differences between the design of corneal topographers and the interpretation of corneal topographic maps as discussed later in this chapter. Recommended reading in this respect is the classic article by Mandell,[14] "The Enigma of the Corneal Contour."

Reflection Topography

Reflection follows the simple rules of Snell's law, where the incidence ray of light and the reflected ray of light form equal angles with the normal to the surface. In corneal topography, a picture is analyzed, from which it is known that the incident rays are coming from the Placido disk and the reflected rays are coming from the cornea. The advantage over keratometry is that with a flat Placido disk, a two-dimensional object is created so that more points can be evaluated. The problem is, however, that it is unknown where the image exactly was and where in space the reflection occurred. So, finding "the normal" for multiple rays, which is essential for reconstruction of the corneal surface, becomes difficult. Furthermore, it is desired to measure as large an area of the cornea as possible. For this, the use of a large disk would be indicated. However, with large disks, the peripheral rays will be incident on a very skewed angle compared to the rays more centrally, and also most of these rays will be obscured by the eyelids. Even more complicated is that the image of a large disk is not flat but curved, so the image space becomes three-dimensional. For all of these reasons, modern corneal topographers use a curved or cone-shaped pattern of rings and try to diminish the working distance as much as possible. If the cornea happened to have a spherical shape, its shape would be easy to measure and actually keratometry would be satisfactory. The ironic fact is that the normal cornea is not spherical and that our specific aim is to actually measure the deviations from the sphere. To do so, the data must be fit to mathematically assumed shapes. The assumed shapes could be a sphere, an ellipse using *e*-values, various polynomials, or splines.

To measure the shape of the cornea with high resolution, one would think that as many as possible rings in the target would be beneficial. This is true, but as can be observed from Figure 3.6 compared with Figure 3.5, both the contrast and the order of the rings (lost rings or ring jam) in the image become problematic for software analysis. Some topographers analyze Placido ring borders by using different colors for the outer and the inner boundary of the ring. This way, confusion of rings may be reduced.

Another serious problem, as can be recognized from Figure 3.6, is alignment of the ring target with the center of the cornea. Slight decentration would give an entirely different picture of the rings in the image. A normal cornea could, with decentered imaging, present as a keratoconus pattern. Also, shape algorithms do need a central reference point (with the exception of splines to some extent). In Placido ring imaging, the real center is not imaged. This is not a problem for normal corneas, where it can be estimated, but in a keratoconic eye, where the top of the cone is usually not at the geometric center of the cornea, it can be problematic. Also, there is no such concept as a spherical apex area in keratoconus. Odd topographic maps may be seen as a result of this. More on this topic will be discussed later in this chapter under Indexes for Irregularity.

A problem in interpretation of topographic maps is that via viewing a map, one could determine that the radius of curvature somewhere on the cornea is, for example, 7.5 mm (or if a dioptric map is used, 45.00 D). But what does this mean? Is the cornea steep, or is it a local steepness, or maybe a flatter area on a very steep cornea? Even more, what is the position of this steeper or flatter area on the slope of the cornea? It is like walking in an area with hills. You see the curve and you might feel the slope while walking, but are you on a mountain at 6,000 feet high, or on the hill next to your house at the beach? To have access to that knowledge, a height map is needed to really know where you are. The same is true with local corneal curvature data. Here the problem is that a Placido disk inherently estimates radii of curvature, where ideally a height map would be desired. Therefore, most modern corneal topographers also present *height maps*. Although these maps are still derivatives from curvature, by using fast and smart algorithms combined with logical iterative/interpolation/extrapolation processes, they can (given a reasonable starting point in the Placido disk image) be reasonably accurate. These data are ideal when designing and manufacturing custom contact lenses.

Reading of a height map is quite different from a curvature map. A height map representing the total, absolute sagittal height of the cornea actually would not give any detail at all. All it would show is that the central cornea is higher than the periphery, which is not really a surprise. It becomes useful only after matching the corneal surface with a so-called "best-fit sphere" (or sometimes "a best-fit oval"). Everything that is higher (meaning being closer to the observer) is color coded with warmer colors; everything that is positioned farther away from that shape is presented with cooler colors. Therefore, what the exact (and actual) shape of the cornea is can be immediately observed.

In summary, reflection corneal topographers, compared to keratometry, are ideal in obtaining more information on an extended area of the cornea, but still do not measure the complete corneal surface. They are not difficult to use, but care should be taken in obtaining both proper alignment and focusing. Looking at the image before processing is recommended, and proper interpretation of the different maps is a key consideration. This topic will be further discussed later in this chapter under How to Use a Corneal Topographer.

Projection Topography

Appreciating the disadvantages of reflection systems, alternatives to the Placido disk-based corneal topographers have been developed.[15-17] Although some of these systems are more complicated in use, can be more expensive, or are more used in research settings than in routine clinical settings, some of these devices are increasingly finding their place in (advanced) contact lens practices. To explain the principles of using a projecting light source, three different possibilities are described here. The first is projecting a set of lines on the cornea (Maastricht Shape Topographer [MST], or eye surface profiler [ESP]); the second is the use of a scanning slit such as that used in Orbscan (Rochester, NY), Pentacam (Oculus, Germany), and Galilei (Ziemer, Zwitserland) systems. The ESP, based on Fourier profilometry, is able to present a height map of the total area composed to the instrument (Fig. 3.8A). The system projects from two directions, a line pattern on the front surface of the eye in which fluorescein acts as diffusing medium. Because the line patterns are viewed by a central camera, they become, depending on the shape of the eye, curved in the image (Fig. 3.8B). Fourier analysis can transform this information to height data, and from there it is possible to create cross sections of the cornea and sclera, including limbal topography (Fig. 3.8C). As with Placido disk devices, a good image is essential. Advantages of the ESP include that it measures shape directly and—especially important in contact lens designing—presents height information of the entire eye's front surface. This instrument has now become available to practitioners.

The principle of a scanning slit, as in the Orbscan, Pentacam and Galilei devices,[15] can be easily appreciated from a cross-section view of the cornea (Fig. 3.9A), routine for eye care practitioners. In the slit image, the profile of the cornea front and back surface can be observed. Unfortunately, this is only one meridian and if the incidence angle of the slit were changed, a dramatic change would be observed. In the Orbscan device, a scanning slit is used to obtain multiple images over the horizontal meridian. To overcome distortion by different incidence angles, a Scheimpflug correction system is built in (Fig. 3.9B). From the many imaged slits, the

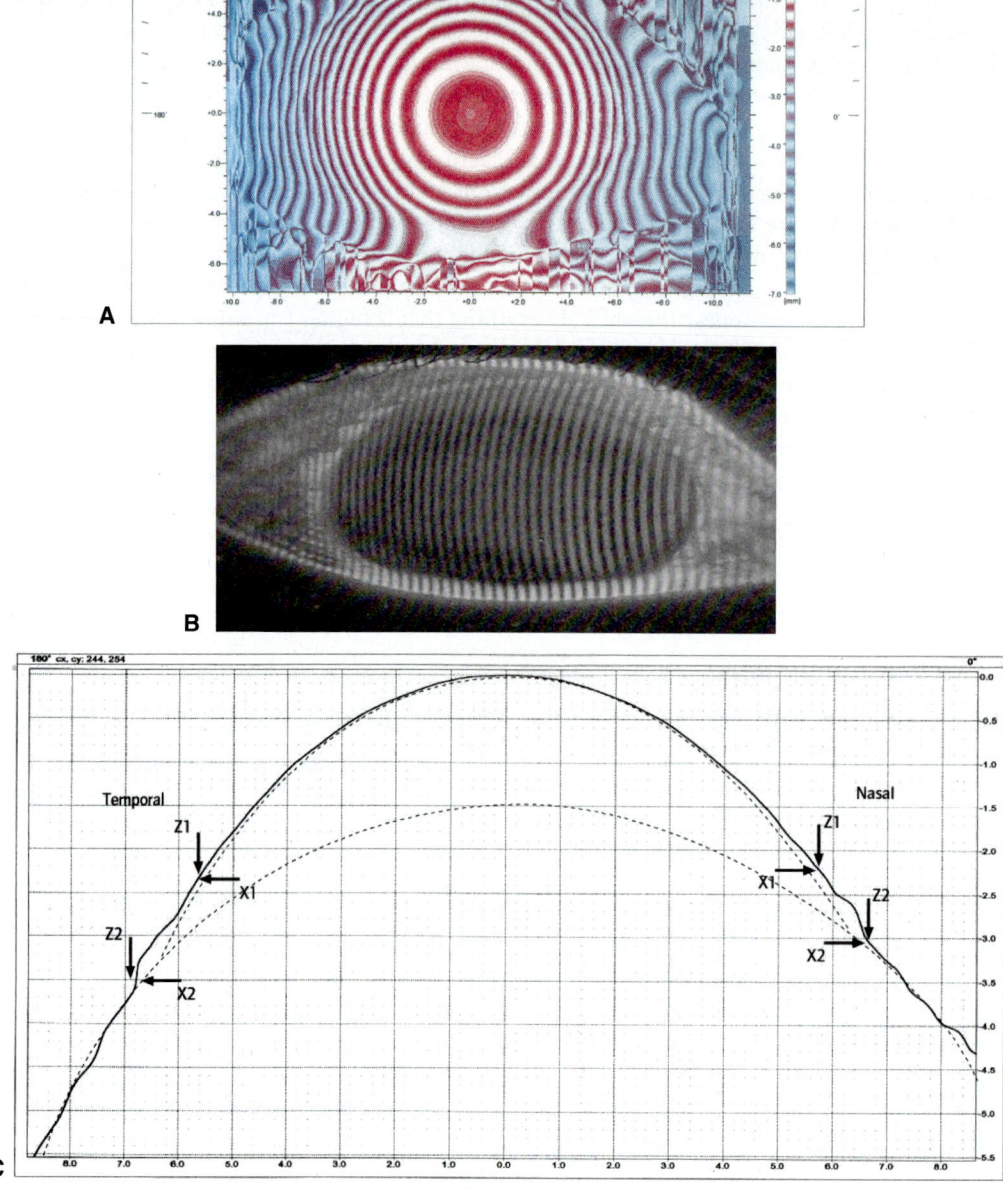

FIGURE 3.8 (A) Height contours obtained with the MST. The contours represent lines of equal height that can be translated into x, y, and z coordinates to describe the complete eye surface as exposed to the device. **(B)** Projected lines at the eye surface with the MST device. **(C)** Cross section of a horizontal true height profile of a normal eye (OD) as obtained with the MST device. Topography of the entire eye surface, including the limbal area and part of the sclera, can be obtained.

corneal shape, both front and back surface, can be computed. So, actually indirect pachymetry is performed. The results are presented in color-coded maps, including corneal thickness data (Fig. 3.9C). Advantages of the Orbscan device are that it is able to present height data on both the front and back surface of the cornea. In the Pentacam device, a rotating slit is used, resulting in an image of the cornea and the anterior chamber. With available software, the anterior

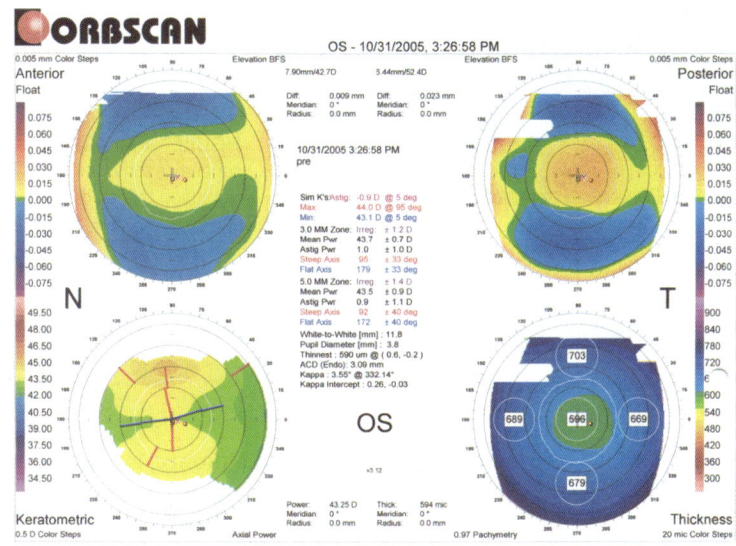

FIGURE 3.9 (A) Image cross section as obtained with the slit lamp, including the profile of the cornea front surface, gas-permeable contact lens back surface, and fluorescent tear layer. **(B)** Schematic view of a Scheimpflug correction. The tilted object plane (S) is conjugated with the projection plane when the tilted lens plane meets the object plane and projection plane at the same point (R). **(C)** Presentation of data with the Orbscan including corneal pachymetry.

chamber and the cornea can be described in detail using Zernike terms. In combination with aberrometry, this gives a very complete and detailed picture of the optics of the eye.

Optical Coherence Tomography

Devices have been developed that are able to image the front segment of the eye based on OCT. The principle behind these devices is a Michelson interferometer, in which time differences using two imaging paths from the same target are used to compute distance data. One imaging path is calibrated for the device, and the other path contains the object to measure (in this case, the eye). Next to the front segment of the eye (Fig. 3.10A), the cornea can also be measured using so-called high-resolution imaging (Fig. 3.10B) using Fourier domain analysis techniques. Although this is a zoom function rather than higher resolution, from these images, real corneal height topography can be obtained. At present, not much information on the accuracy and

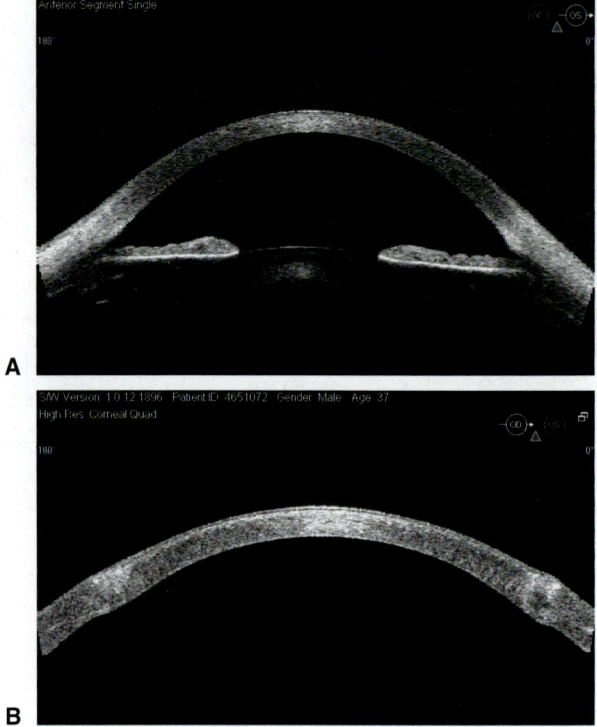

FIGURE 3.10 (A) Front segment optical coherence tomography (OCT). **(B)** Corneal high-resolution meridian topography with OCT.

reproducibility of OCT to function as a corneal topographer is available, but it appears to be a promising device in the future. The first commercially available OCT providing corneal topography data, with 360 degrees representation, has now entered the market.

CLINICAL POTENTIAL OF DEVICES

The question about which one of all the technologies mentioned is the best cannot be easily answered. It largely depends on the aim of the application. Corbett et al.[18] mentioned four considerations regarding this question: the kind of required measurement, the kind of eye surface, the kind of situation, and the kind of required presentation. If the corneal surface is considered to be an optical surface, a parametric measurement might be indicated with the advantage that considerable sensitivity is gained. Most devices based on specular reflection, including the Placido disk-based corneal topographers, measure parametrically. If the local corneal anatomy is important in the diagnosis, devices based on scattering can offer interesting modalities (e.g., pachymetry). Should it not be the optical performance but the shape that is the object of the diagnosis (e.g., pre- and postoperative evaluation or contact lens fitting), devices based on diffuse reflection offering direct height measurements can be more useful. Sometimes a diffusing membrane or simply a thin soft contact lens may be beneficial. Dry corneas, for example, exclude effective use of specular reflection, whereas during surgery, no fluorescein can be used as this penetrates the stromal tissue.

For corneas with a regular surface, a mirrored image, which is easily acquired with a Placido disk-based corneal topographer, is adequate. For irregular corneas, of which the shape is to be determined, detailed height mapping might be more accurate when obtained with a nonparametric measurement using projection principles.

In general, any topographer will be a valuable instrument, providing substantially more information for the practitioner, and may prove to be a crucial and indispensible device in the contact lens practice of the future.

HOW TO USE A CORNEAL TOPOGRAPHER

A corneal topographer is a very powerful tool, and the primary limitation appears to be the amount of data that is provided, which might be too overwhelming to be of practical use. This part of the chapter on corneal topography will discuss the necessary insights on how to use the tools available in the giant toolbox that a topographer is, and how to optimize usage of the instrument.

Measuring Procedure

Most of the topographers, especially so in contact lens practices, are the reflection systems, and these will be further discussed in detail here. One of the primary disadvantages of a reflection system topographer is the limited area that typically can be measured. To measure the maximal surface area of the cornea, it is important to first minimize the upper eyelid interference, which can cause shadows on the cornea, leading to missing data points. This is typically accomplished by asking the subject to make "large eyes." If this is not sufficient, the eyelid can be held up by a cotton swab. However, it is important for there to be an absence of pressure on the eyeball, as pressure can easily cause corneal curvature changes. It is preferable to use the orbital rim as a resting point. The subject's nose also can cause shadows on the cornea, which may lead to missing data points. To avoid this, the patient can be asked to move his or her head slightly; if the right eye is being measured, ask the patient to rotate his or her head slightly to the left, while emphasizing the importance of fixation straight ahead. This way the nose will have a lesser impact on the topography picture that is taken.

In general, reflection system topographers have difficulty measuring the periphery of the cornea, and the area that is measured is limited. The more irregular a cornea is, the more data points are missing in the periphery.

Figure 3.11A shows a typical map of a keratoconus eye, with limited data points available. Figure 3.11B also shows a map of a keratoconus, but with the missing data points extrapolated. The topographer simply assumes that the cornea will continue farther out in the periphery in the same manner. As these are not actually measured data, but rather mathematically generated points, caution should be taken. In clinical practice, extrapolation can still be of value as calculated data might be preferable to no data at all. Some topographers (see Fig. 3.11C) will

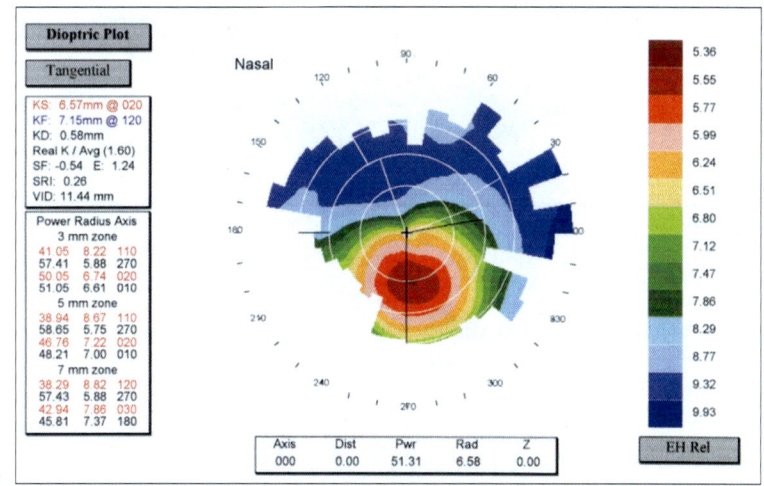

FIGURE 3.11 (A) Topography map of a keratoconus eye with limited data points available. **(B)** Topography map of a keratoconus eye with the missing data points extrapolated. **(C)** Some topographers will show the extrapolated data (*dashed*) and the real measured data in the same picture.

(continued)

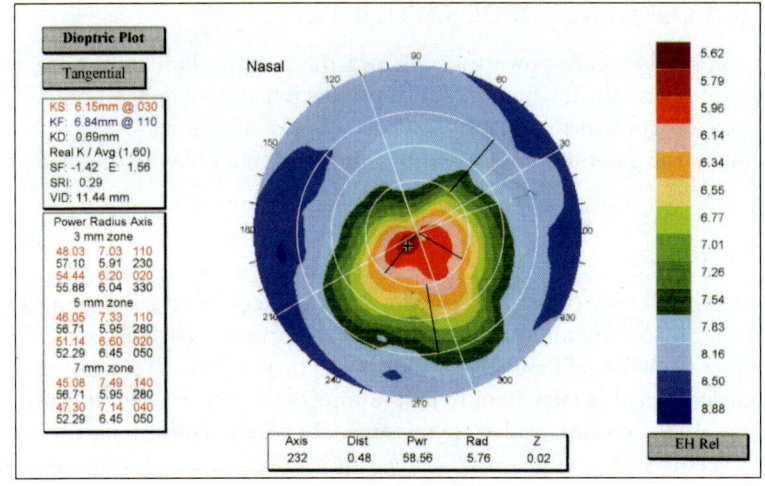

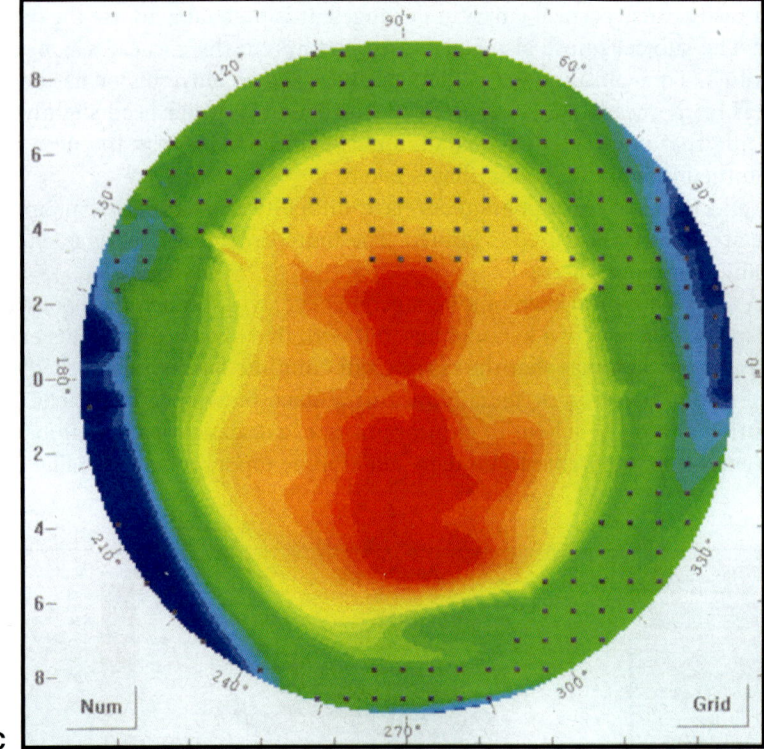

FIGURE 3.11 *(Continued)*

show the extrapolated data (*dashed*) and the real measured data in the same picture, so that the practitioner knows exactly what the origin of all data points is.

In addition to this, it is crucial when using reflection systems to have a well-wetting ocular surface. Having the subject blink several times before measurement can help in achieving this. If this does not provide a well enough wetting ocular surface, tear supplements can be used to overcome the problem. It is suggested not to use viscous drops, as they can mimic corneal irregularities. Liquid eye drops or saline can alleviate the dryness issue. If the cornea is still not wetting properly, this could lead to an increase of missing data points in the dry areas. Conversely, excessive meibomian gland secretions can also alter corneal topography.[19]

While the clinical implications are still a question mark, researchers in Brisbane, Australia, have found, using dynamic corneal topography, that the upper eyelid can also induce changes to the corneal topography.[20] While reading, the composition of the eyelids is different than when looking in primary eye gaze. The refractive power change to the cornea caused by the upper eyelid while reading was found to be significant: as a general rule, it takes the cornea as long to recover to normal after reading as the length of time that was devoted to reading. Based on this, at least theoretically, it would be worth considering having patients not read in the reception room immediately before performing corneal topography.

Corneal staining and corneal scarring can also cause erroneous or missing topography data points. If corneal reflection rings overlap, corneal topographers can get confused and may assume that what started off as one ring will continue in a next ring, which is referred to as ring *jam*. It can occur with corneal staining and with dry spots, but also sometimes if the cornea is simply too irregular itself. That is why, a higher ring density in a corneal topographer is not always better. As a result of these risks involved when performing corneal topography, it is advised to always take more than one picture and to compare the maps (which may include the original Placido image). In fact, taking three or four measurements is suggested, and maps that do not match the others should be excluded from further analysis. If the distortion of the rings is too severe and cannot be overcome, sometimes placing a thin, hydrogel contact lens over the cornea might help. Over this thin hydrogel lens, corneal topography can be performed and, although the curvatures might not be very accurate, a good impression about the shape of the cornea can be achieved.[21]

Ring jam can also occur near the upper and lower eyelid margins. The tear prism present on these margins can cause such steep curves that the topographer is easily misled (Fig. 3.12). An increase in peripheral corneal astigmatism, which will be discussed in more detail later in this chapter, can sometimes be exaggerated this way. Some topographers will allow the practitioner to manually erase the areas of confusion to alleviate the problem. Again, trying to avoid interference of the eyelid (and its tear prism) by taking measurements with larger eyes is very important in performing topography.

Different Topography Maps

What Does a Map Tell Us?

On a typical curve map (Fig. 3.13), usually the following information is displayed: the simulated keratometry values, different colors representing the corneal curves, a representation of the pupil zone, and sometimes a millimeter grid overlapping the corneal map. The latter is

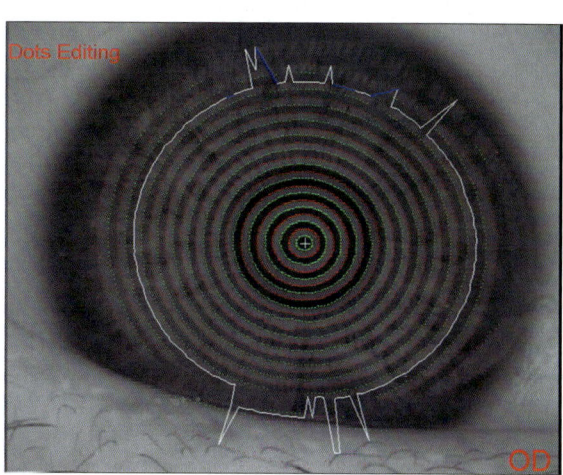

FIGURE 3.12 Tear prism on the eyelid margins have steep curves that can mislead the corneal topographer.

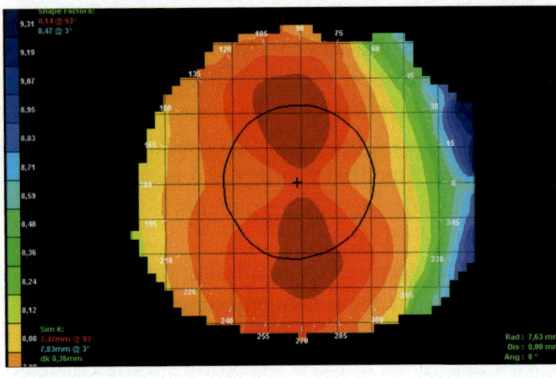

FIGURE 3.13 A typical curve topographic map.

useful to keep track of the size of the actual measured area of the cornea and the location of certain corneal distortions.

The pupil size is of limited value in most instruments, as certain light levels are required to perform the corneal topography (e.g., it is a reflection system, which requires light to be reflected off of the cornea). These lighting conditions will influence pupil diameter. Some instruments added infrared pupillometers that can measure the pupil diameter under various light conditions, which then can be assessed in relation to the topography data. Especially in ortho-k and refractive surgery, this can be a valuable tool, but also in normal rigid gas-permeable (GP) lens fitting and, for example, bifocal lens fitting, this can be very beneficial in creating a successful fit.[22] With a normal topographer without an infrared pupillometer, the pupil diameter representation can give some idea about the pupil size relative to previously measured pupils if this is always measured under the exact same light conditions. This way it is rather a subjective tool than an objective instrument.

The simulated keratometry values are of questionable value. They might be of use to practitioners, who are accustomed to using a keratometer, and perhaps to compare these values to previously measured keratometry values, but they generally are not ideal since there is such a large amount of data points that are potentially available. They give no information about corneal shape and do not identify the top of the cornea. Notably in more irregular corneas, it is misleading to use the simulated keratometry data.

Instead of presenting all the individual curves of a cornea, colors are used to visualize the large amount of data. Cooler colors represent flatter curves, warmer colors steeper curves. Generally speaking, cooler colors are visible toward the periphery of the cornea, as the average cornea flattens in this region. Toward the center, warmer colors are present, but it is quite common that the warmest color is not necessarily the geometric center of the cornea. Another common finding is that the cornea nasally is flatter than peripherally, even after correcting for the angle kappa.

The display of colors depends on the scale that is used. First of all, the steps representing different colors are typically set to 0.25 D. For irregular corneas, it can be beneficial for the scale to be set to 0.50 D or 1.00 D steps to obtain a better general overview of the corneal shape.

Relative versus Absolute Scale

Whether an absolute or relative scale is used is critical to know for practitioners who are evaluating topography maps. Absolute scales are a representation of all curves available in normal corneas, and the available colors are evenly distributed over that range (in some topographers, a customized absolute scale can be set by the practitioner). The relative scale represents curves that are available for that particular cornea, and the colors available represent a much smaller range of curves. This means that much more detail is visible with this type of scale than with an absolute scale, which is usually preferred in contact lens practice. However, the relative scale will not allow practitioners to compare one cornea to another cornea, or even allow comparison of the same cornea over time, as the scale may vary. A "red" cornea on a relative scale does not mean this is a steep cornea. It only means that there is a relatively large steep (red) area within that particular cornea. Both parts of Figure 3.14 are post corneal-graft maps that, at first glance, look very similar. However, Figure 3.14A represents a 0.74-mm difference horizontally and vertically (or 3.7 D corneal astigmatism), whereas Figure 3.14B has a 3.46-mm difference or 17 D astigmatic cornea. This difference is not immediately obvious by simply viewing the images as they are both relative scales. Typically, a normal cornea in a contact lens practice is best viewed on a relative scale as it provides the most details, as long as practitioners understand its limitations.

Tangential versus Sagittal Scale

Also of importance is the tangential versus sagittal representation of data. Sagittal curves make the assumption that the center of the radius of that curve is always on the central axis, hence the alternative name for this setting: an axial map. This will represent best the optical characteristics of a cornea. The tangential (or instantaneous) setting will typically show more detail than the sagittal setting of the same eye (Fig. 3.15). Tangential maps are sometimes referred

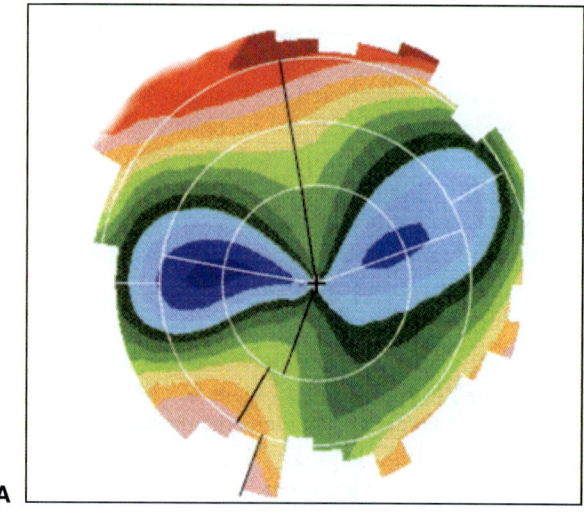

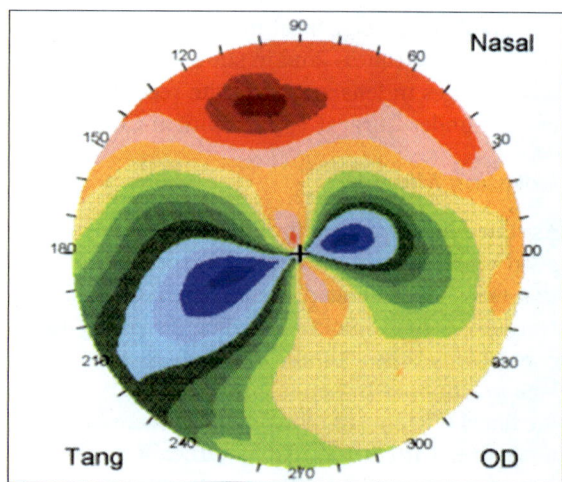

FIGURE 3.14 (A) Post corneal-graft cornea with 3.7 D astigmatism. **(B)** Post corneal-graft cornea with 17 D astigmatism.

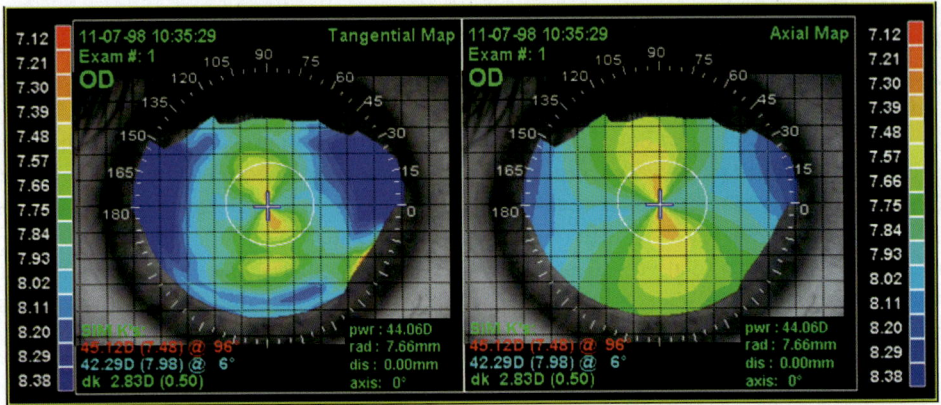

FIGURE 3.15 Tangential map **(A)** and sagittal map **(B)** of same eye.

to as true curve data. Tangential curves do not make an assumption about where the center of the radius might be. They simply look at a certain part of the cornea and measure the radius of that point under 90 degrees (as a tangent), of which the center of the radius could be anywhere. This will give, especially in the periphery of the cornea, a much more detailed representation. In contact lens practice, where the periphery is of special interest, this is usually the preferred option. However, as with absolute versus relative scales, the sagittal map is more suitable for comparison between corneas as it has a standard reference point. In refractive surgery, axial maps are usually preferred over tangential maps for that reason.

Viewing both maps could be beneficial in some cases. In ortho-k, for example, tangential maps are used to determine the overnight centration of the lens (as lens centration while sleeping cannot be evaluated behind a slit lamp), but to assess the optical state of a cornea and to follow the progression of the refractive change, axial maps are used. More on ortho-k and reading ortho-k topography maps will be covered in Chapter 22 of this book.

Difference Maps

Difference maps are desired when evaluating the effect that lenses have on the cornea and are among the most useful of all maps in clinical practice. Difference maps take the original topographic data before contact lens fitting and subtract the topographic data of a certain time after lens fit. This could be 1 day, 1 week, or 1 month after lens fit (typically to evaluate the lens fit of normal GP or hydrogel lenses), or even years later (to evaluate the long-term effects of any lens and to evaluate the risk of developing corneal warpage and spectacle blur). Corneal topographers are beneficial in the initial fitting of the contact lenses—which can be somewhat confronting at times—and in showing how well the lens respects the shape of the cornea. Corneal changes in lens wear and the recovery of corneal changes will be discussed later in this chapter under Corneal Topography in Contact Lens Practice.

Elevation Maps

As stated before, a height or elevation map of the cornea may be one of the best ways to get a good representation of corneal shape to really know "where you are"—whether these elevation maps are generated from a height topographer or are derived from Placido disk ring data. Not only is elevation crucial when designing and manufacturing custom contact lenses (as the contact lens lathes "think" in height data), they also can be of tremendous help for the contact lens practitioner to better visualize the true shape of the cornea and therefore better predict the likely outcome in terms of fluorescein fit. This is especially true for (but not limited to) the more irregular cornea, like in corneal ectasia. In the right eye of the keratoconus patient represented in Figure 3.16, the small red area on the axial map (Fig. 3.16A) looks like a localized area of elevation midperipherally, inferior on the cornea. But all that the red area here really means is that there is "steepness" in that area. In this case, the steepness actually may mean "a drop" instead of an elevation. In the elevation map (Fig. 3.16B), this can be seen, which is confirmed when an actual GP lens (an aspheric GP lens with an eccentricity of 0.98, BCR of 7.40, and a 10.2-mm diameter in this case) is placed on the eye (Fig. 3.16C). So this cornea represents a general "high" area over a large surface, with a significant depression just inferior of the elevated area. This case clearly shows that "red" on the axial map is not always an elevation,

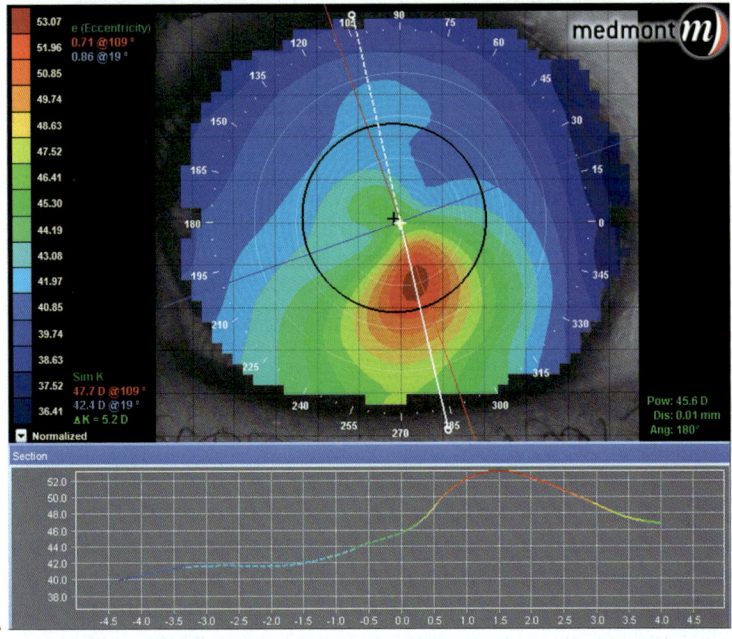

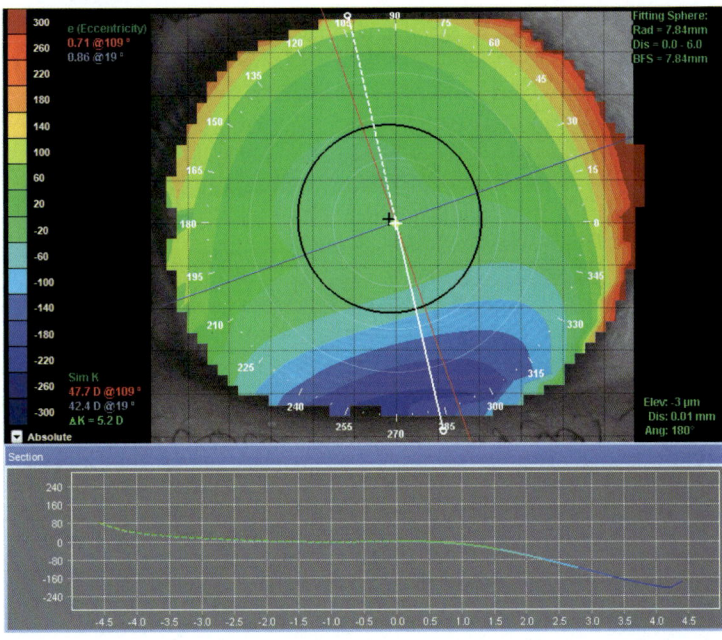

FIGURE 3.16 (A) Axial topography map, right eye of a keratoconus patient. **(B)** Elevation map of the same eye. **(C)** GP lens fluorescein pattern for the same eye. (Courtesy of Patrick Caroline and Randy Kojima, Pacific University College of Optometry.)

(continued)

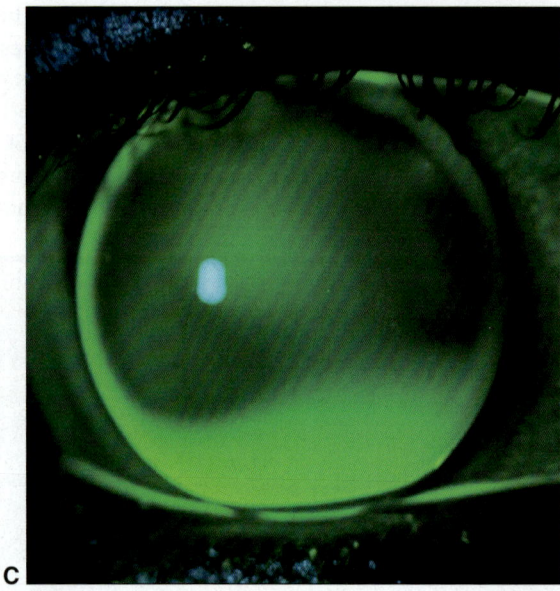

FIGURE 3.16 *(Continued)*

but rather can also be a transition to a depression. Some have suggested that using the elevation maps would actually be a good way to distinguish a keratoconus from a pellucid marginal degeneration (PMD).[23] In PMD, the curve maps sometimes show artificial "red" areas centrally on the cornea, which may be interpreted as elevation, while in reality they represent a drop-off. In addition, the assumptions the topographer makes with regards to the normal cornea, which do not apply to irregular corneas like PMD, may lead to a partly erroneous representation of the actual situation. In other words, the classical "kissing doves" pattern seen in PMD may be a (partial) artifact and not necessarily represents true corneal shape. Figure 3.17 shows the left

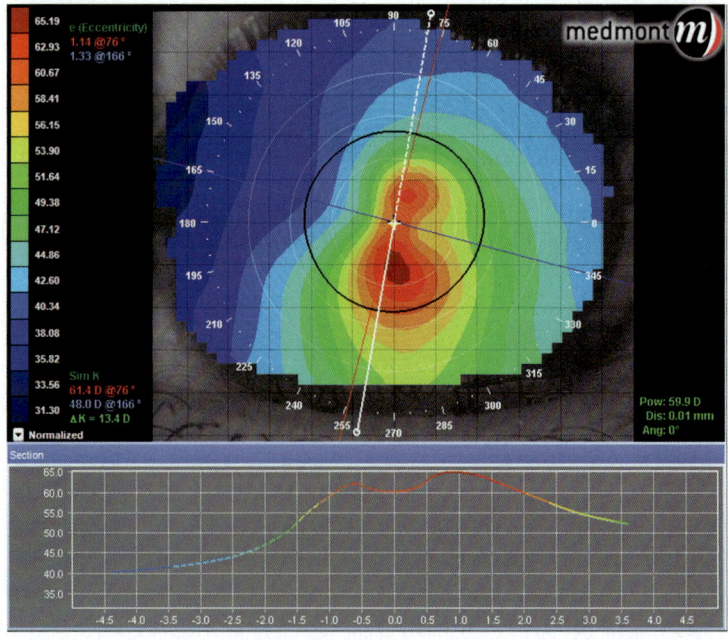

FIGURE 3.17 **(A)** Axial topography map, left eye of a keratoconus patient. **(B)** Elevation map of the same eye. **(C)** GP lens fluorescein pattern for the same eye. (Courtesy of Patrick Caroline and Randy Kojima, Pacific University College of Optometry.)

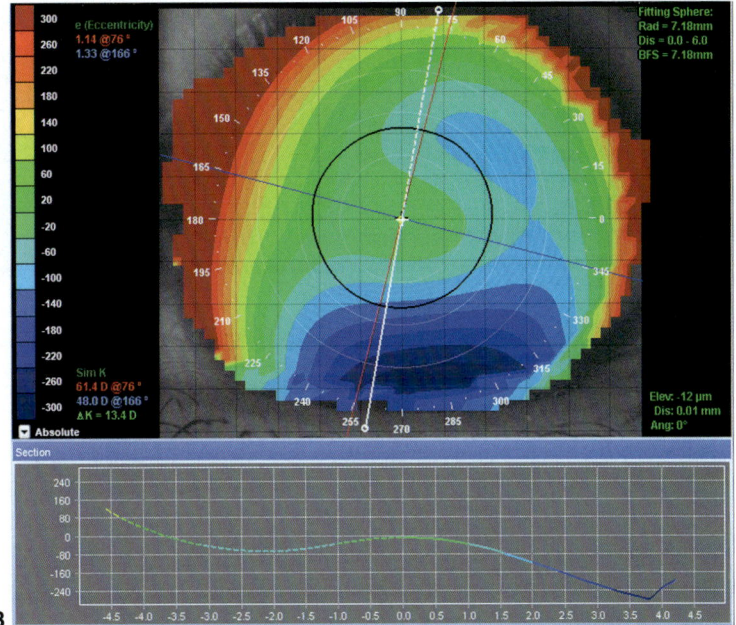

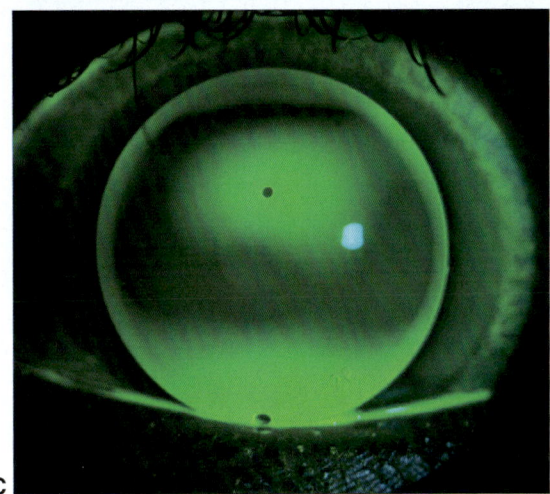

FIGURE 3.17 *(Continued)*

eye of the same patient as in Figure 3.16. Again, the elevation map much better represents and mimics the actual fluorescein pattern with the GP lens on the eye (an aspheric GP lens with an eccentricity of 1.3, BCR of 6.20, and a 10.2-mm diameter). Also to better "image" corneal astigmatism to see what areas are "deeper" (not steeper) than other areas, elevation maps can be useful. In Figure 3.18, it becomes evident that the "blue" areas on the elevation map correspond with the "green" areas in the fluorescein pattern, representing pooling; for example, space between the lens' back surface and the cornea. Thus, elevation maps can be a powerful tool in contact lens practice, especially in—but not limited to—the irregular cornea.[24–26]

Indices for Corneal Irregularity

When evaluating topographic maps, practitioners should not focus too much on differences in colors, but primarily look for symmetry to determine whether or not a particular cornea is distorted. Figure 3.14 shows a standard topography map with warmer colors in the vertical

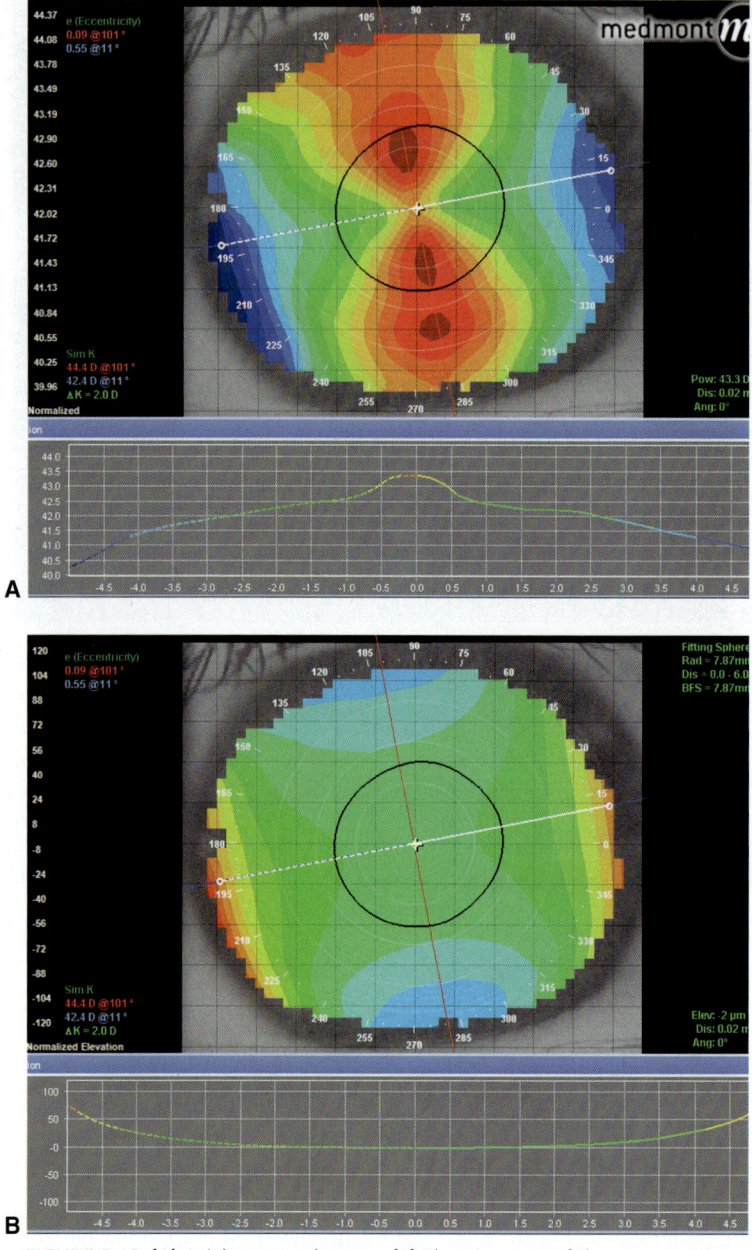

FIGURE 3.18 (A) Axial topography map. **(B)** Elevation map of the same patient. **(C)** GP lens fluorescein pattern for the same eye. (Courtesy of Patrick Caroline and Randy Kojima, Pacific University College of Optometry.)

meridian than in the horizontal meridian, representing corneal astigmatism. This is represented as a typical eight-shape pattern, which in this case shows symmetry. As the warmer colors represent steeper curves, this map represents with-the-rule corneal astigmatism. The differences between the horizontal and the vertical meridian are 0.36 mm or 2.13 D. In Figure 3.19, approximately the same difference between horizontal and vertical curves is seen (0.34 mm or 2.38 D), but within the vertical meridian alone, there is also a 1.55 D difference. This topography map is not symmetric. This is an indication that this cornea is potentially irregular, whether existing or acquired. Corneas with a difference of 1.4 to 1.9 D within one meridian are moderately irregular

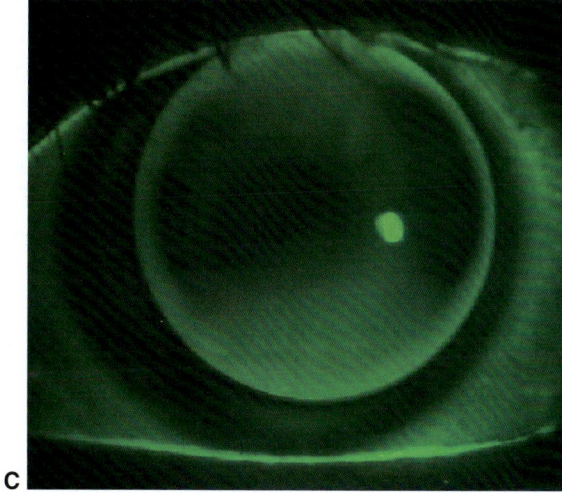

FIGURE 3.18 *(Continued)*

but suspect for having keratoconus, while corneas with more than 1.9 D of asymmetry in one meridian are considered irregular and are highly suspect for having keratoconus.[27]

As it is not always obvious whether asymmetry of the corneal surface is clinically significant, corneal topographers provide indices that can help the practitioner in analyzing the corneal surface. The most commonly used index for the detection of irregularity and keratoconus is the I–S value (the inferior–superior value). It typically compares the cornea on five points in the superior half of the cornea, with five points in the inferior half. Some topographers use the SAI value (surface asymmetry index), which evaluates the difference between opposite semi-meridians, which is another way of comparing one part of the cornea with the opposite site. The modified Rabinowitz/McDonnell test that is used with some topographers does, in essence, the same (it uses the I–S value), but it adds the difference in corneal power between the right and the left eye. In keratoconus, one eye is usually more progressed than the other, and if there is more than 1 D of difference between the two corneas, this is also considered a risk for the condition.[28]

In addition to this, to detect irregular corneas, it is also of interest to analyze the angle within one of the principal astigmatism axes. Astigmatism axes are usually fairly straight, although even in corneas that are considered normal, deviations from this can be observed. But if the angle within the astigmatism axis has a large deviation from straight, then the probability of an irregular cornea increases. The SRAX index considers a cornea to be irregular and keratoconus suspect if the astigmatism axis angle is more than 21 degrees diverged from straight, and combines this with the I–S value to give a prediction for the risk of keratoconus.[29]

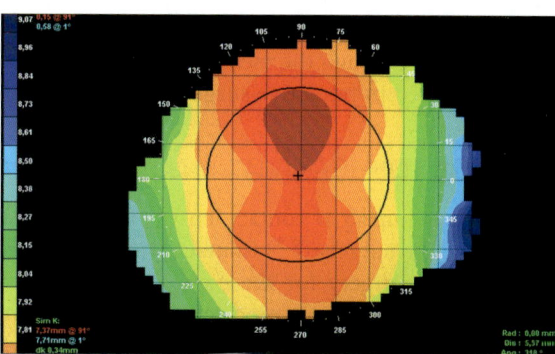

FIGURE 3.19 Asymmetry in vertical meridian.

KISA is another index, which is based on the just-described astigmatism angle together with the I–S value, but this also takes the absolute keratometry values into account. Typically, steeper curves are seen in patients with keratoconus than in normal corneas.[30]

Another way of detecting keratoconus is looking at *e*-values that corneal topographers provide (see more on this under Corneal Topography in Contact Lens Practice, Corneal Shape in this chapter). High *e*-values are common in keratoconus. Dao et al.[31] found that if the *e*-value of eyes was ≥0.8, the specificity (98%) and sensitivity (97%) were high for dealing with a keratoconus cornea. This abnormal *e*-value was observed in keratoconus eyes with a visual acuity of 1.0, whereas slit-lamp examination showed no abnormalities.

PMD is another corneal degeneration that can mimic many of the clinical signs and symptoms observed in keratoconus. The topography map of a PMD is different than that of keratoconus, in that the steeper curves are typically visible in the periphery of the cornea, sometimes shaped like a band of steepening parallel to the limbus. Centrally, this arc comes together toward the center of the cornea. This has been described as a pattern of two doves kissing. Confusingly, this pattern can also be found in decentered oval cones in keratoconus patients. See "elevation maps" earlier in this chapter for using these elevation maps to potentially be able to differentiate between this and PMD. Typically, the distance from the center of the cornea (apex) to the steepest part of the cornea (the peak elevation index, PEI) is 1.95 mm in keratoconus, while it is, on average, 3.5 mm in eyes with PMD.[32] Differentiation between PMD and keratoconus can be important as contact lens-fitting approaches may be different in the two conditions.[33] In addition to topography, it is apparent that wavefront aberrometry, especially if combined with corneal topography, can be a valuable tool to predict early stages of keratoconus and/or PMD as well.[34]

When fitting contact lenses to keratoconus eyes, it is often difficult to obtain accurate curve data on the top of the cone. Typically, the top of the cone is not in the center of the cornea and central corneal curvatures (including simulated *k*-values) are not accurate. Moving the cursor to the top of the cone on the map and reading off the local *k*-values will provide a better idea. But this still has its limitations as corneal topographers assume that the top of the cornea is close to or on the geometric center of the cornea. As this is typically not the case in keratoconus, practitioners can ask the patient to look in the opposite direction of where the top of the cone is located to artificially create a situation where the top of the cone is centered in the map. Obviously this does not provide the real representation of the corneal geometry, but it will give the best possible curve values of the top of the cone.

When fitting bi- or multifocal contact lenses, it is also of importance to have information about the location of the exact top of the cornea. If this is not in line with the geometric center of the cornea, as in keratoconus, simultaneous lenses might be better avoided since the optical center of the lens needs to match the optical center of the cornea. If this is not the case, translating lenses might be preferred.

Other indices to evaluate corneal regularity are the SRI value (surface regularity index), which compares the power of each point within the central 4.5 mm (the pupil zone) to the points immediately surrounding it. This index correlates best with visual acuity. Normal corneas have low SRI values (<1.0). Other indices that attempt to do the same are the CIU (corneal uniformity index) and the PVA (potential visual acuity) index. The Holladay index fits a best-fit ellipse through the measured cornea, also to give a prediction of the PVA. These indices are widely used in refractive surgery management.

CORNEAL TOPOGRAPHY IN CONTACT LENS PRACTICE

Recently, the impact of contact lenses on the cornea has become clear within the framework of laser refractive surgery.[35,36] Contact lens wearers frequently need to cease lens wear for many weeks before surgery for the cornea to return to its baseline shape. One refractive surgery center in the Netherlands reported that 95% of all retreatments for refractive reasons were performed on previous contact lens wearers. (Lafeber R. Personal communication, 2004).

Corneal Changes in Gas-Permeable Lens Wear

Alterations of corneal topography in GP contact lens wearers have been reported by many researchers.[37,38] With GP lenses, it is more the mechanical pressure of the lens on the cornea rather than hypoxic stress that causes topographic changes. Hypoxic stress was a significant problem with polymethylmethacrylate (PMMA) lenses (causing up to 98% of corneas to have corneal edema),[39] which very often resulted in corneal distortion and corneal warpage. Still, patients who are wearing PMMA lenses are among the most difficult to be refitted with other lenses or to be treated with refractive surgery, but fortunately these cases are becoming rare today. First, refitting PMMA lens wearers with GP lenses before temporary cessation of lens wear seems advised in these cases. Currently, it is advised to stop GP lens wear for at least 8 weeks prior to laser surgery. After this, the cornea needs to be evaluated at 2-week intervals until a stable topography is reached, which is usually defined as 0.50 D change or less compared to the last visit. This also shows the importance of performing a baseline corneal topography before every single contact lens fit in your practice.

To avoid induced corneal changes, it is of importance to assess the fit of every GP lens wearer regularly, using fluorescein. Steep lens fits should be avoided at all times. It has been shown that GP lenses that are fitted 0.3-mm steeper than the flattest meridian induce corneal steepening after short-term lens wear.[40] In a recent ortho-k study, patients showed significant central corneal flattening (-0.61 ± 0.35 D) within 10 minutes of open-eye lens wear, showing the vulnerable nature of the epithelium and the speed with which it can be altered.[41] Flat lenses can cause corneal changes as well and are, in addition, more prone to lead to decentration. A GP lens is designed and fitted on the central cornea. This means that decentration of the lens will cause a situation in which the lens and cornea are not in alignment with each other. Therefore, it is important to avoid decentration of lenses as much as possible as well. A map of a decentered GP lens can easily be confused for a keratoconus map. Typically, if a lens is decentered to a position lower on the cornea (a low rider), then in the inferior part of the cornea, flatter curves will be observed while steeper curves will be present in the opposite direction of the cornea (superior).[38,42]

Another way the cornea might be altered by the GP lens is if a spherical lens geometry is used on a toric cornea. Mechanical pressure nasally and temporally in with-the-rule corneal astigmatism can cause significant corneal changes. The cornea always tries to mimic the shape of the back surface of the lens, which works as a mold. A corneal topography map that is taken immediately after GP lens removal is often quite inaccurate. Corneal astigmatism might be present, but suppressed by the GP lens. Typically, within a few days, the original corneal astigmatism begins to reappear.

Some of the back aspheric bi- and multifocal contact lenses are an example of the GP lens fits that cause a lot of corneal distortion. They are suggested to be fit 1 D, 2 D, or sometimes even 3 D steeper than K because of the nature of the high eccentricity of the back surface of the lens. While, generally, in GP lens wear fitting, practitioners try to avoid steep fitting lens patterns, with these lenses it is interesting to note that apparently it is accepted to fit lenses steep. Corneal topography changes can be induced by this, and epithelial cells are typically suppressed in the midperiphery of the cornea and an increase in corneal thickness may even be observed centrally. Basically, this is hyperopic ortho-k, but with lenses that are not suitable for that purpose. Therefore, they can decenter and can cause severe corneal distortion. For corneas like this, it can take several months to return to their baseline values. Luckily, these lenses are becoming less common in today's contact lens practice.

Changes in Hydrogel Lens Wear

Less known than the GP changes during lens wear, and therefore more neglected, are the topographic changes underneath hydrogel lenses. If monitored closely, however, many changes can be detected. Schornack[43] estimated that 27% of all cases of corneal warpage are in patients wearing hydrogel lenses. These topographic changes are thought to be primarily the result of hypoxia, and indeed are observed more in patients wearing conventional lenses and especially in lenses that are thick and made of a low oxygen permeability (Dk) material. Topographic changes are, for example, regularly observed in prism-ballasted toric hydrogels made out of conventional materials. Generally, a minimum of 2 weeks of discontinuation of hydrogel contact lenses is advised, followed by 2-week-interval checkups to assess the corneal stability, before laser surgery can be considered. A change of <0.5 D is generally accepted as being within the margins of a stable cornea. A study by Ng et al.[44] showed that it, respectively, took 10.7 days ($\pm$10.4 days) on average for the manifest refraction to stabilize after soft lens wear, 16.2 $\pm$ 17.5 days using keratometry and 28.1 $\pm$ 17.7 days with corneal topography. With pachymetry (using a 7-micron criterion), it took 35.1 $\pm$ 20.8 days for the cornea to stabilize.

The case at the end of this chapter is a good example of a patient exhibiting soft lens-induced corneal distortion, which dissipated after 2 weeks of non-lens wear. However, as a result of this ordeal, the patient decided not to return to contact lens wear.

The topographic changes under a hydrogel lens are often subtle and these patients also should be monitored on a routine basis. Distortion of keratometer mires can be the initial clinical sign, but these are limited to a small (usually 3 mm) central portion of the cornea and the changes cannot be classified.

Corneal topography covers a large, if not the total, area of the cornea and a difference map can identify subtle topographic changes promptly and accurately. Figure 3.20 shows a patient exhibiting an unusual case of severe peripheral corneal disruption underneath a conventional toric hydrogel lens, which is even visible without the use of a corneal topographer.

With the arrival of silicone hydrogel contact lens materials, the hypoxia-related corneal warpage cases have been reduced or essentially eliminated. However, the early versions of silicone hydrogel lenses brought on a different type of distortion because of the higher modality of the material compared to conventional hydrogels. Peripheral corneal changes, in particular, were not uncommon.

In order to best respect the shape of the cornea in each individual, and to minimize corneal distortion underneath soft lenses, soft contact lenses may best classified into different groups. The first and largest group is the "Inventory" or "off the rack" lenses. These are the lenses found in traditional diagnostic sets and all disposable lenses. Group two is represented by soft lenses with expanded parameters: these are lenses that go beyond the traditional standard diagnostic set, but are generally limited by factors such as design, and so forth. The third group consists of custom-made lenses: these lenses are made to order for the individual cornea, based on corneal topography data. In the latter category would surely fall custom-made lenses for keratoconus, for instance. Technically, manufacturing of these lenses almost have no limitations.

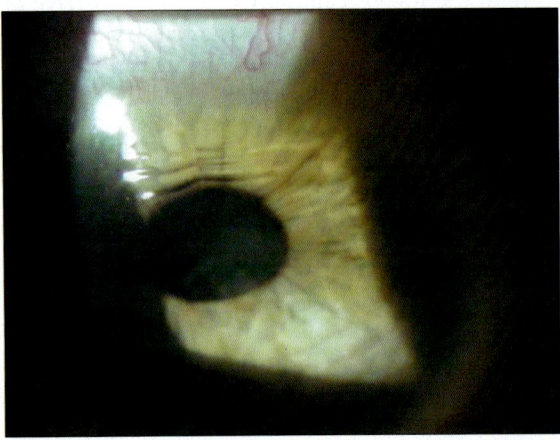

FIGURE 3.20 Unusual case of severe peripheral corneal disruption underneath a conventional toric hydrogel lens. (Courtesy of Hans Kloes, Kloes Eye Kliniek, the Netherlands.)

Back-surface quadrant-specific soft lenses for keratoconus, in any prescription (sphere or cylinder), are currently available, even in silicone hydrogel materials.[45]

Interestingly, topographic changes to the cornea can also be used to the advantage of the lens wearer. Hydrogel lenses also have shown to be able to create ortho-k-like patterns. Patients who accidentally wore silicone hydrogel lenses inside out reported changes in refraction, often leading to a decrease in myopia. This phenomenon was first described by Patrick Caroline at the British Contact Lens Association Meeting in June 2003. Practitioners should be aware of this effect, as apparently, no decrease in lens-wearing comfort is noted when the silicone hydrogel lenses are worn inside out. The effect is found to be more pronounced in higher myopes wearing silicone hydrogel lenses, and the topographic effect is very difficult to distinguish from a (successful) ortho-k lens fit with GP lenses.

Figure 3.21 shows a CIBA Focus Night & Day lens (base curve 8.4, −10.00 D, diameter 13.8 mm) that has been worn inside out purposely on a continuous-wear basis for 30 days. The difference map that is shown on the right of this figure shows a 3.12 D reduction in myopia in the center of the topography. Research is under way to investigate whether these lenses can be used to purposely change the shape of the cornea to temporarily reduce myopia.

Contact Lens Fitting Based on Corneal Topography

Careful lens selection while respecting the shape of the cornea with every lens fit is the basis for every successful lens wearer. This is true for silicone hydrogel lenses and in conventional lens wear, as shown in the previous section. With regard to fitting GP lenses, respecting the shape of the cornea is of even more importance. Corneal topography can be a major help in achieving this.

Respecting Corneal Shape

The primary goal in fitting GP lenses is to respect the shape of the cornea as much as possible and to distribute pressure equally over the entire corneal epithelium. If the surface area of contact is maximized, the weight of the lens is distributed over the largest possible area of cornea.[46] In this situation, the force per unit of surface area applied to the cornea by the lens is minimized, and the likelihood of corneal distortion is reduced.

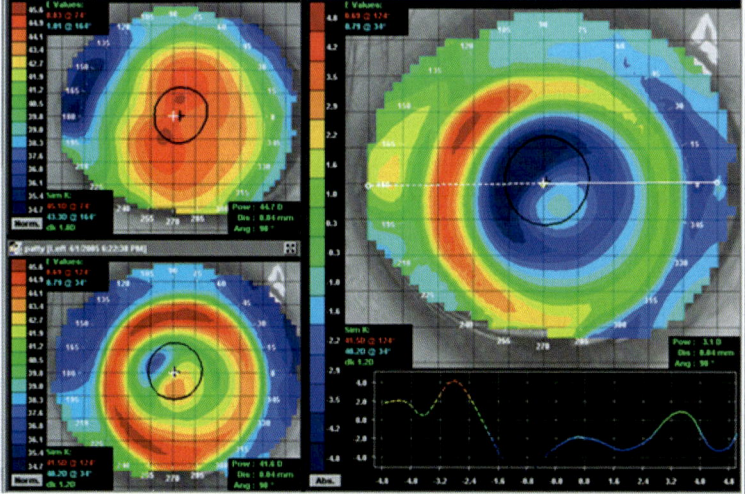

FIGURE 3.21 A high minus silicone hydrogel contact lens that has been worn inside out purposely on a continuous-wear basis for 30 days, showing an orthokeratology-like difference map. (Courtesy of Patrick Caroline, Pacific University College of Optometry.)

The goal in normal GP lens wear is to avoid the induction of corneal change as much as possible. To do so, knowledge of the shape of the cornea is essential. By far, the best instrument to analyze this shape is the corneal topographer. Several attempts to modify manual keratometers to carry out this analysis have proven to be of limited use. Although many of the Placido disk systems are not able to measure curves in the far periphery of the cornea, they are usually able to measure up to the point where the resting point of the lens will be positioned.

The shape of the average corneal surface is usually described as prolate ellipse, indicating a gradual flattening from center to periphery. This is one of first things that is obvious when looking at an average corneal topography map: relatively cooler colors in the periphery of the corneal map represent this flattening. The amount of flattening is traditionally designated as eccentricity, mostly noted as the e-value. The e-value of an ellipse can be calculated from the central curvature and the peripheral curvature plus the distance (angle) from the center where that peripheral curve was measured. The average cornea has been described as roughly 0.43, and typically is between 0.40 and 0.57.[47–49] But the e-value varies widely among individuals, and ideally, it should be measured and evaluated on every single eye before fitting contact lenses. As an example, the Ohio State University looked at the corneal shape of 683 children's eyes (aged 8–15): the vast majority flattened toward the periphery, but two corneas actually steepened.[50] There seems to be a small correlation between ametropia and eccentricity (higher myopia showing reduced eccentricity).[47,51]

Not all meridians of the cornea have the same e-value. Most corneal topographers and automated keratometers will provide the average e-value of all meridians, although some will give e-values per meridian or quadrant. A major drawback with regard to e-value measurement is that manufacturers of topographers are very secretive about the way they calculate the e-value: it should be taken off the axial map, but neither the distance from the center nor the meridian used is usually revealed, which means that differences in e-values between topographers may occur. Unfortunately, there is no standard for defining corneal shape.

Besides this, another disadvantage of the e-value is that it can only describe prolate shapes. In corneas that are steeper in the periphery by default or in corneas that are reshaped that way by ortho-k or laser surgery, an oblate shape is present. In these cases, the e-value is useless, since mathematically it can only define shapes larger than zero (spherical). This problem can be overcome by using what has been called the p-value, which can be derived directly from the e-value: $p = 1 - e^2$. By using the p-value, the exact same shape is described, but it should be borne in mind that a circle's value is now 1 instead of 0.[52] The p-value of all prolate shapes is <1, and in the case of peripheral steepening, the p-value is larger than 1, which is exactly the opposite of the e-value. Practitioners may be confronted with p-values as an alternative to e-values in the international literature, and should be aware of the opposite effect compared to the e-value.

Another approach to describe the asphericity of the cornea is to use the Q-value. This value can be derived as follows: $Q = p - 1$, or $Q = -e^2$. A negative Q-value describes prolate shapes and positive values an oblate shape, but the Q-value of a sphere remains 0, the same as the e-value.[51,52] Therefore, the Q-value has advantages over both the other shape descriptors and may be considered as a standard index for describing corneal shape,[53] especially in ortho-k and refractive surgery practice.

In reality, however, the actual corneal shape is not as easily defined as a standard ellipse. Especially toward the periphery, it becomes more complex and less predictable. The corneal shape is usually more spherical near the apex and it may flatten at a variable (usually progressive) rate toward the periphery. Zernike polynomials are often used to describe the corneal shape in more detail, but even these complex mathematical formulations have their limitations, and newer mathematical definitions of the corneal shape are being developed. However, the clinical usefulness of these complex formulations when manually fitting GP lenses seems limited. Therefore, to describe corneal eccentricity, shape parameters are still preferred and provide a good idea about the flattening of the cornea. The e-value is still the parameter most used in contact lens practice, and most topographers and automated keratometers currently use this.

As a rule of thumb, practitioners may square the *e*-value that was provided by the topographer or automated keratometer to have some idea of the amount of flattening in the periphery of average corneas. An *e*-value of 0.4 means that the flattening in the periphery at 30 degrees from the center is about 0.16 mm. An *e*-value of 0.6 describes a flattening of 0.36 mm, and a cornea with an *e*-value of 0.8 is 0.64 mm flatter in the periphery. From this, it can be concluded that, as the *e*-value goes up, flattening increases progressively. This also means that small *e*-values are clinically of little importance, but the importance of *e*-values increases rapidly as the value gets higher.

To respect the shape of the cornea, the amount of flattening should be followed as much as possible. A spherical lens (tricurve, tetracurve, etc.) on an aspheric cornea could give friction in the midperiphery of the cornea. As most corneas flatten toward the periphery, theoretically, most lenses should also be aspheric in nature.[46,54] In practice, this usually means choosing a lens with an *e*-value closest to the *e*-value of the cornea. If the exact *e*-value is not available, use a higher *e*-value lens (flatter lens fit appearance) rather than a smaller *e*-value lens. Usually, aspheric GP lenses are manufactured with an *e*-value between 0.4 and 0.8 for normal corneas and higher *e*-values for keratoconus eyes. The common interval between *e*-values of available lenses is 0.15 or 0.2, but some manufacturers allow the practitioner to order the *e*-value in as little as 0.05 steps if desired.

By using aspheric lenses, the shape of the lens is followed accurately in an annular fashion. Also, in fitting bi- and multifocal contact lenses, it is essential to know the *e*-value of the cornea. Back aspheric simultaneous lenses are designed for the average cornea (e.g., an *e*-value of 0.43). The lens is designed with a very high *e*-value (meaning more flattening toward the periphery). Because of this, the lens needs to be fitted steeper (as discussed before). However, if a cornea has an exceptional small or large *e*-value, then this can lead, respectively, to an exceptionally poor lens fit and/or to no near addition for the lens wearer.

Some lens design software programs allow the practitioner to choose different *e*-values for different zones. In this way, the shape of the cornea can be followed even more closely (since the cornea is not usually a perfect ellipse). This can be very valuable when fitting keratoconus eyes, in which the differences in *e*-value in different meridians can be substantial.

In GP lens wear, 3 and 9 o'clock staining is one of the most often reported problems, and this complication is difficult to remedy. Several authors[55–58] have suggested that in theory, an aspheric lens design could be beneficial in managing 3 and 9 o'clock staining. First, this is because aspheric back surface designs may follow the corneal shape closely, lessening areas of contact between the lens and (peripheral) cornea, and thus enhancing tear fluid exchange and corneal wettability. Furthermore, aspheric lens designs are able to minimize lid–lens interaction, thereby decreasing discomfort and interference with blinking habits. Also, decreased edge lifts in aspheric lenses could lead to a reduction of the bridge effect (upper eyelid bridging the gap between lens edge and cornea) and tear meniscus formation around the edge of the lens[52]— all thought to be beneficial in 3 and 9 o'clock staining management.

To summarize, to avoid the induction of corneal topographic changes by GP lenses, the shape of the cornea should be followed as closely as possible. Matching the corneal shape with the lens shape by using aspheric lenses can be helpful in achieving this and also may aid in the management of 3 and 9 o'clock staining. Corneal topography is very useful for this purpose.

Corneal Astigmatism

The other major factor with regard to respecting the shape of the cornea is corneal toricity. Dealing with corneal toricity follows the same principle as dealing with corneal shape: the lens pressure should be evenly distributed over the corneal surface. Nontoric lenses on with-the-rule corneas will create pressure in the horizontal meridian.

Devising a general rule for the degree of corneal toricity that should be fitted with a toric back surface is not easy. Textbooks generally consider that toric designs are indicated when the corneal toricity is 2.5 to 3.0 D or more.[59] However, this could easily lead to topographic changes and spectacle blur. As stated above, 0.3-mm steep lenses (accounting roughly for a 1.5 D steep fit) can give significant corneal changes. In addition to this, corneal toricity may increase or decrease toward the periphery and thus influence fitting characteristics.[54] Szczotka et al.[60] found peripheral corneal toricity to be one of the major factors determining the success of toric hydrogel lens fitting. Since GP lenses rest mostly peripherally, this influence should not be neglected in GP lenses either. Central corneal astigmatism is easier to deal with than limbal-to-limbal corneal astigmatism when fitting GP lenses (Fig. 3.22). Corneal topographers can aid in assessing the degree of peripheral astigmatism. Researchers at the University of Brisbane, Australia[61] looked at peripheral corneal astigmatism and found that 38% of cases showed a spherical central cornea with a spherical periphery. In 21% of cases, a toric cornea was found with a stable astigmatism toward the periphery. However, 15% showed a spherical center with a toric periphery, 22% showed a toric center with a decrease of astigmatism toward the periphery, and in 4%, the toricity increased toward the periphery. Although this was a small sample size, it clearly shows that different types of corneal astigmatism can be present. In addition to normal (GP and hydrogel) lens fitting, this is extremely important in ortho-k practice and in bi-and multifocal lens fitting. In these cases, it can predict the risk of lens decentration, and therefore, it influences lens fit to a large degree. If a corneal topographer is not available, as

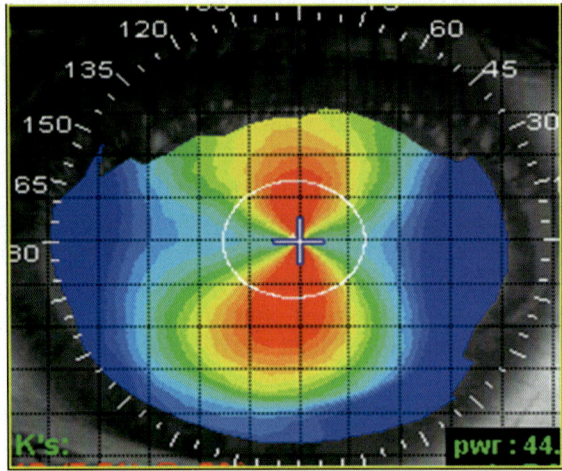

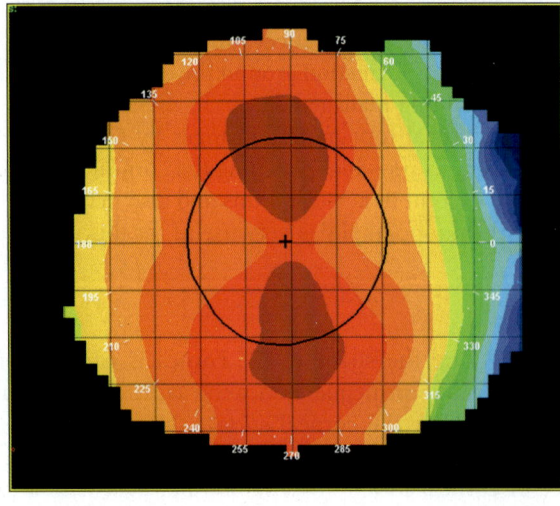

FIGURE 3.22 Central (A) versus peripheral (B) corneal astigmatism.

an alternative, a standard nontoric trial lens can be placed on the eye and the fluorescein pattern will tell the practitioner how much corneal toricity is present and whether or not this is acceptable.

When significant corneal toricity is noted, the first option is often to choose a full back toric lens design. The flattest meridian is usually fitted in alignment with the cornea or slightly flatter, taking radius of curvature and the e-value into account. The other meridian is generally fitted flatter than alignment to create a lens that moves well, but also to compensate for the difference in refractive index between tears and lens material and thus to prevent induced astigmatism. A popular rule of thumb is to take two-thirds of the corneal astigmatism and add this to the flattest meridian to calculate the steepest meridian. However, with the highly sophisticated lathing technology currently available, it is technically no problem to compensate the induced astigmatism on the front surface of the lens. Hence, practitioners should not worry about induced astigmatism when fitting the lens. Still, a slightly flatter back optic zone radius in the steepest meridian than alignment is desirable to promote movement, but should be limited to about 0.75 D.

Newly developed peripheral or edge toric back surface geometries with one spherical and one aspheric meridian can be used in lower degrees of corneal toricity, in particular when peripheral corneal toricity is present. Usually, one meridian is fitted with a low or zero e-value, while the flattest meridian is fitted with an e-value between 0.6 and 0.8. Practical tips are to use fairly high e-values that provide more flattening and therefore more peripheral toricity. Also, use large diameters since the toric effect increases toward the periphery. It is important to be aware that, when evaluated with a radiuscope, these lenses are spherical centrally and only start to diverge toward the periphery. Some corneal topographers provide a lens holder, to be placed on the chin rest, to evaluate contact lens surfaces. However, most topographers use assumptions about the shape of the cornea and, since the back surface of a contact lens is hollow in contrast to the convex corneal shape, this could lead to erroneous values. The lenses are marked in the flattest meridian to make evaluation of the position of the lens on the eye possible; these lenses typically show very limited signs of rotation during lens wear. Another reason for using back-surface toric geometries on toric corneas is that this improves lens centration. Especially in with-the-rule toricity, there is a tendency for the lens to ride high or low.[59]

In summary, to reduce the influence of the contact lens on the corneal epithelium, corneal toricity should be respected. Textbooks generally advise practitioners to use back toric lens designs on corneas with an astigmatism of 2.5 or 3 D and higher, but this could easily lead to topographic corneal changes and spectacle blur. When fitting back toric lens designs, the amount of peripheral astigmatism should also be taken into account. Different types of back toric surface geometries are available to the practitioner to respect the shape of the cornea at all times.

Comfort, Corneal Topography, and Lens Fit

A study initiated by the University of Maastricht in the Netherlands[62] looked at the relation between GP lens fitting and comfort of wear. The first question this study sought to answer was what percentage of lens fits was acceptable when only central k-readings were used to fit the lenses. The second question in this study was related to corneal topography: can information derived from this technique be beneficial in finding the optimal lens fit? Finally, does accurate GP lens fitting improve comfort of wear?

Of all initial fits based on traditional computation, only 40% were acceptable (optimal or suboptimal). From the unacceptable fits, 15% needed an adaptation of the back optic zone radii to be acceptable. In 28%, it was necessary to switch from a multicurve (MC) to an aspheric (AS) lens design to create an acceptable fit, and in 17% a toric back surface was necessary since the fluorescein pattern happened to be too toric. This was despite the fact that the maximum degree of central corneal astigmatism was only 1.83 D. The influence of peripheral astigmatism on lens fit was evident in these cases.

When the changes in lens fit that were made based on keratometry alone are compared with the topographic data, it can be concluded that in 88% of cases, the reasons for changing the lens parameters originated from midperipheral differences between corneal shape, as established with corneal topography height data, and lens shape, as predicted from keratometry readings. In other words, in 88% of cases, the lens fit could have been optimized before fitting by making use of corneal topography data.

The next question in the study was: does accurate lens fitting improve comfort? At the initial visit and at 2 weeks, there was no statistically significant difference between optimal versus suboptimal fits. In other words, initially (up to 2 weeks), the accuracy of the lens fit is not important for wearing comfort.

However, after 3 months of lens wear, the group of optimal fits scored 7.7 on the comfort scale, whereas comfort in the suboptimal group was 5.7. Also, the gain in comfort between the initial visit (5.2) and the visit 3 months later (7.7) was statistically significant in the group of optimal fits. In the group of suboptimal fits, there was only a small temporary increase in comfort from dispensing (6.1) to the visit 2 weeks later (6.3), while after 3 months, comfort had even slightly (but not statistically significantly) decreased to 5.7.

To analyze the aspect of comfort further, patients were subdivided into three groups on the basis of the lens geometry worn at 3 months. No relationship between comfort and lens geometry was found at the initial visit. Within the aspheric lens geometry group (AS group), comfort increased significantly from dispensing (5.6) to the follow-up visit after 2 weeks of wear (7.5). Although there was also an increase in comfort over that same period in the multicurve lens geometry group (MC group) from 5.9 to 6.7, this increase was statistically not significant. Both groups did also show a significant increase in comfort between the initial visit and the follow-up visit 3 months later.

In contrast to the other two groups, comfort scarcely increased between dispensing (4.8) and a follow-up visit after 2 weeks (5.0) in the group with unacceptable toric fluorescein patterns with standard lens design. At this point, the lens design was changed to a back toric lens. Because of the relatively low central difference in keratometry readings, a peripheral toric lens was chosen (two different *e*-values in two meridians). This resulted in an increase in comfort from the moment the lenses were introduced at the 2-week visit to the follow-up visit at 3 months. This increase (2.3 points) was statistically significant and resulted in a final comfort rate of 7.3, which is equal to the average comfort scores obtained with the other two lens designs.

In conclusion, there seems to be no difference in comfort within the first 2 weeks between optimally fitted lenses and suboptimally fitted lenses. However, after 3 months, there is a 2-point difference on a 10-point scale between these two groups, which is a statistically and clinically significant difference. This implies that even small improvements in GP lens fits could influence comfort of wear.

Another interesting result of this study is that corneas with lesser degrees of central corneal astigmatism can show toric fluorescein patterns because of an increase in corneal astigmatism toward the periphery and would therefore benefit from modern back toric lens designs, leading to improved comfort compared to nontoric designs.

SUMMARY

The assessment of corneal topography is integral to successful contact lens design and wear. While keratometry provides some information—albeit quite limited—that can assist in determining the design to be used and in assessing corneal distortion, the use of a corneal topographer is invaluable in providing corneal shape information and allowing the examiner to observe subtle changes in topography over time. The continual improvements in corneal topography instrumentation have resulted in lens design software programs that can design contact lenses to fit even the most challenging corneas. The future in corneal topography assessment appears to be even more exciting.

CLINICAL CASE

A 49-year-old woman who wears hydrogel lenses came in for an eye examination, complaining of decreased visual acuity in her left eye. She was referred by an optician because her poor visual acuity could not be explained. She was wearing spherical monthly replacement lenses made of a conventional lens material. Figure 3.23A shows the topographic map of the left eye soon after lens removal. Her maximal visual acuity with lens was 20/50 and refraction without lenses did not improve her vision:

$$OS: -4.75 - 1.75 \times 040 \ 20/50$$

The cornea looked unremarkable behind the biomicroscope, but the irregularities in the center of the map easily explain her decrease in visual acuity.

Two weeks after lens removal, the cornea returned to baseline (Fig. 3.23B), showing a symmetric topographic map with limited central corneal astigmatism, and her visual acuity returned back to 20/20. Unfortunately, this patient discontinued contact lens wear because of this incident, which could have been prevented.

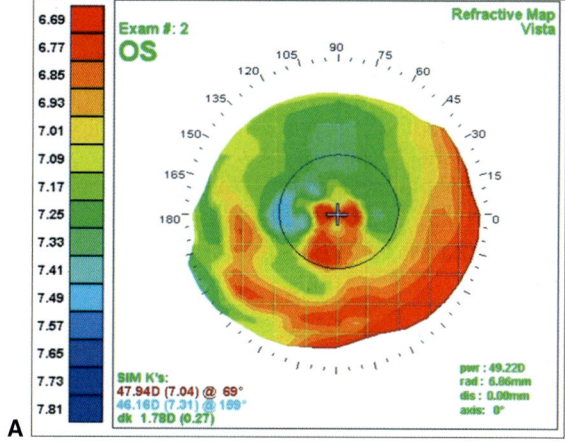

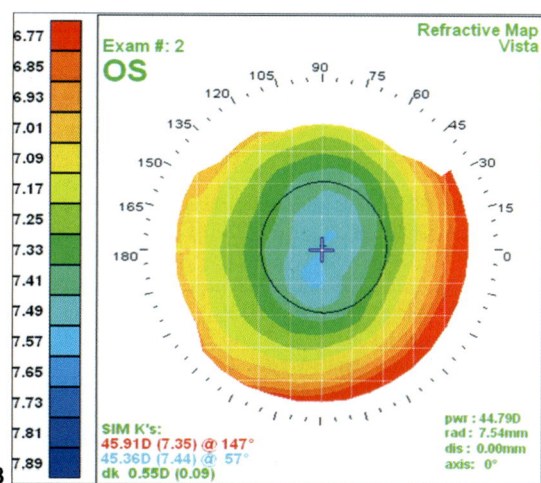

FIGURE 3.23 **(A)** Corneal warpage in hydrogel lens wear. **(B)** Same eye 2 weeks later. (Courtesy of Marco van Beusekom.)

CLINICAL PROFICIENCY CHECKLIST

- Many advances have occurred recently with corneal topographers. They can now be integrated with wavefront aberrometers, which can be a major advantage in contact lens practice.
- The keratometer can provide information that can be used for initial decisions for GP fitting as well as information—via assessment of distortion of imaged mires—on corneal irregularities, tear quality and, indirectly, the fit and front surface quality of soft contact lenses.
- Reflection corneal topographers, as compared to keratometry, result in much more information from an extended area of the cornea.
- When using a reflection corneal topographer, it is critical to have the patient blink several times immediately before the measurement to have a well-wetting ocular surface (i.e., no dry spots).
- Ring jam can occur near the upper and lower eyelid margins. The tear prism present on these margins can cause such steep curves that the resultant topography can be misleading.
- Sagittal maps are beneficial for comparison between corneas. Tangential maps represent true curve data and typically show more detail than a sagittal map. They have applications in ortho-k to assess lens centration during sleep and in keratoconus.
- If topographic changes occur under a silicone hydrogel lens, this can often be observed (mid-) peripherally.
- Corneal topography systems provide rate of flattening information (e-value or eccentricity). To avoid the induction of corneal topographic changes by GP lenses, the shape of the cornea should be followed as closely as possible. Matching the corneal shape with the lens shape by using aspheric lenses can be helpful in achieving this and also may aid in the management of 3 and 9 o'clock staining.
- It is important to assess peripheral corneal toricity before determining whether a back toric GP lens is indicated.

REFERENCES

1. Von Helmholtz H. Ueber die Accomodation des Auges. *Graefes Arch Clin Exp Ophthalmol.* 1854:3.
2. Javal E, Schiötz I. Un opthalmomètre practique. *Ann Oculis.* 1881;84:5.
3. Placido A. Novo instrumento de exploracao da cornea. *Periodico d'Ophthalmol Pract Lisbon.* 1880;5:27–30.
4. Gullstrand A. *Photographisch-ophthalmometrische und klinische Untersuchungen ueber die Hornhautrefraction.* Kongliga Svenska Vetenskap-Akademiens Handlinger; 1896;28:7.
5. Klyce SD. Computer-assisted corneal topography. High-resolution graphic presentation and analysis of keratoscopy. *Invest Ophthalmol Vis Sci.* 1984;25:1426–1435.
6. Jongsma F, de Brabander J, Hendrikse F. Review and classification of corneal topographers. *Laser Med Sci.* 1999;14:2–19.
7. Iskander DR, Collins MJ. Applications of high-speed videokeratoscopy. *Clin Exp Optom.* 2005;88:223–231.
8. Read SA, Collins MJ, Carney LG, et al. The topography of the central and peripheral cornea. *Invest Ophthalmol Vis Sci.* 2006;47:1404–1415.
9. Sicam VA, van der Heijde RG. Topographer reconstruction of the nonrotation-symmetric anterior corneal surface features. *Optom Vis Sci.* 2006;83:910–918.
10. de Brabander J, Chateau N, Marin G, et al. Simulated optical performance of custom wavefront soft contact lenses for keratoconus. *Optom Vis Sci.* 2003;80:637–643.
11. Mandell R. Methods to measure the peripheral corneal curvature. *J Am Optom Assoc.* 1962:889–892.
12. Wilms K, Rabbetts R. Practical concepts of corneal topometry. *Optician.* 1977 Sept; 16:7–11.
13. Meyer N. RGP-auswahl der ersten messlinse. *Die Kontaktlinse.* 2001;27–33.
14. Mandell RB. Everett Kinsey Lecture. The enigma of the corneal contour. *CLAO J.* 1992;18:267–273.

15. Swartz T, Marten L, Wang M. Measuring the cornea: the latest developments in corneal topography. *Curr Opin Ophthalmol.* 2007;18:325–333.
16. Jongsma FH, de Brabander J, Hendrikse F, et al. Development of a wide field height eye topographer: validation on models of the anterior eye surface. *Optom Vis Sci.* 1998;75:69–77.
17. Vos F, van der Heijde G, Spoelder H, et al. A new PRBA-based instrument to measure the shape of the cornea. *IEEE Trans Instrum Meas.* 1997:794–797.
18. Corbett M, Marchall J, O'Brart D, et al. New and future technology in corneal topography. *Eur J Implant Refr Surg.* 1995;7:372–386.
19. Markomanolakis MM, Kymionis GD, Aslanides IM, et al. Induced videokeratography alterations in patients with excessive meibomian secretions. *Cornea.* 2005;24:16–19.
20. Buehren T, Collins MJ, Carney L. Corneal aberrations and reading. *Optom Vis Sci.* 2003;80:159–166.
21. Kojima R. Validating corneal topography maps. *Contact Lens Spectrum.* 2007;22:42–44.
22. Chateau N, De Brabander J, Bouchard F, et al. Infrared pupillometry in presbyopes fitted with soft contact lenses. *Optom Vis Sci.* 1996;73:733–741.
23. Sindt, C. GP lens management of keratoconus. GPLI webinar, March 15, 2011.
24. Van der Worp E. Raising the bar. I-site newsletter (www.i-sitenewsletter.com); May 15 2012.
25. Jackson, JM. Elevation: key to right design. *Contact Lens Spectrum.* 2010;25:56.
26. Caroline P, Andre M. Elevating your knowledge of corneal topography. *Contact Lens Spectrum.* 2012;27:56.
27. Maeda N, Klyce SD, Smolek MK. Comparison of methods for detecting keratoconus using videokeratography. *Arch Ophthalmol.* 1995;113:870–874.
28. Rabinowitz YS, McDonnell PJ. Computer-assisted corneal topography in keratoconus. *Refract Corneal Surg.* 1989;5:400–408.
29. Li X, Rabinowitz YS, Rasheed K, et al. Longitudinal study of the normal eyes in unilateral keratoconus patients. *Ophthalmology.* 2004;111:440–446.
30. Rabinowitz YS, Rasheed K. KISA% index: a quantitative videokeratography algorithm embodying minimal topographic criteria for diagnosing keratoconus. *J Cataract Refract Surg.* 1999;25:1327–1335.
31. Dao CL, Kok JH, Brinkman CJ, et al. Corneal eccentricity as a tool for the diagnosis of keratoconus. *Cornea.* 1994;13:339–344.
32. Anderson D, Kojima R. Topography: a clinical pearl. *Optom Manage.* 2007;42:35–41.
33. Miller W. Treating PMD with contact lenses. *Contact Lens Spectrum.* 2007;22:31.
34. Buhren J, Kuhne C, Kohnen T. Defining subclinical keratoconus using corneal first-surface higher-order aberrations. *Am J Ophthalmol.* 2007;143:381–389.
35. Budak K, Hamed AM, Friedman NJ, et al. Preoperative screening of contact lens wearers before refractive surgery. *J Cataract Refract Surg.* 1999;25:1080–1086.
36. Wang X, McCulley JP, Bowman RW, et al. Time to resolution of contact lens-induced corneal warpage prior to refractive surgery. *CLAO J.* 2002;28:169–171.
37. Ruiz-Montenegro J, Mafra CH, Wilson SE, et al. Corneal topographic alterations in normal contact lens wearers. *Ophthalmology.* 1993;100:128–134.
38. Wilson SE, Lin DT, Klyce SD, et al. Topographic changes in contact lens-induced corneal warpage. *Ophthalmology.* 1990;97:734–744.
39. Tomlinson A. *Complications of Contact Lens Wear.* St. Louis: Mosby Year Book; 1992.
40. Swarbrick HA, Hiew R, Kee AV, et al. Apical clearance rigid contact lenses induce corneal steepening. *Optom Vis Sci.* 2004;81:427–435.
41. Sridharan R, Swarbrick H. Corneal response to short-term orthokeratology lens wear. *Optom Vis Sci.* 2003;80:200–206.
42. Wilson SE, Lin DT, Klyce SD, et al. Rigid contact lens decentration: a risk factor for corneal warpage. *CLAO J.* 1990;16:177–182.
43. Schornack M. Hydrogel contact lens-induced corneal warpage. *Cont Lens Anterior Eye.* 2003;26:153–159.
44. Ng LT, Lee EM, Nguyen AL. Preoperative assessment of corneal and refractive stability in soft contact lens wearing photorefractive candidates. *Optom Vis Sci.* 2007;84:401–409.
45. Lampa M, Andre M. What is a Custom Soft Contact Lens? Soft Special Edition newsletter (www.softspecialedition.com). Fall 2010 edition.
46. Edwards K. Contact lens problem-solving: aspheric RGP lenses. *Optician.* 2000;219:28–32.
47. Carney LG, Mainstone JC, Henderson BA. Corneal topography and myopia. A cross-sectional study. *Invest Ophthalmol Vis Sci.* 1997;38:311–320.
48. Eghbali F, Hsui EH, Eghbali K, et al. Oxygen transmissibility at various locations in hydrogel toric prism-ballasted contact lenses. *Optom Vis Sci.* 1996;73:164–168.
49. Guillon M, Lydon DP. Tear layer thickness characteristics of rigid gas permeable lenses. *Am J Optom Physiol Opt.* 1986;63:527–535.
50. Walline JJ, Mutti DO, Jones LA, et al. The contact lens and myopia progression (CLAMP) study: design and baseline data. *Optom Vis Sci.* 2001;78:223–233.
51. Horner DG, Soni PS, Vyas N, et al. Longitudinal changes in corneal asphericity in myopia. *Optom Vis Sci.* 2000;77:198–203.

52. Lindsay R, Smith G, Atchison D. Descriptors of corneal shape. *Optom Vis Sci.* 1998;75:156–158.
53. Swarbrick HA. Mind your P's and Q's Rodger Kame Award Lecture. In: *Symposium on Global Orthokeratology*. Toronto, Ontario, Canada; July 23–25, 2004.
54. Kok J. *New Developments in the Field of Contact Lenses*. Amsterdam, Netherlands: University of Amsterdam; 1991.
55. Barr J. Aspheric update. *Contact Lens Spectrum.* 1988:56–62.
56. Bennett E. DW investigation of aspheric posterior Boston IV lens design. *Contact Lens Forum.* 1987;12:65–69.
57. Holden T, Bahr K, Koers D, et al. The effect of secondary curve lift-off on peripheral corneal desiccation. Poster presented at: Annual Meeting of the American Academy of Optometry; December 1987; Denver, Colorado.
58. van der Worp E, De Brabander J, Swarbrick H, et al. Corneal desiccation in rigid contact lens wear: 3-and 9-o'clock staining. *Optom Vis Sci.* 2003;80:280–290.
59. Grosvenor T. Fitting the astigmatic patient with rigid contact lenses. In: Ruben M, Guillon M, eds. *Contact Lens Practice*. London: Chapman & Hall; 1994:623–647.
60. Szczotka LB, Roberts C, Herderick EE, et al. Quantitative descriptors of corneal topography that influence soft toric contact lens fitting. *Cornea.* 2002;21:249–255.
61. Franklin RJ, Morelande MR, Iskander DR, et al. Combining central and peripheral videokeratoscope maps to investigate total corneal topography. *Eye Contact Lens.* 2006;32:27–32.
62. van der Worp E, de Brabander J, Lubberman B, et al. Optimising RGP lens fitting in normal eyes using 3D topographic data. *Cont Lens Anterior Eye.* 2002;25:95–99.

Chapter 4

Gas-Permeable Material Selection

Edward S. Bennett

Prior to the fitting, evaluation, and patient education procedures, it is important to select the most appropriate lens material for a given patient. An understanding of gas-permeable (GP) advantages and applications, as well as material properties and composition are important in assisting in this decision.

GAS-PERMEABLE LENS BENEFITS, APPLICATIONS, AND LIMITATIONS

It is evident that GP lenses still have an important role in eye care practices today and will likely continue to have an important role in the future. Although the use of spherical lens designs continues to decline, specialty lens use for myopia control, irregular corneas, and presbyopia continues to increase with a notable increase in scleral lens design use.[1] Therefore, GP lens use is staying relatively stable with 9% (including hybrids) of new fits and refits in the United States[2] and 10% internationally.[3]

Benefits

GP lenses have traditionally exhibited many benefits, including quality of vision, ocular health, stability and durability, and patient retention and practice profitability.[4-6]

Quality of Vision

It is evident that—when properly fit—GP lenses will provide the best vision results of any vision correction option and, for the most part, resulting in close to aberration-free vision.[7] Studies comparing hydrogel and GP lenses have found significantly better visual performance with GP lenses. This includes both subjective patient preference[8,9] and contrast sensitivity function.[10,11] The superior optical quality provided by a stable refractive surface with little to no water content is the primary reason for this visual difference between contact lens types. In comparing both soft and GP lenses, it was found that, whereas both soft and GP lenses induce more aberrations for the eyes that have low wavefront aberrations, soft lens wear tends to induce more higher-order aberrations and GP lens wear tends to reduce higher-order aberrations.[12-14] GP lenses also maintain surface wettability better than hydrogel lenses. This can lead to improved long-term comfort and less deposit formation, although this benefit is less with the popularity of disposable lenses, especially daily-disposable lenses. GP lenses represent a very good option if the sphere–cylinder refractive error ratio is ≤2:1. When the corneal cylinder is 2.5 D or greater, a bitoric design often provides a stable and nonfluctuating vision correction.

Ocular Health

The benefits of a small overall diameter (OAD) lens that does not compress the limbus, lens movement typically resulting in good tear exchange and debris with the blink, potentially (depending upon the material) unparalleled oxygen permeability, and good surface wettability have resulted in numerous clinical studies that have found GP lenses to be a safer alternative to soft lenses. GP lenses have resulted in less corneal staining[8,15] and less likely to result in peripheral corneal infiltrates, not uncommon with tight-fitting soft lenses.[16,17] Compared to hydrogel and silicone hydrogel lenses, GPs have resulted in the lowest incidence of corneal inflammatory events.[18] The prevalence of microbial keratitis has been found to be less with GP lenses with an incidence of 1.2 per 10,000 eyes as compared to 1.9 per 10,000 eyes with daily-wear (DW) soft lenses,[19] and 20 per 10,000 eyes with extended wear (EW) soft lenses.[19–23] In several studies conducted in the United States in which the relative risk of wearing EW lenses was evaluated, GP lenses resulted in the lowest rate of infectious keratitis.[22,24,25] In a recent UK-based study, GP lenses reduced the risk of microbial keratitis by 84% compared to planned replacement soft lenses.[26] There is also less binding of *Pseudomonas aeruginosa*[27,28] and *Acanthamoeba*[29] to GP lenses than soft lenses. In addition, giant papillary conjunctivitis (GPC, also known as contact lens papillary conjunctivitis—CLPC) is less likely to occur with GP than with soft lenses.[30]

Stability/Durability

Unlike soft lenses, GP lenses do not tear or easily change shape or coloration; therefore, frequent lens replacement is not necessary.

In fact, it has been reported that approximately half of GP wearers only replace their lenses every 2 to 3 years.[2]

Patient Retention/Profitability

One of the challenges facing contact lens practitioners today is patient retention and revenue from replacement contact lenses. The Fairness to Contact Lens Consumers Act (FCLCA) mandates that practitioners provide the contact lens prescription to their patients. With the increasing number of Internet sites offering replacement lenses, many patients feel that they can bypass the professional care provided by eye care practitioners. However, as a custom device, GP lenses are much more difficult to obtain through these unconventional channels; in fact, it has been reported that only 1% of mail-order lenses were GP.[31] That percentage may not be any higher via the Internet for the same reason. The variety of parameters specified in a GP lens prescription (including base curve radius, overall and optical zone diameters, peripheral curve widths and radii) helps to demonstrate the specialty nature of the device to patients. Likewise, although the FCLCA requires that every contact lens patient is entitled to his or her prescription, he or she can only be provided this information once it has been determined, which may be as long as 1 to 3 months after dispensing for a GP patient.

There is evidence that GP wearers who successfully overcome awareness associated with adaptation do not discontinue contact lens wear as much as soft lens wearers.[32] In addition, it has been found that contact lens patients are approximately 50% more profitable to the eye care practice than non-contact lens wearers.[33] Further, it has been found that GP wearers generate greater revenue to the practice than soft lens wearers.[34] This was attributed to several factors, including the fact that GP lens patients return more frequently for eye examinations and purchase eyeglasses more often than soft lens patients.

Applications

Myopia Reduction

Several studies have found that GP lenses slow down the progression of myopia,[35–37] although this was not the conclusion of a study by Katz et al.[38] The most comprehensive and best controlled study was the Contact Lens and Myopia Progression (CLAMP) study[37] In this study, children were adapted to GP lenses prior to being randomized to GP or soft lens groups. After 3 years, GP lenses wearing young patients increased by 1.56 D in myopia whereas soft lens wearers increased by 2.19 D. However, most of the refractive error change occurred in the first year, and no difference was found between soft lens and GP lens wearers in axial growth of the eyes. Therefore, it would be safe to conclude that conventional GP lenses may slow down the progression of myopia in young people; however, they do not appear to impact axial length.

A more important benefit of GP lenses, particularly with—but not limited to—young people, pertains to overnight orthokeratology (OOK). Recent studies have found that OOK reduces myopia[39] and slows down axial growth.[40,41] In fact, both the Longitudinal Orthokeratology Research in Children (LORIC)[40] and the Corneal Reshaping and Yearly Observation of Nearsightedness (CRAYON)[41] studies found that OOK subjects resulted in over 50% less axial growth than control subjects (i.e., consisting of spectacle wearers in LORIC and both soft lens and non-OOK GP wearers in CRAYON) over a 2-year period. What is most exciting is the work by Earl Smith in which he has recognized the important role of peripheral retinal hyperopic defocus regarding the growth in axial length that occurs in myopia.[42] OOK has an apparent effectiveness in shifting this hyperopic defocus to a myopic defocus; therefore, eye growth is slowed or halted. More recently, several confirmatory studies have found that changes in relative peripheral refraction after OOK are similar in children as in adults; therefore, induced myopic defocus in the retinal periphery may provide a potential mechanism for myopia control.[43-45] This could ultimately result in young potential myopes never having to wear any correction—until presbyopia—after early intervention with this type of design.[46] More information on this topic is provided in Chapters 18 and 22.

Postsurgical/Irregular Cornea

GP lenses are most often the material of choice when fitting postsurgical and irregular corneas. The optical quality and rigid nature of these lenses allow for a more regular refractive surface due to the ability of these lenses to exhibit some molding ability and sphericalization of an irregular cornea. It has been found in the Collaborative Longitudinal Evaluation of Keratoconus (CLEK) study, with over 1,100 keratoconus subjects, that 73% were GP lens wearers.[47] Patients who have undergone refractive surgery and still require an optical correction benefit from the increased oxygen delivery of GP lenses versus soft lenses. Recent studies have confirmed the benefit of GP lenses in reducing higher-order aberrations and increasing optical quality in keratoconic eyes.[48,49] Numerous types of reverse geometry lens designs—incorporating a steep secondary curve radius—have been developed to allow a GP lens to align better and exhibit satisfactory centration on a postrefractive surgery patient who has a significantly flatter central than mid-peripheral cornea. Likewise, with the use of corneal topography instrumentation, it is possible for laboratories to fabricate a lens to closely match the corneal irregularity resulting from keratoconus, trauma, postpenetrating keratoplasty, postrefractive surgery, and other causes of irregular cornea. The availability of hyperpermeable GP lens materials also allows for optimum oxygen delivery to the cornea.

Presbyopia

Presbyopic patients benefit from any one of several GP presbyopic designs. Aspheric multifocal and segmented and annular translating designs have resulted in success rates of over 75%.[50-54] In addition, when compared to progressive addition lenses, monovision and soft bifocal lenses, aspheric GP multifocal lenses resulted in significantly better high- and low-contrast acuity and contrast sensitivity function as compared to the other contact lens options, and exhibited visual parity to spectacle wear.[55] As a result of improvements in manufacturing technology, higher add aspheric multifocal and segmented translating segmented designs with an intermediate correction have been introduced. The introduction of GP multifocal scleral lens designs has great potential for providing better vision than soft multifocal designs while exhibiting initial comfort that could rival their soft lens counterparts.[56-58]

Astigmatism

GP lenses have the natural ability to correct anterior corneal astigmatism by allowing the tear to compensate for the corneal toricity. In a recent study consisting of 20 high astigmatic subjects (average refractive cylinder = −3.62 D), who wore soft toric lenses for 1 month and GP bitoric lenses for 1 month concluded that—although only two subjects entering the study were GP wearers—11/19 subjects completing the study preferred to continue using GP lenses and 14/19 preferred the vision of the GP lenses.[59]

Soft Lens Refits

It has been reported that patients who failed with soft lens wear due to factors such as poor vision or GPC have been successfully refitted into GP lenses.[60,61] Likewise, individuals who have had a history of eye infections are also good candidates and often are motivated to be refit into a potentially safer modality. Patients who are not satisfied with their vision from soft toric lenses are often successful with GPs. Practitioners who continue to fit a series of soft toric lenses on astigmatic—especially high astigmatic patients or individuals who have <2:1 sphere–cylinder ratio for their refraction—despite reduced vision due to lens rotation are doing a disservice to their patients. These individuals often observe an immediate improvement in vision when refitted into GP lenses. If GPs are presented proactively with the vision benefit emphasized, it is likely they will be successful.[62] As will be discussed in the next chapter, the use of a topical anesthetic prior to the initial lens application will be beneficial in minimizing initial awareness.

Limitations

The applications and benefits listed above would appear to position GP lenses as a primary modality; however, as mentioned previously, in 2011 they consisted of 9% of new fits and refits in the United States.[2] There are several reasons for this low number, including the ease of fitting soft lenses, as well as their disposability and availability of replacement lenses. Certainly, the increasing emphasis on consumerism and a desire to have immediate gratification has had an impact worldwide. However, the primary reason for the increasing use of soft lenses worldwide pertains to the difference in initial comfort between both modalities. This impacts the patients' interest in GP lenses and the confidence (or lack thereof) that a practitioner has in fitting patients into GP lenses.

Initial Comfort

The most commonly reported cause of discontinuation of GP lens wear is discomfort.[8,60,63] The initial sensation experienced by new GP wearers varies from mild awareness to much discomfort and tearing. Conversely, soft lenses are more comfortable initially, primarily a result of their larger OAD resulting in less movement with the blink. Andrasko and Billings[64] evaluated numerous factors in new GP lens wearers after 20 to 30 minutes of wear. If patients reported that they experienced poor comfort, itching (or both) after this time period, they were deemed a poor candidate for GP lenses. Whether discomfort is going to be problematic can sometimes be determined during the prefitting evaluation. If the patient exhibits apprehension during primary care examination procedures such as lid eversion, fluorescein application, or tonometry, soft lenses should be considered or the patient should be provided with a slow buildup schedule for adaptation. The author has a three-step program to minimize initial awareness that consists of how GP lenses are presented to the patient, the use of a topical anesthetic prior to the initial application and, if possible, allowing the patient to see optimally with the first lenses applied (i.e., via fitting empirically or from an inventory).[65] This will be explained in much more detail in the next chapter.

In recent years, the increasing use of 13.5- to 16.0-mm diameter scleral lenses on healthy eyes represents an option that provides similar initial comfort to a soft toric lens in astigmatic wearers while providing better vision.[58,59,66–68] These lenses vault the cornea and rest on the conjunctiva, a less sensitive tissue.[69] When a panel of 33 expert GP fitters were asked what they thought the greatest advancement in GP lenses was in 2012, 29 indicated that it pertained to scleral lenses, with an emphasis on the newer, smaller designs for healthy eyes.[1] They also indicated that this trend should continue for many years.

Lack of Disposability

GP lens wearers should always have a backup pair as lenses can be lost and, on occasion, warped or possibly broken. Soft lenses have the benefit of being available in, at minimum, six to a package in most cases.

Fitting Inventory

The simplicity of soft lens design lends itself very well to fitting from an inventory and being able to make small changes easily and determine if they have successfully improved vision and/or fitting relationship. Patients can be sent home in trial lenses for which they experience good vision and can be assessed afterward to determine the final lenses to be ordered. The custom nature of GP lenses often results in practitioners ordering lenses for the patient and, if changes are indicated, new lenses have to be ordered.

Occasional/Cosmetic Wear

Soft lenses also have the benefit of allowing occasional or intermittent wear with relatively little effect on comfort. Soft lenses also can be used to change or enhance eye color, whereas the smaller OAD of GP lenses all but precludes iris color changes.

Environmental Limitations

Another limitation of GP lenses is increased susceptibility for dust and debris to become trapped underneath the lens. Patients who work exclusively outdoors in a dusty, windy environment may be better candidates for soft lenses. Likewise, individuals who participate in sports often benefit from soft lenses.[70] If GP lenses are indicated in these athletes, the use of a large OAD, low-edge clearance design would be indicated.

Smaller Palpebral Aperture Size

It has been found that GP lenses can result in a smaller palpebral aperture size versus soft lens wearers and non-contact lens wearers.[71] In addition, one study reported 15 cases of long-term rigid lens wearers who presented with blepharoptosis.[72] It was hypothesized that this problem may be the result of chronic lens removal, in which the pulling of the lids laterally over time may lead to levator aponeurosis dehiscence.

MATERIAL PROPERTIES

Oxygen Permeability/Transmission

Oxygen permeability (Dk) is a property of the lens material independent of the size, shape, or surface condition of a lens. Oxygen transmissibility (Dk/t) is a measure of the amount of oxygen transmitted through the lens. It is dependent on the Dk value of the material and thickness (typically center thickness [CT] for GP lenses), and is essentially equal to the Dk divided by the CT in millimeters $\times 10$. For example, lenses manufactured in identical materials and Dk values with different thicknesses will result in a difference in oxygen transmission; the greater the lens thickness, the lower the oxygen transmission. For example, if the Dk value is 40 and the

CT is 0.10 mm, the Dk/t is equal to 40; if the CT of this material is instead 0.20 mm, the Dk/t decreases in half to a value of 20 (the respective units are [10^{-11} cm^2 × mL O_2] [sec × mL × mm Hg] for Dk [which has also been termed "Fatt" units] and 10^{-9} × same units for Dk/t). Another method of evaluating oxygen transfer through a rigid lens is equivalent oxygen percentage (EOP). EOP is a measure of the amount of oxygen in the tears between the lens and the cornea and is determined in vivo; essentially, it is a predictor of how much oxygen will reach the anterior corneal surface with a particular lens material and design, the maximum value equaling 21%.[31]

Historically, there have been many methods to assess the Dk of a GP lens material. Early measures did not compensate for inaccuracies that could result from the so-called "boundary layer" and "edge effect."[73,74] As these effects often resulted in inflated Dk values, the marketing and promotion of contact lenses was often not consistent with the research behind these materials.[75,76] In addition, calibrations were often not performed via similar testing of reference lenses. These effects were resolved via the work of Benjamin and Cappelli[76] in 1998, which was funded by the Contact Lens Manufacturers Association (CLMA) and is often referred to as the "CLMA Method."

Certainly, there are advantages in potential oxygen transmission with GP versus hydrogel lenses. As a rule, GP lenses are able to deliver two to three times more oxygen to the cornea than hydrogel lenses of equal thickness.[77] This is a result of both the availability of higher-Dk materials and the fact that these lenses exchange up to 20% of the tear volume per blink.[78,79] Conversely, hydrogel lenses can exchange only approximately 1% of the tears per blink.[80] GP lenses having Dk values in the range of 18 to 25 have exhibited an amount of overnight corneal swelling (10%–12%) similar to that of many hydrogel EW lenses.[81,82] However, upon awakening, the cornea deswells much faster with a rigid lens, and unlike hydrogel lenses, the cornea typically returns to the zero swelling level. The introduction of hyperpermeable silicone hydrogel lenses has closed the gap between the two modalities; however, research has found that a GP lens with a Dk/t of 90 is equivalent to a silicone hydrogel lens with a DK/t of 125.[83] In addition, the tear film between the cornea and scleral GP lens reduces oxygen transmission, necessitating the use of very highly oxygen-permeable materials for these larger and thicker lens designs.[84]

How much oxygen is necessary for corneal physiological success? Research has shown that a Dk/L equal to 24 (10% EOP) should satisfy the DW oxygen requirements of every patient.[85] Therefore, this value should be the goal of clinicians. A 30-Dk lens with a CT of 0.12 mm would meet this requirement, as would a 60-Dk material with a CT of 0.25 mm. For EW, however, this value is much higher. Originally established as a Dk/t of 87 (17.9% EOP),[85] it has more recently been increased to 125.[86–88] This makes it imperative to use hyperpermeable silicone hydrogel and GP materials for EW. It has been found that fitting plus power hydrogel lenses on a hyperopic, EW patient results in providing much less than half of the oxygen demand of the cornea.[89]

There have been several classifications of GP lens materials. Benjamin[90] has divided GP lenses into five categories based on Dk and using a standard thickness of 0.12 mm. The author simply divides the materials into three categories: low Dk (25–50), high Dk (51–99), and hyper Dk (≥100).[91] These classifications are shown in Table 4.1. The bottom line, however, is that oxygen transmission, although important to successful lens wear, should not be viewed apart from other lens performance factors, such as adequate movement, comfortable edge design, resistance to deposit buildup, flexural resistance, and dimensional stability.

Surface Wettability

Surface wettability is the ability of the blink to spread tear film mucin across the anterior contact lens surface. The mucin layer is essential for this purpose and its presence in the tear film raises the surface tension of the cornea to allow the spreading of tears. Good wetting properties

TABLE 4.1 GP Oxygen Permeability/Transmission Classifications

BENJAMIN[90,a]	BENNETT[91]
Low Dk: <15	Low Dk: 25–50
Medium Dk: 15–30	High Dk: 51–99
High Dk: 31–60	Hyper Dk: ≥100
Super Dk: 61–100	
Hyper Dk: >100	

[a]Assuming a center thickness of 0.12mm

are important for patient success as it enhances visual acuity, comfort, and corneal integrity.[92] This is of major importance to polymer chemists, manufacturers, and clinicians. In fact, a desire to have better wettable materials has been expressed as the number one request for desired rigid lens improvements in a nationwide survey of optometrists.[93] If the tear film over the lens surface evaporates rapidly after the blink, the mucin dries out and becomes more mucus-like, ultimately resulting in a mucoprotein film. Although the tear film wets the lens via three types of surface interactions: hydrogen bonding, hydrophobic interaction, and electrostatic interaction, the latter is the strongest of these forces.[94] The GP lens surface is negatively charged, making it a perfect compliment for the positively charged tear protein, lysozyme.

Wetting agents within the lens enhance surface wettability and assist in overcoming the hydrophobic properties of silicone. The material polymer chemistry has to be carefully formulated as the excessive use of wetting agents can result in a material that is too soft and possibly too brittle. Wetting agents have included methacrylic acid, polyvinyl alcohol, hydroxyethylmethacrylate (HEMA), and N-vinyl pyrrolidone. Representative management of these wettability-related problems is discussed in Chapter 6.

A clinical predictor of how well a GP contact lens anterior surface spreads the tear film mucin has been via wetting angle measurements. In theory, the lower the wetting angle, the better the on-eye wetting performance will be. Methods that have been used to assess wetting angle have included Wilhelmy plate, sessile drop, and captive bubble. The difficulty has been the fact that different methods have been used and if low values result, these values are heavily promoted by the manufacturer. In reality, these tests have proven to truly have a correlation with on-eye wetting and comfort.[95] The tear components, notably mucin, form a biofilm on the surface, which acts as a natural wetting agent to coat the lens within a few blinks. This reduces the lens wetting angle, contributing greatly to the surface wettability. Therefore, laboratory wetting angle measurements are typically not representative of on-eye performance.

Flexural Resistance

Flexural resistance pertains to the ability of a GP lens to resist the bending or flexing forces when a rigid lens is on a toric cornea. In other words, a lens with poor flexural resistance will tend to flex during the blinking process and therefore inadequately correct the patient's corneal astigmatism, resulting in reduced vision.[96] Factors that can influence flexure include amount of corneal toricity, lens material, optical zone diameter, CT, and lens-to-cornea fitting relationship. If the lens design increases in sagittal depth via a steeper BCR[97–99] or larger optical zone diameter,[100] flexure is increased. Material flexibility via a high- or hyper-Dk material or from a thin CT in minus power lenses can contribute to lens flexure.[101,102] Modulus is another term that has been ascribed to the stiffness—or resistance to flexure—of a material. Higher-Dk GP lens materials have a much lower modulus rating than polymethyl methacrylate (PMMA).[95] Typically, flexure can be problematic for patients with corneal toricity ≥1.50 D.[103]

Specific Gravity

Specific gravity (SG) refers to the weight of a GP lens at a given temperature divided by the weight of an equal volume of water at the same temperature. It is often compared to water that has a SG of 1.00. SG values for rigid lens materials can be divided into low (1.10 or less), medium (1.11–1.20), or high (>1.20) values. These values can play an important role in the success of GP lenses as it is possible that the higher SG (i.e., "heavier") lens materials may have more of a tendency to decenter inferiorly because of the forces of gravity.[104] In fact, if all other parameters are held constant, changing to a different lens material, with a different SG, can produce as much as a 20% change in lens mass; therefore, potentially impacting the lens-to-cornea fitting relationship.[105] This problem can be overcome by making higher SG lenses thinner, thus resulting in an overall decreased lens weight. This should be particularly applicable in plus-power and prism-ballasted GP lenses.

The recent introduction of high refractive index (RI) lens materials (to be discussed) with values between 1.51 and 1.54, in combination with low SG values (i.e., as low as 1.04), allows for designs that can be made thinner and potentially result in less risk of inferior decentration.[106,107] They have also been found to result in higher add powers with aspheric multifocal designs than what was found with these designs in conventional GP lens materials.[108]

Hardness

Other properties pertain to the so-called "softness" of a given material. Such factors as hardness value, scratch resistance, and optical quality have been described and compared. Hardness has been defined as resistance to penetration. If an indicator is pressed on the surface of the material being tested, the extent to which it compresses for a given pressure and time is an inverse measure of the hardness.[109] The Rockwell R hardness method is commonly used for testing the hardness of GP buttons; the Shore D hardness method is commonly used on finished lenses.

MATERIAL TYPES AND COMPOSITION

The materials in use today include (a) silicone/acrylate (S/A) and (b) fluoro-silicone/acrylate (F-S/A).

Silicone/Acrylate (S/A)

The first successful GP lens materials were of S/A (also termed siloxane–methacrylate) composition. Also referred to as "silicone"-based, these copolymers actually contained the element silicon as siloxane bonds in side branches of the main carbon–carbon polymer chain. The silicon-containing side branches increases the free volume (space between the polymer chains), which allows the passage of oxygen.

The introduction of silicone-based copolymers in 1979 was a major breakthrough, because silicone can greatly enhance the Dk characteristics of the material. Unlike PMMA lens materials, which are made up of a single component, S/A materials contain "silicone" methacrylate, wetting agents, and cross-linking agents. The latter two ingredients are important because their purpose is to neutralize both the hydrophobicity and the flexibility of the silicone component. Wetting agents, as previously indicated, achieve their effect by their strong affinity for water molecules. Most cross-linking agents strengthen the material, increasing its rigidity, and making the material less sensitive to solvents.

However, the hydrophobicity of silicone resulted in a lens surface that was likely to attract both lipid and, notably, bound protein deposits.[96] This rapid drying of the tear film over the lens surface often resulted in patient complaints of redness, dryness, and fluctuating vision. The introduction of higher-Dk S/A lens materials often resulted in increased (or potential to increase) surface deposits,[95] warpage,[110–112] crazing,[113–114] and brittleness.[115]

Even with the aforementioned problems, there are several S/A materials in common use today. These include Boston II and Boston IV (Bausch + Lomb), Optacryl 60, Paraperm O2, and Paraperm EW (Paragon Vision Sciences), SA-18 and SA-32 (Lagado), and SGP and SGP II (LifeStyle).

Fluoro-Silicone/Acrylate (F-S/A)

F-S/A lens materials are similar to S/A, with the notable exception of the addition of fluorine. Fluorine, known for its nonstick properties in Teflon-coated cooking materials, increases the deposit resistance of the lens material, which is accomplished by fluorine, promoting a tear film mucin interaction with the lens surface. In addition, low surface tension (energy) is present; in other words, there is a reduced affinity of polarized tear components to become adherent to the contact lens surface.[116] Therefore, the primary problem experienced with S/A lens materials, dryness, should be reduced with F-S/A materials. This has, in fact, been the case. Several comparison studies have concluded that F-S/A lenses are more wettable and are perceived as more comfortable by patients than S/A lenses.[111,117,118] In addition, it has been found that these materials are less prone to deposit buildup[119,120] and the rate of tear breakup is slower with the fluorinated material.[121]

The fluorinated component also assists in the transmission of oxygen through the lens material. This is accomplished by oxygen's preference to dissolve into fluorinated materials (i.e., oxygen transmission is achieved by solubility, not diffusion).[115,121] It is very apparent that, although the ability of "silicone" to promote diffusion of oxygen through the lens material is very important, the additional permeability provided by fluorine will reduce the need for using excessive amounts of "silicone." Therefore, it has been found that the F-S/A materials are more dimensionally stable than S/A materials as well.[111,115]

As mentioned previously, F-S/A lenses can be divided into low-, high-, and hyper-Dk materials. All of the commonly available GP lens materials and their properties are provided in Table 4.2.[76,122] Low-Dk materials have become the lens of choice for most myopic DW patients as a result of the benefits of surface wettability and dimensional stability.[123–126]

High-Dk F-S/A lens materials are typically the lens of choice with patients in need of higher oxygen transmission, although from a Dk level, they could be prescribed (if FDA-approved for overnight wear) for all but those individuals desiring EW or hyperopes desiring EW.[127] As mentioned before, the thickness of scleral lens designs—in combination with the tear film between lens and cornea—mandates that a high- or hyper-Dk lens material is indicated to meet the corneal oxygen needs. Hyper-Dk lens materials can be worn by all patients interested in GP wear but are definitely indicated for EW and represent the only option (i.e., Menicon Z, Menicon) for 30-day continuous wear. Menicon Z has been found to be successfully worn for close to 30 days and nights by most wearers over a 2-year period.[128] These applications are summarized in Table 4.3. It is not uncommon for practitioners to offer some form of annual replacement program for hyper-Dk lens materials as they often have a shorter life span than lower-Dk materials.

Improved material composition and manufacturing processes have resulted in the production of higher-Dk lenses that are durable and flexible resistant, and maintain good wettability.[62] Bausch + Lomb developed the Boston series of materials (ES, EO, XO) using the unique AERCOR technology, introduced in the mid-1990s. These materials contain an oxygen-permeable backbone and AERCOR O cross-linking agents, allowing more free volume within the lens and thus allowing more oxygen to reach the cornea. This allows the lens to be manufactured with a low level of silicone, thus potentially enhancing surface wettability. Soon thereafter, Paragon Vision Sciences introduced their hyperpurification process, which, in effect, sorts silicone molecules to select more oxygen-efficient silicone.[91,128] This resulted in the introduction of Paragon Thin, Paragon HDS, and Paragon HDS 100. Not long after the new Paragon lenses were introduced, both Contamac and Lagado introduced F-S/A lenses with hydrophilic claims.[129] Contamac introduced the Optimum series of lens materials, which are polymerized via a proprietary new technology process that claims to not induce stress into the

TABLE 4.2 Commonly Available Gas-Permeable Lens Materials and Their Properties

NAME	MANUFACTURER	MATERIAL	DK	DK METHOD	REFRACTIVE INDEX	SPECIFIC GRAVITY
AccuCon	Innovision	F-S/A	25(19.6)	Revised Fatt	1.458	1.16
Boston XO_2	B+L	F-S/A	141	ISO/Fatt	1.424	1.19
Boston XO	B+L	F-S/A	100	ISO/Fatt	1.415	1.27
Boston Equalens II	B+L	F-S/A	85(93–114.6)	ISO/Fatt	1.423	1.24
Boston EO	B+L	F-S/A	58	ISO/Fatt	1.429	1.23
Boston Equalens	B+L	F-S/A	47(58)	ISO/Fatt	1.439	1.19
Boston RXD	B+L	F-S/A	24	ISO/Fatt	1.435	1.27
Boston IV	B+L	S/A	19(20.8)	ISO/Fatt	1.469	1.10
Boston ES	B+L	F-S/A	18(27.3)	ISO/Fatt	1.443	1.22
Boston II	B+L	S/A	12(16.3)	ISO/Fatt	1.471	1.13
FLOSI	Lagado	F-S/A	26	ISO/Fatt	1.455	1.12
FluoroPerm 151	Paragon	F-S/A	151(99.3)	Revised Fatt	1.422	1.1
FluoroPerm 92	Paragon	F-S/A	92(64)	Revised Fatt	1.453	1.1
FluoroPerm 60	Paragon	F-S/A	60(42.7)	Revised Fatt	1.453	1.15
Fluoroperm 30	Paragon	F-S/A	30(30.3)	Revised Fatt	1.466	1.14
Hybrid FS	Contamac	F-S/A	31	Revised Fatt	1.4465	1.183
$Hydro_2$	Innovision	F-S/A	50	Revised Fatt	1.463	1.145
Menicon Z	Menicon	F-S/A	163(175.1)	ISO/DIS	1.436	1.20
ONSI-56	Lagado	F-S/A	56	ISO/ANSI	1.452	1.206
Optacryl 60	Paragon	S/A	18	Revised Fatt	1.467	1.13

Optimum Extreme	Contamac	Roflufocon E	125	ISO/Fatt	1.4332	1.155
Optimum Extra	Contamac	Roflufocon D	100	ISO/Fatt	1.4333	1.166
Optimum Comfort	Contamac	Roflufocon C	65	ISO/Fatt	1.4406	1.178
Optimum Classic	Contamac	Roflufocon A	26	ISO/Fatt	1.4527	1.189
Paragon HDS 100	Paragon	F-S/A	100	ISO/ANSI	1.442	1.1
Paragon HDS	Paragon	F-S/A	58	Revised Fatt	1.449	1.16
Paragon Thin	Paragon	F-S/A	29	Revised Fatt	1.463	1.14
Paraperm EW	Paragon	S/A	56	Revised Fatt	1.467	1.07
Paraperm O_2	Paragon	F-S/A	16	Revised Fatt	1.473	1.12
SA-32	Lagado	S/A	32	Fatt	1.467	1.101
SA-18	Lagado	S/A	18	Fatt	1.469	1.126
SGP 3	LifeStyle	F-S/A	43.5(33.5)	CLMA	N/A	1.13
SGP II	LifeStyle	S/A	43.5(31.9)(13.8)	CLMA	N/A	1.13
SGP	LifeStyle	S/A	22(14.9)	CLMA	N/A	1.13
TYRO-97	Lagado	F-S/A	97	ISO/ANSI	1.440	1.187

Data from Benjamin WJ, Cappelli QA. Oxygen permeability (Dk) of thirty-seven rigid contact lens materials. *Optom Vis Sci.* 2002;79(2):103–111; Rah MJ. A GP materials guide. *Contact Lens Spectrum.* 2007;22(7):19; www.gpli.info, and www.bausch.com.

TABLE 4.3 Gas-Permeable Material Selection (In General)

LOW DK	HIGH DK	HYPER DK
• Myopia	• Hyperopia	• Hyperopia
• Daily ear	• Flexible wear (hyperopia)	• Extended wear (myopia and hyperopia)
• Optimal wettability	• Extended wear (myopia)	
• Optimal stability	• Prism-ballasted lens design	

Adapted from Bennett ES, Johnson JD. Material selection. In: Bennett ES, Weissman BA, eds. *Clinical Contact Lens Practice*. Philadelphia, PA: Lippincott Williams & Wilkins;2005:243–253.

finished product. The "modified" F-S/A materials incorporate HEMA into the lens in an effort to optimize surface wettability and have been found to be successful in over 80% of GP wearers being refit into the Optimum lenses.[130] Lagado Corporation introduced the Onsi-56 and Tyro-97 lens materials. These lens materials also contain HEMA and are modified F-S/A lens materials. They achieve their surface wettability via a combination of HEMA and a high proportion of fluoromonomer within the polymer formulation. Water is attracted to the lens surface but not absorbed into the interior of the lens.

The current generation of hybrid lens materials from SynergEyes utilizes a central hyper-Dk GP core surrounded by a hydrogel skirt with the SynergEyes family of lenses and a silicone hydrogel skirt for the Duette HD and Duette multifocal designs. These designs represent a very welcome addition to the contact lens selection toolbox while also representing an upgrade from previous hybrid designs due to much higher-Dk materials, as well as a much stronger connection between GP and soft lens polymers, making lens tearing at that junction much less common. The Duette designs use a high modulus hyper-Dk GP(MaxVu) center,[128] incorporating a class II ultraviolet (UV) blocker surrounded by a low modulus silicone hydrogel 32% water skirt with a Dk of 84. These hybrid designs are a viable option for anyone desiring the vision of a GP lens and the initial comfort of a soft lens. Commonly fit to patients with irregular corneas, they are also beneficial for athletes due to the stability of fit, and anyone experiencing difficulty adapting to a standard diameter GP lens.

Other Material Factors

Ultraviolet Blockers

Several GP lenses have UV blockers in the lens to reduce UV radiation exposure and the potential long-term complications such as cataracts, photokeratitis, and retinal degenerative changes.[95] UVB (200–300 nm) are the rays that can be most problematic, and UV absorbers in contact lenses do assist in providing some—but not total—protection to the eye. Sunglasses are still recommended for optimum protection. GP lenses with UV blockers also reduce fluorescence when evaluating the fluorescein pattern; therefore, an adjunct yellow filter over the observation system is recommended.

Plasma Treatment

The challenges involved in maintaining a clean surface as new—and higher Dk—polymers are being introduced has resulted in the FDA approval of plasma treatment of almost all of the GP materials in common use today. This process is not a coating—like a wax—but is truly a treatment in which the front surface of the lens is sterilized via exposure to cold plasma gas in a reaction chamber.[67,131–133] Plasma is matter consisting of neutrons, positive ions, and electrons in a highly energized state. As the effect is localized to the surface, this form of plasma treatment does not adversely affect the material properties.

There are several benefits of plasma treatment. As it is not uncommon for polish residues to be attracted to the lens surface during the manufacturing process, plasma treatment results in removing all of these residues, resulting in an extremely clean and wettable surface. Although the clinical relevance of wetting angle measurements is debatable, it is evident that plasma treatment does greatly reduce the wetting angle of GP lenses while increasing surface hydrophilicity.[134] Paragon Vision Sciences, via their FDA-approval process, has been able to claim that plasma treatment results in improved initial comfort. Therefore, the value of this process is not necessarily long-term comfort as it is not known how long the process lasts.[62] It is also evident that the use of abrasive cleaners as well as in-office polishing can both negatively impact this treatment and are not recommended with plasma-treated lenses. In addition, the cost of this technology to the laboratory is quite high. However, with the benefits of initial wettability and perhaps better initial comfort, an increasing number of laboratories are providing plasma-treated lenses, often for a small additional fee.

High Refractive Index

GP lens materials in common use today have a refractive index (RI) varying from 1.42 to 1.47. Recently, new materials have been introduced in both a high RI and a low SG.[103] These materials include the OptimumHR Hirafocon A (SG = 1.04; RI = 1.51) and Hirafocon B (SG = 1.04; RI = 1.53), both from Contamac, and the Paragon HDS HI (SG = 1.12; RI = 1.54) from Paragon Vision Sciences. The higher RI value results in a lens that can be manufactured thinner; the lower SG values indicate that these materials are lighter than conventional materials. Therefore, these materials have the potential advantage of optimizing lens centration and, potentially, comfort. There is much interest in using these materials for front surface aspheric multifocal designs as it has been found that as much as between 0.50 and 0.75 D, higher add is predicted with a front surface add with a high RI material versus a back surface add with a conventional RI material.[107,108]

MATERIAL SELECTION

The availability of all of these different rigid (or semirigid) lens materials presents a myriad of choices to the practitioner. What GP material is preferable to our patients? The answer depends on the particular patient to be fitted. In other words, it is recommended to use diagnostic sets of several different materials.

Figure 4.1 shows the author's recommendations for material selection. It can be divided into five categories: (a) refractive error, (b) corneal topography, (c) refits, (d) occupation/hobbies, and (e) age.

Refractive Error

Because of the thin CTs typically available in minus power lenses, most myopic patients would benefit from the dimensional stability provided by low-Dk F-S/A lenses while still meeting (or approximating) the cornea's DW oxygen requirements. However, if edema is present with a low-Dk lens material, often the result of either a high corneal oxygen need (which varies between individual patients) or a tight-fitting lens, the patient should be refit into a higher-Dk material. Hyperopic patients will benefit most from a high-Dk lens material because of the greater CTs present in these lens powers. For the same reason, dimensional stability problems with high-Dk materials are less with plus (vs. minus) powers.

Corneal Topography

Patients with moderate astigmatism (i.e., >1.50 D) benefit from the flexural resistance provided by low-Dk F-S/A lens materials. High astigmatic (i.e., 2.50 D and greater) patients often benefit from bitoric designs, which benefit from the rigidity of low-Dk materials unless the patient is hyperopic. Likewise, for patients exhibiting high astigmatism associated with an irregular cornea, notably keratoconus, the greater rigidity of lower-DK lens materials can be beneficial. However, the decision-making process also has to take into consideration the amount of existing corneal compromise and fragility, as well as patient compliance with wearing schedule

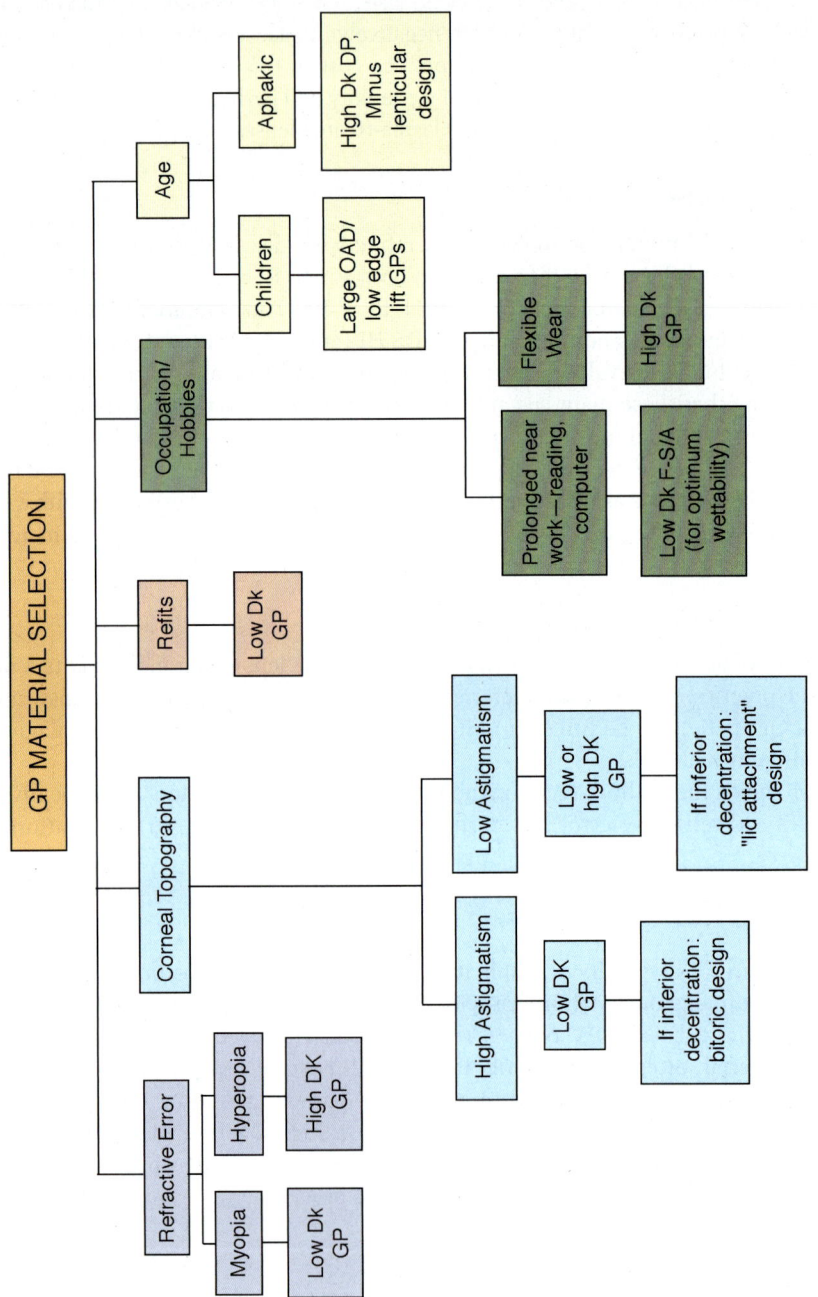

FIGURE 4.1 Gas-permeable material selection nomogram.

(i.e., very compromised and fragile corneas, as well as noncompliant patients would benefit from a higher-DK lens material). In addition, the increasing use of scleral lenses—not only for irregular corneas but also for healthy astigmatic and presbyopic eyes—mandate the use of high and hyper-Dk materials due to the greater CTs of these materials.

Refits

Former PMMA and first-generation GP lens wearers should be refit into low-Dk rigid lenses. Typically, these individuals have established care habits that could be damaging to the new softer lens materials. Surface scratches and warpage could occur (see Chapter 8), especially if these patients are not properly educated.

Previous soft wearers, who have experienced deposit-related problems (redness, itching, decrease in wearing time) resulting in papillary hypertrophy, would benefit from being refit into essentially any GP material, preferably the most wettable available material. This may include a low-Dk F-S/A or any plasma-treated material. Patients with a history of eye infections and peripheral soft lens-induced complications often benefit from the oxygen transmission and smaller diameter of GP lenses. These materials would also be recommended for all borderline dry-eye patients and mild allergy sufferers. In addition, spherical soft and soft toric lens wearers who are not satisfied with their vision are often good candidates for GP lenses.

Occupation

Individuals who perform much near work would benefit from the highest wettability materials available (similar to those for the aforementioned papillary hypertrophy patients), supplemented by the frequent application of rewetting/reconditioning drops. Athletes benefit most from soft lenses; however, if this option is not satisfactory, a large hybrid material, such as Duette (SynergEyes), which would less likely be displaced, or scleral lenses would be recommended.[135] Individuals who desire (or have a need) to wear their lenses on a flexible schedule or EW basis (such as nurses, police, firefighters) would benefit from a high-Dk F-S/A material. Likewise, pilots and flight attendants, who are often exposed to less than optimum oxygen levels, would benefit from the higher-Dk materials.

Age

Pediatric aphakic children often benefit by being fitted with a silicone hydrogel lens. Phakic children would benefit from larger diameter GP lenses, which should be less likely to dislodge. Initial comfort could be optimized by achieving an underneath-the-upper-lid fitting relationship and by the use of a rolled, tapered edge design. Aphakic patients would benefit from a high-Dk F-S/A material in a minus lenticular design and large (9.2–9.6 mm) OAD.

The bottom line is that the lens materials today are better than the ones we had yesterday and they continue to improve. With the concurrent advancements in lens design and manufacturing technology, the decision to select a material is often unnecessary as more and more designs are available in a specific compatible material. However, any questions about what lens material would be optimum for a given patient can always be answered by your laboratory consultant.

SUMMARY

GP lenses have numerous applications and benefits and, in fact, differentiate the novice practitioner from the practitioner who considers all options prior to making the decision as to what type of contact lens to fit for any given patient. It is important to determine the patient's level of motivation, sensitivity to something approaching the eyes, and factors such as desired wearing time, occupation, and refractive error. Although no one GP material will be successful on every patient, the process for material selection does not have to be overly complicated as well.

A close relationship with the independent GP fabricating laboratory consultant will be invaluable in deciding which material to use for any given patient.

CLINICAL CASES

CASE 1

A previously successful PMMA (12 years) and Polycon II (11 years) wearer is in your office complaining of blur through spectacles and a need to replace the contact lenses because they are "old and scratched." The patient has a tear breakup time (TBUT) equal to 7 seconds and a refraction equal to the following:

$$OD: -5.00 - 1.75 \times 170 \quad 20/25$$
$$OS: -5.50 - 1.50 \times 005 \quad 20/25$$

Keratometry was as follows:

OD: 42.75 @ 170; 44.25 @ 080

OS: 43.25 @ 005; 44.75 @ 095

SOLUTION: This patient is an ideal candidate for a low-Dk F-S/A material for several reasons: (a) Former PMMA wearers (and first-generation GP wearers) would benefit from the dimensional stability of a low-Dk material. If the corneal edema is not eliminated with the new material, a higher-Dk material can then be used. (b) Patients with borderline tear quality would benefit from the wettability provided by relatively low "silicone-containing" materials unless the material has a surface that has effectively neutralized the polarity and overcome the hydrophobicity of "silicone." (c) Myopic patients usually achieve sufficient oxygen transmission through the lens to meet the DW requirements. (d) The presence of a moderate amount of corneal astigmatism would best be corrected by a low-Dk material to minimize the effects of flexure.

CASE 2

A first-time contact lens wearer desires good visual acuity since she is a nurse and has many critical demands on her vision. In addition, she works 18-hour shifts and would desire a lens that would be optimum for long periods of wear. Her refraction was

$$OD: +4.25 - 1.00 \times 180$$
$$OS: +3.75 - 1.25 \times 175$$

SOLUTION: This patient would benefit from rigid lenses, in general, because of her critical vision demands. A high-Dk material (preferably F-S/A, although any other high-Dk lens materials with good surface wettability properties would be possible options) would be recommended for the following reasons: (a) she would benefit from the Dk and possible flexible-wear schedule allowed with these materials, and (b) as a result of the large CTs required in her lenses, a high-Dk material would be necessary to provide sufficient oxygen through the center of the lens to meet the cornea's oxygen requirements.

CASE 3

A college baseball player comes to your office with complaints of foggy vision, itching, and redness from his hydrogel lenses, which have been bothering him for the past 6 months, gradually increasing in severity. He has decreased from a maximum of 14 to 8 hours of wearing time. He has been wearing his hydrogel lenses for a period of 12 months and has never been satisfied with his comfort or vision. The examination reveals the following:

VA (with CLs): OD: 20/20   OS: 20/25 + 1
SLE (OU): With lenses on
        Mucoprotein film
        <0.5-mm lens lag
    With lenses off
        6-second TBUT
        Grade 1 + conj. injection
        Grade 2 + papillary hypertrophy
Refraction: OD: $-1.50 - 0.50 \times 020$
             OS: $-1.25 - 0.50 \times 172$

SOLUTION: This patient would be a good candidate for a GP lens material, preferably a large-diameter wettable lens material that does not exhibit excessive lens lag after the blink. A large (10.0–11.2 mm) diameter low-Dk F-S/A material would be recommended, although a hybrid or corneo-scleral design can be considered as well. Ordinarily, most athletes would be better hydrogel candidates; however, this patient would benefit from GPs because of (a) his dissatisfaction with hydrogels, (b) marginal tear quality, (c) surface deposits/papillary hypertrophy, (d) uncorrected refractive astigmatism, and (e) the limited amount of physical contact in baseball (typically much less than that of other major sports such as football and basketball). Initially, the patient will need to decrease or preferably discontinue wearing time to decrease the clinical signs of papillary hypertrophy and eliminate existing symptoms.

CASE 4

A 39-year-old woman who is a long-term GP wearer complains of dryness and redness with her GP lenses, especially late in the day. Her comfortable wearing time has decreased from 15 to 10 hours per day, although the current lenses are only 12 months old. She is wearing a high-Dk F-S/A lens material. Her TBUT was 8 seconds OU and her refraction and keratometry values were as follows:

        OD: $-3.25 - 1.25 \times 180$ 20/20 + 2   43.25 @ 180; 44.25 @ 090

        OS: $-3.00 - 1.00 \times 173$ 20/20 + 1   43.00 @ 180; 43.75 @ 090

SLE (OU): Good centration and an alignment fluorescein pattern OU; mucoprotein film OU VA (with CLs): OD: 20/25 + 1 OS: 20/20 − 2

SOLUTION: This patient could potentially benefit from being refitted into a plasma-treated low-Dk F-S/A lens material. The lens material may result in prolonging tear film interaction with the lens surface, and the plasma treatment should optimize short-term surface wettability. The patient was also provided with a combination (nonabrasive) cleaning/disinfection solution, as well as a wetting solution. The wetting solution could also be used as a rewetting agent if needed.

CASE 5

An 8-year-old girl is interested in contact lenses. She has been a 2-year spectacle wearer and she does not enjoy wearing her spectacles for sports (she plays soccer and softball) and at school. Her refraction was as follows:

        OD: $-2.00 - 0.75 \times 175$ 20/20 + 2

        OS: $-2.25 - 0.50 \times 006$ 20/20

Her parents are highly myopic and they are concerned about the progression of her refractive error.

SOLUTION: It is important that the child has been a spectacle wearer first and that she—not just her parents—is motivated to wear contact lenses. There are two viable options for this young lady:

1. DW GP lenses. The GP modality may slow down the progression of her myopia. It would also be important to design the lenses such that they would have a large OAD (>10 mm) and low edge clearance to minimize the risk of displacement and loss during sports activities.
2. OOK. She would be an excellent candidate for OOK. This topic will be discussed in Chapter 20.

CASE 6

A 16-year-old high school student has been a soft toric lens wearer for 3 years. She indicates that she has never been satisfied with her vision. She has been refitted by three different practitioners, all of whom were determined for her to be successful with this modality. She indicated that she has probably worn six to seven different types of soft toric lenses, but that they all resulted in fluctuating vision and her doctors all commented that the lenses tended to rotate on her eyes. Her mother had read about GP lenses on the Internet and mentioned this to her previous eye doctor; however, her doctor indicated that he does not fit GP lenses. Her refraction and keratometry readings were as follows:

$$OD: -1.50 - 1.75 \times 168 \quad 20/20 \qquad 43.50 @ 165; 45.00 @ 075$$

$$OS: -1.00 - 2.00 \times 011 \quad 20/20+1 \qquad 43.75 @ 180; 45.25 @ 090$$

SOLUTION: This patient is an excellent candidate for GP lenses. Although she will experience some initial awareness and will need to adapt to the lenses, the quality of vision she should experience with the GP lenses should result in a very satisfied patient.

CASE 7

A 25-year-old, long-term highly myopic GP wearer expresses an interest in wearing EW lenses. He's frustrated at how blurry his vision is when he awakens and his friends have discussed how satisfied they are with continuous wear of some of the new soft lenses. His refraction was as follows:

$$OD: -6.75 - 1.25 \times 004 \quad 20/15$$

$$OS: -7.00 - 1.00 \times 173 \quad 20/15-2$$

His tear film and ocular health are normal.

SOLUTION: This patient would be a good candidate for continuous-wear GP lenses. A material that would be consistent with this desire would be Menicon Z.

CASE 8

A 23-year-old hyperopic patient enters your office and is greatly motivated to wear contact lenses. He is currently wearing spectacles, although he did have a history of wearing contact lenses. He indicated that he was fitted into spherical soft lenses when he was 12 but that he was never satisfied with his vision. He was fitted into soft toric lenses when he was 15 but he experienced an infection on two separate occasions, one of which was central and resulted in a slight loss of best corrected vision. Therefore, at age 19, he decided to return to spectacle wear. However, he is not pleased with the weight and the cosmetic appearance of spectacles. His refraction was as follows:

$$OD: +4.50 - 1.50 \times 010 \quad 20/25+1$$

$$OS: +4.25 - 1.75 \times 173 \quad 20/25+1$$

SOLUTION: A high-Dk F-S/A lens material would be a viable option for this patient. A low-Dk material would not meet the patient's corneal oxygen demands, but a high (or hyper)-Dk material would meet or exceed this requirement. The new generation of silicone hydrogel toric lenses would also represent a good option for this patient. However, due to the patient's history and expressed concern about soft lenses, the GP option would be recommended.

CLINICAL PROFICIENCY CHECKLIST

- It is important to verify if the lens material and design selected for a given patient meets the cornea's oxygen requirements. A minimum Dk/t (oxygen transmission or oxygen permeability/CT) of 24 is recommended for DW.
- Recommended rigid lenses can be divided into low Dk (25–50), high Dk (51–99), and hyper Dk ($\geq$100).
- Although good oxygen permeability is possible with these materials, S/A materials can be compromised by the hydrophobic properties and flexibility of "silicone." This can result in desiccation, deposits, warpage, flexure, and subjective symptoms of dryness and decreased vision.
- The addition of F-S/A-based copolymer materials promotes tear film mucin interaction with the lens surface. These materials—especially the low-Dk group—have become the lens of choice for most rigid lens-wearing patients.
- The SynergEyes family of hybrid lenses is revolutionary in that, via molecular bonding, combines an outer hydrogel skirt with a hyper GP center. It has the benefits of good initial comfort, astigmatic correction, and centration. The latter is especially important with patients having irregular corneas. Its problems include cost, adherence, tearing, and handling.
- Hyperopes, individuals desiring extended/flexible wear and those exhibiting edema with low-Dk lenses would all benefit from being fitted into high-Dk lens materials, preferably F-S/A.
- Former PMMA wearers, borderline dry-eye patients, and myopes would all benefit from the dimensional stability and wettability of low-Dk F-S/A lens materials.
- Athletes, unable to wear soft lenses, would benefit from a large diameter, low-edge clearance GP lens, or a hybrid design.

REFERENCES

1. Bennett ES. GP annual report 2012. *Contact Lens Spectrum*. 2012;27(10):26–33,39.
2. Nichols JJ. Contact lenses 2011. *Contact Lens Spectrum*.2012;27(10):20–25.
3. Morgan PB, Woods CA, Tranoudis IG, et al. International contact lens prescribing in 2011. *Contact Lens Spectrum*. 27(1):26–31.
4. Bennett ES. Patient selection, evaluation, and consultation. In: Bennett ES, Hom MM, eds. *Manual of Gas Permeable Contact Lenses*. 2nd ed. St. Louis, MO: Elsevier Science; 2004:58–85.
5. McMahon TT. The case for rigid lenses. *Eye Contact Lens*. 2003;29(1S):S119–S121.
6. Van der Worp E, de Brabender J. Contact lens fitting today. *Optom Today*. 2005;27–32.
7. Kollbaum P. Aberration correction part two. *Rev Cornea Contact Lenses*. 2009;34–37.
8. Johnson TJ, Schnider C. Clinical performance and patient preference for hydrogel versus RGP lenses. *Int Cont Lens Clin*. 1991;18(7,8):130.

9. Fonn D. Gauthier CA, Pritchard N. Patient preferences and comparative ocular responses to rigid and soft contact lenses. *Optom Vis Sci* .1995;72(12):857.
10. Ziel CJ, Gussler JR, Van Meter WS, et al. Contrast sensitivity in extended wear of the Boston IV lens. *CLAO J.* 1990;16:276.
11. Timberlake GT, Doane MG, Bertera JH. Short-term low contrast visual acuity reduction associated with in vivo contact lens drying. *Optom Vis Sci.* 1992;69(10):755.
12. Hong X, Himebaugh N, Thibos LN. On-eye evaluation of optical performance of rigid and soft contact lenses. *Optom Vis Sci.* 2001;78(12):872–880.
13. Joslin CE, Wu SM, McMahon TT, et al. Higher-order wavefront aberrations in corneal refractive therapy. *Optom Vis Sci.* 2003;80(12):805–811.
14. Dorronsoro C, Barbero S, Llorente L, et al. On-eye measurement of optical performance of rigid gas permeable contact lenses based on ocular and corneal aberrometry. *Optom Vis Sci.*2003;80:115–125.
15. Goldberg EP, Bhatia S, Enns JB. Hydrogel contact lens-corneal interactions: a new mechanism for deposit formation and corneal injury. *CLAO J.* 1997;23:243.
16. Sucheki JK, Ehlers WH, Donshik PC. Peripheral corneal infiltrates associated with contact lens wear. *Trans Am Ophthalmol Soc.* 1996;22:41.
17. Dart JK. The epidemiology of contact lens-related diseases in the United Kingdom. *CLAO J.* 1993;19:241.
18. Efron N, Morgan PB, Hill EA, et al. The size, location, and clinical severity of corneal infiltrative events associated with contact lens wear. *Optom Vis Sci.* 2005;82(6):519–527.
19. Stapleton F, Keay L, Edwards K, et al. The incidence of contact lens-related microbial keratitis in Australia. *Ophthalmology.* 2008;115(10):1655–1662.
20. Cheng KH, Leung SL, Hoekman HW et al. Incidence of contact lens-associated microbial keratitis and its related morbidity. *Lancet.* 1999;354:181–185.
21. Dart JK, Stapleton F, Minassian D. Contact lenses and other risk factors in microbial keratitis. *Lancet.* 1991;338(8768):650–653.
22. Poggio EC, Glynn RJ, Schein OD, et al. The incidence of ulcerative keratitis among users of daily-wear and extended-wear soft contact lenses. *N Engl J Med.* 1989;321(12):779–883.
23. Schein OD, McNally JJ, Katz J, et al. The incidence of microbial keratitis among wearers of a 30-day silicone hydrogel extended-wear contact lens. *Ophthalmology.* 2005;112(12):2172–2179.
24. Schein OD, Buehler PO, Stamler JF, et al. The impact of overnight wear on the risk of contact lens-associated ulceratitis keratitis. *Arch Ophthalmol* .1994;112(2):186–190.
25. Schein OD, Poggio EC. Ulcerative keratitis in contact lens wearers: incidence and risk factors. *Cornea.* 1990;9:S55–S58; discussion S62–S63.
26. Dart JK, Radford CF, Minassian D, et al. Risk factors for microbial keratitis with contemporary contact lenses: a case control study. *Ophthalmology.* 2008;115(10):1647–1654.
27. Ren D, Yamamoto K, Ladage P, et al. Adaptive effects of 30-night wear of hyper-O2 transmissible contact lenses on bacterial binding and corneal epithelium: a 1-year clinical trial. *Ophthalmology.* 2002;109:27–40.
28. Ren DH, Petroll WM, Jester JV, et al. The relationship between contact lens oxygen permeability and binding of Pseudomonas aeruginosa to human corneal epithelial cells and after overnight and extended wear. *CLAO J.* 1999;25(2):80–100.
29. Seal DV, Bennett ES, McFayden AK, et al. Differential adherence of *Acanthamoeba* to contact lenses: effects of material characteristics. *Optom Vis Sci.* 1995:72:23.
30. Donshik PC. Giant papillary conjunctivitis. *Trans Am Ophthalmol Soc.* 1994;92:687–744.
31. Bennett ES, Johnson JD. Material selection. In: Bennett ES, Weissman BA, eds. *Clinical Contact Lens Practice.* Philadelphia, PA: Lippincott Williams & Wilkins; 2005:243–253.
32. Morgan PB, Efron N, Maldonado-Codina C, et al. Adverse events and discontinuations with rigid and soft hyper-Dk contact lenses used for continuous wear. *Optom Vis Sci.* 2005;82(6):528–535.
33. Ritson M. Which patients are more profitable? *Contact Lens Spectrum.* 2006;21(3):38–42.
34. Ames K. Rethink your approach to RGP lenses. *Contact Lens Spectrum.* 1993;8(12):24–27.
35. Perrigin J, Perrigin D, Quinteros S, et al. Silicone-acrylate contact lenses for myopia control: 3-year old results. *Optom Vis Sci.* 1990;67(10):764.
36. Khoo CY, Chong J, Rajan U. A 3-year study on the effect of RGP contact lenses on myopic children. *Singapore Med J.* 1999;40:230–237.
37. Walline JJ, Jones LA, Mutti DO, et al. A randomized trial of the effects of rigid contact lenses on myopia progression. *Arch Ophthalmol.* 2004;122(12):1760–1766.
38. Katz J, Schein OD, Levy B, et al. A randomized trial of rigid gas permeable contact lenses to reduce progression of children's myopia. *Am J Ophthalmol.* 2003;136:82–89.
39. Walline JJ, Rah M, Jones LA. The Children's Overnight Orthokeratology Investigation (COOKI) Pilot Study. *Optom Vis Sci* .2004;81(6):407–413.
40. Cho P, Cheung SW, Edwards M. The Longitudinal Orthokeratology Research in Children (LORIC) in Hong Kong: a pilot study on refractive changes in myopic control. *Curr Eye Res.* 2005;30:71–80.
41. Walline JJ, Jones LA, Sinnott LT. Corneal reshaping and myopia progression. *Br J Ophthalmol.* 2009;93:1181–1185.

42. Smith EL III, Kee CS, Ramamirtham R, et al. Peripheral vision can influence eye growth and refractive development in infant monkeys. *Invest Ophthalmol Vis Sci.* 2005;46:3965–3972.
43. Kang P, Swarbrick H. Peripheral refraction in myopic children wearing orthokeratology and gas-permeable lenses. *Optom Vis Sci* .2011;88(4):476–482.
44. Charman WN, Mountford J, Atchison DA, et al. Peripheral refraction in orthokeratology patients. *Optom Vis Sci.* 2006;83:641–648.
45. Quieros A, Gonzalez-Meijome JM, Jorge J, et al. Peripheral refraction in myopic patients after orthokeratology. *Optom Vis Sci.* 2010;87:323–329.
46. Walline JJ. Current and future developments in myopia control. *Contact Lens Spectrum.* 2012;27(10):34–39.
47. Zadnik K, Barr JT, Edrington TB, et al. Baseline findings in the Collaborative Longitudinal Evaluation of Keratoconus (CLEK) study. *Invest Ophthalmol Vis Sci.* 1998;39(13):2537–2546.
48. Jinabhal A, Charman WN, O'Donnell C, et al. Optical quality for keratoconic eyes with conventional RGP lens and simulated, customized contact lens corrections: a comparison. *Ophthalm Physiol Opt.* 2012;32(3):200–212.
49. Shi YH, Wany LY, Lu TB, et al. Changes of ocular higher order aberration in keratoconic eyes wearing rigid gas-permeable contact lens. *Chinese J Ophthalmol.* 2011;47(7):601–606.
50. Lieblein JS. Finding success with multifocal contact lenses. *Contact Lens Spectrum.* 2000;14(3):50–51.
51. Byrnes SP, Cannella A. An in-office evaluation of a multifocal RGP lens design. *Contact Lens Spectrum.* 1999;14(11):29–33.
52. Remba MJ. The Tangent Streak rigid gas-permeable bifocal contact lens. *J Am Optom Assoc.* 1988;59:212.
53. Gussler JR, Lin ES, Litteral G, et al. Clinical evaluation of the Anterior Constant Focus (ACF) annular bifocal contact lens. *CLAO J.* 1993;19:222.
54. Smith VM, Koffler BH, Litteral G. Evaluation of the ZEBRA 2000 (Z10) Breger Vision bifocal contact lens. *CLAO J.* 2000;26(4):214–220.
55. Rajagopalan AS, Bennett ES, Lakshminarayanan V. Visual performance of subjects wearing presbyopic contact lenses. *Optom Vis Sci.* 2006;83(8):611–615.
56. DeNaeyer GW. Today's scleral lens. *Rev Cornea Contact Lenses.* June 2012; 18–22.
57. Bennett ES, Henry VA. Contemporary contact lens multifocal primer. *Contact Lens Spectrum.* 2012;27(2):24–32.
58. Potter RT. Toric and multifocal lens options. *Contact Lens Spectrum.* 2012;27(2):34–39.
59. Michaud L, Barriault C, Dionne A, et al. Empirical fitting of soft or rigid gas-permeable contact lenses for the correction of moderate to severe refractive astigmatism: a comparative study. *Optometry.* 2009;80:373–383.
60. Connelly S. Why do patients want to be refit? *Contact Lens Spectrum.* 1992;7:39.
61. Andrasko G, Smiley T, Nichold L, et al. Clinical recommendations for the management of symptomatic soft contact lens wearers. *Contact Lens Spectrum.* 1993;8:24.
62. Potter R. The road to GP comfort. *Contact Lens Spectrum.* 2008;23(10):37–41.
63. Hewitt TT. A survey of contact lens wearers. Part II: behaviors, experiences, attitudes and expectations. *Am J Optom Physiol Opt.* 1984;61:73.
64. Andrasko GJ, Billings R. A simple nomogram for RGP fitting success. *Contact Lens Spectrum.* 1993;8:28.
65. Jedlicka J, Malooley MM, Reeder RE. Semi-scleral applications for healthy eyes. *Contact Lens Spectrum.* 2011;26(11):34–42.
66. Herzberg CM. Technology to optimize GP comfort and success. *Contact lens Spectrum.* 2011;26(6):34–39.
67. Michaud L, Woo SL, Bennett ES, et al. Correction of low to moderate astigmatism with large diameter rigid gas permeable lenses versus soft: a clinical study. Paper presented at: Global Specialty Lens Symposium; January 2013; Las Vegas, NV.
68. Michaud L. The modern RGP lens revolution. *Rev Cornea Contact Lenses.* www.reviewofcontactlenses.com/content/d/rgp_lenses/c/34148. Accessed May 5, 2012.
69. Bennett ES. Be flexible about rigid lenses. *Rev Cornea Contact Lens.* 2007;38–40.
70. Schwartz CA. New strategies for screening RGPs. *Rev Optom.* 1994;131:29.
71. Fonn D, Pritchard N, Garnett B, et al. Palpebral aperture sizes of rigid and soft contact lens wearers compared with nonwearers. *Optom Vis Sci.* 1996;73(3):211–214.
72. Thean JH, McNab AA. Blepharoptosis in RGP and PMMA hard contact lens wearers. *Clin Exp Optom.* 2004;87(1):11.
73. Fatt I, Chaston J. Measurement of oxygen transmissibility and permeability of hydrogel lenses and materials. *ICLC.* 1982;9:76–88.
74. Fatt I, Rasson JE, Melpolder JB. Measuring oxygen permeability of gas permeable hard and hydrogel lenses and flat samples in air. *ICLC.* 1987;14:389–401.
75. Benjamin WJ. "Wiggle room" and the traditional Dk statistic. *ICLC.* 1998;25(7&8):118–120.
76. Benjamin WJ, Cappelli QA. Oxygen permeability (Dk) of thirty-seven rigid contact lens materials. *Optom Vis Sci.* 2002;79(2):103–111.
77. Mandell RB, Liberman GL, Fatt I. Corneal oxygen supply: RGP versus soft lenses. *Contact Lens Spectrum.* 1987;2(10):37–39.
78. Bennett ES, Ghormley NR. Rigid extended wear: an overview. *Int Cont Lens Clin.* 1987;14(8):319–332.
79. Machara JR, Kastl PR. Rigid gas-permeable extended wear. *CLAO J.* 1994;20:139.
80. Polse KA. Tear flow under hydrogel contact lenses. *Invest Ophthalmol Vis Sci.* 1979;18:409.

81. O'Neal MR, Polse KA, Sarver MD. Corneal response to rigid and hydrogel lenses during eye closure. *Invest Ophthalmol Vis Sci.* 1984;27(7):837–842.
82. Tomlinson A, Armitage B. Closed-eye corneal response to a tertiary butyl styrene gas-permeable lens. *Int Eyecare.* 1985;1(4):320–323.
83. Ichijima H, Cavanagh HD. How rigid gas-permeable lenses supply more oxygen to the cornea than silicone hydrogels: a new model. *Eye Contact Lens.* 2007;33(5):216–223.
84. Michaud L, van der Worp E, Brazeau D, et al. Predicting estimates of oxygen transmissibility for scleral lenses. *Cont Lens Anterior Eye.* 2012;35(6):266–271.
85. Holden BA, Mertz GW. Critical oxygen levels to avoid corneal edema for daily and extended wear contact lenses. *Invest Ophthalmol Vis Sci.* 1984;25:1161–1167.
86. Sweeney DF, Keay L, Jalbert I, et al. Clinical performance of silicone hydrogel lenses. In: Sweeney DF, ed. *Silicone Hydrogels: The Rebirth of Continuous Wear Contact Lenses.* Oxford: Butterworth-Heinemann; 2000:90.
87. Harvitt DM, Bonanno JA. Re-evaluation of the oxygen diffusion model for predicting minimum contact lens Dk/t values needed to avoid corneal anoxia. *Optom Vis Sci.* 1999;76:712–719.
88. Papas E. On the relationship between soft contact lens oxygen transmissibility and induced limbal hyperemia. *Exp Eye Res.* 1998;67:125–131.
89. Gordon JM, Bennett ES. Dk revisited: the hypoxic corneal environment. Presented at: Annual Meeting of the American Academy of Ophthalmology; November 1993; Chicago, IL.
90. Benjamin WJ. EOP and Dk/L: the quest for hypertransmissibility. *J Am Optom Assoc.* 1993;64:196.
91. Bennett ES. Gas permeable materials. In: Bennett ES, Hom MM, eds. *Manual of Gas Permeable Contact Lenses.* 2nd ed. St. Louis, MO: Elsevier Science; 2004:48–56.
92. Benjamin WJ. Wettability. In: Bennett ES, Grohe RM, eds. *Rigid Gas-Permeable Contact Lenses.* New York, NY: Professional Press; 1986:118–136.
93. Maruna C, Yoder M, Andrasko GJ. Attitudes toward RGPs among optometrists. *Contact Lens Spectrum.* 1987;12(11):57.
94. Hom MM, Bruce AS. Material properties. In: Bennett ES, Hom MM, eds. *Manual of Gas Permeable Contact Lenses.* 2nd ed. St. Louis, MO: Elsevier Science. 2004:30–47.
95. Cannella A, Bonafini JA. Polymer chemistry. In: Bennett ES, Weissman BA, eds. *Clinical Contact Lens Practice.* Philadelphia, PA: Lippincott Williams & Wilkins; 2005:233–242.
96. Sorbara L, Fonn D, MacNeil K. Effect of rigid gas permeable lens flexure on vision. *Optom Vis Sci.* 1992;69:953–958.
97. Corzine JC, Klein SA. Factors affecting rigid contact lens flexure. *Optom Vis Sci.* 1997;74(8):639–645.
98. Herman JP. Flexure. In: Bennett ES, Grohe RM, eds. *Rigid Gas-Permeable Contact Lenses.* New York, NY: Professional Press; 1986:137–150.
99. Herman JP. Flexure of rigid contact lenses on toric corneas as a function of base curve fitting relationship. *J Am Optom Assoc.* 1983;54(3):209–213.
100. Brown S, et al. Effect of the optic zone diameter on lens flexure and residual astigmatism. *Int Cont Lens Clin.* 1984;11(12):759–766.
101. Bennett ES, Egan DJ. Rigid gas-permeable lens problem-solving. *J Am Optom Assoc.* 1986;57:504–512.
102. Egan DJ, Bennett ES. Trouble-shooting rigid contact lens flexure - a case report. *Int Contact Lens Clin.* 1985;12:147.
103. Bennett ES. Problem solving. In Bennett ES, Hom MM, eds. *Manual of Gas Permeable Contact Lenses.* 2nd ed. St. Louis, MO: Elsevier Science; 2004:190–211.
104. Levitt AO. Specific gravity and RGP lens performance. *Contact lens Spectrum.* 1996;11(10):43.
105. Ghormley NR. Specific gravity - does it contribute to RGP lens adherence? *Int Cont Lens Clin.* 1991;18:125.
106. Bennett ES. How high index GP materials will impact your practice. *Contact Lens Spectrum.* 2009;24(2):23.
107. Watanabe RK. When to go high-index. *Contact Lens Spectrum.* 2010;25(6):17.
108. Norman C, Caroline P, Koch T, et al. Do we need high index materials? Presented at: 47th Annual Meeting of the Contact Lens Manufacturers Association; 2008; Hoover, AL.
109. Tighe BJ. Contact lens materials. In: Phillips AJ, Speedwell L, eds. *Contact lenses.* 5th ed. London, Elsevier: Butterworth-Heinemann; 2007:59–78.
110. Ghormley NR. Rigid EW lenses: complications. *Int Cont Lens Clin.* 1987;14:219.
111. Bennett ES, Tomlinson A, Mirowitz MC, et al. Comparison of corneal overnight swelling and lens performance in RGP extended wear. *CLAO J.* 1988;14:94.
112. Henry VA, Bennett ES, Forrest JF. Clinical investigation of the Paraperm EW rigid gas-permeable contact lens. *Am J Optom Physiol Opt.* 1987;64:313–320.
113. Grohe RM, Caroline PJ, Norman CW. RGP surface cracking. Part I: Clinical syndrome. *Contact Lens Spectrum.* 1987;2(5):37–45.
114. Grohe RM, Caroline PJ, Norman CW. RGP surface cracking. Part II: Clinical syndrome. *Contact Lens Spectrum.* 1987;2(9):40–46.
115. Weinschenk JI. A look at the components of fluoro-silicone/acrylates. *Contact Lens Spectrum.* 1989;4(10):61.
116. Feldman G, Yamane SJ, Herskowitz R. Fluorinated materials and the Boston Equalens. *Contact Lens Forum.* 1987;12:57.
117. Gelnar PV, Behnken BH. Paraperm EW vs. Fluoroperm 90 gas-permeable contact lens study. *Contact Lens J.* 1989;17:15.

118. Andrasko GJ. Comfort comparison between silicon acrylates and the Boston Equalens. *Contact Lens Spectrum.* 1988;3(6):61.
119. Bark M, Hanson D, Grant R. A guide to rigid gas-permeable contact lens materials. *Optician.* 1994;207:17.
120. Doane M, Gleason W. Tear film interaction with RGP contact lenses. Presented at: First International Material Science Symposium; March 1988; St. Louis, MO.
121. Caroline PJ, Ellis EJ. Review of the mechanisms of oxygen transport through rigid gas-permeable lenses. *Int Eyecare.* 1986;2:210.
122. Rah MJ. A GP materials guide. *Contact Lens Spectrum.* 2007;22(7):19.
123. Quinn TQ. Clinical experience with Fluoroperm 30 lenses. *Contact Lens Spectrum.* 1989;4(2):63.
124. Quinn TQ. Base curve stability of a fluoro-silicone-acrylate material of moderate permeability. *Contact Lens Spectrum.* 1989;4(3):52.
125. Bennett ES. Basic Fitting. In: Bennett ES, Weissman BA, eds. *Clinical Contact Lens Practice.* Philadelphia, PA: Lippincott Williams & Wilkins; 2005:255–275.
126. Jackson JM. Prescribing GP lenses in a material world. *Contact Lens Spectrum.* 2006;21(4):19.
127. Laurenzi A. Choosing the right GP material for each patient. *Contact Lens Spectrum.* 2009;24(3):25.
128. Schachet JL, Rigel LE, Reeder KM, et al. Rethinking the link between RGP lens performance. *Contact Lens Spectrum.* 1998;13(9):43–47.
129. Bennett ES. Optimizing GP wettability and performance. *Contact Lens Spectrum.* 2006;21(2):21.
130. Knutson E, Young R, et al. Assessing a new GP lens family. *Contact Lens Spectrum.* 2005;20(5):50–52.
131. Bennett ES. To plasma treat or not to plasma treat? *Rev Cornea Contact Lenses.* November 2006;9.
132. Schafer J. Plasma treatment for GP contact lenses. *Contact Lens Spectrum.* 2006;21(11):19.
133. Pence NA. Plasma treatment facts: no sugar coating. *Contact Lens Spectrum.* 2008;23(5):19.
134. Gu Z, Han Y, Pan F, et al. Surface hydrophilicity improvement of RGP contact lens material by oxygen plasma treatment. *Materials Science Forum.* 2009;1268:610–613.
135. Pence N. Scleral GPs: more indications? *Contact Lens Spectrum.* 2012;27(10):21.

Chapter 5

Gas-Permeable Lens Design, Fitting and Evaluation

Edward S. Bennett, Luigina Sorbara and Randy Kojima

The ability to successfully fit rigid gas-permeable (GP) contact lenses is often what separates the good contact lens practitioner from the average one. Certainly, there are numerous patients who benefit from the quality of vision and ocular health provided by GP lenses. This chapter will discuss the importance of fitting GP lenses, and the lens design, fitting, evaluation, and ordering procedures.

HOW TO OPTIMIZE INITIAL COMFORT

The first time a patient experiences contact lens wear can be quite traumatic. This is especially true with GP lenses because of the smaller diameter and greater lens movement with the blink as compared to soft lenses. This experience, in itself, can affect the fitting habits of practitioners who may decide to fit soft lenses—even when they are not the best option for patients—in an effort to provide a more initially comfortable and less time-consuming experience.

It is important, if not imperative, for the initial patient experience to be positive for the patient to be successful. The common perception by patients is that the initial comfort with GP lenses is poor, and this represents the primary reason why patients discontinue GP lens wear.[1] It is evident that if the patient has a poor initial experience with GP lenses, he or she will influence others away from considering this option. If the clinician—via his or her educational background (or lack thereof) or employment environment—is not motivated to fit GP lenses, it is likely that, despite the many benefits of GP lenses, patients will not be fitted into the mode of correction that would be indicated because of quality of vision, eye health, or some other reason.

The authors have recommended a fourfold approach to optimizing initial comfort.[2] These factors include: (a) presentation, (b) topical anesthetic, (c) initial vision, and (d) lens design.

Initial Presentation

Most contact lens patients rely on their practitioner to recommend an appropriate lens material and design. It is important for practitioners to recognize that when presenting patients with a choice, they may, without realizing it, bias that choice. The doctor's language creates and colors patient perceptions. Such terms as *discomfort, pain,* or *always seems to feel like there is something on the eye* set up strong negative expectations.[3] Prescribing practitioners are powerful authority figures. What they say and how they say it can easily influence patients.

Simple words like *soft, hard,* or *rigid* can influence a patient's contact lens preferences. Even nonverbal cues such as facial expression and eye contact can communicate an attitude to the patient. It is always important to begin with the assumption that a new patient has somewhere been given the impression that rigid lenses are uncomfortable. GP lenses can then be described in the following way: "GP lenses typically provide excellent vision and eye health. They are also quite wettable and durable. However, they do not feel the same way a soft lens does at first. Because they are smaller, they move more on the eye. The lids sense this movement initially and gradually adapt, typically resulting in comfortable lens wear." The use of the term *gas permeable* as compared to the previous *rigid gas permeable* terminology was recently proposed by the Contact Lens Manufacturers Association (CLMA) to minimize the focus on "rigid" lenses.

The impact of presentation methods was confirmed by a study in which subjects who were not previous contact lens wearers were divided into three groups before initiating GP lens wear.[4] Group 1 subjects, as part of the diagnostic fitting process, observed a videotape of a doctor discussing GP lenses with a new wearer using terms such as *discomfort, possible pain, intolerance,* and *failure* when describing GP lenses. Group 2 subjects observed a videotape of a doctor discussing GP lenses using neutral terms such as *lens awareness* and *initial lid sensation*. However, this doctor did not appear to be particularly positive about the GP lens option. In Group 3, the doctor discussing GP lenses used the same terminology as in the videotape observed by Group 2 but exhibited a positive attitude toward GP lenses. Eight subjects in this 1-month study discontinued lens wear; six of these subjects were in Group 1, and the other two were in Group 2. No subject provided with a neutral content and enthusiastic presentation discontinued lens wear. Likewise, the Group 3 subjects were significantly more compliant in returning daily questionnaires than the other two groups.

It is important for patients to know the benefits of GP lenses, that they will adapt over time, and that good comfort is a very realistic goal.[5] An effective presentation has been recommended by Quinn[6] (Table 5.1). Certainly experienced GP fitters do not have a problem with the comfort issue, and as one acquires more experience in fitting GP lenses, greater confidence in presenting this option in a positive but realistic manner results.

Topical Anesthetic Use

A second important technique for obtaining initial GP patient comfort and satisfaction is the use of a topical anesthetic during contact lens fitting. This has been considered somewhat controversial because of concerns pertaining to its potential for softening the epithelium, resulting in a greater incidence of corneal staining.[7–9] In addition, there is always the potential for misleading the patients who will ultimately experience the typical lens awareness with GP lenses. Fortunately, although these are legitimate concerns, they have not been confirmed by clinical research with GP lenses.[9,10]

With these issues in mind, an 80-subject multicenter study was performed to evaluate the effect of topical anesthetic use on initial comfort and patient satisfaction among first-time GP lens wearers.[9] Forty subjects were administered a topical anesthetic at the fitting visits, while a second group of 40 received a placebo. One month later, 70 of the 80 subjects were still wearing lenses. Eight of the 10 who discontinued lens wear were in the placebo group. In addition,

TABLE 5.1 GP Presentation Pearls

1. Rather than presenting a list of lens options, recommend GP lenses with confidence.
2. Prepare patients for the adaptation process by using the Sandwich Approach (necessary information communicated between two positive statements).

    Opening positive statement: "I recommend we fit you with GP lenses. They will provide you with excellent vision, superior safety, and easy handling."
    Key message: "There will be some initial awareness of the lens, much like adapting to a new watch or ring."
    Closing positive statement: "GP lenses are a great fit for your needs."

3. Practice the no-surprise approach to lens care.
    a. Make patients aware of the initial awareness with GP lenses, but don't dwell on it!
    b. Utilize anesthetic for initial lens application. Tell the patient, "I am going to put a drop in your eye to help you with the initial adjustment to the lenses. It will help me assess your vision and fit more accurately."

Reprinted with permission from Quinn TG. GP versus soft lenses: Is one safer? *Contact Lens Spectrum.* 2012;27(4):34–39,58.

at the completion of the study, subjects who had been given anesthetic rated their experience during adaptation, their comfort, and their overall satisfaction significantly higher than those subjects who had received placebo.

The benefits of topical anesthetic are significant. All patients are, at minimum, mildly apprehensive about the initial application of contact lenses. If the first few minutes of lens wear are acceptable, it makes sense that patient satisfaction, and the potential for successful long-term wear, will be greatly enhanced. The topical anesthetic should be allowed to wear off, and the patient will gradually experience lens awareness. In addition, in busy clinical practice environments, where time is a precious resource, the ability to evaluate the fluorescein pattern soon after diagnostic lens application is invaluable.[10] This is also important because of the fact that soft lenses often require little chair time during the fitting process and GPs benefit from being competitive with soft lenses whenever possible.

Nonsteroidal anti-inflammatory drugs (NSAIDs) have also been used to reduce awareness during adaptation.[11,12] Because NSAIDs reduce production of prostaglandins, which are mediators of pain, reducing their production reduces pain. The most effective drug within this class at inhibiting prostaglandin synthesis appears to be Voltaren. A recommended NSAID dosage for GP lens adaptation is as follows[12]:

- Instill one drop of Voltaren in each eye 30 minutes and then 15 minutes before lens insertion.
- Instill a third drop just before lens insertion.
- A fourth drop can be instilled 1 hour after insertion.
- This regimen can be maintained for 3 to 5 days or until adaptation is completed.

Topical anesthetic use is certainly not a requirement for GP fitting. However, for apprehensive practitioners as well as patients—particularly young people, people with keratoconus, and soft lens refits—anesthetic use can mean the difference between success and failure.

Initial Vision

Providing patients with an important benefit from GP lenses, good quality of vision, can be very important for initial patient satisfaction. When a patient is fitted with GP lenses in their correct power—either via empirical fitting or from an inventory—the resulting "wow" factor may reduce apprehension about lens awareness.[13]

Lens Design

This will be discussed in more detail later in this chapter; however, a well-designed, alignment fitting lens with an optimal edge design and shape will contribute to a more positive initial patient experience. GP lens designs in common use today tend to be larger and thinner with back surface geometries that are more in alignment with corneal shape.

FITTING AND EVALUATION

There are numerous important components to fitting lenses successfully. These include such factors as diagnostic fitting, fluorescein application and evaluation, and an accurate and compatible lens design.[14]

Methods of Fitting

Empirical Fitting

Empirical fitting refers specifically to designing lenses empirically or without using diagnostic lenses. Practitioners who utilize empirical fitting methodologies claim that manufacturers' recommendations (supplying the laboratory with such minimal prefitting information as keratometry values and refraction) and fitting guides provide effective means to obtain maximum lens performance and fit. Empirical fitting also means that a new, unworn lens will be fitted to one patient only. Empirical fitting has the attraction of eliminating a fitting visit and, consequently, enabling a simplistic fitting approach, which is both efficient and patient-friendly by simulating a soft-lens-fitting approach.[15,16] As indicated previously, however, empirical fitting often provides a very important benefit, good initial vision. The newer automated manufacturing equipment makes the success of empirical designs more likely than 10 to 20 years ago because of higher-quality lenses, aspheric and pseudoaspheric peripheries, thinner center thicknesses (CTs), and more consistent edge designs. Likewise, topography software programs allow the practitioner to better match corneal shape with the recommended computer-assisted design.[17–20] A representative empirical design is the Visions Ultra Thin lenses (X-Cel Contacts). These lenses can be ordered in a pack of two such that patient always has a spare pair.[21] Likewise, the fabricating laboratory typically has nomograms and calculators to determine the specific parameters if they are provided with refractive and keratometric/topographical information. Both eyedock.com and the GP Lens Institute have online calculators to design spherical lenses.

Diagnostic Fitting

Diagnostic fitting is still a popular method of fitting GP lenses. It allows the practitioner to feel confident in the final lenses to be ordered as multiple diagnostic lenses can be applied (if necessary), and those that result in the best lens-to-cornea fitting relationship will be ordered. Greater patient compliance with the follow-up schedule in addition to significantly fewer re-ordered lenses have been found with diagnostic fitting versus empirical fitting.[22] Although a fitting visit and a sufficient number of diagnostic lenses are required, diagnostic fitting allows practitioners the opportunity to evaluate the lens-to-cornea fitting relationship and to make the changes necessary to obtain a good fit and provide acceptable vision to the patient. It is also apparent that the fitting visit provides patients with an opportunity to become familiar with their particular lenses. Finally, such factors as lens centration and residual astigmatism can be evaluated.[23] The primary limitations pertain to (likely) not leaving the office with lenses, as compared with most soft lens patients, and the fact that, in most cases, satisfactory vision will not be obtained with the first pair of GP lenses applied. The 6 D myopic patient who is fitted with 3 D power diagnostic GP lenses will not only experience initial awareness, but also blurred vision. Nevertheless, with most special design GP lenses, including bifocal, keratoconic, and postsurgical designs, it is important to use diagnostic fitting sets because of the greater challenges involved in the fitting process and the more custom nature of the designs. When diagnostic fitting sets are to be used, it is important that the lenses are in the same design and material as the lenses to be ordered. A comparison of the factors involved in deciding between empirical and diagnostic fitting is provided in Table 5.2.

TABLE 5.2 Diagnostic Fitting versus Empirical Fitting
Diagnostic Fitting Advantages
Fewer reorders
Practitioner confidence in fitting relationship
Greater patient satisfaction
Better patient compliance
Empirical Fitting Advantages
Good initial vision experience
Easier method
Minimizes transfer of diagnostic lens contaminants
Less initial chair time
Allows topography software to assist in lens design

Diagnostic Fitting Sets/Inventories

Specific Fitting Sets

Having available several different diagnostic fitting sets is important, if not essential. For example, 20 lens diagnostic fitting sets in a −3.00 D power would be beneficial in materials of both low (<50) and high (≥50) oxygen permeability (Dk). An example of such a fitting set is provided in Table 5.3. In addition, similar diagnostic sets in a +3.00 D power in a high-Dk material with a minus lenticular edge design and in a −8.00 D power in a low-Dk material and a plus lenticular edge design would be recommended. Keratoconic, bitoric, aphakic, and bifocal diagnostic sets are also recommended and are discussed in other chapters of this text (Chapters 14, 15, 17, and 18).

For the diagnostic fitting sets, a good average overall diameter (OAD) is 9.4 mm with an 8.0-mm optical zone diameter (OZD). However, for steeper than 44.50 D, you may find a 9.0/7.6-mm design to provide an optimum fitting relationship. Base curve radii (BCRs) can range from 40.75 D (8.28 mm) to 45.50 D (7.42 mm) in 0.25 D steps. A relatively constant

TABLE 5.3 Recommended Parameters for a 20-Lens Diagnostic Set, Low- and High-Dk Gas-Permeable Materials

OAD		9.2 mm		
OZD		7.8 mm		
CT		0.14 mm		
Power		−3.00 D		
LENS	BCR (mm)	SCR/W	ICR/W	PCR/W
1.	7.42	8.00/.3	8.80/.2	10.00/.2
2.	7.46	8.10/.3	8.90/.2	10.10/.2
3.	7.50	8.20/.3	9.00/.2	10.20/.2
4.	7.54	8.20/.3	9.00/.2	10.20/.2
5.	7.58	8.30/.3	9.10/.2	10.30/.2
6.	7.63	8.30/.3	9.20/.2	10.40/.2
7.	7.67	8.40/.3	9.30/.2	10.50/.2
8.	7.71	8.50/.3	9.40/.2	10.60/.2
9.	7.76	8.50/.3	9.50/.2	10.60/.2
10.	7.81	8.60/.3	9.60/.2	10.70/.2
11.	7.85	8.60/.3	9.60/.2	10.80/.2
12.	7.89	8.70/.3	9.70/.2	10.80/.2
13.	7.94	8.70/.3	9.70/.2	10.90/.2
14.	7.99	8.80/.3	9.80/.2	11.00/.2
15.	8.04	8.80/.3	9.90/.2	11.10/.2
16.	8.08	8.90/.3	10.00/.2	11.20/.2
17.	8.13	8.90/.3	10.10/.2	11.30/.2
18.	8.18	9.00/.3	10.20/.2	11.40/.2
19.	8.23	9.10/.3	10.30/.2	11.50/.2
20.	8.28	9.20/.3	10.40/.2	11.60/.2

BCR, base curve radius; ICR/W, intermediate curve radius/width; PCR/W, peripheral curve radius/width; SCR/W, secondary curve radius/width.

edge lift of 0.09 to 0.11 mm is recommended for the diagnostic lenses; therefore, the flatter BCRs will have a greater flattening of the PCRs, and steeper BCRs will have a greater steepening. Finally, the appropriate CT should be ordered. For example, a low-Dk material may have a CT of approximately 0.14 mm in a −3.00 D power, although this can vary from material to material. All of the diagnostic lenses of the same power should have equal and appropriate CTs; these parameters—and especially edge shape—should be verified upon receiving them from the laboratory. With the increasing popularity of ultrathin designs, a diagnostic set of this design in a minus power (i.e., −3.00 D) would be recommended as well.

Inventories

The use of a large (100- to 200-lens) inventory system, which has been very popular with hydrogel lenses, is also an alternative available to practitioners. The advantages of using a large inventory to fit rigid lenses are many and include the following: (a) some patients can be fitted out of stock; (b) lens replacements can be provided to patients without delay, so patient satisfaction is enhanced; and (c) lens parameter changes can be made in the office without delay. Unlike hydrogel lenses, because of the custom or multiparameter design—especially BCR—inherent with successful fitting of GP lenses, a minimum of 200 lenses is necessary to directly fit the majority of patients without having to order the lenses from a laboratory. Such a 200-lens inventory is given in Table 5.4.

Some of the manufacturers, including those who manufacture the Boston Envision lens design (Bausch + Lomb) and the Naturalens (Advanced Vision Technologies; Fig. 5.1), can provide smaller inventories because of the philosophy that their respective designs can be successfully fitted to the great majority of patients with fewer BCRs.[2]

Some GP lens manufacturers are unwilling to manufacture such large inventories because of the labor and expense necessary to do so. However, they are often available to practitioners who fit a high volume of GP lenses. As with soft lenses, the initial expense to the practitioner is minimal; however, the laboratory usually requires the practitioner to meet the following agreement provisions[24]: (a) maintain an inventory of lenses equal to the original consignment, (b) fit a certain number of lenses within a specified period, and (c) use manufacturer's lens design parameters. Nevertheless, it is a valuable alternative that can increase your success with GP lenses while also providing a valuable service to many GP patients.

Storage of Diagnostic Lenses

Storing diagnostic lenses in the hydrated state has the advantage of providing good initial wettability while maintaining the lenses in a somewhat sterile state. However, depending on the frequency with which the solution is changed, there are many advantages to keeping the lenses in the dry state.[25,26] It is both efficient and convenient to store the lenses dry because they can be kept in flat-pack cases that occupy very little space in the office. If the lenses are stored in the hydrated state, it is possible for the solution to either dry up in the case or leak out, both of these problems resulting in a lens that may adhere to the case or even change in BCR because of variation between the hydrated and unhydrated states. No contact lens disinfecting solution is approved for storage for greater than 30 days. Diagnostic lenses (and storage cases) must be recleaned and disinfected at least every 30 days if stored in a wet state. In addition, the dried solution may be difficult to remove from the lens surface. Whenever a diagnostic lens has been applied, however, it is recommended to carefully clean the lens and blot it dry with a soft tissue prior to disinfection and placement in the case and into the appropriate diagnostic lens set. The Centers for Disease Control and Prevention (CDC) recommends ophthalmic-grade hydrogen peroxide for GP lenses; therefore, AOSept or Clear Care (Alcon Laboratories) for a 5- to 10-minute soak has been recommended.[27] Before reuse, the diagnostic lens should be

TABLE 5.4 Parameters for Gas-Permeable Inventory Lens Set

BASE CURVE RADIUS (mm)

RX	7.42	7.50	7.54	7.58	7.63	7.67	7.71	7.76	7.80	7.85	7.89	7.94	7.99	8.04	8.13
−1.25									110	123	136	149	162	175	188
−1.50							79	94	111	124	137	150	163	176	189
−1.75							80	95	112	125	138	151	164	177	190
−2.00	1	14	27	40	53	66	81	96	113	126	139	152	165	178	191
−2.25	2	15	28	41	54	67	82	97	114	127	140	153	166	179	192
−2.50	3	16	29	42	55	68	83	98	115	128	141	154	167	180	193
−2.75	4	17	30	43	56	69	84	99	116	129	142	155	168	181	194
−3.00	5	18	31	44	57	70	85	100	117	130	143	156	169	182	195
−3.25	6	19	32	45	58	71	86	101	118	131	144	157	170	183	196
−3.50	7	20	33	46	59	72	87	102	119	132	145	158	171	184	197
−3.75	8	21	34	47	60	73	88	103	120	133	146	159	172	185	198
−4.00	9	22	35	48	61	74	89	104	121	134	147	160	173	186	199
−4.25	10	23	36	49	62	75	90	105	122	135	148	161	174	187	200
−4.50	11	24	37	50	63	76	91	106							
−4.75	12	25	38	51	64	77	92	107							
−5.00	13	26	39	52	65	78	93	108							

OAD = 9.4
OZD = 8.2
SCR = BCR + 1.0 mm/0.3 mm wide; PCR = BCR + 3.0 mm/0.3 mm wide

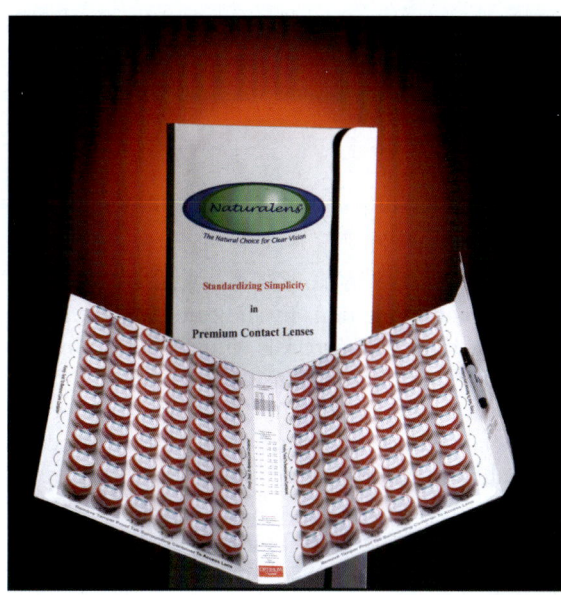

FIGURE 5.1 The Naturalens inventory (Advanced Vision Technologies).

cleaned with an approved cleaner, then rinsed prior to application of the wetting solution. GP lenses that are going to be dispensed to a patient should be hydrated for a minimum of 24 hours prior to application to enhance surface wettability and maintain the BCR in the hydrated state (similar to the "on-eye" condition as the back surface rests against the tear film). Obviously, patients should likewise be advised to maintain the lenses in the appropriate soaking/disinfecting solution upon removal (see Chapter 6).

Fluorescein Application and Evaluation

Description

Sodium fluorescein is an organic compound that is inert and harmless to tissue.[28] The application of fluorescein enables the practitioner to evaluate the lens-to-cornea fitting relationship. In fact, it would be appropriate to indicate that fluorescein has an invaluable, if not essential, role in rigid lens fit assessment.

To perform the procedure, the fluorescein strip is wetted with an ophthalmic irrigating solution. The strip is then gently applied against the superior bulbar conjunctiva with the patient viewing inferiorly. It is important to reassure the patient that this procedure is painless. In addition, the thumb should carefully pin back the upper lid to prevent the possibility of the lid pushing the strip toward the superior cornea, which could result in superior corneal staining and accompanying subjective discomfort.

The use of an ophthalmic irrigating solution has numerous advantages for wetting the fluorescein strip, including the following:

- Sterility.
- Slightly alkaline in pH, which assists in fluorescence.
- Reduced risk of burning and stinging caused by pH.
- Less viscous than use of a wetting solution (which may result in an abnormally thick tear layer).

However, for optimum fluorescence, the use of liquid fluorescein has been recommended.[29]

Methods of Observation

The fluorescein pattern can be evaluated with both a Burton lamp and a biomicroscope.

Burton Lamp: The traditional method of evaluating the fluorescein pattern is by use of an ultraviolet (UV) fluorescent lamp that utilizes a +5.00 D magnification lens to assist in viewing (Fig. 5.2). This method has the following advantages:

- Inexpensive.
- Easy to use.
- Overall field of view (FOV) and ability to directly compare fluorescein pattern of both eyes simultaneously.

However, the Burton lamp is very limited in its abilities. It does not allow for variable magnification or illumination. In addition, it is an ineffective method of observing the fluorescein pattern of rigid lens materials with UV-absorbing capabilities. Therefore, it would not be advantageous or appropriate to use this as the only method to evaluate a fluorescein pattern. However, it is a useful adjunct to the biomicroscope because of the overall FOV. This is especially beneficial in observing some of the more distinctive patterns, such as those pertaining to high corneal toricity and keratoconus.

Biomicroscope: The most popular method of evaluating the fluorescein pattern of a rigid lens is with the biomicroscope. The primary advantage of this over other observational methods is flexibility. It allows the practitioner the opportunity to vary the magnification, illumination, and slit-beam width while observing the fluorescein pattern. Proper use of a biomicroscope for GP fitting and evaluation is essential for patient success.

As biomicroscopes vary considerably from manufacturer to manufacturer, it is important for a good illumination source and variable magnification to be present to effectively evaluate the fluorescein pattern. In fact, it has been determined that with many biomicroscopes, it is not possible to use >10× magnification and still retain an adequate FOV.[30]

Once fluorescein has been properly instilled, the patient should be instructed to blink several times for adequate distribution on the eye. The fluorescein pattern should be initially observed under low magnification with a wide (diffuse) slit-beam and high-intensity illumination. The central and peripheral fluorescein pattern should be relatively easy to determine after several seconds. An optic section with the angle of illumination equal to 45 to 60 degrees can also be used to observe the pooling of tears in relation to the contact lens. It will appear as a green layer representing the outer layer of tears on the lens; then a wider dark layer, which is the contact lens; next another green layer, which represents the tear layer between the lens and

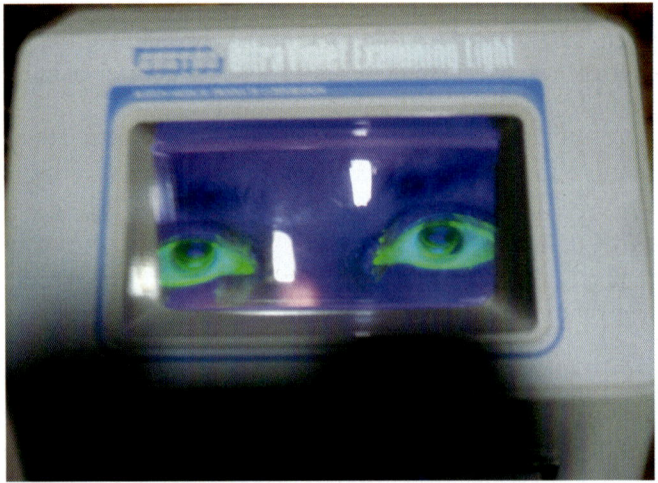

FIGURE 5.2 The Burton lamp for fluorescein pattern evaluation.

cornea; and finally a bright grayish layer, the cornea.[28] The lens-to-cornea fitting relationship can be evaluated by viewing the thickness of the tear layer along the optic section.

Typically, the fluorescein pattern is viewed with the assistance of a cobalt blue filter, which, in effect, transmits blue light that will activate the fluorescein dye. It is important to use a Wratten number 12 yellow filter (or equivalent) that can be attached to the observation system to serve as a barrier filter, screening out all but the wavelengths of interest.[31] The importance of the yellow filter cannot be underestimated since it makes an easily observable improvement in fluorescein pattern evaluation. The use of a yellow filter, in combination with a good illumination source, is especially important in the evaluation of GP materials that contain UV inhibitors because, as the material absorbs wavelengths that correspond to the illumination source, there is an apparent reduction or even absence of fluorescence behind the lens unless the appropriate filters and illumination source are used. It is hoped that biomicroscopic manufacturers will begin to incorporate the yellow filter into their respective instruments.

Pattern Evaluation: The fluorescein pattern assumes a variety of forms. Areas of fluorescein pooling appear green; areas in which fluorescein is absent or where the tear layer is too thin to detect, having the contact lens in direct contact with the cornea, appear as dark or black. In between these extremes, the varying thickness of the tear layer is observed as varying shades of green.

An alignment fit is observed when the lens evenly contours the cornea with a light, even tear pooling (Fig. 5.3). Apical clearance exists when a steep central fit with excessive fluorescence or central tear pooling is present (Fig. 5.4). This can result in midperipheral bearing and seal-off with a reduced ability to remove cellular debris and mucus that may be an important precursor to rigid lens adherence to the cornea. Apical clearance has also been found to induce corneal steepening, even after short-term wear.[32] Apical bearing exists when there is direct contact of the lens against the central cornea or the amount of tear pooling is too shallow to detect with the instillation of fluorescein (Fig. 5.5). Excessive apical bearing can potentially result in corneal molding with resultant distortion or warpage. In addition, the gradual formation of a central corneal abrasion is also possible.

With corneal astigmatism greater than one diopter, a dumbbell-shaped fluorescein pattern will be observed (Fig. 5.6). Typically, along the steeper meridian of the cornea, the tear layer thickness gradually increases toward the edge and the lens does not touch the cornea.

Along the flatter meridian, however, the tear layer thickness decreases toward the periphery and the lens comes in contact with the cornea at the edge of the optical zone. As corneal astigmatism increases, the difference in tear layer thickness between the two primary meridians becomes greater, the area of alignment becomes smaller, and the astigmatic, or dumbbell-shaped

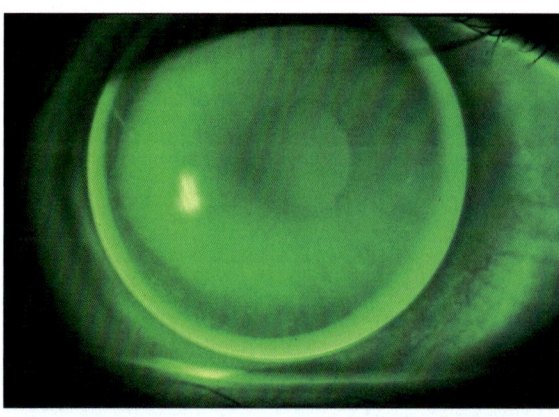

FIGURE 5.3 An alignment fluorescein pattern.

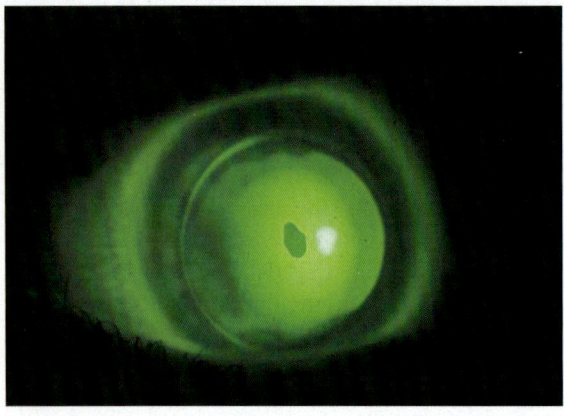

FIGURE 5.4 An apical clearance fluorescein pattern.

fluorescein pattern becomes exaggerated.[33] If the cornea exhibits with-the-rule corneal astigmatism, the pooling is in the vertical meridian with alignment or bearing in the horizontal meridian. If the cornea exhibits against-the-rule astigmatism, the opposite is true: the pooling is in the horizontal meridian with alignment or bearing in the vertical meridian. In high corneal astigmatism—typically >2 D—the use of a high-Dk material with a steeper-than-K BCR will result in excessive flexure and reduced visual acuity. In addition, the "rocking" of the lens during the blink process may result in discomfort, mechanical corneal staining, and possible lens adherence. The selection of a lower oxygen-permeable material, and perhaps a flatter BCR, is recommended. Another option would be a bitoric design, especially if the high amount of corneal toricity results in inferior decentration of the lens (see Chapter 14).

It is important to evaluate the fluorescein pattern after the blink since the amount of pooling and bearing will vary during the blink process. If the lens is decentered, the position of the lens relative to the cornea must be considered prior to evaluating the fluorescein pattern. For example, an inferior decentering lens will typically exhibit excessive superior pooling since the flatter peripheral bevel is adjacent to the steeper central cornea.

The evaluation of the fluorescein pattern at the lens periphery is also beneficial. There should be sufficient clearance peripherally—typically greater than apically—to allow sufficient tear exchange and debris removal while avoiding mechanical irritation as the lens moves across the cornea. If fluorescein pooling is minimal or absent peripherally and seal-off exists, the peripheral curve(s) should be flattened.

Fluorescein pattern evaluation of the rigid lens-to-cornea fitting relationship should be performed both at the fitting visit and at all subsequent follow-up visits. A practitioner's ability to properly assess fluorescein patterns occurs with experience and frequent evaluation. There

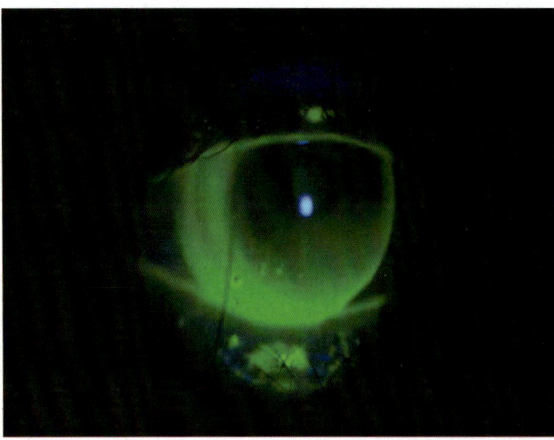

FIGURE 5.5 An apical bearing fluorescein pattern.

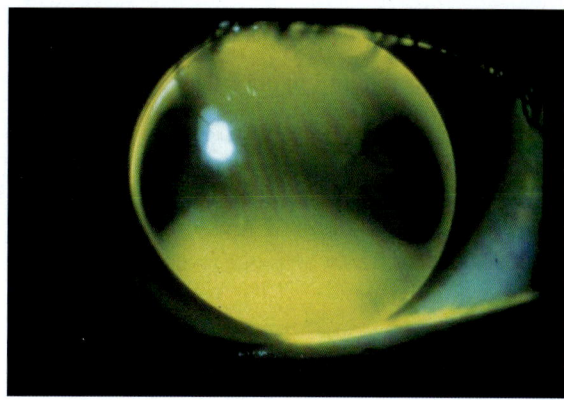

FIGURE 5.6 The dumbbell-shaped fluorescein pattern present with a highly astigmatic patient.

are several educational resources available from the GP Lens Institute (GPLI; www.gpli.info), including an educational CD-ROM entitled "GP Fitting, Evaluation, and Problem-Solving," a GP Lens Management Guide, and a Fluorescein Pattern Identification laminated card. It would be erroneous to believe that fluorescein pattern evaluation is not as important with GP materials as with polymethylmethacrylate (PMMA), as a result of the reduction in edema-related complications. The lens material is only as good as the practitioner's ability to properly evaluate it; a poor lens-to-cornea fitting relationship can result in numerous problems, including desiccation, adhesion, and abrasion. In particular, the fluorescein pattern evaluation is invaluable in the difficult-to-fit cases such as high corneal toricity, irregular/distorted corneas, and keratoconus.[34]

False Fluorescein Patterns: Occasionally, the fluorescein pattern is contrary to the expected appearance. This phenomenon can occur as a result of a variety of causes:

1. Corneal topography. This varies between patients; for example, a patient with a small corneal cap (defined as the region within 0.50 D of the corneal apex) will exhibit a somewhat steeper fluorescein pattern than a patient with a larger-than-average cap.[35,36]
2. Selection of a steep BCR may result in poor tear exchange and a misleading small amount of fluorescein centrally.
3. If the peripheral curve is too steep, peripheral seal-off can occur and the fluorescein pattern can exhibit apical clearance.
4. In certain individuals—particularly dry-eye patients—the fluorescein will dissipate quickly and may create a "pseudoapical flat" relationship; therefore, the pattern should be evaluated immediately after fluorescein instillation.
5. A "pseudosteep" pattern has been reported in high minus fluoro-silicone/acrylate (F-S/A) lenses.[37] Apparently, the edge thickness blocks the fluorescence, giving an appearance of central pooling. Likewise, one would expect that a high plus lens may demonstrate a flatter-than-actual base curve fitting relationship because the thick center would attenuate the light more.

Designs/Fitting Philosophies

There are numerous available methods for determining the rigid lens design parameters for diagnostic fitting. In this section of the chapter, two fitting philosophies will be presented.

There are two primary fitting philosophies for designing and fitting GP lenses, both based on lens position on the eye. The first approach is to design a lens so that it positions consistently under the upper eyelid (i.e., a lid-attached fit), and the second is to design a lens that achieves an interpalpebral fit on the eye.

Studies have been done to compare these two lens designs with respect to comfort, vision, and physiologic response.[38–40] Results are mixed as to which design performs the best because of individual variation in corneal topography, lid/cornea interaction, and lid tension.

Lid-Attachment Fitting and Design

Overall/Optical Zone Diameter: The OAD of a rigid lens should be large enough to allow for a sufficient optical zone while providing good lag with the blink. The OZD typically encompasses anywhere from 65% to 80% of the lens diameter.[41] The size of both OAD and OZD depends on the following factors:

Palpebral Aperture Size/Lid Position: The palpebral aperture size refers to the vertical separation of the lids in the normal state. An average amount of separation is 9.0 to 10.5 mm. If the difference is greater, a larger-diameter lens should be considered; if less, a smaller-diameter lens can be used.

The position of the lids, however, is more important. This varies between patients, and it has been demonstrated that if the upper edge of the lens rides underneath the upper lid when gazing straight ahead, it will be more comfortable than an interpalpebral fitting relationship.[42,43] The reason for this is that the initial rigid lens sensation is usually the result of the lid margin.[44,45] During the blink process, the upper lid moves over the upper edge of the lens; if the position of the upper lid is above the edge of the lens, there will be contact between the two, creating an initial awareness or sensation. However, if the upper lid is positioned at or above the superior limbus, a position not easily obtainable, it may be preferable to select a smaller-diameter lens and a fit steeper than K, and to obtain a well-centered lens that positions, at minimum, 1 mm below the upper lid.

Pupil Size: The diameter of the pupil should be measured in both high and low illumination. Assuming a good lens-to-cornea fitting relationship, the OZD should be greater than the pupil size in dim illumination to minimize the risk of subjective symptoms of flare at night.

Refractive Power: It is often necessary to select a larger OAD/OZD with hyperopic lens powers to provide adequate pupil coverage with the thicker, higher-mass lens. This large OAD, however, should be in combination with a minus lenticular edge design. In addition, although not always the case, it is not uncommon for hyperopia to be accompanied by flatter keratometry values (and myopia by steeper K values); therefore, the same principle as indicated in the following section holds true.

Corneal Curvature: It is recommended to select a larger-than-average OAD with flatter corneal curvatures (e.g., flatter than 41 D) and a smaller-than-average OAD with steeper curvatures (e.g., steeper than 45 D) to maintain an optimum centering lens. A good rule of thumb has been proposed by Caroline and Norman[40]: select an OZD equal to the BCR in millimeters. In other words, a 41.75 D (8.09 mm) BCR would be accompanied by an OZD equal to 8.1 mm, and a 45.50 D (7.42 mm) BCR would be accompanied by an optical zone equal to 7.4 mm.

Lid Tension: The amount of lid tension will play a prominent role in diameter selection. Lid tension can be determined by lid eversion. As this should be performed both at the prefitting evaluation and at all subsequent follow-up visits, one can obtain a good idea of which patients have loose lids (i.e., upper lid everts very easily) and which have tight lids (i.e., upper lid everts with much effort, if at all). Since a loose upper lid will provide little assistance in raising a lens during the blink process, a larger-than-average OAD is recommended in this case.

What are good OAD/OZDs to use? Average values are typically in the 9.4- to 9.6-mm range for an OAD and 7.6- to 8.2-mm range for an OZD. A 9.4/8.0-mm design is a good starting point in many custom-designed lenses. When a larger OAD/OZD is indicated, a 9.8/8.4-mm design is recommended; when a smaller OAD/OZD is indicated, a 9.0/7.6-mm design is recommended.

Bottom Line: The current trend with new GP materials is for manufacturers to recommend larger OADs (i.e., typically in the 9.6-to 10.2-mm range) to optimize initial comfort. This often occurs because of less initial lens movement and good centration.[46] A word of caution is indicated here. A larger lens tends to exhibit more of an effect on the cornea, possibly resulting in molding and distortion. In addition, in a highly flexible material, the potential for limited lens lag and adherence exists; therefore, debris removal and additional oxygen flow are limited. Likewise, selecting a large OZD may result in limited lateral lens movement with the blink since the junction between the BCR and the SCR is located at a more peripheral region of the cornea. This may encourage peripheral corneal desiccation since the lens does not move over the peripheral cornea.[44] Some practitioners prefer to use a large OAD (e.g., 9.6 mm) with a small OZD (e.g., 7.4 mm) for the purpose of creating an optimum midperipheral corneal alignment. This design would be acceptable, assuming that both sufficient lens lag and pupil coverage exist. In addition, when making a change in diameter, it is important that this change is a significant one, which has been found to be a minimum of 0.4 mm in OAD and 0.3 mm in OZD.[47]

It is also important to emphasize that several semi-scleral designs (i.e., 14- to 15-mm OAD) are being introduced for astigmatic patients with healthy eyes.[48] These designs tend to exhibit initial comfort that rivals soft lenses while being much more initially comfortable than standard diameter GP lens designs.[49] It is evident that the future of GP lens applications on healthy eyes could be in some form of scleral design.[50]

Base Curve Radius: The primary purpose of the BCR is to optimize the fitting relationship of the lens to the central and midperipheral cornea. The BCR to be selected depends on several factors, including corneal curvature, the observed fluorescein pattern, and the desired lens-to-cornea fitting relationship. It can be specified in diopters or millimeters (see Appendix 1).

It is important to emphasize that the selection of a given BCR (e.g., "on K") on several patients will result in differences in the observed fluorescein patterns because of differences in corneal topography (apical area, rate of flattening, etc.) and lens design. Typically, a lens fit "on K" will provide an apical clearance fitting relationship since the optical zone is often much larger than the corneal cap or apex (Fig. 5.7).[44] Therefore, to maintain an alignment fitting

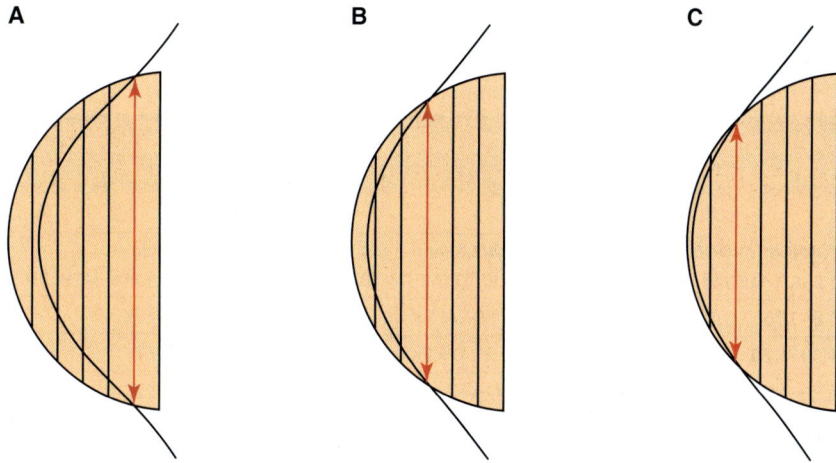

FIGURE 5.7 The fitting relationship of various OZDs. If OZD **(A)** or **(B)** is chosen, a steep fitting relationship will result. The smaller optical zone **(C)** will provide an alignment fitting relationship. (Reprinted with permission from Caroline PJ, Norman CW. A blueprint for rigid lens design. I. *Contact Lens Spectrum.* 1988;3(11).)

relationship, it is necessary in most cases to select a BCR flatter than K. In addition, a flatter BCR will minimize both lens-induced flexure and the potential for seal-off of tear exchange, which can potentially occur with an "on K" fit on a spherical cornea.[51]

What BCR should you select? A philosophy for diameter and BCR selection is provided in Table 5.5.[14]

It is important to mention that if the OZD is smaller than normal, a slightly steeper BCR is necessary. For example, with steeper than 45 D corneal curvatures, a smaller OZD is necessary to maintain alignment. Conversely, if the OZD is larger than normal, a slightly flatter BCR than recommended in Table 5.5 may be indicated. For example, with flatter than 41 D corneal curvature values, a larger OZD is necessary to maintain alignment; in addition, patients with large pupil diameters will need a larger OZD to minimize flare. A simple rule to remember: Flatten the BCR 0.25 D for each increase in OZD of 0.5 mm and steepen the BCR 0.25 D for each decrease in OZD equal to 0.5 mm.[40] Of course, the specific BCR to be selected will depend primarily on the fluorescein pattern, especially if an instrument to measure eccentricity or shape factor of the cornea (i.e., from central to, at minimum, midperipheral cornea) is not available.

A steeper BCR may be necessary with high rather than low astigmatic patients because of many factors, the most important of which is to increase the probability of obtaining an optimum lens-to-cornea fitting relationship. Typically, with high astigmatic patients (i.e., corneal astigmatism >2 D), the BCR has to be steepened, or a bitoric design can be used to obtain the best distribution of lens alignment over the largest area.[28] An "on K" BCR fitted on a highly astigmatic cornea will not only provide very little corneal alignment and subsequent decentration, but the resulting areas of bearing and excessive clearance may also result in lens "rocking" on the cornea with the blink, discomfort caused by an increase in edge contact with the upper lid, and corneal desiccation.

A steeper-than-K BCR is also often necessary with hyperopic patients since the CT is greater and the center of gravity is located more anteriorly; therefore, the lens would have a greater tendency to drop inferiorly after the blink. A steeper-than-K BCR would be more likely to provide a well-centered lens position.

The geometric center of the lens should coincide or be positioned slightly above the patient's line of sight. A slightly superiorly positioned (tucked underneath the lid) lens-to-cornea fitting relationship should maximize patient comfort by minimizing the interaction of the lens edge with the upper lid. This is the basis behind the "lid-attachment" design philosophy developed by Korb and Korb.[42] In addition, this fitting relationship has been found to result in less corneal desiccation than interpalpebral and inferiorly positioned lenses.[52]

TABLE 5.5 Gas-Permeable Diameter and Base Curve Selection Criteria (Lid Attachment)

	OAD/OZD	
CORNEAL CYLINDER (D) (KERATOMETRY)	9.4/8.0 mm (LID ATTACHMENT)	9.8/8.4 mm (LARGE PUPILS/ATHLETES)
0.0–0.75	0.50 D FTK	0.75 D FTK
1.00–1.25	0.25 D FTK	0.50 D FTK
1.50–1.75	"On K"	0.25 D FTK
2.00–2.25 D	0.25 D STK	"On K"
≥2.50	Bitoric design	Bitoric design

FTK, flatter than K; OAD, overall diameter; OZD, optical zone diameter; STK, steeper than K.

The amount of lens lag or downward movement after the blink should be, at minimum, 1 mm and, at maximum, 3 mm. A larger amount of lens lag may result in fluctuation in vision because of flare and possible lens awareness, while a smaller amount of lag could cause adherence with resultant trapped debris and edema. Good pupillary coverage by the OZD should be present throughout the blink process.

What is the bottom line? Although recommendations have been made, it is important to mention that no single BCR selection philosophy can accurately predict the resultant lens positioning on a given patient. Therefore, trial and error, supplemented by fluorescein pattern evaluation, is an important factor in deciding on the appropriate BCR.

Peripheral Curve Radii/Width: The PCRs, which typically encompass the outer 20% to 35% of the lens, surround the OZD of the lens. Designs in common use have either one (i.e., bicurve), two (i.e., tricurve with a SCR and a PCR), or three (i.e., tetracurve with an SCR and ICR and a PCR) peripheral curves. In addition, some lens designs utilize an aspheric periphery with a continuous flattening of the peripheral region of the lens. Each curve must be progressively flatter than the adjacent, more centrally positioned curve to provide proper lens clearance from the cornea. The peripheral curve, in particular, serves the following three functions[53]:

- To prevent the edge of the lens from digging into the corneal surface during lens movement.
- To permit proper circulation of the tears beneath the lens to maintain the metabolism of the cornea.
- To support a meniscus at the edge of the lens to provide forces that cause the lens to center.

The peripheral curves serve no optical purpose. If the contact lens is decentered such that the peripheral curves are directly in front of the visual axis, flare will result.[54]

The application of peripheral curves creates a sharp ridge between the curves. This ridge can prevent adequate circulation of tears to the central cornea and can also impair the removal of metabolic debris from under the lens. Therefore, the application of a blend will result in more even tear flow. Typically the blend, which is performed with a radius tool midway between the PCRs values (see Chapter 9), can either be light, medium, or heavy. At minimum, a medium blend should be performed to enhance debris removal. Blending the PCRs junction will increase lens lag caused by the smoother surface and may also increase initial comfort.[55]

The distance from the lens edge perpendicular to the peripheral cornea is termed *edge clearance*. A geometrical and therefore quantifiable term, *edge lift,* has also been used to approximate edge clearance; this pertains to the distance between the lens edge and an extension of the BCR of the lens (therefore, it is a slightly larger value than clearance). If the PCR is flattened and/or the PCW is increased, edge clearance will increase, all other lens parameters being held constant. Changing the PCR and/or width has more of an effect on edge clearance than changing the secondary or intermediate curves.[56]

Lens positioning can be influenced by the amount of edge lift. Essentially, as the edge lift increases, the interaction with the upper lid will increase.[57] A high edge-lift/clearance design will result in excessive interaction with the upper lid and a superiorly decentered lens. An excessively low edge-lift/clearance design will result in very little, if any, interaction with the upper lid and potentially position inferiorly. To provide good tear circulation and debris removal, the use of a flat, wide peripheral curve has been customarily used in traditional PMMA lens design because of enhanced oxygen flow to the cornea. These philosophies typically used either a bicurve design or a tricurve design, with an SCR approximately 1.0 to 1.5 mm flatter than the BCR and a PCR equal to 12.00 to 12.25 mm. For example, a lens design equal to 7.8-mm BCR, 9.2/0.3-mm SCR/SCW, and 12.25/0.4-mm PCR/PCW was not uncommon. However, excessive edge clearance may result in lens decentration, lens awareness, and corneal desiccation.[44,58–61] The latter problem may result from a combination of a receding tear meniscus as it is pulled underneath the lens edge from the adjacent peripheral cornea and a possible alteration in the normal blink pattern caused by the upper lid contacting the anteriorly positioned edge.[53,62,63] The decentration may result from either inferior displacement caused by the increased contact between edge and lid or actually superior displacement caused by an alignment of the flatter part of the lens with the flatter corneal region.[44]

What peripheral curve system should we use? As GP lenses are not as dependent on the tear pump as PMMA and since many of these materials are silicone-based, presenting the possibility of a short over-the-lens tear breakup time[64] and evaporation of the peripheral tear pool,[62] a lower edge-clearance design should be advantageous. Most aspheric designs (to be discussed later in this chapter) align well with the paracentral and midperipheral cornea and, therefore, have a relatively low edge clearance. If such an option is not feasible, the following peripheral curve system, tetracurve, is recommended by the first author:

$$SCR/W = BCR + 0.8/0.3 \text{ mm}$$

$$ICR/W = SCR + 1.0/0.2 \text{ mm}$$

$$PCR/W = ICR + 1.4/0.2 \text{ mm}$$

For example, if the BCR = 7.8 mm:

$$\frac{SCR}{W} = 7.8 + 0.8 = 8.6/0.3 \text{ mm}$$

$$\frac{ICR}{W} = 8.6 + 1.0 = 9.6/0.2 \text{ mm}$$

$$\frac{PCR}{W} = 9.6 + 1.4 = 11.0/0.2 \text{ mm}$$

However, to maintain a fairly constant edge clearance, the peripheral curve system must be flattened at a greater rate with flat BCRs and flattened at a lesser rate for steep BCRs. Therefore, the aforementioned peripheral curve design philosophy can be used for the average BCRs; however, slightly flatter than recommended values should be used with flatter BCRs and slightly steeper values with steeper BCRs.

Lenses having steeper than recommended PCRs (i.e., low edge clearance) are often more difficult to remove and may also trap debris.[65] In addition, increased risk of lens adherence[66,67] and vascularized limbal keratitis (VLK)[68] have been associated with the use of low edge-lift designs.

What is the bottom line? It is important to avoid excessively flat/wide peripheral curves and especially a limited curve design (i.e., bicurve), which can provide poor midperipheral alignment with the cornea. Likewise, it is important to verify the number and width of the peripheral curves (radius is extremely difficult to verify) and the quality and accuracy of the blends.

Center Thickness: CT is dependent on many other lens parameters, but primarily lens power and OAD. The CT is greater and the center of gravity more anterior for plus lenses, while the edge thickness is greater and the center of gravity more posterior for minus lenses.[41]

There is a fine line between a lens that is too thin and a lens that is too thick. A lens that is too thin will likely be too unstable and could flex significantly on the eye as well as be prone to warpage. Therefore, standard-thickness designs are recommended in moderate-to-high corneal astigmatism (i.e., >1.50 D). A lens that is too thick, however, may result in inferior decentration, with accompanying variable vision, corneal desiccation, and injection.[69]

The introduction of ultrathin lenses in many of the new lower-Dk lens materials has resulted in reducing the incidence of decentration and increasing patient satisfaction,[70–73] although initial comfort may not be better.[74] These lenses are as much as 50% thinner than standard designs. For example, a −3.00 D lens may be made as thin as 0.10 mm in a −3.00 D power as compared to a standard thickness of approximately 0.14 mm.

What CT should be ordered? Recommended CT values for standard (not ultrathin) designs are given in Table 5.6. The recommended CT values vary from material to material and from manufacturer to manufacturer.

What is the bottom line? It is extremely important to verify CT because an inaccurate value may affect lens performance. Often, it is easier for the laboratory to manufacture a thicker-than-necessary lens to reduce the probability of breakage during the procedure. In fact, in a study in which center and edge thickness values were the only parameters not provided to the laboratory (lenses of four different powers were ordered from eight laboratories selected at random), the differences in CT, overall thickness, and lens mass were significant for a given power.[75] A decision on CT should not be made on the basis of Dk alone but on factors such as vision, lens stability, and positioning. For example, increasing CT by 0.04 mm will increase mass by 24% but will only decrease equivalent oxygen percentage by <1%.[76]

The sign of a good laboratory is the ability to consistently manufacture thin lens designs. Likewise, although Table 5.6 is a recommended guide, it is a good idea to obtain the recommended CT table from the manufacturer for every GP material to be used in your practice.

Edge Thickness/Design: The edge design is an extremely important and often underestimated parameter that can be the primary variable affecting comfort and lens positioning. A thin, tapered, rolled-edge design is desirable. The edge can be divided into three zones.[77] The anterior zone interacts with the upper lid during blinking. The posterior zone is often a narrow reverse curve that is placed onto the posterior lens surface to flare the edge away from the cornea. This assists in allowing free movement of the lens across the cornea. The junction between the anterior and posterior zones is the lens apex, which must be well rounded to minimize lens awareness during the blink.

The shape of the lens edge is important as well. As indicated previously, Korb and Korb[42] recommend an edge design that has its apex anteriorly to assist the upper lid in lifting and attaching to the upper lens edge. Likewise, it has been found that lenses with well-rounded anterior edge profiles were significantly more comfortable than lenses with square anterior edges; there was no significant difference between a rounded and square posterior edge profile.[78] Therefore, it was concluded that the interaction of the edge with the eyelid is more important in determining comfort than edge effects on the cornea.

Several studies have demonstrated the inconsistency of edge design with GP materials.[78–80] One study found that not only was there much inconsistency between materials, but also there

TABLE 5.6 Custom Design Gas-Permeable Center Thickness Values (mm)[a]

POWER (D)	DK VALUE	
	20–49	50 +
−1.00	0.18	0.19
−2.00	0.16	0.18
−3.00	0.14	0.16
−4.00	0.14	0.15
−5.00	0.13	0.14
≥−6.00	0.13	0.14

[a]Standard thickness.
Dk, oxygen permeability.

were large differences within lenses of the same material from the same manufacturer with identical parameters.[79] Typically, as a material increases in Dk, it also increases in softness and potential for chipping and breakage. If, in fact, an unverified lens is defective from an edge that is too sharp, too blunt, or chipped, but is nevertheless dispensed to the patient, the result may be a dissatisfied patient who may never again desire to wear GP lenses. However, because of the advanced manufacturing and polishing methods in common use today, inconsistent and defective edges are much less common. Nevertheless, edge verification, as recommended in Chapter 7, is important. One device that is commercially available only to evaluate the edge is the Contact Lens Edge Profile Analyzer (CLEPA, from Valley Contax, Springfield, OR) (Fig. 5.8).

What about the interaction of CT and edge thickness? Both CT and edge thickness change with changes in OAD and with different lens powers.[81] Edge thickness is greater in medium-to-high minus powers and CT is greater in low minus and all plus powers. Edge and CT are not equal at plano but at approximately -2.00 D power.[44,81]

What are lenticular designs? As a result of the variation in edge thickness with lens power and OAD, the use of a lenticular design is sometimes indicated. In a lenticulated lens, the front surface consists of a central optical portion surrounded by a peripheral carrier portion that is thinner and flatter.[54] The thickness of the lens at the junction of the optic cap and carrier portion should equal 0.12 to 0.14 mm.[43,82] If it is thicker, lens mass is unnecessarily added to the lens; if thinner, the lens can break at this junction.

In high minus powers, either an anterior CN bevel (Fig. 5.9) or plus lenticular design (Fig. 5.10) can be used to reduce edge thickness, with the latter option most often used. Plus lenticular designs are often used because they minimize problems associated with thick edges such as lens awareness, inferior positioning caused by lid–lens interaction, and corneal desiccation resulting from compromise in the normal blinking process. In addition, plus lenticular designs reduce CT and overall lens mass. Typically, minus lens powers of ≥5 D are lenticulated because the edge thickness is ≥0.20 mm without this modification.[38] A minus lenticular design to increase edge thickness is also very important to enhance lid interaction with the edge and

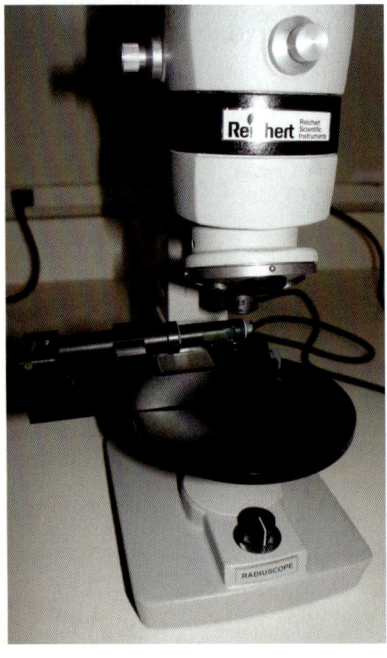

FIGURE 5.8 The Contact Lens Edge Profile Analyzer (Valley Contax, Springfield, OR).

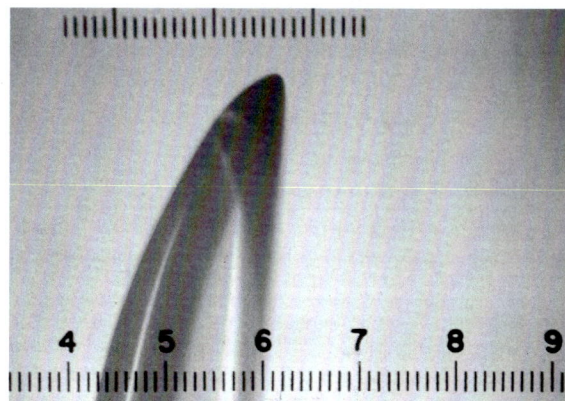

FIGURE 5.9 Anterior CN bevel.

minimize inferior decentration. A minus lenticular design is recommended with minus powers ≤ −1.50 D and all plus power lenses. A summary of minus versus plus lens design parameters is given in Table 5.7.

What is the bottom line? The importance of verifying every lens edge cannot be emphasized enough. This is the number one means of reducing the initial discomfort while also ensuring that your laboratory has good quality control. The hallmark of any given laboratory is its ability to fabricate a good edge. The use of a lenticular edge design, when appropriate, is a win-win situation as it typically improves lens centration while increasing oxygen transmission.

What is the bottom line on lens design? A summary of important factors in GP lens design and fitting is given in Figure 5.11.

One factor that is especially important to adhere to is as follows: Whenever you make a change in lens design, make sure it is a significant one. In other words, merely increasing the diameter 0.1 to 0.2 mm, decreasing the CT by 0.01 mm, or changing the base curve by 0.25 D will rarely have the desired effect on the lens-to-cornea fitting relationship. The parameter changes necessary to have a significant effect on the fitting relationship are given in Table 5.8.[47]

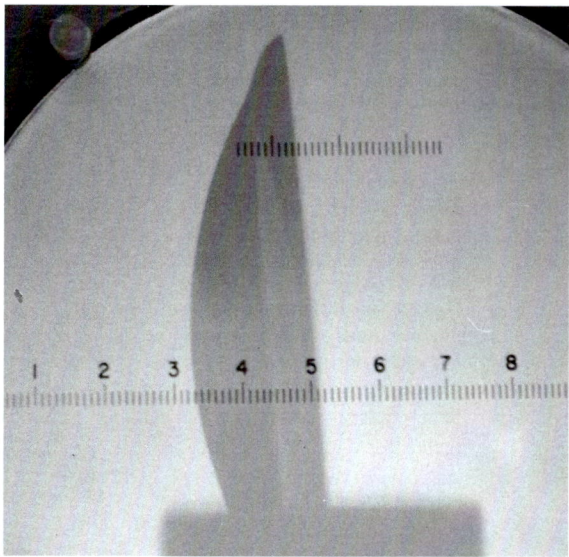

FIGURE 5.10 Plus lenticular design.

TABLE 5.7 Minus versus Plus Lens Design Parameters

PARAMETER	MINUS POWER	PLUS POWER
BCR	Flatter than K	Steeper than K
OAD	Smaller (8.8–9.6 mm)	Larger (9.2–9.8 mm)
CT	Lesser (<0.20 mm)	Greater (>0.20 mm)
Edge design	Thicker—plus lenticular for all high (>−5 D) powers; minus lenticular for all powers with low (<1.50 D) powers	Thinner—minus lenticular necessary

BCR, base curve radius; CT, center thickness; OAD, overall diameter.

Interpalpebral Fitting

There are many similarities to lid-attachment fitting in selecting the proper lens design to achieve a between the lids or interpalpebral fitting relationship. Some of the candidates for such a design would be individuals with an upper lid positioned at or above the superior limbus, plus

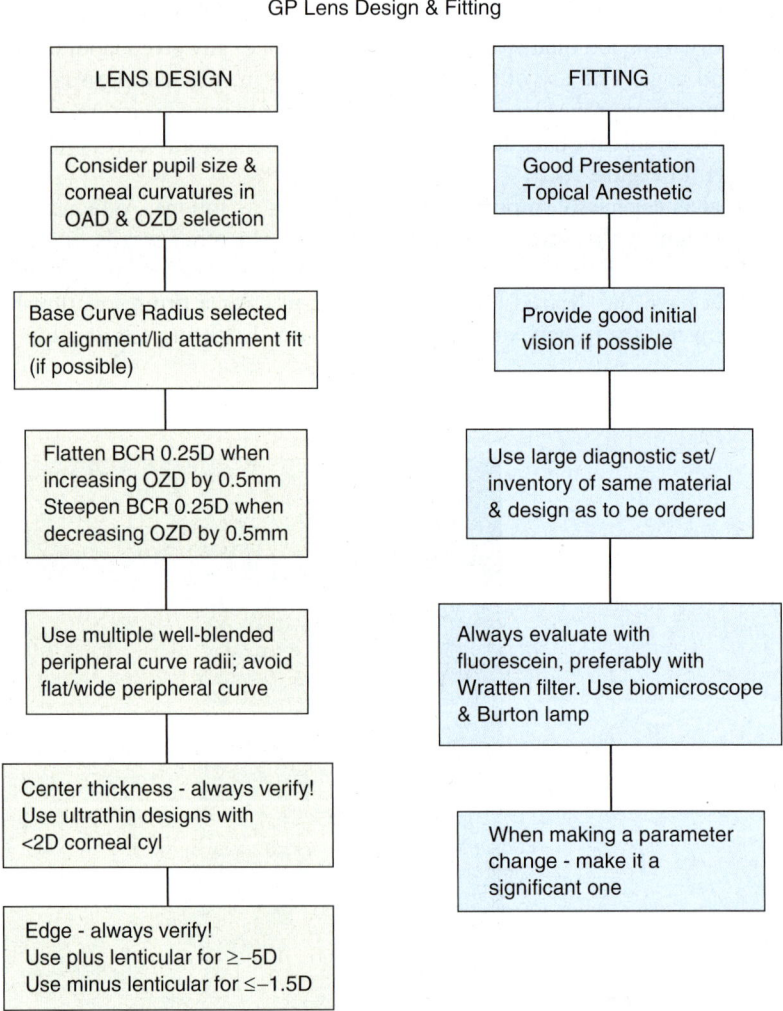

FIGURE 5.11 Lens design/fitting nomogram.

TABLE 5.8 Clinically Significant Parameter Changes

PARAMETER	CHANGE FOR CLINICAL SIGNIFICANCE
BCR	0.50 D (approximately 0.1 mm)
OAD/OZD	0.4/0.3 mm
PCR	0.5 mm
CT (high Dk)	0.02 mm

Dk, oxygen permeability.

Reprinted with permission from Szczotka LB. RGP parameter changes: how much change is significant? *Contact Lens Spectrum*. 2001;16(4):18.

powers designs in which gravity tends to bring the lens more inferiorly, and Asian eyes in which a small diameter may position better on the eye.[83] Particular differences are detailed below.

Overall Lens Diameter: The overall lens diameter is determined by the average corneal diameter (horizontal visible iris diameter [HVID]) of the patient, the interpalpebral aperture height, and the contact lens power. These factors affect the contact lens center of gravity and thus lens position, lens stability, the option to have larger back and front optic zone diameters (BOZDs and FOZDs), lens comfort, and the physiologic response to the lens (i.e., 3 and 9 o'clock staining and palpebral conjunctival response).

The center of gravity of contact lenses and thus the lens position can be moved anteriorly (lower position) with smaller-diameter lenses and posteriorly (higher-riding lens position) with larger-diameter lenses. Selection of overall lens diameter is based on Table 5.9, taking into account interpalpebral aperture height, HVID, and pupil size. Normally, the selection for an interpalpebral fit is based on the HVID, unless the interpalpebral aperture height is unusually small or if the pupil size is unusually large.

Adjustments to the lens diameter can be made based on the contact lens power. The power has an effect on lens position because of the location of the center of gravity (CG). Generally, plus lenses whose CG is forward because of thick CT result in a low lens position. Plus lenses should be designed with larger OADs (with lenticulated minus carriers and thinner CT designs) to move the CG back and toward a more centered interpalpebral position. Conversely, high minus lenses tend to be high riding because of the CG being too far backward and so should be designed with a smaller diameter (with lenticulated plus carriers and slightly thicker CT designs) to move the CG forward to achieve an interpalpebral lens-fitting relationship.

TABLE 5.9 Gas-Permeable Lens Diameter Selection (Interpalpebral)

FACTOR	MEASUREMENT	PREDICTED DIAMETER
PA	<8.0 mm	9.0–9.3 mm
	8.5–11.0 mm	9.4–9.6 mm
	>11.5 mm	9.7–9.9 mm
HVID	10.0–11.0 mm	9.2–9.4 mm
	11.5–12.5 mm	9.5–9.7 mm
	>12.5 mm	9.8–10.0 mm
PS	PS + (3.5–4.0 mm) = BOZD	BOZD + (1.2–1.4 mm)

BOZD, back optic zone diameter; HVID, horizontal visible iris diameter; PA, palpebral aperture; PS, pupil size.

What is the bottom line? A lens that is too small may result in decentration and exposure of the pupil (especially in the dark), causing flare, a visual disturbance resulting in visual discomfort. A lens that is too large may initially feel more comfortable but may result in conjunctival (CT) staining if the lens overlaps the limbus in any position with movement on the blink.

Base Curve Radius Selection: In interpalpebral fitting lens design, an aligned lens-to-cornea relationship needs to be achieved. Corneal topography, to check for regularity of the corneal astigmatism, whether the astigmatism is centrally located or extends out to the limbus, the eccentricity values (*e*-value), and the simulated K readings, are essential to determine the base curve (or back optic zone radius [BOZR]) that will result in an aligned fluorescein pattern according to the amount of corneal astigmatism and lens diameter. Figure 5.12 shows corneal

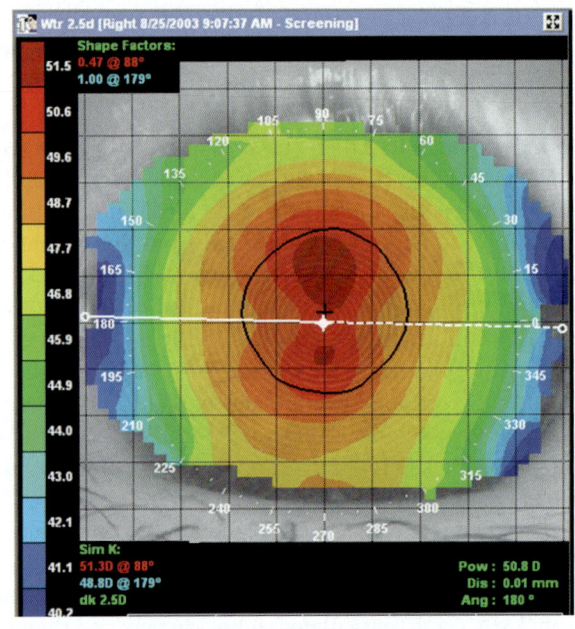

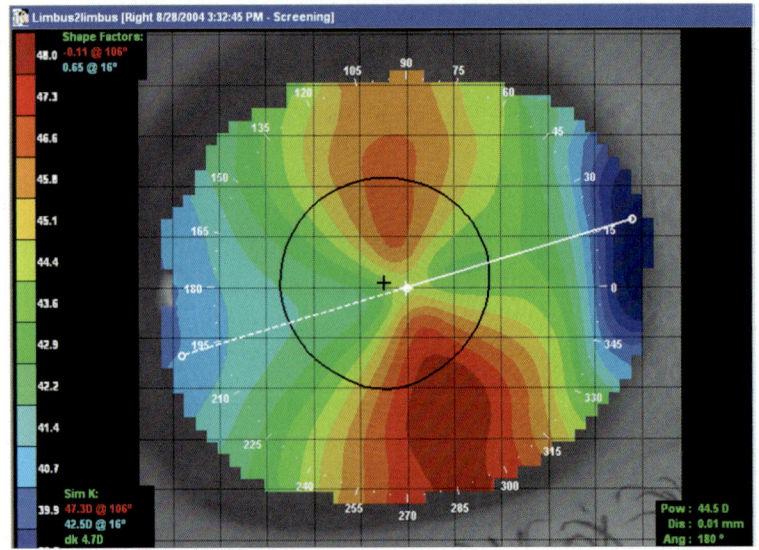

FIGURE 5.12 Corneal topographies demonstrating regular astigmatism that is only located centrally **(A)** versus regular astigmatism extending from limbus to limbus **(B)**. (Photographs courtesy of Randy Kojima, Precision Technology, BE Enterprises.)

topographies demonstrating regular astigmatism that is only located centrally versus regular astigmatism extending from limbus to limbus.

It is important to note that the shape of the cornea resembles a prolate ellipse. The e-value is a measure of the rate of flattening from the center of the cornea to the periphery.

The selection of the BCR varies with the lens diameter that was initially chosen and depends on the amount of corneal astigmatism. Table 5.10 shows the relationship between the amount of corneal astigmatism and the BCR to choose for an interpalpebral, aligned fitting relationship for lens diameters of 9.2 to 9.4 mm.

If the lens diameter that was chosen was <9.2 mm (i.e., 8.8–9.1 mm), then the rules of thumb based on the ΔK from Table 5.10 can be used and the BCR that was calculated can be steepened by an additional 0.25 D. If the selected OAD is >9.6 mm (i.e., 9.7–9.9 mm), then the calculated BCR from the table can be flattened by 0.25 D. These adjustments for smaller and larger lens diameters will ensure that an aligned fitting relationship is still maintained to result in an interpalpebral positioned lens by maintaining the same sag. One will know that the proper lens-to-cornea fitting relationship has been achieved by instilling fluorescein and interpreting the fluorescein pattern. An aligned fitting relationship in the central pattern must be achieved. Lenses that are either fitting too flat or too steep cannot be accepted and adjustments must be made.

What is the bottom line? Proper selection of the BCR according to the amount of corneal astigmatism that is present and with an average lens diameter will ensure that the lens-to-cornea fitting relationship will result in an interpalpebral fitting lens as the BCR steepens with increasing astigmatism. In addition, proper assessment and interpretation of the fluorescein pattern in ensuring that the lens-to-cornea relationship is neither too steep nor too flat will result in an ideal interpalpebral fitting relationship.

Peripheral Curve Radii/Width and Optical Zone Diameter: The selection of the widths and radii of the peripheral curves and resultant BOZDs will strongly determine the amount of peripheral edge clearance that determines the lens position (and final comfort) and the central lens-to-cornea fitting relationship (from OZD), respectively.

To achieve an interpalpebral lens positioning, one must design the periphery (and BOZD or BOZR) to maintain an axial edge lift (AEL) and resultant axial edge clearance (AEC) of 0.10 to 0.12 mm and >0.08 to 0.10 mm, respectively.[74] These values assume that the average cornea has an e-value between 0.45 and 0.55.

As defined earlier, AEL is the vertical distance from the lens edge to an extension of the BOZR of the lens. Radial edge lift is the extension of the lens edge perpendicular to the extension of the BCR. AEC is the vertical distance from the lens edge to the peripheral cornea and is usually less than the AEL (Fig. 5.13).

Regardless of the diameter of the lens and the BCR, a constant amount of AEL/AEC is desired and is to be maintained when fitting the average patient. On average (i.e., for an average e-value), this amount is 0.10 to 0.12 mm for AEC (usually reported in micrometers). This amount of AEC should result in a 0.50-mm-wide band around the lens periphery as seen with fluorescein instilled in the eye.

TABLE 5.10 Base Curve Radius Selection for a 9.2- to 9.4-mm Overall Diameter Lens

CORNEAL CYLINDER	BCR
0.00 to −1.00 D	On K
−1.12 to −2.00 D	1/4 delta K + flat K
−2.12 to −2.87 D	1/3 delta K + flat K
>−3.00 D	Back surface/bitoric lens

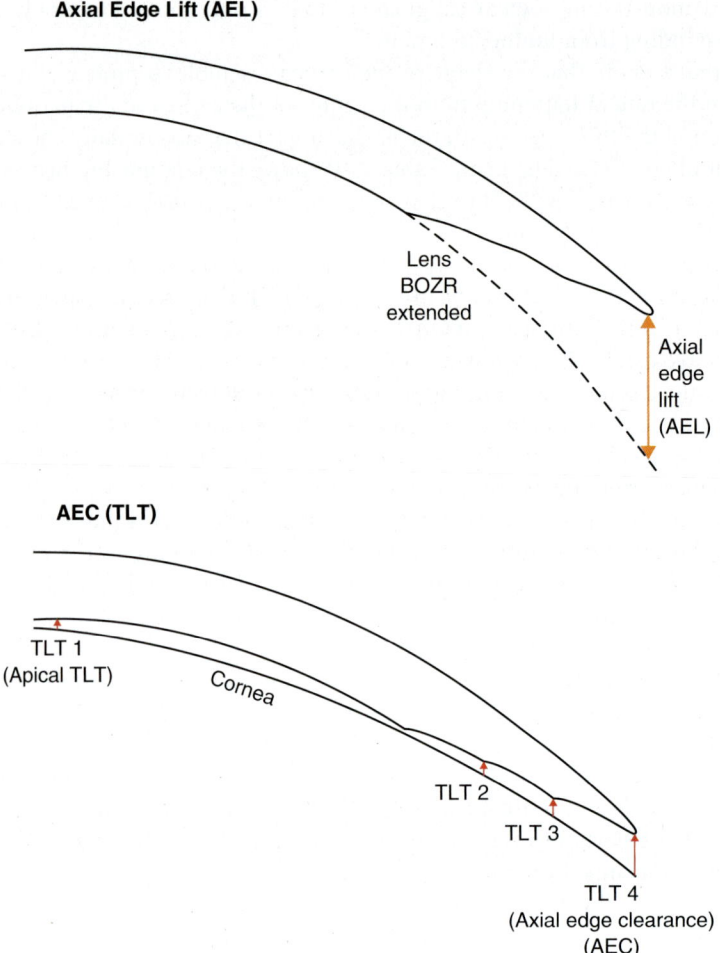

FIGURE 5.13 Axial edge lift and axial edge clearance.

Constant Axial Edge Lift: If the same radius value is added to the BCR for the SCR and PCR, the resulting AEL will not be a constant but will be higher for steep lenses (6.5–7.3 mm) and lower for flat lenses (7.9–8.3 mm). Thus, a computer program aids the practitioner and the laboratories in manufacturing lenses with constant AELs regardless of the BCR. Most diagnostic lens sets have made the adjustments in SCR and PCR to maintain a constant AEL.

Once the lens is inserted, the subject's individual corneal topography in the periphery will determine the appearance of the fluorescein pattern in the periphery (i.e., the AEC). Adaptations in AEL can then be made to either increase or decrease the AEL to achieve the ideal AEC after central alignment is achieved. Also, when changes in OAD, OZD, and BCR are made, care must be taken to first maintain the AEL/AEC. Once these new parameters are ordered and, with this new trial lens, an alignment fit is achieved, then adjustments to the periphery can be made.

Changes in AEL/AEC are made only after the central fluorescein pattern demonstrates an alignment fitting relationship.

Table 5.11 provides an average selection amount for the SCW and PCW and BCR. Table 5.12 outlines the average amount that the BCR needs to be flattened to result in the radii of the secondary and peripheral curves to maintain an approximate AEL of 0.12 mm.

What is the bottom line? Only adjust the AEC as seen with the fluorescein pattern by adjusting either the SCR or PCR or SCW or PCW after an aligned central fluorescein pattern is achieved. These average values of AEL (plus AEC) are based on an average corneal eccentricity

TABLE 5.11 SCW, PCW, and BCR Selection to Maintain an Approximate AEL of 0.12 mm

LENS DESIGN	WIDTHS
Tricurve (lens diameter: 9.0–9.6 mm)	SCW = 0.25–0.35 mm
	PCW = 0.30–0.40 mm
Tetracurve (lens diameter: 9.7–10.2 mm)	SCW − 1 = 0.20 mm
	PCW − 2 = 0.30 mm
OZD	= OAD −1.1 − 1.6 mm

AEL, axial edge lift; BCR, base curve radius; OAD, overall diameter; OZD, optical zone diameter; PCW, peripheral curve width; SCW, secondary curve width.

(as measured via a corneal topographer). Corneal e-values that are well outside that average will result in an aligned central fluorescein pattern but may demonstrate an AEC that is either insufficient (if e-value is much higher, 0.65–1.0) or excessive (if e-value is much lower, 0.25–0.40).

Center Thickness: As a general rule of thumb for lenses of high-Dk values, Table 5.13 offers some further suggestions to select CT.

What is the bottom line? In choosing the most appropriate CT of a lens, consideration of the material Dk and thus resultant transmission of oxygen must be considered along with the factors that control lens flexure, including the amount of corneal astigmatism, lens-to-cornea fitting relationship, and material rigidity.

Edge Thickness Design: To maintain comfort with an interpalpebral lens design, the edge contour must be as thin and as smooth as possible. All plus lenses and high (>−4.00 D) minus lenses are lenticulated with minus or plus carriers, respectively, to achieve the proper lens positioning to counter the forces of the CG. This will allow plus lenses to sit up and more centrally and minus lenses to sit lower and more centrally from their usual positions on the eye. Excessively flat minus carriers (combined with excessive edge clearance) will result in superior lens positioning.

What is the bottom line? Look at the comfort of the patient and lens position to determine if an interpalpebral fitting has been achieved. If not, the FOZD that controls the size of the lenticular carrier and the edge thickness to improve both comfort and centration can be adjusted. The smaller the FOZD for a plus lens, the larger the effect that the minus carrier will have in lifting the lens position. Conversely, the larger the FOZD for a minus lens, the larger the effect of the plus carrier in lowering the lens position. Parameters of a typical interpalpebral fitting set are provided in Table 5.14.

TABLE 5.12 SCR and PCR to Maintain an Approximate AEL of 0.12 mm

LENS DESIGN	SCR/PCR
Tricurve (lens diameter = 9.0–9.6 mm)	SCR = BCR + 0.8–1.0 mm (flatter)
	PCR = BCR + 1.5–2.5 mm (flatter)
Tetracurve (lens diameter = 9.7–10.2 mm)	SCR −1 = BCR + 0.8–1 mm (flatter)
	SCR −2 = BCR + 1.5–2.5 mm (flatter)
	PCR = BCR + 2.5–3.5 mm (flatter)

AEL, axial edge lift; BCR, base curve radius; PCR, peripheral curve radius; SCR, secondary curve radius.

TABLE 5.13 Center Thickness (DK >50)

POWER	CT
Plano	0.20 mm
Minus	Subtract 0.02 mm per diopter of power from initial 0.20 mm up to a limit of CT = 0.10 mm
Plus	Add 0.02 mm per diopter of power from initial 0.20 mm up to a limit of CT = 0.30 mm, then lenticulate to keep CT low

CT, center thickness; Dk, oxygen permeability.

Corneal Topography Based

Corneal topography, to check for regularity of the corneal astigmatism, whether the astigmatism is centrally located or extends out to the limbus, the eccentricity values (e-value) and the simulated K readings, is essential to determine the base curve (or [BOZR]) that will result in an aligned fluorescein pattern according to the amount of corneal astigmatism and lens diameter. The shape of our cornea resembles a prolate ellipse. The e-value is a measure of the rate of flattening from the center of the cornea to the periphery. For an average eye, this value is between 0.40 and 0.57.[85–87]

The use of corneal topography instrumentation can be a valuable asset for any practitioner desiring to increase contact lens patient satisfaction and success. This is especially important as it has been found that only 40% of lenses fit empirically, using keratometry and refraction only,

TABLE 5.14 Parameters of a Representative Interpalpebral Fitting Set

BCR	SCR/W	PCR/W	OAD/OZD	RX	AEL	REL	CT
8.55	9.44/.3	12.00/.4	9.8/8.4	−3.00	0.115	.094	.14
8.44	9.24/.3	11.75/.4	9.8/8.4	−3.00	0.114	.093	.14
8.33	9.10/.3	11.50/.4	9.8/8.4	−3.00	0.115	.093	.14
8.23	9.00/.3	11.50/.4	9.6/8.2	−3.00	0.115	.094	.14
8.13	8.90/.3	11.15/.4	9.6/8.2	−3.00	0.114	.093	.14
8.08	8.85/.3	11.00/.4	9.6/8.2	−3.00	0.114	.092	.11
8.04	8.80/.3	10.89/.4	9.6/8.2	−3.00	0.115	.092	.14
7.99	8.78/.3	10.70/.4	9.6/8.2	−3.00	0.114	.092	.11
7.94	8.75/.3	10.60/.4	9.6/8.2	−3.00	0.115	.092	.14
7.90	8.65/.3	10.50/.4	9.6/8.2	−3.00	0.114	.091	.11
7.85	8.55/.3	10.45/.4	9.6/8.2	−3.00	0.114	.091	.14
7.80	8.45/.3	10.40/.4	9.6/8.2	−3.00	0.115	.091	.11
7.76	8.50/.3	10.35/.4	9.4/8.0	−3.00	0.114	.091	.11
7.67	8.37/.3	10.15/.4	9.4/8.0	−3.00	0.114	.090	.11
7.58	8.20/.3	10.00/.4	9.4/8.0	−3.00	0.114	.090	.10
7.50	8.00/.3	9.95/.4	9.4/8.0	−3.00	0.114	.087	.11
7.42	8.32/.3	10.30/.3	9.2/8.0	−3.00	0.111	.087	.10
7.34	8.15/.3	10.45/.3	9.2/8.0	−3.00	0.116	.091	.11
7.18	7.87/.3	10.20/.3	9.2/8.0	−5.00	0.122	.094	.12
7.03	7.85/.3	9.95/.3	9.2/8.0	−5.00	0.128	.097	.12

AEL = 0.11 mm. Rx is in diopters; all other parameters are in millimeters.

AEL, axial edge lift; BCR, base curve radius; CT, center thickness; OAD, overall diameter; OZD, optical zone diameter; PCR/W, peripheral curve radius/width; REL, radial edge lift; SCR/W, secondary curve radius/width.

resulted in first fit success.[88,89] However, it was also found that in 88% of the cases in which lenses were changed, the change in lens parameters originated from midperipheral differences between corneal shape as originated with corneal topography and lens shape as predicted from keratometry readings. In other words, the great majority of lens-to-cornea fitting relationships could have been optimized before fitting if corneal topography data would have been used.

Corneal topography instrumentation can provide the practitioner with much more information about the cornea (apex location, rate of flattening, irregularity) while simplifying the fitting process via obtaining recommended lens design information based upon corneal topography. The lens design parameters can be changed and their effect on a simulated fluorescein pattern viewed. These software programs typically have a recommended design philosophy, which should result in an alignment or near alignment simulated fluorescein pattern. The practitioner often has the option of custom designing the lenses as well. One of the most important benefits of all such programs is the ability to view a simulated fluorescein pattern prior to diagnostic lens application. The proximity of the posterior lens surface to the anterior surface of the cornea and the thickness of the layer of tear fluid in between can be viewed in various shades of green. This allows lens fitting with a preevaluation of the actual lens base-curve-to-cornea fitting relationship via the tear lens thickness, rather than a numerical estimate provided by keratometry. Often it is possible to make lens design changes and then, by recalculating, the revised simulated fluorescein pattern can be observed. Therefore, changes in PCRs and PCWs (i.e., edge clearance), diameter, and BCR can be made and the revised fluorescein pattern determined prior to lens application. There have been reports of 90% or more patients having a similar fluorescein pattern with their actual lens as that simulated with topography-based contact lens software.[90–92] When differences do exist, they may be attributed to software limitations such as an absence of simulated lens movement, flexure, lid position and tension, and corneal periphery topographical data inaccuracy.[93,94] However, the programs continue to improve and some programs provide the ability to simulate such factors as lens decentration and tilt. Several software programs have the capability of sending information, including contact lens orders, topography information, etc. to contact lens laboratories or other practitioners. In addition, several manufacturers are interfacing their computer numerical control (CNC) computer-driven lathes with topography software programs so that the practitioner can send topography information and lens parameters directly to the manufacturer.

There are several corneal topographers available today with the capability of successfully and accurately developing empirical fitted GP lens designs. Representative programs include the OrthoTool (www.orthotool.com)[95] and the WAVE system, which is associated with the Keratron Corneal Topographer.[96] Both of these systems allow the fitter to design spherical, toric, multifocal, keratoconic, or reverse geometry design.

Another such design has been developed by Randy Kojima and Patrick Caroline and is available with the Medmont E300 Corneal Topographer from Precision Technology, Vancouver, BC. The rules they have established designing GP lenses from corneal topography are provided in Table 5.15.[97] A representative case is provided to illustrate the applications of this software.

TABLE 5.15 Rules for Designing GP Lenses from Corneal Topography

1. **Diameter selection:** The optimum diameter should be large enough to stabilize the lens along the horizontal meridian while smaller than the visible iris diameter to allow for 1 mm of movement vertically.
2. **Apical clearance:** The central base curve should be steep enough to clear the corneal apex (definite apical clearance—approximately 20 microns).
3. **Horizontal alignment:** The GP lens should be steep enough to land midperipherally along the horizontal meridian.
4. **Vertical channel of tears:** The lens should exhibit unobstructed movement along the vertical meridian.

Reprinted with permission from Kojima R, Caroline P. Designing GPs from corneal topography. *Contact Lens Spectrum.* 2009;24(10).

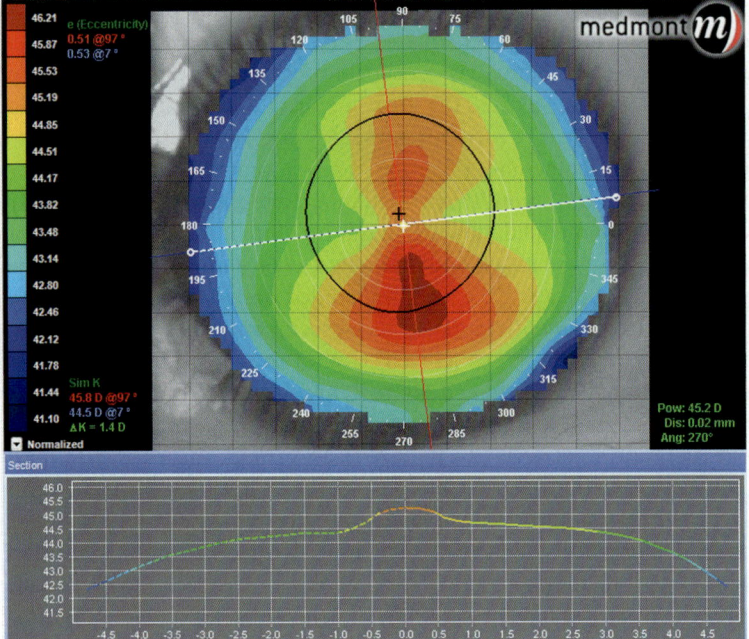

FIGURE 5.14 Axial/sagittal/power map.

This patient has sim K readings of 44.50 @ 007; 45.8 @ 097. The axial map (Fig. 5.14), tangential map (Fig. 5.15), and elevation maps (Fig. 5.16) are provided. Elevation or height maps are especially beneficial for both the design and manufacture of custom GP lenses.

Determining Overall Lens Diameter (OAD): In this design, the OAD is selected to be 2 mm less than the measured visible iris diameter (VID). In Case 1, the VID was approximately 11 mm; therefore, a 9.0-mm diameter was selected.

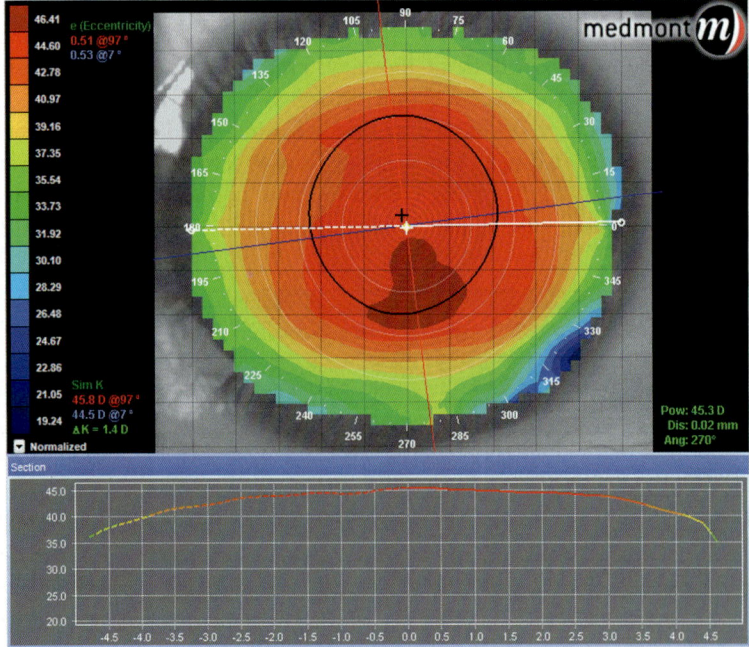

FIGURE 5.15 Tangential/instantaneous map.

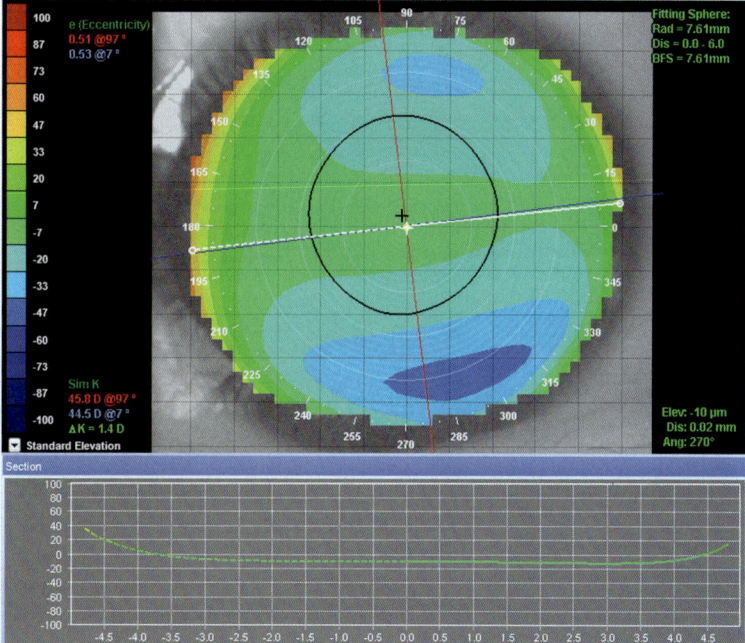

FIGURE 5.16 Elevation map.

Determining the Base Curve Radius (BCR): An advantage of topography-based fitting is the ability to design lenses with a specific number of microns of clearance. The designers recommend a BCR resulting in 20 to 30 microns of central clearance. In the above case, the calculated design with a 9.0-mm OAD, a 7.59-mm BCR, and a 7.50 OZD resulted in a central clearance of only 9 microns (Fig. 5.17). However, increasing the OAD to 9.50 and the OZD to 8.0, while keeping the same BCR, resulted in an increase in sagittal depth to 24 microns (Fig. 5.18).

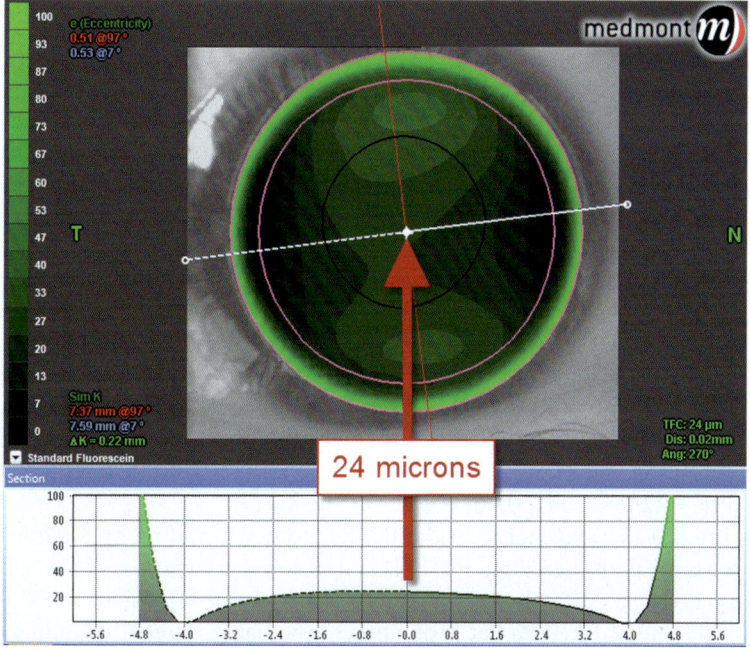

FIGURE 5.17 Software selected lens with 9.0 mm OAD fit "On K" resulting in only 9 microns of central clearance

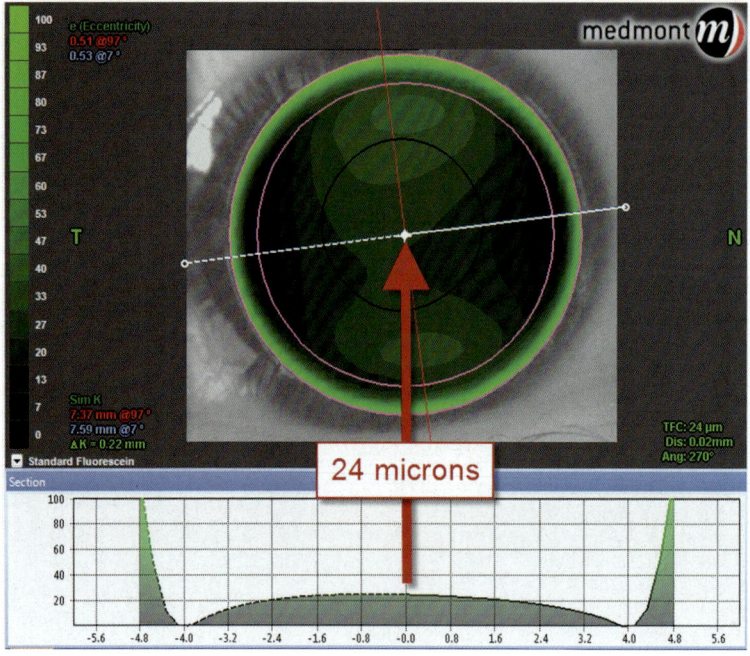

FIGURE 5.18 Changed OAD from 9.0–9.5 mm to produce 20–25 μm apical clearance.

Horizontal Alignment and Vertical Clearance: With the best-fitting simulated design, the flattest meridian of the cornea, and therefore the axis of lowest sagittal depth, will exhibit the greatest lens bearing in the midperiphery (Fig. 5.19). In other words, the GP lens should bear along the flattest axis, creating a "fulcrum" of contact with the peripheral cornea. Conversely, the steeper meridian would exhibit clearance in the midperiphery resulting in a channel of tears under the vertical meridian (Fig. 5.20).

The resulting fluorescein pattern of the lens designed with this program is shown in Figure 5.21.

Power Determination and Lens Order

Once the proper lens design and an optimum lens-to-cornea fitting relationship have been achieved, determination of the final lens power can occur. This is obtained by a comprehensive overrefraction and an understanding of both tear layer optics and vertex distance.

Tear Layer Power: Tear layer power effects are important when a rigid contact lens is fitted either flatter or steeper than flat K. If a rigid lens is fitted flatter than flat K, a minus tear lens power is created; therefore, a correcting plus power is necessary. If a lens is fitted steeper than flat K, a plus tear lens power is created; therefore, a correcting minus power is indicated. For example, if a lens is fitted 0.50 D flatter than flat K on a cornea with a flat keratometry reading of 43.50 D, the tear layer power is equal to -0.50 D; therefore, $+0.50$ D is necessary to correct for the tear layer. If the spherical refractive value is equal to -2.00 D, the final predicted lens power is equal to $-2.00 + (+0.50) = -1.50$ D (Fig. 5.22).

If a lens is fitted 0.25 D steeper than the flat keratometry reading on a patient, a $+0.25$ D tear layer power is created; therefore, -0.25 D is necessary to correct it. If the spherical refractive value is equal to -2.00 D, the final predicted lens power will equal $-2.00 + (-0.25) = -2.25$ D. If a rigid lens is fitted on flat K or equal to the flat keratometry reading, the tear lens

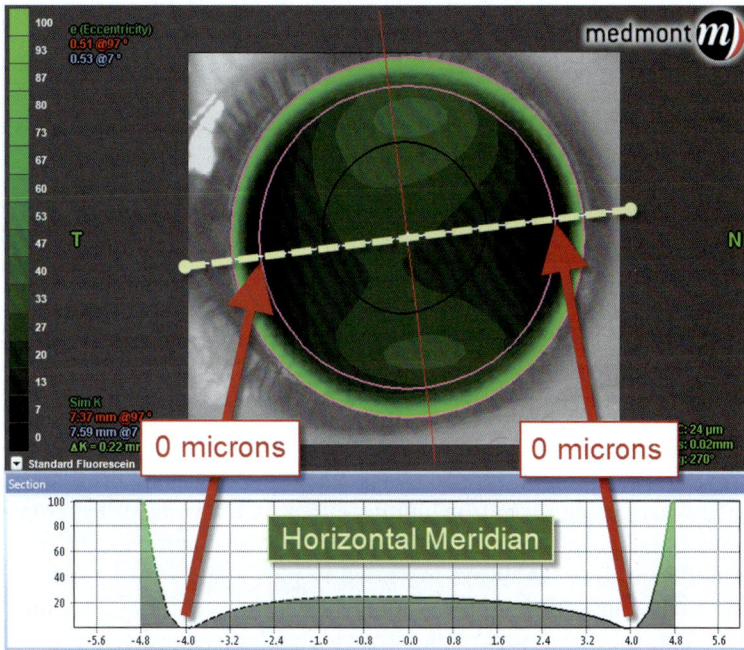

FIGURE 5.19 Horizontal meridian showing points of bearing at the optical zone junction (on the flat meridian).

power is equal to zero. The predicted lens power is then equal to the spherical refractive value if the latter is <±4 D. It is *incorrect* to assume that the final predicted lens power will be equal to the spherical equivalent (as is often true with soft lenses), unless the lens is being fitted one-half of the difference steeper than flat K.

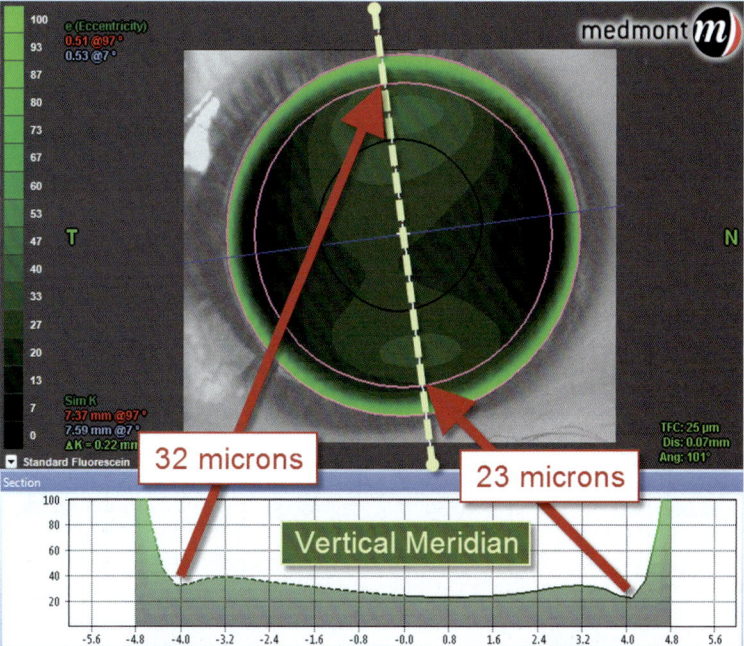

FIGURE 5.20 Vertical meridian showing lift at the optical zone junction (on the steep meridian).

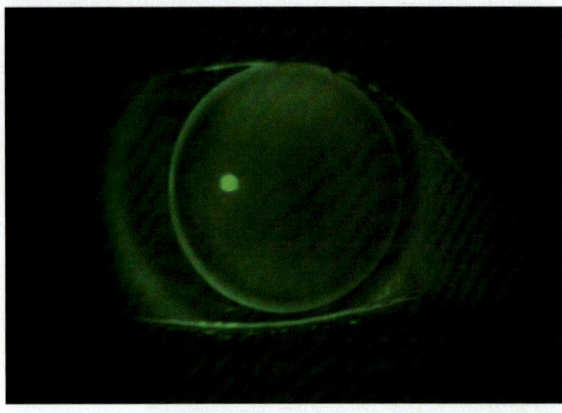

FIGURE 5.21 Photo of 7.50-mm BCR, 9.5-mm OAD lens on this patient.

Vertex Distance: Determination of the effective power at the corneal plane is another important factor to consider when fitting patients exhibiting either high myopia or hyperopia; specifically, the effective power difference becomes significant at ≥4 D of ametropia. The effective power at the corneal plane, in all cases, is always increased in plus relative to the spectacle plane. The first step in any contact lens–fitting process is to vertex the powers of both the flat and steep meridians to the corneal plane, assuming either a standard vertex distance or measuring it precisely.

Appendix 2 presents the difference in effective power from the spectacle to the corneal plane, assuming a 12-mm vertex distance. The formula for determining the effective power is as follows:

$$Fc = \frac{Fs}{1 - d(Fs)}$$

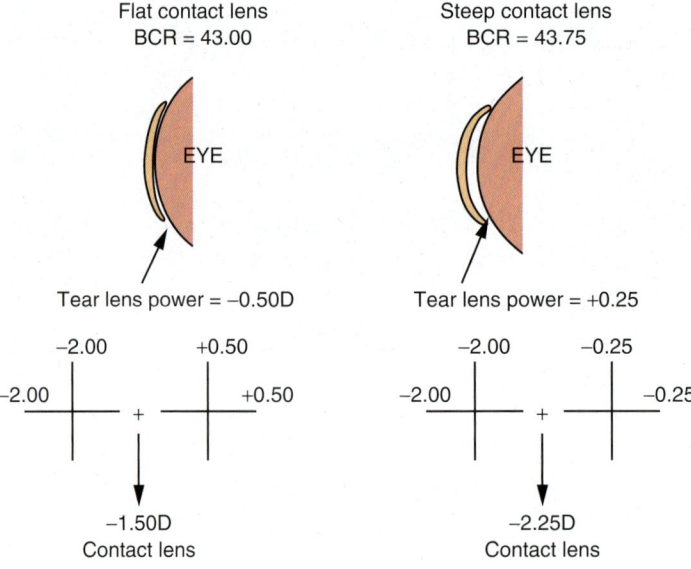

FIGURE 5.22 Tear lens calculations in determining the final lens power.

where

    Fc = contact lens power
    Fs = spectacle lens power
    d = distance between the spectacle lens and the contact lens in meters

If, for example, a 12-mm vertex distance is present and the patient's refractive error is equal to $-6.50 - 1.00 \times 180$, at the corneal plane this will equal the following:

$$\frac{-6.50}{1 - (0.012) \times -6.50} = -6.03 D$$

$$\frac{-7.50}{1 - (0.012) \times -7.50} = -6.88 D$$

Therefore, the spectacle prescription at the corneal plane is equal to $-6.03 - 0.85 \times 180$ or $-6.00 - 0.75 \times 180$. Especially for aphakic patients, this effective power difference becomes quite significant. For example,

$$\frac{+14.50}{1 - (0.012) \times +14.50} = +17.55 D$$

$$\frac{+11.50}{1 - (0.012) \times +11.50} = +13.34 D$$

It is important to measure vertex distance because it can vary between patients; this factor increases in importance as the ametropia increases.

Ordering: Before fitting GP diagnostic lenses, it is desirable to indicate the predicted vertexed lens powers on the fitting form. In addition, information pertaining to the diagnostic lens parameters, lens-to-cornea fitting relationship, and overrefraction should also be provided. Table 5.16 shows an example of the fitting information and resultant order for a high myopic patient.

The predicted lens power can be obtained from simply adding the best sphere overrefraction value to the contact lens power. For example,

Keratometry	42.50 @ 180; 42.75 @ 090
Spectacle refraction	$-6.50 - 0.25 \times 180$
Effective power	$-6.00 - 0.25 \times 180$
BCR	42.00 D or 0.50 D flatter than K (using aforementioned lid attachment philosophy)
Predicted lens power	Spherical refractive value at the corneal plane − tear lens power $= -6.00 - (-0.50)$ $= -5.50$ D

In the previous example, the overrefraction values equaled the predicted. In many cases, this does not occur because of several factors, including the following:

1. Inaccurate refraction.
2. Inaccurate keratometry values.
3. BCR not equal to desired.

TABLE 5.16 Fitting Form and Final Lens Order

Patient data (OD only):	
Keratometry readings: 42.50 @ 180/42.75 @ 090	
Spectacle refraction: −6.50−0.25 × 180 20/20	
Vertexed to corneal plane: −6.00 − 0.25 × 180	
Predicted Lenses (OD only): BCR 8.04, OAD 9.4, Power −5.50	
Diagnostic lens	FP 30
BCR/OAD/Rx/CT	8.04/9.4/−4.00/.14
Fluorescein pattern	Mild apical touch/alignment pattern
Position and lag	Superior central with 2-mm lag
Retinoscopy/VA	−1.50 20/20
Best sphere/VA	−1.50 20/20
Final Design and Order (OD only)	
BCR	8.04 mm
SCR/W	8.9/.03 mm
ICR/W	9.9/0.2 mm
PCR/W	11.3/0.2 mm
OZD	8.0 mm
OAD	9.4 mm
Power	−5.50 D
CT	0.14 mm
Blend	Medium
Lenticular	Plus
Tint	Blue
Material	FP 30

BCR, base curve radius; CT, center thickness; ICR/W, intermediate curve radius/width; OAD, overall diameter; OZD, optical zone diameter; PCR/W, peripheral curve radius/width; SCR/W, secondary curve radius/width; VA, visual acuity.

4. Lens power not as ordered.
5. Flexure.
6. Lens decentration.

If this discrepancy is only 0.25 D, it is probably not significant; if it is a higher amount, the other factors should be ruled out prior to ordering the lenses. This is one of many important reasons for using diagnostic lenses as opposed to fitting empirically since the final power derived from adding the overrefraction with the diagnostic lens power will usually be more successful than selecting the lens power based on the predicted values. In addition, in some cases, a large amount of residual astigmatism is predicted; therefore, spherical rigid lenses may not be desirable. However, on performing an overrefraction, if very little or no cylinder is present and the patient is satisfied with the vision obtained with a spherical overrefraction, success should be achieved.

Other Important Design/Fitting Considerations

Standard Versus Custom Lens Design

Many practitioners order lenses using a standard design. Typically, the BCR, OAD, and power are ordered with the manufacturer using its own design to determine such parameters as thicknesses, peripheral curves, and optical zone. This method has the advantage of being less time consuming, and if difficulty is experienced by the practitioner in determining what other parameter specifications to provide, an experienced laboratory should be able to assist in developing an effective design for a given GP material. The disadvantages of this option versus custom lens design are that it takes some control away from the practitioner and no one parameter such as OAD, OZD, CT, or peripheral curve system will be successful on every patient. Nevertheless, with the ability to manufacture thin designs in aspheric and pseudoaspheric designs, the current generation of standard designs has been quite successful and practically every laboratory has, at minimum, one standard design available to practitioners.

Aspheric Design

Although knowledge of the role and design of specific BCRs, PCRs, and OZD is important, the use of aspheric designs is increasing in popularity. This section will discuss the benefits, applications, and fitting considerations of the various types of aspheric lens designs.

Definitions: The term *aspheric* can simply be described as "not spherical" as it pertains to the cornea. In other words, the cornea is not a sphere but gradually flattens from center to periphery. Therefore, an aspheric lens design typically consists of a design that gradually flattens, often at a similar—if not greater—rate than the cornea.

The term *eccentricity*, which has been loosely defined as the rate of corneal flattening, is actually the deviation from a circular path. A circle has an eccentricity value equal to zero. A value between zero and one is termed an *ellipse*. With this definition, the cornea would be an ellipse as it has an average eccentricity value of about 0.4.[98] Some corneas exhibit a greater rate of paracentral flattening, therefore having a higher eccentricity (or *e*) value. An eccentricity value >1.0 is termed a *hyperbola*. Some presbyopic lens designs, as a result of the greater plus power generated with higher than 1.0 eccentricity, use hyperbolic aspheric designs. In addition, some single-vision aspheric designs have a hyperbolic periphery to allow for good tear exchange.

Benefits/Disadvantages: The benefits of aspheric designs include the following:

- An alignment lens-to-cornea fitting relationship resulting from the posterior lens design shape approximating the corneal shape.[99,100]
- Better initial comfort resulting from the elimination of both localized bearing areas on the cornea and peripheral curve junctions.[101,102]
- Better centration on against-the-rule and irregular astigmatic corneas.[102]
- Easier to fit and design because of the reduced number of parameters and the reduced importance of the BCR in most aspheric designs.[103]

Some of the perceived/experienced problems with aspheric designs include the following[101]:

- Reduced vision because of poor-quality optics.
- Variable vision if lens decentration is present.
- Difficult to verify because of variable optical quality.

Applications: There are numerous applications for aspheric designs, including the following[102,103]:

- Patients experiencing decentration with other spherical lens designs.
- Patients with irregular corneas or against-the-rule astigmatism.
- Pre-presbyopic and incipient presbyopic patients.
- Computer users.
- Myopic patients with a poor accommodation convergence/accommodation (AC/A) relationship.

Lens Designs: There are many types of aspheric and "pseudoaspheric" lens designs.[103] It is important for practitioners to understand the differences between these designs, which can be placed into the following four categories:

Pseudoaspheric: These designs typically consist of a series of well-blended peripheral curves. If well manufactured, these designs have benefits over other more conventional spherical lens designs. These designs tend to vary in their effectiveness, and a recent study found no difference in performance between a conventional design and a pseudoaspheric design.[104] It is important for practitioners to use good judgment when considering use of these designs, which are often advertised as being "aspheric-like."

Spherical Optical Zone/Aspheric Periphery: These are typically designs in which the aspheric periphery is tangential to the spherical OZD (in other words, the transition from the optical zone to the periphery is a continuous curve). The optical zone is rarely larger than 6 mm in these lenses, and the clinical performance is typically superior to blended bicurve and tricurve lens designs. An aspheric periphery, while similar to a well-blended spherical periphery, provides a more uniform edge lift and can be maintained with greater consistency and accuracy on replacement lenses.

Aspheric Optical Zone/Aspheric Periphery: These lenses have a totally aspheric posterior surface; however, the optical zone and the periphery are two different curves. This design should, in theory, provide more uniform alignment by means of a more uniform tear layer, both centrally and midperipherally.

The EnVision (Bausch + Lomb) has an elliptical optical zone equal to approximately 0.4 and a hyperbolic periphery that is tangential to the optical zone. The term *bi-aspheric* has been used to describe this design configuration. The clinical results with the EnVision and its early generation predecessors have been favorable. It is apparent that the selection of BCRs in 0.1-mm steps is sufficient. It has provided better initial comfort than spherical lens designs,[100] and it is claimed to have excellent centration characteristics.[99] In addition, as a result of the limited parameters necessary with this design, the ability to inventory this lens is easily obtained.

Single Aspheric Curve Posterior Surface: These conicoid lenses are typically elliptical in design. More information about these designs will be forthcoming in the future.

Fitting Considerations: Several lens design and fitting considerations are important:

- The importance of using a diagnostic set is essential as a result of the design characteristics of every type of aspheric lens.
- Dependence on central keratometry readings is not recommended with these designs as the fitting relationship of a lens of any given BCR is determined by the shape of the paracentral, not the central, cornea.
- Because of the proximity of posterior lens design to cornea and the corresponding uniform tear layer thickness, small incremental changes in BCR are usually unnecessary.
- As a result of all of the differing types of aspheric designs with variations in posterior surface geometry, eccentricity, and manufacturing methods, one should not make generalizations about aspheric designs without referring to a specific aspheric design.[100]

Design and Fitting Resources

Online Resources: There are many online clinical resources when managing different types of GP patients. Eye-Dock (www.eyedock.com) offers lens databases and design calculators to assist in GP lens design.[105] The GPLI (www.gpli.info), the educational division of the CLMA, has a searchable database for GP designs and the CLMA member laboratories who manufacture those designs. There are also a number of clinical resources provided by the GPLI, most of which can be accessed online (Table 5.17).[105–107] These resources include an online case grand

TABLE 5.17 Spherical GP Lens Design and Fitting Resources

- "Click n" Fit to GP Click 'n' Fit
- How to Optimize Initial Comfort (narrated PowerPoint)
- Contact Lens Clinical Pearls Pocket Guide
- Fluorescein Pattern Identification Guide
- GP Lens Management Guide
- GPLI Toric and Spherical Lens Calculator
- GP Case Grand Rounds Troubleshooting Guide
- Monthly GP webinars

rounds book with over 70 unique cases, videos on how to fit and troubleshoot GP lenses, a spherical and toric empirical lens design calculator, and a clinical pearls pocket guide. "Click n" Fit to GP Click 'n' Fit is an interactive simulated fitting and fluorescein evaluation resource that allows the user to select lenses from a virtual trial set, and evaluate the lens-to-cornea fitting relationship and make changes if indicated. The GP Eye Care Professional Locator allows GP fitting practitioners to be listed in a directory such that patients desiring GP lenses can seek someone with expertise to fit them.

Most laboratories have websites with a large and increasing number of practitioner resources. This includes fitting guides and calculators pertaining to their GP lens designs as well as problem-solving information and publications. In addition, many laboratories provide online webinars to assist in the understanding of the fitting and problem-solving of their designs.

The Laboratory Consultant

One of the greatest underutilized resources is the GP laboratory consultant. These individuals can assist in such factors as advising on which material(s) to recommend, providing diagnostic fitting sets and inventories, and offering lens design advice on specific cases.[108,109] An experienced consultant will often provide an opinion based on the experience of designing thousands of lenses for similar patients and essentially serve as the "decision-making tree" for an potential GP wearer. The specialty lens designs and custom fits are typically the consultant's specialty. However, questions pertaining to the so-called routine fittings that may be perceived as challenging by the novel fitter are welcomed by the consultant. Similarly, with increasing use of corneal topography to assist in GP specialty fittings, many laboratories are set up to assist practitioners in interpreting the maps and making recommendations. Many consultants are familiar with the software and pertinent data from multiple topographers, and those data are influential in choosing a specific design. Likewise, with the increasing use of photography and video to document the lens-to-cornea fitting relationship, laboratories welcome these forms of photo documentation to help in custom designing a lens for a specific patient.

SUMMARY

The importance of diagnostic fitting, comprehensive fluorescein evaluation, and selection of the appropriate lens design parameters for a given material are paramount to successful fitting of GP lenses. As shown in Figure 5.10, there are several important factors to consider when determining the final lens parameters for a given patient. If careful attention is devoted to proper design and evaluation, a high success rate with GP lenses should be expected.

CLINICAL CASES

CASE 1

A 12-year-old progressive myopic patient had complaints of peripheral corneal ulcers as well as blurred vision from her (nonsilicone hydrogel) soft toric lenses. She had been fitted into soft torics 2 years previously because that was the recommendation of her practitioner. In addition, she plays soccer throughout the year. Her manifest refraction was the following:

$$OD: -3.25 - 2.25 \times 007$$
$$OS: -2.75 - 2.00 \times 177$$

Slit-lamp evaluation: Both lenses tended to rotate approximately 10 to 15 degrees with the blink and were slow to return to a set position.

SOLUTION: GP lenses were mentioned as a viable option. The patient commented that she has heard that "hard lenses hurt." She was reassured that there is some initial lid awareness because of the smaller size and the greater movement present with the blink, but that she will adapt and should achieve total comfort with the lenses. In addition, she was advised that this is both a healthier alternative and one that should provide improved, and more consistent, vision. A topical anesthetic was applied immediately before fitting her from the Naturalens inventory. This type of design is very good for young athletes because of the large OAD and low edge lift, both combining to minimize decentration and loss. Fitting from an inventory also allowed the patient to experience good vision after the initial application of GP lenses. If an inventory is not available, empirical fitting would be recommended to provide the same benefit, good initial vision.

CASE 2

The practitioner uses PMMA lenses of the following design for diagnostic fitting purposes, and a good lens-to-cornea fitting relationship is obtained OU:

BCR: 7.81 mm
OAD/OZD: 8.8 mm/7.4 mm
PCR/W: 12.25 mm/0.7 mm
CT: 0.12 mm

The lenses are ordered with only BCR, power, and diameter indicated to the laboratory. When the lenses arrive, they decenter inferiorly on the patient.

The laboratory has provided lenses in a 60-Dk material in the following parameters:

BCR: 7.81 mm
OAD/OZD: 8.8 mm/7.8 mm
SCR/W: 9.0 mm/0.3 mm; PCR/W: 11.00 mm/0.2 mm
CT: 0.17 mm

SOLUTION: This is an example in which the use of a different material and design for diagnostic fitting from what was ordered occurred, resulting in a less than desirable fitting relationship.

The lenses received from the laboratory were much thicker, which contributed to a change in the fit. In addition, the OZD was larger and the edge clearance was less. Diagnostic fitting of GP lenses should be with the same (or similar) material and design as that to be ordered. In this particular case, another diagnostic fitting with the same material is indicated.

CASE 3

An alignment lens-to-cornea fitting relationship and good centration has been achieved with the following lens design:

BCR: 7.89 mm
OAD/OZD: 8.8 mm/7.2 mm

However, good pupillary coverage is not present because of the patient's large pupil size. A larger diagnostic lens in this material is not available. An approximate 0.5-mm larger optical zone should be necessary to avoid subjective complaints of flare.

What BCR should be ordered?

SOLUTION: To maintain an alignment lens-to-cornea fitting relationship, for every 0.5-mm increase in optical zone, a 0.25 D flatter BCR should be selected. Therefore, the following design should be ordered:

BCR: 7.94 mm
OAD/OZD: 9.3 mm/7.7 mm

CASE 4

What material, diagnostic lens, and predicted overrefraction would you expect with the following daily-wear patient?

$$\text{OD Keratometry: } 42.00 @ 180; 42.50 @ 090$$
$$\text{Refraction: } -2.50 - 0.50 \times 180$$

SOLUTION: A low-Dk (25–50) lens material is recommended. According to the authors' recommended design philosophy, a BCR 0.50 D flatter than K or equal to 41.50 (8.13 mm) should be used. If this diagnostic lens has a power equal to -3.00 D, the predicted overrefraction is equal to the following:

$$[-2.50 \text{ D (sphere value)} - (-)0.50 \text{ D (tear lens)}]$$
$$-(-)3.00 \text{ D (diagnostic lens)} = +1.00 \text{ D}$$

CASE 5

What material, diagnostic lens, and predicted overrefraction would you expect with the following daily-wear patient?

$$\text{OS Keratometry: } 41.00 @ 180; 42.25 @ 090$$
$$\text{Refraction: } +3.00 - 1.25 \times 180$$

If the overrefraction equals the predicted values and an optimum fitting relationship is obtained, using the authors' recommended design philosophy, what final lens design parameters would you recommend?

SOLUTION: Since hyperopic patients benefit from a higher-Dk material for optimum oxygen transmission, selecting a >50-Dk GP lens material is recommended. A slightly steep BCR equal to 0.25 D steeper than K or 41.25 (8.18 mm) is recommended for diagnostic purposes. If this lens has a power equal to +3.00 D, the predicted overrefraction is equal to the following:

$$[+3.00 \text{ D (sphere value)} - (+)0.25 \text{ D (tear lens)}]$$
$$(+)3.00 \text{ D (diagnostic lens)} = -0.25 \text{ D}$$

The lens power would equal the diagnostic lens + overrefraction = +3.00 D + (−)0.25 D = +2.75 D. The final order would be the following:

Material	BCR	OAD/OZD	Power	SCR/W	ICR/W	PCR/W	CT	Edge
Fluoroperm 60	8.18 mm	9.4/8.0 mm	+2.75 D	9.00/0.3	10.00/0.2	11.40/0.2	Min.	−Lent.

CASE 6

What diagnostic lens and predicted overrefraction would you expect with this patient?

$$\text{OD Keratometry: } 43.50 \text{ @ } 180; \; 44.50 \text{ @ } 090$$
$$\text{Refraction: } -6.75 - 1.25 \times 180$$

If the overrefraction equals the expected values and an optimum fitting relationship is obtained, using the authors' recommended design philosophy, what are the recommended final lens design parameters?

SOLUTION: The first step is to vertex the refraction to the corneal plane:

$$\text{Vertexed refraction: } -6.25 - 1.00 \times 180$$

Next, select a BCR 0.25 D flatter than K or equal to 43.25 (7.81 mm). The predicted overrefraction for a −6.00 D diagnostic lens power would equal the following:

$$[-6.25 \text{ D (sphere value)} - (-)0.25 \text{ D (tear lens)}]$$
$$- (-)6.00 \text{ D (diagnostic lens)} = \text{plano}$$

The final lens parameters would equal the following:

BCR	OAD/OZD	Power	SCR/W	ICR/W	PCR/W	CT	Edge
7.81 mm	9.2/7.8 mm	−6.00 D	8.60/0.3	9.60/0.2	11.00/0.2	0.13	+Lent.

CASE 7

A 45-year-old female came in for a progress check on her GP lenses. She has been a GP lens wearer for many years, and her current pair of Boston ES is 2 years old. She wears her lenses 14 hours a day, 7 days a week. Her vision has always been better in her left eye than right eye when wearing contact lenses. Lenses off:

$$\text{Keratometry: OD } 41.50 \text{ @ } 180; \; 42.00 \text{ @ } 090 - 0.50 \times 180$$
$$\text{OS } 42.50 \text{ @ } 180; \; 42.12 \text{ @ } 090 - 0.62 \times 180$$
$$\text{Subjective refraction: OD } -2.75 - 0.75 \times 0.90$$
$$\text{OS } -3.00 \text{ DS}$$

Present GP parameters

Material	BCR	SCR/W	PCR/W	OZD	OAD	Power	CT	AEL	Blend
OD Boston ES	8.15	9.10/0.3	11.60/0.4	8.2	9.6	−3.00	0.16	0.12	med
OS Boston ES	8.15	9.10/0.3	11.60/.04	8.2	9.6	−2.50	0.16	0.12	med

Biomicroscopy:

Current lens appearance (OD and OS)
Lag = 1.5 mm
Well centered; held in place with upper lid
Some scratches and film observed on lens surface
Fluorescein pattern: center thin, even layer of fluorescein; midperiphery has slight bearing; edge clearance of approximately 0.5 mm
Visual acuity (VA): OD 6/7.5 − 1 OS 6/6

OVERKERATOMETRY (GP):

OD: 39.50 @ 180/39.00 @ 090

OS: 39.87 @ 180/39.50 @ 090 Ret (sph/cyl)

OD: pl − 1.25 × 090 VA 6/4.5

OS: +0.25 − 0.50 × 090 VA 6/4.5

Problems include the following:
1. Reduced visual acuity OD because of uncorrected residual astigmatism

OD: CRA = spectacle cyl − delta K
$$= -0.75 \times 090 + (-0.50 \times 180) = -1.25 \times 090$$
OS: CRA = spectacle cyl − delta K
$$= 0.00 + (-0.62 \times 180) = -0.62 \times 090$$

2. Scratched and deposited lenses OU

SOLUTION:
1. Correct for the residual astigmatism by ordering new lenses with decreased CT to increase flexure.
2. Order new lenses.

Final lens parameters

Material	BCR	SCR/W	PCR/W	OZD	OAD	Power	CT	AEL	Blend
OD Optimum Extreme	8.15	9.10/0.3	11.60/0.4	8.2	9.6	−3.00	0.13	0.12	med
OS Optimum Extreme	8.15	9.10/0.3	11.60/0.4	8.2	9.6	−2.50	0.14	0.12	med

CLINICAL PROFICIENCY CHECKLIST

- It is important to discuss GPs with all new patients in a neutral, nonthreatening manner.
- Topical anesthetic use can be very beneficial in assisting the patient over the initial psychological hurdle of wearing GPs while accelerating the fitting process.
- The use of GP diagnostic lenses will reduce lens replacement and increase both patient compliance and patient confidence in the practitioner. However, many patients, especially those apprehensive about GP lenses, would benefit from experiencing the clear vision obtained from lenses received via empirical fitting or from an inventory.
- Standard GP diagnostic fits should include −3.00 D power lenses in both low-Dk (<50) and high-Dk (>50) materials, +3.00 D power lenses with a minus lenticular edge in a high-Dk material, and −8.00 D power lenses with a plus lenticular edge in a low-Dk material. A good average OAD/OZD is 9.2 mm/7.8 mm; a BCR range from 40.75 to 45.50 D in 0.25 D steps is also recommended.
- The use of fluorescein is essential for rigid lens assessment. Educational resources are available from the GP Lens Institute, the educational division of CLMA.
- The use of a larger OAD with flatter BCR (i.e., <41 D) and a smaller OAD with steeper BCR (i.e., >45 D) is recommended. In addition, the BCR should be flattened by 0.25 D for each 0.5-mm increase in OZD; likewise, the BCR should be steepened by 0.25 D for each 0.5-mm decrease in OZD.

(continued)

- The use of several PCRs (i.e., tetracurve or aspheric design) is recommended to better align the lens periphery with the cornea. Prevent possible corneal desiccation and edge awareness by the use of a wide, flat peripheral curve with the traditional PMMA bicurve design.
- It is important to verify CT; often the contact lenses may be thicker than requested, which results in increased lens mass and possibly inferior decentration.
- Edge verification is essential as a rolled, tapered edge will optimize patient comfort.
- The use of a minus lenticular edge design is recommended for <-1.50 D and all plus powers; a plus lenticular edge design is recommended for all lenses with -5.00 D and higher lens powers.
- The tear lens power and vertex distance must be considered when determining contact lens power.
- Modern low eccentricity single-vision aspheric designs have the potential benefits of enhancing centration, better initial comfort, and ease of fit.
- Topography-assisted designs have several benefits, including making the design process simpler, simulating lens-fitting characteristics on the eye, and online transmission of order and topography information to the laboratory.
- The laboratory consultant can be invaluable in assisting with GP lens design, material, and fitting.

REFERENCES

1. Polse KA, Graham AD, Fusaro RE, et al. Predicting RGP daily wear success. *CLAO J.* 1999;25:152–158.
2. Bennett ES. Be flexible about rigid lenses. *Rev Cornea Contact Lenses.* 2007;144:38–40.
3. Rinehart JM. Tackle comfort issues in GP wearers. *Rev Cornea Contact Lenses.* Nov 2010;7.
4. Bennett ES, Stulc S, Bassi CJ, et al. Effect of patient personality profile and verbal presentation on successful rigid contact lens adaptation, satisfaction and compliance. *Optom Vis Sci.* 1998;75(7):500–505.
5. Quinn TG. Presenting the GP lens option. *Contact Lens Spectrum.* 2004;19(10):41.
6. Quinn TG. GP versus soft lenses: is one safer? *Contact Lens Spectrum.* 2012;27(4):34–39,58.
7. Jervey JW. Topical anesthetic for the eye: a comparative study. *South J Med.* 1989;48:770–774.
8. Lyle WM, Page C. Possible adverse effects from local anesthetics and the treatment of these reactions. *Am J Optom Physiol Opt.* 1975;52:736–744.
9. Bennett ES, Smythe J, Henry VA, et al. The effect of topical anesthetic use on initial patient satisfaction and overall success with rigid gas permeable contact lenses. *Optom Vis Sci.* 1998;75:800–805.
10. Schnider CM. Anesthetics and RGPs: crossing the controversial line. *Rev Optom.* 1996;133:41–43.
11. Gordon A, Bartlett JD, Lin M. The effect of diclofenac sodium on the initial comfort of RGP contact lenses: a pilot study. *J Am Optom Assoc.* 1999;70:509–512.
12. Caroline PJ, Andre MP. NSAIDs in RGP adaptation. *Contact Lens Spectrum.* 2001;16(5):56.
13. Bennett ES. The GP decision-making process. *Contact Lens Spectrum.* 26(11):44–48.
14. Bennett ES. Basic fitting. In: Bennett ES, Weissman BA, eds. *Clinical Contact Lens Practice.* 2nd ed. Philadelphia, PA: Lippincott Williams & Wilkins; 2005:255–275.
15. Ames K. Rethink your approach to RGP lenses. *Contact Lens Spectrum.* 1993;8:24–27.
16. Benoit DP, Ames KS. Diagnostic versus empirical fitting. *Contact Lens Spectrum.* 2010;25(4):12–13.
17. Lebow KA. Fitting accuracy of an arc step-based contact lens module. *Contact Lens Spectrum.* 1997;12(11):25–30.
18. Soper B, Shovlin J, Bennett ES. Evaluating a topography software based program for fitting RGPs. *Contact Lens Spectrum.* 1996;11(10):37–40.
19. Szczotka LB. Clinical evaluation of a topographically based contact lens fitting software. *Optom Vis Sci.* 1997;74:14–19.
20. Evardson WT, Douthwaite WA. Contact lens back surface specification from the EyeSys videokeratoscope. *Cont Lens Anterior Eye* 1999;22:76–82.
21. Bennett ES. A closer look at lens comfort. *Contact Lens Spectrum.* 2010;25(2):17.
22. Bennett ES, Henry VA, Davis LJ, et al. Comparing empirical and diagnostic fitting of daily wear fluoro-silicone/acrylate contact lenses. *Contact Lens Forum.* 1989;14:38–44.
23. Davis R, Keech P, Dubow B, et al. Making RGP fitting efficient and successful. *Contact Lens Spectrum* .2000;15(10):40–47.
24. Keech P. The top 10 reasons to inventory RGPs. *Contact Lens Spectrum.* 1996;11(10):32–36.

25. Snyder C, Daum KM, Campbell JB. Rigid contact lens base curve constancy between wet and dry lens storage conditions. *J Am Optom Assoc.* 1990;61(3):184–187.
26. Ward MA. In-office care and disinfection of diagnostic GP lenses. *Contact lens Spectrum.* 2011;26(9):25.
27. Szczotka LB. In-office RGP lens disinfection. *Contact Lens Spectrum.* 2001;16(11):17.
28. Mandell RB. Trial lens method. In: Mandell RB, ed. *Contact Lens Practice.* 4th ed. Springfield, IL: Charles C. Thomas; 1988:243–264.
29. Herman JP. Managing the delayed allergic response in CL patients. Presented at: Annual American Optometric Association Contact Lens Section Symposium; October 1990; Williamsburg, VA.
30. Korb DR. Recent developments in the observation of the cornea lens relationship. In: *Encyclopedia of Contact Lens Practice*, vol. 3. South Bend, IN: International Optics; 1959–1963:Appendix B:98 101.
31. Courtney RC, Lee JM. Predicting ocular intolerance of a contact lens solution by use of a filter system enhancing fluorescein staining detection. *Int Cont Lens Clin.* 1982;9(5):302–310.
32. Swarbrick HA, Hiew R, Kee AV, et al. Apical clearance rigid contact lenses induce corneal steepening. *Optom Vis Sci.* 2004;81(6):427–435.
33. Young G. Fluorescein in rigid lens fit evaluation. *Int Cont Lens Clin.* 1988;15(3):95–100.
34. Bennett ES, Barr JT, Johnson J. Unmasking the RGP fit with fluorescein. *Contact Lens Spectrum.* 1998;13(10):31–38.
35. Edmund C. Location of the corneal apex and its influence on the stability of the central corneal curvature. a photokeratoscopy study. *Am J Optom Physiol Opt.* 1987;64(11):846–852.
36. Rowsey JJ, Reynolds AE, Brown R. Corneal topography. *Corneascope Arch Ophthalmol.* 1981;99:1093–1100.
37. Davis LJ, Bennett ES. Fluorescein patterns in UV-absorbing rigid contact lenses. *Contact Lens Spectrum.* 1989;4(8):49.
38. Sorbara L, Fonn D, Holden BA, et al. Centrally fitted versus upper lid-attached rigid gas permeable lenses. Part I. Design parameters affecting vertical decentration. *Int Cont Lens Clin.* 1996;23(5&6, pt 1):99–104.
39. Sorbara L, Fonn D, Holden BA, et al. Centrally fitted versus upper lid-attached rigid gas permeable lenses. Part II. A comparison of the clinical performance. *Int Cont Lens Clin.* 1996;23(7&8, pt 2):121–126.
40. Caroline PJ, Norman CW, A blueprint for RGP design *Contact Lens Spectrum.* 1988;3(11, pt 1):39–49.
41. Bennett ES. Lens design, fitting and troubleshooting. In: Bennett ES, Grohe RM, eds. *Rigid Gas Permeable Contact Lenses.* Boston, MA: Butterworths; 1986:189–224.
42. Korb DR, Korb JE. A new concept in contact lens design. I and II. *J Am Optom Assoc.* 1970;41(2):1023–1032.
43. Bier N, Lowther GE. Lens design. In: Bier N, Lowther GE, eds. *Contact Lens Correction.* London: Butterworths; 1977:207–225.
44. Lowther GE. Review of rigid contact lens design and effects of design and lens fit. *Int Cont Lens Clin.* 1988;15(12):378–389.
45. Lowther GE, Hill RM. Sensitivity thresholds of the lower lid margin in the course of adaptation to contact lenses. *Am J Optom.* 1968;45:587–594.
46. Hazlett R. Custom designing large-diameter rigid gas permeable contact lenses: a clinical approach intended to optimize lens comfort. *Int Cont Lens Clin.* 1997;24(1):5–9.
47. Szczotka LB. RGP parameter changes: how much change is significant? *Contact Lens Spectrum.* 2001;16(4):18.
48. Jedlicka J. Malooley MM, Reeder RE. Semi-scleral applications for healthy eyes. *Contact Lens Spectrum.* 2011;26(10).
49. Bennett ES. GP corneal and scleral lens update. Presented at: University of Houston 28th Annual Cornea, Contact Lens, and Contemporary Vision Care Symposium; December 2011; Houston, TX.
50. Bennett ES. GP annual report 2011. *Contact Lens Spectrum.* 2011;26(10);28–33,48.
51. Herman JP. Flexure of rigid contact lenses on toric lenses as a function of base curve fitting relationship. *J Am Optom Assoc.* 1983;54(3):209–213.
52. Henry VA, Bennett ES, Forrest JF. A clinical investigation of the Paraperm EW rigid gas permeable contact lens. *Am J Optom Physiol Opt.* 1987;14(8):313–320.
53. Bibby MM. Factors affecting peripheral curve design. *Am J Optom Physiol Opt.* 1979;56(1):2–9.
54. Honan PR, Morgan JF, Dabezies OH. Nomenclature, lens design, and fitting parameters. In: Dabezies OH, ed. *CLAO Guide to Contact Lenses.* Orlando, FL: Grune & Stratton; 1984:22.1–22.17.
55. Picciano S, Andrasko GJ. Which factors influence RGP lens comfort? *Contact Lens Spectrum.* 1989;4(5):31–33.
56. Young G. The effect of rigid lens design on fluorescein fit. *Cont Lens Anterior Eye.* 1998;21(2):41–46.
57. Atkinson TCO. The design of the back surface of gas permeable lenses. *J Br Contact Lens Assoc.* 1982;5(1):16–30.
58. Bennett ES. Silicone/acrylate lens design. *Int Cont Lens Clin.* 1985;12(1):45–53.
59. Jackson JM. We have (edge) liftoff. *Contact Lens Spectrum.* 2005;20(4):21.
60. van der Worp E, de Brabander J. Contact lens fitting today part one: modern RGP lens fitting. *Optom Today.* July 2005;27–32.
61. Edrington T, Barr JT. We have edge lift. *Contact Lens Spectrum.* 2002;17(10):49.
62. Stone J. Designing hard lenses in the 1980s. *J Br Contact Lens Assoc.* 1982;4(4):130–137.
63. Poster MG. Clinical evaluation of the Polycon 8.5 design. *J Am Optom Assoc.* 1981;52(3):243–246.
64. Doane M, Gleason W. Tear film interaction with RGP contact lenses. Presented at: First International Material Science Symposium; March 1988; St. Louis, MO.
65. Williams CE. New design concepts for permeable rigid contact lenses. *J Am Optom Assoc.* 1979;50(3):331–336.

66. Swarbrick HA, Holden BA. Rigid gas permeable lens binding: significance and contributing factors. *Am J Optom Physiol Opt.* 1987;64(11):815–823.
67. Zabkiewicz KR, Terry R, Holden BA, et al. The frequency of rigid lens binding in extended wear increases with time. *Am J Optom Physiol Opt.* 1987;64:110P.
68. Grohe RM, Lebow KA. Vascularized limbal keratitis. *Int Cont Lens Clin.* 1989;16(7,8):197–209.
69. Andrasko G. Center thickness: an important RGP parameter. *Contact Lens Forum.* 1989;14(6):40–41.
70. Toscano F, Bridgewater B. A comparative study of RGP materials in thin lens designs. *Contact Lens Spectrum.* 1997;12(10):25–28.
71. Croatt C, Wing F. An RGP lens with a soft lens fit. *Contact Lens Spectrum.* 2000;15(6):49–52.
72. Norman C. Today's RGPs: better performance through innovative technology. *Contact Lens Spectrum.* November 1996.
73. Achiron LR. Custom-designed ultra-thin RGP lenses. *Contact Lens Spectrum.* 2001;16(5):40–45.
74. Cornish R, Sulaiman S. Do thinner rigid gas permeable contact lenses provide superior initial comfort? *Optom Vis Sci.* 1996;73(3):139–143.
75. Nelson JM, Huff J, Bennett ES, et al. Evaluation of variation in oxygen transmission in rigid contact lens extended wear. *CLAO J.* 1989;15:125–133.
76. Hill RM, Brezinski SD. The center thickness factor. *Contact Lens Spectrum.* 1987;2(10):52–54.
77. Campbell R, Caroline P. Don't take RGP lens edge design for granted. *Contact Lens Spectrum.* 1997;12(7):56.
78. Andrasko GJ. Keeping your eye on edge quality. *Contact Lens Spectrum.* 1991;6(9):37–39.
79. Morris DS, Lowther GE. A comparison of different rigid contact lenses: edge thickness and contours. *J Am Optom Assoc.* 1981;52(3):247–249.
80. LaHood D. The edge shape and comfort of rigid lenses. *Am J Optom Physiol Opt.* 1988;65(8):613.
81. Andrasko GJ, Stahl B. Hard choices made easy. *Rev Optom.* 1986;123(4):85–86.
82. Snyder C. Designing minus carrier RGP lenses. *Contact Lens Spectrum.* 1998;13(12):20.
83. Hom MM, Bruce AS, Consider lid geometry when fitting RGP lenses, Ocular Surgery News, US Edition, June 1, 2000.
84. Atkinson, TCO, A computer assisted and clinical assessment of current trends in gas-permeable lens design. *Optician.* January 1985;16–22.
85. Carney LG, Mainstone JC, Henderson BA. Corneal topography and myopia: a cross-sectional study. *Invest Ophthalmol Vis Sci.* 1997;38:311–320.
86. Eghbali F, Yeung KK, Maloney RK. Topographic determination of corneal asphericity and its lack of effect on the refractive outcome of radial keratotomy. *Am J Ophthalmol.* 1995;119:275–280.
87. Guillon M, Lydon DP, Wilson C. Corneal topography: a clinical model. *Ophthalmol Physiol Opt.* 1986;6:47–56.
88. van der Worp E. Respecting the shape of the cornea in RGP fitting. *Optom Pract.* 2004;5:153–162.
89. van der worp E, de Brabander J, Lubberman B, et al. Optimising RGP fitting in normal eyes using 3D topography data. *Cont Lens Anterior Eye.* 2002;11:1–5.
90. Dubow B. Corneal topography and RGP fitting in a managed care world. *Eyecare Technol.* 1996;6(1):61–63.
91. Soper B, Shovlin J, Bennett ES. Evaluating a topography software based program for fitting RGPs. *Contact Lens Spectrum.* 1996;11(10):37–40.
92. Szczotka LB. Clinical evaluation of a topographically based contact lens fitting software. *Optom Vis Sci.* 1997;74(1):14–19.
93. Roberts C. Characteristics of the inherent error in a spherically-biased corneal topography system in mapping a radially aspheric surface. *J Refract Corneal Surg.* 1994;10:103–116.
94. Szczotka LB, Reinhart W. Computerized videokeratoscopy contact lens software for RGP fitting in a bilateral postkeratoplasty patient: a clinical case report. *CLAO J.* 1995;21(1):52–56.
95. Caroline PJ, Andre MP. Designing your own GP lenses. *Contact Lens Spectrum.* 2010;25(2).
96. http://www.wavecontactlenses.com. Accessed April 2012.
97. Kojima R, Caroline P. Designing GPs from corneal topography. *Contact Lens Spectrum.* 2009;24(10).
98. Editorial staff. Hard gas permeable elliptical lenses. Optician 1986;5075(192):19–20.
99. Bennett ES, Henry VA, Seibel DB, et al. Clinical evaluation of the Boston Equacurve. *Contact Lens Forum.* 1987;12(4):65.
100. Andrasko GJ. A comfort comparison. *Contact Lens Spectrum.* 1989;4(4):49–52.
101. Ames KS, Erickson P. Optimizing aspheric and spheric rigid lens performance. *CLAO J.* 1987;13(3):165–170.
102. Goldberg JB. Aspheric corneal lenses for nonpresbyopic and presbyopic patients. *Contact Lens Spectrum.* 1990;5(4):71–74.
103. Feldman GE, Bennett ES. Aspheric lens designs. In: Bennett ES, Weissman BA, eds. *Clinical Contact Lens Practice.* Philadelphia, PA: JB Lippincott;1991;16:1–10.
104. Snyder C, Poling T. Does the Starlens clinically differ from a conventional tricurve design? *Contact Lens Spectrum.* 1990;5(4):33–38.
105. Bennett ES. Obituary for GPs premature. *Contact Lens Spectrum.* 2011;26(2):16.
106. Newman CD. Let the GPLI help you set your practice apart. *Contact Lens Spectrum.* 2011;26(11).
107. Jedlicka J. A vital GP resource. *Rev Cornea Contact Lenses.* November 2011:5.
108. Bennett ES. Laboratory consultants: your most valuable GP resource. *Contact Lens Spectrum.* 2010;26(6).
109. Bennett ES. Use your no. 1 GP resource: your laboratory consultant. *Contact Lens Spectrum.* 2012;27(1).

Chapter 6

Gas-Permeable Lens Care and Patient Education

Edward S. Bennett and Heidi Wagner

The ability to care for and handle rigid gas-permeable (GP) contact lenses properly depends on several factors. First, the patient must be provided with several methods of insertion and removal, and proficiency in these methods must be demonstrated before leaving the office. Second, the patient must be aware of the function of each solution in the recommended care regimen, the importance of performing each function properly and regularly, and the basis for which other solutions are not compatible with the particular material. Third, several methods should be provided to both educate the patient and reinforce the education. The patient must know the "do's and don'ts" of the newest GP lenses; in other words, the patient must recognize the limitations of the lenses and the problems that can occur through noncompliance. The purpose of this chapter is to provide an overview of the ways in which these important factors can be satisfied, thereby enhancing the probability of patient success.

CARE REGIMEN

Wetting and Soaking

The majority of solutions used for wetting and soaking GP lenses combine several functions into one solution. These solutions have four major functions[1]:

1. To temporarily enhance the lens surface wettability.
2. To maintain the lens in a hydrated state similar to that achieved on the eye.
3. To disinfect the lens.
4. To act as a mechanical buffer between the lens and cornea.

The specific formulation of the ingredients in these solutions, especially the preservatives and wetting agents, is very important.

Preservatives

Preservatives are capable of either killing microorganisms (bactericidal agents) or inhibiting their growth (bacteriostatic agents).[2] They are the active ingredients in these solutions (and all other GP care solutions) that should perform the following functions[3]:

- Provide the necessary degree of disinfection.
- Preclude toxic reactions.
- Avoid adverse effects on lens surface wettability and parameters.
- Enhance compatibility with the tear film.

There are numerous preservatives currently in common use, all differing in their mode of action and effectiveness. The most common preservatives include benzalkonium chloride (BAK), chlorhexidine, thimerosal, ethylenediamine tetraacetate (EDTA), polyaminopropyl biguanide (PAPB), polyquarternium-1 (polyquad), and benzyl alcohol (Tables 6.1 and 6.2).

TABLE 6.1 Storage and Disinfection Solutions

MANUFACTURER	NAME	PRESERVATIVE(S)
Bausch + Lomb	Boston Advance Comfort Formula Conditioning Solution	Chlorhexidine gluconate, polyaminopropyl biguanide
Bausch + Lomb	Original Formula Boston Conditioning Solution	Chlorhexidine

Benzalkonium Chloride: BAK is a quaternary ammonium compound that is effective against a wide spectrum of bacteria and fungi and normally is used at a concentration of 0.004%. It was first introduced as a preservative in the late 1940s and is currently used in the majority of ophthalmic preparations. The effectiveness of BAK is enhanced when it is used in combination with EDTA, allowing a lower concentration than otherwise necessary.[4] It is not used as a preservative with soft lens solutions because the soft polymer will bind the preservative and actually concentrate it, thereby allowing it potentially to reach toxic levels and cause ocular injury.[5]

Chlorhexidine: Chlorhexidine is bactericidal in action and traditionally has been used in a concentration of 0.0005% in soft lens chemical disinfection solutions. However, unlike soft lenses, the binding capacity of chlorhexidine to GP lenses appears to be limited because of the wettability of GP lenses and chlorhexidine's large molecular structure.[6] Although chlorhexidine has been reported to have an excellent spectrum of antimicrobial activity, it has limited effectiveness against yeast and fungi; therefore, it often has been combined with EDTA for greater effectiveness. In addition, chlorhexidine has been found to be relatively ineffective against *Serratia marcescens*.[7]

Thimerosal: Thimerosal is a bactericidal organic mercurial compound that at one time was a commonly used soft lens solution preservative. However, some patients are sensitive to organic mercurial compounds and experience a burning sensation and associated clinical signs of redness and superficial punctate keratitis.[8,9] In addition, it is slow-acting in nature and, in low concentrations, may be ineffective against *Pseudomonas*.[2,10] Although thimerosal has been found to be compatible with GP lenses, exhibiting only rare sensitivity reactions, for optimal antimicrobial effectiveness, it should be used in combination with another preservative such as chlorhexidine.[11] It has largely been eliminated from contact lens care systems.

Ethylenediamine Tetraacetate: EDTA is a chelating agent and not a true preservative. However, it is commonly used in combination with BAK and other preservatives in GP contact lens solutions because of its synergistic ability to enhance the bacterial action of pure preservatives against *Pseudomonas*.[12]

Polyaminopropyl Biguanide: PAPB has been used as a preservative in soft disinfection regimens because of its low sensitivity rate. It has supplemented chlorhexidine as a preservative in one of the GP care systems because it exhibits greater antimicrobial effectiveness, notably against *Serratia marcescens*.[7] However, in the concentration used in GP lens solutions, which is 30 to

TABLE 6.2 Combination Solutions

MANUFACTURER	NAME	PRESERVATIVE
Menicon	Unique pH Multipurpose Solution	Polyquaternium-1
Lobob	Optimum by Lobob	Benzyl alcohol
Bausch + Lomb	Boston Simplus Multi-Action Solution	Chlorhexidine gluconate, polyaminopropyl biguanide
Menicon	Menicare	Benzyl alcohol

50 times the concentration used in soft lens solutions, the potential for toxicity reactions has been documented.[13,14] However, when reduced in concentration by one-third, it has demonstrated excellent antimicrobial activity in comparison with other systems.[15] It has also demonstrated effectiveness against *Acanthamoeba*.[16]

Polyquaternium-1: Polyquaternium-1 is a large cationic (+) polymer that also is similar in molecular structure to chlorhexidine. The quaternary ammonium group has a lower cationic (+) charge than polyhexamethylene biguanide and, as a result, is used at higher concentrations.[17] It is less likely to produce toxic or allergic reactions than previously developed preservatives such as benzalkonium chloride and thimerosal.[17]

Benzyl Alcohol: Benzyl alcohol originally was considered for use as a solvent for contact lens materials; however, it was also found to have good disinfection capabilities. Pure benzyl alcohol possesses certain physicochemical characteristics that are regarded as ideal for an ophthalmic preservative, including low molecular weight, bipolarity, and water solubility.[18] Benzyl alcohol exhibits negligible binding to the surface of GP lenses, especially fluoro-silicone/acrylate (F-S/A) lens materials.[19] In addition to its properties as a disinfectant, benzyl alcohol is effective in lipid removal.[18]

All commonly used preservatives in GP lens solutions appear to be safe and exhibit far fewer sensitivity reactions than soft lens disinfecting solutions. Certainly, it is possible for an occasional patient to exhibit a sensitivity reaction to any one of the aforementioned preservatives. This sensitivity is manifested, as with any allergic reaction, in the form of itching, burning, and redness. If this reaction occurs, it is often eliminated by switching to a care regimen using a different preservative.

Wetting Agents

Wetting/soaking solutions typically contain either polyvinyl alcohol (PVA) or a methylcellulose derivative as a wetting agent.

PVA has several properties that make it a beneficial additive to GP lens solutions.[2] It is water soluble and is relatively nonviscous and nontoxic to ocular tissues. It has good viscosity-building properties and exhibits good spreading and wettability on the eye and lens surfaces.[20,21] Also, unlike methylcellulose, PVA does not retard regeneration of corneal epithelium.[22] Methylcellulose derivatives have been used successfully as wetting agents in more viscous GP lens solutions.

Cleaning

Several types of cleaners are available for use by GP lens wearers, including nonabrasive surfactants, abrasive surfactants, surfactant-soaking solutions, enzymes, and laboratory cleaners.

Nonabrasive Surfactants

GP cleaners and traditional hard lens cleaners may contain nonabrasive surfactant (detergent) cleaning agents to remove contaminants (e.g., mucoproteins, lipids, and debris) from the lens surface. The use of digital pressure or friction during the cleaning process is important in removing deposits from rigid lenses. Optimum Extra Strength Cleaner (Lobob Laboratories, Inc.) is an example of a nonabrasive surfactant lens cleaner.

Abrasive Surfactants

Abrasive particulate matter has been used in cleaners as an effective adjunct in removing adherent mucoproteinaceous deposits from the lens that may be resistant to use of the surfactant alone. The daily use of abrasive cleaning regimens has been demonstrated to be more effective than the use of nonabrasive cleaners.[23] However, two problems have been described with abrasive cleaners. First, small surface scratches have been observed under high magnification.[24] Second, inducing minus lens power while reducing center thickness can result.[25-27] These problems have been minimized by the introduction of small-particle abrasive cleaners;

however, abrasive lens cleaners may be contraindicated for lens materials with hyper-oxygen permeability (hyper-Dk), as well as for lens materials that have been plasma treated (discussed below). Examples include Boston Cleaner and Boston Advance Cleaner (Bausch + Lomb) and Opti-Free Daily Cleaner (Alcon Laboratories, Inc.).

Surfactant-Soaking Solutions

GP lens care systems have traditionally embraced two-bottle regimens composed of separate cleaning and soaking solutions. One-bottle GP systems, combining these procedures, are a more recent innovation. These solutions use surfactant soaking, intended to dissolve deposits during the overnight soaking cycle; therefore, little digital pressure is necessary and warpage is less likely.[28] Optimum by Lobob C/D/S (Lobob Laboratories, Inc.) and MeniCare GP CDS (Menicon) contain nonabrasive surfactants; they are used for both cleaning and disinfection. They should be rinsed prior to insertion to remove the benzyl alcohol and facilitate the mechanical removal of lens debris. Boston Simplus Multi-Action (Bausch + Lomb) and Opti-Free GP (Alcon Laboratories, Inc.) are examples of multipurpose lens care products that do not require rinsing before insertion.

The lens care system should be prescribed for the needs of the patient. For example, Boston Conditioning Solution (Bausch + Lomb) was formulated specifically for silicone/acrylate (S/A) lens materials that are predisposed to protein deposition. Boston Advance Comfort Formula Conditioning Solution (Bausch + Lomb) was designed for F-S/A lens materials that are more likely to attract lipids. Multipurpose lens care systems may be most appropriate for patients who do not tend to deposit lenses or who are not compliant with two-bottle lens care regimens. Patients who exhibit sensitivity to one formulation may be better served by a system using a different preservative.

Enzyme and Protein Removers

The use of a weekly enzymatic cleaning regimen for GP lens wearers has been proven to be a beneficial adjunct to surfactant cleaning in protein removal from the lens surface.[29] In addition, enzyme use has not been reported to cause any adverse effects for GP lens wearers.[30]

Unlike their more cumbersome tablet predecessors, protein removal products are in liquid form and may be used with the manufacturers' accompanying storage solution. Boston One-Step Liquid Enzymatic Cleaner (Bausch + Lomb) is added to the storage solution weekly, whereas SupraClens (Alcon Laboratories, Inc.) is added to the storage solution daily. Both products should be rinsed before insertion. Boston One-Step is composed of subtilisin; SupraClens is a pancreatin derivative. Both products are designed to promote patient compliance and meet the patient's desire for convenience.[31,32] Other extra-strength cleaners include Progent Protein Remover (Menicon) and Walgreen's Extra Strength Daily Cleaner.

Progent Protein Remover is a biweekly protein remover and disinfectant approved for home use in 2010. The lenses are soaked for 30 minutes (5-minute disinfectant; 30-minute protein removal). It exhibits strong oxidative activity and decomposes protein deposits on the lens surface. Walgreen's Extra Strength Daily Cleaner (Sereine), although not approved for routine GP lens use, is an excellent restorer of lens surface wetting. Since prolonged and repeated exposure to alcohol-based cleaners such as the recently discontinued MiraFlow (Ciba) may result in parameter changes,[33] brittleness, and cracking,[34] it should be used for no more than 30 seconds and then thoroughly rinsed off. Walgreen's Extra Strength Daily Cleaner has the same ingredients as MiraFlow: isopropyl alcohol, purified water, poloxamer-407, and amphoteric-10.[35]

Available GP lens cleaners are listed in Table 6.3.

Laboratory Cleaners and Solvents

The use of laboratory-approved, extra-strength cleaners such as the Boston Lens Laboratory Cleaner (Bausch + Lomb) or Fluoro-Solve (Paragon Vision Sciences) can be beneficial. The Boston Lens Laboratory Cleaner, a solution consisting of several surfactants, can be beneficial

TABLE 6.3 Daily Cleaners

MANUFACTURER	NAME
Alcon	Opti-Free Daily Cleaner
Bausch + Lomb	Original Boston Formula Cleaner
Bausch + Lomb	Boston Advance Cleaner

for in-office cleaning of lenses that either exhibit poor initial wettability or have acquired a heavy film over time. However, surface debris that is more tenacious and difficult to remove, such as pitch or wax, can be removed only with Fluoro-Solve, which is a mild solvent. Walgreen's Extra Strength Daily Cleaner can be an excellent restorer of lens surface wetting. Since prolonged and repeated exposure to isopropyl alcohol may result in permanent damage because of parameter changes[33] brittleness and cracking,[34] it should be used for no more than 30 seconds and then thoroughly rinsed off. Menicon Progent Intensive Protein Remover is a further example of lens care products intended for professional in-office use. Available GP lens cleaners are listed in Table 6.3.

Plasma Treatment

Plasma treatment for GP lenses removes residue from the manufacturing process and imparts an ultra-clean lens surface. This can enhance lens wettability and patient comfort and vision, particularly upon initial dispensing and early lens wear. Certain lens materials (Menicon Z) are routinely manufactured with plasma treatment, whereas other materials (Boston and Paragon) utilize plasma treatment at the discretion of the laboratory or practitioner.[36]

Rewetting and Relubricating

A solution that is used to rewet a GP lens surface while it is still on the eye should perform the following functions[37]:

1. Rewet the lens surface.
2. Stabilize the tear film.
3. Rinse away trapped debris.
4. Breakup loosely attached deposits.

Ideally, this solution should clean the lenses of any debris while rewetting them for an extended period. Essentially, these are surface-active chemical substances that increase the spreading and penetrating properties of a liquid by lowering its surface tension.[38] Because the key to rewetting a GP lens is contact time, PVA often is added to increase the length of contact time. Some solutions contain hydroxyethylcellulose, methylcellulose, or other cellulose derivatives to aid surface wetting by increasing viscosity. Several rewetting solutions also contain a mild, nonionic detergent to loosen and solubilize mucus and debris, and keep it from adhering tenaciously to the lens surface.[37] Available rewetting/relubricating drops formulated specifically for GP lenses are listed in Table 6.4.

TABLE 6.4 Wetting and Lubrication Solutions

MANUFACTURER	NAME
Bausch + Lomb	Boston Rewetting Drops
Lobob	Optimum by Lobob Wetting and Rewetting Drops
Menicon	Menicare GP WRW Wetting & Rewetting Drops

DISPENSING VISIT

Procedures

Knowledge about the available care regimens and their respective functions, applications, and benefits becomes especially important at the dispensing visit. Before dispensing new lenses to a patient, it may be beneficial to apply fluorescein dye to the tear film to rule out any baseline staining with the biomicroscope. Once GP lenses have been inserted, an adaptation period is necessary before performing any test procedures. When the patient's awareness has decreased and he or she is able to gaze in the straight-ahead position with minimal difficulty (a variable period, typically 10–45 minutes), visual acuity and lens evaluation can be performed. The use of a topical anesthetic immediately before initial lens application may result in the ability to assess both vision and the lens-to-cornea fitting relationship much more readily.

Visual Acuity

The patient's vision should be assessed. Biomicroscopy should then be performed to evaluate lens position and surface wettability. If both good lens centration and surface wettability are present, an overrefraction can be performed to determine the necessary additional correction.

Overrefraction

If the visual acuity is equal to the expected value, typically, only a spherical overrefraction is indicated. If a reduction of one line or greater is present, a sphero–cylindrical overrefraction should be performed. Just as the diagnostic fitting is imperative, both for obtaining a proper fit and for enhancing patient motivation (by the knowledge that contact lenses can be tolerated), the dispensing visit is important in continuing this momentum toward eventual patient success by the ability to see, handle, and care for the new GP lenses.

If an uncorrected cylinder that is not residual in nature is causing reduced visual acuity, overkeratometry should be performed to determine if the lens is flexing. If the keratometry readings are not spherical, flexure is present. This induced flexure can be minimized by selecting a flatter base curve radius (e.g., 0.50 D minimum) or increasing center thickness by a minimum of 0.02 mm.[39]

Slit-Lamp Biomicroscopy

The use of a biomicroscope is essential for evaluating lens centration, lag, fluorescein pattern, and surface wettability (although a Burton lamp would be a valuable adjunct for assessing fluorescein pattern). The lens-to-cornea fitting relationship should be evaluated initially using a wide beam with low-intensity white light and low magnification to scan the lens surface. In addition, the lens can be evaluated for regions of poor wettability or hazing. If the patient experiences variable visual acuity in combination with poor initial wettability, this problem can be minimized by presoaking the lenses for at least 24 hours to precondition the surface before insertion.

If poor wettability is present after presoaking the lenses, an in-office cleaner can be used or approved laboratory solvents should eliminate the problem. Polishing the front surface of the lens also may be beneficial; however, this should be performed after the lens is initially cleaned with an in-office cleaner and only if the lens has not been plasma treated.

Comprehensive evaluation of the fluorescein pattern is also important. Is the pattern similar to that observed at the diagnostic fitting visit? The use of high illumination, low magnification, and a moderate-to-wide beam width with cobalt filter should be beneficial when observation is made by biomicroscope. If there is difficulty in observing the pattern, a Wratten number 12 or similar filter can be used, especially if the lens material contains an ultraviolet inhibitor. In addition, if lower magnification is necessary to evaluate the pattern accurately, or to view both eyes simultaneously, a Burton lamp can be used.

Patient Education

Handling

The key to teaching patients to handle GP lenses successfully is *reassurance*. No matter how frustrating it is to the person performing the instruction, that feeling of frustration must not be conveyed to the patient. The instructions must be provided slowly and one at a time. Performing group instruction is distracting and denies the patient the necessary one-on-one personal instruction. The patient should not have the perception that the eye care provider or assistants have lost confidence in the patient's ability to learn how to handle the lenses properly; otherwise, feelings of failure and surrender may arise, possibly leading to the attitude that contact lenses will never be worn again. Conversely, if the patient feels confident about handling the lenses, a perception of satisfaction and success is often present. A minimum of three successful insertions and removals is recommended, although the number depends on how confident the patient feels. If it takes two or three visits (closely spaced to maximize memory of techniques and to minimize further anxiety) for the patient to master lens handling, it is often worth the effort. This is more often a problem with presbyopic patients, who not only are experiencing blurred vision at near, but also may have lived 40 or more years without having a foreign body placed on their eye, thereby increasing anxiety.

Patients should be instructed to insert and remove the lenses over a cloth or paper towel spread on a table (not over a sink drain). In addition, patients should be asked and reminded to avoid oily substances such as hand creams, lotions, or cosmetics, and their hands should be washed and rinsed thoroughly and dried with a lint-free towel. It is important for both practitioner and staff members to set a good example by washing hands before handling lenses in the office and requiring patients to do likewise. Use of an antimicrobial soap is recommended to prevent the transfer of pathogens from hand to lenses during the insertion and removal process. Hands should be washed for a total of 30 seconds using two pumps of an antimicrobial pump prior to handling the lenses.[40,41]

Insertion by the Patient: Insertion of lenses by the patient is a three-step procedure.

Positioning: The patient should be encouraged to use an adjustable mirror when inserting the lenses. This will help to ensure that the lens is positioned properly on the finger and to view the position of the lens; the latter is especially important because patients may consistently bring the lens in contact with the upper or lower lid.

Lid Retraction: For the right eye, the lens should be placed on the right index finger. The middle finger of the left hand should be placed *over* the upper lashes to lift up the upper lid. The middle finger of the right hand should be placed directly *over* the lower lashes to depress the lower lid (Fig. 6.1). The ability to retract the lashes successfully is essential.

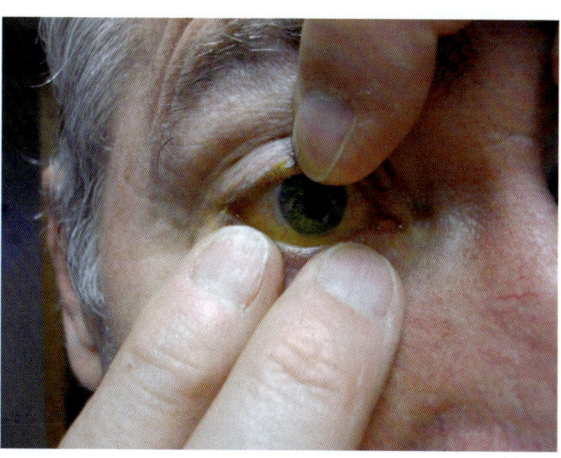

FIGURE 6.1 Proper lid retraction for insertion of a gas-permeable lens.

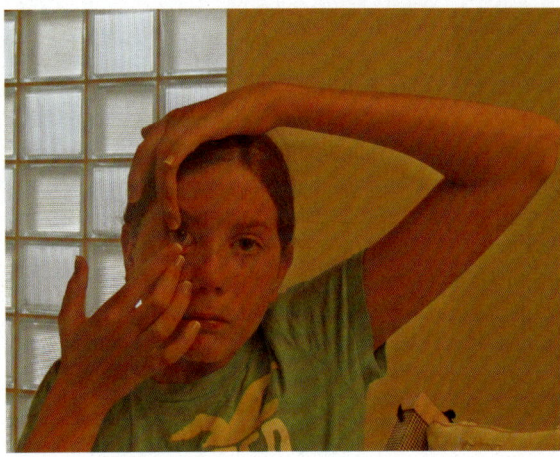

FIGURE 6.2 Proper insertion of a gas-permeable lens by the patient.

Placement: The patient should be looking straight ahead (Fig. 6.2), typically at a mirror on a table or counter. Often, the new rigid lens patient will experience difficulty maintaining proper fixation as the lens approaches the eye; therefore, it is important to assure the patient that the lens will not damage the eye. Finally, once the lens has made contact with the eye, the patient should be instructed first to release the finger holding the lens, then the lower lid, and finally the upper lid. This procedure can then be performed in reverse for the other eye (i.e., use the index finger of the left hand for holding the lens, the middle finger of the right hand for holding the upper lid, and the middle finger of the left hand for holding the lower lid).

Insertion by the Practitioner or Assistant: The procedure is similar if performed by an office member. If the lens is to be placed on the right eye, the lens will be placed on the index finger of the right hand, with the left middle finger holding the upper lid and the right middle finger holding the lower lid (Fig. 6.3). Because the patient may become especially apprehensive with someone else inserting the lens, it is very important to apply pressure underneath the lashes to ensure that they will not move during this process. In this case, the patient can be instructed to view a distant target, for example, a letter on the acuity chart.

Removal by the Patient: There are at least three methods of removing a GP lens. Which method is used depends on factors such as lid tension, lens design, and personal preference.

The easiest method is to use the index finger of the same hand as the eye from which the lens is to be removed to eject the lens. The finger is placed at the junction of the lateral edge of the lids

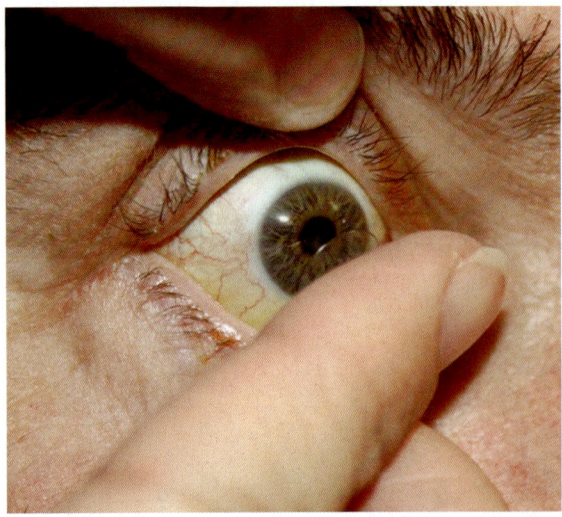

FIGURE 6.3 Proper insertion of a gas-permeable lens by the practitioner.

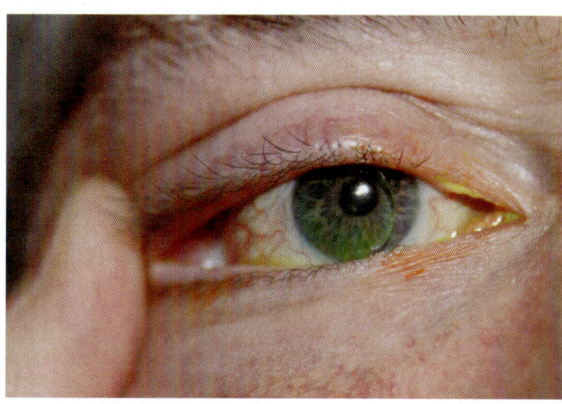

FIGURE 6.4 Removal of a gas-permeable lens by having the patient place the index finger at the lateral edge of the lids.

(Fig. 6.4). With the eye opened wide, the lids are pulled laterally; at the same time, the patient blinks and the lens should be ejected. This procedure can be performed with both the middle and index fingers of the same hand to enhance the possibility of lens ejection. The other hand can be positioned underneath the eye to catch the lens if it fails to adhere to the lower eyelashes.

With today's larger-diameter, lower–edge-clearance GP lens designs, the first method is often unsuccessful; therefore, a more forceful method to remove the lens is to use both hands. The middle and index fingers of the same hand are positioned over the lower lid; the middle and index fingers of the opposite hand hold up the upper lid. As with the first method, the lids are pulled laterally and, while the patient blinks, the lens is ejected (Fig. 6.5). As with all methods of removal, the most important factor is allowing the lid margins to eject the lens. Figure 6.6

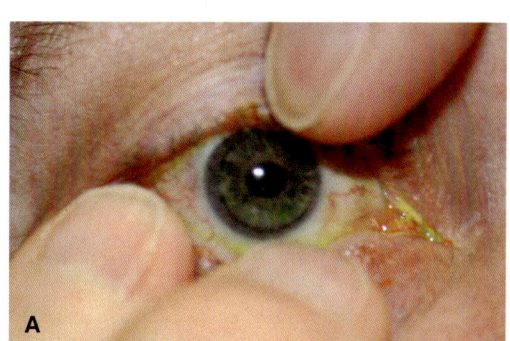
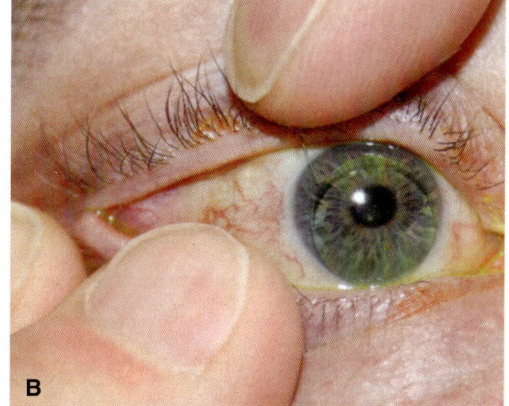
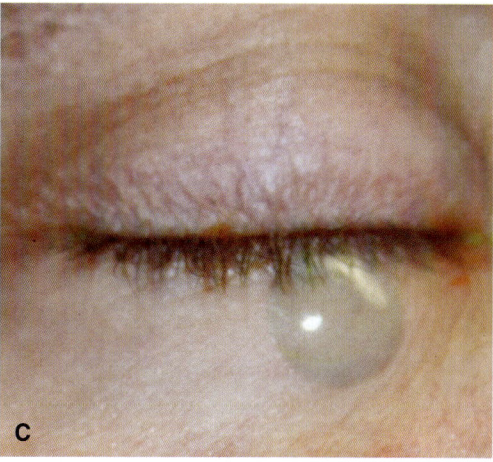

FIGURE 6.5 **(A)** With proper position of fingers over lid margins, **(B)** as the lids are pulled laterally, and **(C)** the lens is ejected.

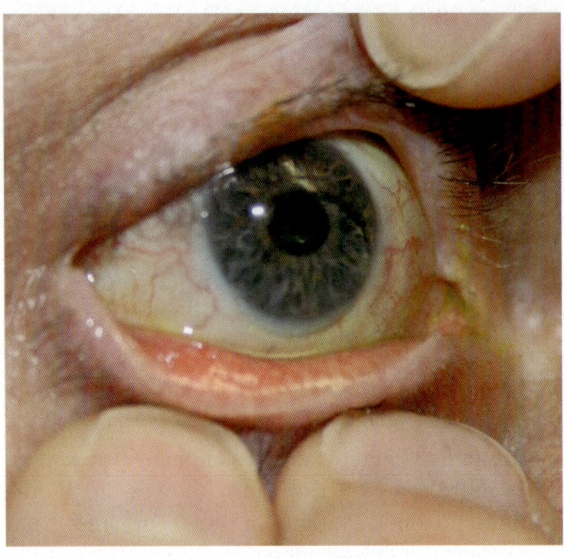

FIGURE 6.6 Improper lid retraction can result in lid eversion and inability to remove the lens.

shows that if the lids are not retracted properly (i.e., if the finger is not placed *over* the lashes), the lid can evert and, therefore, apply very little pressure toward ejecting the lens.

Another forceful method of removing the lens is to eject the lens with a vertical (not lateral) motion. The fingers are positioned as in the second method (i.e., fingers of the opposite hand holding the upper lid, fingers of the same hand positioned on the lower lid). The lower lid is pushed superiorly and the lens is then ejected.

Removal by the Practitioner: The methods used for lens removal by the patient can also be used by the practitioner. In the first method, the lids are pulled laterally (Fig. 6.7). In the second method (i.e., fingers of one hand holding the upper lid, fingers of the other hand positioned on the lower lid), the lens is ejected with a vertical motion (Fig. 6.8).

The fear of being unable to remove a GP lens is perhaps the greatest cause of anxiety with a new wearer. Every patient should be able to remove his or her lenses easily before leaving the office. Although practitioners may be tempted to allow the patient to practice at home, this

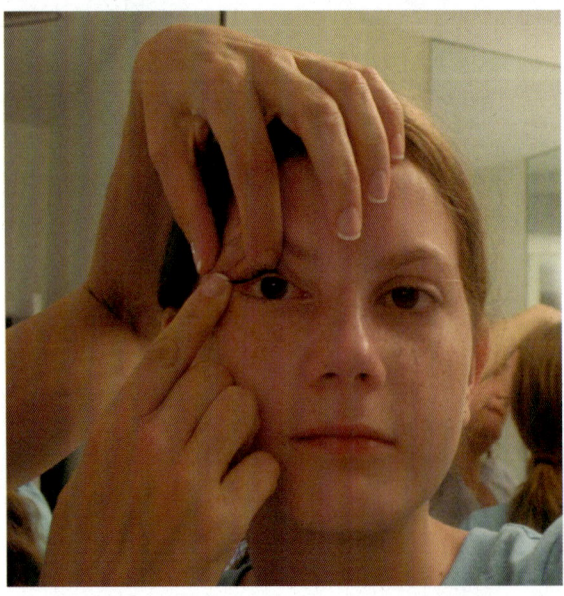

FIGURE 6.7 removal by practitioner or office staff member by pulling laterally with the index finger and having the patient blink.

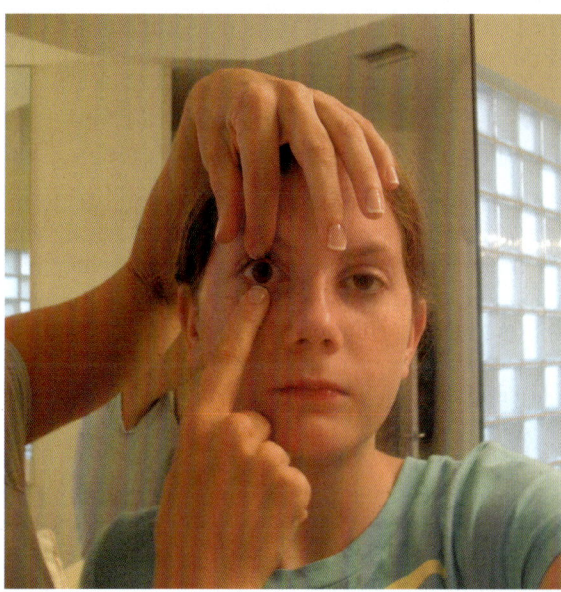

FIGURE 6.8 Another effective removal method of gas-permeable lens is for the practitioner or assistant to push the lids in a vertical motion.

may eventually result in a frustrated and dissatisfied patient. Both practitioners and assistants should be skilled in all of these removal methods.

A suction cup should not be used as a crutch for patients unless the practitioner deems it essential. However, in an emergency situation in which a suction cup is unavailable, the patient's head can be placed in sink filled with water and his or her eyes opened, allowing the lenses to dislodge from the eye.

Recentration: It is extremely important to demonstrate, to new GP lens wearers, how to recognize when a lens has decentered off the cornea and how to reposition it. This often occurs during adaptation, when lenses tend to drop further on the cornea after the blink.

If the patient notices a unilateral blurring of vision, the eye should be evaluated for the possibility of a decentered lens. Location can be determined by the use of a mirror, or if this is not possible, a finger can be placed gently over different regions of the lids to feel any region that may be overlying the lens. Once the lens has been located, it can be manipulated through the lids. The patient should look away from the lens and, after placing a finger on the opposite side of the lens, should look toward the direction of the lens, repositioning it on the cornea (Fig. 6.9). Often, the patient will develop the confidence to reposition the lens gently without

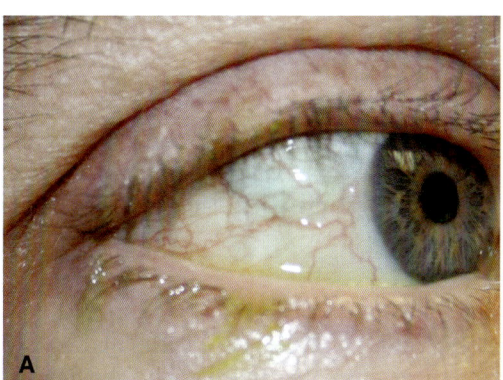
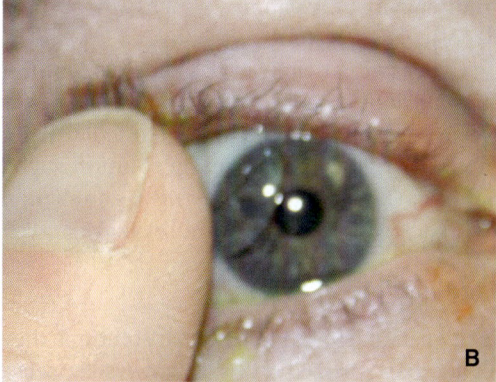

FIGURE 6.9 **(A)** To properly recenter a gas-permeable lens, the patient must first look in the opposite direction of the lens. **(B)** Next, the lens is gently nudged onto the cornea as the patient shifts his or her gaze toward the lens.

the benefit of the lids. If the lens is difficult for the patient to locate, it most likely is superior. If the lens is decentered during the dispensing/educational session, fluorescein can be applied to determine the specific location.

Cleaning

Patients should be told what specific brand of cleaning solution(s) should be used, when to use it, and how to clean the lens properly. Cleaning with a surfactant cleaner should be performed *immediately* upon removal at the end of the day, not before insertion the next morning. This is important in maintaining good surface wettability, because the lens is inserted directly from the wetting/soaking solution and debris is removed more easily after the lens has been in recent contact with the tear film. It is difficult for any patient to exhibit compliance if the lenses are placed in an empty case instead of cleaning upon removal. Any mucoproteinaceous and other deposits may adhere to the lens surface if the lenses are stored dry; therefore, deposit removal will become more difficult.

Cleaning should be performed carefully in the palm of the hand (not between the fingers). Excessive digital pressure can result in lens warpage or lens fracture, especially with the more flexible hyper-Dk lens materials.[25] This has been shown to be a much greater problem in former polymethylmethacrylate (PMMA) wearers.[42] These patients may be accustomed to lens care habits (i.e., cleaning between the fingers, storing in a dry state, carelessness in handling). An exception to the rule may, in fact, be the Menicon Z lens, which has been found not to exhibit greater warpage when cleaned digitally versus in the palm of the hand.[43] Patients should also be advised to rub their lenses, with the recommended cleaner or multipurpose solution, for a minimum of 20 seconds after removal.[44] In general, patients should be warned about what can occur with noncompliance, and the proper cleaning techniques should be reviewed at the follow-up visits.

It is also important to note that patients should be told what *not* to use in cleaning the lenses and why. Former PMMA wearers may have used such products as baking soda, toothpaste, baby shampoo, or dishwashing liquid to clean their lenses. It should be emphasized that these products are not approved for use with GP lenses and may be both irritating and harmful to surface wettability.

Patients should also be warned of the so-called "left lens syndrome." This pertains to the problem of patients who clean the right lens first and more thoroughly than the left. Eventually, the left lens becomes more deposit bound and problematic to the patient. Simply bringing this potential problem to the patient's attention should be sufficient to prevent its eventual occurrence.

In addition to a surfactant cleaner, the use of an enzymatic cleaner for one 2-hour cycle every week should be recommended for some patients. Both extended-wear (EW) and borderline dry-eye patients should be started with an enzyme cleaner. Other patients also may benefit from enzymatic cleaning, which can be provided once it has been established that surface deposits have become problematic.

Hyperopic patients can also benefit from a more aggressive cleaning process. Mucoproteinacous "bevel plaque" tends to occur on plus power lenses where the anterior power curve is markedly steeper compared to the flatter lenticular flange.[45] Use of an abrasive cleaner followed by soaking in a surfactant-disinfecting solution such as Optimum Cleaning, Disinfecting and Storage Solution (Lobob Laboratories) is recommended; this is also less invasive than the use of a cotton swab, which can result in breakage.

Care Regimen

Every patient should know what solutions they can and cannot use with their lenses and why. It should be explained that the care system selected for them is unique, and that all solutions are not alike. Patients should realize that this regimen was selected to be most compatible with their contact lenses, as well as optimizing their eye health. It must be emphasized that although other

NEW PATIENT INFORMATION

We appreciate your choice of the Eye Institute for your contact lens needs. Contact lens wear can improve the quality of your life. However, you must take proper care of your lenses and know what to do in the event of a problem. This information sheet provides important instructions and information. Please read it completely and refer to it if you have any questions.

EMERGENCY INFORMATION
- In an emergency we can be reached at (954) 262-4200 for 24 hours a day.
- Remove your lenses and call our office for assistance if you experience any of the following:
    - ☏ EYE PAIN
    - ☏ SENSITIVITY TO LIGHT
    - ☏ REDNESS OF YOUR EYES
    - ☏ EXCESSIVE TEARING OR DISCHARGE
    - ☏ CLOUDY, FOGGY OR REDUCED VISION

GENERAL INFORMATION
- Contact lenses are medical devices that are regulated by the U.S. Food and Drug Administration. The recommended wearing, replacement and follow-up schedules are indicated below.
- Different types of lenses have varied risk. For example: lenses worn overnight have a higher risk of complications than do lenses removed on a nightly basis. This risk is greater after swimming with lenses.
- For all types it is best to remove contact lenses before swimming in fresh, salt or pool water. If lenses are mistakenly worn during this period, they should be removed and disinfected as soon as possible.
- It is best not to wear lenses during periods of illness or in situations where you will not be able to properly care for your lenses.
- Contact lenses must never be shared. Glasses and sunglasses should be maintained for wear as needed.
- As with prescription medications, contact lenses can only be dispensed pursuant to a prescription of an eye care practitioner, with a limit on the supply of lenses to be purchased before an expiration date.

LENS WEAR SCHEDULES AND REPLACEMENT INFORMATION
- Maintaining healthy eyes and proper vision includes regular evaluations by your doctor every:
    ❑ 3 mos ❑ 6 mos ❑ 12 mos ❑ other _____   ❑ Please wear your lenses into your next visit
- Your lenses are designed to be worn on the following schedule:
    ❑ Daily wear, up to ___ hours with removal before sleeping   ❑ Continuous wear, up to ___ nights
- Your lenses are designed to be replaced on the following basis:
    ❑ daily ❑ weekly ❑ biweekly ❑ monthly ❑ every 3 mos ❑ every 6 mos ❑ every 12 mos ❑ other _____

IMPORTANT: Wearing your lenses beyond this schedule may expose you to additional risk. Should you purchase your contact lenses elsewhere, your lens wear schedule, care regimen, lens replacement cycle, and periodic examinations will remain unchanged.

LENS CARE INFORMATION
To a large extent, lens wear success will depend on carefully following the care instructions we reviewed, and following common-sense instructions concerning hand-washing prior to lens handling, and lens case cleaning or frequent replacement.
To best meet your needs we have recommended the following lens care products:

❑ Care System: _____   ❑ Contact Lens Cleaner: _____
❑ Rewetting Drop _____   ❑ Other _____

IMPORTANT: Please do not change care products unless you are specifically instructed to do so by our office, as products are not all the same. Some may be incompatible with your lenses/eyes, thus substitution without approval from your doctor is discouraged.

ACKNOWLEDGEMENT
I have read this document carefully, and fully understand the importance of the doctor's recommendations. I have been trained in the care and handling of my contact lenses. I understand the policies of this office and understand that I am free to purchase lenses from a dispenser of my choosing. I understand the importance of following all directions, caring for my lenses as instructed and returning for all recommended, periodic examinations. I have been given the opportunity to have all of my questions answered and concerns addressed.

_____   _____
Patient Name (Print)   Doctor/Assistant Signature

_____ _____   _____ _____
Patient Signature   Date   Parent/Guardian Signature Date

FIGURE 6.10 A form from Nova Southeastern used for providing important information to new contact lens patients.

solutions may cost less and appear to have similar functions, changing to such a solution may cause redness, burning, and reduced surface wettability. The specific recommended solutions and any acceptable alternative solutions should be provided as part of the patient instruction materials (Fig. 6.10). In addition, the progress evaluation forms should have a space for solutions such that patients can be asked to provide the brand names of their care regimens at each visit.

Every product in the care kit provided to a new GP lens patient should be explained to the patient as they pertain to everyday use (i.e., inserting, removing, cleaning and disinfection, etc.). The patient should then repeat the care instructions to ensure understanding and aid compliance. What the assistant and practitioner believe is common sense may be confusing to the patient. It cannot be assumed that every patient will carefully read and understand product labels and care instructions. If each product is explained and the patient still appears to be confused, the specific care instructions for each care product can be provided in written form. In addition, the function(s) of each bottle can be applied on a large label taped to the solution. The latter is especially beneficial for presbyopic patients who may experience difficulty with small print.

Rewetting or relubricating drops do provide some important functions with GP lenses. Specifically, these solutions can be used on an as-needed basis to rewet the lens surface while also rinsing loosely adherent debris off the lens surfaces.

Patients should be advised *always* to soak the lenses in the recommended disinfecting solution, not in the dry state. Soaking the lenses overnight has numerous benefits, including the following:

1. Disinfection.
2. Enhanced surface wettability because these solutions contain wetting agents.
3. Maintenance of hydrated state—the lenses are in this state during wear because they are in contact with the tear film.
4. Minimization of "case" scratches—a dry, dirty case can result in damage to a GP lens surface.

Patients should not allow their disinfecting solution to remain in the case for longer than 30 days without replacement.[46] It has been found that not only is contamination an issue, but also solutions lose their effectiveness over time.[47] In addition, the patients should be advised against "topping off" their disinfecting solution. Instead of replacing the solution every night, the patient simply adds a small amount to top off what is already in the case. The resulting contaminated solution may cause potential sight-threatening ocular complications (Fig. 6.11).

Overall, the appropriate sequence to follow for a patient for lens removal is an eight-step process. This is shown in Table 6.5.

Lens Case

The lens case should have several important features to be effective for GP lens storage. It should easily differentiate left from right lenses. Many cases have an "L" and an "R" in the lens well or on the cap (Fig. 6.12). A hard plastic, ribbed, and deep-welled case is recommended, both to allow sufficient solution in the wells and to minimize leakage. The more flexible, hyper-Dk lens materials can adhere to a smooth-welled case if placed improperly in the case (e.g., convex side up), possibly resulting in warpage caused by the force required to remove the lens from the case. In addition, lenses that adhere to the bottom of a smooth-surface case may

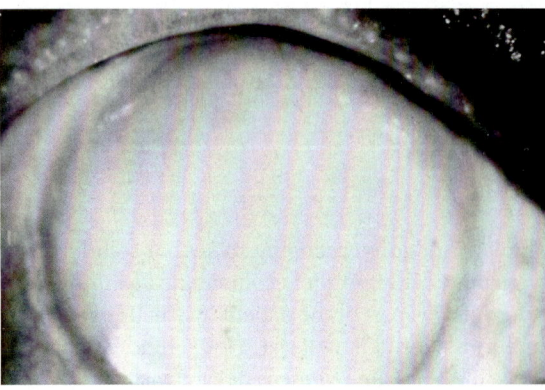

FIGURE 6.11 A *Pseudomonas* ulcer in which "topping off" of solution was implicated as the probable cause. (Courtesy of Larry J. Davis, OD.)

TABLE 6.5 Proper Steps for Gas-Permeable Lens Removal

1. Wash hands with an antimicrobial soap (30 s).
2. Always begin with the same lens every time.
3. Remove the lens and place it in the palm of the hand.
4. Apply contact lens solution/lens cleaner and rub the lens for 30 s.
5. Rinse the lens with contact lens solution; never use tap water.
6. Place the contact lens into a clean lens case and completely fill the case well with the recommended multipurpose/disinfection solution.
7. Soak the lens according to the manufacturers' recommended soaking time.
8. Read the solution packaging thoroughly for instruction about lens cleaning and always follow the recommended procedures.

experience edge chipping from the excessive digital pressure needed to dislodge the lens. Both these problems can be eliminated by using a case that has ridges or holes in the wells. As the lens case is an excellent source of microorganisms (Fig. 6.13), it should be washed every morning and allowed to air dry face down with caps off. Immediately after the lenses are removed from the case, the case wells should be rubbed with clean fingers for at least 5 seconds, rinsed with contact lens disinfection solution, then wiped clean with a clean cloth.[48] Patients should be encouraged to replace their case on a regular basis (i.e., every 1–3 months). To reinforce the importance of a clean case, a new one can be provided at every progress evaluation.

Scratches

Every patient should be warned about the softness of these materials, especially the hyper-Dk lens materials. Lenses should be handled over a towel or soft tissue. If the lens is exposed to a hard surface, a drop of wetting solution can be placed on a finger and the lens can be gently lifted off the surface to minimize scratches. In addition, bathroom floors, in particular, may harbor significantly high numbers of microorganisms; therefore, it is important to clean the lens anytime it has been dropped on the floor.[49]

Foreign-Body Particles

GP lens patients should be informed about the possibility of dust or debris becoming trapped underneath the lens and irritating the cornea. Using rewetting drops in this situation is very beneficial. If it results in greater than momentary discomfort, the patient should be told to remove the lens and clean it. If discomfort persists, the patient should call the practitioner's office.

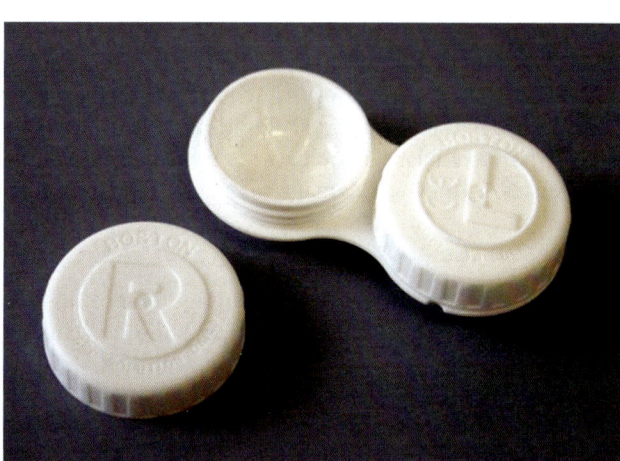

FIGURE 6.12 Easy differentiation of "L" versus "R" results from having these initials on the lens caps and within the wells of the case.

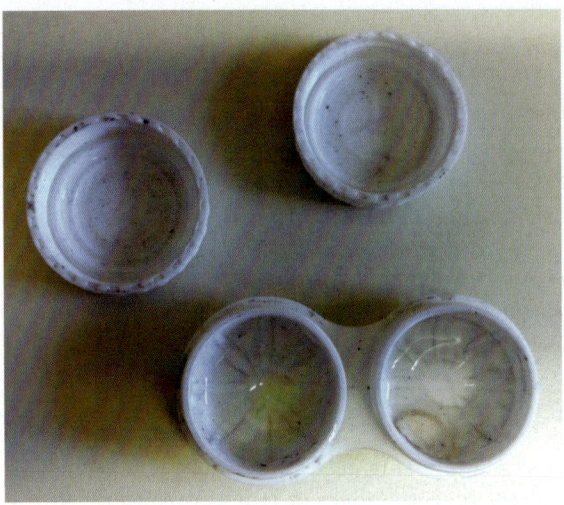

FIGURE 6.13 A contaminated gas-permeable lens case.

Cosmetics

Every contact lens patient should be thoroughly educated about the proper use of cosmetics. Cosmetics can be the cause of lens discoloration, damage, and surface deposition. Because many popular cosmetics contain ingredients such as preservatives, pigments, oils, and solvents, subjective discomfort and eye infection can result from their use.[50]

Cosmetics should be applied after lenses have been inserted. Mascara—notably lash-extending mascara that contains fibers that can irritate the eye—can flake off into the tear film, resulting in corneal abrasion. This is especially problematic with rigid EW patients in whom these flakes are trapped underneath an adherent lens during sleep.[51] Likewise, the application of solvent-based mascaras may lead to irritation of the skin around the eye.[52]

Bacterial infection is also a problem.[53] A patient may transfer infectious organisms from the lashes to the mascara wand and then to the mascara tube, where they colonize. In addition, eyeliner should not be applied to the inner lid margin because it may clog the meibomian glands, possibly resulting in blepharitis, hordeolum, or chalazion.

Numerous cosmetic products on the market are recommended for contact lens wearers. They are water soluble and contain little, if any, fragrances or fillers. It is important to note again that cosmetics should be applied after lenses have been inserted.

Any cream or oil that is used on the face or hands can be transferred to the contact lenses, resulting in discomfort and blurred vision; therefore, these substances should be applied after the lenses have been inserted. Any contaminant or residual oils on the hands can be transferred to the lens and possibly be absorbed into the lens matrix. Hand soaps contain additives such as oils, perfumes, dyes, deodorants, and abrasives that can complicate the problem.[54] The addition to the care regimen of an optical-compatible hand cleaner developed specifically for contact lens wearers will minimize discoloration and deposit buildup on contact lenses. In addition, it is important to advise female patients to keep false eyelash cement, perfume, and cologne away from lenses, as they can damage the plastic.[55]

Medication Use and GP Wear

Although GP lenses have the advantage of not absorbing a significant amount of topical medications, as with soft lenses drops, should be instilled 15 or 20 minutes before application of contact lenses or after they are removed.[56,57] If instilled with lenses on, the presence of the lens may limit the effectiveness of the drops.[58] Likewise, contact lenses should not be applied after application of an ointment as the viscosity of this medication can film up the lenses.

Swimming

The United States Food and Drug Administration (FDA) has recommended that contact lenses not be exposed to any form of water.[59] GP lens patients in particular should be advised not to swim with their contact lenses unless they wear goggles. If a patient swims with the GP lenses but without goggles, he or she should know not only about the likelihood of lens ejection but also that it may place them at risk for infection. *Acanthamoeba keratitis*, in particular, is caused by an organism present in all forms of impure water (i.e., swimming pools, tap, saunas, well, and showers).[60,61] Therefore, patients should be advised to insert their contact lenses after showering or, if lenses are to be worn while showering—to keep their eyes firmly closed.[62]

Adaptation

Patients should be told that adaptation varies from person to person with an average of 10 to 14 days before the achievement of no lens awareness. This period can be estimated by how much awareness is experienced at the dispensing visit. However, the patient should also know that it could last as long as 4 weeks in some patients. The patient should be reassured that comfort will typically improve on a daily basis. Avoiding the use of sensitizing words like pain and discomfort is helpful in reassuring the patient. Normal and abnormal adaptation symptoms are described for the patient in Table 6.6.

In addition, the patient should be told that, if lens wear must temporarily be discontinued (e.g., because of irritation or a lost lens), wearing time will need to be rebuilt gradually. A typical wearing schedule is given below:

Day 1 4 hours
Day 2 4 hours
Day 3 6 hours
Day 4 6 hours
Day 5 8 hours
Day 6 8 hours
Day 7 10 hours
Day 8 10 hours

Current all-day rigid lens wearers should be able to go into a full 12-hour wearing schedule immediately after receiving their new GP lenses. New patients who exhibit little awareness initially—often the same individuals who have little difficulty with procedures such as drop

TABLE 6.6 Normal and Abnormal Gas-Permeable Lens Adaptation Symptoms

Normal Adaptation Symptoms (Diminish Gradually)
Tearing
Minor irritation
Intermittent blurry vision
Light sensitivity as well as extra sensitivity to wind, smoke, and dust
Mild redness
Abnormal Symptoms (Occur Suddenly)
Sudden pain or burning (greater than minor irritation)
Severe or persistent haloes seen around lights
Severe redness or irritation
Blurry vision through spectacles for over 1 hr
Increasing eye discharge or mattering

instillation, tonometry, and lid eversion—can increase their wearing time 2 hours per day. Some practitioners prefer to have daily-wear patients wear their lenses a minimum of 4 hours prior to their scheduled progress evaluation; therefore, it is important to schedule these visits in the afternoon or evening. Exceptions to this are GP EW patients, who should be seen in the morning. Typically, orthokeratology patients are evaluated in the morning after the first night of wear and then later in the day for subsequent visits to monitor residual refractive error at the end of the day.

Progress visits for a new daily-wear patient should be scheduled as follows:

Visit one	1 week after dispensing
Visit two	1 month after visit one
Visit three	6 months after visit two

After the 6-month visit, patients should be scheduled at regular 6-month intervals.

For continuous-wear patients, visits should be scheduled as follows:

Visit one	1 week after dispensing (daily wear)
Visit two	24 hours after initiating EW
Visit three	1 week after initiating EW
Visit four	1 month after visit three
Visit five	3 months after visit three

After the initial five visits, progress evaluations should be scheduled every 3 months for the EW patient.

Educational Methods

The educational process should be a four-step process: written, verbal, audiovisual, and reinforcement.

Written: A patient instructional manual is beneficial in the educational process. It should be comprehensive and should contain the information provided in Table 6.7. In addition, it should be written in layperson's language with a print quality that makes it easy for a patient to read, understand, and comply with the information presented. The manual can also have a patient agreement form that has important information such as the after-hours contact information and care regimen (see Fig. 6.10). This should be signed in duplicate; for example, the second form can be attached by perforation and easily removed for the patient's permanent record. This manual can include customized inserts on such information as a fee or compliance agreement, cosmetic use, and continuous wear. The assistant can discuss the most important information with the patient and encourage the patient to ask questions. It should also be noted that, from a medical–legal point of view, an informed consent document listing wearing schedule and solution brands should be signed and dated by the patient.[63]

Verbal: The verbal educational process is much more important than the written process because patients cannot be expected to understand all the information provided and, on occasion, the manual may not be read at all. In addition to handling information, a well-trained assistant can review important care information provided in the manual.

Audiovisual: A more innovative and effective method of patient education is the use of audiovisual materials. For example, an instructional DVD produced by the Contact Lens Manufacturers Association (CLMA) and the GP Lens Institute (GPLI) is available from the CLMA (1-800-344-9060). Video segments demonstrating lens handling as well as a care and handling patient brochure are also available on the GPLI website (http://www.gpli.info). If any reservations pertaining to a patient's ability to handle or care for contact lenses exist, audiovisual

TABLE 6.7 Checklist for Gas-Permeable Patient Instruction Manual

- Composition, benefits, and applications of a GP lens
- Insertion, removal, and decentration
- Cleaning techniques
- Normal and abnormal adaptation symptoms
- Importance of adhering to prescribed wearing schedule
- Causes of reduced wear (e.g., colds, hay fever, medications)
- Importance of using the recommended care regimen (not saliva or other brands); alternative acceptable solutions
- How to minimize loss and surface damage
- Benefits of a spare pair of lenses or spectacles
- Swimming and showering
- Cosmetic use
- Caring for the lens case
- Possible contact lens-induced complications (i.e., redness, reduced vision, pain, etc.) and what to do
- Visit schedule
- Fee and refund policy

materials reviewed together in the office or for frequent viewing at home would be an excellent supplement to the instruction manual.

Reinforcement: Important care instructions should be reviewed with the patient at *every* progress evaluation visit. They can include such information as the following:

1. What solutions are being used? Are the solutions the same as originally dispensed?
2. How often is the patient cleaning the lenses?
3. What method is being used for cleaning?
4. What is the current wearing schedule?
5. What is the current condition of the lens case?
6. Does the patient have any questions?

Studies have found that patient awareness of the need for proper care can be improved by regular reinforcement.[64,65] In one large clinical study, asymptomatic contact lens wearers who did not have their lens care instructions reinforced at progress visits over a 3-month period ended up with over 50% contamination of their solution samples.[51] A second group, who had their care instructions reviewed with them at every follow-up visit, ended up with only 6% contamination of their solution samples.

IMPORTANT ISSUES

Compliance

Several recent studies have found a low patient compliance rate with contact lenses in general.[66,67] In fact, when over 1,400 lens wearers were asked to complete a 14-question compliance questionnaire, only 0.3% admitted compliance with all steps.[67] This was validated more recently when it was found that—although 85% of patients reported that they perceived themselves as compliant, only 2% demonstrated good compliance and only 0.4% perfect compliance.[68] Ocular complications associated with noncompliance are more common with soft lens wearers.[69–71] However, GP lens wearers who do not comply with the recommended care guidelines may experience problems as well. Some of the more frequent causes of noncompliance problems with GP lens wearers include the following:

1. Patient does not clean the lenses as often or as comprehensively as desired (if at all).
2. Patient does not adhere to the prescribed wearing schedule.
3. Patient does not use disinfection solution or, if used, does not replace it regularly.
4. Patient does not wash hands before handling the lenses.
5. An inappropriate wetting solution such as saliva or tap water is used.
6. Expired solutions are used.
7. Case is not cleaned regularly.
8. Patient substitutes originally recommended solution with another brand.

One study found that approximately 50% of rigid lens care solutions were contaminated.[70] In addition, a much higher percentage of patients who admitted noncompliance were found to have contaminated care regimens than compliant patients. It is important to note that all solutions that were <21 days old were uncontaminated.

It is evident that patients exhibiting poor case hygiene are at greater risk of having an infection.[72] A 2009 study found that only 26% of patients clean their cases every night, with one-third cleaning the cases monthly or even less.[73] Case contamination is not uncommon and often occurs from failure to clean and store cases properly, dirty fingers, climate, "topping off," tap water, and variable storage times.[74] The most common pathologic organisms found in lens cases include *Pseudomonas, Serratia marcescens, Staphylococcus, Acanthamoeba*, and *Fusarium*.[74] There is evidence that adherence occurs at a greater frequency in used cases than in new cases.[75]

One important problem resulting from poor compliance is the development of a *microbial biofilm* within the case, attached to the lenses or the solutions.[76-78] Bacteria in a nutrient-deprived environment, such as the contact lens case, initiate a survival strategy to make them more resistant to disinfectants. The principal strategy is the development of a bacterial (although fungi, algae, and protozoa may also be present) biofilm, which is a collection of bacterial cells in an exopolysaccharide glycocalyx slime secreted by the bacterial cell (Fig. 6.14).[79]

This glycocalyx slime can serve as protection for the bacteria against certain preservatives. A notable example is the resistance of *Serratia marcescens* against chlorhexidine. It has been found that PAPB's performance is superior to that of chlorhexidine- and benzalkonium-preserved solutions with respect to preservative efficacy and prevention of biofilm formation in contact lens cases.[80] In addition, the combination of benzyl alcohol and a surfactant mixture should provide good effectiveness against biofilm formation. To minimize biofilm formation, cases should be designed with minimal hard-to-clean areas and replaced every 1 to 3 months, as noted before. Disposing of cases on a regular basis may be as—or more—important than

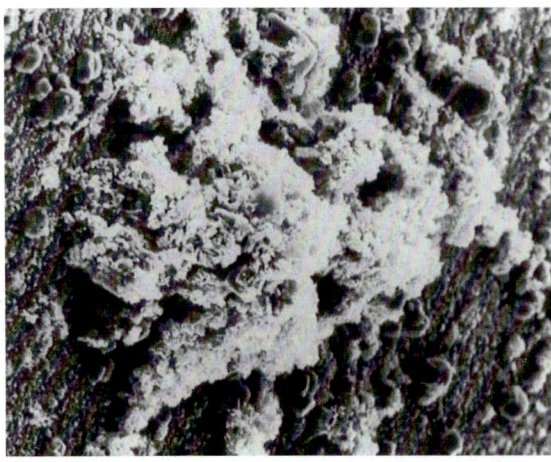

FIGURE 6.14 Bacteria biofilm formation. (Courtesy of Patrick J. Caroline.)

disposing of lenses as recommended. Ideally, every bottle of multipurpose solution should have a case enclosed; if so, four of five wearers would replace their case with each purchase.[81] Finally, another method of reducing contaminated case-related complications would be to add two steps to the case cleaning regimen: fill the empty case with solution, rub with the finger for 5 seconds, discard the solution, and then wipe the case with a clean tissue[82] as the mechanical wiping action will significantly reduce the lens case bioburden.[76,83]

The introduction of silver-impregnated cases such as Pro-Guard (Alcon Labs) result in less biofilm formation due to a lower potential for developing bacterial resistance than standard polypropylene cases.[84,85] As moisture helps activate the silver, however, these cases should be stored with the caps on. Another innovative case is LensAlert (Watchdog Group, LLC, www.lensalert.com). These cases are placed in the LensAlert holder, and a digital countdown timer for contact lens case replacement can be set for 1, 2, or 3 months.[86]

In a recent international analysis of contact lens compliance, the most important factors were found to be importance of case cleaning, hand washing, and rubbing and rinsing, especially in young male wearers.[87] Appropriate cleaning and disinfection practices should also be executed on a daily basis. Certainly, by optimizing patient compliance, the probability of ocular complications and liability problems will be minimized. A three-step approach has been recommended.[88]

1. Inspect the lens care products that you use in your office or sell—look for contamination, tampering, and expired bottles.
2. Assume patients know nothing; document your instructions and warnings in patient files.
3. Inspect patient's solutions at follow-up visits, and question patients about any solution substitutions while reinforcing proper care procedures. A summary nomogram on management of patient noncompliance is provided in Figure 6.15.

Tap Water

Just as saliva should not be used as a wetting agent because it contains an estimated 109 bacteria per milliliter,[89] the use of tap water with GP lenses remains a contentious issue because of the association of contact lens wear with *Acanthamoeba* keratitis.[90–93] Although the condition is rare, the prognosis for visual rehabilitation is poor, and the treatment regimen expensive and prolonged.[94,95] *Acanthamoeba* is a ubiquitous, free-living protozoan organism that is present in water, soil, sewage systems, and air.[96] The scientific literature first documents case reports of *Acanthamoeba* keratitis in 1974.[97] Disease incidence increased slightly over the following decade, with an outbreak in the mid-1980s associated with homemade saline and inconsistent hydrogel contact lens disinfection practices.[90,98] In the most recent outbreak, the Centers for Disease Control and Prevention determined that the risk for *Acanthamoeba* keratitis was seven times greater for consumers who used a multipurpose solution, which was soon after withdrawn from the market.[99,100] Recent research implicates other environmental factors, such as contaminated water.[101] Hence, contact lens wear appears to be a primary risk factor with inappropriate contact lens cleaning or disinfection practices, swimming or showering with contact lens wear, improper lens case care, and preexisting corneal compromise predisposing factors. Furthermore, a number of recent cases are in conjunction with GP lenses prescribed for overnight orthokeratology.[102–104] Therefore, it is beneficial to avoid the potential for contamination through good lens care practices, with the use of tap water contraindicated in GP, as well as soft lens regimens.[105] The mechanical effect of digital rubbing, accompanied by rinsing, has been found to dislodge *Acanthamoeba* from the lens surface.[106,107] Likewise, as the FDA has not, to date, required solutions to demonstrate efficacy against *Acanthamoeba* to be introduced to the market, this recommendation has been made by both the American Academy of Optometry and the American Optometric Association.[108] Another option to reduce noncompliance via tap water use to reduce costs would be to prescribe the same unit dose 0.9% sodium chloride inhalation/irrigation vials used with scleral lenses to rinse off the cleaner from smaller diameter

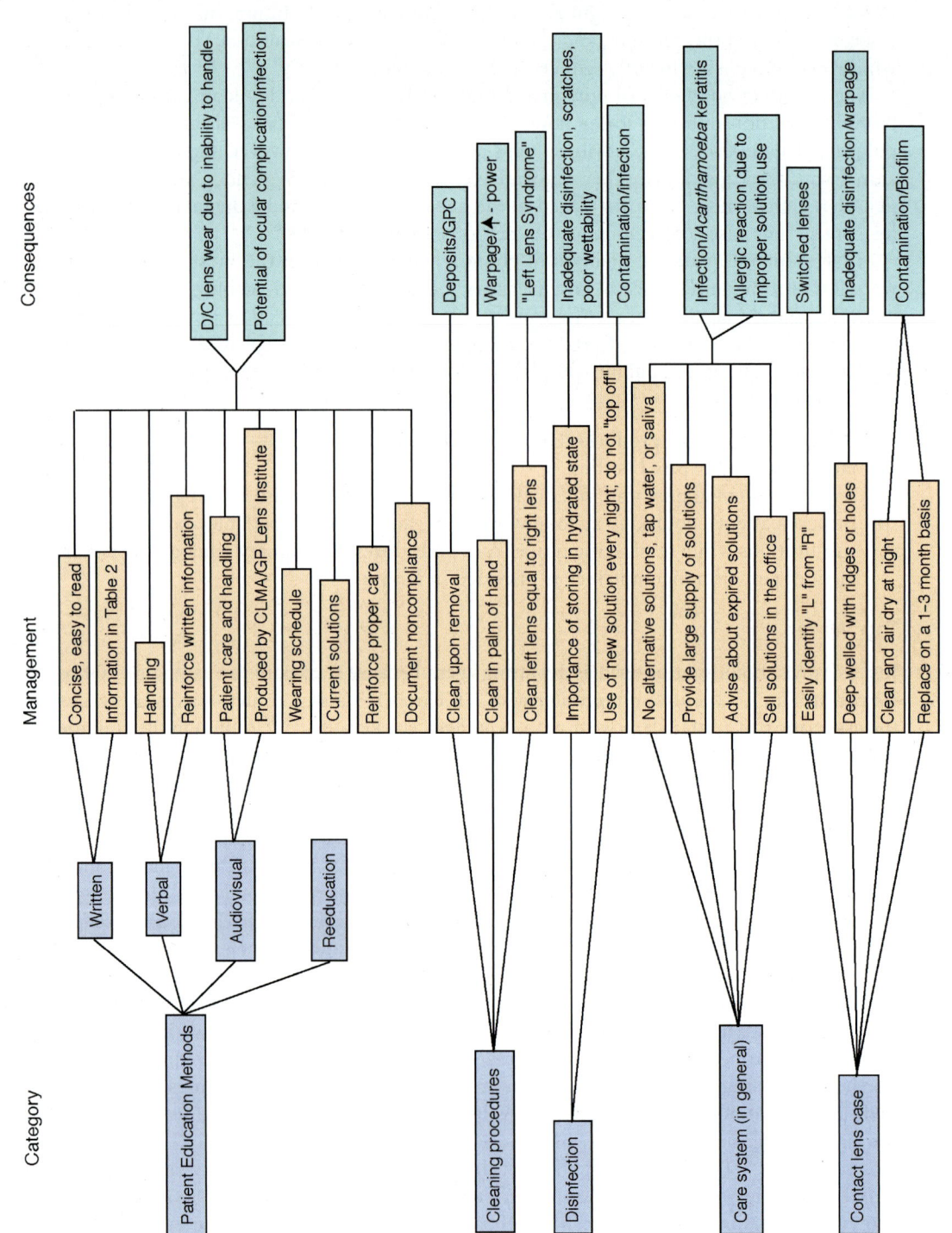

FIGURE 6.15 Compliance summary nomogram.

TABLE 6.8 Guidelines to Minimize Risk of *Acanthamoeba* Keratitis

Solution Use

- Use fresh disinfecting solution every day. Do not reuse or top off solution.
- Use only products recommended by your eye care practitioner. The use of saline solution (not intended for disinfection) and rewetting drops should be used for soaking the lenses.
- Tap water should not be used in the wetting, rewetting, or soaking of contact lenses.

Care and Compliance

- Always wash your hands before handling contact lenses.
- Unless daily disposable lenses are being worn, always clean the lenses or—at minimum—utilize a rub-and-rinse action upon removal.

Lens Case

- Replace the lens case, at minimum, every 3 months, although preferably every month.
- Rinse the case every day with sterile disinfecting solution, and allow to air dry (exception: Proguard lens case with Aquify solution has antimicrobial properties with lens caps on).
- The lens case should be sterilized on a regular basis (weekly recommended); either by boiling the case in hot water or microwaving the case (in dry form) for 3 min.

Environment

- Do not swim while wearing your contact lenses. If so, dispose of the lenses immediately after swimming (use rewetting drops to loosen lenses first). It would be preferable to wear airtight goggles over the lenses if they are to be worn during swimming.
- Do not wear contact lenses while showering, while in a hot tub, or during exposure to well water.

GP lenses.[109] This application is an off-label use. Important steps in optimizing compliance and minimizing the incidence of *Acanthamoeba* keratitis are provided in Table 6.8.[110]

Solution Confusion

The large number of currently available GP and soft lens care products also makes patient compliance more challenging. In one study, 40% of patients could not recall the name of their prescribed product(s).[111] This could result in their inadvertently selecting a similar-appearing but incorrect (and possibly ill-advised) solution. The situation may be further confused by competitive contact lens solution marketing, which may result in companies' adopting similar-appearing label colors, print styles, and bottle sizes and shapes.[112] Finally, solution substitution may simply be a result of pricing—the patient may buy the solution simply because it is less expensive. Certainly, generic solution use has increased and over 25% of patients do switch solutions within the first year.[113,114] This is important as it has been found that patients using generic solutions are at a higher risk for ocular complications.[115]

Solution confusion can be minimized by the following steps:

1. Thoroughly educate patients about what solutions they can use, including alternatives.
2. Emphasize *why* you are recommending specific solutions to discourage price shopping.
3. Inquire about what solutions are being used at progress evaluation visits to ensure that solution switching has not occurred. To obtain an honest response, it is important for the practitioner or assistant to use neutral questioning, such as "What is the name of the solution you are using?" Otherwise, if patients are asked if they are still using the recommended solution, they may sheepishly answer "yes."
4. Provide a large (3 months) supply of solutions, initially, to minimize solution substitution.
5. Sell solutions in the office or provide them at no extra cost—put the cost into the office fees, for example.

One system that satisfies both points 4 and 5 above is the newly introduced Menicon WebStore (http://store.meniconamerica.com). The eye care practitioner (ECP) can register online and order Deluxe Care Systems. It can be dispensed to the patient who can then register online and order solutions. The ECP can track patient purchases while also benefitting financially from each purchase.

WHEN TO CALL THE DOCTOR

Patients should be advised to call their ECP if problems arise. According to the FDA, it is important not to ignore symptoms of eye irritation or infection, which can include discomfort, excess tearing or other discharge, unusual sensitivity to light, itching, burning, gritty feelings, unusual redness, blurred vision, swelling, and pain.[116] Patients should be told to remove their lenses immediately and keep them off, contact their ECP immediately, and keep their lenses as their ECP may want to evaluate them. If an eye infection exists, and they wait 2 days or longer before contacting their ECP, there is a 4.5 times greater risk of experiencing permanent loss of vision,[117] and therefore, it is important for them to seek treatment immediately when these symptoms are present.[118] In addition, it is important for the patient to be advised to always have a pair of glasses to wear when contact lens wear needs to be discontinued.

Consumer Resources

There are some excellent consumer-based resources that can help educate both patient and practitioner about proper lens care.

1. www.contactlenssafety.org. This website represented a collaboration of leaders from the American Optometric Association Contact Lens and Cornea Section and the American Academy of Optometry Cornea, Contact Lenses, and Refractive Technologies Section. It consists of 50 commonly asked questions asked by consumers with the accompanying answers. There are questions pertaining to contact lens replacement compliance, common causes of infection, when to call a doctor if a contact lens-induced problem has occurred, what to do if the contact lenses are filmy and uncomfortable, the importance of the solution expiration date, storing lenses that are not currently being worn, lens case care and compliance, tap water implications, showering and swimming with contact lenses on, and appropriate use of cosmetics while wearing contact lenses. This is not only a beneficial site to direct patients in an effort to educate them about proper contact lens care, but as all questions have the appropriate references to support each answer, this is a valuable site for practitioners and students as well.[119]
2. www.contactlenses.org. This is the consumer-based website of the CLMA. The emphasis of this site pertains to GP lenses, with an entire section on GP lens care and handling. Included in this area are videos on GP lens care insertion and removal. There is also an opportunity for consumers to submit questions, which are answered by an optometrist who is a consultant to the CLMA.
3. www.allaboutvision.com. The most popular consumer vision website, this site has a very large section on contact lenses. This includes information on contact lens tips and frequently asked questions, GP lens care, use of tap water, and contact lens complications.

SUMMARY

GP lenses provide less risk of surface contamination and preservative sensitivity than soft lenses. Nevertheless, comprehensive and effective patient education is extremely important for the eventual success of the patient.

CLINICAL CASES

CASE 1

A GP patient enters your office for her 1-week progress evaluation with her 45-Dk GP lenses. She has complaints of mild itching, burning, and redness that occur for a few minutes after insertion of her lenses. She is using a PAPB-preserved care system. The slit-lamp examination reveals mild diffuse punctate staining and grade 1+ conjunctival injection in both eyes.

SOLUTION: Most likely, this is the result of an allergic reaction to the preservative in this system. This patient can be switched to another preserved system such as BAK, chlorhexidine, or benzyl alcohol.

CASE 2

Your patient returns for a 1-month evaluation of his 60-Dk F-S/A lenses. He complains of "foggy vision," which began in the past week. Your slit-lamp evaluation shows a mucoprotein film on the lens surface. In addition, he has grade 1 conjunctival injection and mild (grade 1+) papillary hypertrophy. He is currently using a nonabrasive surfactant cleaner, although he admits that the lenses are not being cleaned every night.

SOLUTION: Review proper lens care procedures with the patient and indicate why these procedures are important. Emphasize proper cleaning upon removal every night followed by storage of the lens in the recommended soaking solution. In addition, an abrasive cleaner supplemented by liquid enzymatic cleaning (as often as every night) should be recommended (unless the lens is plasma treated or manufactured from a hyper-Dk lens material).

CASE 3

Your patient is motivated for GP lenses and you are able to achieve a successful fit, although some difficulty is experienced with placing the lenses on the patient's eyes because she is apprehensive about anything touching her eyes; in addition, her eyes are somewhat deep set. The lenses have arrived from the laboratory, and the patient is in your office for the dispensing visit. Your assistant is experiencing difficulty with teaching the patient proper lens insertion. How do you handle this situation?

SOLUTION: In this case, emphasizing the importance of lid retraction accompanied by *much* reassurance is very important. It should be demonstrated to the patient how to pin back the lashes to minimize the lid closure effect not uncommon with new patients. Likewise, with removal, the lashes should be pinned back to eliminate the possibility of lid eversion. The use of an instructional video, which can be viewed repeatedly, if desired, would also be beneficial. If the patient is still experiencing difficulty, she can be asked to return for a second visit to continue learning how to handle the lenses; in the interim, she can practice bringing her finger (with a warm drop of water, which will have a numbing effect) up to her eye. The patient can also be provided with an educational DVD to reinforce proper handling.

CASE 4

A patient enters your office for a 3-month GP lens evaluation. It is readily apparent that the patient's hygiene is less than ideal; in addition, upon removal of the lenses, it is observed that his case is contaminated.

SOLUTION: Comprehensive patient reeducation and a regular case replacement program are important in this case. If his case is contaminated, it is very likely his solutions are as well (e.g., cap off the bottle, hands not washed before handling lenses, "topping off" solution). It is important to review proper care procedures and the possible ramifications if noncompliance continues. Reviewing daily and weekly case cleaning methods is important. The patient can be provided with several new cases to reinforce the importance of using clean cases. A photo album illustrating compliance-induced complications would be very beneficial in this case as well.

CASE 5

Your GP lens patient enters for his 6-month progress evaluation. His only complaint is intermittent blurred or foggy vision in his left eye. Slit-lamp evaluation shows a good lens-to-cornea fitting relationship in both eyes; however, the left lens shows a mucoprotein film. In addition, the left bulbar conjunctiva is slightly injected, whereas it is clear in the right eye. Upon lid eversion, the right upper tarsal conjunctiva exhibits a grade 1—papillary hypertrophy, whereas the left lid is grade 2.

SOLUTION: Very likely, this is "left lens syndrome." The patient will need to be educated to clean the left lens as well as the right. In addition, in-office cleaning with a compatible laboratory cleaner or solvent should assist in cleaning the left lens.

CASE 6

Your long-term PMMA and very-low-Dk S/A lens wearer, who has been refit into high-Dk F-S/A GPs, is in your office for dispensing of his new lenses. During the patient education process, he admits to your assistant that he often uses tap water as a wetting solution for insertion of the lenses. In addition, when asked, he also admitted to occasionally rewetting the lenses with saliva. What do you tell this individual?

SOLUTION: This patient is similar to many former PMMA patients who developed poor care habits with their hard lenses. Since the durability and wettability of hard lenses typically are superior to GP lenses, the patient needs to be told to adhere to the recommended care instructions to minimize the incidence of problems such as warpage, scratches, and deposits. In addition, the possibility of ocular infection (e.g., corneal ulcer, *Acanthamoeba* keratitis) should be mentioned as well, especially if an inappropriate wetting solution is used. The fact that the incidence of *Acanthamoeba* keratitis has increased recently, often resulting in vision loss and a corneal transplant, should be indicated as well.

CASE 7

A GP lens patient enters your office complaining of redness, itching, and burning, which began right after she purchased her new solutions. Upon questioning, she admitted that she bought a generic brand of solution, which was on sale at the pharmacy. In addition, she admitted some difficulty in remembering the specific solutions she is supposed to use. Upon performing slit-lamp evaluation, she exhibited the same signs of a preservative-induced solution reaction as experienced by the patient in Case 1.

SOLUTION: Patient reeducation is important in this case. She can (once again) be provided with a form giving the specific recommended solutions. In addition, the possible problems resulting from the use of inappropriate (including "bargain") solutions should be discussed. If she is experiencing much difficulty in remembering the solution names, she can be provided with a generous supply of the solutions. If she also admits difficulty with using a solution appropriately (e.g., using wetting/soaking solution for cleaning the lens), large labels can be placed over the bottles, each indicating the specific function of that particular solution.

CASE 8

A patient returns to the office for a 1-week follow-up visit for scleral GP lenses. Your patient reports vague symptoms of discomfort that worsened over the week. You observe diffuse punctate corneal staining with biomicroscopy.

SOLUTION: Review lens care to ensure that the patient is using preservative-free saline to fill the lens bowl prior to lens insertion. Scleral lenses have limited tear exchange. This characteristic results in an increased contact time between the lens care products and the corneal epithelium. It should be noted that some patients report enhanced comfort with the use of preservative-free lens care products with a higher viscosity.

CLINICAL PROFICIENCY CHECKLIST

- PAPB and benzyl alcohol are examples of GP lens preservatives that have demonstrated an ability to minimize microbial biofilm formation.
- The use of a small particulate abrasive cleaner (unless a plasma-treated lens) or surfactant-soaking regimen, supplemented by liquid enzyme use, is effective for deposit-prone patients.
- In-office use of a laboratory cleaner, compatible solvent, or alcohol-based cleaner is recommended for both poor initial wettability and long-term acquired deposit buildup problems.
- Patients should clean their lenses immediately upon removal in the palm of the hand and then place them in the recommended disinfecting solution.
- At the dispensing visit, visual acuity, overrefraction, and a comprehensive slit-lamp examination (i.e., lens position and lag, fluorescein pattern, and surface wettability) should be performed.
- As GP lenses typically have a lower edge lift design, patients need to be educated about alternative methods of lens removal, with an emphasis on lid pressure against the lens edge.
- Comprehensive patient education is essential. A four-step approach is recommended: verbal instruction, written education manual, audiovisual observation, and reinforcement of care at follow-up visits. Patients should be advised to restate the important care instructions.
- The lens case is an important component of the care regimen. Patients should be instructed to clean the case every night and dispose it on a regular (every 1–3 months) basis.
- Tap water should not be used with GP lenses, especially for wetting/rewetting purposes. *Acanthamoeba* keratitis has been implicated with tap water use when caring for GP lenses.

REFERENCES

1. Bennett ES, Grohe RM. Lens care and solutions. In: Bennett ES, Grohe RM, eds. *Rigid Gas-Permeable Contact Lenses*. New York, NY: Professional Press; 1986:225–244.
2. Mandell RB. Lens care and storage. In: Mandell RB, ed. *Contact Lens Practice*. Springfield, IL: Charles C. Thomas; 1988:326–351.
3. Hopkins GA. The formulation of rigid lens care systems. *Optician*. 1986;191(5038):18–22.
4. Brown MRW, Richards RME. Effect of ethylenediamine tetraacetate on the resistance of *Pseudomonas aeruginosa* to antibacterial agents. *Nature*. 1965;207:1391–1393.
5. MacKeen GD, Bulle K. Buffers and preservatives in contact lens solutions. *Contacto*. 1977;21(6):33–36.
6. Lieblein JS. Overview of soft contact lens hygiene. *Rev Optom*. 1978;115(4):29–32.
7. McLaughlin R, Barr JT, Rosenthal P, et al. The new generation of RGP solutions meet increasing demands. *Contact Lens Spectrum*. 1990;5(1):45–50.
8. Witten EM, Molinari JF. Allergic keratoconjunctivitis from thimerosal in soft contact lens solutions. *South J Optom*. 1981;23(7):12–20.
9. Binder PS, Rasmussen DM, Gordon M. Keratoconjunctivitis and soft contact lens solutions. *Arch Ophthalmol*. 1981;99(1):87–90.
10. Erikson S, et al. Suitability of thimerosal as a preservative in soft lens soaking solutions. In: Bitonte JL, Keates RH, eds. *Symposium on the Flexible Lens*. St. Louis, MO: Mosby; 1972.

11. Huth S, et al. Care products for silicone-copolymer lens materials. *Optician.* 1981;181(4701):16–18.
12. Mac Gregor DR, Elliker PR. A comparison of some properties of strains of *Pseudomonas aeruginosa* sensitive and resistant to quaternary ammonium compounds. *Can J Microbial.* 1968;4:449–503.
13. Begley CG, Weirich B, Benak J, et al. Effects of rigid gas permeable contact lens solutions on the human corneal epithelium. *Optom Vis Sci.* 1992;69(5):347–353.
14. Begley CG, Waggoner PJ, Hafner GS, et al. Effect of rigid gas permeable contact lens wetting solutions on the rabbit corneal epithelium. *Optom Vis Sci.* 1991;68(3):189–197.
15. Keeven J, Wrobel S, Portoles M, et al. Evaluating the preservative effectiveness of RGP lens care solutions. *CLAO J.* 1995;21:238–241.
16. Hiti K, Walochnik J, Haller-Schober E, et al. Efficacy of contact lens storage solutions against different acanthamoeba strains. *Cornea.* 2006;25(4):423–427.
17. Hom MM. Current multi-purpose solution concepts. *Contact Lens Spectrum.* 2001;16(9):33–39.
18. Feldman GL. Benzyl alcohol: new life as an ophthalmic preservative. *Contact Lens Spectrum.* 1989;4(5):41–44.
19. Gasson A, Morris J. Care systems. In: *The Contact Lens Manual.* Oxford, England: Butterworth-Heinemann; 1992:234–244.
20. Weisbarth RE. Hydrogel lens care regimens and patient education. In: Bennett ES, Weissman BA, eds. *Clinical Contact Lens Practice.* Philadelphia, PA: Lippincott Williams & Wilkins; 1993:34-1–34-27.
21. Hill RM, Terry JE. Ophthalmic solutions: viscosity builders. *Am J Optom Physiol Opt.* 1974;51:847–851.
22. Krishna N, Brow F. Polyvinyl alcohol as an ophthalmic vehicle. *Am J Ophthalmol.* 1964;57:99–106.
23. Chou MH, Rosenthal P, Salamone JC. Which cleaning solution works best? *Contact Lens Forum.* 1985;10(8):41–47.
24. Doell GB, Palombi DL, Egan DJ, et al. Contact lens surface changes after exposure to surfactant and abrasive cleaning procedures. *Am J Optom Physiol Opt.* 1986;63(6):399–402.
25. Carrell B, Bennett ES, Henry VA, et al. The effect of abrasive cleaning on RGP lens performance. *J Am Optom Assoc.* 1992;63(3):193–198.
26. Boltz KD. The overzealous contact lens cleaner. *Contact Lens Spectrum.* 1989;4(12):53–56.
27. Bennett ES, Henry VA. RGP lens power change with abrasive cleaner use. *Int Cont Lens Clin.* 1990;17(3):152–154.
28. Feldman G. Manufacturer's report: a new system for RGP lens care. *Contact Lens Forum.* 1989;14(6):48.
29. Lasswell LA, Tarantino N, Kono D. Enzymatic cleaning of extended-wear lenses: papain vs. pancreatin. *Int Eyecare.* 1986;2(2):101–105.
30. Lowther GE. Caring for hard GP lenses. *Int Cont Lens Clin.* 1984;11(2):75.
31. Morgan P. A new liquid enzyme cleaner for daily use. *Optician.* 1998;215(5654):30–33.
32. Misel JP. Reviewing today's lens care systems. *Optom Today.* 1998;6(6):32–34.
33. Lowther GE. Effect of some solutions on HGP contact lens parameters. *J Am Optom Assoc.* 1987;58(3):188–192.
34. Rakow PL. Solution incompatibilities and confusion: observations and caveats. *Contact Lens Forum.* 1989;14(9):60–66.
35. Gromacki S. Contact lens care update. Presented at: Global Specialty Lens Symposium; January 2012; Las Vegas, NV.
36. Schafer J. Plasma treatment for GP contact lenses. *Contact Lens Spectrum.* 2006;21(11):19.
37. Greco A. Lubricating drops for hard and soft contact lenses. *Int Cont Lens Clin.* 1985;12(4):205–211.
38. Ward MA. Approved GP wetting drops. *Contact Lens Spectrum.* 2011;26(1):23.
39. Herman JP. Flexure of rigid contact lenses on toric corneas as a function of base curve fitting relationship. *J Am Optom Assoc.* 1983;54(3):209–213.
40. Fuls JL, Rodgers ND, Fischler GE et al. Alternative hand contamination technique to compare the activities of antimicrobial and nonantimicrobial soaps under different test conditions. *Appl Environ Microbiol.* 2008;74(12):3739–3744.
41. Szczotka-Flynn LB. Hand washing and contact lens contamination. *Contact Lens Spectrum.* 2011;26(5):15.
42. Henry VA, Bennett ES, Forrest J. Clinical investigation of the Paraperm EW rigid gas-permeable contact lens. *Am J Optom Physiol Opt.* 1987;64(5):313–320.
43. Cho P, Ng H, Chan I, et al. Effect of two different cleaning methods on the back optic zone radii and surface smoothness of menicon rigid gas permeable lenses. *Optom Vis Sci.* 2004;81(6):461–467.
44. Walline JJ, Rah MJ. Emphasizing lens care. *Contact Lens Spectrum.* 2008;23(1):51.
45. Caroline PJ, Andre MP. Preventing GP bevel plaque. *Contact Lens Spectrum.* 2010;25(4). http://www.clspectrum.com/articleviewer.aspx?articleID=104107.
46. Ward MA. Maintaining and disinfecting GP diagnostic lenses. *Contact Lens Spectrum.* 2006;21(9):24.
47. Boost M, Cho P, Lai S. Efficacy of multipurpose solutions for rigid gas permeable lenses. *Ophthalm Physiol Opt.* 2006;26(5):468–475.
48. Wu YT, Zhu H, Willcox M, et al. Removal of biofilm from contact lens storage cases. *Invest Ophthalmol Vis Sci.* 2010;51(12):6329–6333.
49. Gerba CP, Wallis C, Melnick JL. Microbiological hazards of household toilets: droplet production and the fate of residual organisms. *Appl Microbiol.* 1975;30(2):229–237.
50. Baldwin JS. Cosmetics: too long concealed as culprit in eye problems. *Contact Lens Forum.* 1986;11(6):38–41.
51. Bennett ES, Ghormley NR. Rigid extended wear: an overview. *Int Cont Lens Clin.* 1987;14(8):319–331.
52. Lodén M, Wessman C. Mascaras may cause irritant contact dermatitis. *Int J Cosmet Sci.* 2002;24(5):281–285.

53. Ng A, Mostardi B, Mandell RB. Adherence of mascara to soft contact lenses. *Int Cont Lens Clin.* 1988;15(2):64–68.
54. Hoffman WC, Cook SA. Reducing lens spoilage via CL wearers' hand soap. *Contact Lens Forum.* 1986;11(5):44–45.
55. American Optometric Association website. Contact lenses and cosmetics. http://www.aoa.org/x5236.xml. Accessed May 2012.
56. Bennett ES, Watanabe RK, Begley CG. Preliminary evaluation. In Bennett ES, Henry VA, eds. *Clinical Manual of Contact Lenses.* 3rd ed. Philadelphia, PA: Lippincott Williams & Wilkins; 2009:2–28.
57. Weisbarth RE, Henderson B. Hydrogel lens care regimens and patient education. In Bennett ES, Weissman BA, eds. *Clinical Contact Lens Practice.* Philadelphia, PA: Lippincott Williams & Wilkins; 2005:381–419.
58. Bartlett JD. Medications and contact lens wear. In: Silbert JA, ed. *Anterior Segment Complications of Contact Lens Wear.* New York, NY: Churchill-Livingstone, Inc.; 1994:474–482.
59. US Food and Drug Administration. http://www.fda.gov/medicaldevices/productsandmedicalprocedures/homehealthandconsumer/consumerproducts/contactlenses/default.htm. Accessed February 20, 2011.
60. Joslin CE, Tu EY, Shoff ME, et al. The association of contact lens solution use and Acanthamoeba keratitis. *Am J Ophthalmol.* 2007;144:169–180.
61. Butcko V, McMahon TT, Joslin CE, et al. Microbial keratitis and the role of rub and rinsing. *Eye Contact lens.* 2007;33(6):421–423.
62. Sweeney D, Holden B, Evans K, et al. Best practice contact lens care: a review of the Asia Pacific Contact Lens Care Summit. *Clin Exp Optom.* 2009;92(2):78–89.
63. Harris MG. Is your CL practice vulnerable to legal action? *Contact Lens Forum.* 1990;5(1):51–52.
64. Wilson LA, Sawant AO, Simmons RB, et al. Microbial contamination of contact lens storage cases and solutions. *Am J Ophthalmol.* 1990;109(2):193.
65. Cho P, Boost M, Cheng R. Non-Compliance and microbial contamination in orthokeratology. *Optom Vis Sci.* 2009;86(11):1227–1234.
66. Donshik PC, Ehlers WH, Anderson LD, et al. Strategies to better engage, educate, and empower patient compliance and safe lens wear: compliance what we know, what we do not know, and what we need to know. *Eye Contact Lens.* 2007;33(6):430–434.
67. Morgan P. Contact lens compliance and reducing the risk of keratitis. *Optician.* June 2007;20–25.
68. Robertson DM, Cavanagh HD. Non-compliance with contact lens wear and care practices: a comparative analysis. *Optom Vis Sci.* 2011;88(12):1402–1408.
69. Ky W, Scherick K, Stenson S. Clinical survey of lens care in contact lens patients. *CLAO J.* 1998;24(4):216–219.
70. Donzis PB, Mondino BJ, Weissman BA, et al. Microbial contamination of contact lens care systems. *Am J Ophthalmol.* 1987;104(4):325–333.
71. Smith RE, MacRae SM. Contact lenses: convenience and complications. *N Engl J Med.* 1989;321(12):824–826.
72. Stapleton F, Keay L, Edwards K, et al. The incidence of contact lens-related microbial keratitis in Australia. *Ophthalmology.* 2008;115(10):1655–1662.
73. Radford CF, Minassian D, Dart JK, et al. Risk factors for nonulcerative contact lens complications in an ophthalmic accident and emergency department: a case-control study. *Ophthalmology.* 2009;116:385–392.
74. Szczotka-Flynn L, Pearlman E, Ghannoum M. Microbial contamination of contact lenses, lens care solutions, and their accessories: a literature review. *Eye Contact Lens.* 2010;36(2):116–129.
75. Boost M, Shi GS, Cho P. Adherence of *Acanthamoeba* to lens cases and effects of drying on survival. *Optom Vis Sci.* 2011;88(6):703–707.
76. Caroline PJ, Campbell RC. Strategies of microbial cell survival in contact lens cases. *Contact Lens Forum.* 1990;15(9):27–36.
77. Campbell RC, Caroline PJ. Inefficacy of soft contact lens disinfection techniques in the home environment. *Contact Lens Forum.* 1990;15(9):17–25.
78. Caroline PJ, Andre MP. Searching for an antimicrobial contact lens case. *Contact Lens Spectrum.* 2005;20(1):56.
79. www.contactlenssafety.org. Accessed May 2012.
80. Chou MH, DeCicco BT, Keeven JK, et al. The mechanism of survival of bacteria in contact lens cases. Presented at: Annual Meeting of the Contact Lens Association of Ophthalmologists. January 1989; New Orleans, LA.
81. Cho P. Biofilms, noncompliance, and the contribution of the contact lens case. Presented at: Global Specialty Lens Symposium; January 2011; Las Vegas, NV.
82. Wu YT, Teng YJ, Nicholas M, et al. Impact of lens case hygiene on Contact lens case contamination. *Optom Vis Sci.* 2011;88(10):E1180–E1187.
83. Abengózar-Vela A, Pinto FJ, González-Méijome JM, et al. Contact lens case cleaning procedures affect storage solution pH and osmolality. *Optom Vis Sci.* 2011;88(12):1414–1421.
84. Amos CF, George, MD. Clinical and laboratory testing of a silver-impregnated lens case. *Cont Lens Anterior Eye.* 2006;29:247–255.
85. Dantam J, Zhu H, Stapleton F. Biocidal efficacy of silver-impregnated contact lens storage cases in vitro. *Invest Ophthalmol Vis Sci.* 2011;52(1):51–57.
86. Hall B, Jones L. Countering noncompliance with lens care and case technology. *Contact Lens Spectrum.* 2010;25(12):50.
87. Morgan PB, Efron N, Toshida H, et al. An international analysis of contact lens compliance. *Cont Lens Anterior Eye.* 2011;34(5):223–228.

88. Harris MG. Save yourself from lens care lawsuits. *Rev Optom*. 1990;127(4):69–71.
89. Dawes C. Salivary flow pattern and the health of hard and soft oral tissues. *J Am Dent Assoc*. May 2008; 139(suppl):18S–24S.
90. *Acanthamoeba* keratitis associated with contact lenses—United States. *Morb Mortal Wekly Rep*. 1986;35:405–408.
91. Stehr-Green JK, Bailey TM, Visvesvara GS. The epidemiology of *Acanthamoeaba* keratitis in the United States. *Am J Ophthalmol*. 1989;107:331–336.
92. Stehr-Green JK, Bailey TM, Brandt FH, et al. *Acanthamoeba* keratitis in soft contact lens wearers: a case-control study. *JAMA*. 1987;258:57–60.
93. Shoff ME. Joslin CE, Tu EY, et al. Efficacy of contact lens systems against recent clinical and tap water *Acanthamoeba* isolates. *Cornea*. 2008;27(6):713–719.
94. Kumar R, Lloyd D. Recent advances in the treatment of *Acanthamoeba* keratitis. *Clin Infect Dis*. 2002;35:434–441.
95. Mathers W. *Acanthamoeba*: a difficult pathogen to evaluate and treat. *Cornea*. 2004;23:325.
96. Kilvington S, Larkin DF. *Acanthamoeba* adherence to contact lenses and removal by cleaning agents. *Eye*. 1990;4:589–594.
97. Naginton J, Watson PG, Playfair TJ, et al. Amoebic infections of the eye. *Lancet*. 1974;2:1537–1540.
98. *Acanthamoeba* keratitis in soft-contact-lens wearers. *Morb Mortal Wkly Rep*. 1987;36:397–398.
99. *Acanthamoeba* keratitis—multiple states. *Morb Mortal Wkly Rep*. 2007;56:1–3.
100. Advanced Medical Optics voluntarily recalls Complete MoisturePlus contact lens solution. *FDA News*. May 26, 2007.
101. Joslin CE, Tu EY, Shoff ME, et al. The association of contact lens use and *Acanthamoeba* keratitis. *Am J Ophthalmol*. 2007;144:169–180.
102. Xuguang S, Lin C, Yan Z, et al. *Acanthamoeba* keratitis as a complication of orthokeratology. *Am J Ophthalmol*. 2003;136:1159–1161.
103. Yepes N, Lee SB, Hill V, et al. Infectious keratitis after overnight orthokeratology. *Cornea*. 2005;24:857–860.
104. Wilhelmus KR. *Acanthamoeba* keratitis during orthokeratology. *Cornea*. 2005;24:7.
105. Davis L. Lens hygiene and care system contamination of asymptomatic rigid gas permeable lens wearers. *Int Cont Lens Clin*. 1995;22:217–221.
106. Snyder C. Lens care complications where's the rub? *Cont Lens Anterior Eye*. 2006;29:161–162.
107. Shih KL, Hu JC, Sibley MJ. The microbiological benefit of cleaning and rinsing contact lenses. *Int Cont Lens Clin*. 1985;12(4):235–242.
108. Benjamin WJ, Bennett ES, Sindt CW, et al. Closing statement of the American Optometric Association and the American Academy of Optometry. FDA workshop on microbiological testing of contact lens care products. Jan 23, 2009. http://www.aaopt.org/content/docs/closing%20Statement%20AOAAAO%20FDA%20Micro%20Workshop.pdf. Accessed April, 2012.
109. Sindt CW. Going off-label. *Rev Cornea Contact Lenses*. March 2011:6.
110. Bennett ES. Contact lens care and compliance: has it changed since the *Fusarium* scare? *Rev Optom*. 2007;144(5):34–42.
111. Dumbleton K, Woods C, Jones L, et al. How compliant are today's wearers? *Contact Lens Spectrum*. 2010; 25(6):32–36.
112. Berenblatt AJ. Lens care systems: a practitioner's wish list. *Contact Lens Forum*. 1988;13(3):37–38.
113. Claydon BE, Efron N, Woods C. A prospective study of the effect of education on non-compliant behavior in contact lens wear. *Ophthal Physiol Opt*. 1997;17(2):137–146.
114. Miller J, Powell S, Espejo L, et al. Solution recommendations for soft contact lens wearers. Poster presented at: AOA; June 2010; Orlando, FL.
115. Forister JF, Forister EF, Yeung KK, et al. Prevalence of contact lens-related complications: UCLA contact lens study. *Eye Contact Lens*. 2009;35(4):176–180.
116. FDA Consumer Health Information. Focusing on contact lens safety. www.fda.gov/consumers/features/contactlens1107.html. Accessed April 8, 2011.
117. Edwards K, Keay L, Naduvilath T, et al. Characteristics of and risk factors for contact lens-related microbial keratitis in a tertiary referral hospital. *Eye*. 2009;23:153–160.
118. Keay L, Edwards K, Naduvilath T, et al. Microbial keratitis predisposing factors and morbidity. *Ophthalmology*. 2006;113:109–116.
119. Sindt C. Providing a safety net. *Rev Cornea Contact Lenses*. November 2011;12.

Chapter 7

Verification of Gas-Permeable Lenses

Vinita Allee Henry

VERIFICATION OF RADIUS

Base Curve Radius

The base curve radius (BCR) is one of the most important lens parameters to verify because it affects the lens-to-cornea fitting relationship. The most commonly used method of determining the BCR is the radiuscope or radiusgauge. The BCR is determined by the distance between the real and aerial images observed in the radiuscope (Fig. 7.1).

Following are the steps for determination of the BCR.

1. Place a small amount of water or saline in the depression of the lens mount. Gas-permeable (GP) solutions that are viscous should not be used, but multipurpose soft solutions can be used.
2. The lens should be clean and dry when placed in this depression, concave side upward. Caution should be taken to avoid submerging the entire lens or allowing any fluid on the concave surface as this will result in an inaccurate reading or a poor-quality image (Fig. 7.2).
3. Center and position the lens mount so that a small green beam of light can be observed reflected in the lens. The aperture selector should be in the large aperture position at the back of the instrument.
4. Viewed in the oculars, the real and aerial images will be observed as a spoke or star pattern (Fig. 7.3). The real image will appear at the lower end of the scale at approximately zero and will be centered; however, the aerial image will be located approximately 6 to 9 mm on the scale and may not be centered. This aerial image should be centered, and the lens mount should not be moved again before setting the instrument at zero and a reading is taken. Note that between the two images, the light filament (Fig. 7.4) will be observed.
5. On obtaining a clear, sharp spoke pattern of the real image at the lower end of the scale, place the needle on zero. This can be accomplished by using the knob located at the left side of most radiuscopes and the back of most radiusgauges (Fig. 7.5). The manual provided with the instrument should provide this information.
6. The objective should be adjusted with the coarse adjustment knob to obtain a clear, sharp image of the aerial image. As the scale increases in value, the light filament will be observed before the aerial image is viewed. The BCR will be the reading taken from the zero point to the clear, sharp image of the aerial image.
7. The BCR is read off the millimeter scale to the nearest hundredth. The millimeter scale is located in the ocular of the radiuscope and on a clock dial at the back of the radiusgauge. For example, a typical BCR would be recorded as 8.20 mm.

If the needle of the instrument will not position at zero when the real image is in focus, the nearest whole number should be used. This whole number will be added or subtracted from the final reading. For example, if the real image is in focus at +1.0 and the final reading is 7.0 mm, the BCR is 8.0 mm.

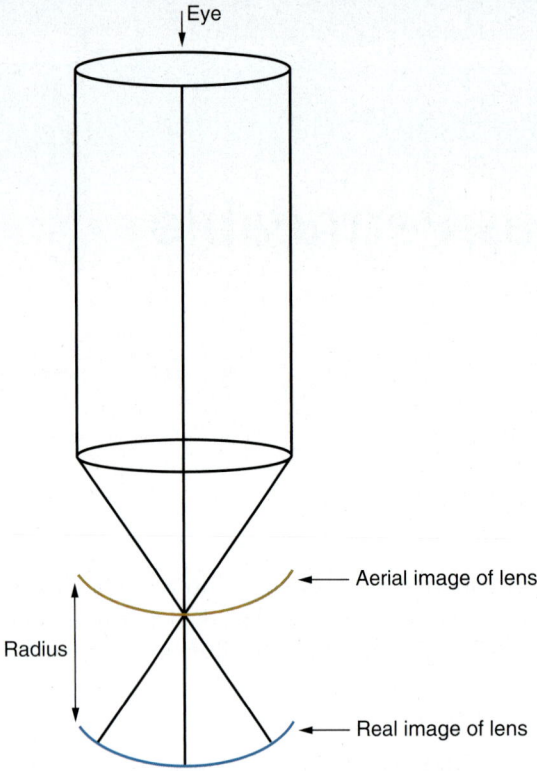

FIGURE 7.1 Diagram demonstrating that base curve radius is the difference between real image and aerial image.

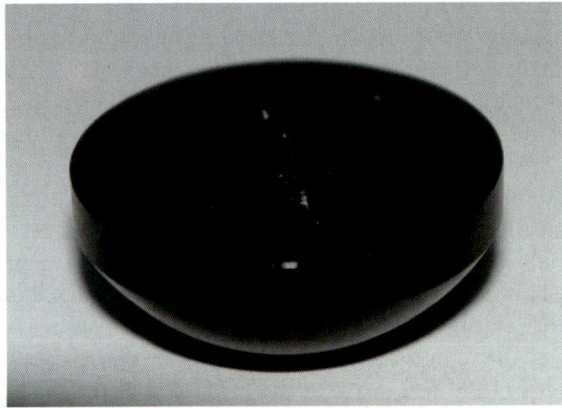

FIGURE 7.2 Lens mount for determining base curve radius.

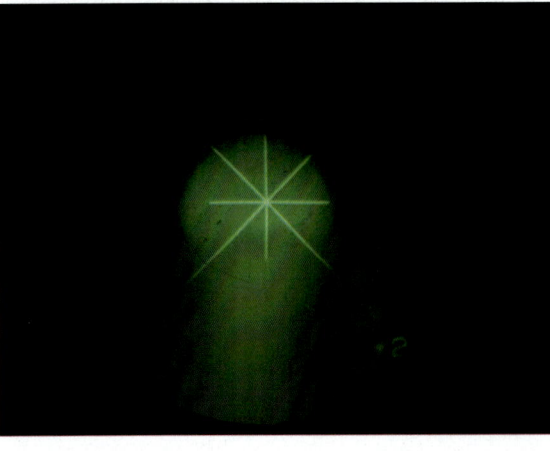

FIGURE 7.3 Spoke pattern observed in the radiuscope.

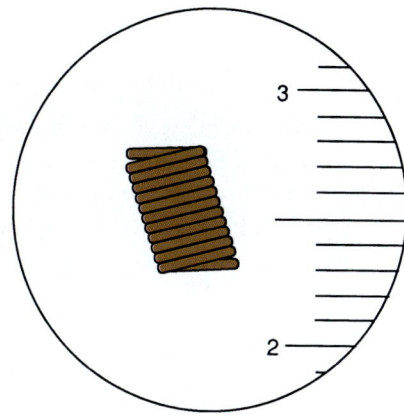

FIGURE 7.4 Diagram of light filament observed in the radiuscope.

Verification of the BCR of GP contact lenses is also possible with several automated keratometers. These devices have been found to accurately measure the BCR within tolerance.[1]

Verification of the BCR should be performed before dispensing and after 12 to 24 hours of soaking the lenses in an approved disinfecting solution. GP lenses may flatten on hydration, and verification is necessary to determine if the lens is still within tolerance.[2,3]

Front (Convex) Curve Radius

In addition to measuring the BCR, it may be necessary to measure the convex radius—for example, with front toric and bitoric lenses. A different lens mount is used to determine the convex radius (Fig. 7.6). The procedure is similar to determining the BCR with the exception that the real image is now the upper image and the aerial image is now the lower image. The needle should be set at the nearest whole number when the real image is in focus. When the

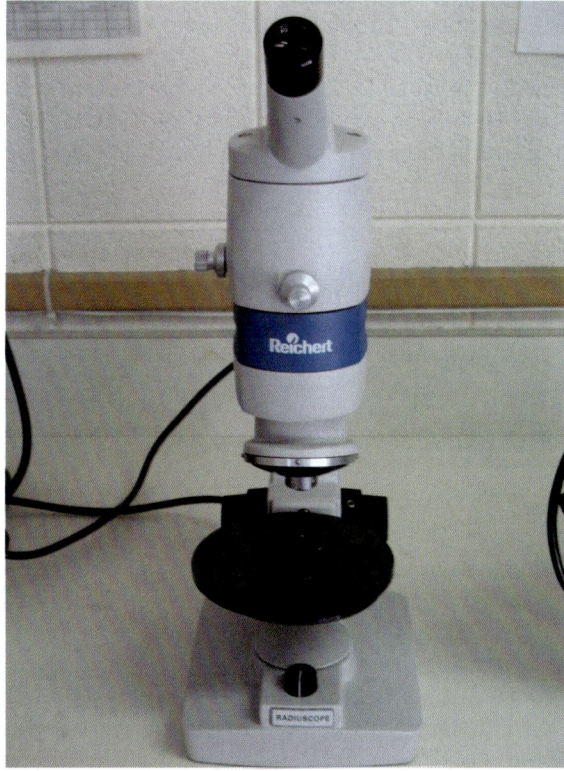

FIGURE 7.5 Radiuscope.

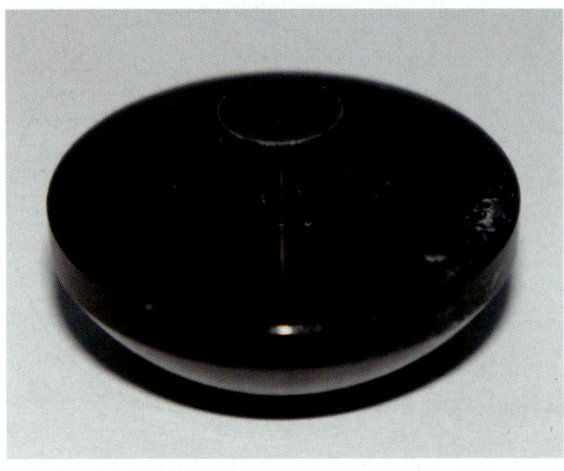

FIGURE 7.6 Lens mount used to measure the convex surface.

aerial image is in focus, the number is read from the scale and subtracted from the whole number. For example, if the real image is in focus at 8.00 mm and the aerial image is in focus at 1.00 mm, the resulting front curve radius would be 7.00 mm.

Toric or Warped Lenses

The steps for determining a toric or warped lens are similar to those for determining the BCR; however, the spokes of the image will not all be in focus at the same time. First, one set of spokes will come in sharp focus; this will represent the steeper curve. The spokes 90 degrees away from the first set of spokes will next come in focus, and this is the flatter curve. The symptoms of a patient wearing a warped lens will vary from no subjective symptoms but slightly reduced visual acuity to subjective symptoms of blur and decreased visual acuity, accompanied by a sphero–cylindrical over-refraction. These symptoms alone will not indicate a warped lens. Verification of the BCR is necessary as lens flexure may also produce these symptoms. A lens that is flexing may appear warped immediately on removal; however, typically it will return to the original spherical state soon after removal. Patients exhibiting lenses that are warped will require reeducation in the proper care and handling of GP lenses because poor care habits, such as cleaning the lenses between the index finger and thumb instead of the palm of the hand, will greatly increase the likelihood of lens warpage.

Peripheral Curve Radius

The peripheral curve radius can be determined by the same method as BCR. The lens mount should be tilted such that the beam is located on the peripheral curve that is to be measured. If the peripheral curve is not ≥1 mm in width, it is unlikely that it can be obtained. Typically, this is not a parameter that the practitioner can verify.

VERIFICATION OF LENS POWER

Spherical Lenses

Back vertex power (BVP) is typically the method by which power is determined for contact lenses. For low-power lenses, there is very little difference in back and front vertex power; however, there can be as much as 1 D difference in back and front vertex lenses in high prescriptions.[4] If there is doubt about which surface power to verify, it would be best to check with the laboratory that supplies the lenses.

BVP of contact lenses is determined similarly to spectacles. The lensometer should be adjusted for the individual user before the lens power is verified as specified in the instrument manual. The lens is placed concave side against the lens stop of the lensometer, and the power drum is adjusted until a clear image is achieved. The lens should be clean and dry. It will be necessary to tilt the lensometer upward into a vertical position to allow the lens to rest on the lens stop or for the lens to be gently held on the lens stop with the thumb and forefinger. Caution should be taken not to flex the lens. Most lensometers have a contact lens accessory device that can be placed on the lens stop to aid in more accurate measurements.

Prism

To measure prism on a contact lens, the lens must be centered with the concave side against the lens stop. The reticule inside the ocular consists of concentric black rings designating one to five prism diopters. For example, when the center of the target is on the first concentric ring of the reticule, it corresponds to one prism diopter (Fig. 7.7). Prism is primarily used in front toric lenses to reduce rotation.

Toric Lenses

Front toric lenses should be placed on the lensometer with the prism in the base-down direction. The resulting power will be recorded in a sphero–cylindrical notation. For example, if the lens is positioned so the prism indicates one prism diopter base down and the power drum indicates powers of -1.00 and -3.00 D at 90, the power would be recorded as $-1.00 - 2.00 \times 90$.

In toric lenses with no prism, such as bitorics and back torics, the power is not recorded in the sphero–cylindrical form, but as the values found in each meridian. An example of this is as follows:

BCR: 7.50/8.04 mm
Powers: Pl/-3.00 D

VERIFICATION OF CENTER/EDGE THICKNESS

A dial gauge is the most frequently used method of determining lens thickness. The lens is positioned on the gauge, and a plunger is lowered onto the lens with the thumb (Fig. 7.8). The center thickness (CT) or edge thickness can be measured by changing the portion of the lens beneath the plunger. The thickness is read directly off the gauge; for example, if the needle is on 23, then the thickness is recorded as 0.23 mm. Lens thickness can also be determined with the Marco radius-gauge because a thickness gauge is incorporated into the instrument itself. It is important to verify this parameter in cases pertaining to flexure, oxygen transmission, comfort, and lens position.[5]

INSPECTION OF THE LENS EDGE

The shape and condition of the lens edge can represent the most important factor in providing patient comfort. If the edge is not inspected before the lens is dispensed to the patient, symptoms of foreign-body sensation or scratchy, irritated eyes, for example, may result from edge

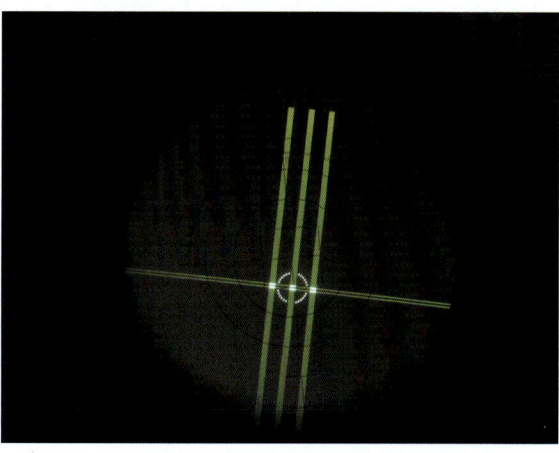

FIGURE 7.7 Prism as shown on a lensometer.

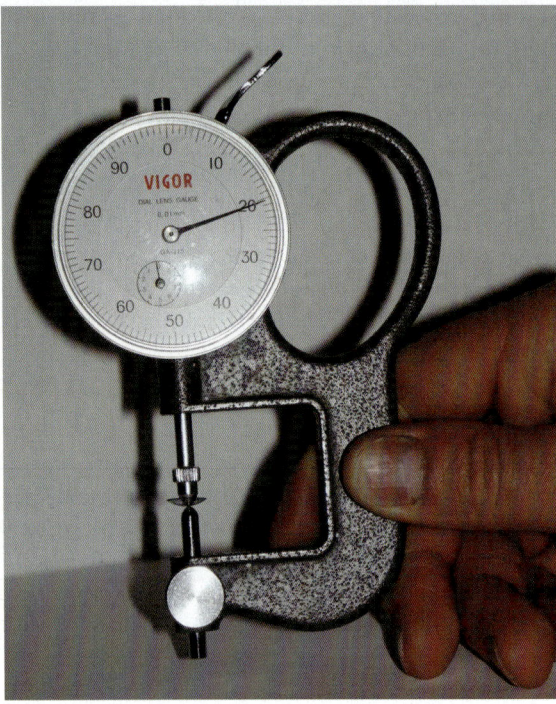

FIGURE 7.8 Center thickness gauge.

defects. The use of the "palm test," in combination with one of the methods of projection magnification, makes this parameter relatively easy to inspect. To perform the palm test, the lens is placed concave side down in the palm of the hand and gently pushed across the palm (Fig. 7.9). A good edge will glide easily and feel smooth. A poor edge will feel scratchy, will show resistance to movement, and may make an audible scratchy sound. A projection magnifier provides

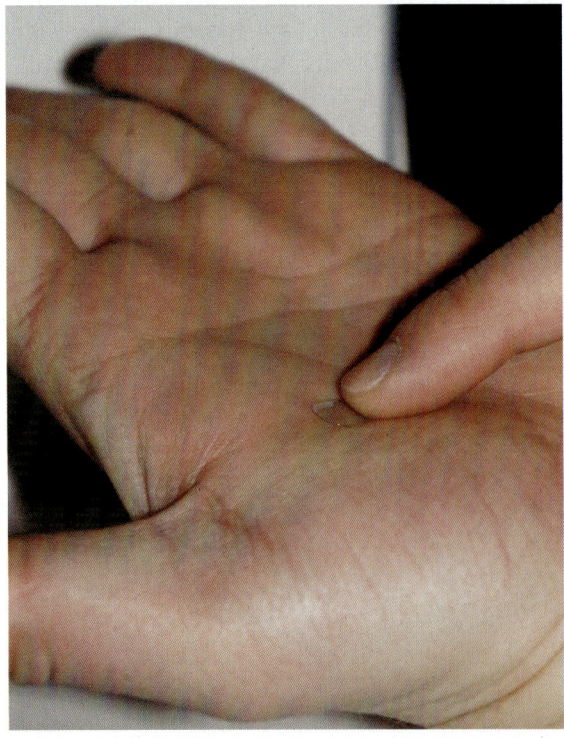

FIGURE 7.9 Palm test used to determine the quality of the edge.

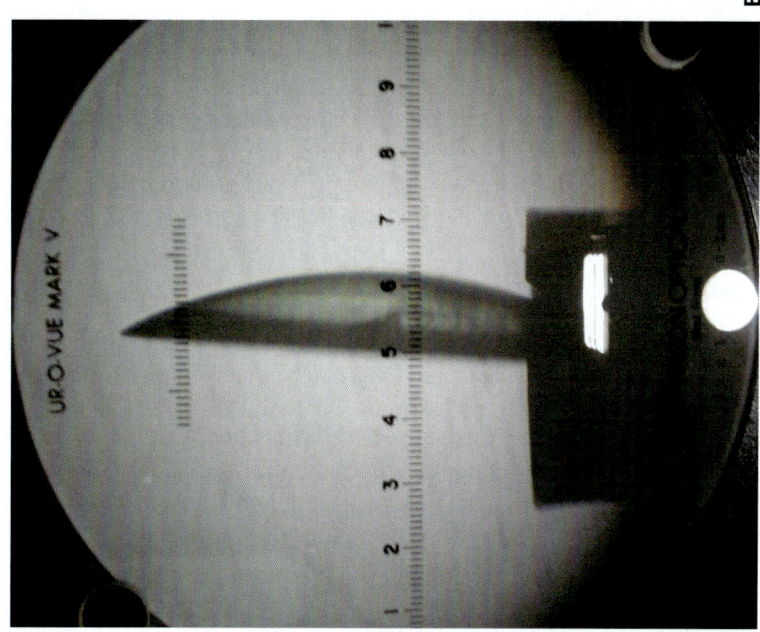

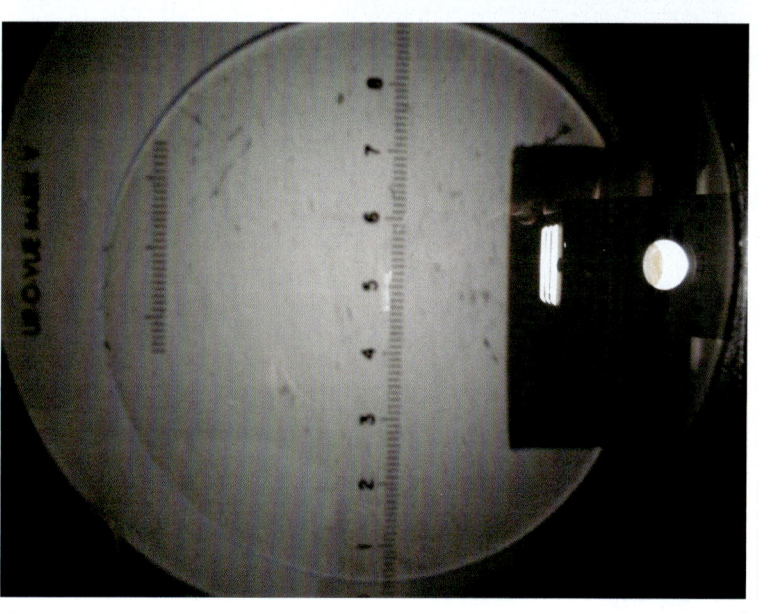

FIGURE 7.10 (A) Front view of edge with projection magnifier. (B) Side edge profile.

193

a magnified image of the lens, allowing inspection of the edges. The lens is positioned so that it can be viewed from both the straight-ahead and the profile positions (Fig. 7.10).

VERIFICATION OF LINEAR DIMENSIONS

Overall Diameter

The overall diameter (OAD) of a lens can be determined by several methods. The projection magnifier, a PD stick (used to measure interpupillary distance), a V-channel gauge, and a dial gauge can all be used to determine OAD (Fig. 7.11). The most common and practical method, as it can be used for measuring other parameters and for inspection, is the use of the measuring magnifier or reticule. On the back of the measuring magnifier, there is a scale ranging from 0 to 20 mm. The lens is placed on the measuring magnifier and held up to a background light source (Fig. 7.12A). By positioning the lens on the scale, the diameter can be easily measured (Fig. 7.12B).

Optical Zone Diameter

The optical zone diameter (OZD) is the area between the innermost peripheral curve on each edge of the lens (Fig. 7.13). Like the OAD, the OZD can be determined by using the measuring magnifier. It can also be determined by the formula OZD = OAD − 2(PCW), PCW is the total width of the peripheral curves on one side of the lens. With some lens designs, the optical zone will be oval, making it necessary to rotate the lens and check the OZD 90 degrees away. Some examples of this are a spherical base curve with toric peripheral curves, a toric base curve with spherical peripheral curves, and a toric base curve and toric secondary curve in which the differences in curvature of the major meridians are not equal.[6]

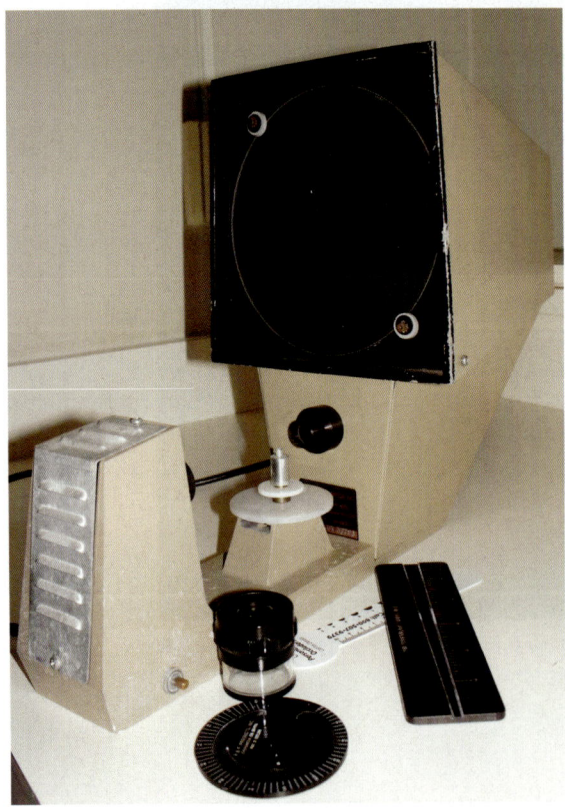

FIGURE 7.11 Methods to determine overall diameter: Measuring magnifier, V-channel gauge, dial gauge, projection magnifier, and PD stick. The blend is notated by B.

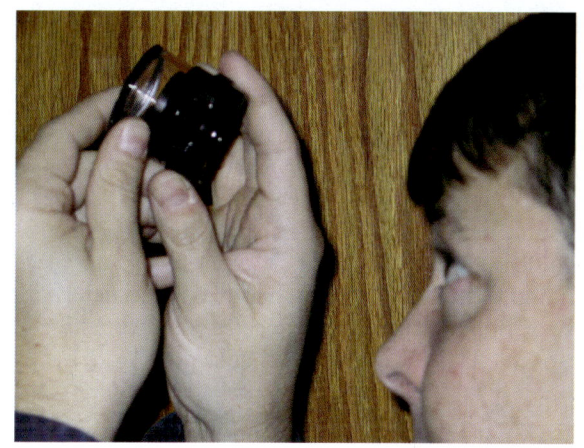

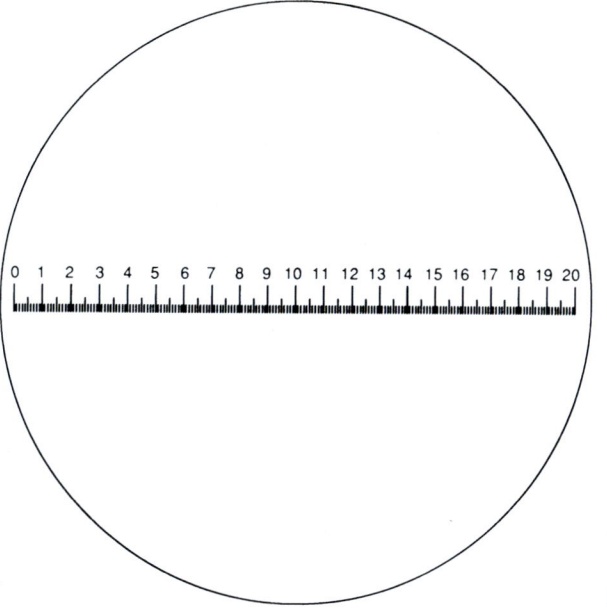

FIGURE 7.12 **(A)** Demonstration of viewing a lens through a measuring magnifier. **(B)** Diagram of measuring magnifier scale.

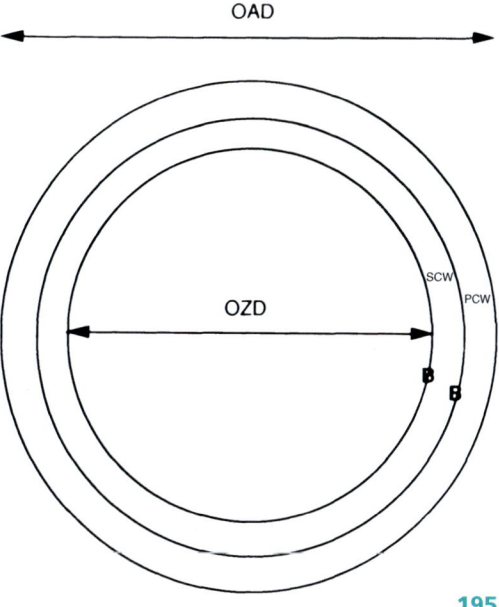

FIGURE 7.13 Diagram showing overall diameter (OAD), overall zone diameter (OZD), and peripheral curve widths.

Peripheral Curve Widths

Contact lenses are typically manufactured in a bicurve (base curve and peripheral curve), a tricurve (base curve, secondary curve, and peripheral curve), or tetracurve (base curve, secondary curve, intermediate curve, and peripheral curve) design. The measuring magnifier is the preferable method to measure the widths of these curves. The lens is placed on the measuring magnifier as specified for the OAD; however, the measuring magnifier may need to be moved back and forth slightly in the light source to determine where the curve exists. The junctions of the peripheral curves are typically blended. As the blend time is increased, determination of the specific PCW becomes more difficult (Fig. 7.14).

SURFACE QUALITY

The surface quality of a lens is best determined by the projection magnifier or the biomicroscope. A measuring magnifier can be used; however, the magnification may not be high enough to reveal small surface defects. Examination of the lens surface may reveal surface scratches, cracking/crazing, residual pitch, deposits, or film (Fig. 7.15).

VERIFICATION OF SOFT LENSES

Because of the challenges of verifying soft lenses, this process is often overlooked. When soft lenses are ordered and arrive packaged in sterile vials or blister packs, the parameters should be verified from the package label. However, there are times when being able to verify a soft lens is beneficial to the practitioner. The parameters that are simplest to verify are power, OAD, surface and edge inspection, and any identification markings. Other parameters that can be verified but are more difficult and may require special equipment are BCR and CT.[7]

Lens Power

The power of a soft lens can be verified either in a dry or wet state. The simplest method is to blot the lens dry on a lint-free tissue and place the lens concave side against the lensometer stop, identical to the method used for GP lenses. The power is read from the lensometer. A wet cell can also be used in the same manner, except the lens is floating in saline to keep it hydrated (Fig. 7.16). With this method, a correction factor must be used to find the correct power because of the lens being immersed in saline, which has a similar index of refraction as the lens. For low-water-content lenses, the correction factor is 4.6.[8] The correction factor is higher for high-water-content lenses.

Diameter

The diameter of a soft contact lens can be measured on a measuring magnifier or reticule. The lens should be blotted gently with a lint-free tissue and quickly measured on the reticule concave side down before dehydration occurs. Dehydration will cause the diameter to be smaller than the actual OAD.

Surface and Edge Inspection

Inspection of the surface and edge of a soft contact lens will be performed each time the lens is examined on the patient's eye with a slit-lamp biomicroscope. This is the easiest way to inspect the lens. The lens may also be held with soft lens tweezers behind the slit lamp while off the eye. Other methods of inspecting the lens surface are holding the lens up behind the light source of a projection magnifier or viewing the lens through a measuring magnifier. During the inspection of the lens surface, any identification markings on the lens can be viewed and recorded. The markings may identify the manufacturer, type of lens, inversion indicators, or toric lens laser marks.

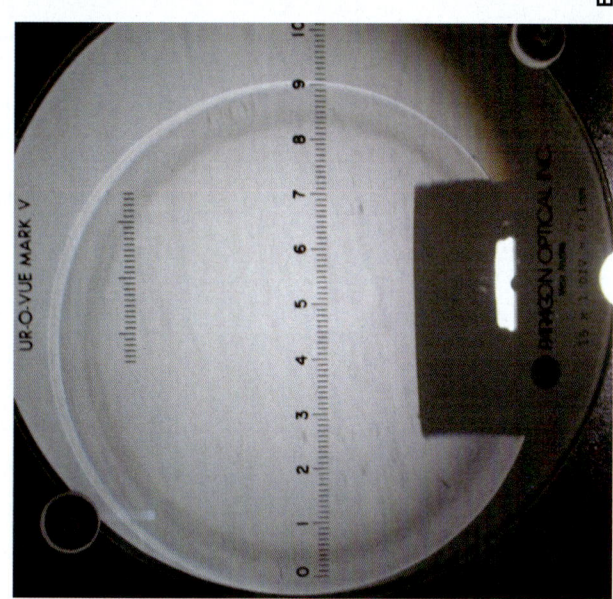
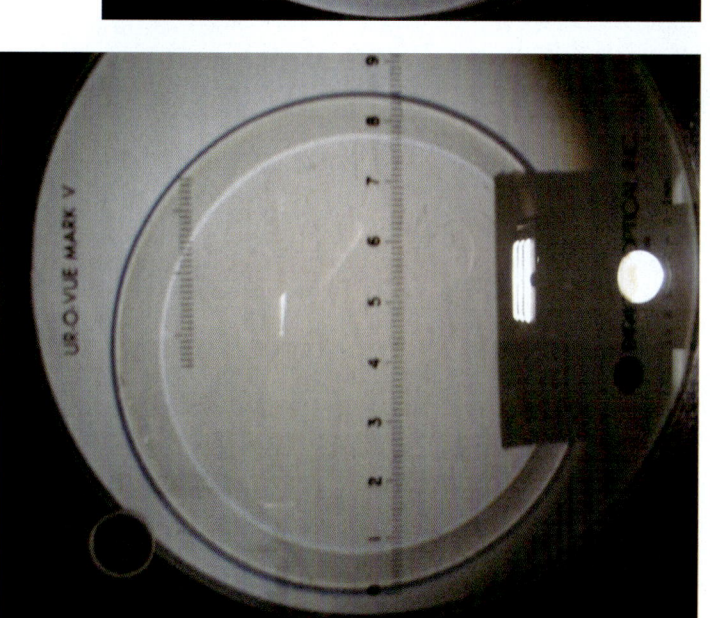

FIGURE 7.14 **(A)** Light blend of the peripheral curves. **(B)** Medium blend of the peripheral curves.

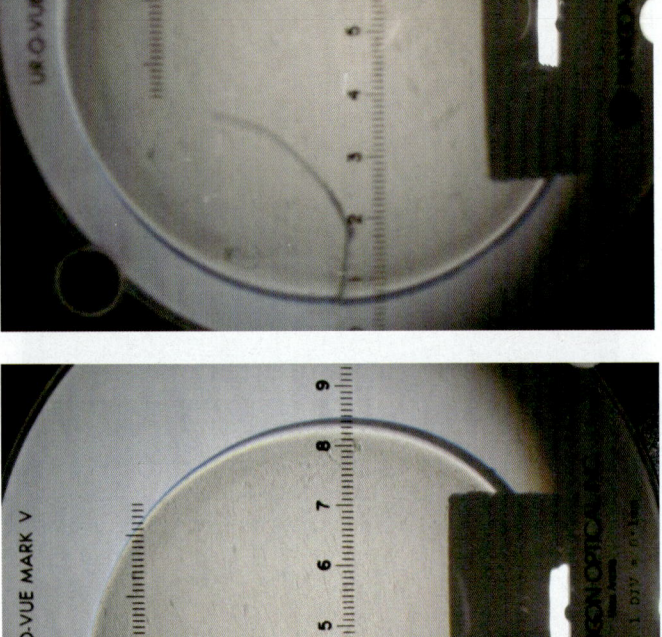

FIGURE 7.14 (*Continued*) **(C)** Heavy blend of the peripheral curves.

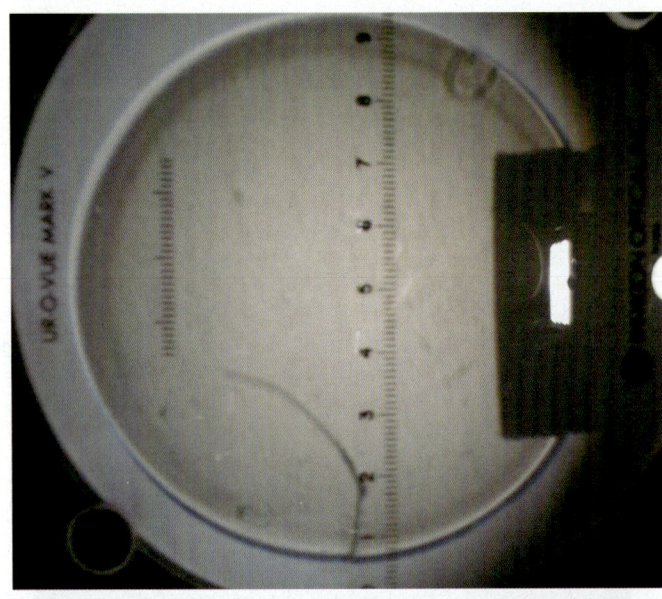

FIGURE 7.15 Lens crack as observed on a projection magnifier.

Chapter 7 • Verification of Gas-Permeable Lenses   **199**

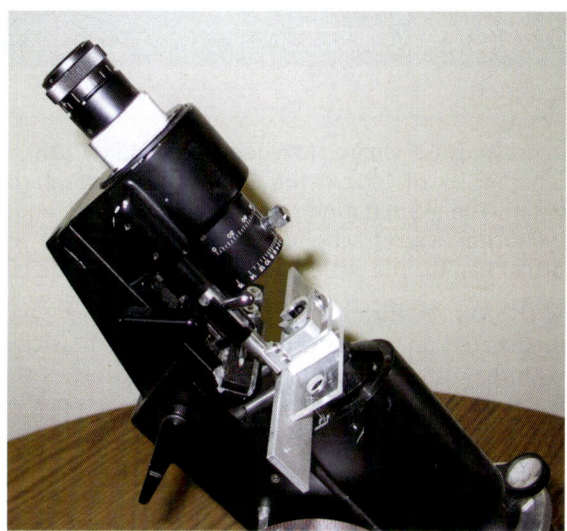

FIGURE 7.16 Soft lens wet cell power verification on lensometer.

SUMMARY

A summary of verification procedures is provided in Figure 7.17.

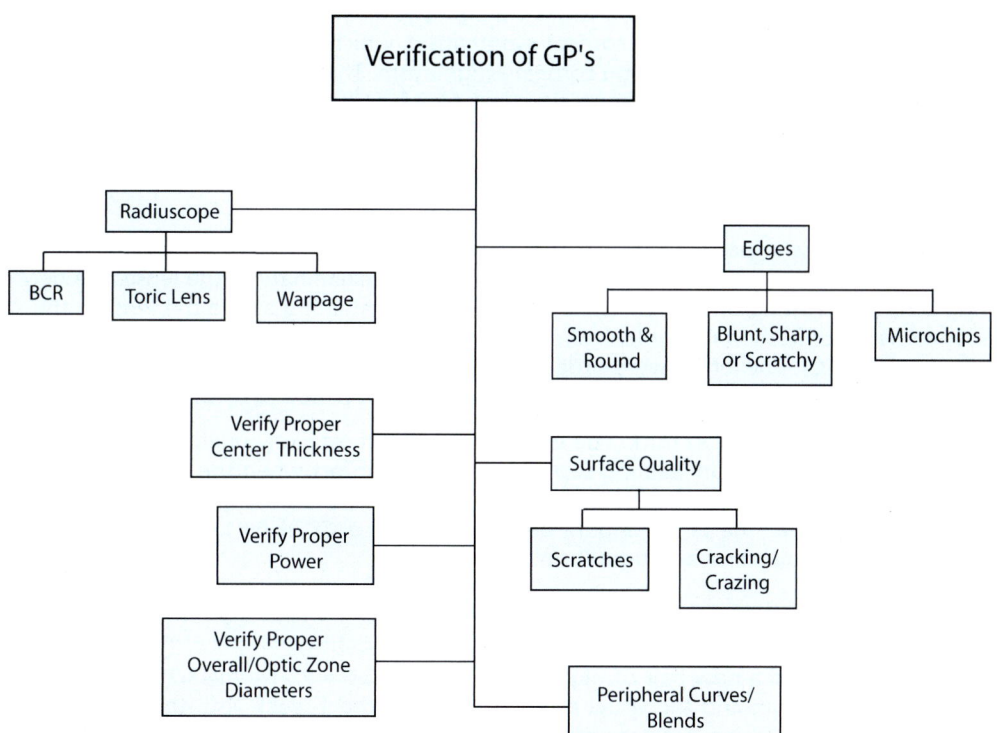

FIGURE 7.17 Summary nomogram of gas-permeable verification.

CLINICAL CASES

CASE 1

A previous GP wearer (oxygen permeability [Dk] = 18) is refit into a GP lens material with a higher Dk of 100. At the 6-month visit, the patient returns, complaining of slightly blurry vision. The examination reveals a visual acuity equal to 20/40 (OD) and 20/30 (OS), a sphero–cylindrical overrefraction (OU) that improves the visual acuity through the lenses, and normal ocular health. The patient admits to cleaning the lenses between the index finger and thumb.

SOLUTION: Verification of the BCR of the lens reveals warpage for both eyes. The patient is reeducated on proper care procedures such as cleaning the lenses in the palm of the hand with the little finger and, if tap water is used, it should be used prior to disinfection and the water temperature should be lukewarm. It is preferable not to use tap water at all, however.

CASE 2

A patient is dispensed a GP extended-wear lens material with a Dk of 151. The lens parameters (OU) include an OAD of 9.2 mm, Rx of −3.50 D, CT of 0.15 mm, and BCR of 7.50 mm. The patient's keratometry readings are OU 44.50 @ 180/47.00 @ 90. At the 1-month visit, the patient's visual acuity is decreased to 20/25−3. The overrefraction is +0.50 − 1.00 × 180 OU, and overkeratometry is 44.00 @ 180, 45.00 @ 90. Verification of the BCR reveals no toricity.

SOLUTION: The reduced visual acuity is caused by flexure. Typically, a flatter base curve may be used to reduce flexure; however, in this case, a flatter base curve would most likely compromise the fit. Lens materials with the higher Dk values used for extended wear are prone to flexure and need to be made slightly thicker than a low-Dk lens of the same power. This patient may have been fitted with a low-Dk diagnostic lens that did not exhibit flexure. In addition, this patient has 2.50 D of corneal astigmatism, which warrants a thicker lens than is required for a patient with little to no corneal astigmatism. The lens should be reordered with an increase in CT or at least 0.03 mm thicker, or a CT of 0.18 mm, which is recommended for this lens power with this amount of corneal astigmatism.[9]

CASE 3

A previously successful patient is refitted with a new pair of 30-Dk GP lenses and returns 2 weeks later complaining of discomfort. On biomicroscopic examination, the lenses are decentering inferiorly, resting on the lower lid, with superficial staining above the lens on the superior cornea. Verification of the lenses results in parameters identical to those ordered with the exception of CT. The lenses were ordered "ultrathin," which is typically about 0.11 mm in this material and design (power = −5.50 D OU), and were verified as 0.15 mm.

SOLUTION: The lenses are too thick. The increased mass is most likely pulling the lenses to an inferior position, resulting in staining superiorly and discomfort when the lenses contact the lower lid after a blink. If the lenses had been verified before dispensing, this problem would have been prevented. The lenses should be returned and a CT of 0.11 mm ordered, as the patient has little to no corneal astigmatism.

CASE 4

A patient is dispensed a new pair of high-Dk GP lenses (BCR = 7.71 mm/43.75 D OU). The fit appears to be optimum and the visual acuity is good. At the 1-week visit, the lenses appear to exhibit an apical bearing pattern with a lag of approximately 3 to 4 mm. The lenses were not soaked before dispensing.

SOLUTION: The lenses have flattened on hydration. The BCR was found to be within tolerance before dispensing; however, the lenses were not hydrated. Now the lenses are too flat (i.e., verified as 7.89 mm/42.75 D), and they exhibit an apical bearing pattern and excessive movement. The lenses need to be reordered in the correct BCR. Although this is most likely the result of excessive heat generated during the manufacturing process, CT should also be verified to rule out that the lenses are too thin.

CASE 5

A patient is dispensed GP lenses for the first time. The patient returns at the 1-week visit complaining of discomfort. The patient is told that an adaptation period is normal; generally, at minimum, 2 weeks is necessary. The patient returns at 2 weeks, requesting a refund as the lenses are intolerable.

SOLUTION: Inspection reveals sharp, "scratchy" edges with small edge defects or microchips in both lenses. If the lenses had been verified before dispensing, the edges could have been polished or the lenses returned to the laboratory. At this time, the only option is to explain the problem to the patient and to indicate that it can be easily solved.

CASE 6

A patient comes for a follow-up examination on his Menicon Z lenses. Upon slit-lamp examination, the practitioner observes scratches on the lens surface. The patient had depleted his supply of the solutions dispensed and purchased Boston Original Formula.

SOLUTION: The Boston Cleaner is too abrasive for use on the Menicon lenses and it is not a recommended cleaner. The lens material is a hyper-Dk, soft material; therefore, the abrasive cleaner scratches the lenses. The recommended care regimen is a nonabrasive system—for example, MeniCare GP or Unique pH (Menicon), Optimum (Lobob), or Boston Simplus (Bausch + Lomb/Boston). The patient should be reeducated on proper care and handling of his lenses.

CASE 7

A patient is fitted with a new pair of soft contact lenses. The powers and brand of his previous lenses are unknown. At the follow-up examination, he complains of poor vision. His vision is 20/20 OU. The new lenses are -1.50 D OU.

SOLUTION: The powers of his previous lenses are verified. The previous lenses verify as -2.00 D OU. The red–green test shows that he is overminused in the previous lenses. The patient is educated to try the new powers, and if he does not adapt, a compromise between the old and the new powers will be attempted.

CASE 8

A patient comes for an examination reporting discomfort in the left eye with her soft lens on. The discomfort has been present for about 1 week.

SOLUTION: Inspection of the soft lens on the eye reveals a central tear in the left lens, which has caused superficial corneal staining upon lens removal.

CASE 9

A new patient comes to your office to be fit with soft lenses. She does not remember what her previous soft lenses are, but she thinks they are some kind of Vistakon lens.

SOLUTION: When the lenses are viewed with the slit-lamp biomicroscope, the marking "AV" is found on the lenses. "AV" was an inversion indicator manufactured onto Acuvue lenses. The other Vistakon lenses have a "123" on the lens.

CLINICAL PROFICIENCY CHECKLIST

- It is imperative that GP lenses be verified before dispensing to ensure that, at minimum, the appropriate BCR, power, OAD and OZD, CT, and edge design have been received.
- It is necessary to soak GP lenses in an approved disinfecting solution for at least 12 hours before base curve verification and dispensing.
- Overkeratometry readings, BCR, and power verification are all necessary procedures to determine the difference between a lens that is flexing and one that is warped.
- It is important for the lens edge to be inspected in both the frontal and side (profile) views on a projection magnifier before dispensing or whenever the edge design or condition may be in question. In addition, the "palm test" may be used as an initial screening procedure before the aforementioned method of projection magnification is performed to determine the condition of the edge.
- With toric lens designs, it is possible to differentiate between spherical and toric designs and front, back, and bitoric designs by verifying the BCR, the front curve, and the power of the lens.
- If a patient complains of soft lens irritation, the soft lens should be inspected on or off the eye for tears, deposits, or other lens damage.
- The easiest parameters to verify on a soft lens are power, OAD, surface inspection, and identification markings.

REFERENCES

1. Jurkus JM, Kelly SA. Automated and manual base curve assessment of rigid gas permeable contact lenses. *Int Cont Lens Clin.* 1996;23(7–8):138–141.
2. Henry VA, Bennett ES. Inspection and verification of gas-permeable contact lenses. In: Bennett ES, Weissman BA, eds. *Clinical Contact Lens Practice.* Philadelphia, PA: Lippincott Williams & Wilkins; 2005:294–305.
3. Barr JT, Hettler DH. Boston II base curve changes with hydration. *Contact Lens Forum.* 1984;9:65–67.
4. Sarver MD. Verification of contact lens power. *J Am Optom Assoc.* 1963;34(16):1304–1306.
5. DeKinder JO, Henry VA. Verifying GP contact lenses. *Contact Lens Spectrum.* 2005;20(4):51.
6. Lowther GE. Inspection and verification. In: Lowther GE, ed. *Contact Lenses: Procedures and Techniques.* Boston, MA: Butterworth-Heinemann; 1982:153–192.
7. Jameson M. Verifying soft contact lens parameters. *Contact Lens Spectrum.* 2003;18(8):47.
8. Janoff LE. Hydrogel lens verification. In: Bennett ES, Weissman BA, eds. *Clinical Contact Lens Practice.* Philadelphia, PA: JB Lippincott Co; 1991:37-1–37-13.
9. Bennett ES. Hydrogel versus rigid gas permeable lenses for extended wear: criteria and difference. *J Am Optom Assoc.* 1986;57(7):500–502.

Chapter 8

Gas-Permeable Lens Problem Solving

Edward S. Bennett, Terry Scheid, and Bruce W. Morgan

Renewed interest in gas-permeable (GP) lenses has been fueled in no small part by their advantage of having a relatively high safety profile. The continued development of material and manufacturing technology has only enhanced this benefit over time, with the result that the incidence of problems with GP lenses is further reduced and sight-threatening problems are particularly rare. However, as with any contact lens wear, the presence of some risk remains and the purpose of this chapter is to discuss the management of the potential problems or problematic patients related to GP lens wear.

THE EVALUATION PROCESS

As discussed in Chapter 5, it is important for GP wearing patients to be evaluated at 1 week, 1 month, 3 months, and every 6 months thereafter. At each visit, it is recommended for practitioners to perform the procedures provided in Table 8.1.

Case History

The value of a comprehensive case history cannot be overestimated. At each visit, it is important to explore the areas of wearing time, comfort, vision, and compliance.[1,2] When determining wearing time, be sure to ask the patient how long they can *comfortably* wear their lenses as opposed to when they typically remove them. Patients often continue to wear their lenses beyond this comfort point due to a variety of reasons.[3] Patients in this situation are more likely to have existing or potential contact lens complications. At each and every visit, patients should be asked about the care and handling of their lenses. Potential problems with handling issues or the misuse of the prescribed care regimen can often be limited with routine patient education in this area. In addition, the patient should be asked about their vision, comfort, and overall satisfaction.

Procedures before Lens Removal

It is important to perform certain procedures such as the fit of the lens and visual acuity before the lens is removed upon follow-up. If the lens is removed and then replaced later in the exam, the accuracy of these measurements is compromised. A quick spherical overrefraction, preferably with loose lenses, will rule out any errors of under- or overcorrection. If additional minus power is indicated, this can be added in-office if modification capabilities are available. If the visual acuity is not optimal with a spherical overrefraction, then a sphero–cylindrical overrefraction via retinoscopy becomes important. There may be residual astigmatism present, the lens could be warped or in some cases, corneal distortion may be the cause of reduced acuity.

A biomicroscopic evaluation of the lens position and movement with the blink, as well as the lens-to-cornea relationship via fluorescein should be assessed at every visit. At the same time,

TABLE 8.1 Progress Evaluation Procedures (Gas-Permeable Lens Wearers)

Before Lens Removal

1. Case history: symptoms, wearing time, level of satisfaction, care system, review handling (if necessary)
2. Visual acuity
3. Retinoscopy for sphero–cylindrical overrefraction
4. Best sphere overrefraction
5. Biomicroscopic evaluation (before removal):
   a. Surface quality (deposits, scratches)
   b. Centration and movement with the blink
   c. Fluorescein pattern
6. Overkeratometry[a]

After Lens Removal

1. Biomicroscopic evaluation (after lens removal):
   a. Corneal staining
   b. Vascularization
   c. Edema
   d. Papillary hypertrophy
2. Manifest refraction[a]
3. Keratometry/corneal topography[a]
4. Verification (base curve radius [BCR], surface, edge)[a]

[a]Not necessary at every visit.

the surface quality can be evaluated for any deposits, scratches, or edge defects. If flexure is suspected, keratometry or topography should be performed over the lenses.

Procedures after Lens Removal

After lens removal, the cornea should be evaluated for signs of vascularization (360-degree evaluation) and staining. Central corneal clouding (CCC), which is rare with the current generation of GP lens materials, can be evaluated by using sclerotic scatter of split-limbal illumination and viewing the presence of any haze against the black pupil background. The lids should be everted to observe any possible changes in papillary hypertrophy.

Although not mandatory at every visit, it is always recommended to check the patient's manifest refraction and corneal curvature values at progress evaluation visits. Corneal topography instrumentation, if available, can assist in detecting if there are any regions of corneal distortion or large curvature change (i.e., inferior steepening via a superiorly decentered lens). Lens inspection procedures such as radiuscopy (warpage) or edge inspection (discomfort) should be performed as needed.

REDUCED VISION

When a contact lens patient complains of reduced vision, it is helpful to ask the secondary question: "is the reduced vision present only when wearing the contact lenses or does it persist when wearing spectacles as well." The answer to this question should pinpoint this problem as a "lens problem" or a "cornea/eye problem." If the patient responds that the reduced vision is only present when wearing his or her lenses, then there are five likely causes: flexure, warpage, decentration, poor surface wettability, or power change.

Flexure

Flexure of a GP lens results from the bending force of the upper lid during the blink process. This bending force induces a certain amount of toricity within the lens. For example, on a high, with-the-rule astigmatic patient, this induced toricity will reduce the amount of astigmatic correction provided by the lens. There are several causes for this problem, including a steep fitting relationship, reduced center thickness (CT), large optical zone diameter (OZD), and material flexibility.[4-6] Flexure can be diagnosed by performing keratometry over the patient's lenses (preferably during the diagnostic fitting process). The values obtained should be spherical; the presence of any toricity in this measurement is typically the result of flexure. If undiagnosed, patients will typically report asthenopic complaints indicative of inadequate astigmatic correction.

Flexure can be managed by changing the lens design. The most important design change would be to flatten the BCR by, at minimum, 0.50 D, assuming this modification does not compromise the lens-to-cornea fitting relationship.[4] Increasing the CT by 0.02 mm per diopter of corneal astigmatism has also been recommended[7]; however, this change should only be considered if option one is not possible, since the increased lens mass may compromise the fitting relationship. Other secondary, but effective, management options include reducing the OZD of the lens by, at minimum, 0.3 mm or changing materials (typically from a higher to a lower oxygen permeability [Dk]).

Warpage

Another common GP-induced problem is warpage or permanently induced toricity within the lens. This problem differs from flexure in several ways:

1. It is diagnosed by verifying the BCR and will verify as toric with the radiuscope, whereas in flexure-related decreased visual acuity, the warpage will verify as spherical.
2. This problem is acquired over time, whereas flexure-induced problems can be evident immediately.
3. The induced toricity is permanent.

The primary cause of warpage is the application of excessive digital pressure during the cleaning process. In fact, it has been determined that cleaning the lenses between the fingers will result in over three and one-half times more warpage than cleaning in the palm of the hand.[8] In addition, the incidence of warpage is higher in former polymethylmethacrylate (PMMA) wearers[9] (primarily, a result of customary use of the digital cleaning method) and is proportional to Dk of the material.[10] Finally, warpage and, possibly, an inverted lens may result from placing the lens upside down in a smooth-welled case.[6]

Warpage can be minimized by adherence to the following recommendations:

1. Routinely verify the BCR at all patient progress evaluation visits; therefore, if a small increase in toricity is detected, the patient can be properly educated before further change and resulting possible dissatisfaction with rigid lenses.
2. Educate all patients and especially former PMMA wearers to clean the lenses carefully in the palm of the hand.
3. Always provide patients with a case having ridges or holes within the wells.
4. If warpage persists (and some patients are truly "warpers" as a result of possessing thick, rough fingers or an inability to clean the lenses gently), changing to a lower-Dk material and to a multipurpose system that has surfactant cleaning agents is recommended as well.

Decentration

GP lens decentration can result in numerous problems, including corneal desiccation,[9] corneal warpage,[11] poor corneal alignment,[12] and reduced vision. The poor alignment results in a space underneath the lens as it rests on the flatter, more peripheral region of the cornea;

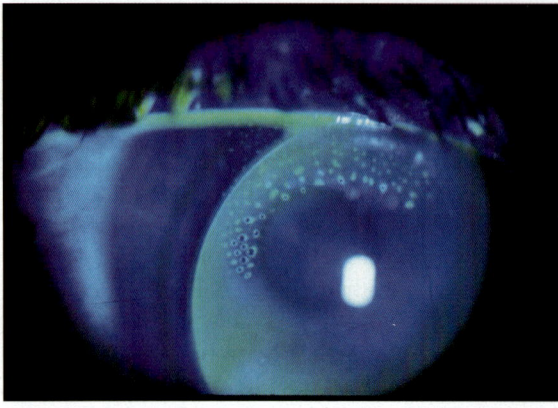

FIGURE 8.1 Dimple veiling.

therefore, poor tear exchange and even adherence can result.[13] Likewise, some region under the lens will exhibit excessive clearance, with a dimple veil pattern possible with fluorescein (Fig. 8.1). However, the vision changes, including fluctuating visual acuity and flare, are typically the most frustrating to both patient and practitioner. Any form of decentration can result from a decentered corneal apex, an unusual corneal topography, lid characteristics, a less than optimum lens design, or the specific lens material. Ideally, as much of the corneal topography as possible should be evaluated. As keratometry is often the only option, lens design and, particularly, fluorescein pattern evaluation become very important. Inferior, superior, and lateral decentration are discussed below.

Inferior

Lens design plays an important role in reducing the incidence of a rigid lens decentering inferiorly. An "on K" to "flatter than K" fitting relationship appears to be preferable to steep fitting designs, especially in minus powers.[4] If the lens decenters, it is recommended to change the BCR by, at minimum, 0.50 D to improve the fit.[14] CT should be maintained to a minimum; in fact, recommended CT values for any given material should be available from the manufacturer. This parameter should be routinely verified; however, verification of CT only occurs in approximately one-half of contact lens fitting practices.[15] It has been found that increasing CT typically has only a slight effect on oxygen transmission but can have a large effect on lens mass and, therefore, centration characteristics.[16,17] The use of ultrathin lens designs, recommended for all patients with <2 D of corneal cylinder, should assist with centration.[18,19]

Perhaps, the most important parameter affecting centration is lens edge. The effect of using a minus lenticular to "lift up" a lens of plus or low minus power is very dramatic.[17] Likewise, the use of a plus lenticular on high minus lenses minimizes the likelihood of inferior decentration resulting from the increase in lens mass and the effect of the upper lid on the thick lens edge. The anterior optic cap is generally designed 0.1 to 0.2 mm larger than the back optic zone diameter. The larger the anterior cap, the thicker the CT of the lens for a given lens overall diameter (OAD). In addition, the use of a "lid attachment" lens design with an anteriorly positioned edge[20] is also beneficial in cases of inferior decentration. However, if excessive edge clearance is present, either via an excessively flat BCR, a flat peripheral curve radius (PCR), a wide peripheral curve width (PCW), or a combination of these factors, the resulting lid interaction could result in an inferiorly positioned lens.[21]

It has also been found that specific gravity may also play a role. Materials of high specific gravity have greater lens mass than do equal volumes of materials with lower specific gravities.[22] Material-specific gravities range from approximately 1.05 to 1.27. It has been found that, for inferior positioning lenses, changing to a lower specific gravity material resulted in a greater effect on centration than reducing CT.[23]

Therefore, to minimize inferior decentration:

1. Consider a flatter BCR for myopic patients.
2. Keep CT to a minimum without inducing flexure.
3. Use a lenticular design when indicated (typically with all plus and <-1.50 D lens powers for a minus lenticular and >-5 D for a plus lenticular).
4. Consider use of a lid attachment design.
5. Consider use of a scleral design.[24]
6. If options 1 to 5 are unsuccessful, changing to a lower specific gravity material, if possible, may be of benefit.

Superior

If slight superior decentration is present, this can be beneficial for both vision and comfort as a result of a "tucked under the lid" fitting relationship. However, if the decentration is excessive, lens adherence can result. In addition, the use of corneal topography instrumentation has confirmed that corneal distortion is possible in the region of bearing superiorly.[11,25-27] Therefore, these patients need to be carefully monitored. For lenses that decenter superiorly, the opposite types of changes are indicated, including the use of a thinner edge design, a greater CT, and a steeper BCR. Changing CT, in particular, has been found to be more effective than changing to a higher specific gravity material.[22] The use of a scleral design, as with any decentration, will also offer a solution.[23]

Lateral

Lenses decentering laterally can be especially frustrating. This often results from either a decentered corneal apex or an against-the-rule astigmatic patient. In the latter case, the lens tends to move more in a lateral motion after the blink with a tendency (as in with-the-rule astigmatism) to transverse the steeper corneal meridian. Some options have enjoyed limited success, including selecting a larger OAD, including sclera designs, or a steeper BCR. However, a viable alternative is to fit an aspheric lens design in an effort to provide better alignment and possibly improve centration. If these options fail, a soft toric lens may be indicated.

Poor Surface Wettability

The importance of good GP lens surface wettability or the ability of the blink to spread tear film mucin across the anterior contact lens surface cannot be underestimated. In fact, good surface wettability may be the most desirable rigid lens property. Poor wettability can be divided into two separate categories: initial and acquired.[28]

Initial

Poor initial wettability is almost always a manufacturing problem and could result from the following:

1. Too much heat buildup during the manufacturing process.
2. Poor polishing techniques.
3. Improper or old diamond used for cutting.
4. Residual pitch polish left on the lens surface.

This problem is typically not diagnosed by the appearance of a film, but by the breakup of the tear film on the lens surface during biomicroscopic evaluation (Fig. 8.2). This is an especially frustrating problem to the patient who expected excellent visual acuity but instead is experiencing fluctuations in vision.

Many GP lenses are shipped from the laboratory dry in a flat pack. If dispensed directly from the pack, the lens often exhibits poor initial wetting and hazy vision. This problem can

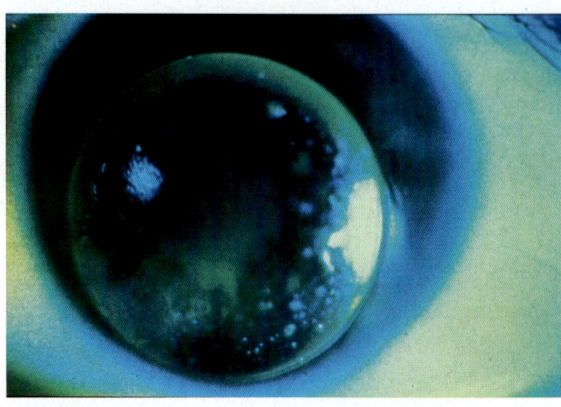

FIGURE 8.2 Poor initial surface wettability.

often be prevented by presoaking the lenses for a minimum of 24 hours prior to dispensing in the recommended soaking solution. This solution typically contains wetting agents that can condition the surface to be initially compatible with the tear film. If the wettability is still not optimum, a compatible laboratory cleaner (e.g., The Boston Laboratory Cleaner, Bausch + Lomb) or solvent (e.g., FluoroSolve, Paragon Vision Sciences) can be used. After laboratory cleaning, the lens should be conditioned by rubbing wetting solution onto the surface using the same technique as when cleaning the lens. As a final procedure, light surface polishing of the lens can be performed, although this is rarely necessary and only if the lens is not plasma treated.

Many GP lenses today are available with wet shipping. This should usually allow for better and more consistent initial wettability. As discussed in Chapter 3, new plasma treatments are available for Boston, Paragon, Contamac, and Menicon lens materials. The treatment of GP lenses with plasma is an effective method to remove any remaining lens-manufacturing residues. An outcome of this treatment process is a dramatic reduction in wetting angle, maximizing initial lens wettability, and possibly increasing initial lens comfort. Plasma coating may also repel protein, cell, and bacterial adhesion.[29] Plasma-treated lenses should be shipped wet. The treatment effects will diminish over weeks to months, but aid in initial GP lens wettability and patient adaptation.

Acquired

The more commonly experienced problem is acquired mucoprotein film or haze on the anterior lens surface. Typically, this occurs over a period of several weeks to several months. The thick, film-like appearance is easily diagnosed by biomicroscopy (Fig. 8.3). There are several causes of the formation of this film, including poor tear quality, improper blinking, inadequate compliance, use of improper solutions, foreign contaminants, and surface scratches.

Patients having a borderline tear quality should be placed on an aggressive care regimen, including daily use of either an abrasive cleaner (if the lens is not plasma treated) or a surfactant cleaning/disinfecting regimen supplemented by both daily liquid enzymatic cleaning and rewetting drops several times each day. Patients should be educated about the importance of cleaning the lenses thoroughly immediately after lens removal followed by placement in the appropriate soaking solution; otherwise, any fresh deposits in contact with the tear film while on the eye will dry out and become more difficult to remove. Patients should also be advised to wash their hands thoroughly with a non–lanolin-containing hand soap (i.e., most bar soaps and all optical hand soaps) before handling their lenses because hand creams and other substances on the hand can adhere to the lens surface and compromise wettability.[30] In addition, patient compliance with the proper care regimen can be evaluated by having a space on the progress evaluation form for listing the solutions; therefore, this can be asked at every patient visit. To

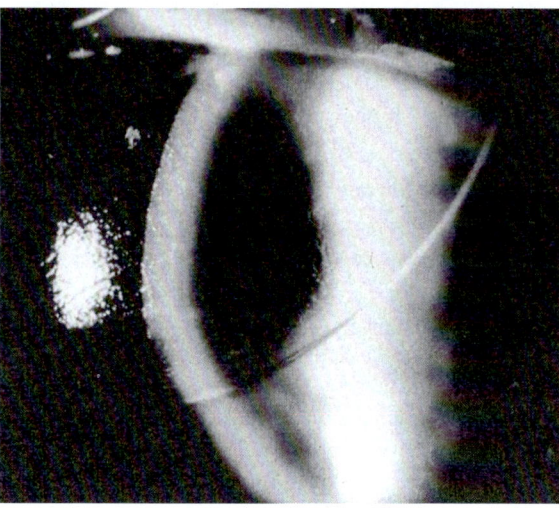

FIGURE 8.3 Mucoprotein film.

clean a heavily deposited lens in the office, the aforementioned laboratory cleaners or solvents should be used. In cases of heavy lens deposits, even in the presence of plasma-treated lenses, the Menicon Progent (Menicon Inc.) system—now approved for patient use—is valuable. Lenses are placed in a sodium hypochlorite–potassium bromide mixture for 30 minutes, then cleaned and rinsed (Fig. 8.4). Optimum Extra Strength Cleaner (Lobob) is also a very good cleaner for use by patients prone to deposits.[31,32]

If scratches or deposits are present on the posterior surface of the lens, a light polish should be beneficial. Finally, if all else fails, a change in lens material is recommended. Changing from a silicone/acrylate (S/A) to a fluoro-silicone/acrylate (F-S/A) material or from a high-Dk to a lower (i.e., 25–50)-Dk F-S/A material should provide an improvement in deposit resistance as a result of a higher over-the-lens tear breakup time (TBUT).[33] To summarize, acquired surface wettability can be minimized by the following steps:

1. An aggressive cleaning regimen should be used for the heavily depositing patients.
2. Proper patient cleaning should be supplemented by frequent monitoring of the care regimen; lanolin-containing products should be avoided.

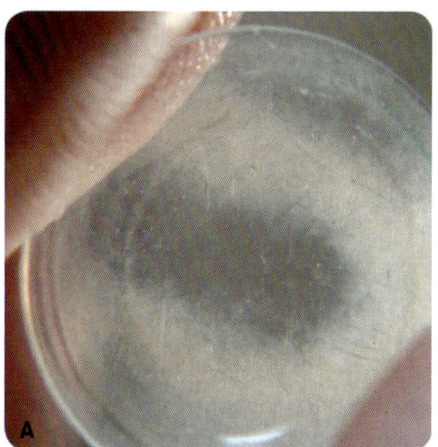
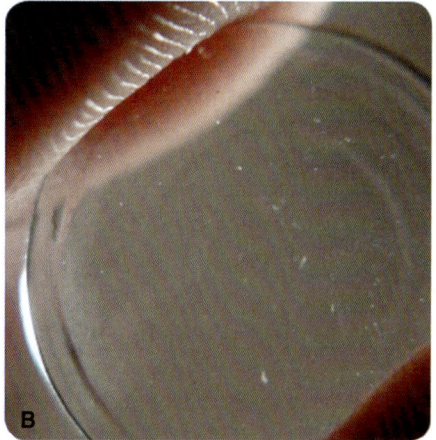

FIGURE 8.4 A lens with heavy deposits before **(A)** and after **(B)** cleaning with Progent (Menicon, Inc.), now available for at-home use. (Courtesy of Stephen P. Byrnes, OD, Londonderry, NH.)

3. In-office cleaning with a laboratory cleaner or solvent is often indicated in these cases; a light polish may be necessary in some cases.
4. Changing to a low-Dk F-S/A lens material will maintain the tear film in contact with the lens surface for a longer period.

Power Change

Another problem pertains to an increase in minus power over time accompanied by a decrease in CT in some GP lens wearers using an abrasive cleaner.[34–38] This change has been reported to be as much as −2.00 D.[31] The use of an abrasive cleaner, in combination with forceful digital cleaning in a circular manner, has been implicated as the cause of these changes. In particular, former PMMA wearers have been implicated in these reports. One study found that the greatest changes were exhibited by the Boston Cleaner (Bausch + Lomb), less change with a milder abrasive cleaner (Opticlean II [Alcon]), and the least change with a nonabrasive cleaner (Resolve [Allergan Optical]) in a three-cleaner comparison study.[8] This problem can be minimized by complying with the following recommendations:

1. Patients should clean the lenses gently in the palm of the hand with their "pinky" finger.
2. A circular motion while cleaning should be avoided versus cleaning in a linear "spoke-like" pattern.
3. For patients prone to warpage, the use of a mild abrasive cleaner or a hands-off regimen is recommended.
4. Practitioners should consider verifying lens power, CT, and BCR at follow-up visits, particularly when the patient is symptomatic.

REDUCED COMFORT

Initial

Methods of minimizing initial awareness are discussed in Chapter 5. These include how lenses are presented to the patient, the use of a topical anesthetic, and having the patient's first experience with GP lenses be a positive one (whenever possible) by providing lenses in his or her correct power. In addition, if the patient is especially apprehensive about wearing contact lenses in general (i.e., reacted negatively to such tests as lid eversion, tonometry, and dilation), a slow build-up schedule would be indicated to gradually adapt the patient's lids to the sensation of the lens edge.

As a result of improvements in manufacturing quality, a defective edge is only an occasional problem. However, every lens should be inspected before dispensing to the patient as a defective edge will likely drastically affect initial comfort. Decentration, as discussed in the previous section, may also impact initial comfort and should be managed accordingly. One design change that does appear to improve comfort, in addition to changes that improve centration (i.e., ultrathin design, lenticular use), would be to increase the OAD,[39] although a minimum change of 0.4 mm is recommended to have a significant effect.[40] Patients should also be warned that they may occasionally have a foreign body trapped behind the lens, causing momentary discomfort until the blink washes it away (Fig. 8.5).

Acquired

Lens awareness can be acquired, either from dryness-related causes such as corneal desiccation and vascularized limbal keratitis (VLK) (to be discussed), from papillary hypertrophy, or from damage to the lens edge. As mentioned earlier, if papillary hypertrophy is problematic, lens wear should be discontinued, often up to several weeks, while the prescribed mast cell stabilizer/anti-inflammatory medications are being used. If the edge would happen to become abraded or mildly chipped, in-office modification is invaluable. As discussed in Chapter 9,

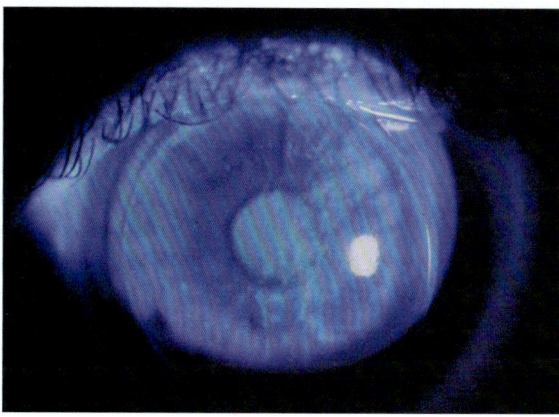

FIGURE 8.5 Foreign body tracks.

modification tools are available from many of the Contact Lens Manufacturers Association (CLMA) member laboratories.

DRYNESS

Corneal Desiccation

Corneal desiccation, or "3- and 9 o'clock" staining, refers to the drying or dehydration of the peripheral cornea. The staining results from a disruption in the tear film, adjacent to the lens edge.[41–43] This is a very common lens-induced complication, occurring in over 40% to 90% of patients wearing GP contact lenses.[9,44–46] Initially, and in most cases, the desiccation consists of isolated punctate stains (Fig. 8.6). However, in certain cases, the staining can coalesce with engorgement of the adjacent conjunctival blood vessels.[47] It has been found to be clinically significant in 10% to 15% of cases.[21,44,48] Extended-wear (EW) GP wearers have greater than two times the incidence of corneal desiccation than daily wearers.[49] In most severe cases, peripheral corneal thinning occurs with ulceration, neovascularization, and scarring.[6,50] The term *dellen* has been ascribed to a well-circumscribed oval area of peripheral thinning, occasionally resulting from desiccation in this region.[51] If symptoms are present, they are typically dryness and redness, with the latter often representing the first subjective symptom.[52,53] The following scale has been used to classify corneal desiccation[54]:

0 = No staining.
1 = Diffuse, superficial, noncoalesced staining.
2 = Superficial coalesced staining.
3 = Marked coalescence with some deep epithelial penetration.
4 = Complete coalescence with extensive loss of epithelial cells.

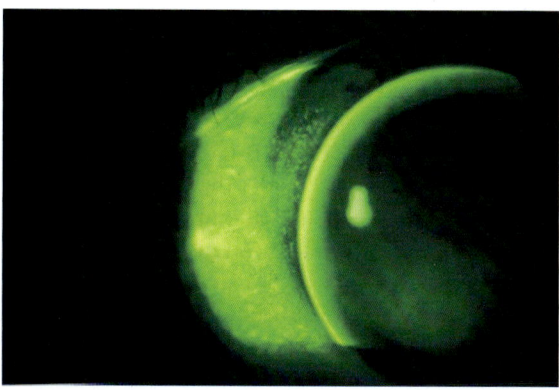

FIGURE 8.6 A corneal desiccation (3- and 9 o'clock) staining.

Factors to consider in the management of corneal desiccation include the lens material, lens centration, edge clearance, and tear film stability.

Lens Material

As mentioned previously, the most successful lens materials for minimizing the incidence of corneal desiccation are those that can maintain the tear film on the lens surface for the longest period. Therefore, the evaporation of the tear film peripheral to the lens edge may not occur during the interblink period. A low-Dk F-S/A material may be optimum for accomplishing this goal, although newer hyper-Dk lens materials such as the Menicon Z, and Boston XO$_2$ have appeared to demonstrate excellent short-term surface wettability.[55,56] If severe desiccation persists, a soft lens material may be necessary.

Lens Centration

A superior lens-to-cornea fitting relationship, with the lens tucked underneath the upper lid, is important in minimizing the incidence of moderate-to-severe cases of corneal desiccation. This position allows the lid and lens edge interaction to be at a minimum; therefore, interference with the normal blinking pattern is reduced.[28] Intrapalpebral and, especially, inferiorly positioned lenses encourage lens edge interaction with the upper lid, resulting in irritation and alteration of the normal blink reflex. This was confirmed in a 12-month GP extended-wear study in which the incidence of corneal desiccation was almost twice as high with inferiorly positioned versus superiorly positioned lenses.[9] A more recent study found that an interpalpebral fitting relationship resulted in fewer complete eyeblinks and more eyeblink attempts than a lid attachment fitting relationship.[57] To minimize this problem, the same design principles mentioned in the decentration section of this chapter apply here, namely, the use of an "on K" to "flatter than K" BCR (a steeper BCR may be necessary for plus power lens designs to obtain centration); CT at a minimum; a thin, rolled, tapered edge design (a thick, sharp, or chipped edge may increase desiccation by inducing a partial blink response); and the use of a minus lenticular edge design in all plus and low minus lens powers and a plus lenticular design for all high minus (≥−5.00 D) power designs. It is evident that a thick edge can compromise blink quality, resulting in corneal desiccation.[58] Diameter is a controversial parameter. It is safe to assume that increasing the OAD will decrease the area of staining because of the greater amount of corneal coverage; however, this increase in diameter will also increase the overall mass, and the possibility of a more inferiorly decentered lens should be evaluated. The use of a properly fitted scleral lens will all but eliminate corneal desiccation with its constant tear reservoir, and significant decentration is unlikely due to its very large size and "grip" of the conjunctiva.[59]

Edge Clearance

Edge clearance is another controversial parameter. It is important to avoid excessively high edge lift designs to reduce the peripheral tear volume, to decrease the gap in the periphery between the lid and the cornea, and to minimize the potentially compromising effect on the blink caused by the interaction between the upper lid and the lens edge[4,20,60–63] (Fig. 8.7).

This can be achieved by using a tricurve or tetracurve design with a PCW no greater than 0.3 mm and a PCR no flatter than 11.0 mm. In addition, an aspheric design may be advantageous because of better alignment of the posterior surface with the cornea.[64] However, insufficient edge clearance can also result in corneal desiccation because of insufficient tear exchange and peripheral seal-off.[65] Therefore, the most effective method of determining if the edge clearance is appropriate is via fluorescein application and pattern evaluation. The peripheral band of fluorescein should be slightly deeper or more dense (brighter fluorescence) than centrally.[66]

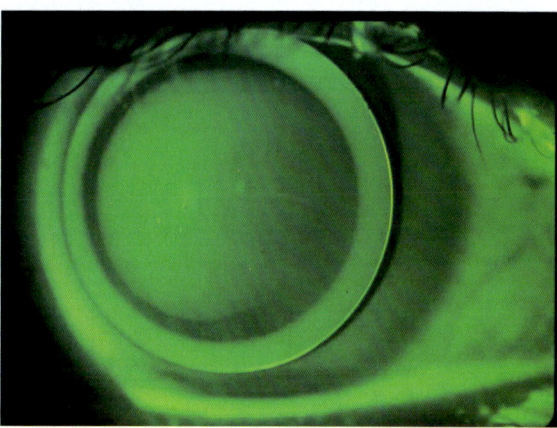

FIGURE 8.7 A high-edge clearance design, which often ultimately results in corneal desiccation.

Tear Film Stability

As the interblink interval is typically 4 to 6 seconds, patients should have a TBUT equal to, at minimum, 5 seconds to be fit with contact lenses. Patients with low- to borderline-tear quality (i.e., TBUT of 5–9 seconds), fit with GP lenses, typically will have subjective symptoms of dryness accompanied by corneal desiccation caused by evaporation of the peripheral tear pool. The use of rewetting drops, as often as every hour, accompanied by a highly wettable lens material will somewhat help in increasing the number of hours of daily lens wear.

The Bottom Line

It is evident that optimizing centration, material, and tear film will likely minimize the incidence and severity of corneal desiccation. In fact, with today's materials and lens designs, it is likely that the incidence of this condition is much less than 10 to 25 years ago. In the worst-case scenario, soft lenses would likely be a viable option.[52] A summary management nomogram is provided in Figure 8.8.

Vascularized Limbal Keratitis

Associated with limbal desiccation is the presence of a more acute complication of the peripheral cornea in the 3- or 9-o'clock regions termed *vascularized limbal keratitis*.[67] With this condition, a raised translucent inflamed area is present, which is accompanied by vascularization and adjacent bulbar conjunctival injection[68] (Fig. 8.9). It is more common in, but not limited to, GP EW. Patients typically report increasing lens awareness over the previous few weeks and often notice the "white spot" on their eye. It is often present in long-term rigid lens wearers—notably S/A lens materials—with a steep lens-to-cornea fitting relationship and peripheral seal-off. It is best managed by having the patient discontinue lens wear until the affected region is no longer elevated and the vessels have receded. A combination antibiotic–steroid should be prescribed (i.e., Tobradex or Zylet OS q.i.d.) and the patient should be evaluated after 24 hours. Typically, after 4 to 5 days, this region is no longer elevated and the patient can taper the medication (Fig. 8.10).

If the patient is wearing a S/A lens material, refitting into a F-S/A lens material would be recommended to provide enhanced surface wettability and, therefore, improved peripheral corneal lubrication. A new lens should be ordered with a flatter peripheral curve system to allow better tear exchange or the present lens modified to achieve the same result. In addition, reducing the patient to a flexible-wear or even a daily-wear (DW) schedule would be recommended. Table 8.2 shows GP-induced problems and their management.

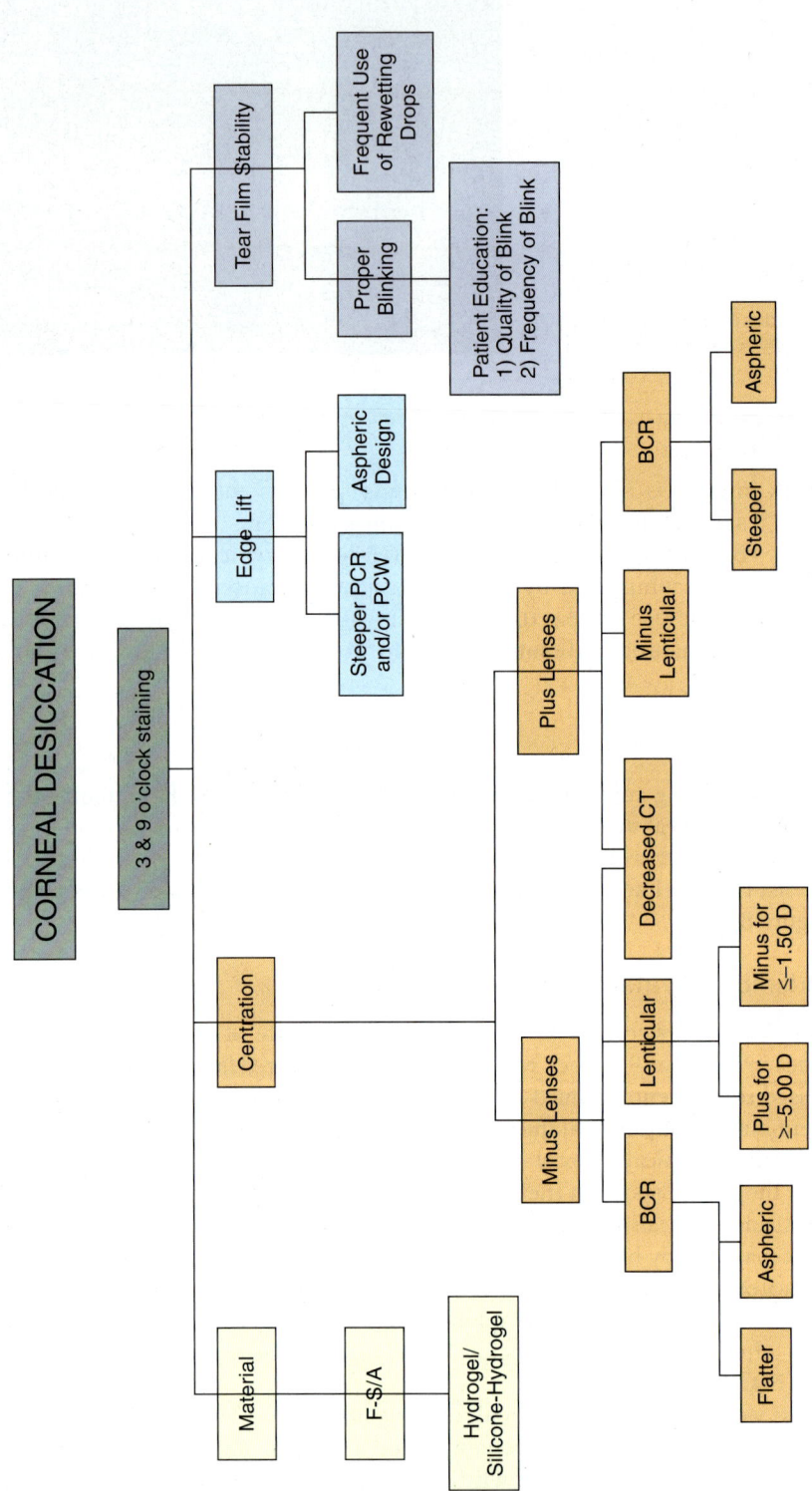

FIGURE 8.8 Corneal desiccation management nomogram.

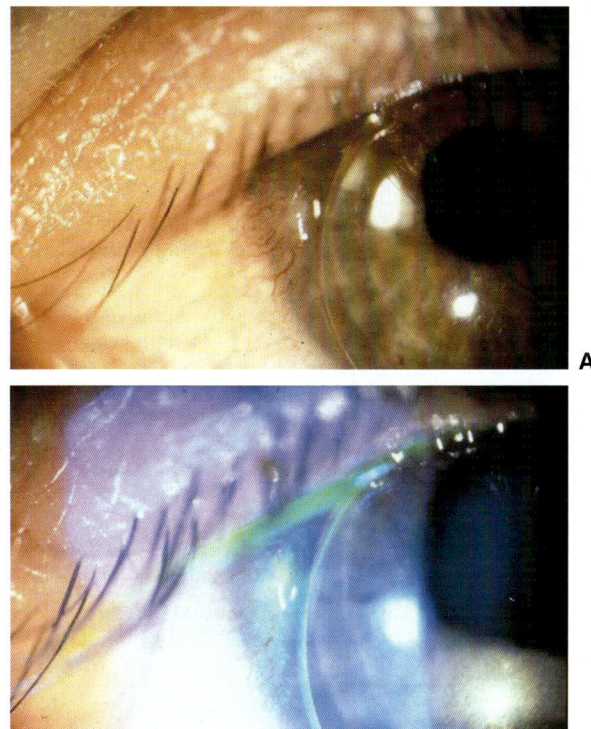

FIGURE 8.9 (A) Vascularized limbal keratitis showing the elevated, opacified, raised peripheral region. **(B)** This same area exhibits staining with fluorescein.

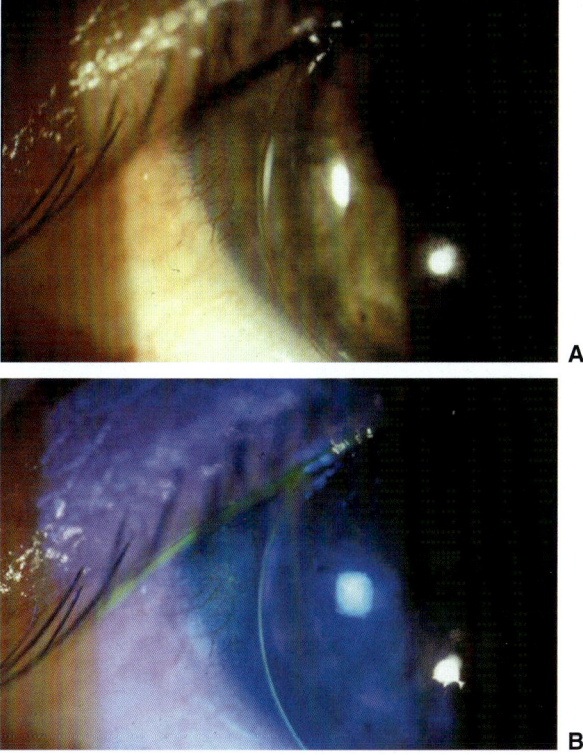

FIGURE 8.10 (A) The same patient in Figure 8.9 after 7 days of lens discontinuation. Notice the reduction in elevation of this region. **(B)** Reduced corneal staining.

TABLE 8.2 Gas-Permeable Problem Solving Based Upon Condition

CONDITION	SYMPTOMS	CAUSES	DIAGNOSIS	MANAGEMENT
Flexure	Poor initial and variable vision	High (often ≥2 D) corneal cyl, steep BCR, Thin design, steep BCR	Toric over-K's Sph–Cyl OR	Flatter BCR, CT, Decr OZD Lower Dk
Warpage	Vision gradually decreases	High-/hyper-Dk Digital cleaning	Toric radiuscope values Sph–Cyl OR	Clean in palm "Hands-off" care system
Power change	Vision reduced @ near (pre-presbyopic); may be asymptomatic	Abrasive cleaner Digital cleaning	Minus power with lensometer	Clean in palm Nonabrasive cleaner
Decentration				
Inferior	Variable vision with blink Lens awareness	Thick lens High WTR cyl Inferior apex Plus power lenses Loose lid tension	Inferior decentration Excessive movement	Ultrathin design + Lent ≥ −5.00 D −Lent for all + & low − (≤−1.50 D) Bitoric: ≥2.50 D cyl
Superior	Flare around lights Lens awareness	Flat BCR Ultrathin design	Superior position Possible adherence	Steepen BCR CT[a] + Lent if high − power
Lateral	Flare around lights Lens awareness	ATR cyl Lateral apex	Lateral decentration Movement along horizontal meridian	Steeper BCR OAD Aspheric design Soft toric design
Reduced Surface Wettability				
Initial	Poor initial/fluctuating vision	Manufacturing problems (pitch, residues) Use of lanolin	Beading up of tear film/haze	Use plasma treatment lab cleaner/solvent Presoak lens
Acquired	Gradual reduction in vision	Noncompliance with cleaning Use of lanolin creams/soaps Poor tear quality/volume Use of medications	Mucoprotein haze/film Papillary hypertrophy	Reeducate on care and avoid lanolin soaps before insertion Use liquid enzyme
Discomfort				
Initial	Lens awareness	Defective edge Decentration	Edge inspection Biomicroscopy	Polish edge/new lens As noted above
Acquired	Lens awareness	Chipped edge GPC Staining	Edge inspection Lid eversion Biomicroscope	Polish edge/reorder lens D/C lens wear and anti-inflammatory meds If 3- & 9 o'clock staining or VLK, treat as indicated below

TABLE 8.2 Gas-Permeable Problem Solving Based Upon Condition (Continued)

CONDITION	SYMPTOMS	CAUSES	DIAGNOSIS	MANAGEMENT
Dryness				
Corneal desiccation	Dryness Redness Low-grade awareness	Poor tear quality Inferior decentration Thick edge/CT High edge lift Poor lid hygiene Poor blink quality	3- & 9 o'clock staining Injection Possible vascularization/opacification	Ignore if diffuse only Decr center/edge thickness, add lent Decr edge lift, steepen PCR/decr PCW lid hygiene; if MGD, warm compresses/lid massage Frequent use of rewetting drops
VLK	Acute awareness Reduced wearing time Red eye Observable opaque area at corneal periphery	Prolonged dryness S/A material Low edge lift Steep BCR EW schedule	Opaque, elevated vascularized region @ 3- & 9 o'clock region	D/C lens wear: 5–7 D Ab/steroid combination F-S/A material DW only Flatter/wider periphery Flatter BCR Reduce diameter

Ab, antibiotic; BCR, base curve radius; CT, center thickness; cyl, cylindrical; D/C, discontinue; decr, decreased; Dk, oxygen permeability; EW, extended wear; F-S/A, fluoro-silicone/acrylate; GPC, giant papillary conjunctivitis; Lent, lenticular; MGD, meibomian gland dysfunction; OAD, overall diameter; OR, overrefraction; OZD, overall zone diameter; PCR, peripheral curve radius; PCW, peripheral curve width; S/A, silicone/acrylate; sph–cyl, sphero–cylindrical; VLK, vascularized limbal keratitis.

REFITTING INTO GAS-PERMEABLE LENSES

There are numerous cases in which patients can benefit by refitting from another lens material into GP lenses. This includes PMMA, very-low- and high-DK GPs, and soft lens wearers.

Polymethylmethacrylate/Very-Low-Oxygen Permeability Gas-Permeable Lens into Higher-Oxygen Permeability Gas-Permeable Lens Materials

Why Refit Polymethylmethacrylate/Very-Low-Oxygen Permeability Gas-Permeable Lens Wearers?

There are, at minimum, three important considerations when refitting PMMA wearers into GP lenses. The first pertains to PMMA-induced complications. The philosophy often associated with allowing patients to continue wearing their PMMA lenses is "if it ain't broke, don't fix it." In other words, if no symptoms and clinical signs exist, then the PMMA or very-low-Dk (<25 Dk) GP lens wearer should not be refit into a higher-Dk lens material. However, the cornea needs an oxygen level of approximately 10% (equivalent to an oxygen transmission value of 24 Dk/t) to avoid corneal swelling in the DW situation.[69] Therefore, with a comprehensive evaluation, it is very likely that any one or a combination of the following hypoxia-related complications will be present.[70]

Central Corneal Clouding: CCC is a circumscribed region of epithelial edema that appears as a grayish haze against the dark background of the pupil when sclerotic scatter/split-limbal illumination with biomicroscopy is used. Although the patient ordinarily experiences acceptable visual acuity with contact lens wear, vision is usually unsatisfactory through spectacles. In addition, an increase in myopia and steepening of the keratometer readings are also associated with CCC. This condition has been observed in almost every PMMA wearer.[71]

Edematous Corneal Formations: Edematous corneal formations (ECFs) are subepithelial arborized or dendritic-appearing formations located in the central cornea. ECFs reflect low-grade edema and develop gradually in the long-term wearer.[72] They are difficult to detect; using indirect illumination is recommended.

Polymegethism: Alteration or variation in the endothelial cell area is termed *polymegethism*. Since the endothelium controls corneal hydration, any disruption of this layer of cells may encourage edema or swelling. This is best observed during biomicroscopy with a parallelepiped using high magnification and illumination, or with an automated specular microscope. It has been determined that a significant variation in the endothelial cell area occurs with long-term PMMA wear.[73] It has also been demonstrated in low-to medium-Dk GP lens wear as well.[74]

Corneal Warpage Syndrome: Prolonged corneal edema can result in corneal distortion and unpredictable keratometric and refractive changes in as many as 30% of long-term PMMA wearers.[75] Refitting this corneal warpage syndrome patient can be extremely difficult since the cornea tends to exhibit keratoconus-like changes (although often reversible) with the development of irregular astigmatism and reduced vision through the best spectacle correction (Fig. 8.11).

Corneal warpage syndrome is most likely caused by a sequence of events resulting from a combination of corneal hypoxia, leading to typically central corneal steepening and irregular astigmatism, and the mechanical effects of a rigid lens on the cornea. Eventually, a change in the lens-to-cornea fitting relationship can occur, resulting in decentration. Studies by Wilson have concluded that once decentration has occurred, significant changes in corneal topography typically result.[11,26,27,76] The topographic abnormalities that result correlate with the decentered resting position of the contact lens on the cornea. For example, superior decentered lenses produced superior flattening with a relatively steeper contour inferiorly, simulating the topography of early keratoconus. In one study, 21 eyes of 12 predominantly PMMA-wearing patients with contact lens-induced warpage were followed with topography.[26] The corneal topography of these patients was characterized by central irregular astigmatism, loss of radial symmetry, and frequent reversal of the normal topographic pattern of progressive corneal flattening from center to periphery. Detection of the presence of corneal warpage that persisted for months was attributable to the increased sensitivity of computer-assisted topographic analysis relative to keratometry and other previous techniques.

Another important consideration pertains to convincing the asymptomatic PMMA or very-low- Dk GP lens wearer—who may only desire a new spectacle prescription—about the need

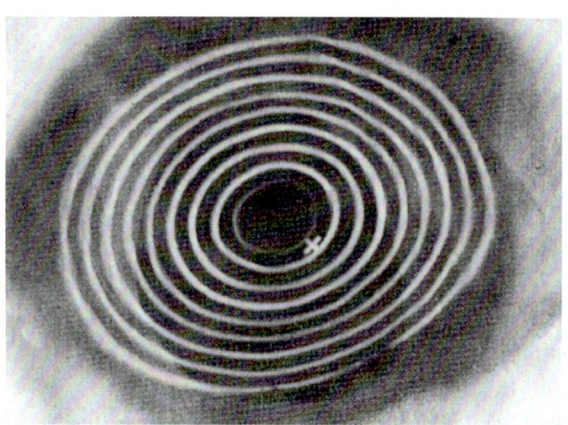

FIGURE 8.11 Corneal distortion present in a patient with corneal warpage syndrome.

to be refit into higher-Dk GP lenses. With few exceptions, patients will accept this change if a comprehensive explanation is provided of why a refit is necessary and what they should expect during the rehabilitation period.[77]

Refitting Strategy

It is important to perform a comprehensive evaluation of the patient while the patient is still wearing his or her lenses, preferably for several hours. This will allow observation of the amount and types of corneal edema and the level of difficulty in determining the refractive and keratometric values. A good case history should be performed, including questions pertaining to length of rigid lens wear per day, years of lens wear, and incidence of corneal abrasion. Patients who have worn their lenses all their waking hours for more than 15 years and are prone to overwear abrasions are prime candidates for corneal warpage or corneal exhaustion syndrome.[78,79]

The most effective strategy is to immediately refit the patient into higher-Dk GP lenses without loss of wearing time. This has the benefits of limiting excessive refractive change and enhancing patient satisfaction.[80] When refitting a patient immediately, the procedure used will depend on the effects of hypoxia on the cornea. If there is minimal or no compromise, the patient can be refit with no change in wearing time. If corneal distortion is present, the patient should be advised to reduce the wearing time to the minimum number of hours possible. Typically, this equals 8 to 12 hours per day. The patient should be advised to return for a visit in 1 week. At this time, much improvement in mire quality, postrefraction visual acuity, and corneal integrity is usually present, and the patient can be refit. Although uncommon, if the corneal compromise continues to make it difficult to have usable keratometric and refractive information, either the patient can maintain a reduced wearing schedule for a longer period or fluorescein pattern analysis can be used for determining the optimum BCR of the lenses to be ordered. In all cases, spectacles can be prescribed once refractive stability in the new GP lenses has been achieved.

Material, Lens Design, and Fitting

The first fitting decision is choosing which lens material is preferable. Although the initial temptation is to select the highest-Dk material available, especially for corneal warpage syndrome patients, low-to medium-Dk (i.e., 25–50) lens materials would provide greater rigidity. This results in less corneal sensitivity and refractive change during the stabilization period when compared to higher-Dk materials. In addition, former PMMA wearers appear to experience warpage-related problems with high-Dk GP lenses.[9] If clinical signs of hypoxia continue with GP lens wear, the patient can later be refit into a higher-Dk material. If the patient has an optimum lens-to-cornea fitting relationship, the parameters can typically be duplicated in a GP lens material, although it is not unusual to refit into a larger OAD and lower–edge-clearance design.

Soft into Gas-Permeable Lenses

Why Refit into Gas-Permeable Lenses?

There are many reasons why soft lens wearers would benefit by being refit into GP lenses. This need is confirmed by a study that evaluated the results of 200 consecutive refits from one material to another at the Park-Nicollet Medical Center in Minneapolis, perhaps the largest contact lens practice in the United States at that time.[81] The largest number of refits were in the category of being refit from hydrogel into GP lenses (92 patients, or 46%), whereas only 9% were refit from GP into hydrogel lenses. The most common reasons cited for refitting into GP lenses were reduced vision and GPC, and a 98% success rate was present after 6 months of GP lens wear. Reduced vision can result from several causes, including uncorrected refractive astigmatism, surface deposits, corneal edema, and a poorly fitting, soft toric lens. Other reasons for considering refitting a patient from soft into GP lenses include persistent edema, infiltrative keratitis, neovascularization, and difficulty in handling the larger-diameter lenses.

Soft lens wearers deserve a comprehensive explanation of why GP lenses will be more beneficial for them. In addition, they should be provided with a realistic idea of the adaptation period associated with GP lenses. Some individuals believe they are "semi-soft" lenses and will necessitate a similar adaptation schedule as soft lenses. It is essential to indicate that GP lenses do not feel the same as soft lenses at first, but that over time, they should reach a point where they are very comfortable. As indicated in Chapter 5, terms such as *discomfort* and *pain* should be avoided. If the soft lens wearer is not experiencing any symptoms or clinical signs but is simply inquiring about GP lenses (e.g., a friend may be wearing them successfully or perhaps he or she is simply interested in what is new), realistic expectations about the initial lens sensation and adaptation period need to be provided. In most cases, these patients should not be refit unless motivation is high.

Refitting Procedure

Unless severe corneal compromise or lid inflammation is present, necessitating soft lens removal, these patients can be refit and can gradually increase GP lens wear while simultaneously decreasing soft lens wear. The refitting is similar to a new GP lens patient, with the exception that even more encouragement than usual is necessary during the adaptation (i.e., "awareness") phase. If, for example, the patient is an "excessive reactor" and tears for a lengthy period, and becomes disillusioned, it would be preferable to continue the use of soft lenses in this patient, if possible. If GPC is the cause for refitting into GP lenses, the symptoms must be eliminated and the clinical signs markedly reduced (i.e., grade 1 papillary hypertrophy) before refitting into the new material.[82] In all cases, topical anesthetic use is important during the initial fit process. Patients are often apprehensive about making the transition into "hard" lenses. However, this transition is often quite easy if the first few minutes of lens wear are comfortable ones.

Patients also need to be educated about properly caring for these lenses. Each patient must be aware of the differences in lens handling and care, and must demonstrate a knowledge and competence in these procedures before leaving the office.

SUMMARY

The types of problems described in this chapter are typically minor in nature, often necessitating a change in lens design or material. In most cases, these changes result in the lessening, if not elimination, of the indicated problem. With advances in material, design, and manufacturing technology, these problems should become fewer in the years to come.

CLINICAL CASES

CASE 1

A new GP patient has the following refractive information at the time of examination:

Keratometry: 42.25 @ 180; 44.25 @ 090 OU
Spectacle Rx: $-4.00 - 1.75 \times 180$ OU

As it was a hectic day in the office, the lenses were ordered empirically in the following parameters:

OU: OAD/OZD = 9.2 mm/7.8 mm
BCR = 7.85 mm
Secondary curve radius/width (SCR/W) = 9.0 mm/0.4 mm
PCR/W = 11.0 mm/0.3 mm
Power = -4.50 D

CT = 0.14 mm
Material: Fluoroperm 60

Upon dispensing, the visual acuities were 20/25 − 1 (fluctuating) OU, with an overrefraction equal to +0.25 − 0.75 × 180. Overkeratometry also resulted in some toricity: 42.75/43.50. Slit-lamp evaluation (SLE) revealed good surface wettability, and no toricity was verified with the radiuscope.

SOLUTION: This is a flexure-induced problem that can be managed by changing lens design—preferably by selection of a flatter BCR, for example, 7.94 mm (42.50 D)—and reevaluating visual acuity and overkeratometry. This problem could have been prevented by diagnostically fitting lenses of similar design and material. It is important to rule out warpage and poor surface wettability in making the diagnosis, which can then be confirmed by the presence of toric overkeratometric readings. Additional management alternatives to consider if the change in BCR does not solve the problem include increasing CT 0.02 to 0.03 mm minimum, reducing OZD, and changing to a lower-Dk material.

CASE 2

The following GP lenses were ordered for a new patient:

OAD/OZD = 9.4 mm/7.8 mm
BCR = 7.89 mm
SCR/W = 8.7 mm/0.3 mm
Intermediate curve radius/width (ICR/W) = 9.8 mm/0.3 mm
PCR/W = 11.2 mm/0.2 mm
Power = −4.00 D
CT = Minimum
Material: Fluoroperm 30

On dispensing, the lenses decentered inferiorly. The patient was advised to gradually increase wearing time. However, after the 1-week and 1-month visits, the patient was still unable to achieve full-time wear, complaining of poor vision and lens awareness. Verification of the lens at that time resulted in a CT equal to 0.15 mm, and the lenses were still decentered in an inferior position.

SOLUTION: Reorder the lenses in a thinner design (i.e., always make the change a significant one; therefore, a thickness of 0.11 mm can be ordered). If the original diagnostic lens was available, what was the CT of that lens? Do not ever assume that merely indicating "minimum" on the order form will provide you with the thinnest possible design; some laboratories are able to make a particular lens material in a thinner design than others. As mentioned previously, it is beneficial to obtain the manufacturer's recommended CT values and confirm that your laboratory can make the lenses to those specifications. It is important to always verify CT of all incoming lenses; in addition, this information should be provided on all of the diagnostic lenses.

CASE 3

This case is identical to Case 2, with the exception that the lens power is equal to +4.00 D OU. The lens was verified as ordered; however, after 1 month, the patient was still symptomatic, and the lenses were decentered inferiorly.

SOLUTION: A minus lenticular (or similarly designed) edge design should be ordered with these lenses. The center of gravity of a plus lens is decentered anteriorly, and this factor, in combination with a thin edge, often results in an inferiorly decentered lens. The addition of a lenticular will often have a dramatic effect on improving lens centration and should always be ordered with all plus (and low minus) lens powers. Never assume the laboratory will automatically manufacture a lenticulated lens design; this typically involves a slightly higher fee, and the laboratory may have the opinion that you would prefer not to have this particular type of design. Secondary alternatives would include a steeper BCR or a smaller OAD (to decrease lens mass). In some cases, fitting a larger scleral design may be indicated in order to provide centration.

CASE 4

A patient has the following refractive information:

OD: $-2.00 - 1.25 \times 085$

42.50 @ 085; 44.00 @ 175

The following three diagnostic lenses attempted on this eye all decentered nasally, all of which positioned such that reduced visual acuity and flare would be likely if ordered:

Dx Lens No. 1	Dx Lens No. 2	Dx Lens No. 3
BCR = 42.75 D	BCR = 42.25 D	BCR = 42.25 D
OAD/OZD = 9.0 /7.8 mm	OAD/OZD = 9.2/7.8 mm	OAD/OZD = 8.8/7.4 mm

All of these lenses were of tricurve construction, with the SCR 1 mm flatter than the BCR and the PCR 3 mm flatter than the BCR.

SOLUTION: Against-the-rule astigmatism of any amount is a great challenge to the contact lens practitioner. Often the trial and error process can be exhausted in attempting to achieve an optimum fitting relationship; in fact, we often have to be satisfied with some amount of displacement. A good alternative in this situation would be an aspheric design. However, since visual compromise can be even greater when an aspheric design decenters, other design options should be considered if this option fails—for example, the use of a steeper BCR or a larger OAD. The use of a bitoric lens can be used in slightly greater astigmatic cases (i.e., ≥2 D).

CASE 5

A former PMMA wearer had been refit into the Paragon HDS100 lens material (Paragon Vision Sciences) over 1 year previously. He was not provided with any instructions pertaining to caring for the new lenses since he has been a hard lens wearer. In addition, he was provided with the Boston care regimen (Bausch + Lomb). He was in the office for the first time in 9 months, complaining of blurred vision and eyestrain, especially after prolonged near work (he is a 39-year-old attorney). The lenses, originally ordered in a -5.25 D power OU, now verified as -6.50 D. In addition, the lenses exhibited 0.50 D of toricity with the radiuscope. Since the lenses had never previously been verified, an apology is given to the patient and the lenses are reordered and eventually dispensed. However, 6 months later, he has the same complaints.

SOLUTION: This is a typical case of a patient who has unintentionally added minus power to the lenses by forceful cleaning with an abrasive cleaner on a high-Dk GP lens material. In addition, if asked, it is likely he is cleaning the lenses between the fingers ("digitally"), not in the palm of the hand. Obviously, the most important factor is to be aware that this problem can occur. The management approach is essentially threefold:

1. Educate all GP lens patients to clean the lenses gently in the palm of the hand with the "pinky" finger; if the patient cleans very forcefully in the palm of the hand or, similarly, if the lenses are cleaned between the fingers, minus power can be added. These harsh cleaning methods, especially when a circular motion is applied, are similar to adding minus power and can result in both a power change and a reduction in CT. These changes are enhanced by the use of an abrasive cleaner on the softer, high-Dk materials. Former PMMA wearers are especially prone to this problem, and they need to be educated about the differences in care and handling between this material and their previous hard lenses.

2. Always verify GP lens parameters after arrival of the lenses from the laboratory (after soaking in the recommended soaking solution for, at minimum, 24 hours).

3. Verify these lens parameters at progress evaluation visits—especially BCR, power, and CT. As a secondary option, the patient can be switched to a multipurpose solution or a separate, nonabrasive cleaner.

CASE 6

On dispensing the patient's new Optimum Extra (Contamac) lenses, poor surface wettability is present. In addition, the patient's visual acuity is two lines worse than at the diagnostic fitting. The lenses had just arrived from the laboratory and were stored in the dry state.

SOLUTION: GP lenses should be soaked, at minimum, 24 hours prior to dispensing as a preventative measure. To manage this case, some wetting/conditioning solution should be rubbed onto the surfaces of the lenses, and they should be reinserted by the patient. If poor wettability persists, it is most likely a manufacturing problem and the lenses should be cleaned with a laboratory cleaner or approved solvent followed by conditioning with the wetting solution. As a final resort, a light surface polishing can be performed.

CASE 7

A patient was dispensed Boston XO (Polymer Technology Corporation) lenses and was quite satisfied. At the 1-month visit, however, the tears are "beading" up on the lens surface. After extensive questioning, the patient mentions her frequent use of a hand lotion before lens insertion in the morning.

SOLUTION: Obviously, this is an example of either poor patient compliance or inadequate patient education since lanolin-based soaps, hand lotions, and even facial tissues with lanolin added can coat contact lenses, resulting in a reduction in surface wettability. Use of a laboratory cleaner, an approved solvent, or Menicon Progent will most likely remove the residue. The patient should then be instructed not to use any lanolin-based soaps or hand creams when handling the lenses. Liquid soaps often contain lanolin; therefore, it is necessary for the patient to examine labels and use a bar soap or special optical hand soap. Hand lotions should be used after lens insertion and then thoroughly washed off before handling the lenses.

CASE 8

The patient has been wearing Boston XO (Bausch + Lomb) lenses on a DW basis for 6 months and is complaining of blurred vision, mild redness, and reduced wearing time. On biomicroscopic evaluation, the lenses have decreased surface wettability resulting from a thick adherent mucoprotein film. When the patient is asked about his lens care routine, it is evident that he does not adequately care for his lenses. He is cleaning the lenses, at most, two times per week with the prescribed cleaner and is not using an enzymatic cleaner.

SOLUTION: The same steps for in-office cleaning, as recommended in Case 7, should be performed (i.e., laboratory cleaner or approved solvent and possibly a light surface polish). The patient needs to be reeducated about the importance of cleaning the lenses upon removal every night before placement in the recommended soaking solution. A secondary option would be to switch the patient to either the Boston Simplus solution system (Bausch & Lomb) or Optimum (Lobob) such that the lenses would soak in the cleaning/disinfecting solution. In addition, daily enzymatic cleaning should be performed. Frequent use of rewetting drops to both rinse off debris from the lens surface and rewet the lens surface should be recommended. Finally, this patient may need a brief lecture on how noncompliance can eventually result in, at minimum, a temporary discontinuation of lens wear. Upper lid eversion, not performed in this particular case, should be routinely performed on contact lens patients. It may have revealed mild-to-moderate papillary hypertrophy, commonly associated with lens surface contamination, which may have necessitated a reduction or discontinuation in lens wear.

CASE 9

The patient is returning for a 12-month follow-up visit wearing Boston IV S/A contact lenses on a DW basis. He is complaining of dryness and redness, especially toward the end of the day. SLE reveals a good lens-to-cornea fitting relationship with mild surface deposit formation. With lens removal, a grade 2 (mild coalescence) peripheral corneal staining is present.

SOLUTION: In this case, simply changing to a F-S/A material should provide an improvement in over-the-lens TBUT; therefore, the peripheral tear film would not break up as quickly, and the probability of desiccation-induced symptoms and clinical signs would be minimized. Neither a reduction in wearing time nor a change in lens design is warranted, since the fitting relationship is good and the staining is not severe. The patient's cleaning regimen should be reviewed. Are the lenses being cleaned in the palm of the hand every night upon removal? Is the appropriate cleaning regimen being used?

CASE 10

A patient presented with symptoms of a gradual reduction in lens comfort in the left eye over the last 3 weeks. In addition, her eyes were red, and she noticed a small white area on that eye. She had been a 10-year Boston IV lens wearer, who had been refit first into Paraperm EW for extended wear 13 years previously and then, 7 years ago, into Fluoroperm 92. She is currently wearing the lenses about 8 hours per day. SLE revealed VLK. A raised area was present in the peripheral cornea at the 3 o'clock position. This area was translucent and was accompanied by vascularization. The adjacent bulbar conjunctiva was very injected. The left lens exhibited good centration, although peripheral seal-off was observed.

SOLUTION: This patient should be discontinued from lens wear until the affected region is no longer elevated and the vessels have receded. A combination antibiotic–steroid should be prescribed (i.e., Tobradex or Zylet OS q.i.d.) and the patient should be evaluated after 24 hours. Typically, after 4 to 5 days, this region is no longer elevated and the patient can taper the medication. A new lens should be ordered with a flatter peripheral curve system to allow better tear exchange. In addition, reducing the patient to a flexible-wear or even a DW schedule would be recommended.

CASE 11

A 23-year-old PMMA wearer is in your office to obtain an updated spectacle prescription. The patient is very satisfied with the vision, comfort, and wearing time obtained with his hard lenses. He has not "had a doctor who could give him glasses he could see out of in many years." He is also concerned about the fees for an examination and new spectacles. The following information was obtained during the examination (the patient had been advised to wear his rigid lenses before the examination):

Visual acuity: OD: 20/20−1   OS: 20/20−2 (with contact lenses)
SLE (OU): inferior decentration, 1-mm lag, CCC grade 2+
Refraction: OD: −3.50 − 1.25 × 022 20/40−2
OS: −3.25 − 1.00 × 155 20/50 + 1
Keratometry: OD: 42.25 @ 020; 43.75 @ 110 (distorted mires)
OS: 41.75 @ 160; 43.00 @ 070 (distorted mires)

Lens parameters:

	OD	OS
BCR:	7.85 mm/43 D	7.94 mm/42.50 D
OAD/OZD:	8.8 mm/7.0 mm OU	
Power:	−3.25 D	−3.00 D
CT:	0.13 mm	0.13 mm

SOLUTION: This is a typical corneal warpage syndrome case in which the patient is a long-term PMMA wearer who has worn the lenses during all waking hours. Although he may have been told in the past that his eyes are not receiving sufficient oxygen, he is not motivated for change because, in his opinion, the contact lenses are performing very well.

The examination reveals good visual acuity through the contact lenses, but as a result of the severe edema, the best spectacle-corrected visual acuity is reduced by several lines; in addition, this is accompanied by an increase in myopic refractive error, since the patient tends to accept minus power to compensate for the edema-compromised cornea. Although small OAD/OZD (typical of a 1970s PMMA design that minimizes the amount of corneal area covered by a non–oxygen-transmitting lens material) were employed, the lenses were also fit steep to enhance centration, while at the same time minimizing lens movement and transfer of oxygenated tears. The end result was long-term chronic hypoxia resulting in irregular astigmatism and corneal distortion which, in turn, compromised the lens-to-cornea fitting relationship. Corneal topography showed mild central and paracentral regions of corneal distortion. The patient should be refit into a low-to medium Dk GP material; however, as a result of the corneal distortion, the following "loaner" lenses were provided to the patient:

Material: Boston ES
BCR: OD 7.94 mm (42.50 D) OS 8.04 mm (42.00 D)
Power: OD −2.75 D OS −2.50 D
OAD/OZD: 9.4 mm/7.8 mm OU
CT: 0.14 mm OU

The patient was advised to initiate full-time wear of these lenses and to return for a progress evaluation in 1 week. The corneas should rehabilitate underneath the GP lenses, and the patient should be monitored on a weekly basis until the corneas have stabilized and distortion is absent or minimal. If it is not possible to provide loaner lenses, the patient should be instructed to reduce the number of hours of PMMA lens wear and to return for an evaluation in 1 week. The corneal health may have improved sufficiently to refit at that time, using lens parameters similar to the loaner lenses recommended above.

The most difficult task, however, may be convincing the patient of the need to be refit into a GP material. The effects of insufficient oxygen to the eyes must be thoroughly explained, and the possibility of eventual loss of contact lens tolerance and reduction in vision should be mentioned. Usually, mentioning the condition (i.e., "corneal warpage syndrome") has a startling effect on the patient's concern about the health of the eyes. The use of audiovisuals to illustrate the PMMA-induced complications would be invaluable. Why they are unable to see out of spectacles and how this problem can be corrected with GP lenses (although no time frame should be provided) can be explained. If the patient still refuses to be refit because of such factors as fees or satisfaction with his present lenses, his reasons for refusal and your recommendations should be thoroughly documented in the record.

CASE 12

This patient is a 5-year DW hydrogel lens wearer who is complaining of redness, itching, and a reduction in wearing time. She had been using a 55%-water-content hydrogel lens material for 4 years, and these lenses had to be replaced frequently because of lens deposits. She was then diagnosed as having GPC, and after the condition had lessened, she was placed on a 1-month planned replacement program with a low-water-content hydrogel lens material. Initially, this was successful, but after 12 months, she is symptomatic once again. The examination reveals the following (all results OU):

Visual acuity: 20/25−1 (fluctuates)
Overrefraction: plano −0.25 × 180
SLE (lenses on): Good centration, 0.5-mm lag
                Heavy mucoprotein film
SLE (lenses off): diffuse staining
TBUT = 6 seconds
Grade 3 papillary hypertrophy

SOLUTION: The first step would be to discontinue contact lens wear until the papillary hypertrophy has greatly reduced (grade 1+ or better). The patient should be monitored on a regular basis (i.e., every 1–2 weeks) until recovery has occurred. The patient should be provided realistic expectations of when a refit can occur (typically, this could be a range of anywhere from 2 weeks to 3 months). At that time, the patient should be refit into GP lenses, which should result in fewer complications in the borderline dry-eye patient as a result of the more wettable surface. This type of patient is usually motivated because of the hydrogel-induced problems; nevertheless, the adaptation schedule should be thoroughly explained. In addition, a topical anesthetic should be used at the refitting visit. Alternatively, the use of a sclera design will provide comfort similar to their hydrogel lenses.

CASE 13

This patient has been a soft lens wearer for over 1 year and has been quite satisfied with the comfort and wearing time provided by these lenses. However, he has never been satisfied with his vision through the lenses. He is an accountant who obviously performs an immense amount of near work. He was originally fit with spherical soft lenses at a local optical establishment, and as a result of vision-related complaints, he was eventually fit into soft torics. At the time he visits your office, he has been in soft torics for 3 months and thinks his vision is no better than he achieved with his previous soft lenses and desires a change. You find the following information:

Visual acuity: OD: 20/25 OS: 20/25 − 2
SLE: both lenses are rotating excessively with the blink
Refraction: OD: −1.50 − 0.75 × 172 20/20 + 2
OS: −1.75 − 1.00 × 010 20/15 − 1

SOLUTION: This patient is an excellent candidate for GP lenses because of his need for critical vision, which has not been possible with soft lenses. He is actually a challenging soft lens patient as a result of the low ametropia in combination with a small but significant amount of refractive astigmatism for someone who performs many near-work tasks. Since he is very satisfied with the comfort of soft lenses, both the benefits of GP lenses—especially vision—and the lens awareness present during adaptation should be strongly emphasized. As in Case 12, a topical anesthetic should be used at the refitting visit. Again, a scleral design with its hydrogel-like comfort may also be considered.

CLINICAL PROFICIENCY CHECKLIST

- Causes of reduced vision in GP lens-wearing patients include flexure, warpage, lens decentration, poor surface wettability, and power change.
- Flexure-related reduced visual acuity can be minimized by selecting a flatter BCR (by an amount equal to, at minimum, 0.50 D flatter) and, secondly, by selecting a greater CT.
- An improvement in fitting relationship with inferior decentering lenses can often be obtained by decreasing CT and, when indicated, by the use of a lenticular edge design or a scleral lens design.
- Poor initial surface wettability can be minimized by presoaking the lenses for a minimum of 24 hours and by rubbing wetting solution into the lens surface. Ordering lenses that have been plasma-treated will also minimize the incidence of this problem.
- Poor acquired surface wettability can be managed by the use of a laboratory cleaner or approved solvent. Patients should be educated to clean the lenses regularly, immediately upon removal, and to avoid lens contact with lanolin-containing substances.
- Minus power change over time can be minimized by educating patients to clean the lenses gently in the palm of the hand, supplemented by frequent verification of the lens parameters by the practitioner.
- Corneal desiccation can be minimized by obtaining a lid attachment fitting relationship (if possible), selecting an F-S/A lens material, avoiding excessively high edge clearance designs, and keeping CT to a minimum. Scleral designs will also alleviate this issue.
- PMMA and very-low-Dk GP patients with corneal edema—but no distortion—can be refit immediately into higher-Dk GP lenses without loss of wearing time. A low-to medium-Dk (i.e., 25–50) material is recommended.

- The most common reasons why soft lens-wearing patients are refit into GP lenses are poor vision and GPC. It is important for these patients to understand both the benefits of GP lenses and the need for a gradual adaptation period.

REFERENCES

1. Bennett ES. Problem solving. In: Bennett ES, Hom MM, eds. *Manual of Gas Permeable Contact Lenses*. 2nd ed. St. Louis, MO: Elsevier Science; 2004:190–222.
2. Fonn D, Sorbara L. Progress evaluation procedures. In: Bennett ES, Weissman BA, eds. *Clinical Contact Lens Practice*. Philadelphia, PA: Lippincott Williams & Wilkins; 2005:325–339.
3. Gasson A. Aspects of hard lens aftercare. *Contact Lens J*. 1979;8:4–11.
4. Bennett ES. Silicone/acrylate lens design. *Int Cont Lens Clin*. 1985;12(1):45.
5. Herman JP. Flexure. In: Bennett ES, Grohe RM, eds. *Rigid Gas-Permeable Contact Lenses*. New York, NY: Professional Press; 1986:137–150.
6. Bennett ES, Egan DJ. Rigid gas-permeable lens problem-solving. *J Am Optom Assoc*. 1986;57(7):504–512.
7. Egan DJ, Bennett ES. Trouble-shooting rigid contact lens flexure—a case report. *Int Cont Lens Clin*. 1985;12(2):147.
8. Carrell BA, Bennett ES, Henry VA, et al. The effect of rigid gas permeable lens cleaners on lens parameter stability. *J Am Optom Assoc*. 1992;63(3):193–198.
9. Henry VA, Bennett ES, Forrest JF. Clinical investigation of the Paraperm EW rigid gas-permeable contact lens. *Am J Optom Physiol Opt*. 1987;64(3):313–320.
10. Ghormley NR. Rigid EW lenses: complications. *Int Cont Lens Clin*. 1987;14(6):219.
11. Wilson SE, Lin DTC, Klyce SD, et al. Rigid contact lens decentration: a risk factor for corneal warpage. *CLAO J*. 1990;16(3):177–182.
12. Kikkawa Y, Salmon TO. Rigid lens tear exchange and the tear mucous layer. *Contact Lens Forum*. 1990;15(12):17–24.
13. Schnider CM, Bennett ES, Grohe RM. Rigid extended wear. In: Bennett ES, Weissman BA, eds. *Clinical Contact Lens Practice*. Philadelphia, PA: JB Lippincott; 1991;56:1–14.
14. Laurenzi-Jones A. Centering a decentered GP lens. *Contact Lens Spectrum*. 2010;25(11):22.
15. Bennett ES, Grohe RM. RGP quality control: the results of a national survey. *J Am Optom Assoc*. 1995;66(3):147–153.
16. Hill RM, Brezinski SD. The center thickness factor. *Contact Lens Spectrum*. 1987;2(10):52–54.
17. Bennett ES, Gibbons G. Clinical grand rounds. *Video-aided presentation given at RGP Lens Practice Today and Tomorrow*. St. Louis, MO; July 1990.
18. Bennett ES. Be flexible about rigid lenses. *Rev Cornea Contact Lenses*. May 2007;38–40.
19. Quinn TG. Avoiding the low riding lens. *Contact Lens Spectrum*. 2000;15(7):21.
20. Korb DR, Korb JE. A new concept in contact lens design I and II. *J Am Optom Assoc*. 1970;40(12):1–12.
21. Fonn D, Sorbara L. Rigid gas-permeable lens problem solving. In: Bennett ES, Weissman BA, eds. *Clinical Contact Lens Practice*. Philadelphia, PA: Lippincott Williams & Wilkins; 2005:341–354.
22. Levitt A. Specific gravity and RGP performance. *Contact Lens Spectrum*. 1996;11(10):43–45.
23. Carney L, Mainstone J, Quinn T, et al. Rigid lens centration: effects of lens design and material density. *Int Cont Lens Clin*. 1996;23(1):6–11.
24. Hartstein J, Ward M, Lipson M, et al. Scleral and mini-scleral lenses: a case series. *Contact Lens Spectrum*. 2010;25(10):40–47.
25. Kalin NS, Maeda N, Klyce SD, et al. Automated topographic screening for keratoconus in refractive surgery candidates. *CLAO J*. 1996;22(3):164–167.
26. Wilson SE, Lin DT, Klyce SD, et al. Topographic changes in contact lens-induced corneal warpage. *Ophthalmology*. 1990;16:177–182.
27. Ruiz-Montenegro J, Mafra CH, Wilson SE, et al. Corneal topographic alterations in normal contact lens wearers. *Ophthalmology*. 1993;100:128–134.
28. Grohe RM, Caroline PJ. RGP non-wetting syndrome. *Contact Lens Spectrum*. 1989;4(3):32–44.
29. Brown M. Gas permeable lens options continue to expand. *Primary Care Optom News*. July 2007;25–26.
30. Bennett ES, Grohe RM, Brown MJ, et al. Resolving filmy GPs, part 2. *Contact Lens Spectrum*. 2011;26(12):21.
31. Ward MA. GPC and GP lens care. *Contact Lens Spectrum*. 2010;25(9):23.
32. Bennett ES. Dry eye and GP lens wear, part 2. *Contact Lens Spectrum*. 2009;24(12).
33. Doane M, Gleason W. Tear film interaction with RGP contact lenses. Presented at: First International Material Science Symposium; March 1988; St. Louis, MO.
34. Friedman DM. Too much lens cleaning can also be destructive. *Contact Lens Forum*. 1989;14(9):80.
35. Boltz KD. The overzealous contact lens cleaner. *Contact Lens Spectrum*. 1989;4(12):53–54.
36. Bennett ES, Henry VA. RGP lens power change with abrasive cleaner use. *Int Cont Lens Clin*. 1990;17(3):152–153.
37. Caroline PJ, Andre MP. Inadvertent patient modification of RGP lenses. *Contact Lens Spectrum*. 1999;14(1):56.
38. O'Donnell JJ. Patient-induced power changes in rigid gas permeable contact lenses: a case report and literature review. *J Am Optom Assoc*. 1994;65(11):772–773.

39. Williams-Lyn D, MacNeill K, Fonn D. The effect of rigid lens back optic zone radius and diameter changes on comfort. *Int Cont Lens Clin.* 1993;20:223–229.
40. Szczotka LB. RGP parameter changes: how much change is significant? *Contact Lens Spectrum.* 2001;16(4):18.
41. Andrasko G. Peripheral corneal staining: incidence and time course. *Contact Lens Spectrum.* 1990;5(7):59–62.
42. Businger U, Treiber A, Flury C. The etiology and management of three and nine o'clock staining. *Int Cont Lens Clin.* 1989;16(50):136–139.
43. Scheid T, Bennett E. 3&9 o'clock staining/peripheral corneal desiccation. Cornea and Contact Lens Living Library. http://www.aocle.org/livingL/3-9stain.html. Accessed June 20, 2008.
44. Solomon J. Causes and treatments of peripheral corneal desiccation. *Contact Lens Forum.* 1986;11:30–36.
45. Edrington TB, Barr JT. Peripheral corneal desiccation. *Contact Lens Spectrum.* 2002;17(1):46.
46. Bennett ES. Lens design and troubleshooting. In: Bennett ES, Grohe RM, eds. *Rigid Gas-Permeable Contact Lenses.* New York, NY: Professional Press; 1986:189–224.
47. Van der Worp E, de Brabander J, Swarbrick HA, et al. Evaluation of signs and symptoms in 3- and 9-o'clock staining. *Optom Vis Sci.* 2009;86(3):260–265.
48. Ghormley N, Bennett E, Schnider C. Corneal desiccation clinical management. *Int Cont Lens Clin.* 1990;17:5–8.
49. Schnider CM, Terry RL, Holden BA. Effect of patient and lens performance characteristics on peripheral corneal desiccation. *J Am Optom Assoc.* 1996;67:144–150.
50. Bennett ES. How to manage the rigid lens wearer. *Rev Optom.* 1986;123(10):102–110.
51. Fonn D, Gauthier C. Aftercare of RGP lens wearers. *Contact Lens Spectrum.* 1990;5(9):71–81.
52. van der Worp E, de Brabander J, Swarbrick H, et al. Corneal desiccation in rigid contact lens wear: 3-and 9-o'clock staining. *Optom Vis Sci.* 2003;80(4):280–290.
53. Lowther GE. Dryness, tears, and contact lens wear. *Clinical Practice in Contact Lenses.* Boston, MA: Butterworth-Heinemann; 1997:84–90.
54. Schnider C. Rigid gas permeable extended wear. *Contact Lens Spectrum.* 1990;5(9):101–106.
55. Ghormley NR. New guy on the block. *Int Cont Lens Clin.* 1995;22(pt 1):139–140.
56. Norman C. A new hyper-dk option for gp lenses. *Contact Lens Spectrum.* 2007;22(10):44–47.
57. van der Worp E, de Brabander J, Swarbrick H, et al. Eyeblink frequency and type in relation to 3- and 9-o'Clock staining and gas permeable contact lens variables. *Optom Vis Sci.* 2008;85(9):857–866.
58. Rinehart JM. The balancing act. *Rev Cornea Contact Lenses.* 2010;7. Available at: http://www.reviewofcontactlenses.com/content/d/gas-permeable_strategies/i/1244/c/23404/
59. DeNaeyer G. Large diameter lenses to the rescue. *Rev Cornea Contact Lenses.* 2009;146(3):14–17.
60. Edrington T, Barr JT. We have edge lift. *Contact Lens Spectrum.* 2002;17(10):49.
61. Musset A, Stone J. *Contact Lens Design Tables.* London: Butterworths; 1981:1–12.
62. Bennett ES. The effect of varying axial edge lift on silicone/acrylate lens performance. *Contact Lens J.* 1986;14(4):3–7.
63. Lowther GE. Review of rigid contact lens design and effects of design on lens fit. *Int Cont Lens Clin.* 1988;15(12):378–389.
64. Ames KS, Erickson P. Optimizing aspheric and spherical rigid lens performance. *CLAO J.* 1987;13(2):165–169.
65. Schnider CM, Terry RB, Holden BA. Effects of lens design on peripheral corneal desiccation. *J Am Optom Assoc.* 1997;68(3):163–170.
66. Bennett ES. Corneal desiccation: how to manage the most common GP problem. *Rev Cornea Contact Lenses.* 2005;(suppl):10.
67. Grohe RM, Lebow KA. Vascularized limbal keratitis. *Int Cont Lens Clin.* 1989;16(7&8):197–209.
68. Edwards K, Hough T. Contact lens related case studies: vascularized limbal keratitis. *Optician.* 1998;216(5680):36–37.
69. Holden BA, Mertz GW. Critical oxygen levels to avoid corneal edema for daily and extended wear contact lenses. *Invest Ophthalmol Vis Sci.* 1984;25:1161.
70. Bennett ES. Refitting PMMA and hydrogel lens wearers into RGPs. In: Harris MG, ed. *Contact Lens Problem-Solving* vol 2, *Special Contact Lens Procedures.* Philadelphia, PA: JB Lippincott; 1990:201–209.
71. Finnemore VM, Korb JE. Corneal edema with polymethacrylate versus gas permeable rigid polymer contact lenses of identical design. *J Am Optom Assoc.* 1980;51(3):271–274.
72. Kame RT. Clinical management of edematous corneal formations. *Rev Optom.* 1979;116(4):69–71.
73. Stocker E, Schoessler JP. Corneal endothelial polymegathism induced by PMMA contact lens wear. *Invest Ophthalmol Vis Sci.* 1985;26:857–863.
74. Bourne WM, Holtan SB, Hodge DO. Morphologic changes in corneal endothelial cells during three years of fluorocarbon contact lens wear. *Cornea.* 1999;18(1):29–33.
75. Rengstorff RH. The Fort Dix report: longitudinal study of the effects of contact lenses. *Am J Optom Arch Am Acad Optom.* 1965;42(3):153–163.
76. Wilson SE, Klyce SD. Advances in the analysis of corneal topography. *Surv Ophthalmol.* 1991;35:269–277.
77. Henry VA, Campbell RC, Connelly S, et al. How to refit contact lens patients. *Contact Lens Forum.* 1991;16(2):19–30.
78. Holden BA, Sweeney DF. Corneal exhaustion syndrome (CES) in long-term contact lens wearers: a consequence of contact lens-induced polymegethism? *Am J Optom Physiol Opt.* 1988;65:95P.
79. Sweeney DF. Corneal exhaustion syndrome with long-term wear of contact lenses. *Optom Vis Sci.* 1992;69(8):601–608.
80. Bennett ES. Immediate refitting of gas permeable lenses. *J Am Optom Assoc.* 1983;54(3):239–242.
81. Connelly S. Why do patients want to be refit. *Contact Lens Spectrum.* 1992;7(5):39–41.
82. Henry VA, Bennett ES, Sevigny J. Rigid extended wear problem solving. *Int Cont Lens Clin.* 1990;17(3):121–133.

Chapter 9

Modification of Gas-Permeable Lenses

Edward S. Bennett and Keith Parker

The in-office modification of gas-permeable (GP) lenses is a well-established art that has existed for many decades. The ability to change the lens design to result in an immediate improvement in the fitting relationship, vision, or comfort is quite integral to the long-term success of all GP lens wearers and, as with verification, should be performed in any office where GP lenses are being fit.

WHY MODIFY?

Modification of GP lenses is essential for long-term patient satisfaction. The procedures are easy to perform, require little time or expense, and result in both patient satisfaction and a lower dropout rate.

In-office modification of rigid lenses enables any contact lens practice to increase its efficiency and provides a valuable service to the patient. Every student, assistant, and practitioner should be proficient at performing the modifications discussed in this chapter. Almost any material can be modified, including the superpermeables, if the modifier exercises care in the procedures. These valuable skills are acquired easily through practice, and the benefits derived easily will justify the effort.[1]

If a patient's lenses need modification, the inconvenience of sending the lenses to the laboratory and interrupting the patient's wearing schedule can result in a very dissatisfied patient. Patients place a high value on their time and appreciate receiving personalized custom services. It also reduces practice expenditures incurred by purchasing additional lenses. The returned lenses may not be satisfactory to the practitioner or the patient, which leads to further delays and the need for readaptation. In-office modification not only provides for uninterrupted lens wear, but also allows the practitioner to correlate the applied lens modifications with the desired fitting results and, therefore, to develop techniques that allow the best lens-to-cornea fitting relationship. This gives the practitioner optimum control over the fit of the lenses, and saves time for patient and practitioner by reducing the number of patient visits.

The ability to modify GP lenses is a powerful in-office problem-solver. GP quality is improving because of technological advancements in manufacturing. Nevertheless, there will be that occasional defective edge, or poorly wettable lens. For example, a patient experiencing symptoms of lens awareness can often be managed by a simple edge polish.[2] Dryness or fluctuating vision can be managed by surface polishing. A lens that feels dry and exhibits very little movement with the blink can be managed by blending or flattening the peripheral curves. If the addition of a slight amount of power will provide the patient with better vision and eliminate the need for reordering the lens, this can be performed in the office as well. Solving these problems in the office will not only result in a much more satisfied patient, but will also minimize the resulting negative effects of a dissatisfied patient who may communicate his or her feelings to other people and, as a result of frustration, give up on contact lens wear in general.

Modifying rigid lenses is simple and requires little time. The procedures discussed in this chapter all take no more than a few minutes to perform. As will be discussed, there are several ways for practitioners to gain proficiency in performing common modification procedures. In addition, technicians in the office can easily be trained to perform these procedures. The expense for equipment is, at most, a few hundred dollars; this is not much to ask to keep patients satisfied while enhancing the lens performance. Some modifications, such as a clean and polish, can be provided as an annual service to patients who have a service agreement.

THE MODIFICATION UNIT

Modification of GP contact lenses begins with the modification unit. Cost is not a factor since most units are very reasonably priced and pay for themselves over a short period. The basic modification unit consists of a small, electric, motor-driven spindle mounted below a steel or plastic bowl. Some units also have multiple spindles and a variable spindle speed. The latter option has become a very desirable feature with the introduction of newer, softer materials. Many units have fixed spindle speeds in the range of 1,200 to 1,600 rpm, whereas the new materials require speeds of only 1,000 rpm or less.[3] High spindle speed causes polish to be removed very quickly, which results in a dry tool. As the tool dries, excess heat is built up, resulting in lens surface defects that will affect surface wettability.[4,5] A variable speed modification unit would be preferable, although the spindle speed of a unit can be monitored with a rheostat system purchased at a local hardware store. Caution is needed when using variable speed units. These units are easily inadvertently set to the fastest speed, greatly increasing the risk of lens damage.

The spindle base may be encased in a wood, plastic, or metal protective covering, or may be built directly into a table (Fig. 9.1). The splash bowl prevents water and polish from splashing onto the operator and gives the operator room to place his or her hands and tools near the spindle. A plastic bowl is less likely to scratch or chip a lens that may be thrown from the spindle and is therefore a safer option.[6] A table-mounted bowl is a desirable feature because it provides a place for the operator to rest his or her elbows and steady his or her hand during modification procedures.

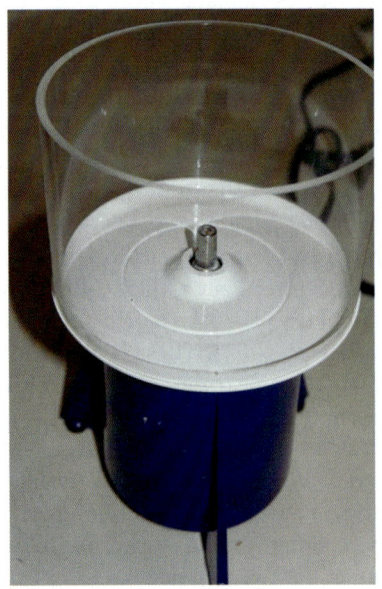
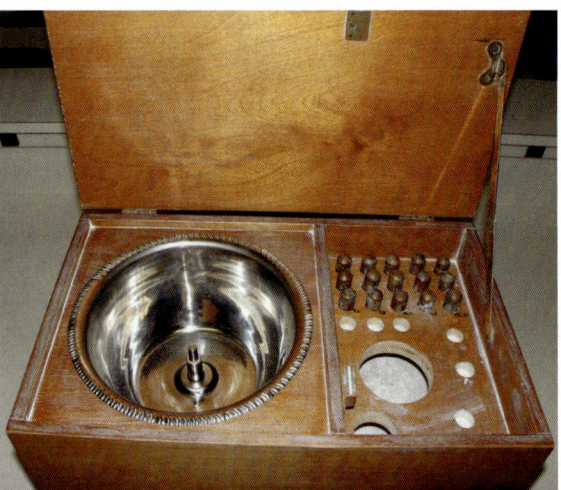

FIGURE 9.1 **(A)** Free-standing bowl modification unit. **(B)** Duffens modification unit (no longer available).

LENS ATTACHMENT DEVICES

Holding the contact lens firmly with good centration without altering the lens parameters is crucial for all modification procedures. The most common type of lens holder is a suction cup, sometimes incorporated into a spinning holder device.

Most modification procedures involve using the suction cup as a lens holder. It is very helpful to use one that has interchangeable ends, such as the R&F Stronghold suction cup (DMV Corporation), so that both the concave and convex surfaces of the lens may be attached. It is suggested that although the concave and convex ends can be reversed, two separate holders are used to allow easy conversion from one to another. DMV now offers larger-headed suction cup tips for both convex and concave surfaces, providing increased stability of holding increasingly more common larger GP lenses. The suction cup should be wet when the lens is attached, and special care should be taken to ensure lens centration (Fig. 9.2). Failure to center the lens will result in an oval optical zone diameter and uneven edge or surface polishing and will possibly compromise the lens optics.[4] Minimum pressure should be used during application to prevent lens warpage. The suction cup should be held by the operator as close to the lens as possible to impart maximum control during the modification process.

Spinner tools are very beneficial for certain procedures requiring care in maintaining optical quality, such as front surface polishing and power changes. The exact style of spinner may vary, but all types work similarly. Most utilize a suction cup for lens attachment, which is preferable over one requiring double-sided tape. Double-sided tape often leaves a residue on the surface of the lens, which must be removed by a compatible solvent. Once the lens is attached to the spinner, it is free to spin along with the spindle while the handle is held stationary. This allows power changes or polishing to be performed slowly and evenly, resulting in little or no optical distortion.

OTHER EQUIPMENT

Several accessories are required in addition to the modification unit and lens attachment devices, including radius tools, polishing sponges, and polish (Table 9.1). The radius tools used for polishing and grinding are often included with the unit and commonly attach to the spindle

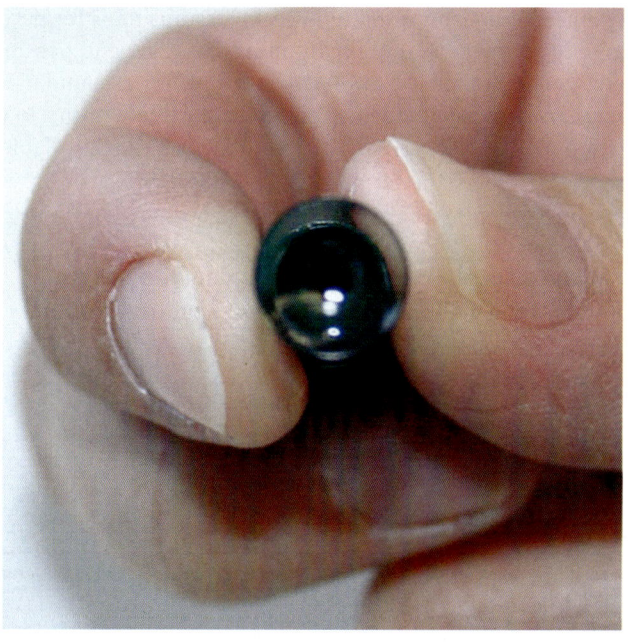

FIGURE 9.2 Lens centered on a suction cup.

TABLE 9.1 In-Office Modification Equipment
Required
Modification unit (variable speed or low single speed)
Edge and surface sponge polishing tools
Suction cups
Polish
Strongly Recommended
7× or 10× magnifying loupe
CLEPA or projection magnifying device
Recommended
Suction cup spinner
Radius tools
90-degree anterior bevel cone tool
CLEPA, contact lens edge profile analyzer.

by a form fit. The tool contains a tapered hole drilled along its axis that matches the tapering of the spindle. Friction then holds the tool in place as it is spinning. Although some tools are interchangeable with other units, taper size may vary for both units and tools. It is important to keep in mind that the tapers must match exactly. Incorrect taper size can result in tool wobble and improper modification. Some Contact Lens Manufacturers Association (CLMA) laboratories where you can obtain modification equipment are listed in Table 9.2.[7]

The amount of cost for modification equipment varies depending on the number of procedures that are performed. For basic edge and surface polish procedures, many laboratories have economical packages ranging from $225 to $350.[8] This typically includes a single-speed modification unit in addition to sponge or velveteen tools for polishing procedures. Suction cups and polish are also typically provided. A deluxe package (often $300–$500) allows the practitioner or staff to perform peripheral curve procedures such as blending and flattening, in addition to changing the power of the lens. This package typically includes a suction cup spinner for polishing and repowering, radius tools for peripheral curve procedures, a 90-degree anterior bevel cone tool for thinning the edge, and possibly a 7× magnifying loupe or a diameter gauge. As most CLMA laboratories either manufacture or distribute modification equipment, it is recommended to contact a local laboratory to determine if it provides modification equipment and, if so, what types of packages are available.

TABLE 9.2 Where to Obtain Modification Equipment		
MANUFACTURER	HOW TO CONTACT	EQUIPMENT/SUPPLIES
Advanced Vision Technologies	Keith@avtlens.com	Units and all tools
Boston/Bausch + Lomb	www.bausch.com	Polish
Conforma Contact Lenses	info@conforma.com	Units and all tools
DMV Corporation	www.dmvcorp.com	Suction cups
Larsen Equipment Design	www.larsenequipment.com	Units and all tools
Misupco	MikeF@misupco.com	Units, tools, and polish
Polychem	PolychmUSA@aol.com	Units, tools, and polish

Modified from DeKinder J, Bennett ES. Equip yourself for modifying GP lenses. *Contact Lens Spectrum.* 2005;20(2):48.

POLISHING COMPOUNDS

The importance of polishing compounds used for modification should not be overlooked. *Liberal* use of polish specifically designed for GP lenses is necessary for all modification procedures. These solutions contain a mild abrasive—typically a grit aluminum base—that erodes lens material along with surfactants and detergents to lubricate and cool the lens during modification. They all appear to be successful in modifying GP lens materials. One study evaluated the effectiveness of seven commonly used polishes in repowering GP lenses.[9] The polishes used included the following premixed liquid solutions: Boston White Finishing Polish (Polymer Technology Corporation, Wilmington, MA), Evergreen (R&F Products, Denver, CO), Mirapolish (ABBA Optical, Stone Mountain, GA), Nu-Care 2000 (Polychem, Gaithersburg, MD), and Sil-O2-Care (Polychem, Gaithersburg, MD). Two dry powder polishes were used (which can be mixed with water or saline): Al-Ox 721 (Transelco Ferro, Cleveland, OH) and X-Pal (Davison Chemical, Chattanooga, TN). It was found that all seven polishes were effective in adding 0.50 D of power to a 92-oxygen permeable (Dk) GP lens material. The powder forms were faster, taking 35 to 40 seconds, whereas the premixed solutions took up to 2½ minutes to add the desired amount of power. Therefore, it is advisable to practice with a particular polishing compound to ensure predictable results with future modifications. Products containing ammonia are not suitable for use with GP lenses since they can adversely affect surface wettability. Silvo was a popular polish with polymethylmethacrylate (PMMA) lenses, but it contains ammonia and therefore is not recommended for GP lenses.

MODIFICATION PROCEDURES

Introduction

It is important to obtain some baseline parameter information on the lenses before performing any modification procedure. An educated decision about how to modify a lens can only be made after first knowing what the specifications are. Be sure to record all verifications of the optical and structural quality of the lens before beginning *any* procedure, since modification of one parameter can often affect another.

Obtaining the original specifications of the lens is very beneficial. It is, therefore, important to verify parameters of all new lenses from the laboratory before they are dispensed to the patient. This information becomes quite pertinent should the lens need modifying in the future. Note that some laboratories still measure front vertex power instead of back vertex. It becomes critical to know which was used when working with aphakic contact lenses, where the power can vary up to 2 D depending on the method.

Blending/Flattening Peripheral Curves

In-office blending or flattening of the peripheral curve radii allows the practitioner to adjust the fit of the lens and immediately observe an improved lens-to-cornea fitting relationship and, more than likely, an improvement in lens performance. If limited lens movement is present with the blink accompanied by tear stagnation, blending the junctions between peripheral curve radii should result in increased movement and better tear exchange. In addition, blending the peripheral curve junctions can also increase patient comfort.[10] If peripheral or midperipheral bearing is present, seal-off and possibly lens adherence—more common in GP extended wear—can result. Once again, only limited, if any, tear exchange will result. Flattening the peripheral curve radius should resolve the problem and result in greater clearance peripherally. If these problems are not promptly managed, edema and dryness-related problems can result.[11]

The radius tools used to apply peripheral curves are customarily made of brass, plastic, or Delrin (Conforma). Some brass tools may or may not be impregnated with an abrasive, such as diamond dust (Fig. 9.3). These diamond-coated tools are used to abruptly change the existing

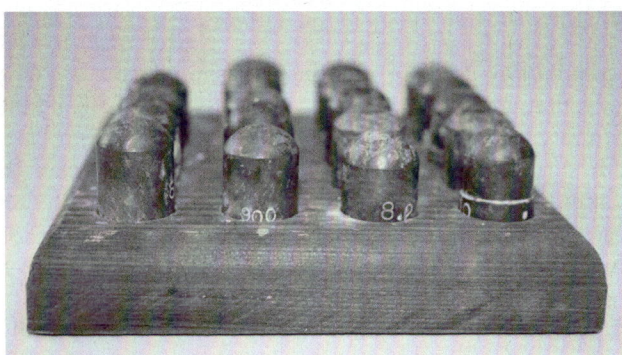

FIGURE 9.3 Radius tools.

curve to reestablish a desired radius of peripheral alignment. The radius blending tools are normally available in 0.10- to 0.25-mm steps, with a minimum set consisting of the following radii: 7.50, 8.0, 8.5, 9.0, 10.50, and 12.00 mm. A more complete set for advanced modification could possibly include 7.6, 7.8, 8.0, 8.2, 8.4, 8.6, 8.8, 9.0, 9.3, 9.6, 10.0, 10.5, 11.2, 12.0, 12.5 and 13.0 mm.[4] Steeper tools such as 6.0, 6.25, 6.5, and 6.75 mm may be required and prove very useful in modifying steeper keratoconus designs. Radius diamond-coated tools are fairly expensive and are usually intended in grinding the outer peripheral curve. Hard-pad radius tools, although slower to change radii than a diamond radius tool, are recommended when establishing a change in the secondary or intermediate radii.

A peripheral curve is applied to a lens modified by first attaching the lens to a suction cup or spinner tool, concave side out. The appropriate radius tool is chosen, and either a square of waterproof adhesive tape or a precut velveteen soft pad or cotton hard pad is attached smoothly over its surface. Some practitioners prefer the softer velveteen pads for obtaining a more gradual peripheral curve or for blending. The soft pad will create a smoother blending area, whereas the hard pad will create a more abrupt change where contacted with the contact lens. The velveteen pad is approximately 0.4 mm thick, and the adhesive tape is 0.2 mm; therefore, either pad on a radius tool will actually be a flatter radius than the actual tool radius. Note: It is recommended to never use a radius blending tool with a soft or hard pad no less than 0.50 mm flatter than the central base curve of the contact lens to avoid pad marks in the optical surface area of the base curve. If a 9.0-mm curve is needed, an 8.6-mm tool should be used with velveteen and an 8.8-mm tool with adhesive tape.[6]

The soft pad on the radius tool is first thoroughly made wet with fresh clean water, and then the tool is placed on the spindle, the motor is turned on, and polish is applied to the tool surface.[4] Note that the appropriate polishing compound must be applied to the tool *before* use and throughout the modification procedure. In addition, the tool surface and polish must be kept free from all dirt and other abrasive materials, or scratches will appear on the posterior peripheral lens surface (Fig. 9.4A). Once the spindle is spinning, the lens is held lightly against the tool with the concave surface facing the tool (Fig. 9.4B). If a suction cup is used, the lens should be held at a 30-degree angle to the vertical, and the entire outer edge should be in contact with the covered tool at all times. The suction cup is rotated smoothly and evenly with the fingers in the opposite direction of the spindle rotation. Since the spindle rotates clockwise in most units, the suction cup should be turned counterclockwise. Alternatively, rather than holding the suction cup at a 30-degree angle, the lens may be held vertically to the radius tool and rotated in a figure-eight design (Fig. 9.4C). The lens should be lifted from the tool every 5 to 10 seconds and a drop of polish added to the surface every time the lens is touched to the tool. Insufficient polish, as well as excessive pressure, can lead to heat build-up and lens damage.

This procedure may also be performed utilizing a spinner tool. The lens is centered on the spinner, again with the concave surface facing the tool. The spinner is held at a 45- to 60-degree angle off the center of the radius tool. The lens must be spinning at all times during the procedure and polish continually applied as previously discussed.

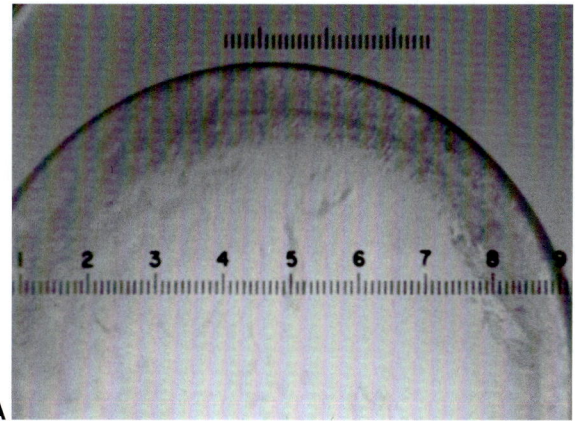
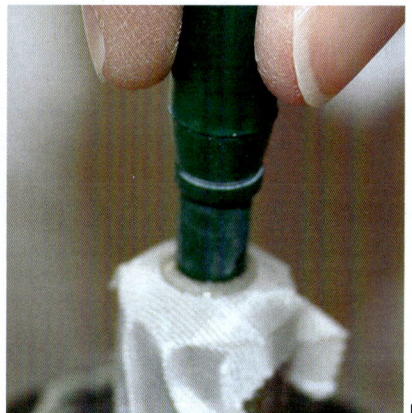
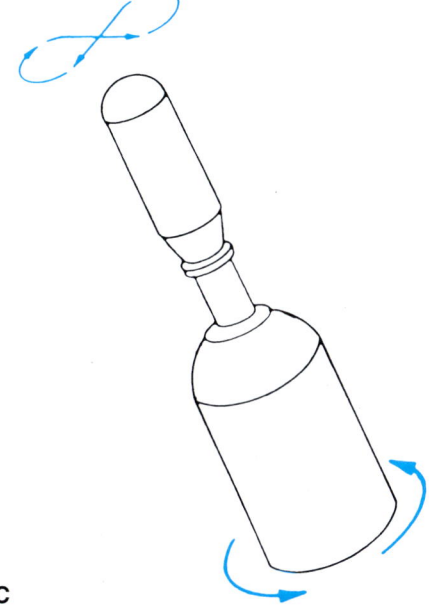

FIGURE 9.4 (A) "Bull's-eye" effect from scratches on the posterior lens surface caused by excessive pressure or dirty polish. **(B)** Peripheral curve application with lens and suction cup. **(C)** Figure-eight design is used to apply peripheral curve.

Practice and experience are necessary to obtain confidence in producing consistent results with peripheral curves. The amount of bevel obtained depends on numerous factors, including spindle speed, pressure of the lens against the pad, consistency of the polish, and flatness of the radius tool (in relation to the base curve of the lens). After a little experience, the operator will be able to quickly determine the length of time needed to produce a peripheral curve of desired radius and width. It is recommended that records should be made of all adjustments made to the lenses, including peripheral curves applied, spindle speed, and time for each curve.[12] These records will enable the operator to duplicate a lens adjustment, if necessary, in the future.

The width and quality of the peripheral curve should be monitored periodically during the procedure. The lens is removed from the lens holder, cleaned thoroughly, and viewed through a magnified reticule graduated in 0.10-mm divisions. A projection magnifier can also be used to verify peripheral curves.

Blending

Following peripheral curve application, the junction between curves consists of a significant ridge of material that can inhibit tear exchange and cause discomfort to the patient. Blending of this transition zone is necessary to remove this ridge and, therefore, increase lens movement and promote tear exchange.[6] The tear exchange is accompanied by increased oxygen, as well as flushing of debris that may deposit on the back surface of the lens.

The tool selected for blending typically has a radius approximately halfway between the radii of the two adjacent curves. Again, the thickness of the tape or pad must be taken into consideration. Generally, only the peripheral curves are blended, but the optical zone junction also may be blended if it is unusually sharp or if the clinician desires to lower a high-fitting lens. The tool used to blend the optical zone junction, however, should never be less than the base curve radius of the lens. Otherwise, the base curve radius could be flattened or warped quickly.

The following is an example of how to determine the radius tool necessary for blending. All figures are in millimeters.

Base curve radius: 7.80 mm
Secondary curve radius: 9.00 mm
Peripheral curve radius: 12.00 mm

First blend:
7.80 + 9.00
16.80/2 = 8.40
8.40 blend radius
− .40 pad thickness
8.00-mm tool

Second blend:
9.00 + 12.00
21.00/2 = 10.50
10.50 blend radius
− .40 pad thickness
10.10-mm tool

In many cases, the exact radius tool needed to create a blend is not available. The tool most approximating the desired one should be used in these instances. In the above example, a 10.00-mm radius tool would be used for the second blend. The desire to blend the junction more toward the base curve versus more toward the lens edge will determine whether a tool slightly steeper or flatter than the best designated tool is used.

The methods for blending are the same as those discussed for peripheral curve fabrication. However, the ridge of plastic is removed easily, and therefore only a gentle touch for a short time is necessary to obtain the desired blend. There are three types of blends most commonly used. A light or *touch* blend is achieved with only a few seconds of blending, and the transition zone is still readily observable with a measuring magnifier. In a medium blend, the junction between curves is less distinct and measurement of the curves is more difficult. A heavy blend blurs but does not remove the transition zone completely. However, the measurement of curve widths can only be estimated (Table 9.3).

Excessive pressure should be avoided when creating or blending peripheral curves. The GP materials, particularly the newer ones, are relatively flexible, and increased pressure will likely produce steeper or slightly more distorted curves than desired. In addition, excessive pressure may produce a *bull's-eye* effect in the lens periphery, which appears as concentric scratches or scorch marks (see Fig. 9.4A). Fine scratches may also result from material particles contaminating the polish during the procedure. The finish of the peripheral curves should be examined with a projection magnifier or biomicroscope to confirm the optical quality of the lens surface.

TABLE 9.3 Blending Guidelines

BLEND	TIME (S)	APPEARANCE
Light	5	Transition easily seen
Medium	10	Transition seen, but shadows begin forming at peripheral junction
Heavy	15–20	Very difficult to read accurately; nothing is observed but shadows

From Tracy D, Sanford M. *Modification Procedures, Guidelines and Tips.* Norfolk, VA: Conforma Laboratories.

Edge Shaping and Polishing

Arguably, the most important component of a comfortable and well-centered GP lens fit is the shape and quality of the lens edge.[13,14] Modification of the lens edge has become a common procedure as a result of the difficulty in consistently fabricating the newer, softer materials, although recent advances in manufacturing technology has resulted in more consistency in edge quality.

Both the anterior and posterior edges should be rolled and tapered, since the posterior edge is in near alignment with the cornea and the anterior edge is often in contact with the upper lid. A poor edge will most often result in the patient complaining of persistent lens awareness or discomfort (usually monocular). Even if the edge appears acceptable on inspection, it should be polished to rule out the possibility of a defect.

Verification of the lens edge is essential before initially dispensing the lens to the patient. One simple initial method of determining if a lens edge is defective is using the palm test.[14] The lens, concave side down, is placed in the palm of the hand and then pushed across the palm by the forefinger of the other hand. If it fails to glide easily across the palm (i.e., does not tend to move or, if movement is present, the lens feels rough), the edge is defective. The edge should then be observed both frontally and in profile with some type of projection magnifier. It cannot be assumed that a replacement lens will have the same edge as the original or that the left lens will have the same edge as the right. Initial discomfort is very detrimental to the success of future lens wear, especially in the case of a first-time GP wearer. However, in recent years, edge quality has been consistently high. Most GP laboratories now use computerized lathes that generate a consistent edge thickness, and some lathes will generate a uniform apex on the lens. However, the lens edge should always be inspected whenever discomfort is suspected to be problematic.

There are several methods for shaping and polishing the lens edge. To thin the edge, or create an anterior bevel, a cone tool is most commonly used. Slight shaping and polishing of the edge may be performed with a sponge tool containing a central hole or with a flat sponge and the aid of a spinner tool.

Finger Polishing

A simple edge polishing technique using two fingers and a drop of polish will improve the polished edge quality of any GP lens. This procedure is quick and simple and will not affect any other parameters of the lens. A special tool holder is needed to hold the suction cup, or inserting the holder end of the suction cup holder through a hole in a sponge tool will work to hold the suction cup holder as it spins on the polisher spindle.

Cone Tool

A 90-degree cone tool is usually used to add an anterior or CN bevel to the lens edge. Alternatively, a 60-degree tool may be used to create a narrower bevel or a 120-degree tool for a wider bevel.[6] The CN bevel serves to decrease the edge thickness in an attempt to align the edge most comfortably with the cornea posteriorly and with the lid anteriorly. This procedure also is beneficial in lowering a high-fitting lens. To begin the procedure, the lens is mounted on a suction cup so that the convex surface faces the cone tool (Fig. 9.5A). A pellon or velveteen pad with a one-quarter section cutout is placed within the tool so that it conforms to the cone surface. The lens is then placed within the cone while it rotates and is gently rocked forward and backward and left and right to a slight degree. This rocking motion enables the modifier to apply a bevel with a smoother transition zone. The rocking should not be excessive, since this can alter the peripheral lens surface quality. The appropriate polish must be continually applied throughout the procedure. The lens should be examined approximately every 4 to 6 seconds until the desired edge thickness is reached (Fig. 9.5B). After the application of an anterior bevel, the edge will be quite sharp and somewhat rough. Therefore, it will be necessary to accompany this procedure with a thorough edge polish.

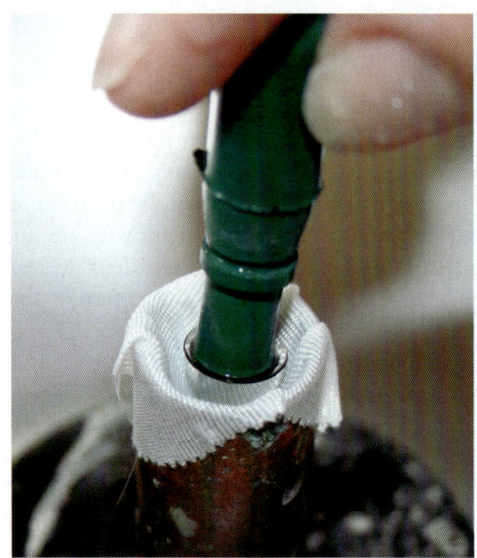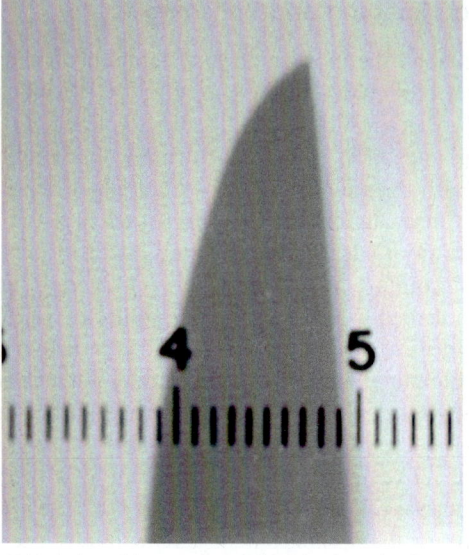

FIGURE 9.5 **(A)** Ninety-degree tool used in creating a CN bevel or thinner edge. **(B)** Lens edge after being thinned with a 90-degree tool (CN bevel).

Sponge Tool (Central Hole)

A small, flat sponge tool containing a central hole is very effective for routine polishing and minor edge shaping. The lens is positioned on a suction cup with the concave surface out. The sponge should be thoroughly moistened with water and placed on the spindle. As the sponge rotates, polish is applied and the suction cup is held vertically to the tool. The lens is then pushed into the central hole of the sponge and moved up and down in the sponge for 30 to 60 seconds (Fig. 9.6). Polish is again applied throughout the procedure. It is important to maintain good suction on the lens during this procedure because a large-diameter lens may become lodged in the sponge. It should be noted that this procedure will reduce the overall diameter of the lens.

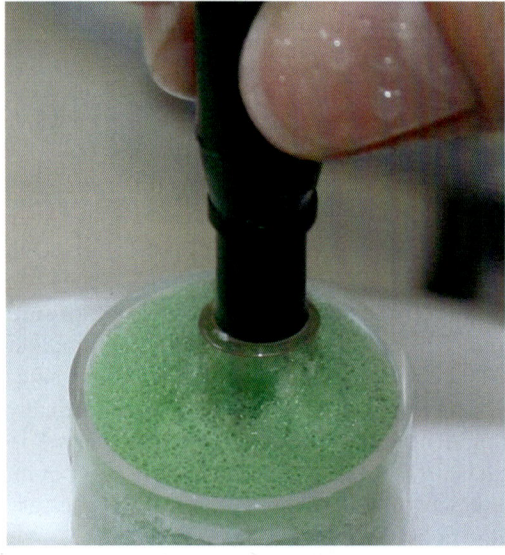

FIGURE 9.6 Sponge tool with central hole used for edge polishing.

Flat Sponge

Alternatively, a large, flat sponge tool may be used to gently shape and polish the lens edge.[15,16] In this case, the lens is mounted on a spinner tool concave side out. The sponge is moistened with water and placed on the spindle. The spinner is then held at an approximately 30-degree angle to the rotating tool with the lens in contact with the sponge approximately halfway between the center and the edge of the sponge (Fig. 9.7A). The lens is then traversed back and forth across the sponge tool from approximately the 4 o'clock position to the 8 o'clock position for 30 to 60 seconds (Fig. 9.7B,C). Polish is continuously applied, and the lens should be

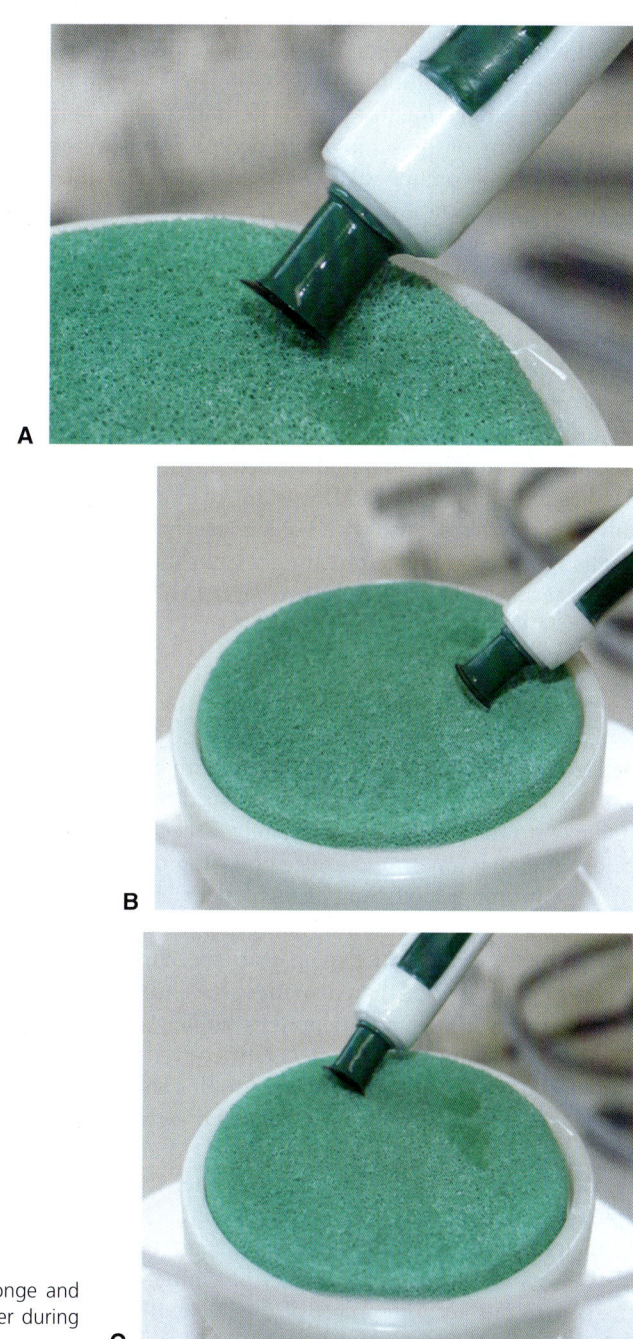

FIGURE 9.7 (A) Edge polish with flat sponge and spinner. **(B, C)** Proper movement of spinner during edge polish.

spinning at all times while in contact with the tool. The edge is preferentially polished posteriorly while the lens is on the left side of the 6 o'clock position of the sponge tool and anteriorly on the right side of 6 o'clock. This allows the clinician to concentrate the effort more on the anterior or posterior surface of the edge as needed.

Surface Polishing

Surface polishing is one of the most commonly performed in-office modification procedures. The new, higher-Dk materials are more susceptible to surface scratches and accumulate more deposits, which necessitates, in many cases, polishing these lenses at least once a year.[17] Surface scratches will often interfere with the wetting performance of a GP lens. The patient will report "foggy" vision when the accumulation of debris in the crevices of the scratches and the subsequent surface filming occur. Unfortunately, to remove all the scratches completely could render the surface quality poor. The objective of polishing the surface of a GP lens is to remove the burrs of the scratches to decrease the awareness of a rough surface because of heavy scratches. These scratches are polished easily from the lens with the use of various sponge tools on the modification unit without risk of damaging the optical quality. The only exception for polishing—or adding power to—the front surface would pertain to plasma-treated lenses, as the surface wettability may be degraded if this surface is altered.

If a lens exhibits poor initial wettability, it is important to first use a laboratory cleaner or solvent to clean the lens, followed by rubbing in wetting solution to help condition the lens before reinsertion. Polishing the front surface should be a last resort because of the possibility of the poor initial wettability being caused by residual pitch polish left on the lens during the manufacturing process. If so, the pitch may just simply be further distributed on the lens surface and the problem is not alleviated. If the problem is an acquired mucoprotein film, which has become plaque-like and resistant to normal cleaning, once again a laboratory cleaner or solvent approved for use with GP lens materials should be used initially. If the deposits are not totally removed, a mild front surface polish should then be considered. Only occasionally does the posterior surface attract sufficient debris/deposits to warrant polishing.

Convex Surface

As previously mentioned, for removing thick adherent mucoprotein deposits and very light scratches, a hand polishing pad such as the Cleaner Accessory Pad (Eaton Medical Corp.) can be used.[18] The pad is wetted with preservative-free saline followed by six to eight drops of a rigid daily cleaning solution. The lens is placed on the tip of the thumb or index finger and gently rubbed into the pad for approximately 20 seconds. The lens power should be verified and noted before and after any front surface polishing to ensure optical quality and proper prescription.

More thorough polishing of the convex surface of the lens requires the use of a flat sponge tool and the modification unit. Many sponge tools allow for a small piece of velveteen or silk cloth to be placed over the sponge surface. This tool is referred to as a *drum tool*. The cloth will hold the polish better than a sponge, lessening the burning effect to the surface of the lens. A spinner tool with a suction cup lens holder is preferred for this method. The lens is centered on a suction cup of the spinner tool, convex side out. The sponge tool is wetted thoroughly and placed on the spindle. Once the tool is rotating, polish is continually applied to the center of the tool and the lens is placed halfway between the center and the edge of the sponge. The exact position of the lens depends on the diameter of the polishing sponge, as the further out on any spinning tool it is placed, the faster it spins, which increases the polishing action. The spinner tool should be slightly oscillated back and forth about 30 degrees while the lens stays in the center of the drum tool or flat sponge tool. A uniform polishing of the convex surface of the lens is desired. If too much polishing occurs either in the center or peripheral area of the convex surface, the power of the lens will be distorted and changed. The lens should only stay in contact with the polishing tool surface for 1 to 2 seconds at a time to minimize burning.

Polish should be applied in between touches to the tool. Remember to apply the polish in the center of the polishing tool because the polish applied will spin away from the center of any spinning tool surface. Usually, only three or four touches of the lens to the polishing tool are needed to remove the burrs from the scratches and debris built up on the lens surface. The lens surface should be examined after this process for remaining scratches with a projection magnifier and the power verified with a lensometer (Fig. 9.8). Frequent polish application and minimal pressure will ensure good lens optical quality following surface polishing.

Another method would pertain to using a suction cup held at a 45-degree angle and rotated in a direction opposite the rotation of a flat sponge tool (Fig. 9.9). This rotation of the lens may be accomplished with the manipulation of the fingers or by the use of a spinner tool, which requires less dexterity. The lens is depressed into the sponge about one-eighth of an inch during the procedure and continued for 3 or 4 seconds. The very center of the lens is polished by holding the suction cup perpendicular to the sponge and depressing the lens in and out of the center of the sponge four or five times. During this step, the lens should be in contact with the sponge for only 1 second at a time to prevent optical distortion or power changes.

An alternative method would be to use a spinner in combination with a rounded sponge tool. In this method, the spinner rolls the lens from edge to center and back until the desired surface quality has been obtained. As long as the spinner continues to rotate, the optical quality should not change. This will be discussed further during the section on repowering.

The lens surface should be examined every 10 seconds for remaining scratches with a projection magnifier and the power verified with a lensometer. Low spindle speed (1,000 rpm or less), frequent polish application, and minimal pressure will ensure good lens optical quality following surface polishing. In addition, it is not recommended to attempt to totally polish out deep scratches, as the optical quality could be compromised from frequent polishing.

Concave Surface

It is necessary to polish the concave surface of a lens, primarily to remove deposits resulting from trapped tear debris behind the lens. These deposits may inhibit lens movement and centration, particularly in extended wear.

A cone-shaped sponge is used to polish the concave lens surface. The cone is ideal for forming a convex surface to match the concave surface of the lens during this procedure. The lens is mounted on a suction cup concave side out, and the cone sponge is moistened and placed on the spindle. After the spindle is rotating, polishing compound is added and the suction cup is tilted slightly, with the lens placed just off the center of the sponge (Fig. 9.10). The lens is depressed into the sponge about one-eighth of an inch and rotated opposite the spindle rotation for 3 or 4 seconds. This may be repeated, if necessary, after inspection. A circular sponge tool may be substituted using the same technique; however, the suction cup should be held at a 30-degree angle from the vertical.

Nonpolishing Alternatives

Progent Contact Lens Cleaner and Protein Remover (Menicon) is an excellent product for thoroughly cleaning a GP lens surface. It is a very strong "bleaching" type of solution and needs to be handled correctly for maximum results. Originally sold only for in-office use, it is now available for direct sales to patients. Make sure the instructions are followed to avoid any exposure to the eye.

Repowering

A significant advantage to fitting GP contact lenses is the ability to modify the power of the lens in the office to provide an immediate improvement in the patient's visual acuity. As a new lens would otherwise need to be ordered, repowering proves to be a very cost-effective procedure. A change in power may be necessary—particularly with lenses ordered empirically—as factors

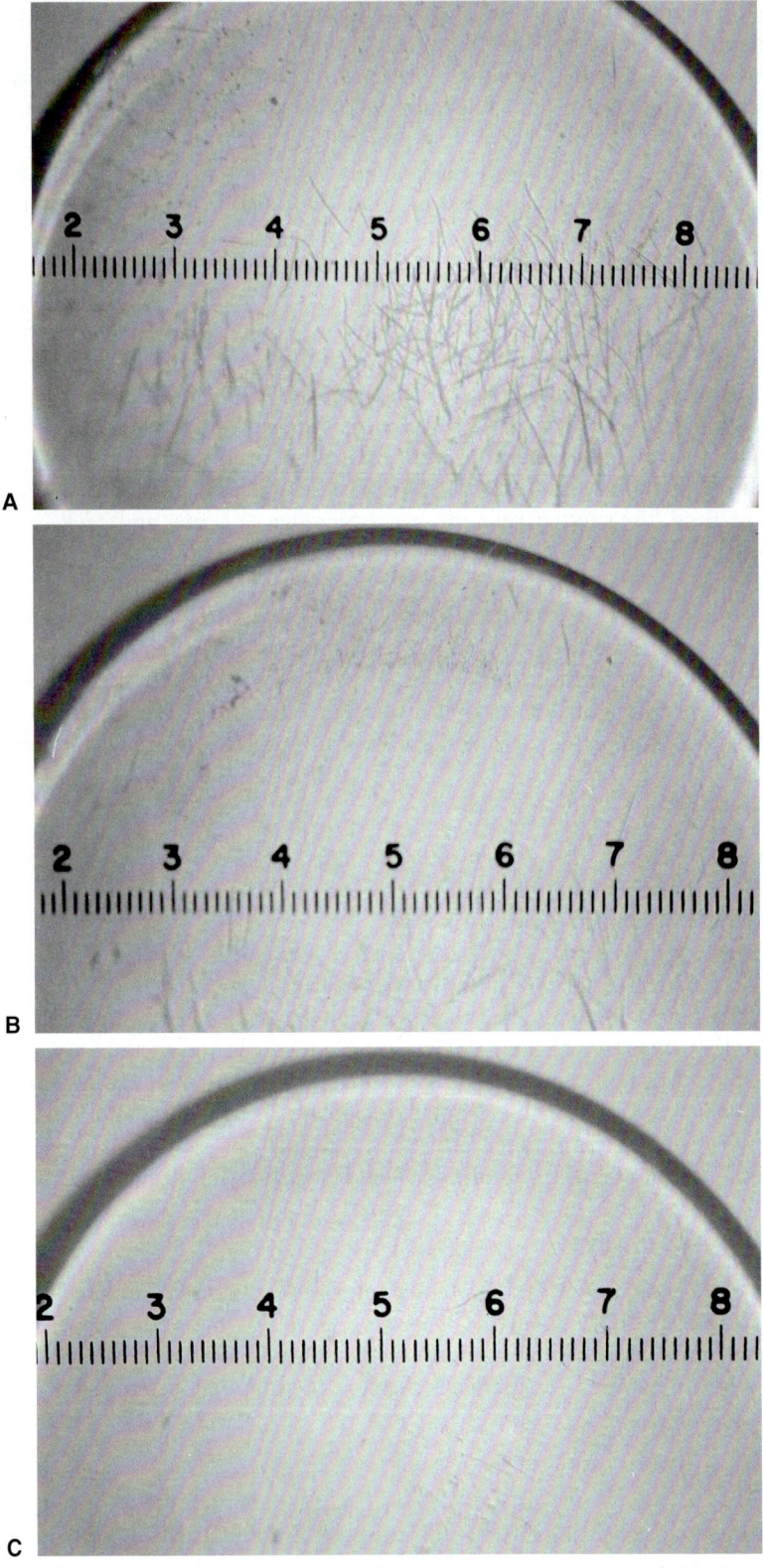

FIGURE 9.8 **(A)** Excessive front surface scratches on a gas-permeable lens. **(B)** Thinned scratches following initial front surface polishing (30 seconds). **(C)** Scratches remaining following 1 minute of front surface polishing.

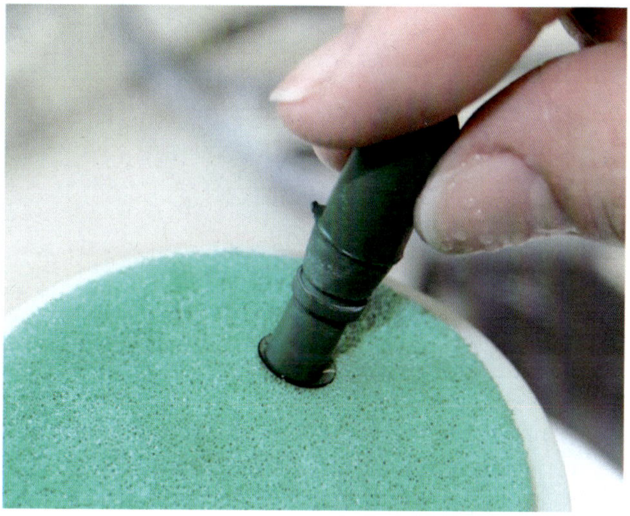

FIGURE 9.9 Demonstration of front surface polish with the use of a flat sponge tool.

such as the corneal curvature, refraction, and lens design may result in a slightly inaccurate power. Normal refractive changes in a young patient and changes in the lens-to-cornea fitting relationship also may necessitate repowering.

Adding Minus

The addition of minus power is more often necessary than the addition of plus power because of patients' visual symptoms. Fortunately, adding minus is the easier of the two procedures to perform. Although many techniques are used to add minus power, a very effective method involves the use of either a rounded sponge tool or the cone sponge tool in combination with a spinner. The sponge tool is mounted vertically on the spindle and wetted thoroughly with water and polish. The lens is mounted convex side out and well centered on a spinner tool that enables the lens to spin freely and rapidly. As the sponge tool rotates, the lens is first held with

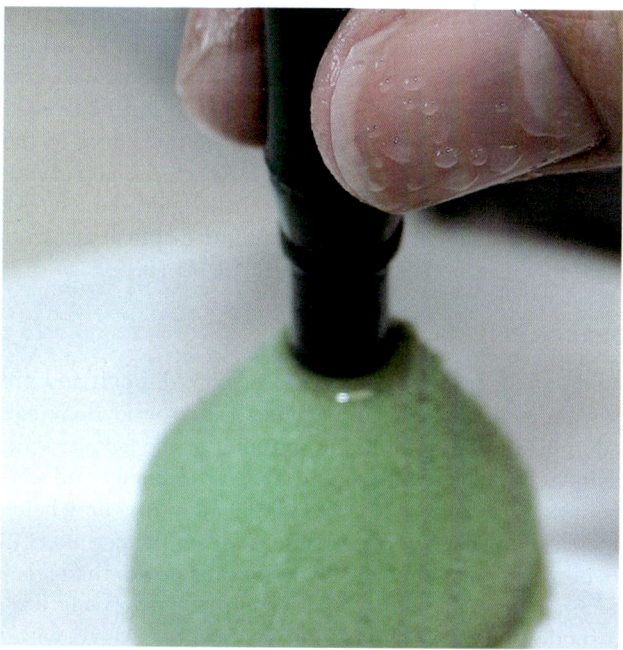

FIGURE 9.10 Polishing the concave surface of a gas-permeable lens with a cone-shaped sponge tool.

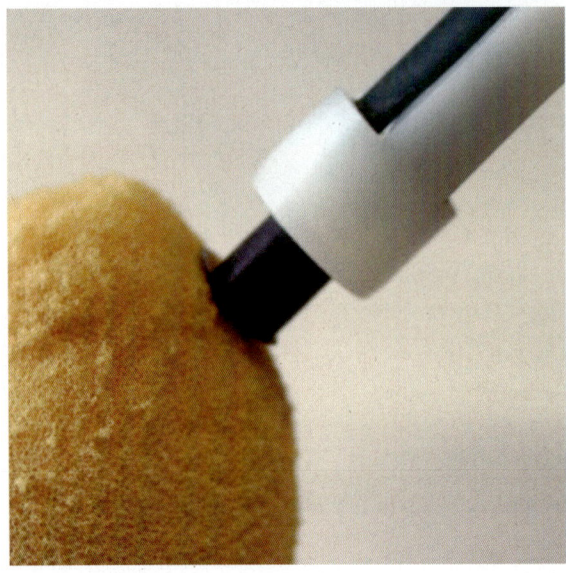

FIGURE 9.11 The use of a rounded sponge pad and spinner for the addition of minus power.

the edge adjacent to the side of the pad to begin the spinning action. Once the lens is spinning freely, the spinner is rotated so that the lens is perpendicular to the sponge pad, approximately 1 to 1.5 cm from its apex (Fig. 9.11). The lens should be turning freely on the spinner at all times when in contact with the sponge tool, and as the position and pressure are held constant, polishing compound is liberally applied. Proper position allows the center of the lens to be in direct contact with the pad while the periphery receives less friction. This, in turn, creates a flatter front curvature, resulting in increased minus power. The amount of minus power added with this technique depends on the amount of pressure, time, and polishing compound used. The power should be monitored every 10 to 15 seconds and as much as 1 D can be added without causing optical distortion.

An alternate method to add minus involves the use of a large, flat sponge tool. The lens is mounted convex side out on a suction cup, with special care to ensure centration. With the flat sponge spinning on the spindle and thoroughly wetted, the lens is placed approximately 1 inch from the peripheral edge. The lens must be held perpendicular to the tool surface at all times. With very slight pressure, the lens is revolved around the tool counterclockwise (if the spindle turns clockwise). The lens should not be twisted about the axis of the suction cup.[14] Polish should be added throughout the procedure to the center of the tool (centrifugal force will spread polish out to the edge). Again, the power must be checked every 10 to 15 seconds to prevent overcorrection and to ensure that the lens is rotated to a different position on the suction cup, which will help to minimize optical distortion. The limit of minus power addition with this method is approximately −0.75 D.

Adding Plus

Adding plus power to GP lenses is more difficult and presents a greater chance of optical distortion compared to adding minus. The rounded sponge tool and spinner may be utilized to add plus power by initiating spinning of the lens, as with adding minus, but then rotating the spinner out of vertical alignment with the sponge pad so that only the periphery of the lens is in contact with the tool (Fig. 9.12). Plus power is now being added as the front surface curvature increases by material being removed from the periphery of the lens and not the center. The rate of power change is much slower for plus power than it is for minus power with the sponge pad.

An alternative method of adding plus power is to use a flat drum tool in combination with a suction cup. The drum tool is typically covered with velveteen or suede cloth.[14] With the

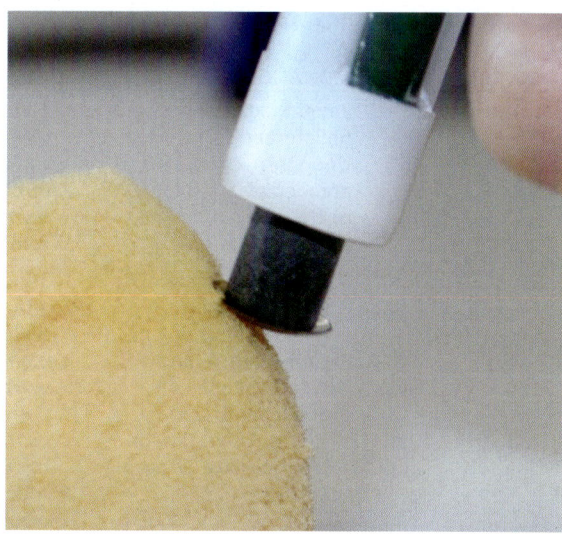

FIGURE 9.12 The use of a rounded sponge pad and spinner for the addition of plus power.

motor running, a small amount of polish is added to the tool. The lens, convex side out on the suction cup, is brought in contact with the center of the drum tool with a perpendicular orientation. With mild pressure, the lens is rotated both clockwise and counterclockwise. As with all other methods, polish should be applied liberally. Only about 0.5 D of plus power can be added with these procedures.

The type of lens material should always be considered whenever power changes are indicated. The time required to change the power of a high-Dk material is less than that for a low-Dk material or PMMA.[2] Failure to allow for different lens materials can lead to improper amounts of power change or distortion of optics.

A summary of commonly performed modification procedures is provided in Table 9.4.[8]

MODIFYING SPECIAL DESIGNS

It is apparent that modification procedures can be the difference between success and failure in bifocal/multifocal patients as well as with keratoconic lens designs. In keratoconus, it is not uncommon to need to reduce the optic zone diameter or flatten the peripheral curve radii to reduce adherence and increase tear flow. Blending the peripheral curves can likewise have a dramatic effect. As a result of the high minus powers often required for keratoconus correction, edge polishing and thinning are not uncommon procedures.[1] The application of an anterior bevel, followed by an edge polish, is very beneficial in thinning a high minus edge.

As many bifocal designs are prism ballasted and truncated and are designed to rest on the lower lid, thinning the upper edge to minimize the lifting effects of the upper lid is a beneficial procedure. To accomplish this, all but the upper edge can be covered by velveteen or a similar material. The edge can be rolled against a sponge using a suction cup spinner. Polishing the occasional sharp thin edge of a plus-powered bifocal/multifocal design can be beneficial, and although we have not done so, some practitioners have found it useful to modify the truncation angle of translating bifocal designs.

SHOULD HIGH-OXYGEN PERMEABILITY LENS MATERIALS BE MODIFIED?

In recent years, the concern over in-office modification of the newer high-Dk materials has increased. Some in-office procedures have been demonstrated to cause microcracks and scorching of the lens surface.[5] These surface defects are clinically unobservable, but may affect wettability and long-term integrity of the lens.

TABLE 9.4 Gas-Permeable Lens Modification Procedures

PROCEDURE	INDICATION(S)	TOOLS	PRECAUTIONS
1. Edge polish	Patient experiences unilateral discomfort. Upon inspection, lens is abraded, sharp, blunt, or chipped	1. 1-inch center hole sponge with suction cup or spinner 2. Inspect with an edge profile analyzer or comparator	Use polish liberally
2. Surface polish	1. Patient has transient blurred vision 2. Patient reports redness or reduced wearing time. Scratches and mucoprotein film on front surface or back surface	1. 3-inch flat sponge tool 2. 3-inch polishing disc or drum tool in combination with velveteen or Delrin 3. Cone or convex sponge tool to polish back surface 4. All of the above in combination with spinner or suction cup	1. <1,200 rpm 2. Use polish liberally 3. Check optical quality with lensometer after 20–30 s
3. Repower	1. Patient has blurred vision that is managed by a change in lens power	1. 3-inch polishing disc or drum tool in combination with velveteen or Delrin with suction cup or spinner 2. Cone or convex sponge tool with spinner	1. <1,200 rpm 2. Use polish liberally 3. Check optical quality with lensometer after 20–30 s
4. Blend/flatten peripheral curves	1. Tear stagnation under lens because of midperipheral or peripheral bearing 2. Insufficient lens lag with the blink	1. 10 tools ranging from 7.5 to 13 mm in radius 2. Diamond-coated tools preferable; brass tools most often used because of reduced cost 3. ¼-inch velveteen or Delrin pad to cover tool 4. All procedures performed with either suction cup or spinner	1. <1,200 rpm 2. Use polish liberally 3. Be careful with high-Dk materials

Dk, oxygen permeability.

One procedure that should not be performed on contemporary GP lens materials is diameter reduction. As these materials are softer and are more likely to chip or break, it is not worth the time and effort to reduce the diameter and then reshape the edge and reapply peripheral curves. Likewise, prolonged surface polishing (i.e., several minutes) is not recommended, especially with high-Dk and hyper-Dk lens materials. Some of the defects that result are not evident with biomicroscopy. The effect of front surface polishing was evaluated on 20 GP lenses.[5] The modified lenses were then evaluated under high-magnification (100−500+) scanning electron microscopy. Several microscopic surface abnormalities were observed, including microcracks, splitting, scorching, and bleaching. It was concluded that prolonged polishing, diameter reduction, and repowering would be unacceptable in-office modification procedures for high-Dk GP lens materials. Walker[19] found similar results. If fluoro-silicone/acrylate lenses were surface polished for longer than 2 minutes, poor surface wettability leading to patient awareness of the lens over time often resulted.

Repowering appears to be rather controversial. Whereas Grohe et al.[5] contraindicated it with high-Dk lens materials, the studies by Reeder et al.[9] and Morgan et al.[3] appear to support it, although some precautions may be necessary depending on the polish used and the specific procedure. It has been found that repowering, even at a high (1,600 rpm) spindle speed with a high-Dk lens material, did not result in optical distortion or reduced quality of vision if a spinner tool was used in combination with a rounded sponge tool.[3] Likewise, under scanning electron microscopy, the lens surface was free of defects. However, use of a velveteen-covered tool resulted in significant optical distortion and reduced vision of the high-Dk lens material, even with the use of a low (550 rpm) spindle speed. Numerous surface defects were typically present under scanning electron microscopy.

Overall, it appears that the use of low spindle speeds (≤1,000 rpm), sponge tools, and minimal pressure are safest when polishing the front surface, modifying the edge, or repowering GP lenses in the office. A summary of the do's and don'ts of modifying GP lenses is given in Table 9.5.[1]

OBTAINING PROFICIENCY AT MODIFICATION

Anyone can modify, and staff members can be of tremendous assistance in performing these procedures. Numerous organizations (GP Lens Institute, Contact Lens Association of Ophthalmologists, Contact Lens Society of America, Heart of America Contact Lens Society, to name a few) provide modification workshops, as do many CLMA member laboratories. Lenses to practice with should not be difficult to obtain, and GP contact lens laboratories are excellent about assisting in these activities.

SUMMARY

A summary nomogram of the modification of GP lenses is given in Figure 9.13. The ability to modify GP lenses is of great benefit to both patient and practice. It takes little time and can solve a problem without losing a patient. In a time when managed care and disposable lenses put a premium on efficiency, it makes good sense to be able to perform in-office modification procedures.

TABLE 9.5 Modification "Do's" and "Don'ts"

DO	DON'T
Procedures	
Edge polish	Diameter reduction
Surface polish	Prolonged surface polish
Peripheral curve blending/flattening (low-/high-Dk)	Blending/flattening (hyper-Dk)
Repowering	Repowering (velveteen pad/suction cup with high-/hyper-Dk); consider proper polish
Techniques	
Keep lens cool	Allow heat to build
Add polish frequently	
Dip lens in water	
Keep sponge tools saturated with water	
Low spindle speed	
Optimize surface wettability	Dispense lens immediately after procedure
Clean lens after procedure	
Condition surface before dispensing	

Dk, oxygen permeability.

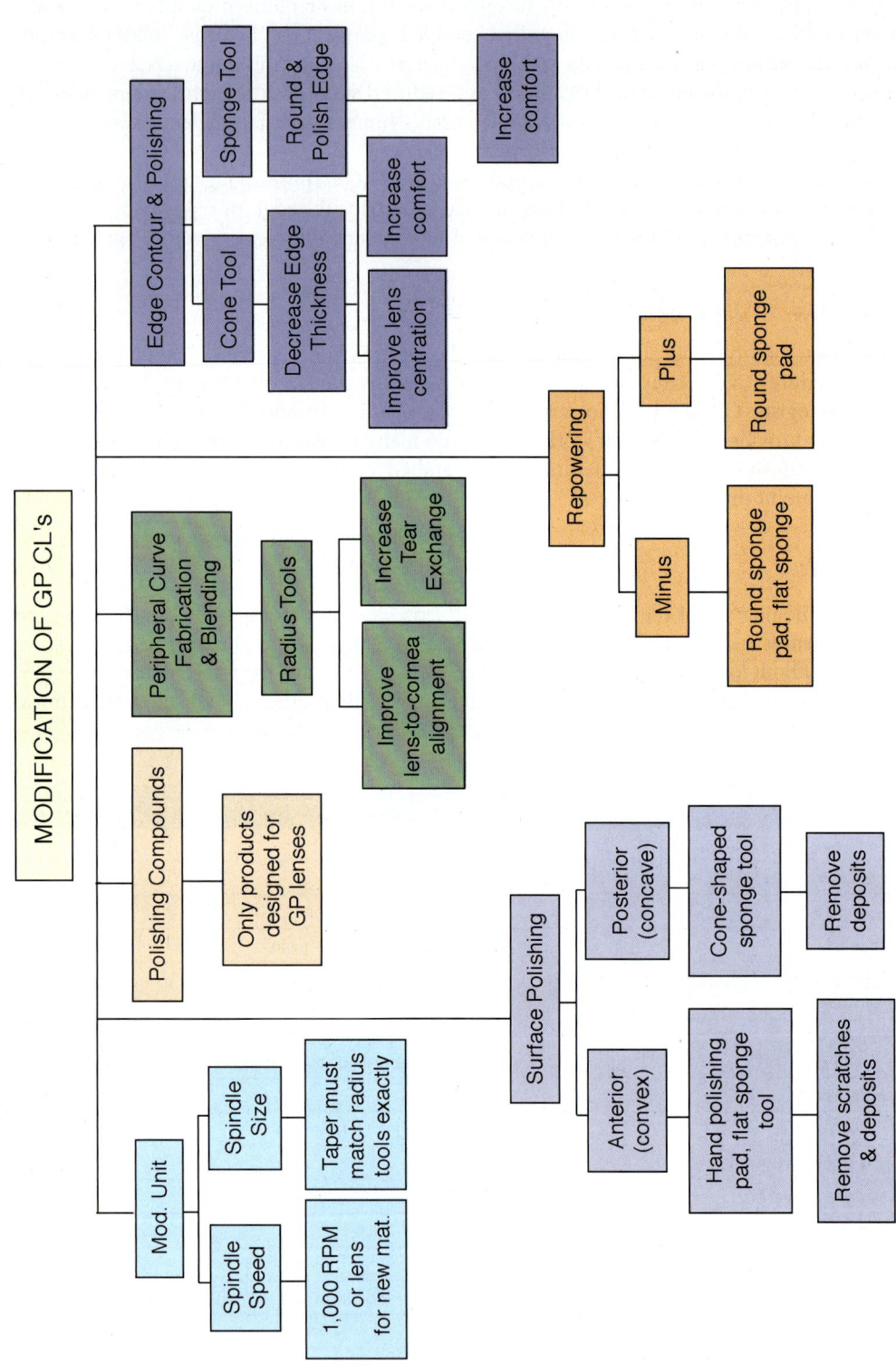

FIGURE 9.13 Modification summary nomogram.

CLINICAL CASES

CASE 1

A 14-year-old patient, currently wearing daily-wear GP contact lenses, returns for a 6-month follow-up visit complaining of slightly blurred vision in both eyes. Examination reveals a visual acuity of 20/30 OD and OS correctable to 20/20 with an overrefraction of −0.50 DS OU. A postrefraction of −3.75 DS OU to 20/20 was found, compared to −3.25 OU 6 months ago. Lens fit, fluorescein pattern, keratometry, and ocular health were unremarkable and unchanged from the previous visit.

SOLUTION: Progressive myopia in a young patient has increased the refractive error. The lenses should be repowered in the office utilizing a minus power addition technique (i.e., rounded sponge pad and spinner). The addition of −0.50 D to the lenses in the office will improve the patient's visual acuity to 20/20 in a matter of minutes and prevent an interruption of the patient's wearing schedule.

CASE 2

A patient is dispensed replacement lenses with the same parameters as the previous pair. The patient returns in 1 week complaining of discomfort in the left eye only. Examination reveals a good lens fit and 20/15 vision OU, unchanged from previous examinations.

SOLUTION: Monocular discomfort is a sign of a possible edge problem. Verification of the left lens with a projection magnifier reveals a slightly blunt edge. Therefore, a routine edge polish (i.e., sponge tool with central hole) is indicated for the left lens, to create a smoother, more rounded edge for greater comfort.

CASE 3

A patient wearing GP lenses for approximately 1 year returns to the office complaining of slightly blurred vision and dryness. Visual acuity measures 20/25 OD and OS with no improvement with overrefraction. The ocular health is normal, and the lens fit is adequate and unchanged from the previous visit. However, fine surface scratches and a quick surface haze after the blink are observed.

SOLUTION: Current GP materials often need routine surface polishing every 6 months to 1 year, and this procedure is indicated in this case. A front surface polish will not only remove the scratches, but will also most likely increase wettability by creating a smoother surface for the tear film and decreasing the affinity for deposit formation. The patient's cleaning regimen should also be reviewed to rule out inappropriate procedures that may be causing excessive front surface scratching.

CASE 4

A patient is dispensed a pair of daily-wear GP lenses. At the 1-month visit, the patient reports that everything is well; however, the lenses occasionally feel "stuck" to the eye, and they are sometimes difficult to remove. Visual acuity has remained stable. The fluorescein pattern shows minimal edge clearance, and the lag after the blink is 1 mm.

SOLUTION: It is not uncommon for the lens-to-cornea fitting relationship to change slightly over the first few weeks of rigid lens wear. The lens fit has apparently tightened with this patient after 1 month of wear, and steps need to be taken to increase edge lift and increase movement. Flattening the peripheral curve should indeed achieve these goals and may be performed in the office in just a few minutes with the proper radius tool.

CLINICAL PROFICIENCY CHECKLIST

- When considering modification units, keep in mind that 1,000 rpm is recommended for safe modification of newer materials.
- It is essential that the taper size of the modification tools exactly matches the spindle size to prevent wobble during modification.
- Remember to use only polish that is specifically designed for use with GP lenses.
- Good centration is absolutely imperative when attaching a contact lens to a lens holder (i.e., suction cup) for modification.
- Spinner tools are very beneficial for certain procedures requiring care in monitoring optical quality, such as power changes and front surface polishing.
- It is important to obtain baseline parameter data on the lenses before performing any modification procedure.
- When applying peripheral curves or blending, be sure to allow for the thickness of the adhesive tape or velveteen when selecting the radius tool (0.2 mm for adhesive tape, 0.4 mm for velveteen).
- When using sponge tools, always moisten the sponge with water before beginning the procedure.
- The use of a rounded sponge tool and spinner is most effective in repowering the newer materials.
- Frequent polish, minimal pressure, and low spindle speed provide the best results with any modification procedure.

REFERENCES

1. Bennett ES. Successfully modifying contemporary RGP materials. *Optom Today.* 1997;5(10):27–34.
2. Bennett ES, Clompus DJ, Hansen DW. A hands-on approach to RGP modification. *Rev Optom.* 1998;135(1):88–103.
3. Morgan BW, Henry VA, Bennett ES, et al. The effect of modification procedures on silicone/acrylate versus fluoro-silicone/acrylate lens materials. *J Am Optom Assoc.* 1992;63(3):193–198.
4. Mandell RB. Modification procedures. In: Mandell RB, ed. *Contact Lens Practice.* 4th ed. Springfield, IL: Charles C. Thomas; 1988:475–501.
5. Grohe RM, Caroline PJ, Norman C. The role of in-office modification for RGP surface defects. *Contact Lens Spectrum.* 1988;3(10):52–60.
6. Bennett ES, Egan DJ. Modification. In: Bennett ES, Grohe RM, eds. *Rigid Gas-Permeable Contact Lenses.* New York, NY: Professional Press; 1986;247–273.
7. DeKinder J, Bennett ES. Equip yourself for modifying GP lenses. *Contact Lens Spectrum.* 2005;20(2):48.
8. Bennett ES. Offer added value with in-office RGP modification. *Contact Lens Spectrum.* 1996;11(10):18–19.
9. Reeder RE, Pate JR, Snyder C. Effectiveness and efficiency of rigid gas permeable lens power modification with various polishes. *Int Cont Lens Clin.* 1996;23(3/4):67–70.
10. Picciano S, Andrasko GJ. Which factors influence RGP lens comfort? *Contact Lens Spectrum.* 1989;4(5):31–33.
11. Meszaros GK. Simplifying lens modification. *Contact Lens Forum.* 1986;11(11):42–49.
12. Gordon Contact Lens. *Contact Lens Adjusting Manual.* Rochester, NY: Division of UCO Optics.
13. Morgan BW, Bennett ES. Modification of RGP lenses. *Contact Lens Forum.* 1990;15(7):33–50.
14. Rinehart JM. Tackle comfort issues in GP wearers. *Rev Cornea Contact Lenses.* November 2010;7.
15. Tracy D, Sanford M. *Modification Procedures, Guidelines and Tips.* Conforma Laboratories.
16. Jurkus JM. Modifying RGPs: a straightforward approach. *Optom Management.* 1996;31(9):54–58.
17. Morgan BW, Bennett ES. Modification. In: Bennett ES, Weissman BA, eds. *Clinical Contact Lens Practice.* 2nd ed. Philadelphia, PA: JB Lippincott; 1991;307–324.
18. Campbell R, Caroline P. New cleaning system for heavy depositors. *Contact Lens Spectrum.* 1997;12(10):56.
19. Walker J. Overpolishing fluoro-silicone/acrylates: the consequence and the cure. *Trans Br Contact Lens Assoc.* 1989;6:29.

Section III

Soft Lenses

Chapter 10

Soft Lens Material Selection

Vinita Allee Henry and Julie Ott DeKinder

Soft contact lenses were introduced in the 1970s, and were essentially hydrogel lenses that were dependent on the water content of the lens to provide oxygen to the cornea. In the late 1990s and early 2000s, a revolutionary new soft lens material, silicone hydrogel, was introduced. This new material incorporated the high oxygen permeability (Dk) of silicone with the benefits of conventional hydrogel lenses.[1] Both types of soft contact lens materials are flexible and made of a plastic that is able to absorb or bind water. Although many similarities exist between hydrogel and silicone hydrogel materials, there are distinct differences between their material properties. When placed on the eye, both forms will conform to the shape of the cornea. Soft lenses have excellent memory; therefore, the lenses can be folded with the edges touching and, when released, will return to the normal shape. The lenses may be inverted and returned to right side out without damaging the optics. Increased water content in the lens, surface treatments, wetting agents, or hydrophilic monomers are used to make this lens surface wettable. This increased wettability also increases the adherence of environmental contaminants (i.e., bacteria, tear lipids and proteins, dust) when the lens is placed in contact with these substances. The purpose of this chapter is to discuss soft lens materials, their similarities and differences, and their properties.

MATERIAL PROPERTIES

Hydrogel contact lens materials are made with a stable, solid polymer component that can absorb or bind with water. Spaces exist in the crossed-linked polymer and are called pores. These pores allow fluid (water) to enter the lens material, thus making it hydrated and soft.

The polymers consist of small building blocks called monomers. Therefore, a sequence of repeating units is created. When more than one monomer is used, the term *copolymer* is more appropriate. Most soft contact lens materials are copolymers. A chemical is added to the monomers to create polymerization. Thus, the backbone of the lens has a series of repeating units that can be arranged, either in a random or nonrandom manner, depending on how the polymerization was initiated.[2] These repeating units are then cross-linked to each other. By varying the amount of cross-linking agents, the copolymer will vary in its ability to absorb fluid, in this case, water.

By polymerizing different combinations of monomers, the physical and chemical properties of the lens material can be created, such as water content, refractive index, hardness, mechanical strength, and Dk. The following monomers are those that are most commonly used to create hydrogel contact lenses[3]:

- 2-Hydroxyethyl methacrylate (HEMA) is the monomer that was used to create the first commercial hydrogel contact lens, and it continues to be the monomer most often utilized. By itself, it will allow a water content of about 38%. When it is combined with other monomers (such as N-vinylpyrrolidone or methacrylic acid), the water content can be increased from

55% to 70%.[2] HEMA is an extremely stable material, and variations in temperature, pH, or tonicity have relatively little effect on its water content. It also offers good wettability.
- Ethylene glycol dimethacrylate (EGDMA) is used primarily as a cross-linking agent. Its primary function is to increase the dimensional stability of the material.[3] Increased use of EGDMA will tend to make the material stiffer, lower in water content, and less stretchable.
- Methacrylic acid (MAA) is used to increase the water content of the lens material. It is extremely hydrophilic because of the presence of a free carboxylic acid group that bonds water. It therefore also tends to impart ionic (charged) properties to a material.
- Methyl methacrylate (MMA) is sometimes used to lower water content or to increase the material hardness or strength of a material. It offers excellent optical clarity and is completely inert and very stable, but does not offer any permeability to oxygen.
- N-vinyl pyrrolidone (NVP) is very hydrophilic and is used to increase water content; it offers excellent wettability, and its high water uptake allows for increased Dk. It generally imparts an ionic property to the material.
- Glyceryl methacrylate (GMA) offers good wettability and helps to increase deposit resistance because it creates smaller pore sizes.[4] Because it also lowers the water content of the material, it imparts a lower Dk.
- Polyvinyl alcohol (PVA) is very hydrophilic, thereby increasing the water content and the Dk of the lens material. It is highly biocompatible and extremely resistant to deposits. It also imparts increased hardness and strength, along with excellent optical clarity. It is completely inert and very stable.

The characteristics of these polymers are summarized in Table 10.1.[5]

Silicone hydrogel lenses were the result of years of research to find a way to combine silicone with conventional hydrogel monomers. Before the introduction of silicone hydrogels, lenses made of silicone elastomers had exceptional oxygen transmission (Dk/t), yet demonstrated poor wettability, poor comfort, manufacturing difficulties, corneal adherence, and were

TABLE 10.1 Common Material Monomers and Their Characteristics

MONOMER	ABBREVIATION	ADVANTAGES	DISADVANTAGES
Hydroxyethyl methacrylate	HEMA	• Hydrophilic • Flexible • Softness • Good wettability	• Low oxygen Permeability
Ethylene glycol dimethacrylate	EGDMA	• Stability	• Low oxygen permeability
Methacrylic acid	MAA	• Hydrophilic	• pH sensitive
Methyl methacrylate	MMA	• Hardness • Machinability • Optical clarity • Stability; inert	• No oxygen permeability
N-vinyl pyrrolidone	NVP	• Hydrophilic • Good wettability • High water uptake • High oxygen permeability	• pH sensitive
Glyceryl methacrylate	GMA	• Good wettability • Good deposit resistance	• Low oxygen permeability
Polyvinyl alcohol	PVA	• Hydrophilic • High water uptake • Deposit resistance	• May be more difficult to manufacture

prone to deposits.[1] Silicone has the ability to link carbon, hydrogen, and oxygen. Silicone-based polymers are composed of long chains of polymers. It is this makeup of long chains and small relative diameter that gives these polymers their elasticity and strength.[6] The properties of silicone have already been observed in gas-permeable (GP) lenses, where silicone was added to increase Dk/t in high-Dk GP lens materials. Finding a method of combining hydrogel properties with silicone—in order to manufacture a high Dk, comfortable, wettable lens with optical clarity and deposit resistance—was the obstacle that was overcome to produce silicone hydrogel materials.

Although contact lens wearers are enjoying the benefits afforded by silicone hydrogels, this does not mean that the material has reached its peak potential. This is demonstrated by the newest silicone hydrogel to come to the marketplace. Delefilcon A is the first water-gradient silicone hydrogel contact lens, which has a change in water content and modulus from the lens core to the lens surface (Fig. 10.1). This new lens structure combines high Dk with a hydrophilic surface. Initial studies have demonstrated that this has a positive impact on wettability and comfort during contact lens wear.[7–9]

Whether a hydrogel or silicone hydrogel material, ideally, material properties are chosen to create a contact lens material that has the following characteristics:

- Safe
- Inert
- Nontoxic
- Biocompatible
- Chemically and physically stable
- Good wettability
- Deposit resistant
- Durable
- Easy to formulate and manufacture
- Good optical clarity

In reality, trade-off between some of these characteristics must be made. The final lens material can then be evaluated in terms of the following properties:

Transparency

Transparency refers to the clearness (clarity) of a material. Among other factors, it is a function of the chemistry, purity, and hydration of the material. No material is completely transparent,

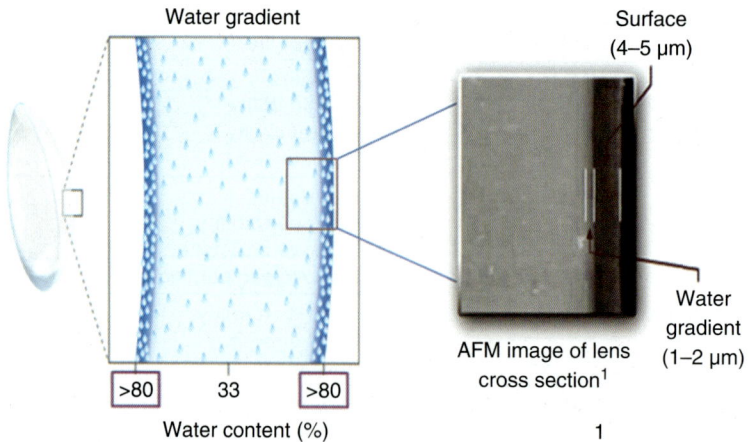

FIGURE 10.1 Dailies Total 1-Lens cross section showing the change from core to surface and relative thickness. (Courtesy of Alcon.)

as some light will always be reflected, absorbed, and scattered. Transparency is often expressed as a percentage of incident light of a certain wavelength that passes through a sample of the material. Values for most clear (nontinted) contact lens materials range from 92% to 98%.

Hardness and Stiffness

The hardness of a lens material is an important quality affecting its ability to be used for the manufacture of contact lenses, and its durability. Generally, hardness is an attribute that is more relevant to rigid lens materials than soft materials. Stiffness is the degree of flexibility of a material, and this can be an important factor when a lens material is selected for a patient. More flexible materials usually result in better initial comfort but do not mask or correct corneal astigmatism, as they tend to drape over the cornea and conform to its shape. Stiffer materials retain their shape during handling and will make insertion and removal of the lens easier.

Tensile Strength

The tensile strength of a material is a value that expresses how much stretching force can be applied before it breaks. Materials with a high tensile strength tend to be more durable, as they are better able to withstand the forces applied during lens handling procedures (i.e., cleaning, inserting) without tearing.

Modulus of Elasticity

The modulus of elasticity is a constant value that expresses a material's ability to keep its shape when subjected to stress and to resist deformation. Materials with a high modulus are stiffer, resist deformation, hold their shape better, are easier to handle, and may provide better visual acuity. Many silicone hydrogel materials have a lens modulus much greater than hydrogel materials. The stiffer lens may have the benefits mentioned previously, or it may adversely affect the lens performance by causing edge lift or fluting, superior epithelial arcuate lesions (SEALs), mucin balls, or giant papillary conjunctivitis (GPC, also called contact lens papillary conjunctivitis [CLPC]).[10–12] Materials with a low modulus of elasticity are less resistant to stress. Most hydrogel materials fall in the low-modulus category. Modulus values can be found in Table 10.2.[1,10,12,13]

TABLE 10.2 Lens Modulus Values

MATERIAL (TRADE NAME)	HYDROGEL OR SILICONE HYDROGEL	MODULUS (MPA)
pHEMA	Hydrogel	0.50
Efrofilcon A (Definitive)	Silicone hydrogel	0.35
Galyfilcon A (AV Advance/AV Advance Plus)	Silicone hydrogel	0.43
Enfilcon A (Avaira)	Silicone hydrogel	0.5
Delefilcon A (Dailies Total 1)	Silicone hydrogel	0.7
Narafilcon B (1 day AV TruEye)	Silicone hydrogel	0.71
Senofilcon A (AV Oasys)	Silicone hydrogel	0.72
Comfilcon A (Biofinity)	Silicone hydrogel	0.75
Balafilcon A (PureVision/PureVision 2)	Silicone hydrogel	1.1
Lotrafilcon B (Air Optix Aqua)	Silicone hydrogel	1.2
Lotrafilcon A (Air Optix N&D)	Silicone hydrogel	1.4

Refractive Index

Refractive index of a lens material is the ratio of the speed of light in air to the speed of light in the material. Materials with higher refractive indices cause more refraction of incident light. For soft lens materials, the index of refraction is related to water content. Generally, increasing the water content lowers the refractive index. A hydrogel lens material with a water content of 80% has a refractive index of about 1.37, and one with a water content of 42% has a refractive index of about 1.44, compared to silicone hydrogel materials (lotrafilcon A and balafilcon A), which have a refractive index of 1.43.[14,15]

Wettability

The surface wettability of a soft lens is an important property. The wettability aids in the closure of the lid over the lens, thereby improving comfort and preventing changes to the papillary surface on the internal surface of the lid.[16] The very wettable surface creates a stable, even tear film. This assists with optimizing comfort, visual acuity, and deposit resistance. As silicone is naturally hydrophobic, its use in soft lenses created a dilemma until the ability to increase the wettability of silicone was discovered.

Early silicone hydrogel materials used a surface treatment to cover up the hydrophobic properties of silicone. Alcon uses a gas plasma technique to apply a uniform plasma coating, approximately 25 nm thick with a high refractive index, on the surface of some of its silicone hydrogel lenses (lotrafilcon A and B) (Fig. 10.2). The gas plasma technique is also used by Bausch + Lomb to apply a plasma oxidation surface treatment to its silicone hydrogel lens (balafilcon A). This surface treatment results in glassy silicate islands on the surface of the lens. The islands leave small areas of exposed hydrophobic regions; however, the wettability of the silicate appears to create a bridge over these areas to produce a net hydrophilic surface.[6] Menicon combines the benefits of plasma coating and plasma oxidation for a plasma surface treatment on its lens (asmofilcon A) called Nanogloss surface modification. The manufacturer reports that this creates a smooth surface with a low contact angle.[10] Silicone hydrogel materials have also used an internal wetting agent, polyvinyl pyrrolidone (PVP), to create wettability (Vistakon, galyfilcon A, and senofilcon A).[1] CooperVision reports that its silicone hydrogel lens (comfilcon A) has no surface treatment or wetting agent. Instead, the lens material contains two silicone-based macromers (a large monomer preassembled to transfer advantageous properties to the final polymer).[6,17] These macromers, when incorporated into the material with hydrophilic monomers, result in a naturally wettable lens (Fig. 10.3). Solution manufacturers are producing new solutions that incorporate surface-active agents with hydrophobic and hydrophilic domains. The hydrophobic portion is attracted to the lens surface, while the hydrophilic portion attracts moisture resulting in a more wettable surface.[13] Newer generations of silicone hydrogels, such as delefilcon A with a water gradient mechanism of action, should enhance the hydrophilic properties of the lens.

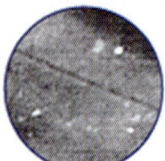

AIR OPTIX® NIGHT & DAY® AQUA contact lenses[3]
A permanent, chemically bonded plasma treatment for a smooth, continuous surface

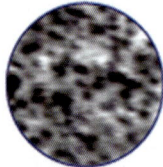

Biofinity® contact lenses[4]
No permanent plasma treatment

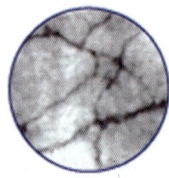

PureVision® contact lenses[3]
Surface made up of silicate islands that do not completely cover the surface

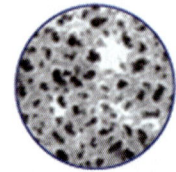

ACUVUE® OASYS™ contact lenses[3]
No permanent plasma treatment

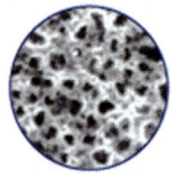

ACUVUE® ADVANCE® contact lenses[3]
No permanent plasma treatment

FIGURE 10.2 Silicone hydrogel surface modifications. (Courtesy of Alcon.)

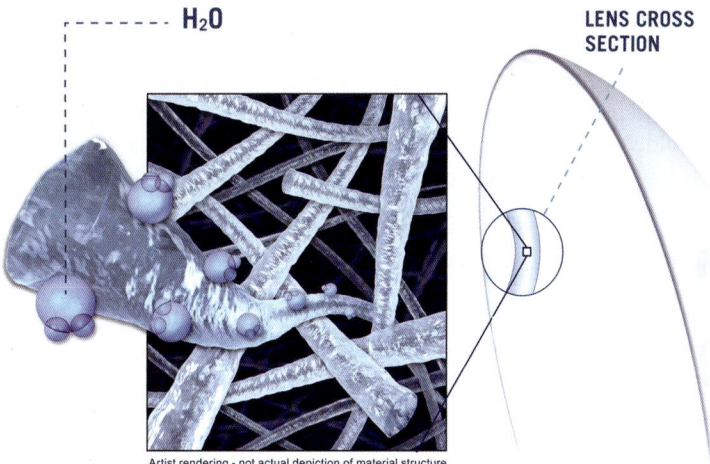

FIGURE 10.3 Biofinity: Siloxane molecules attract and bond to surrounding water molecules, continuously wetting and lubricating the material. (Courtesy of CooperVision.)

Another factor that has changed the wettability of soft contact lenses is the incorporation of PVA or PVP, moisturizing agents, into daily disposable hydrogel lens materials or included in the packaging solution. Potentially, adding these agents to the lens material will result in increased wettability, increased comfort, and enhanced tear film stability. Early results indicate that this may be beneficial to dry-eye patients and provide increased comfort throughout the day, including end-of-the-day comfort.[18–20]

A new hydrogel daily disposable lens material to come to the market, nesofilcon A (Bausch + Lomb), is described by the manufacturer as a "hypergel" material. The outer surface is designed to mimic the lipid layer of the tear film to prevent dehydration and maintain good vision. Potentially, this lens could be very beneficial in maintaining a wettable lens surface (M. Merchea, personal communication, June 10, 2012).

Ionic Charge

Contact lens materials may possess an electric charge, or they may be electrically neutral. This attribute is especially important in soft lens materials, as it affects factors such as solution compatibility and deposit formation. Materials that have an electric charge are said to be ionic. The charge results from the presence of electrically charged groups in their chemical formulation. In most cases, this is an overall negative charge. The presence of a negative ionic charge causes the material to be more reactive, especially in solutions that are acidic. This, in turn, can cause dimensional changes and even material degradation.

An ionic charge may also cause a material to be more prone to deposit formation. Most deposits are positively charged substances from tears that are attracted to the negative ionic charge of the lens material. Materials that are electrically neutral are said to be nonionic. These materials tend to be more inert and less reactive with tear constituents, so they also tend to be more deposit resistant.

Hydration (Water Content)

Most contact lens materials, both GP and soft, absorb some water. The amount absorbed is usually expressed as a percentage of the total weight. When a material absorbs water, it swells, a fact that must be considered during the manufacturing process to achieve precise specifications. Materials that absorb <4% of water by weight are referred to as *hydrophobic materials*; those that absorb ≥4% water are termed *hydrophilic polymers*. With hydrophilic polymers (hydrogels), increasing the water content generally increases Dk. However, this often increases lens fragility and may make the material more prone to deposit formation. Even if it were possible to create a 100% water content lens material, the Dk of water is 80; therefore, this lens would still be unable to meet the Holden–Mertz criterion for extended wear (EW) (87×10^{-9}).[1] Most silicone hydrogel materials have low water contents, because the material is dependent on silicone, not water, to transmit oxygen.

Oxygen Permeability/Oxygen Transmission

Dk usually depends on the water content of the hydrogel lens and is a property of the material.[3,21] Generally, the Dk of a lens increases logarithmically with an increase in water content.[22] Dk/t is defined as the Dk of the lens divided by its thickness (t). Lens power indirectly affects Dk/t. As center thickness (CT) varies considerably in higher powers (both plus and minus), average thickness is typically used for the determination of Dk/t. The highest Dk value obtainable with a HEMA-based hydrogel lens is approximately 40.[23] It is not unusual for a low-water-content, ultrathin hydrogel lens to have a similar Dk/t value as a high-water-content hydrogel lens, which typically has to be manufactured in a greater CT. Decreasing the CT or increasing the water content increases the Dk/t of the lens; however, it also results in a more fragile lens material.

Silicone hydrogel materials have been successful in breaking the dependence on water content for Dk (Fig. 10.4).[24,25] Silicone hydrogel materials tend to have an inverse relationship between Dk and water content; the lower the water content, generally the higher the Dk.[6] However, efrofilcon A deviates from this trend by having a water content of 74% and a Dk value of 60×10^{-11} (cm²/sec) (mL O₂/mL × mm Hg).[13] Silicone hydrogel materials offer Dk/t values in the range of approximately 65 to 175. Many of these lenses meet the Holden–Mertz criterion

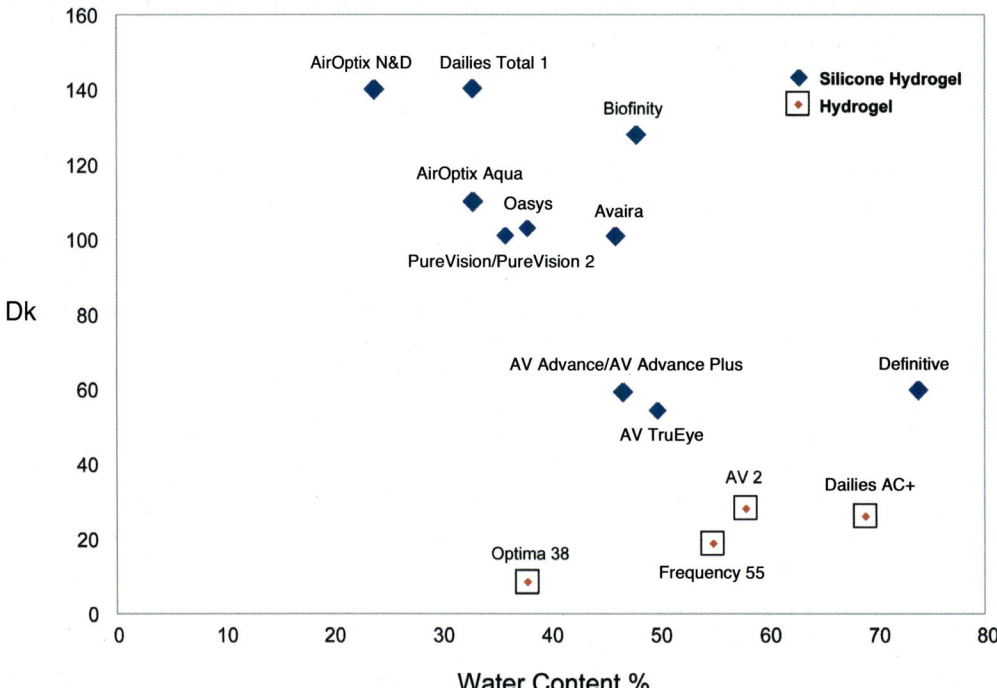

FIGURE 10.4 Oxygen permeablility (Dk) relationship with water content for silicone hydrogel and some hydrogel lenses.

for EW of 87 × 10^{-9} (cm × mL O$_2$)/(s × mL × mm Hg) and Harvitt and Bonanno's suggested Dk/t of 125 × 10^{-9} (cm × mL O$_2$)/(s × mL × mm Hg) to avoid stromal anoxia. These materials make it possible for contact lens patients to wear lenses on a continuous basis overnight for up to 30 days, as silicone hydrogel materials provide up to eight times the Dk/t of conventional hydrogel lenses.[1] Although the estimated value of Dk necessary for daily wear (DW) (24–35)[26] is much lower than the values of silicone hydrogels (Dk values 55–140), these materials are beneficial to the ocular health of patients, who wear their lenses daily and remove them each night, by reducing both epithelial thinning and chronic limbal inflammation (Fig. 10.5).[22] Silicone hydrogel materials dominate hydrogel materials for patient's fit and refit for DW as well as EW.[27] A summary of silicone hydrogel material characteristics can be found in Table 10.3.[1,10,22,28]

Classification of Lens Groups

The U.S. Food and Drug Administration (FDA) has classified soft lens materials according to their water content and ionic charge. This classification has become widely accepted internationally.

This classification simplifies the large number of possible soft lens materials into four groups. This helps to predict the performance of the various lens materials both on and off of the eye. The rationale for this classification is that water content and ionic charge will determine how a soft lens material will interact with contact lens solutions. Additionally, many properties of the material, such as strength, refractive index, deposit resistance, and, generally, Dk, depend on its water content. Lens strength, deposit resistance, and refractive index all decrease as the water content of the material increases. Generally, pore size and Dk will increase as water content increases.

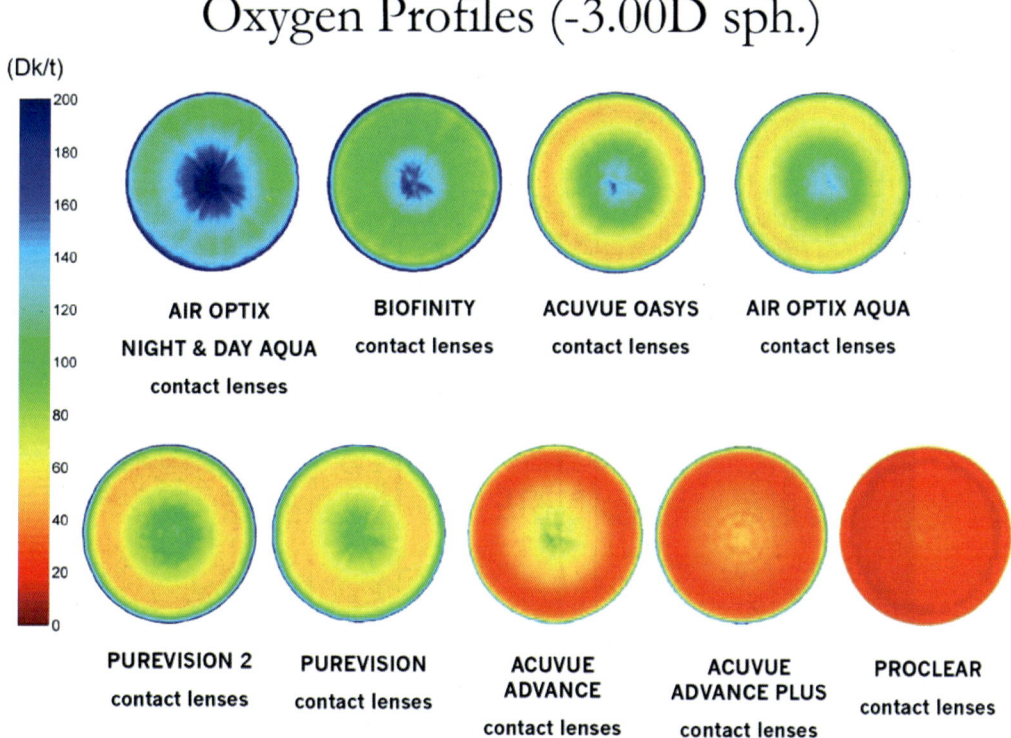

FIGURE 10.5 Oxygen profiles for (−3.00 sphere), Based on in vitro measurement of thickness profiles of unworn lenses. Dk based on manufacturer-published values; Alcon data on file, 2009, 2010. (Courtesy of Alcon.)

TABLE 10.3 Silicone Hydrogel Lenses

BRAND NAME	AIR OPTIX NIGHT & DAY	AIR OPTIX AQUA	DAILIES TOTAL 1	PUREVISION	PUREVISION 2	BIOFINITY	AVAIRA	ACUVUE OASYS	ACUVUE ADVANCE	ACUVUE ADVANCE PLUS	1 DAY ACUVUE TRUEYE	DEFINITIVE
Manufacturer	Alcon	Alcon	Alcon	Bausch + Lomb	Bausch + Lomb	Cooper Vision	Cooper Vision	Vistakon	Vistakon	Vistakon	Vistakon	Contamac (Marketed by other labs)
Material	lotrafilcon A	lotrafilcon B	delefilcon A	balafilcon A	balafilcon A	comfilcon A	enfilcon A	senofilcon A	galyfilcon A	galyfilcon A	narafilcon B	efrofilcon A
Dk	140	110	140	91	91	128	100	103	60	60	55	60
Dk/t	175	138	156	101	130	160	125	147	86	62	65	75
Water Content	24%	33%	33%–80%	36%	36%	48%	46%	38%	47%	47%	48%	74%
Modulus (MPa)	1.4	1.2	.7	1.1	1.1	0.75	0.5	0.72	0.43	0.43	0.71	0.35
Surface Modification	Plasma coating	Plasma coating		Plasma oxidation	Plasma oxidation	None	None	Internal wetting agent	Internal wetting agent	Internal wetting agent	Internal wetting agent	None
Recommended replacement	Monthly	Monthly	Daily	Monthly	Monthly	Monthly	2 wk	2 wk	2 wk	2 wk	Daily	Quarterly
Wear schedule	DW, EW, or CW	DW or EW	DW	DW, EW, or CW	DW	DW or EW	DW	DW or EW	DW	DW	DW	DW
Additional lens modalities	Toric & multifocal	Toric & multifocal		Toric & multifocal	Toric & multifocal	Toric & multifocal	Toric	Toric & multifocal	Toric			Toric & multifocal

In the FDA classification, low water content is defined as <50% water; high water content is defined as >50% water.[8] The five classification groups are:

Group 1: Low-water-content, nonionic polymers
Group 2: High-water-content, nonionic polymers
Group 3: Low-water-content, ionic polymers
Group 4: High-water-content, ionic polymers
Group 5: Silicone hydrogels

Group 1

This group consists of the low-water-content, nonionic polymers. This includes such materials as HEMA and hydrophobic monomers. No lenses with MAA are included in this group. These materials exhibit lower protein deposition because of the lower water content and nonionic nature.[29]

Group 2

This group consists of high-water-content, nonionic polymers. As these lenses have a high water content, they have a potential for greater protein attraction. However, they have the advantage of a nonionic polymer matrix that prevents additional interaction between protein and the lens. Heat disinfection should not be used with these lenses because of the high water content. The preservatives sorbic acid and potassium sorbate should also be avoided with these lenses because of discoloration problems.[29]

Group 3

This group of lenses consists of low-water-content, ionic polymers. The negatively charged surfaces of these lenses show greater attraction for the positively charged tear proteins and lipids. Therefore, they tend to exhibit more deposits than materials in the nonionic groups.[22]

Group 4

This group consists of the high-water-content, ionic polymers. Lenses in this group tend to attract more protein than do those in any other lens group. The high-water-content and ionic properties cause greater absorption of proteins into the lens matrix. Heat disinfection should be avoided in this group of lenses because of the high water content. Sorbic acid and potassium sorbate-preserved solutions should also be avoided. Ionic polymers are more sensitive to change in lens care product composition because added ions in the matrix can change the water content. Changes in pH may alter the lens parameters.[29]

Group 5

Given the differences between hydrogel lens materials and silicone hydrogel materials, it would appear that silicone hydrogel materials would need their own classification. These materials react differently to deposits and solutions, because their basic characteristics (e.g., wettability, water content, Dk) differ from conventional hydrogel materials. A group 5 has been proposed, which would classify silicone hydrogel materials.[30,31] This group is defined as soft materials that have a Dk value >30, which is not explained by their water content. There is continued debate on how to differentiate the materials within this group based on ionicity, water content, differences in the silicone portion of the lens and the lens surface itself (R.P. Stone, personal communication, April 3, 2012). The current FDA classification can be found in Table 10.4.[28]

MANUFACTURING METHODS

Soft lenses can be spun-cast, lathe-cut, cast-molded, or manufactured via a combination of these procedures. The manufacturing of contact lenses involves many different procedures, steps, and technologies. The following section provides a brief overview of the major manufacturing

TABLE 10.4 FDA Classification of Soft Lenses[a]

GROUP 1 (LOW-WATER-CONTENT, NONIONIC POLYMERS)	GROUP 2 (HIGH-WATER-CONTENT, NONIONIC POLYMERS)	GROUP 3 (LOW-WATER-CONTENT, IONIC POLYMERS)	GROUP 4 (HIGH-WATER-CONTENT, IONIC POLYMERS)	GROUP 5 (SILICONE HYDROGEL)
Acofilcon B (49%)	Acofilcon A (58%)	Bufilcon A (45%)	Bufilcon A (55%)	Balafilcon A (36%)
Crofilcon (39%)	Alphafilcon A (66%)	Etafilcon A (43%)	Epsilfilcon A (60%)	Comfilcon A (48%)
Dimefilcon A (36%)	Atlafilcon A (64%)	Deltafilcon A (43%)	Etafilcon A (58%)	Efrofilcon A (74%)
Genfilcon A (48%)	Hefilcon C (57%)	Droxifilcon A (47%)	Focofilcon A (55%)	Enfilcon A (46%)
Hioxiflilcon B (49%)	Hilafilcon B (59%)	Ocufilcon A (44%)	Methafilcon A, B (55%)	Galyfilcon A (47%)
Isofilcon (36%)	Hioxifilcon A (59%)	Phemfilcon A (38%)	Ocufilcon B (53%)	Lotrafilcon A (24%)
Mafilcon (33%)	Hioxifilcon D (54%)		Ocufilcon C (55%)	Lotrafilcon B (33%)
Polymacon (38%)	Lidofilcon B (79%)		Ocufilcon D (55%)	Narafilcon B (48%)
Tefilcon (38%)	Lidofilcon A (70%)		Ocufilcon E (65%)	Senofilcon A (37%)
Tetrafilcon A (43%)	Nelfilcon A (69%)		Ocufilcon F (60%)	Sifilcon A (32%)
	Nesofilcon A (78%)		Perfilcon A (71%)	
	Netrafilcon A (65%)		Phemfilcon A (55%)	
	Ofilcon A (74%)		Tetrafilcon B (58%)	
	Omafilcon A (59%)		Vifilcon A (55%)	
	Scafilcon A (71%)			
	Surfilcon A (74%)			
	Vasurfilcon A (74%)			
	Xylofilcon A (67%)			

[a]The FDA has created the five lens groups to clarify categories of similar polymers for investigating solutions approvals.

methods. All contact lens-manufacturing methods begin with the formulation and preparation of the lens material. In this preparation stage, monomers are added in precise amounts, any impurities are removed, and in some cases, the material is polymerized into rods, buttons, or sheets.

LATHE CUTTING

Lathe cutting is used to manufacture polymethylmethacrylate (PMMA), GP, and many soft contact lenses. This process begins with a long, plastic cylinder of material that is cut into lens buttons. The lathe-cut process is composed of lathing, polishing, hydration, extractions, tinting, finishing, and sterilization.

Lathing

In this procedure, the hard, dry "button" of the lens polymer is ground on a lathe. Computerized, automatic lathes are now available to cut the front and base curves onto the lens, along with any secondary curves and edge bevels.

Polishing

The lenses are then removed from the lathe and polished to remove any lathing marks, improve the optics, and smooth the edges.

Hydration

For soft lenses, the brittle, dry lenses now undergo hydration, where they are immersed in saline until they absorb as much water as their formulation will allow. This is the step where the lens actually transforms from a dry, rigid material to the soft and flexible lens.

During the hydration stage, the lenses swell as they absorb water. For this reason, careful calculations are made regarding the size of the dry lens to achieve the exact dimensions of the fully hydrated lens.

Extraction

Lenses are then moved to the extraction stage. During extraction, lenses are processed to remove all unpolymerized chemicals or materials that may be present.

Tinting

If the lens is to be tinted, the tinting process normally occurs as the next stage in this process.

Finishing

Numerous quality assurance steps occur throughout the manufacturing process. A full quality inspection of the lens is then performed before the lens is finished and the final processing steps are implemented before it is distributed.

Sterilization

The lenses are now sterilized. Trays of lenses are loaded into an autoclave, in which a temperature of 121° to 124°C is maintained for at least 20 minutes. This step inactivates any microorganisms and spores that may be present and ensures the sterility of the packaged lens. Lathe cutting is a relatively labor-intensive and expensive process and is not generally as reproducible as spin casting or cast molding. However, it is a useful method for the manufacture of certain lenses, especially those made in low quantities or with custom parameters.

SPIN CASTING

Spin casting was the first method employed in the manufacture of soft contact lenses. It was invented by Otto Wichterle in 1951 and was further developed by Bausch + Lomb. The process is used to manufacture some hydrogel contact lenses.

Spin casting consists of a liquid form of the lens polymer being injected into a spinning mold. The final shape and power of the resulting lens is due to the combination of temperature, gravity, centrifugal force, surface tension, amount of liquid in the mold, and rate of spin, which is computer controlled. Slower speeds produce flatter posterior curves, and faster speeds produce steeper curves.

The outer (front or anterior) surface of the lens is determined by the curvature of the mold. The inner (base curve) surface of the lens is determined by the factors listed above; because of these forces, the resultant base curves are aspheric.

After spinning for the proper time, the lens material is treated with heat or ultraviolet light. This treatment is called "curing," and causes the liquid polymer to solidify. The lens is then hydrated, extracted, and finished similar to lathe-cut lenses.

Spin casting is an inexpensive manufacturing method. The lenses produced are highly reproducible and have a very thin, comfortable edge. The primary problem when fitting spin-cast lenses is their tendency to decenter on the eye. They often position temporally or in a superior temporal position.

CAST MOLDING

Cast molding is a more reproducible and less labor-intensive process. It is a cost-effective method of production for the high-volume manufacture of contact lenses. Many of the disposable and frequent-replacement lenses are manufactured using this process.

The first step in cast molding is making the molds from which the lenses will be formed. Each different lens design (every possible combination of power, base curve, and diameter) requires a separate master mold. Thousands of plastic molds can be produced from a single metallic master mold.

Liquid polymer is poured into the concave half of the mold. The convex portion of the mold is then applied and clamped into place, and the material is cured with ultraviolet light.

After the lens is removed from the mold, it undergoes the hydration process. Stabilized Soft Molding (Vistakon), Lightstream Technology (Alcon), FormCast (Bausch + Lomb), and Aquaform Molded Science (CooperVision) are proprietary methods of cast molding used to produce high-quality, inexpensive, reproducible soft contact lenses.

LENS TYPES

Wearing Schedules

The FDA approves lenses to be worn for either DW or EW. In DW, the lenses are prescribed to be worn during the day and removed before sleep. EW lenses are currently approved for a maximum of 7 days and 6 nights of wear before removal or for 30 nights of continuous wear (CW) before removal. Some practitioners use the term *flexible wear* to describe the use of EW-approved lenses on an occasional EW basis (i.e., 2 or 3 nights of wear or an occasional nap with the lenses in place).

Generally, EW-approved lenses have a higher DK/t value than DW lenses. The higher DK/t value is generally achieved by using a higher-water-content material, a thinner lens, or both. This may make the lenses more difficult to handle or insert/remove, as well as more fragile. Currently, these conventional hydrogel lenses are discouraged for EW use as silicone hydrogel lens materials provide, as previously mentioned, up to eight times more oxygen to the cornea. Silicone hydrogel lens materials may be used for DW, EW, or CW depending on their FDA approval (see Chapter 16 for more information on EW). When selecting a wearing schedule for a patient, the practitioner must evaluate the patient's ocular health, desires, needs, and lifestyle to determine which schedule is most appropriate for that patient.

Replacement Schedule

The FDA does not directly approve replacement schedules. They classify devices as either disposable (intended for single use) or conventional (cleaned upon removal from the eye and then reused). The FDA does not specify how many times conventional lenses may be reused or how often they should be replaced.

Manufacturers, based on their knowledge of their own lens material's features and attributes, will specify a recommended replacement time. Although the lens may still be usable beyond the recommended replacement time specified by the manufacturer, generally its performance will begin to decline. This is manifested by decreased comfort, increased deposits, decreased vision, increased lens awareness, and increased lens tears or nicks.

In 1989, when the first disposable (true single use) lens was approved by the FDA, it was to be used once and thrown away upon removal from the eye, generally after 7 days of EW use. Because of a variety of factors, the disposable lenses then received approval for "reuse" on a DW basis for up to 2 weeks. Practitioners still referred to these lenses as "disposables," even though they were no longer being used once and then discarded. Currently, most practitioners term any lenses that are used for a month or less "disposable."

In an effort to reduce this confusion, terms such as *frequent replacement, planned replacement,* and *programmed replacement* developed. These terms indicate a lens that is replaced on a practitioner-specified schedule. This schedule may be 2 weeks, 1 month, 3 months, 6 months, or any period within this time frame. It is important to emphasize that this replacement schedule is not dictated or approved by the FDA. Rather, it is only a recommendation by the manufacturer to help maximize lens performance, patient comfort, and patient health. The lenses that most practitioners refer to as "disposable" are really more correctly termed as "frequent-replacement" lenses. Most lenses in vials, which most practitioners refer to as conventional lenses, are recommended to be used on a specified replacement schedule, usually 6 months to 1 year.

Practitioners and the industry have increased their use of disposable and frequent-replacement lenses, virtually eliminating conventional lenses replaced greater than every 3 months.[32] The benefits of this type of lens use are convenience, comfort, health, decreased need for enzyme or separate cleaners, decreased lens deposits, availability of spare lenses, and increased patient satisfaction. Beyond daily disposable use, most lenses are recommended for 2-week or monthly replacement.

With confusion surrounding replacement schedules, how should a practitioner determine what schedule is best for a patient? In general, two rules apply:

1. The more frequent the replacement, the fewer the number of ocular complications.
2. If deposits are ever observed on a patient's lenses, the lens replacement schedule needs to be reduced.

Daily disposable lenses are an affordable reality for most people. In a very large study (almost 46,000 eyes), lenses disposed of on a daily basis had the lowest ocular complication rate of only 2.5%.[33] As a comparison, GP lenses showed a complication rate of 10.5%, PMMA 15.8%, conventional HEMA lenses 8.5%, and weekly disposable EW lenses 4.9%.

Other studies have shown fewer unscheduled office visits with daily disposable lenses, as well as improved visual acuity, comfort, and patient satisfaction.[34,35] Additionally, daily disposable lenses require no lens care, and this is a tremendous convenience for many patients. In a recent contact lens replacement schedule compliance study, daily disposable lens wearers were the most compliant (88%) over monthly (72%) and 2-week (48%) replacement schedules.[36] A separate study found comfort and vision to be the highest upon lens insertion in the morning and in new lenses over end-of-day wear and lenses needing to be replaced. Patients compliant with their replacement schedule had greater comfort and vision at the end of the day and when their lenses needed to be replaced than those who were noncompliant. Monthly replacement wearers were found to be more compliant with replacement frequency than 2-week replacement wearers.[37]

The recommended wearing schedule for silicone hydrogel lens materials is daily, 2 weeks or monthly, depending on the material. Like daily disposable lenses, several studies have shown that silicone hydrogels have improved corneal health and decreased signs of corneal hypoxia[38–40] as compared to conventional hydrogel materials (for more information see Chapter 16). With the introduction of daily disposable silicone hydrogel lenses, contact lens wearers can enjoy a combination of the benefits of daily disposability and increased Dk/t.

Depending on the lens material, different replacement schedules should be recommended. Studies have shown that for group 4 lenses, monthly replacement produces better results, whereas group 2 lenses are able to be replaced quarterly without much change in the lens performance.[41] However, some studies suggest that monthly replacement is easier for patients to maintain and comply with as compared to quarterly replacement.[42,43] Even though many patients are prescribed 2-week replacement of "disposable" lenses, it has been found that the average patient wears these lenses for approximately 1 month, or at minimum stretch the 2-week lenses to a greater replacement interval (in relation to the prescribed replacement interval) than monthly replacement lenses.[44]

Clinically, the only way to observe lens deposits is with a slit lamp. However, studies using scanning electron microscopy have found that by the time lens deposits are visible through the slit lamp, they are already heavy enough to begin to degrade the lens surface. Additionally, these deposits begin to decrease visual acuity long before they are able to be observed with a slit lamp at a clinically significant level.[45] This is why the replacement schedule should be reduced immediately if clinically detectable levels of deposits are ever observed. As with the wearing schedule, the practitioner must evaluate a large number of clinical, health, and patient factors when prescribing a replacement schedule. The schedule should then be monitored for both compliance and health reasons.

SUMMARY

This chapter has summarized the characteristics of hydrogel and silicone hydrogel lens materials. There are many options for the eye care practitioner to select from, including material factors (i.e., Dk/t, modulus, water content, and wettability), wearing schedules (i.e., DW, EW, or CW), and replacement schedules (i.e., daily, every 2 weeks, monthly). Preliminary evaluation of the patient and the desires of the patient will aid the practitioner in finding the material that will provide good vision and ocular health, as well as fit the patient's lifestyle.

CLINICAL CASES

CASE 1

A 28-year-old woman who has worn conventional EW hydrogel lenses (58% water content) for 5 years comes into your office. She wears the lenses for 4 to 6 nights before removing them. Although she does not have any major complaints, you notice limbal engorgement and vascularization, an increase in myopia, and corneal edema grade 1+.

SOLUTION: As the patient desires to stay in EW, she is fitted with a silicone hydrogel lens material approved for EW. She may keep her current wearing schedule of 4 to 6 nights EW. At the follow-up visit, the limbal vessels have emptied, her prescription has stabilized with less myopia, and her cornea is clear.

CASE 2

A patient with refraction and keratometry readings of $-3.00 - 1.00 \times 180$, 43.00 @ 180; 44.00 @ 090 OU is fitted with GP lenses and has a resulting visual acuity of 20/15 OU. The patient appears to be compliant and motivated to wear contact lenses. Two weeks after dispensing, the patient is experiencing difficulty adapting to GP lens wear. The importance of gradually increasing wearing time is emphasized to the patient. At 1 month, the patient is only able to wear the lenses for 2 to 4 hours and reports discomfort.

SOLUTION: Discomfort appears to be the primary factor that is preventing this patient from wearing contact lenses. The patient is fitted into a soft toric lens with a power of $-3.00 - 0.75 \times 180$

and an 8.6-mm base curve radius OU with a visual acuity equal to 20/15 OU. The patient is able to achieve full-day wear.

CASE 3

A patient has been a successful DW GP patient with the exception of chronic lens adherence. The lens design has been changed and no improvements have been observed. Dry eyes or dirty lenses do not appear to be the cause as the patient is very careful and compliant with lens care. Rewetting drops also proved to be unsuccessful.

SOLUTION: Generally, lens adherence in DW GP lenses can be prevented by changing the lens design; however, there are some patients who are prone to lens adherence, and changes in the lens design are unsuccessful. In this case, the patient may be fitted into a soft lens to achieve contact lens wear. While the cornea is rehabilitating, it is possible that there may be a series of lens changes necessary before the lens power and base curve radius are finalized. Using disposable trial lenses, with regular follow-up examinations, will allow the practitioner to make the necessary lens changes before ordering the final lens parameters.

CASE 4

A 30-year-old man who has worn soft lenses for 15 years has been diagnosed in the past as having GPC (or CLPC). He has corneal vascularization of about 1 mm with limbal engorgement. He was refit with a silicone hydrogel lens and noticed improvement in the vascularization and limbal hyperemia within 1 week. However, after wearing the lenses and replacing them every month, he still notices some itching toward the end of the month as the lenses begin to build up deposits.

SOLUTION: There are several ways to manage this case: (a) The patient can be fitted with a daily disposable lens, (b) The patient can be fitted with a daily disposable silicone hydrogel lens, which should give him the benefit of both modalities.

CASE 5

A 20-year-old athlete complains of frequently tearing his contact lenses (high-water-content, group 4). He is in college and his parents want to know if there is a more durable lens than the one he is currently wearing.

SOLUTION: Reeducation on soft lens care and handling should be performed with this patient. Second, he may need to be refitted into a more durable lens, such as a group 1 lens material that is a disposable or frequent-replacement lens (i.e., daily disposable of replacement every 2–4 weeks). This way he not only has a lens that is easier to handle and care for but he also has spare lenses. Another option would be silicone hydrogel lenses, which are typically quite durable for patients because of their higher modulus.

CASE 6

A patient who was previously wearing conventional hydrogel lenses is refitted into a silicone hydrogel lens with a high modulus. The patient is educated that the lenses may require a couple of weeks to adapt to the feel of the lens. At the 3-week follow-up examination, the patient is still unhappy with the comfort despite wearing the lenses for 8 to 12 hours.

SOLUTION: The patient is refitted into a lower-modulus silicone hydrogel lens. This time the patient is satisfied with the comfort. Other issues to address with this patient are the type of solution he is using and if there is any edge fluting. Poor comfort might be the result of not using a recommended care regimen or a preservative sensitivity. If the lens is demonstrating fluting of the edge, using a steeper base curve may solve his symptoms of discomfort.

CLINICAL PROFICIENCY CHECKLIST

- The strength, deposit resistance, and Dk of a hydrogel lens material are all components that generally depend on water content. The Dk of a hydrogel lens material increases logarithmically with an increase in water content.
- Silicone hydrogel lenses do not depend on water content to be permeable to oxygen; generally, the Dk of the material increases as the water content decreases. (There are a few silicone hydrogel lenses that do not follow this rule.)
- Hydrophilic monomers (i.e., NVP, MAA), copolymerized with HEMA, increase the water content of hydrogel lenses.
- Group 1 nonionic/low-water-content lenses demonstrate the lowest rate of protein formation, whereas group 4 ionic/high-water-content lenses tend to develop more protein deposition than the other groups.
- Silicone is hydrophobic; therefore, most silicone hydrogel lens materials require a surface treatment, internal wetting agent, or special design to make the lens hydrophilic.
- Wearing schedules and replacement frequencies must be determined for each patient. In general, more frequent replacement of lenses results in better ocular health and vision.
- Most silicone hydrogel materials have a higher modulus than hydrogel materials. Although this aids in handling and durability, it may result in edge fluting, SEALs, GPC, or lens awareness.
- Silicone hydrogel lenses provide up to eight times higher Dk/t than hydrogel lenses.

ACKNOWLEDGMENT

The authors thank Sally Dillehay, O.D., for her contributions to the Material Selection chapter in the second edition of this book.

REFERENCES

1. Sweeney D, Fonn D, Evans K. Silicone hydrogels: the evolution of a revolution. *Contact Lens Spectrum*. 2006;(special edition):14–19.
2. White P. A complete guide to contact lens materials. *Contact Lens Spectrum*. 1994;9(11):31–44.
3. Winterton LC, Su KC. Chemistry and processing of contact lens materials. In: Bennett ES, Weissman BA, eds. *Clinical Contact Lens Practice*. Philadelphia, PA: Lippincott Williams & Wilkins; 2005:355–362.
4. Hom MH. An inside look at soft lens materials. *Contact Lens Forum*. 1985;10(12):38–39.
5. Dillehay SM, Henry VA. Material selection. In: Bennett ES, Henry VA, eds. *Clinical Manual of Contact Lenses*. Philadelphia, PA: Lippincott Williams & Wilkins; 2000:239–258.
6. Tighe B. Silicone hydrogels: structure, properties and behaviour. In: Sweeney DF, ed. *Silicone Hydrogels Continuous-Wear Contact Lenses*. Edinburgh: Butterworth Heinemann; 2004:1–27.
7. Keir NJ, Richter D, Varikooty J, et al. End of day comfort interpreted using a novel cumulative comfort. Poster presented at: Association for Research in Vision and Ophthalmology; May 9, 2012; Fort Lauderdale, FL.
8. Pruitt J, Qiu Y, Thekveli S, et al. Surface characteristics of a water gradient silicone hydrogel contact lens (delefilcon A). Poster presented at: Association for Research in Vision and Ophthalmology; May 10, 2012; Fort Lauderdale, FL.
9. Davis J, Ketelson HA. Surface characterization of Dailies contact lens material. Poster presented at: Association for Research in Vision and Ophthalmology; May 10, 2012; Fort Lauderdale, FL.
10. Young G. Exploring the relationship between materials and ocular health and comfort. *Contact Lens Spectrum*. 2007;(special edition):37–40.
11. Snyder C. Modulus and its effect on contact lens fit. *Contact Lens Spectrum*. 2007;22(2):36–40.
12. French K. Why is modulus important? [editorial]. October 2007. http://www.siliconehydrogels.org. Accessed January 8, 2008.
13. Szczotka-Flynn L. The many faces of silicone hydrogel contact lenses. *Contact Lens Spectrum*. 2011;(special edition):22–26.

14. Fatt I, Chaston J. The effect of temperature on refractive index, water content and central thickness of hydrogel contact lenses. *Int Cont Lens Clin.* 1980;7:37–42.
15. Yeung KK, Weissman BA. Soft contact lens application. In: Bennett ES, Weissman BA, eds. *Clinical Contact Lens Practice.* Philadelphia, PA: Lippincott Williams & Wilkins; 2005:363–377.
16. Jones L. Understanding the link between wettability and lens comfort. *Contact Lens Spectrum.* 2007;22(6):S4–S6.
17. Tighe B. Trends and developments in silicone hydrogel materials [editorial]. http://www.siliconehydrogels.org, September 2006. Accessed April 10, 2012.
18. Nichols JJ. A look at lubricating agents in daily disposables. *Contact Lens Spectrum.* 2007;22(1):22.
19. Nick J, Winterton L, Lally J, et al. Lubricating lens focuses on patient comfort. *Contact Lens Spectrum.* 2006;21(1):40–41.
20. Watanabe R. Comfort part 2: soft lenses. *Contact Lens Spectrum.* 2011;26(8):21.
21. Holden BA, Stretton S, de la Jara PL, et al. The future of contact lenses: Dk really matters. *Contact Lens Spectrum.* 2006;(special edition):20–28.
22. Brennan N, Efron N, Weissman B, et al. Clinical application of the oxygen transmissibility of powered contact lenses. *CLAO J.* 1991;17:169–172.
23. Mandell RB. Basic principles of hydrogel lenses. In: Mandell RB, ed. *Contact Lens Practice.* 4th ed. Springfield, IL: Charles C. Thomas ; 1988:502–527.
24. Alvord L, Court J, Davis T, et al. Oxygen permeability of a new type of high Dk soft contact lens material. *Optom Vis Sci.* 1998;75(1):30–36.
25. Lowther GE. Will high Dk hydrogel lenses become a reality? *Int Cont Lens Clin.* 1998;251(2):39.
26. Fonn D, Bruce AS. A review of the Holden-Mertz criteria for critical oxygen transmission. *Eye Contact Lens.* 2005;31:247–251.
27. Nichols JJ. Contact lenses 2011. *Contact Lens Spectrum.* 2012;27(1):20–25.
28. Thompson TT. Tyler's Quarterly Soft Contact Lens Parameter Guide. 2012;29(2):1–27.
29. Stone RP. Why contact lens groups? *Contact Lens Spectrum.* 1988;3(12):38–41.
30. Stone RP. A new perspective for lens care-classifying silicone hydrogels [editorial]. June 2007. http://www.siliconehydrogels.org. Accessed April 10, 2012.
31. Hutter JC. FDA group V: is a single grouping sufficient to describe SiH performance? [editorial]. November 2007. http://www.siliconehydrogels.org. April 10, 2012.
32. Morgan PB, Woods CA, Tranoudis IG, et al. International contact lens prescribing in 2010. *Contact Lens Spectrum.* 2012;27(1):30–35.
33. Hamano H, Watanabe K, Mitsunaga S, et al. A study of the complications induced by conventional and disposable contact lenses. *CLAO J.* 1994;20(2):103–108.
34. Freeman M, Dubow B, Lopanik R, et al. A three-year study of the clinical performance of daily disposable contact lenses. *Optician.* 1997;213:36–45.
35. Nason RJ, Boshnick EL, Cannon WN, et al. Multisite comparison of contact lens modalities. Daily disposable wear vs. conventional daily wear in successful contact lens wearers. *J Am Optom Assoc.* 1994;65(11):774–780.
36. Dumbleton K, Woods C, Jones L, et al. Patient and practitioner compliance with silicone hydrogel and daily disposable lens replacement in the United States. *Eye Contact Lens.* 2009;35(4):164–171.
37. Dumbleton KA, Woods CA, Jones LW, et al. The role of compliance with replacement frequency of silicone hydrogel lenses on subjective comfort and vision. Presented at: American Academy of Optometry; November 12, 2009; Orlando, FL.
38. Dumbleton K, Richter D, Simpson T, et al. A comparison of the vascular response to extended wear of conventional lower Dk and experimental high Dk hydrogel contact lenses. *Optom Vis Sci.* 1998;75(12):170.
39. Keay, L, Sweeney DF, Jalbert I, et al. Microcyst response to high Dk/t silicone hydrogel contact lenses. *Optom Vis Sci.* 2000;77(11):582–585.
40. Doughty, MJ, Aakre BM, Ystenaes AE, et al. Short-term adaptation of the human corneal endothelium to continuous wear of silicone hydrogel (Lotrafilcon A) contact lenses after daily hydrogel lens wear. *Optom Vis Sci.* 2005;82(6):473–480.
41. Bleshoy H, Guillon M, Shah D. Influence of contact lens materials surface characteristics on replacement frequency. *Int Cont Lens Clin.* 1994;21(3):82–94.
42. Jones L, Franklin V, Evans K, et al. Spoilation and clinical performance of monthly vs. three monthly group II disposable contact lenses. *Optom Vis Sci.* 1996;73(1):16–21.
43. Pritchard N, Fonn D, Weed K. Ocular and subjective responses to frequent replacement of daily wear soft contact lenses. *CLAO J.* 1996;22(1):53–59.
44. Dumbleton KA, Richter D, Woods CA, et al. Relationship between compliance with lens replacement and contact lens-related problems in silicone hydrogel wearers. Presented at: American Academy of Optometry; November 18, 2010; San Francisco, CA.
45. Gellatly KW, Brennan NA, Efron N. Visual decrement with deposit accumulation on HEMA contact lenses. *Am J Optom Physiol Opt.* 1988;65(12):937–941.

Chapter 11

Soft Lens Fitting and Evaluation

Vinita Allee Henry

PATIENT SELECTION

Soft contact lenses, including conventional hydrogel and silicone hydrogel, are appealing to many patients as a result of both the immediate comfort provided by these materials and the availability of specialty lenses; however, soft lenses are not a viable option for all patients, and careful patient selection will help ensure a successful fit. A comprehensive preliminary evaluation will provide the practitioner with information that will be the key to selecting the type of contact lens suitable for each particular patient, whether it is rigid gas-permeable (GP), soft, extended wear (EW), disposable, or no lens wear at all. Patients may have preconceived ideas about which type of lens they want to wear; however, their selection may not be a viable one. It will be necessary to explain the risks and benefits, advantages and disadvantages, and available options. Only after this has been performed, is it possible to select a particular lens modality.

Indications and Contraindications

Some factors contraindicate contact lens wear of any type, such as inflammation or disease of the anterior segment, any systemic disease that can be complicated by contact lens wear, poor hygiene, poor compliance, and lack of motivation (Table 11.1). Factors that may contraindicate soft lens wear include irregular corneas (i.e., keratoconus, ocular trauma), autoimmune disease, immunocompromised patients, chronic allergies, chronic antihistamine use, and giant papillary conjunctivitis (GPC, also known as contact lens papillary conjunctivitis [CLPC]).

The initial comfort afforded by soft lenses makes this lens type particularly appealing to patients.[1,2] The initial comfort of soft lenses is due to the large diameter, thin edges, limited movement, and minimal resistance to lid closure.[3] Potential contact lens patients often do not want to tolerate the adaptation period that may be present with GP lenses. In addition, the decreased initial reflex tearing and lens awareness help to reduce the time required for the practitioner to fit the lens. Likewise, the practitioner benefits from the ability to dispense new and replacement lenses from inventory.

Patient information to further consider when selecting soft lenses include refractive error, occupation, hobbies, wearing schedule, hygiene, and compliance. Typically, individuals with spherical refractive errors, low astigmatism, and lenticular astigmatism will be the best candidates for soft lens wear. These patients will be able to achieve acceptable visual acuity with a spherical or toric soft lens. Obviously, occupations with tasks that include exposure to fine particles of dust or mist (e.g., sandblasting) are not suitable for contact lens wear unless the recommended protective eye wear, such as safety goggles, is worn. Many occupations and hobbies may be enhanced by contact lens wear (e.g., those of athletes, actors, or models). These groups benefit from improved cosmesis and elimination of spectacle wear, which may decrease the field of view, fog up with precipitation changes, slide down, or possibly break. Soft lenses are preferable for athletes and sports activities as they are more difficult to dislodge than GP lenses.

TABLE 11.1 Soft Lens Wear

INDICATIONS	CONTRAINDICATIONS
Good tear quality and quantity	Inflammation or disease of the anterior segment
Spherical refractive errors	Poor hygiene
Low astigmatism	Lack of motivation
Low lenticular astigmatism	Chronic allergies and antihistamine use
Athletes	Systemic diseases aggravated by contact lens wear
Unable to adapt to GP lenses	Autoimmune disease/immunocompromised
Occasional/flexible wear	Poor tear quality and quantity
Desires tint to enhance or change eye color	Irregular astigmatism
Previous GP adherence	Radial keratotomy
Previous 3- and 9 o'clock staining with GP lenses	Dry, dusty environments
High motivation	GPC

GP, gas-permeable; GPC, giant papillary conjunctivitis.

The minimal movement present with a soft lens aids in initial comfort; provides more stable vision, which may not be present initially with GP lens wear as a result of increased lens movement; and reduces the likelihood of a trapped foreign body. Occasionally, patients desire to wear lenses strictly for sports, such as tennis or basketball, or just for social occasions to improve their appearance. Soft lenses are preferable for these part-time wearers. They are also advantageous for individuals desiring a change or enhancement of eye color, as well as anyone benefiting from a disposable lens.

The disposability and the ability to have multiple lenses readily available is a large advantage for the soft lens patient. Daily disposable lenses provide the patient the ability to be virtually solution-free, which eliminates the cost of solutions and is advantageous when traveling. Many patients with allergies, prone to deposits, or who desire no care regimen, benefit from being able to insert a fresh lens every day and simply discard it at the end of the day. A damaged, lost, or uncomfortable lens can be easily replaced with a new one for those patients who wear some form of disposable lenses as a back-up lens is always available.

Soft lenses are more prone to deposits, and soft lens-wearing patients are more susceptible to infections than GP patients because of the characteristics of the lens. As a result, patients who exhibit poor hygiene, work in an environment that may be unsanitary or dirty, or are noncompliant with their follow-up visits or care regimen are at risk to develop problems resulting from the contamination of their lenses. Extra caution is necessary for both the practitioner and the patient if these patients are to be fitted with any contact lens, in particular, a soft contact lens. Disposable lenses are an excellent choice for these patients.

Other disadvantages of soft lenses are that some patients may experience reduced vision resulting from an inadequate correction of refractive astigmatism, and the lenses are more fragile and more difficult to verify. Hydrogel lenses generally have lower oxygen transmission (Dk/t); however, silicone hydrogel lenses have higher or comparable Dk/t to GP lenses. Advantages and disadvantages are further summarized in Table 11.2.

PATIENT FACTORS AFFECTING MATERIAL SELECTION

Overall, most lens materials can be used for the majority of patients with excellent results. The following recommendations take into consideration certain patient factors when selecting a lens material that will maximize patient health, comfort, compliance, and satisfaction.

TABLE 11.2 Soft Lens Advantages and Disadvantages

Advantages
Excellent initial comfort
Minimal adaptation time
Part-time wearing schedule possible
Risk of corneal distortion minimal
Minimal spectacle blur
Dislocation uncommon
Foreign-body sensation rare
Ability to fit and dispense from inventory
Low incidence of flare
Low incidence of discomfort caused by excessive lens lag
Ability to change or enhance eye color
Simplicity of fit
Rarely causes excessive tearing
Disposable
Replacement of lost or damaged lenses possible
Spare lenses
Therapeutic use possible
Disadvantages
Reduced visual acuity in uncorrected astigmatism
Limited durability
Oxygen transmission with hydrogels
Deposit formation/GPC possible
Greater chance of bacterial contamination/infection
Greater risks with noncompliance
More difficult to verify
Limitations of corrections
Quality of vision may be reduced

GPC, giant papillary conjunctivitis.

Refractive Error

Soft spherical lenses are typically available in powers of ±20 D, but most commonly, the lenses are available in powers of approximately −10.00 to +4.00 D. If in doubt, it is important to check the power availability before fitting the lens. A smaller number of stock lenses and custom lenses are available in high plus, aphakic, and high minus powers (i.e., ±30–50 D). Toric lenses to correct astigmatism are available in cylinder powers up to −1.75 or −2.25 D. A number of lens brands and custom lenses are available in cylinder powers of >−2.25 and up to −5.75 D or higher. Generally, the higher corrections are not available in a variety of materials, tints, or lens designs (i.e., bifocal).

Aspheric lenses, offered by several companies, may be beneficial for patients with low amounts of astigmatism (i.e., ≤−0.75 D). The lenses appear to improve spherical aberration, but not correct astigmatism. Studies have shown that there is little difference between the spherical and aspheric lenses, although patients have reported subjective preferences for aspheric lenses.[4,5]

Handling Issues

First-time wearers will generally benefit from a slightly thicker lens or one with an increased stiffness or modulus of elasticity. Both of these attributes help to make insertion, removal, and handling of the lens easier. Silicone hydrogel lens materials have a higher modulus than most soft contact lenses. Additionally, a handling tint will be beneficial for these patients.

Deposit-Prone Patients

Patients who experience frequent lens deposits, even when using a rigorous care routine, would be best fitted in a daily disposable lens. If this is not used, then a disposable or frequent-replacement lens should be used (i.e., weekly to monthly replacement). Certain lens materials (i.e., Proclear by CooperVision) are more resistant to deposits. With the availability of disposable lenses, deposit issues should not be a problem if the patient is following the recommended replacement schedule.

Marginal Dry Eye

Many contact lens wearers experience dry-eye symptoms with lens wear. As many as 50% of contact lens wearers have reported symptoms of dry eye.[6–8] Factors that affect dry-eye symptoms are wettability, dehydration, contact lens solutions, poor tear film quality, environmental temperature, time of day, humidity, wind, and blink rate.[6,9] With hydrogel lens materials, low-water-content and thicker lenses are thought to dehydrate less than high-water-content or thin lenses. This is thought to be one of the reasons why patients experience more comfortable wear with low-water-content, thick hydrogel lenses. However, a fixed relationship between initial water content and dehydration cannot always be demonstrated.[9] Additionally, some studies have shown that increasing the lens thickness has a greater effect on dry-eye symptoms than the water content.[10]

Recent advances have given practitioners more lens options to aid marginal dry-eye patients. Extreme H_2O (Hydrogel Vision Corp.) is a hydrogel lens that the manufacturer claims retains its water saturation on the eye, thus exhibiting less dehydration and better end-of-the-day comfort. Proclear (CooperVision), mentioned previously, is deposit resistant and contains phosphorylcholine, which aids in hydration of the lens.[11] Dailies Aqua Comfort Plus (Alcon) and 1-Day Acuvue Moist (Vistakon) contain lubricating agents incorporated into the material, which reportedly make the lens more wettable and increase comfort, particularly end-of-the-day comfort. The lubricating agent in the Dailies Aqua Comfort Plus lens is polyvinyl alcohol (PVA), and the lubricating agent in 1-Day Acuvue Moist is polyvinyl pyrrolidone (PVP). In the Dailies lens, the lubricating agent is released from the lens during wear, whereas in the Acuvue lens, the agent is not released. Results of studies comparing these lenses to their predecessors are few and results regarding how much impact they have appear variable.[6] However, they do provide an option to the patient, and after a trial period, the patient can determine whether he or she detects improvement. A new daily disposable material, Biotrue ONEday (Bausch + Lomb) is called a "hypergel" material by the manufacturer because it will reportedly have benefits beyond current hydrogel materials. The lens has 78% water content and its outer surface mimics the lipid layer of the tear film to prevent dehydration (M. Merchea, personal communication, June 10, 2012). Another benefit of daily disposable lenses is that no solutions are necessary, thereby eliminating preservative sensitivities.

Silicone hydrogel lens materials have demonstrated increased comfort for dry-eye patients.[12,13] This may be because of increased Dk/t, decreased water content, and internal wetting agents and natural wettability of some of the lens materials. Two new lenses that may improve the comfort of dry-eye patients by combining silicone hydrogel materials with daily disposability are 1-day Acuvue TruEye (Vistakon) and Dailies Total 1 (Alcon).

In addition to attempting to find the best lens material for a marginal dry-eye patient, the choice of a care system is important. Hydrogen peroxide is beneficial, especially to patients sensitive to a preserved solution. With the newer preservatives, sensitivity symptoms are more subtle and are often manifested by dryness, decreased wear, and superficial staining. Many dry-eye symptoms may be caused by one-bottle lens care symptoms or coated lenses.[14] A good initial step is to use a nonpreserved hydrogen peroxide care regimen. In addition, there are some new preserved solutions that are reported to increase comfort and decrease dryness (e.g., Revitalens [AMO], Biotrue [Bausch + Lomb], Opti-Free PureMoist [Alcon]). If hydrogen peroxide is not beneficial to the patient, the use of one of these solutions should relieve dryness symptoms. In addition, lubricating drops can be used to rehydrate and rinse the lens in the eye.

Therapeutic Use

Only certain lenses are approved by the U.S. Food and Drug Administration (FDA) for therapeutic use (sometimes called bandage lenses). Close monitoring and frequent replacement are required. Silicone hydrogel lenses with high oxygen permeability (Dk) that are FDA approved for therapeutic use are Air Optix Night and Day (Alcon), PureVision (Bausch + Lomb), and Acuvue Oasys (Vistakon).[15,16] Conditions that warrant the use of a therapeutic contact lens include corneal erosions, chronic epithelial defects, bullous keratopathy, mechanical trauma, dry eyes, and filamentary keratitis. Therapeutic lenses are also used following ocular surgery, to aid in sealing a corneal wound, and for drug delivery. These lenses should not be used in the presence of an active ocular infection, in filtering blebs, or for patients who will not return for follow-up evaluation.[17]

Ocular Disease

Obviously, a patient presenting with a serious ocular or systemic disease is not a good candidate for contact lenses, other than those approved for therapeutic use. For example, diabetic patients are at risk when fitted with soft or GP contact lenses because of a decreased wound-healing ability. However, studies have shown that diabetic patients can successfully wear daily-wear (DW) lenses if carefully monitored.[18] For those patients with some form of ocular compromise (i.e., staining, papillary hypertrophy, deficient tear quality), DW is indicated because prolonged lens wear, such as EW, may increase these symptoms. Additionally, daily disposable lenses should be considered for these patients.

Age

Children fitted with a soft lens may experience difficulty inserting a lens of larger diameter. Most contact lenses in stock are available at a minimum of 13.8 mm diameter, but a smaller diameter may aid in lens insertion. Most children who are motivated to wear a soft contact lens will be able to learn to insert and remove the contact lens. There are custom soft lenses available in diameters of 9 to 10 mm. If the contact lens is considered medically necessary (i.e., aphakia, anisometropia) and the child is too young to perform insertion and removal, the parents may be taught to insert, remove, and care for the lens. In addition, disposable lenses are a good modality for children to provide a cost-effective lens, to be used as spare lenses, and to decrease the complications of lens care.

Presbyopes may have difficulty viewing the lens when inserting, removing, or caring for it. A visibility tint or a cosmetic tint is beneficial to these patients when handling the lens. Additionally, they may appreciate a slightly thicker or higher modulus lens, which is easier to handle.

Aphakia

A high-Dk/t lens material is required for aphakic patients. Generally, these lenses are silicone based, available in limited parameters, and very expensive (see Chapter 17 for more information).

Occupation

There are a variety of occupational factors that can affect lens wear and comfort. Generally, a wearing and replacement schedule should be selected to fit the patient's lifestyle. For patients who work unusual hours or travel frequently, lenses that they can sleep in—even for a few nights only—or daily disposable lenses may be beneficial. The ability to take spare lenses along when traveling is advantageous. With airline restrictions on liquids, daily disposable lenses eliminate the need for extra solution.

Pilots, airline attendants, and computer users are examples of occupations that will benefit from a lens that provides good wettability, such as those suggested for dry eyes noted previously. Occupations that require being outdoors or sports that are performed outdoors may benefit from a lens with an ultraviolet (UV) blocker. UV damage to the eye and surrounding tissue will not be eliminated by a contact lens with a UV blocker alone, but it is one more barrier to UV radiation.

Part-Time Wearers

Patients who might not otherwise be good contact lens candidates or have a desire to wear contact lenses for limited periods of time (i.e., golfing, tennis, and social occasions) may be fitted with soft lenses. These patients are excellent candidates for daily disposable lenses. If daily disposable lenses are not used, caution should be taken by these patients in storing lenses for long periods of time. Lenses should be disinfected before wear, and the storage solution should be frequently changed to minimize contamination and dehydration. Any of the newer solutions, such as Revitalens (AMO), Biotrue (Bausch + Lomb), and OptiFree PureMoist (Alcon) may be used to store the lenses for up to 30 days. Likewise, if it is a hydrogel material, caution should be taken not to overwear the lenses when they have not been worn for a long period of time. Soft lens adaptation takes very little time, making this a good choice for part-time wear.

Refits

Typically, caution should be taken when refitting a long-term GP lens wearer into a soft material. There are occasions when a GP lens wearer may require refitting into a soft lens material, such as inability to adapt to GP lenses, chronic staining, or chronic adherence that will not improve with GP lens parameter changes.[19] In these cases, the patient should reduce lens-wearing time or completely de-adapt to determine if the cornea will change or remain stable. Disposable trial lenses are successful for these patients, as the trial lenses can easily be changed if the cornea fluctuates after discontinuing the GP lenses. When the corneal curvature and refractive error stabilize, the final soft lenses can be ordered.

Compliance

If a patient is noncompliant with lens care and disinfection of lenses, a daily disposable lens should be considered. Frequent replacement schedules may also help to improve compliance for certain patients. Patients who occasionally sleep in their lenses should be fitted into an EW silicone hydrogel lens material even if the intention is to wear the lens on a DW basis. Noncompliance creates a real dilemma for the eye care practitioner about whether to fit the patient into contact lenses or not. Patient education and information regarding adverse events that can occur as a result of noncompliance may aid in the patient's willingness to adhere to directions. Patients who refuse to follow proper wear, care, and handling steps should not be fitted into contact lenses.

LENS SELECTION AND FITTING

Once it has been determined that a patient is suitable for soft lenses, the lens selection process begins. Lens materials may be grouped into many different categories. Basically, patients will desire soft lenses that can be placed in one of the following categories: DW lenses, lenses they can wear overnight (EW or continuous wear [CW]), disposable/frequent-replacement lenses, tinted lenses to enhance or change the eye color, toric lenses, and multifocal lenses. Lenses are available in varying powers, base curve radii (BCRs), diameters, thicknesses, water contents, and tints. To select a lens for the patient, it is important to first determine which one of the aforementioned categories of lens wear the patient is most interested in. Although lenses may be fitted empirically, the ability to fit diagnostic lenses is beneficial to both the patient and the practitioner by increasing patient confidence and compliance while also decreasing lens reorders.[20,21] In addition, for most soft lenses, the patient can be dispensed lenses the same day.

Base Curve Radius

Soft contact lenses will typically be available in two to four different BCRs. On average, the selected BCR is approximately 4 D flatter than the flatter keratometry reading (K). Here is a good guideline to follow:

Flat K is >45.00 D   Fit the steeper BCR
Flat K is 41.00–45.00 D   Fit the median BCR
Flat K is <41.00 D   Fit the flatter BCR

If there are only two base curves, the flatter BCR can be used for flat K readings <45.00 D. For example, many soft contact lenses are available in 8.3- or 8.4-mm, 8.6- or 8.7-mm, and 8.9- or 9.0-mm BCR (or radii very close to these). For this example, if a lens is available in 8.4-, 8.7-, and 9.0-mm BCR, a cornea with average keratometric readings should be diagnostically fitted with an 8.7-mm BCR. If the lens is too tight, a flatter BCR should be attempted, in this case 9.0 mm; if the lens is too loose, a steeper BCR can be fitted, in this case 8.4 mm. Likewise, if the keratometric readings are steeper than 45.00 D, the patient can be initially diagnostically fitted with the 8.4 mm or steeper BCR, and if the keratometric readings are flatter than 41.00 D, a 9.0-mm or flatter BCR can be selected. Corneas that have borderline values (e.g., 45.00 D) might be fitted with an 8.7-mm BCR on one eye and an 8.4-mm BCR on the other eye to determine which is the better fit. Some manufacturers recommend fitting the steep BCR on flatter corneas. It is helpful to verify fitting guidelines before fitting the lens.

A tight lens will exhibit <0.3 mm movement, often producing conjunctival drag, in which the conjunctiva moves with the lens and the lens movement, separate from the conjunctival movement, is little to none. When removed, the tight lens may leave an impression ring on the sclera at the position of the lens edge. A flat lens will move 1 to 2 mm, often moving partially off the cornea. On gazing straight ahead, the lens may be decentered inferiorly on the cornea, and on superior gaze, the lens will drop inferior (Fig. 11.1). In addition, edge lift may be observed inferiorly. If the edge is curling out, the lens will decenter superiorly when the patient views inferiorly. A properly fitting soft lens will be well centered over the cornea and exhibit approximately 0.3 to 0.5 mm movement (Fig. 11.2). In superior gaze, the lens may move as much as 1 mm. Generally, lenses that are thinner will move less. A method called the "push-up test"

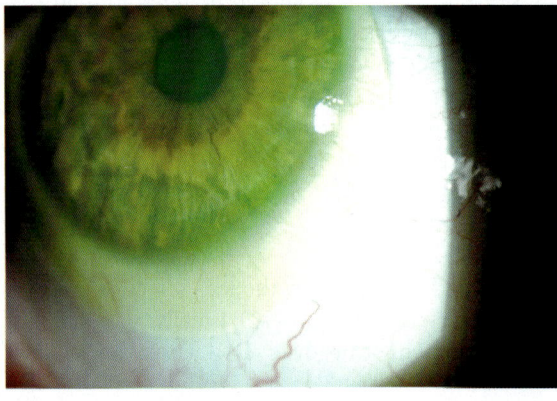

FIGURE 11.1 Lens falling inferiorly when the patient is looking up because of a flat base curve. (Lens is dyed with fluorescein to enhance observation.)

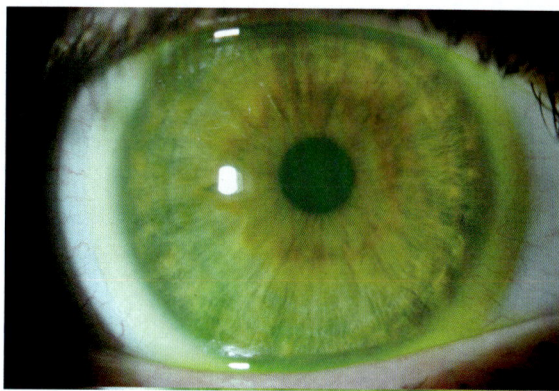

FIGURE 11.2 Well-centered lens with good corneal coverage. (Lens is dyed with fluorescein to enhance observation.)

may be used to judge if the lens is truly tight or just exhibiting minimal movement. This test is performed by gently pushing on the inferior edge of the lens with the lower lid; a tight lens resists movement, whereas an acceptable lens will move when nudged with the lower lid. In one study, the push-up test was found to be the most accurate single test of lens fit acceptability; therefore, it is an important yet simple tool to use in the fitting process.[22] The test is recorded as a positive push-up test when movement is observed and a negative push-up test when the lens shows no movement or there is difficulty in moving the lens with the lid.

Lens Diameter

The overall diameter (OAD) of the soft contact lens is selected to obtain 360 degrees of corneal coverage. Ideally, the lens will extend onto the sclera, at minimum, 0.5 mm in all directions (see Fig. 11.2). By measuring the horizontal visible iris diameter (the diameter across the iris from limbus to limbus) and adding 2 mm, the approximate diameter needed can be obtained (Fig. 11.3). If the lens decenters, a larger-than-predicted OAD may be needed to provide adequate coverage. Lenses are customarily available in diameters of 13.8 to 15.0 mm; however, there are a few manufacturers who produce stock lenses with smaller or larger diameters. Custom lenses with smaller diameters and various BCRs (steep to flat) are available for those difficult-to-fit patients who require parameters outside the normal ranges.

Power

The power of the lens is based on the predicted power and an overrefraction over the diagnostic lens. The predicted power of the lens is determined by the patient's spectacle prescription, which is vertexed back to the corneal plane if the prescription is $>\pm 4.00$ D (Appendix 2). If the patient has a sphero–cylindrical prescription with a low amount of astigmatism, it may be

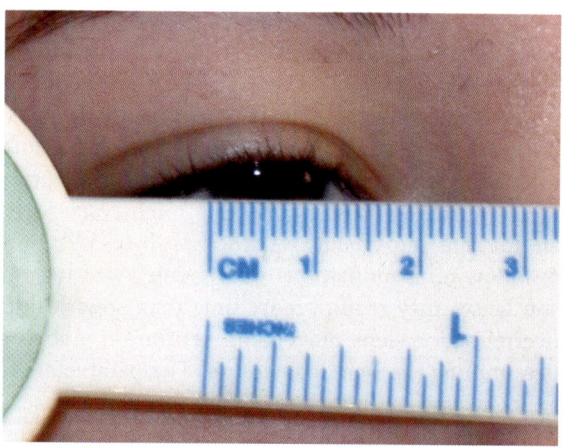

FIGURE 11.3 Demonstration of how to obtain horizontal visible iris diameter.

necessary to use the spherical equivalent to predict the patient's contact lens prescription. The final prescription should be equal to that achieved by the best sphere overrefraction plus the diagnostic lens power, or a close compromise between the predicted power and the overrefraction plus the diagnostic lens power. For example:

Patients 1 and 2

Spectacle Rx: −4.75 D
Vertexed back to corneal plane: −4.50 D
Predicted contact lens (CL) Rx: −4.50 D
Diagnostic CL Rx: −4.00 D

Patient 1

Overrefraction: −0.50 D
Final CL Rx dispensed: −4.50 D

Patient 2

Overrefraction: −1.00 D
Final CL Rx dispensed: −4.75 D

Patient 1 has an overrefraction equal to the predicted Rx. In the case of patient 2, the overrefraction results in a power of −5.00 D; however, the lens dispensed (−4.75 D) is a compromise of the predicted Rx and the overrefraction. The final lens power ordered can be determined after the patient has worn the lens for 1 week and returned for a follow-up evaluation.

Center Thickness

Typically, a center thickness (CT) of a −3.00 D lens will be approximately 0.08 mm. Minus power lenses range from 0.04 to 0.18 mm in CT. Plus lenses range from 0.20 to 0.70 mm in CT.[23] The greater the minus power, the thinner the lens center; likewise, the greater the plus power, the thicker the lens. A thicker hydrogel lens (0.12 mm) is easier for the patient to handle, and thinner hydrogel lenses (0.035 mm) with low water contents may be approved for EW; however, many manufacturers currently provide their standard DW lenses in 0.05 to 0.07 mm thickness for low-minus powers. With the introduction of silicone hydrogel materials, using a hydrogel lens for EW is not recommended. In addition, thicker hydrogel lenses are easier to handle; however, the silicone hydrogel lenses have a higher modulus, which is a benefit for patients who exhibit difficulty in handling a lens.

As a thinner lens tends to drape the cornea more, less lens movement with the blink is commonly experienced. Therefore, these individuals need to be monitored for clinical signs of a tight lens, including absence of lens lag, limbal engorgement, and trapped debris underneath the lens. Likewise, if a thicker, high-water-content lens is used, the patient should be monitored, even if good lens movement with the blink is present initially, as these lenses tend to dehydrate, which will steepen the BCR and reduce lens lag.

After selecting the soft diagnostic lens, the lens should be inserted and allowed to settle. Information varies on how long it takes for a soft lens to settle. One study concluded that evaluating within the first 5 minutes was the optimal time.[24,25] Others have suggested that 10 to 15 minutes is best.[24,25] As this might vary with lens material, practitioners should evaluate the lens movement over the first 5 to 30 minutes and compare that with lens movement at follow-up examinations with greater wearing times (i.e., ≥4 hours). Toric and multifocal soft lenses may require more time than spherical lenses to stabilize on the eye. Visual acuity, overrefraction, lens movement, centration, and coverage should all be evaluated to assist in determining the final lens design. The parameters to specify when ordering a soft contact lens are BCR, power, and name of lens. For some lenses, it may be necessary to additionally specify parameters such as OAD, tint, cylinder with axis, or add power. On lens dispensing, the lenses should be evaluated on the eye, and the patient should be educated on insertion, removal, wearing schedule, normal adaptive symptoms, and lens care (see Chapter 12).

Tinted Lenses

The decision to select a tinted lens depends on the patient's needs and desires (i.e., handling, enhancing, or opaque tints). An enhancing tint enhances the present color of the eye (i.e., a blue eye is made bluer). Opaque tints are used to change eye color. It is not unusual for patients who do not require a refractive correction to desire tinted lenses for the cosmetic effect. Likewise, some patients may desire to wear cosmetic tinted lenses for social occasions. Disposable tinted lenses, especially daily disposable, make occasional social wear a convenient option. Many lenses are available with a handling or visibility tint to make the lens easier to locate.

Disposable/Frequent-Replacement Lenses

Today, it is rare for a patient to wear a conventional soft lens that does not have a predetermined replacement schedule, except for some specialty/custom lenses. Most soft contact lens patients can be fitted with—and will benefit from—a lens that is thrown away, either after a single use, weekly, every 2 weeks, or monthly. Especially beneficial is a disposable, silicone hydrogel lens, which gives the patient the benefits of a clean lens with good Dk/t. More information on disposable and frequent-replacement modalities is presented in Chapter 10.

Silicone Hydrogel Lenses

Silicone hydrogel lenses provide greater amounts of oxygen than hydrogel lenses. The trend in soft lens materials is moving toward the silicone hydrogel materials to improve corneal health. Silicone hydrogel lenses are available in spheres, torics, and multifocals. Most patients will benefit from—and be satisfied with—silicone hydrogel lenses. Silicone hydrogel lenses depend on silicone, not water content, to increase Dk/t through the lens. Patient education will aid in the success of this type of lens. When refitting a hydrogel patient to a silicone hydrogel lens, it is important to discuss the higher modulus of the lens and the improved Dk/t to the cornea. Occasionally, upon refitting from a hydrogel to a silicone hydrogel material, there may be a slight lens sensation after a few days of wear. This may occur due to a hypoxic or edematous cornea that may be less sensitive or "numb." Upon improving Dk/t, the healthier cornea may become more sensitive or less "numb." If the patient continues to wear the lenses for 1 to 2 weeks, an adaptation to the new lens occurs. Additional ways to aid lens comfort include using a lower lens modulus and presoaking the lens in the recommended solution prior to wear. More recent generations of these silicone hydrogel lenses, with improved moisture enhancing packaging solution, have improved initial comfort over the first-generation silicone hydrogels. More information on silicone hydrogel lens materials and care is presented in Chapters 10 and 12.

PROGRESS EVALUATIONS

Lens Evaluation

An optimum-fit soft lens will exhibit good centration, moving 0.3 to 0.5 mm with the blink. In addition, the lens should exhibit complete corneal coverage and extend, at minimum, 0.5 mm onto the sclera. Vision should be 20/25 or better and should be, at minimum, equal to spectacle visual acuity. The lens should be comfortable to be worn 12 to 14 hours for DW, 3 to 7 days for EW, or 30 days for CW, if not worn solely for sports or social occasions. After dispensing of the lenses, evaluations should be performed on a routine basis to ensure that an absence of compromise in corneal physiology is present. For example, follow-up visits for a new daily wearer can be scheduled at 1 week, 1 month, and 6 months after dispensing and every 6 months thereafter. Follow-up visits for a new overnight lens wearer can be scheduled at 1 week, 1 month, 3 months, and 6 months after first wearing the lenses overnight and every 3 months thereafter.

There are complications resulting from soft lens wear; however, with adequate follow-up care and patient compliance, most complications can be prevented. A routine follow-up examination should include the following tests: visual acuity, overrefraction, biomicroscopy (with and without lenses), keratometry, and subjective refraction (Table 11.3). When performing biomicroscopy, the lens should be evaluated for position, coverage, movement, and lens condition. Fingernail tears, edge tears, holes, rust spots, jelly bumps, and protein and lipid deposits can easily be viewed with the lens on the eye by carefully scanning the entire lens surface and the lens edges, including the inferior and superior edges, which may be hidden under the lids. Fingernail tears are generally characteristic slits with a hairlike or lintlike appearance in the central to midperipheral areas of the lens, which result from the lens being pinched off the cornea between the fingernails. Edge tears may appear as an absent wedge-shaped area of the lens or a diagonal slit. Rust spots are orange dots within the lens matrix, which should signal that the patient may be using tap water to rinse the lenses. These can also be caused by the environment or foreign bodies in the eye; however, the most common cause pertains to the use of tap water for rinsing the lenses. Jelly bumps and protein and lipid deposits are all forms of deposits that originate, in part, from the tear film chemistry. Adequate lens care and frequent replacement will help prevent these deposits. When deposits are observed, the practitioner should determine whether the cause is lens age, poor patient compliance, or a tear film predisposed to deposits. Jelly bumps, which can be the result of changes in tear pH, appear as clear-to-white elevations of various sizes and quantity on the front surface of the lens, whereas lipid and

TABLE 11.3 Tests to Perform at Lens Evaluation Visits

Visual acuity
Overrefraction
Overkeratometry
Too steep
Too flat
Clear and undistorted
Biomicroscopy with the lenses on
Lens centration
Lens position
Lens coverage
Lens movement
Condition of the lens (tears, surface deposition)
Biomicroscopy with the lenses off
Limbal vasculature
Fluorescein application
Lid evaluation
Cornea evaluation
Injection
Microcysts
Striae
Polymegethism
Limbal engorgement
Tarsal conjunctiva; follicles, papillae
Keratometry
Subjective refraction

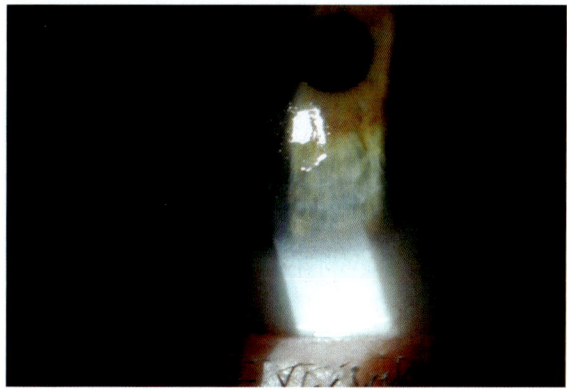

FIGURE 11.4 Lipid deposits on a lens.

protein deposits appear as a film, with lipid deposits exhibiting a greasy film (Fig. 11.4) and protein deposits as a semiopaque white haze.[26,27]

Keratometry can be performed over the lenses to aid in determining if the fit is too flat or too steep. The mires observed when performing keratometry over the lens should be clear and undistorted. A steep fit will exhibit a clear mire image immediately after the blink that then becomes distorted and blurry, whereas a flat fit will exhibit mire distortion that becomes more distorted immediately after the blink.[28]

Ocular Examination

After removing the lens, the cornea and conjunctiva should be inspected for changes resulting from edema (i.e., striae, microcysts, polymegethism), neovascularization, limbal engorgement, and injection (Fig. 11.5A,B). Fluorescein will assist in the evaluation of numerous possible forms of corneal staining, including inferior arcuate staining from lens dehydration,[29] diffuse

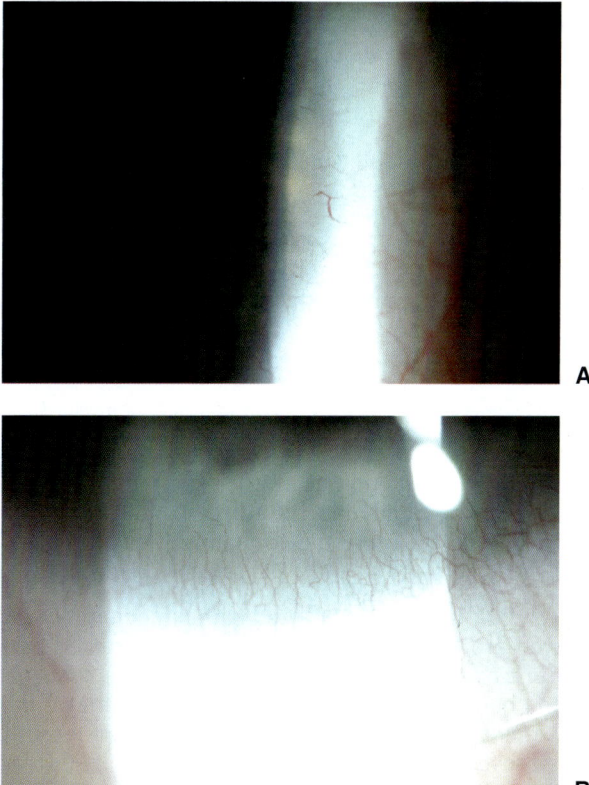

FIGURE 11.5 (A) Limbal vessel engorgement. **(B)** Encroachment.

staining from either an allergic reaction or trapped debris, or a foreign-body stain. In addition, fluorescein aids in the evaluation of lid papillary hypertrophy upon eversion. It is important to evaluate the lids and the cornea with fluorescein at every visit to monitor any subtle changes that may occur with long-term soft lens wear, such as GPC (also known as CLPC) or corneal staining. Care must be taken to rinse the fluorescein from the eye by repeated use of saline or have the patient wear spectacles for 2 to 4 hours afterward to prevent staining of the lens. There are high-molecular-weight fluorescein dyes that will not discolor the soft lens; however, fluorescence is reduced, affecting the ability to view staining. If the soft lens should be discolored by fluorescein, it should be replaced, or the lens may be bleached with repeated cycles of hydrogen peroxide. The author has found that most silicone hydrogel lenses do not stain with fluorescein. This is especially helpful for piggyback designs. In an in-office test at the author's practice, fluorescein was instilled in a case with silicone hydrogel lenses. Air Optix Aqua, Air Optix Night and Day (Alcon) and Acuvue Oasys (Vistakon) cleared within 10 minutes in a multipurpose solution. Biofinity (CooperVision) and PureVision (Bausch + Lomb) were still stained, but after sitting in ClearCare (Alcon), the lenses cleared.

SUMMARY

Soft contact lenses are relatively simple to fit. A well-fitted lens, thorough evaluation, and follow-up examinations will aid in successful lens wear. Soft lenses are popular with patients because of the initial comfort and the ability to fit and dispense lenses from inventory.

CLINICAL CASES

CASE 1

A 45-year-old attorney expresses a desire for contact lenses. In his spare time, he plays golf, basketball, and is involved in numerous other athletic activities. He typically wears bifocal spectacles while at work; however, he would like to wear contact lenses when involved in recreational activities. His refraction is −3.00 − 0.50 × 180 with a +1.25 add OU, and his keratometry readings are 42.00 @ 180/42.37 @ 90 OU.

SOLUTION: Disposable lenses, especially daily disposable, would be beneficial to this patient since he desires lenses he can wear occasionally while participating in sports. Successfully fitting this patient with good near and distance visual acuity may transform him from a part-time to a full-time contact lens wearer.

The benefits of soft lenses for a patient desiring recreational lenses include the opportunity for occasional wear and limited risk of decentration or loss. Most likely, he will need the medium BCR available because his K readings are 42.00 D. The final lens power will depend on the overrefraction; typically, it will equal the spherical equivalent, −3.25 D.

CASE 2

A 12-year-old girl and her mother enter the office to be fitted with contact lenses. The girl appears to be highly motivated for contact lens wear. Her mother says she is very responsible. The girl is interested in making her gray eyes green. The patient's refractive error is OD −4.50 DS and OS −4.25 DS, and the keratometric readings are 42.00 DS OU.

SOLUTION: The patient is fitted with a medium BCR, such as 8.6 or 8.7 mm. The predicted lens powers are OD −4.25 D and OS −4.00 D vertexed back to the corneal plane. A green enhancing tint or a green opaque tint changes the color of the girl's gray eyes in addition to providing her with an automatic handling tint that is beneficial for first-time wearers. This type of patient is generally successful with contact lenses because visually she will think her sight is improved and cosmetically she will think her appearance is improved. As a result of peer pressure to maintain an attractive appearance, the probability of her being successful is quite good. This patient would be an excellent candidate for disposable or frequent-replacement tinted lenses, not only for the improved health, but also for spare lenses in case of lens loss or damage. In addition, using a daily disposable tinted lens would give her the option of wearing clear lenses, plus a variety of tinted opaque lenses that may be discarded after use.

CASE 3

A patient desires to be fitted in soft lenses. Her refraction is OD −5.00 DS, OS −3.00 − 1.00 × 180. The keratometric readings are OD 42.50 @ 180/42.75 @ 90 and OS 43.00 @ 180/43.75 @ 90. The horizontal visible iris diameter (HVID) is 12 mm. All ocular findings, including tear quality and quantity, are normal.

SOLUTION: The BCR selected for the OD is 8.3 mm and the OS is 8.9 mm. The diameter selected is 14.0 mm OD and 14.5 mm OS, which should provide adequate corneal coverage since the HVID + 2 would be 14 mm. The diagnostic lens for the OD is −4.50 D and the OS −3.00 to 0.75 × 180. After evaluating the lenses on the eye, the BCR is changed to an 8.6 mm/−3.00 D OD as the lens appeared slightly tight on the push-up test and conjunctival drag was present with the blink. With good centration and movement of 0.5 mm OU, an overrefraction results in OD −0.25 D and OS Plano with a visual acuity of 20/15 OU. The final lens parameters ordered are OD: 8.6 mm BCR, −4.75 D power and OS: 8.9 mm BCR, −3.00 to 0.75 × 180 power. The lenses are available in a handling tint, which will assist in lens handling.

CASE 4

A 20-year-old woman is prone to jelly bumps and deposits. She replaces her lenses about every 2 to 3 weeks. Changing the care regimen does not appear to solve the problem.

SOLUTION: The patient is fitted into a daily disposable lens. This provides clean, new lenses every day, ensuring good health and convenience. A care regimen is not necessary as the lenses are disposed daily; therefore, even though the lens fees are higher, the patient has reduced cost for solutions.

CASE 5

A 28-year-old man has worn contact lenses for 12 years. He has completed his training as a paramedic and has increased his wearing time from 17 to 20 hours. He states that his eyes become very red and irritated by the end of the wearing period. He is currently wearing a DW hydrogel lens material. Biomicroscopy reveals good centration and lens movement; however, upon lens removal, microcystic edema, conjunctival injection, and incipient superior corneal neovascularization are present.

SOLUTION: This patient needs to be refitted into a silicone hydrogel lens material. Whether he wants to wear the lenses EW or DW, this material will increase the Dk/t six to eight times. Increasing the Dk/t will reduce clinical signs of corneal hypoxia like edema and neovascularization. Educating the patient on some initial adaptation may be necessary, as the hypoxia he is experiencing causes his eyes to be less sensitive. As the health of his eye improves with silicone hydrogel wear, the sensitivity may increase. After 1 to 2 weeks, he should be over any adaptation symptoms. A silicone hydrogel material should make him very comfortable wearing the lenses for 17 to 20 hours while eliminating the edema. Another alternative for him might be a daily disposable silicone hydrogel lens, which he can throw away upon removal; this may be especially beneficial when he is tired.

CASE 6

A 26-year-old woman presents to the office to be fitted with soft contact lenses for the first time. The case history reveals that the patient is 3 months pregnant. All other findings make this patient a good soft contact lens candidate.

SOLUTION: She should be educated on what changes may occur during pregnancy (e.g., dry eyes caused by increased tear viscosity, changes in corneal curvature and vision). It may be beneficial for her to wait to be fitted (e.g., until 6 weeks postpartum or 6 weeks after discontinuation of breast-feeding); however, she should be reassured that she is a good contact lens candidate. Education is imperative, so as not to have her base future contact lens wear success on her current poor experiences due to pregnancy-related ocular symptoms. Many contact lens wearers successfully continue lens wear during pregnancy with no ocular problems.

CASE 7

An 18-year-old man desires to be fitted with soft lenses. He wants to wear the lenses two to three times a week. He desires little care and mentions his busy lifestyle. His demeanor, in addition to his comments, causes the practitioner some concern about potential patient noncompliance.

SOLUTION: The best option for this patient is a daily disposable lens. This type of lens would require no lens care as the lens would be thrown away daily after wear. In addition, concern about proper lens disinfection and storage would not be an issue with daily disposable lenses. Solution cost would be minimal as only the solution in the blister pack to insert the lenses is needed. This patient *must* be educated on the complications that may occur with noncompliance. Photographs or video may be used to demonstrate complications of noncompliance. If this patient appears to be very noncompliant, it may be necessary for the practitioner to refuse to fit him.

CASE 8

A patient is fitted in a soft lens, BCR of 8.4 mm, worn DW. The lenses are available in BCR of 8.4, 8.7, and 9.0 mm. The patient returns in 2 weeks for a follow-up evaluation of the trial lenses. The patient has had the lenses on for 6 hours. Upon the return visit, engorged limbal vessels and conjunctival drag are observed.

SOLUTION: This lens is too tight. The BCR may be flattened to 8.7 mm and the lens movement should be increased. The use of trial lenses and a trial period of wear are helpful to determine lens fit, lens rotation of toric lenses, and visual acuity. Although many times the trial lenses are successful, occasionally a patient returns for follow-up evaluations with a subjective symptom or clinical sign that requires a change in the BCR, diameter, lens material, power change, etc.

CASE 9

A 55-year-old woman complains of her eyes feeling dry all the time. She also thinks the lens will fall out of her eye with quick eye movements. She has used rewetting drops in the past but only experiences relief immediately after using them. She is wearing disposable lenses (medium water content) on a DW basis. She would like to continue wearing disposable lenses. Biomicroscopy results in a tear breakup time (TBUT) of 5 seconds OD and 6 seconds OS.

SOLUTION: If the patient would like to continue with disposable lenses, she has several options. Disposable/frequent-replacement lenses that are recommended for marginal dry eyes are Proclear (CooperVision) and Extreme H_2O (Hydrogel Vision Corp). In addition, silicone hydrogel lens materials may be an alternative (See Chapter 10). Daily disposable lenses like Proclear 1 Day (CooperVision), Soflens Daily Disposable and Biotrue ONEDay (Bausch + Lomb), Dailies with Aqua Comfort Plus (Alcon), and 1-Day Acuvue Moist (Vistakon) may be beneficial in making contact lens wear more successful and comfortable. Two silicone hydrogel daily disposable alternatives would be 1-Day Acuvue TruEye (Vistakon) and Dailies Total 1 (Alcon). Patient education about the composition of her tears and the problems associated with low TBUT should be reviewed. If refitting her into a lens that is recommended for dry eyes does not work for her, she may require more aggressive treatment for her dry eyes (see Chapter 23).

CASE 10

A patient is wearing an EW hydrogel lens EW for 7 to 10 days. She replaces the lenses about once a month. She is satisfied with her vision and comfort. Upon examination with the biomicroscope, neovascularization is observed 360 degrees around the limbus.

SOLUTION: The patient is educated that although her hydrogel lenses were approved for 7-day EW, there are new materials that provide up to eight times more oxygen to the cornea. A digital photo of her cornea is taken to demonstrate the hypoxic condition of the cornea. She is enthusiastic to try a silicone hydrogel lens that she can sleep in. She is refitted in a monthly silicone hydrogel approved for EW and she intends to take the lenses out once a week for overnight disinfection. At her 2-week follow-up examination, digital photos are taken to demonstrate that the increased oxygen has resulted in a whiter eye, with emptying of the limbal vessels.

CASE 11

A 10-year-old myope is brought for a contact lens fitting by her mother. She has a prescription of −1.50 D OU. The mother reports that the girl is a good student and very responsible. All testing is normal and the girl is motivated to wear contact lenses.

SOLUTION: This young girl is a good candidate for contact lenses. Because she plays soccer and basketball, it is decided that a soft lens would be the best option for her. The benefits of a silicone hydrogel lens are discussed with the girl and her mother. The girl is fitted with a 2-week silicone hydrogel lens to be worn DW. This girl is likely to be a long-time contact lens wearer; therefore, fitting her in a silicone hydrogel lens will be beneficial to her long-term ocular health. In addition, the increased modulus of a silicone hydrogel lenses may be easier for a young, first-time wearer to handle.

CLINICAL PROFICIENCY CHECKLIST

- Patient selection is as important to contact lens fitting success as lens selection.
- In selecting patients for soft contact lenses, it is important to evaluate motivation, occupation, compliance, hygiene, and intended use.
- Soft lens advantages versus GP lenses include initial comfort, variable wearing schedule, the availability of daily disposables, and the ability to fit and replace lenses from an existing inventory.
- Lens selection includes selecting the following: BCR, power, OAD, material, tint, wearing schedule, and replacement schedule.
- BCR selection is generally the flattest lens that provides adequate but not excessive movement.
- An ideally fitted soft lens will center well, cover the cornea completely, and move 0.3 to 0.5 mm with the blink.
- The push-up test is a simple but accurate method of determining an optimal lens fit.
- The proper power of the initial lens is determined by calculating the spherical equivalent of the refraction at the corneal plane (i.e., effective power considerations will be necessary for $>\pm 4$ D). Any spherical overrefraction over this lens should then be added to the diagnostic lens power to achieve the final contact lens power.
- Adequate follow-up evaluations are important to reduce the risk of complications.
- Follow-up evaluations should include visual acuity, overrefraction, biomicroscopy with and without lenses, keratometry with and without lenses, lid eversion, and subjective refraction.
- Fluorescein evaluation, an often neglected step in evaluating eyes that wear soft lenses, is an important part of the follow-up evaluation.

REFERENCES

1. Edrington TB, Schornack JA. Initial evaluation. In: Bennett ES, Weissman BA, eds. *Clinical Contact Lens Practice*. Philadelphia, PA: Lippincott Williams & Wilkins; 2005:197–213.
2. Yeung KK, Weissman BA. Soft contact lens application. In: Bennett ES, Weissman BA, eds. *Clinical Contact Lens Practice*. Philadelphia, PA: Lippincott Williams & Wilkins; 2005:363–379.
3. Mandell RB. Basic principles of hydrogel lenses. In: Mandell RB, ed. *Contact Lens Practice*. 4th ed. Springfield, IL: Charles C. Thomas; 1988:502–528.
4. Kollbaum P, Bradley A. Aspheric contact lenses: fact or fiction. *Contact Lens Spectrum*. 2005;20(3):34–38.
5. Vaz TC, Gundel RE. High-and low-contrast visual acuity measurements in spherical and aspheric soft contact lens wearers. *Cont Lens Anterior Eye*. 2003;26(3):147–151.
6. Nichols JJ. Mechanism of contact lens-related dry eye. *Contact Lens Spectrum*. 2007;(special edition):14–20.
7. Doughty MJ, Fonn D, Richter D, et al. A patient questionnaire approach to estimating the prevalence of dry eye symptoms in patients presenting to optometric practices across Canada. *Optom Vis Sci*. 1997;74(8):624–631.
8. Begley CG, Chalmers RL, Mitchell L, et al. Characterization of ocular surface symptoms from optometric practices in North America. *Cornea*. 2001;20(6):610–618.
9. Brennan NA, Efron N. Hydrogel lens dehydration: a material-dependent phenomenon? *Contact Lens Forum*. 1987;12(4):28–29.
10. Orsborn GN, Zantos SG. Corneal desiccation staining with thin high water content contact lenses. *CLAO J*. 1988;14:81–85.
11. Landers RA, Rixon AJ. Contact lens materials update: options for most prescriptions. *Contact Lens Spectrum*. 2005;20(3):24–28.
12. Dillehay SM, Miller MB. Performance of Lotrafilcon B silicone hydrogel contact lenses in experienced low-Dk/t daily lens wearers. *Eye Contact Lens*. 2007;33(6, pt 1):272–277.
13. Schafer J, Mitchell GL, Chalmers RL, et al. The stability of dryness symptoms after refitting with silicone hydrogel contact lenses over 3 years. *Eye Contact Lens*. 2007;33(5):247–252.
14. Caroline PJ, Andre MP. Profession still deciding between preservative free and preserved chemical disinfection. *Primary Care Optometry News*. 1997;1(6):32.
15. Mack CJ. Contact lenses 2007. *Contact Lens Spectrum*. 2008;23(1):26–34.
16. Gromacki, S. The case for bandage soft contact lenses. *Rev Cornea Cont Lens*. January 2012. http://www.reviewofcontactlenses.com. Accessed May 30, 2012.
17. Chan WK, Weissman BA. Therapeutic contact lenses. In: Bennett ES, Weissman BA, eds. *Clinical Contact Lens Practice*. Philadelphia, PA: Lippincott Williams & Wilkins; 2005:619–628.
18. O'Donnell C, Efron N. A prospective evaluation of contact lens wear in diabetes. *Optom Vis Sci*. 1996;73(125):163.
19. Henry VA, Campbell RC, Connelly S, et al. How to refit contact lens patients. *Contact Lens Forum*. 1991;16(2):19–30.
20. Bennett ES, Henry VA, Davis LJ, et al. Comparing empirical and diagnostic fitting of daily wear fluorosilicone/acrylate contact lenses. *Contact Lens Forum*. 1989;14(3):38–44.
21. Benoit DP. Diagnostic fitting is a precise and confident way to fit lenses. *Contact Lens Spectrum*. 2010;25(4):12.21.
22. Young G. Evaluation of soft contact lens fitting characteristics. *Optom Vis Sci*. 1996;73(4):247–254.
23. Thompson TT. Tyler's Quarterly Soft Contact Lens Parameter Guide. 2012;29(3):1–27.
24. Schwallie JD, Bauman RE. Fitting characteristics of Dailies™ daily disposable hydrogel contact lenses. *CLAO J*. 1998;24(2):102–106.
25. Davis RL, Becherer PD. Techniques for improved soft lens fitting. *Contact Lens Spectrum*. 2005;20(8):24–27.
26. Kleist FD. Appearance and nature of hydrophilic contact lens deposits. I. Protein and other organic deposits. *Int Cont Lens Clin*. 1979;6(3):49–58.
27. Kleist FD. Appearance and nature of hydrophilic contact lens deposits. II. Inorganic deposits. *Int Cont Lens Clin*. 1979;6(4):177–186.
28. Mandell RB. Hydrogel lenses with spherical surfaces. In: Mandell RB, ed. *Contact Lens Practice*. 4th ed. Springfield, IL: Charles C. Thomas; 1988:540–553.
29. Zadnik K, Mutti D. Inferior arcuate staining in soft contact lens wearers. *Int Cont Lens Clin*. 1984;12(1):110–115.

Chapter 12

Soft Lens Care and Patient Education

Vinita Allee Henry and Olivia K. Do

DISINFECTION

Many complications of soft lens wear develop after the lenses have been successfully fitted, when patients care for and handle their lenses. Problems arise in numerous ways, such as when patients delete steps in the care regimen, alter the care regimen, or care for and handle the lenses in a careless manner. Because of the nature of soft lens materials, these lenses are susceptible to contamination by bacteria and fungi. Routine lens care, including disinfection and rubbing the lens, is necessary to prevent lens contamination. Soft lens care systems are changed and updated frequently, which makes it difficult for the practitioner to stay updated. This chapter addresses soft lens care and patient education to improve lens care and compliance.

There are three methods of disinfection used with soft lenses: chemical, oxidative (hydrogen peroxide), and thermal. Each has its own advantages and disadvantages. Becoming aware of these advantages and disadvantages will aid the practitioner in selecting the care regimen best suited for each patient and each lens. With a wide variety of care systems available, it is easiest for the practitioner to use only one care system; however, it is beneficial to select a care system appropriate for each individual patient, rather than provide all patients with the same care regimen.

Another issue involved in selecting care regimens is providing a lens that requires no care regimen at all. There are several daily disposable lenses available that allow the contact lens wearer the option to insert a clean, sterile lens each morning and throw it away each night. These wearers only need the solution that is available in the blister pack. If they find that they need to remove the lens during the day and reinsert it, rewetting drop or saline or multipurpose solution (MPS) to aid in inserting the lens may be helpful. This is a viable option for many soft lens wearers. Additionally, other single-use soft lenses worn for 1 week or 30 days continuously and disposed upon lens removal require only a solution for use with inserting the lens.

Chemical Disinfection

Chemical systems (also called MPSs) that combine cleaning, rinsing, and disinfection are extremely popular with patients and practitioners because of their simplicity. MPSs consist of a combination of disinfecting/cleaning/rinsing solution containing one or more preservatives. A separate surfactant cleaner, enzymatic cleaner, or both may be added; however, with disposable/frequent-replacement soft lenses, these additional solutions are rarely necessary. These one-bottle care systems are very popular and are especially beneficial for those patients who tend to be noncompliant when using multiple bottles or are confused by a complicated system.

The problem that originally became apparent with chemical disinfection systems was the use of preservatives, such as thimerosal and chlorhexidine. Although both of these preservatives exhibit excellent preservative action, many patients were sensitive to them. The preservatives currently used cause less patient sensitivity due to their larger molecular weight and difficulty penetrating the lens matrix.[1] Occasionally, some patients may still exhibit sensitivity, reporting symptoms of dryness, itching, burning, injection, decreased wearing time, and discomfort. A condition termed "multipurpose nonkeratitis" has been reported.[2] The soft contact lens wearer using a multipurpose chemical solution presents with normal external findings, but complains of ocular dryness. Changing the patient to a preservative-free, hydrogen peroxide care regimen alleviates the dry-eye symptoms. A study with adolescents found that overall, patients on a hydrogen peroxide system show less staining and inflammatory response than those patients using a chemical care regimen.[3] The Andrasko Staining Grid and the Institute for Eye Research (IER) Matrix both pertained to solution-induced corneal staining (SICS). In the Staining Grid study, staining was assessed after 2 hours of wear and overnight soaking. The IER study investigators looked for the presence of staining three times over a 3-month period. Both studies found a hydrogen peroxide care regimen (ClearCare-Alcon) to perform well with four silicone hydrogel materials (Acuvue Advance & Acuvue Oasys-Vistakon, Air Optix Night and Day-Alcon and PureVision-Bausch + Lomb). The three chemical care regimens resulted in inducing more corneal staining to a small extent in the Staining Grid study and even more in the IER Matrix Study.[4] An updated version of the Andrasko Staining Grid concludes that hydrogen peroxide use with Biofinity (CooperVision) demonstrates similar results versus chemical regimens.[5] Although the sensitivity rate may be lower with the newer preservatives, the practitioner needs to be aware that symptoms of sensitivity to new preservatives may be delayed and somewhat vague. If in doubt, changing the patient to a unpreserved care regimen or a daily disposable contact lens modality may eliminate the symptoms.

Additionally, the preservatives in some, especially earlier generation chemical care regimens, are not as effective against bacteria, fungi, and *Acanthamoeba* as hydrogen peroxide care regimens. Chemical care regimens have been removed from the market due to cases of *Fusarium* (ReNu MoistureLoc) and *Acanthamoeba* (Complete Moisture Plus) that were linked to the use of these solutions. Although patient noncompliance may be partially responsible in these two outbreaks, it is also believed that the disinfection efficacy of these two solutions was decreased, part of the formulation facilitated the pathogen growth, and the solution caused disruption to the corneal surface, creating a portal for the infection to occur.[6] Extended wear (EW), noncompliance, and poor lens hygiene increase the chances of a fungal infection.[7,8] The risk of *Acanthamoeba* keratitis is increased by tap water use, swimming, use of hot tubs and showering with contact lenses on, and improper care. More recent outbreaks of *Acanthamoeba* keratitis were thought to be associated with changes in water purification.[9,10] Digital rubbing in chemical regimens is important in removing *Acanthamoeba* from the lens.[11] Digital rubbing and rinsing have been found to remove up to 99% of *Acanthamoeba* found on a lens prior to chemical disinfection.[12] As would be expected, one study found that the care regimen (chemical or oxidative) is most effective when all steps are performed (i.e., rubbing, rinsing, and disinfecting).[13] The effects of previous chemical disinfection alone on *Acanthamoeba* and the Human immunodeficiency virus (HIV) virus were minimal.[14] Other wearer tips to minimize the risk for *Acanthamoeba* keratitis include if lenses are worn during swimming, airtight goggles should be worn and, if not, the lenses should be disposed immediately after swimming.[15] For more information on diagnosis and treatment of *Fusarium* and *Acanthamoeba*, see Chapter 21.

The past issues of chemical disinfection systems led to updated regulations for lens care systems. The US Food and Drug Administration (FDA) recommended that contact lens MPSs remove "no rub" from labeling and instead emphasize the importance of rubbing and rinsing lenses. In addition, there are recommendations to add *Acanthamoeba* as a test organism.[16] The three most recent MPSs to enter the marketplace (RevitaLens-Abbott Medical Optics or AMO, Opti-Free PureMoist-Alcon & Biotrue-Bausch + Lomb) approach or exceed the disinfection characteristics of hydrogen peroxide for various organisms. All three have some effect against *Acanthamoeba* trophozoites, but RevitaLens is the most effective against *Acanthamoeba* cysts.[17]

Chemical disinfection may be used on all types of lenses and has little effect on lens life. At minimum, 4–6 hours are required for a chemical disinfecting cycle; however, as most patients perform disinfection overnight, this is rarely a disadvantage. Although no rub, rinsing only

MPSs have been promoted to lens wearers in the past, rubbing the lens with the MPS *before* disinfection is an important step to prevent the preservatives from binding to deposits, thus decreasing the effectiveness of disinfection. In addition, cleaning alone has been found to remove >90% of a measured amount of bacteria placed on new and used contact lenses, thus enhancing disinfection.[18] The FDA advises that all patients exercise the rub and rinse method with their lenses in conjunction with their lens care system.[19] The importance of rubbing and rinsing before disinfection cannot be overemphasized, as rubbing is often the first step noncompliant patients eliminate in their lens care systems. The microbial efficacy of these systems is based on the entire regimen (rubbing, rinsing, and disinfection), and when steps are omitted, the efficacy is thus reduced.[20]

SoloCare Aqua (Menicon) is the one chemical disinfection system that can be completed in five minutes. To disinfect a lens in five minutes, the lens should be rubbed on both sides for 10 seconds with three drops of SoloCare Aqua, rinsed and then soaked in SoloCare Aqua for five minutes. This brief disinfection time is helpful if the patient must remove a lens during the day, or used for in-office disinfection, for example, during the eye examination or a lens that has been dropped during insertion. This system is available in Canada and Europe and was previously known as Aquify (CibaVision) in the U.S.[21]

If a patient has a reaction to the preservatives in the solution, the preferable method would be to replace the lens. This is a simple process with a disposable lens. However, if the patient is wearing a conventional-replacement, custom lens that needs to be salvaged, purging the lens may remove the offensive preservative. To purge a lens, it should be placed in a vial of distilled water for 8 hours and this process should be repeated for a total of three cycles. An 8-hour cycle in saline followed by disinfection in a unpreserved system will complete the purging. Purging may also be used to remove fluorescein from a lens that has been stained with fluorescein dye. The author's experience is that most silicone hydrogel materials (Acuvue Oasys-Vistakon, Air Optix Aqua and Air Optix Night and Day-Alcon) that have been stained with fluorescein will return to a clear lens after placement in saline or MPS for a short time (<10 minutes). Biofinity (CooperVision) and PureVision (Bausch + Lomb) will clear after being placed in ClearCare.

A complete listing of available chemical disinfecting solutions is provided in Table 12.1.[22–25]

Oxidative Disinfection (Hydrogen Peroxide)

Another method of disinfection, oxidative disinfection, consists of a 3% hydrogen peroxide solution, neutralizing tablet or disc, case vial, and possibly a saline. Neutralization, by the disc or tablet, takes approximately 6 hours. The neutralizing tablet with Oxysept contains cyanocobalamin, which tints the solution pink to confirm that the tablet has been added to the hydrogen peroxide.[26] The case vial should be replaced every 3 months. Oxidative disinfection can be more complicated and confusing for patients; however, one-bottle oxidative systems have greatly reduced patient confusion over its use. Oxidative disinfection is safe, effective, and preservative-free. Contact lens wearers who use oxidative disinfection typically are very loyal to their system. Patients, particularly those with solution sensitivities, find oxidative disinfection can make the difference between comfortable, all-day wear, and the inability to achieve comfortable wear.

Oxidative disinfection uses hydrogen peroxide which, in addition to disinfection, provides a deep cleaning of the lens via penetration and expansion of the lens matrix. Hydrogen peroxide is hypotonic and has a pH of 4, which makes it effective at removing protein, lipid, and trapped debris.[26–28] Hydrogen peroxide has long been known for its antimicrobial characteristics. A longer exposure time has been recommended to be more effective against fungi and *Acanthamoeba*. This is accomplished by soaking the lenses 45 to 60 minutes in the hydrogen peroxide solution. Hydrogen peroxide is also effective against the HIV virus and against fungal contamination by Aspergillus on soft contact lenses.[29]

Hydrogen peroxide is very acidic and will produce a mild-to-moderate punctate keratitis if it comes in contact with the cornea. No severe damage results if the patient fails to neutralize

TABLE 12.1 Chemical Disinfection Solutions

BRAND NAME	MANUFACTURER	PRESERVATIVE	WETTING AGENT	LONG-TERM STORAGE
Complete Multi-Purpose	Abbot Medical Optics (AMO)	PHMB	Poloxamer 237	30 days
Revitalens OcuTec	Abbot Medical Optics (AMO)	Alexidine dihydrochloride, polyquaternium-1	Tetronic 904	30 days
Opti-Free Express	Alcon	Polyquad & Aldox	Tetronic 1304	30 days
Opti-Free RepleniSH	Alcon	Polyquad & Aldox	TearGlyde (Tetronic 1304 & C9-ED3A)	30 days
Opti-Free PureMoist	Alcon	Polyquad & Aldox	Hydraglyde polyoxyethylene-polyoxybutylene (EOBO)	30 days
SoloCare Aqua	Menicon	PHMB	Dexpant-5, sorbitol	30 days
ReNu Fresh Multipurpose Solution with Protein Remover	Bausch + Lomb	PHMB	Poloxamine, hydranate	30 days
ReNu Sensitive Multi-purpose Solution Gentle Formula	Bausch + Lomb	PHMB	Poloxamine	30 days
Biotrue	Bausch + Lomb	PHMB & Polyquaternium	Hyaluronan, poloxamine	30 days

Polyhexamethylene biguanide (PHMB), also known as polyhexanide and polyaminopropyl biguanide (PAPB).

the hydrogen peroxide before lens insertion or does not fully neutralize the hydrogen peroxide (e.g., old catalytic disc or too brief of a neutralization/dilution soak); however, the patient will experience burning, stinging, moderate discomfort, and injection. Treatment for this keratitis requires proper neutralization or dilution of the residual hydrogen peroxide in the lens and discontinuing lens wear until the symptoms have disappeared (i.e., 2–12 hours). The frequent use of an artificial tear drop will improve comfort and reduce symptoms for a patient with this type of keratitis. To assist in the prevention of hydrogen peroxide being used directly in the eye, the hydrogen peroxide solutions are currently packaged in bottles with red tips, in addition to warning labels on the bottles that direct the patient not to use this solution directly in the eye (Fig. 12.1).

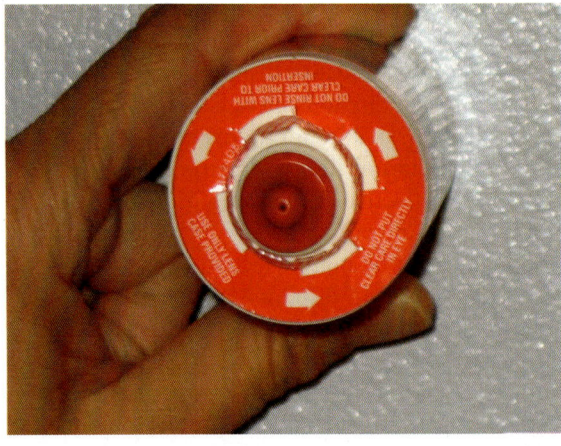

FIGURE 12.1 Red-tipped warning on hydrogen peroxide solution bottle.

An issue with hydrogen peroxide-based systems is the risk of contamination of the lenses stored in the unpreserved solution formed after the period of disinfection. For storage times exceeding those recommended by the manufacturer (typically 7 days), patients should repeat the disinfection step prior to lens wear in order to remove any contaminants that may have found their way into the disinfection chamber. Patients should also remember to disinfect inside of the lens cap by adding fresh hydrogen peroxide and shaking the case a few times.[30]

Removing hydrogen peroxide prior to lens insertion may be accomplished by one of three methods. Two of the three methods are based on a catalyst that is contained primarily in a tablet or platinum disc. AMO has a preservative-free tablet that is placed directly in the vial containing hydrogen peroxide. The neutralizing tablet is coated with a viscosity agent that prevents activation of the tablet for 20 to 30 minutes, thus allowing disinfection with hydrogen peroxide to occur prior to neutralization. This tablet is placed in the vial immediately with the hydrogen peroxide, Oxysept-Ultracare formula (AMO).

The ClearCare vial (identical to the AOSept vial) contains a platinum disc attached to the lens cage that begins neutralizing ClearCare (Alcon) immediately on contact when the lens cage is placed in the vial. The entire vial with the disc should be replaced after approximately 3 months of daily use or 100 cycles if used weekly. When the disc is losing its effectiveness, it will not fully neutralize the hydrogen peroxide, resulting in a mild stinging sensation when the lenses are inserted. The vial also includes an opening in the lid, which should remain upright and unobstructed so that oxygen may escape during the neutralizing step. Sauflon Pharmaceuticals also uses a neutralizing disc to neutralize its hydrogen peroxide solution (Sauflon One-Step Cleaning & Disinfection Solution).

The final method of removing hydrogen peroxide from the lens is dilution of hydrogen peroxide by osmosis with the use of saline solution. Although no commercially available care regimens utilize this method, it might be valuable for the practitioner to be aware of it in cases in which the wearer may need an emergency back-up method for the tablet or disc. The hydrogen peroxide is emptied from the vial after disinfection is completed (10 minutes–12 hours). The lenses and vial are rinsed and agitated with saline solution, followed by standing in fresh saline solution for a specified time period (at minimum 10 minutes). Studies have shown that there is no significant difference in the "sting factor" between this type of method and that of neutralization with a catalyst.[31,32]

Oxidative disinfection systems were previously categorized as one-step or two-step disinfection systems. Currently, only one-step systems are available. Two-step systems have been discontinued, as one-step systems are useful in increasing patient compliance. However, in a one-step system, the concentration of hydrogen peroxide is much reduced and may not provide a long enough exposure time. For example, past studies found that only the two-step systems were effective against *Acanthamoeba* cysts.[11,14,33] A hydrogen peroxide regimen has been found to be significantly more effective against *Acanthamoeba* than chemical disinfection when cleaning and rubbing of the lens were not performed before disinfection.[13] Proper cleaning and rinsing before all types of disinfection will enhance the effects on *Acanthamoeba*. Likewise, hydrogen peroxide has been found to be more effective on *Pseudomonas* than an MPS when cleaning and rubbing were not performed.[34] Evidence shows that hydrogen peroxide is effective against the trophozoite forms of *Acanthamoeba*.[35] ClearCare and AOSept (Alcon) have been found to demonstrate antimicrobial activity against the cyst form of *Acanthamoeba castellani* after 6 hours.[36] In the same study, a multipurpose chemical disinfection solution was shown to have no antimicrobial activity against the cyst form after 6 hours. These findings show protective benefits of hydrogen peroxide for noncompliant contact lens wearers.[34] As mentioned previously, the newer generation of chemical disinfection solutions, RevitaLens, Opti-Free PureMoist, and Biotrue have demonstrated a much higher efficacy against bacteria, fungi, and *Acanthamoeba*. Manufacturers are making the proper attempts to produce effective disinfection systems even for noncompliant patients. Practitioners can reinforce proper lens care with thorough and repeated patient education.

If a daily cleaner is added to a hydrogen peroxide regimen, caution should be taken to ensure that the patient thoroughly rinses the cleaner from the lens prior to disinfection. A chemical reaction between the hydrogen peroxide solution and the catalytic disc will increase the sudsing action of any residual cleaner and may result in all of the hydrogen peroxide pouring out of the opening in the vial, leaving the lenses in an empty vial with inadequate disinfection.

Three percent hydrogen peroxide is commercially available over the counter, typically in brown bottles for nonophthalmic use. The cost of this solution is much less than that of solutions used in contact lens disinfection. Although it is similar to that used for contact lens disinfection, it is not ophthalmically pure and may contain inexpensive stabilizers or heavy metals that may cause lens discoloration. In addition, contamination of the solution may easily occur in these wide-mouthed containers, whereas the narrow openings found in contact lens solution containers decrease the risk of contamination. Available oxidative disinfection systems are listed in Table 12.2.[22–24,26]

Silicone Hydrogel Disinfection and Care

Due to the differences in hydrogel versus silicone hydrogel materials, not all solutions may perform as well with silicone hydrogel lenses. The solutions currently FDA indicated for use with silicone hydrogel lenses are ClearCare, Opti-Free RepleniSH, Opti-Free Express and Opti-Free PureMoist (Alcon), Biotrue (Bausch + Lomb), and RevitaLens (AMO). In addition, silicone hydrogel materials are more prone to lipid deposits due to their hydrophobic nature; therefore, rubbing the lens prior to disinfection is recommended. A daily cleaner such as Sereine Extra Strength Daily Cleaner (Optikem International) is useful for removing lipid deposits if rubbing and frequent replacement of the lenses is not sufficient. In the IER Matrix Study, PureVision lenses were found to exhibit more SICS with Opti-Free RepleniSH, and Opti-Free Express than the other silicone hydrogel materials in the comparison. In the IER and Staining Grid Study, ClearCare performed well with the PureVision material.[4]

Hybrid Lens Disinfection and Care

Hybrid lenses have a rigid gas-permeable (GP) lens center and a soft hydrogel skirt. At this time, SynergEyes makes the only available hybrid lenses. The recommended solution for SynergEyes lens materials is hydrogen peroxide, except for the Duette lens. For the Duette lens material, the recommended solution is Biotrue (Bausch + Lomb). Hydrogen peroxide is not recommended for the Duette lens because some patients will develop an opaque ring around the skirt after approximately 4 to 6 months. The ring is harmless, but is permanent. Opti-Free PureMoist (Alcon) can be used on the Duette lens, but a film occurs on the lens. The film can be removed with 10 to 15 seconds of digital rubbing with saline (J. Sevier, personal communication, June 14, 2012).

Thermal Disinfection

Thermal disinfection is the least expensive and most effective disinfection system in the short term; however, as the heat bakes on the deposits not cleaned off the lens, lens life is shortened and complications such as giant papillary conjunctivitis (GPC, also known as contact lens

TABLE 12.2 Oxidative Disinfection Systems

BRAND NAME	MANUFACTURER	METHOD OF NEUTRALIZATION	RECOMMENDED LONG-TERM STORAGE TIME
Oxysept	AMO	Tablet	7 days
ClearCare	Alcon	Platinum disc	7 days
Sauflon One Step	Sauflon USA	Neutralizing disc	24 hours

*AOSept (Alcon) will be discontinued

papillary conjunctivitis or CLPC) or red-eye reactions may arise from the deposited lens. As a disinfectant, thermal disinfection is effective against all forms of bacteria, including *Pseudomonas*, both cyst and trophozoite forms of *Acanthamoeba*, and the HIV virus. The solutions used with thermal disinfection can be preservative-free for those patients sensitive to preserved solutions. Despite the advantages, the popularity of thermal disinfection has declined to the point where it is not used by contact lens wearers because of electrical requirements and the long-term problem of baked-on deposits. In addition, heat is contraindicated with lenses containing >55% water, and caution must be taken when switching a patient from another type of disinfection to thermal since it is not interchangeable with all systems. Manufacturers no longer support this type of disinfection with heat units for individual use. It can be used for in-office disinfection of vial lenses with the same guidelines mentioned previously for lens materials.

Another alternative method of disinfection that is available is ultraviolet (UV) subsonic disinfection (Purilens UV, Purilens/Lifestyle Co. Inc.).[23]

In-office Disinfection

Most diagnostic soft lenses are used on a one-time basis and discarded. This is the most acceptable method of diagnostic lens use; there is no danger of ocular infection spreading from one patient to the next because the lenses are packaged in sterile containers. At the present time, some diagnostic lenses are reused after being disinfected, which does not produce a sterile lens. Oxidative disinfection, although an excellent method of disinfection, is difficult to use for diagnostic lenses because of the necessity of disinfecting the lens in a special case and transferring the disinfected lens to a glass vial. The lens may become contaminated in the transfer process, or the vial may become contaminated. It is acceptable to store lenses in a glass vial in a chemical disinfecting solution. In addition, it has been recommended, based on study results, that diagnostic lenses disinfected with oxidative or chemical disinfection be redisinfected at least once a month to prevent contamination.[37]

Possibly the best type of in-office disinfection, disregarding disposable diagnostic lenses, is the combination of two disinfection systems. As with any lens worn by the patient, the lens should be thoroughly cleaned and rinsed before disinfection, disinfected in a hydrogen peroxide disinfecting solution for 2 to 12 hours, followed by neutralization, and stored in the glass vial in a chemical disinfection solution. As noted previously, the lenses should be redisinfected every month. The practitioner must keep in mind the limitations of the systems. Any lens used on a known HIV+ patient or a patient exposed to *Acanthamoeba* should be disposed of and not reused, even though at the present time, it is thought that the risk of transmission of HIV via the tears is low.[38,39]

Autoclaving will produce a lens that should be sterile for a year. A procedure for autoclaving includes cleaning the lens with a daily cleaner, rinse with a unpreserved saline, and placing the lens in the glass vial with unpreserved saline. The vial should be sealed and placed in an autoclave. This final method guarantees sterility of the lens.[40]

SALINE

Saline solutions have almost disappeared from the marketplace. Saline solution, which is not toxic to the eye, is a sterile solution used to rinse lenses free of foreign matter and cleaner. In addition, it is used as an in-office rinsing solution or to wet a fluorescein strip. Saline solution is not capable of disinfecting the lens when used alone. Although practitioners are aware of this, it is not always adequately communicated to the patient, and he or she may alter the care system to the use of saline solution alone with no disinfecting solution. The potentially devastating effects of this include vision-threatening complications that can be avoided if the patient is educated initially and the care system is carefully monitored at follow-up evaluations.

When a patient is given a hydrogen peroxide or multipurpose care regimen, a practitioner might feel he or she is benefitting the patient by suggesting he or she use a saline for rinsing.

TABLE 12.3 Salines

BRAND NAME	MANUFACTURER	PRESERVATIVE
Sensitive Eyes Saline Solution	Bausch + Lomb	Sorbic acid & edetate disodium
Sensitive Eyes Plus Saline Solution	Bausch + Lomb	Polyaminopropyl biguanide & edetate disodium
Unisol 4	Alcon	None
PuriLens Solution	PuriLens/Lifestyle	None

Although there is nothing wrong with saline use for rinsing, it sets the patient up for being noncompliant with their care regimen. The saline is really not necessary. The patient is more likely to use the saline for storage, even if only occasionally, than routinely use the disinfectant solution. In addition, it is defeating the purpose of a one-bottle regimen to add saline. Even hydrogen peroxide provides preservative-free saline after neutralization in the vial and this is enough saline to insert and rinse lenses in the morning, making a separate saline unnecessary. A list of available salines is provided in Table 12.3.[23,24]

Saline is available in preserved and unpreserved forms. The first preserved salines were preserved with thimerosal; however, after the sensitivity reactions experienced with thimerosal, less toxic preservatives such as sorbic acid, potassium sorbate, and polyaminopropyl biguanide were used. Currently, the available saline solutions are nonthimerosal preserved or unpreserved. Unpreserved saline solutions are available in aerosol containers and 4 oz. bottles (to be used within 14 days). A benefit of aerosol saline is that the patient is provided with a sterile, unpreserved solution, thus decreasing the risk of solution sensitivity. However, a frustrating problem with aerosol saline occurs when the propellant is depleted before the saline. This results in the inability to use the saline remaining in the container. A few simple tips will prevent this frustration: (a) the nozzle should be turned to match a red dot on the upper rim of the container, and (b) the container should not be tipped below a horizontal position. Both these tips will help prevent the propellant from being used up before the saline solution.[11]

The final type of saline to be discussed is homemade saline made from distilled water and salt tablets. Homemade saline was introduced with the introduction of soft lenses; however, *homemade saline should never be used today*. The sale of salt tablets has been banned by the FDA. There is no benefit to using homemade saline and there are many risks, primarily the possible risk of *Acanthamoeba* keratitis. Sixty percent of reported cases of *Acanthamoeba* keratitis resulted from using homemade saline, swimming with lens wear, or using no disinfection system.[11] The risk presented by homemade saline use is the result of a nonsterile solution that is easily contaminated because the containers used to mix the solution and the large containers of distilled water used to dissolve the tablet may be contaminated.

DEPOSITS

Soft lens-induced complications are largely the result of corneal edema or deposits. The popularity of daily disposable, 1 to 2 week disposable and frequent-replacement soft lenses aid in diminishing the complications found with deposits. When conventional replacement soft lenses are used, proper lens care will aid in maintaining a clean lens surface; however, lens care must be performed routinely as soft lenses are prone to deposits as a result of the hydrophilic surface, patient tear film, environment, and lens handling. A deposited lens will result in a reduction in the effectiveness of the preservatives, oxygen transmission, surface wettability, vision, and wearing time; in addition, the patient is at risk for GPC, red-eye reactions, or corneal ulcers. Silicone hydrogel lenses are more prone to lipid deposits than hydrogel lenses; therefore, rubbing the lens prior to disinfection is important to remove deposits from the lens.

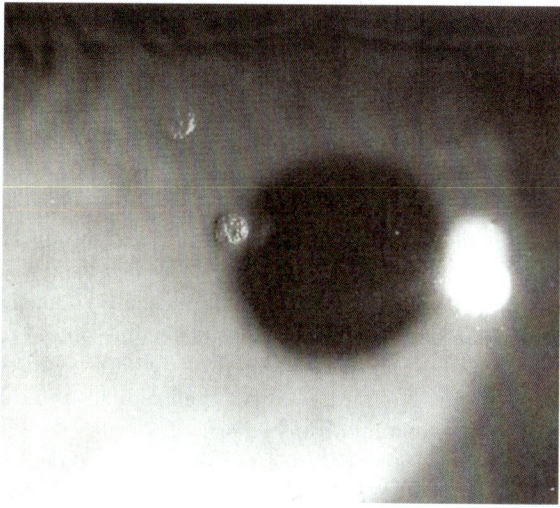

FIGURE 12.2 Jelly bumps on a hydrogel lens.

There are several types of soft lens deposits, which may be identified by the color and appearance of the deposit and categorized as either organic or inorganic deposits.[41,42] The two most common organic deposits are protein, which leaves a white opaque film on the lens surface, and lipids, which have a smeared, greasy appearance. Other organic deposits include pigment deposits, which are a result of melanin polymers in the tears and are increased with the use of thermal disinfection and microorganism growth, which is a result of fungi/yeast appearing in various colors in a filamentary appearance.

"Jelly bumps" are the most common type of inorganic deposit; they occur more frequently in EW. Jelly bumps are named for their characteristic appearance of white to clear elevations on the anterior lens surface (Fig. 12.2). The primary composition is somewhat controversial; however, calcium, lipids, and cholesterol have been found to be a part of the composition.[43,44] Typically, calcium precipitates to form the white base of the deposit. It is then covered with an oily lipid layer and, finally, a mucoprotein outer layer. Jelly bumps become a part of the lens matrix and result in pits in the lens surface if removed. As jelly bumps increase in size and number, vision may be affected and discomfort may be experienced by the patient. Typically, if jelly bumps are observed on a disposable or frequent-replacement lens, the patient is not being compliant with the wear schedule.

Another type of inorganic deposit is a rust spot. The rust spot is generally a circular orange deposit. When a rust spot is observed, the practitioner should immediately question the patient about possible tap water use. Comprehensive patient education and documentation are necessary when rust spots are found. The other possible causes of a rust spot are the environment or a metal foreign body. The concern in the latter case is that the foreign body may still be present in the eye, the lid, or the contact lens; therefore, a careful examination with the biomicroscope is required.

The last type of inorganic deposit observed on soft lenses is the result of contamination with cosmetics, including mascara, hairspray, after-shave lotion, soaps, or suntan lotion. These deposits appear iridescent, filmy, or greasy. Comprehensive patient education will assist in the prevention of these deposits. Simple hand washing before lens handling will greatly reduce this type of contamination.

SURFACTANT CLEANERS

Thorough and routine cleaning will prevent buildup of lens deposition. MPSs contain cleaning agents. If the patient is wearing a conventional lens or prone to deposits, he or she may require a separate surfactant cleaner; however, separate surfactant cleaners are becoming increasingly difficult to find on store shelves. The cleaner, whether in combination with the solution or as a separate cleaner, acts as a soap to remove debris, unbound proteins, lipid deposits, and some microbial contamination. The lens should be placed in the palm of the hand with a few drops of solution or a separate surfactant cleaner and rubbed gently back and forth for 20 to 30 seconds. The back-and-forth motion is less likely to cause lens damage than a circular motion.

After careful cleaning, the lens should be thoroughly rinsed before lens disinfection. The reasons for instructing patients to care for their lenses in this sequence include the following: first, disinfection is greatly enhanced by cleaning and rinsing; secondly, residual cleaner left on the lens will be rinsed off further by the disinfection process, providing a more comfortable lens for the patient on insertion; and finally, deposits will be removed more easily on lens removal than later when the deposits become bound to the lens surface. In addition, the patient should not develop the bad habit of "left lens syndrome" in which the right lens is thoroughly cleaned initially and the patient then reduces the care time given to the left lens, resulting in more contamination of this lens.

Opti-Free Daily Cleaner (Alcon) is an abrasive cleaner preserved with Polyquad. This cleaner has fewer abrasive beads than previous Alcon abrasive cleaners; therefore, rinsing is more effective in removing all the cleaner from the lens. Patients prone to deposits and wearing conventional replacement lenses may benefit from the use of an abrasive cleaner.

Sereine Extra Strength Daily Cleaner (Optikem International), an alternative to MiraFlow (previously produced by Ciba Vision), which has been discontinued contains, among other cleaning ingredients, isopropyl alcohol. Isopropyl alcohol eliminates the need for a preservative because of its broad-spectrum antimicrobial effects. It is also an excellent cleaner, especially for patients with a tendency to lipid deposits, as it dissolves lipids.[11,45,46]

ENZYMATIC CLEANERS

The overwhelming number of contact lens wearers who are fitted in disposable or frequent-replacement soft lenses has almost eliminated the need for enzymatic cleaners. In addition, many MPSs contain ingredients to aid in protein removal. Typically, enzymatic cleaners are reserved for conventional lens replacement patients. For these patients, enzymatic cleaners are to be used once a week to break down peptide bonds, allowing protein to be rubbed off mechanically. The proper care sequence when enzyming soft lenses is to clean and rub, rinse, enzymatically clean and disinfect the lens. Enzyme cleaners are placed in the disinfecting solution and allowed to soak overnight during disinfection. Available enzymatic cleaners are listed in Table 12.4.[23,24]

SupraClens (Alcon) is a daily protein remover. One drop is placed directly in Opti-Free Express or Opti-Free RepleniSH solution in each side of the lens case. The advantages of this cleaner are the convenience it affords the patient, its daily use, and its effectiveness.[47]

LENS LUBRICANTS/REWETTING

The use of lens lubricants or rewetting drops is optional; however, they may be beneficial in cases of dry eyes, foreign-body sensation, irritations, and for morning and evening use in overnight lens wear. Lens lubricants are used directly in the eye with or without the lenses. Patients

TABLE 12.4 Enzymatic Cleaners & Daily Protein Removers

BRAND NAME	MANUFACTURER
Opti-Free Supraclens Daily Protein Remover	Alcon
Ultrazyme Enzymatic Cleaner	AMO

should not substitute artificial tears, GP lens lubricants, or ophthalmic medications for soft lens lubricants because the preservatives are not necessarily compatible with the soft lens materials, the possible result being lens discoloration and toxic reactions. Lubricants that are beneficial to patients by helping clean the lens in the eye are Blink-N-Clean, Opti-Free RepleniSH Rewetting Drop, and Clerz Plus Lens Drops. Blink Contacts, Refresh Contacts, and TheraTears Contact Lens Comfort Drops contain disappearing preservatives to decrease sensitivity reactions.

Contact lens wearers who suffer from symptoms of dryness are especially benefited by a lens lubricant. Lens lubricants initially amounted to little more than a solution similar to saline, but are now carefully formulated to produce solutions that protect and lubricate the eye. The use of disappearing preservatives prevents ocular sensitivities to preservatives (i.e, sodium perborate changes to oxygen and water, and stabilized oxychloro complex changes to sodium chloride and water upon instillation). These preservatives break down when exposed to light, which leaves them preservative-free upon instillation. Wetting agents bind water and aid in spreading the tears between blinks, in addition to retaining the tear film longer. Hyaluronic acid is a viscoelastic component found naturally in the body. Its use in lubricating drops has been found to increase tear breakup time (TBUT), thus improving lens wearing comfort. The potential of these new ingredients to combat dry-eye symptoms is highly useful in lubricating/rewetting drops.[48]

Available lens lubricants or rewetting drops and their manufacturers are listed in Table 12.5.[23,24]

PATIENT EDUCATION AND HYGIENE

Educational Environment

Educating patients about the wearing, handling, and care of soft lenses should be considered as *serious* and *important* to the success of soft lens wear as the fit of the lenses. Patient noncompliance and absence of knowledge are primary causes of soft complications, which may be a result of the patient's lack of concern, the practitioner's lack of seriousness, or both. When patient education becomes secondary, taught by staff members who are less than knowledgeable and with little emphasis, a lack of importance is perceived by the patients that carries over into their lens care routine. Typically, four practitioner factors contribute to patient noncompliance: poor instructions, no instructions, poor example, and overloading the patient with information on the dispensing procedure.[49] Every office should provide the patient with written information

TABLE 12.5 Lens Lubricants/Rewetting Drops

BRAND NAME	MANUFACTURER	PRESERVATIVE	SURFACTANT/WETTING AGENT
Clerz Plus & Opti-Free RepleniSH Rewetting Drops	Alcon	Polyquad	Tetronic 1304 RLM-100
Complete Blink-N-Clean	AMO	Polyhexamethylene biguanide	Tromethamine, tyloxapol, HPMC
Blink Contacts	AMO	OcuPure	Sodium hyaluronate
Theratears CL Comfort Drops	Advanced Vision Research	Sodium perborate	Carboxymethyl cellulose
Refresh Contacts	Allergan	Purite or preservative free	Carboxymethyl cellulose
Sensitive Eyes, ReNu Multiplus, ReNu rewetting drops	Bausch + Lomb	Edetate disodium & Sorbic acid	Povidone

pertaining to insertion and removal, lens care, and lens handling. The Healthy Habits Soft Contact Lens Guide produced by the Association of Optometric Contact Lens Educators (AOCLE) is available for printing at www.aocle.org. Another alternative is for the individual office to personalize an attractive patient booklet. Suggested topics for inclusion (in addition to methods of insertion and removal) are recommended wearing schedule, emergency phone numbers, and consequences of noncompliance. Also, a photograph album or framed poster of contact lens complications (e.g., GPC, ulcers, deposited lenses, *Acanthamoeba* keratitis) that result from noncompliance may be placed in the examination room. These are not to scare the patient away from soft lens wear but to emphasize the seriousness of proper lens wear and care.

The office should provide a good example for the patient. An area that has adequate lighting, capped unexpired solutions, large counter space, and a sink with a drain capable of being closed should be provided for insertion and removal of lenses by patients. A poor example in the office endorses a poor example at home. Likewise, staff and practitioners should set a good example when handling lenses. Even if the practitioner's or staff member's hands have been washed, washing the hands in the patient's presence before handling the lenses reinforces to the patient that this is proper lens care.

The final area where practitioners and staff can be responsible for confusing patients is overloading patients with information on the dispensing procedure. Patient education should be an ongoing process in which the patient's routine is discussed at future visits and bad habits broken before they become routine. Obviously, insertion and removal and lens care must be discussed before the patient takes the lenses home; however, some patients may need more than one visit to learn how to insert, remove, and care for their lenses. Comprehensive written instructions will reassure the patient by reinforcing important points, and patients should be encouraged to phone the office with questions they might have.

Optimum patient education is provided by a trained staff member in an area designed with patient education in mind. This area should include adequate mirrors for teaching insertion and removal, a large counter adjacent to where the patient may be seated, and audiovisual aids. These are a valuable aid in educating both staff members and the patients. If staff members are going to instruct patients in lens care and handling, they should be well-educated in lens care. A checklist of information to be discussed may be helpful to ensure that no information is omitted. An example of a checklist is shown in Table 12.6. In addition, the practitioner may wish to provide the staff member with the opportunity to attend conferences that will train them in contact lens-related topics, such as patient education and lens care.

In addition to new wearers needing education on care and handling of contact lenses, practitioners should never assume that a current contact lens wearer is completing all the steps for proper lens care. The current wearer should be asked to verbally explain their current care regimen. The practitioner should discuss proper lens care with the patient. This should be ongoing at each visit to maintain proper lens care habits.[50] It is also important to review the lens replacement and wear schedule as some patient overwear issues may be the result of patient noncompliance, and others may be related to inadequate or inaccurate education in the past.

Patient Compliance

Even when patient education is optimum, various factors affect patient compliance. Some factors are related to the care system itself, which may be too complex, too time-consuming, or too costly; therefore, a change in the type of lens care system may improve compliance. Manufacturers can assist in this area of noncompliance by a continued effort to develop lens care systems that are simple, effective, and inexpensive. Noncompliance may also occur if the patient takes shortcuts, forms sloppy habits, or is just generally lazy. This type of patient is potentially the most dangerous, and reeducation as well as thorough documentation of noncompliance in the record will be required. It is possible that the patient is using solutions improperly or that substitutions have been made in the lens care regimen. Patients should be

TABLE 12.6 Patient Education Checklist

WAS THE PATIENT TAUGHT THE FOLLOWING TASKS?
Washing hands before handling lenses ____
Lens insertion ____
Lens removal ____
Taco test or other method of determining lens inversion ____
How to open the blister pack ____

WAS THE PATIENT INSTRUCTED IN THE FOLLOWING LENS CARE PROCEDURES?
How to rub/clean a lens ____
How to disinfect a lens ____
When to use saline (optional) ____
When to use a lens lubricating drops ____

WERE THE FOLLOWING TOPICS DISCUSSED?
Hygiene ____
Swimming with lenses ____
Showering in lenses ____
Sleeping in lenses ____
Lens care products to use and not to use ____
Cosmetics ____
Case replacement and cleanliness ____
Lens replacement schedule ____
Normal and abnormal adaptive symptoms ____
Risks of noncompliance ____
Emergency numbers

WAS THE PATIENT REMINDED TO CALL THE OFFICE WITH ANY QUESTIONS REGARDING SYMPTOMS OR LENS CARE? ____

WAS THE PATIENT REMINDED TO WEAR THE LENSES TO FOLLOW-UP EXAMINATIONS? ____

cautioned to consult with their practitioner before changing any solution in their regimen. In the local area, it may be desirable to provide pharmacists with information pertaining to soft lens care and an open invitation to call you if there should be any questions, as pharmacies will at times suggest improper solution substitutions to patients. At each progress visit, it is important to have patients restate their care routine to the practitioner or a staff member to ensure that the care regimen is still accurate. When substitutions have been made, patients may discontinue a step without even realizing it.

Noncompliance was most likely a contributing factor to the outbreaks of *Fusarium* and *Acanthamoeba* keratitis. Despite the fact that most care regimens have returned to the recommendation of rubbing the lens prior to disinfection, the period of "no rub" has resulted in contact lens wearers who believe it is acceptable to place lenses directly in the disinfecting solution without rubbing or rinsing. To aid in patient education of the importance of rubbing a lens, the primary author uses the illustration of a dirty dish that is rubbed and rinsed versus only rinsed. This illustration helps the patient understand the importance of rubbing the lens during the cleaning process.

Past studies evaluating solution cost to the consumer estimated that patients were spending <25% of the amount indicated if they were using the solutions according to directions.[51–53]

This reduction in spending is a perfect example of patient noncompliance. The shortcuts that patients take are easily evident when they are asked about their lens care regimens. One study showed that 82% of 2-week replacement and 53% of 1-month replacement wearers wore their lenses longer than the recommended wearing schedule.[54] Another study found that 7% never clean their case and 48% replace the case annually or less often.[55] Regarding their solution use, a study found that 22% topped off their case and 41% never or almost never rubbed their lenses.[56,57] A survey found that 23% reported soaking or cleaning their lenses with tap water and 12% stored their lenses in something other than a contact lens case.[58]

Private-label solutions create another area of confusion and noncompliance for the lens wearer. In 2011, about 27% of disinfection solution sales were private label.[59] Contact lens wearers believe they are getting identical solutions at a lower price, which is inaccurate. Rather than being identical to the new generation of solutions, many times these solutions are formulations from several generations prior.[60] Great strides have been made to provide effective preservatives that are mild and compatible with the ocular surface and the new solutions are specially formulated for silicone hydrogel lenses. An additional issue with private-label solutions is that it may be purchased in one formulation and be a totally different formulation 6 months later. The complications resulting from these issues with private-label solutions may result in the lens wearers discontinuing wear, not realizing that the real problem is the solution they are using, not the lens or their eye. One study found that complications with soft contact lens wearers using generic solutions were 1.11 complications per eye compared with the lowest value, 0.5 complications per eye found with Opti-Free RepleniSH (Alcon). It is difficult to determine exactly what factors cause an increase in the complications. There are most likely three factors that play a role, or a combination of these factors. It could be that the patient is overall more noncompliant, as demonstrated by discontinuing the use of the doctor's recommended solution, or it could be that the generic solution is incompatible with the lens material or causing a higher rate of corneal staining.[61]

Ten common rules that aid in patient compliance are found in Table 12.7.[62,63]

It is surprising that practitioners do not observe more complications related to patient noncompliance; however, patients often enjoy a period of success, even when they are being noncompliant, and this reinforces their thinking that it is acceptable to continue these poor

TABLE 12.7 Ten Common Rules for Patient Compliance

1. Wash hands with soap and water, and dry thoroughly before handling contact lenses.
2. Store lenses in the recommended disinfecting solution and disinfect at every lens removal.
3. Rub and rinse lenses before disinfection.
4. Wear lenses according to the prescribed wearing schedule (i.e., dispose of lenses according to the recommended replacement schedule, do not sleep in lenses that are DW lenses, and do not sleep in EW lenses longer than the prescribed amount of time).
5. Always discard used solution and start with fresh solution (no topping off).
6. After inserting lenses, dump the solution from the case, rinse the case with disinfecting solution and allow to air dry. Once or twice a week, the lens should be digitally rubbed with disinfecting solution to remove any biofilm, rinsed with solution, and allowed to air dry. The case should be replaced at least every 3 months.
7. Do not use tap water with lenses.
8. Do not swim or shower with lenses on, unless proper precautions are taken.
9. If dissatisfied with current solutions, discuss the care regimen with the doctor to avoid purchasing solutions that are incompatible or cause preservative sensitivities.
10. Solutions become contaminated when old, expired, uncapped, or by repackaging in nonsterile containers.[62,63]

habits. Unfortunately, when problems do occur, they are often vision-threatening and it is too late to manage the problem successfully by simply reinstating proper lens care. The answer to noncompliance is good, intensive patient education, reinforcement of education at each visit, and frequent evaluations to monitor lens wear. Vision is an invaluable sense, and patients must learn not to take it for granted.

Insertion and Removal

Insertion of a soft contact lens may be performed by either of two methods. The first method is to place the lens on the index finger. The index finger should be dry because the lens will stick to the finger instead of the eye if the finger is too wet. While the lids are held apart with the third finger of each hand, the lens is placed on the sclera as the patient looks up (Fig. 12.3A). The second method is performed the same way, except the lens is placed directly on the cornea as the patient looks straight ahead into a mirror (Fig. 12.3B). It is recommended that patients always insert and remove the same lens first; for example, the patient always inserts the right lens first and removes the right lens first.

A patient placing the lens on the index finger before insertion should be able to determine if the lens is right-side or wrong-side out. A lens that is right-side out will appear bowl-shaped (Fig. 12.4A), whereas one that is inverted will appear more like a saucer, with the edges flared out (Fig. 12.4B). If this method does not help the patient, the "taco test" is another method of determining if a lens is inverted. The lens edges are pushed together. If the edges curl toward each other, like the edges of a taco, the lens is correctly positioned (Fig. 12.4C). On the other

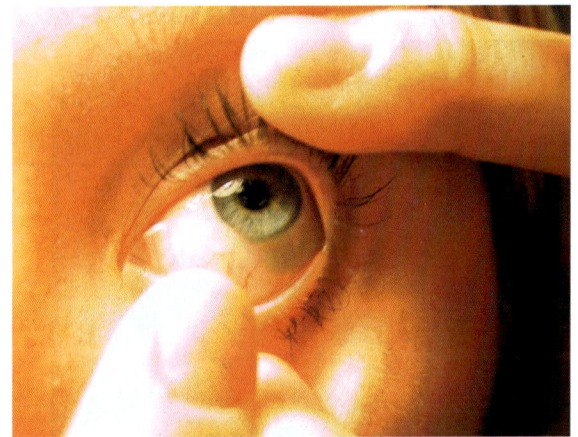

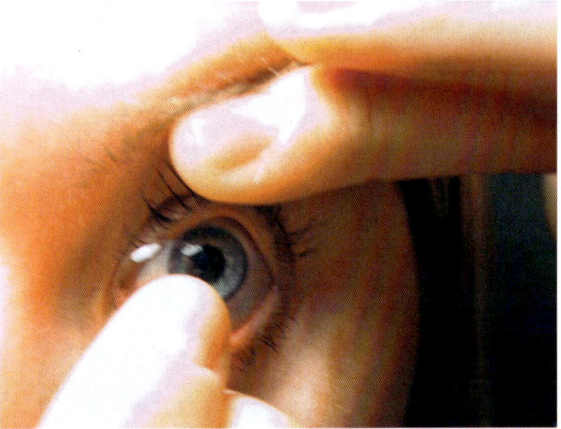

FIGURE 12.3 **(A)** Insertion of lens onto sclera. **(B)** Insertion of lens onto cornea.

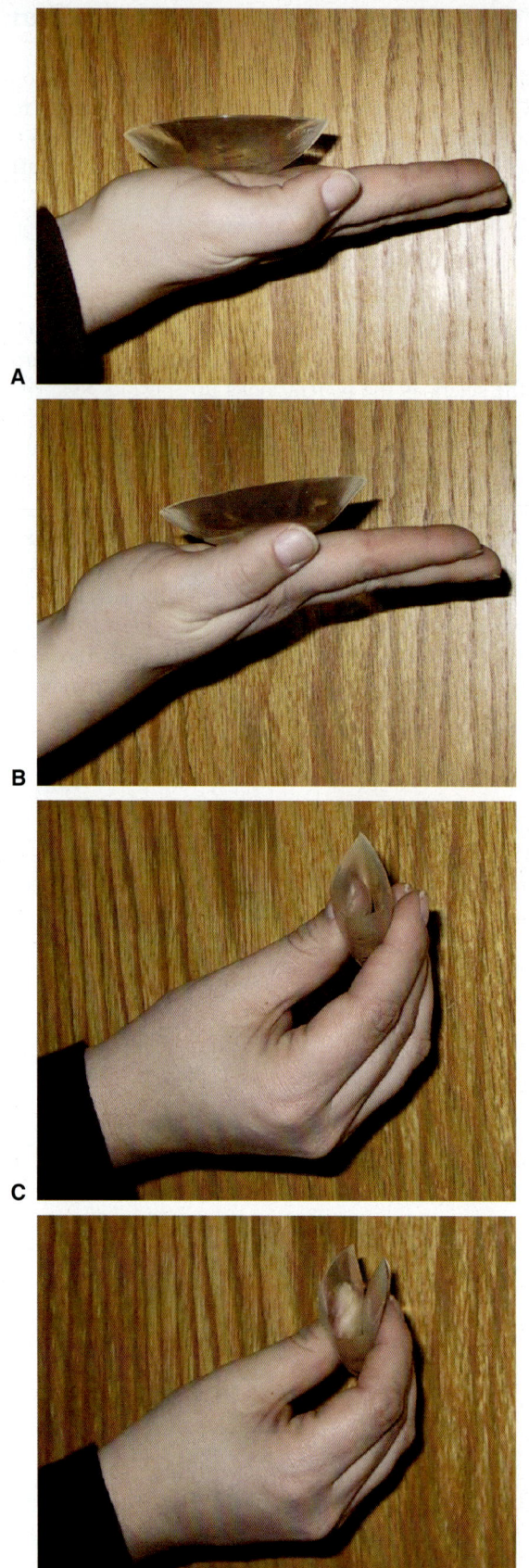

FIGURE 12.4 (A) Lens positioned correctly using large demonstration lens. **(B)** Lens inverted using large demonstration lens. **(C)** Taco test demonstrating a proper lens orientation (using large demonstration lens). **(D)** Taco test demonstrating an inverted lens (using large demonstration lens).

hand, if the edges curl out, the lens is inverted (Fig 12.4D). Typically, an inverted lens will result in mild discomfort, slightly reduced vision, excessive lens movement, or edges flared out from the sclera. If the patient observes any of these symptoms, an inverted lens may be suspected, and the patient should try to insert the lens in the other direction to determine if this corrects the symptoms. The patient may be assured that an inverted soft lens will not damage the eye. In addition, some manufacturers provide inversion indicators, which aid the patient in determining the correct position of the lens.

Soft lens removal is accomplished by holding the lids apart with the third finger of each hand, placing the index finger directly on the cornea, and sliding the lens off onto the sclera as the patient looks up. The lens is gently pinched off the sclera with the pads of the thumb and index finger (Fig. 12.5). Caution should be taken that the lens is not pinched directly off the cornea because this may result in a corneal abrasion. Likewise, the fingernails should not be used to pinch the lens because this may result in fingernail tears in the central portion of the lens. Generally, with practice, patients can learn to insert and remove their lenses without a mirror and without holding both lids open.

Hygiene

Hygiene would seem to be an area that would need little attention in today's society; however, even our cleanest, neatest patients will come to the office with dirty cases, dirty solution bottles, and lenses contaminated by substances on their hands. Simple hand washing before lens handling, with soaps that do not contain lanolin, creams, or oils, will prevent transfer of bacteria and environmental contamination (makeup, suntan lotion) of the lens. Any mild soap that does not have deodorants, creams, lanolin, or oils is compatible.

The second area of hygiene is the case in which the lenses are stored. For years, this component of lens care has been relatively ignored. It is important for cases not to be used for lengthy periods. Not only do they need occasional cleaning; a biofilm develops that remains in the wells of the case. This biofilm is difficult to remove and provides a perfect environment for microorganisms. One study found 27 different types of bacteria plus fungi in the contact lens cases of study subjects.[64] Other studies have shown an 80.95% rate of contamination of cases after 270 days of use[65] and 70% of cases contaminated by bacteria, fungi, yeasts, and amoebae.[66] A new case should be given to the patient, at minimum, every 3 months at follow-up evaluations, or manufacturers often package cases with solutions to encourage frequent case replacement.[67] Practitioner, manufacturer, and FDA recommendations for case replacement vary from 1 to 6 months.[68,69] Between periods of case replacement, the case should be emptied of solution each time the lenses are inserted, rinsed with disinfecting solution, and allowed to air dry. Once

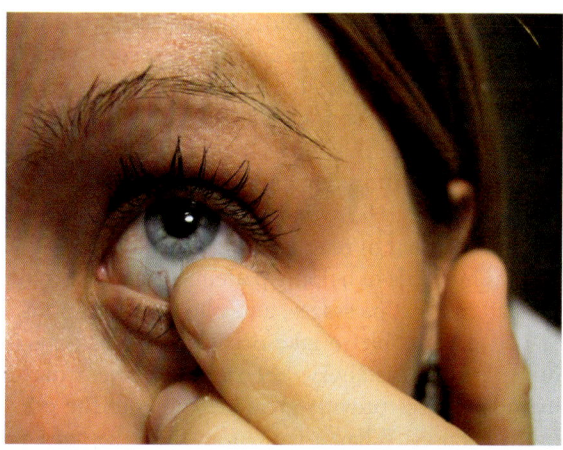

FIGURE 12.5 The lens has been pulled down on the sclera to remove the lens from the eye. The thumb is not yet positioned to pinch the lens.

or twice a week, the case should be thoroughly scrubbed to eliminate biofilm, which can develop within 7 days.[70] This can be achieved by digitally scrubbing with the disinfecting solution and allowing the case to air dry. Rinsing the case in tap water is not recommended, as the risk of *Acanthamoeba* in the cyst form is a possibility. Cases may be boiled in water periodically or microwaved for 3 minutes to sterilize.[15] Alcon has a case called Pro-Guard, which incorporates silver, an inorganic antibacterial agent, into the case to decrease microbial contamination.[22,71] Amcon has a similar case called I-Clean case.

Another area of microbial contamination is the solution bottles. The solution is provided initially sterile; however, microbial contamination may occur if the solution is left uncapped, the tip of the bottle comes in contact with the fingers or lens, the solution is old and expired, or the solution is transferred to another container. Several of the manufacturers have designed new solution lids that are easier to open, close, and less likely for the patient to contaminate the solution tip when manipulating the lid. The new closure completely covers the top of the bottle, creating less bioburden on the top of the solution bottle.

Cosmetics

Cosmetics are associated with women; however, cosmetics may also include suntan lotions, after-shave lotions, acne medications, shampoo, and deodorants.[72] When cosmetics are thought of in this broader sense, all patients, including men, women, and teenagers, are using cosmetics. This is an important area to mention during routine patient education. Washing the hands before handling the lenses will prevent contaminating the contact lens surface with, for example, oils, and creams. Water-soluble cosmetics are preferable for contact lens patients because they can be cleaned from the surface of the lens. Hypoallergenic cosmetics are often suggested for contact lens wearers. Cosmetics will become contaminated with time; thus, it is recommended that cosmetics be replaced every 3 to 6 months. In addition, cosmetics, especially eye makeup, should not be shared as this increases the risk of spreading ocular infections. Cosmetics should be applied around the eyes with caution to avoid blocking the openings to the glands, introducing them into the eye, or producing an abrasion from the application wand or cosmetic particles. Cosmetics should be applied after the lenses are inserted to prevent contamination of the lens surface. Hairspray, however, should be used before the insertion of contact lenses or, if applied during lens wear, the eyes should be kept closed until the patient moves to another room away from the place where the hairspray was applied. Likewise, spray deodorants should be avoided.[73,74]

Miscellaneous Tips

Replacement of lenses on a frequent basis (daily, every 1–2 weeks, monthly, or quarterly) reduces the number of complications that result from old, dirty lenses. *This option is the preferred method of lens wear.* The older the lenses, the more likely the buildup of deposits on the lenses which, in turn, results in decreased oxygen supply to the cornea, reduced vision, and ocular complications. Patients tend to extend the wear of the soft lenses dispensed beyond the time the practitioner recommends; therefore, emphasis should be place on educating the patient thoroughly about the replacement schedule. Generally, daily or monthly replacements are easiest for the patient to remember. When educating a 2-week replacement lens wearer, the author finds it helpful to have the patient replace the lens on the 15th and the 30th day of the month to assist the patient in remembering when the lenses need to be replaced. Technology is providing various methods of helping patients remember to replace their lenses; storage cases that remind the patient, text messages, and phone applications.[69]

It is permissible to take occasional short naps (1–2 hours) while wearing DW soft lenses; however, there is always the risk the patient may sleep much longer than intended. Silicone hydrogel lenses provide greater oxygen to the eye, especially for those who may sleep or nap in their lenses. When a patient awakes, the lenses will likely have dehydrated to some extent, and the application of a few drops of rewetting solution before lens removal is suggested to prevent a corneal abrasion. Likewise, anytime a soft lens becomes dehydrated, the lens should be soaked in solution to restore the lens to its hydrated state. Disinfection prior to wearing the lens is also recommended. Lenses that have been dehydrated for a lengthy period may not be fully restored to their previous condition. Soft lenses become very brittle when dehydrated and may break.

If, for some reason, the patient discontinues lens wear for a period (2 weeks or more), the wearing time may need to be gradually increased when lenses are worn again. This gradual increase in wearing schedule is less important with silicone hydrogel lens materials. Although many MPSs can be used to store lenses for 30 days, it is recommended that spare lenses or lenses that have been stored be placed in a deep-welled case with frequent replacement of the solution. These lenses should be disinfected within 24 hours prior to lens wear. Long-term storage of soft lenses depends on the solution used (see Tables 12.1 and 12.2).

Some very definite areas of potential noncompliance that should be avoided with soft lens wear are tap water, GP lens solutions, use of ophthalmic medications while wearing lenses, shallow lens cases, and swimming with the lenses on. Tap water and swimming place the patient at risk for *Acanthamoeba* keratitis. Ophthalmic medications and GP solutions contain preservatives and ingredients that may discolor the lens or cause a toxic reaction as a result of absorption into the lens. Soft lenses are often damaged by closure of the lens case, particularly lens cases that are shallow and intended for shipping GP lenses.

Patients should always *read* the labels on contact lens solution bottles. Some GP solutions look very similar to soft solutions. In addition, the person stocking the store shelves may not be educated regarding ophthalmic solutions; thus, tear substitutes may be mixed in with rewetting drops, GP solutions may be mixed in with soft solutions, or hydrogen peroxide solutions may be mixed in with saline solutions. The bottles are clearly marked regarding their purpose; however, it is necessary to read the label. Of course, if the patients are purchasing the same solutions given to them by their contact lens practitioner, they should be familiar enough with the solutions to be able to obtain the same ones every time. This makes a case for practitioners' providing solutions for purchase directly from their office.

SUMMARY

Patient education and care of soft lenses are an important part of successful lens wear. Emphasis on education and lens care by the practitioner will aid in producing a serious patient attitude toward this aspect of lens wear. A summary nomogram on lens care and patient education is provided in Figure 12.6.

CLINICAL CASES

CASE 1

A patient has monthly replacement lenses that are 4 months old on the OD and 1 month old on the OS. He wears the lenses on a DW basis. He makes an appointment for his annual examination. He admits that he is overdue for his visit, but as he had extra left lenses, he had procrastinated about coming in. He reports that the right lens feels like it has sand or something under it. Lens removal and cleaning does not improve the condition.

SOLUTION: Upon examination with the biomicroscope, three jelly bumps are observed on the right lens. New lenses are ordered for the patient and the patient is educated on the importance of maintaining the recommended replacement schedule of disposing of his lenses every month. Replacing the lenses each month on the first day of the month is an excellent method of remembering to replace the lenses.

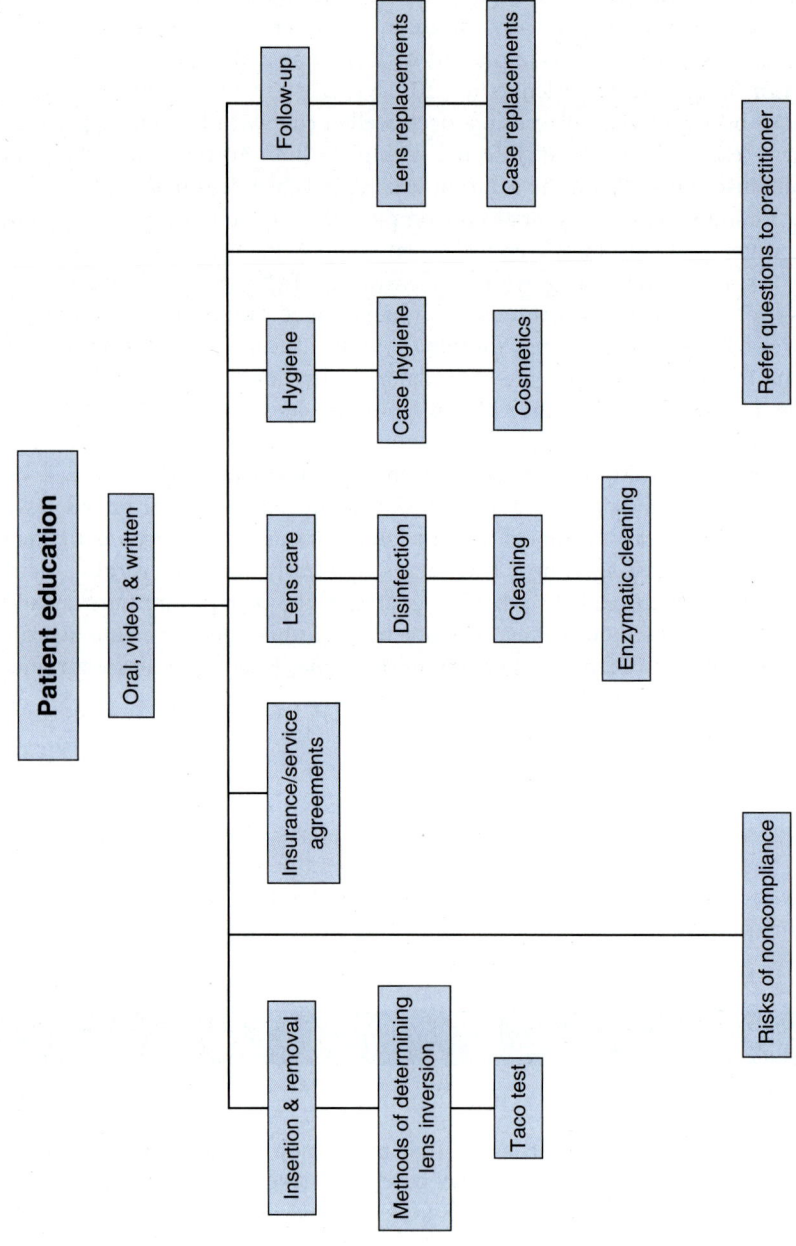

FIGURE 12.6 Summary nomogram for patient education.

CASE 2

A first-time soft lens wearer returns to the office for her 1-month follow-up visit. She feels the lenses and visual acuity are good; however, she admits that her allergies seem to be bothering her slightly because her lenses, primarily her left lens, have been mildly irritating. Slit-lamp examination reveals two superficial slits in the midperiphery of the left lens. On lens removal and fluorescein evaluation, there is mild superficial corneal staining in the region where the slits were visible.

SOLUTION: The patient has fingernail tears in the lens that have penetrated the lens and resulted in irritation to the cornea in that region. Demonstration of the patient's removal technique reveals she is using her fingernails to remove the lens. Reeducation of soft lens removal with the pads of the fingers is demonstrated to her. If her nails are too long, she should be warned that it would be best to cut them to prevent a recurrence of the problem. Treatment for the corneal staining depends on the severity. In most cases where the patient is able to wear the lens and the staining is superficial, the patient only needs to discontinue lens wear for 12 to 24 hours and use a lubricating drop to improve comfort and healing during lens discontinuation.

CASE 3

A patient returns to the clinic for a follow-up visit. He has worn soft lenses for 8 years. His present lenses are 3 months old. Inspection of the lens reveals a small, round orange mark.

SOLUTION: This patient has a rust spot on the lens. The first thought of the practitioner should be that the patient is using tap water on the lenses and should be questioned about this. The rust spot may be the result of frequent tap water use; for example, rinsing the cleaner from the lens. The patient should be cautioned about the dangers of tap water use and educated to never use tap water on the lenses. This should be documented in the patient's file. If the patient has not used tap water on the lens, the eye and lid should be examined for a metal foreign body that may be embedded. The lens should be replaced.

CASE 4

A patient is wearing a daily disposable soft lens. She reports that some days one lens or the other is mildly uncomfortable. Other than this, she is happy with the lenses.

SOLUTION: Most likely she is wearing an inverted lens. Soft lenses, especially some daily disposable lenses, are very thin and many are difficult to determine if they are inverted. The patient denies checking to see if the lens is inverted. The patient is reeducated on how to determine if the lens is wrong-side out, for example, the "taco test" or if the lens looks like a bowl or a saucer. If she is unsure if the lens is inverted and she notices mild lens awareness, she should remove the lens and try inserting it the other direction to see if this makes the lens more comfortable.

CASE 5

A patient is asked at the follow-up evaluation about the solutions she is using. She is not sure of the names but she thinks she remembers the solution bottle.

SOLUTION: A patient will sometimes be unsure of the names of her solutions; however, she will be able to describe the bottle to her practitioner. This indicates two important points: (a) if she is unsure of the name of the solution, then the practitioner must make sure she is purchasing the proper solution at the store, and (b) it will be helpful if the practitioner and staff are up-to-date on the solutions that are commercially available and have samples of these in the office to enable them to determine which solution the patient is using, either by description or by having the patient determine which of the samples she is using. Reeducation of lens care solutions would be appropriate for this patient. In addition, the practitioner may find that patient compliance can be enhanced by dispensing solutions directly from his or her office, eliminating the patient's need to try to find appropriate solutions at the store or to price shop.

CASE 6

A patient comes to your office with mildly irritated eyes. The patient has no discharge of any kind. She complains of dryness. Her wearing time is reduced because of the discomfort. She left her lenses out for 2 days, which seemed to help; however, on wearing lenses again, the irritation returned. TBUT was previously recorded as 12 seconds OU. Mild diffuse punctate staining is noted.

SOLUTION: This patient is likely experiencing a preservative sensitivity. She should be questioned about the solutions she is presently using. The lenses may need to be replaced. She should be given a new solution system, possibly one that is preservative-free or put into a modality such as daily disposable lenses, which requires no care regimen.

CASE 7

A 35-year-old woman desires replacement soft lenses. The patient has worn soft lenses for 2 years, dispensed from another office. The present pair of lenses are 6 months old. The patient wears substantial amounts of eyeliner, mascara, and eyes shadow. Biomicroscopy reveals much debris in the tear layer in addition to surface deposits and pigment spots on the lenses. The patient's eyeliner is present on the lid margins, and it is evident that this is flaking off into the eye. The patient admits to separating her eyelashes with a straight pin, keeping cosmetics for a year or more, and frequent sensations of burning and discomfort as if something is behind the lens.

SOLUTION: Caution should be taken in fitting this patient. Patient education is necessary to avoid serious complications. Abrasions are often caused by trapped debris such as mascara behind the lens. Cosmetics can become contaminated, and it is wise to have patients replace their cosmetics every 3 months. An eye infection or corneal ulcer may occur if this contamination occurs and is introduced to the eye. This patient needs to be cautious that her hands are washed thoroughly prior to handling the lenses, that lenses are inserted before applying makeup, that eyeliner is never placed on the lid margin closest to the eye, and that lenses are properly cleaned and disinfected to clean off any makeup that adheres to the lenses. This patient should benefit from a comprehensive education program and disposable/frequent lens replacement.

CASE 8

A long-time patient comes to the office complaining of decreased wearing time and lens awareness. The patient has been lost to follow-up for 2 years. During that period of time, he admits to extending his lens wear to a period of 4 to 6 months. When asked about the care regimen he uses, he pulls out a plastic bag containing an assortment of private-label solutions.

SOLUTION: Lens replacement schedules are discussed with the patient and he agrees to a monthly replacement lens. The patient is given a new care regimen. Both the care regimen and the replacement schedule are thoroughly discussed and the importance of adhering to both is noted. The patient seems somewhat skeptical that the solutions and replacement schedule are the issue, but agrees to closely follow this recommended plan for the next couple of months. At his 2-month visit, he is pleased with his lens comfort and wearing time. He admits that replacing the lenses monthly and the new care regimen have made the difference.

CASE 9

A patient comes to the office for the first time for an emergency visit. He is experiencing irritation and itching in the left eye. The patient reports sleeping in his lenses for 7 to 10 days. The brand he is using is not approved for EW. When asked about his care regimen, he reports that he is using purified water and sea salt. He does not like to use chemicals in his eyes.

SOLUTION: First the patient's immediate problem must be addressed. This patient is at risk for *Acanthamoeba* keratitis due to the homemade saline use. This patient may never be a good candidate for contact lenses, depending on the diagnosis of his left eye and his ability to be compliant to a proper lens wearing and care regimen. If he is ever to wear lenses again, thorough education about daily wear (DW) and EW lenses, following recommended guidelines and use of proper solutions must be discussed. Some patients are willingly noncompliant and some have been given poor instructions from another source. Differentiating the cause of the noncompliance will be the difference between fitting this patient again in lenses and refusing to fit on the basis that he is a poor candidate. Of course, all this is based on the diagnosis and recovery of the left eye.

CASE 10

A young college student comes to see you and is concerned with irritation and dryness with her contact lenses. She has been wearing lenses since she was 12 years old and had been successful until the last few months. She is using a MPS chemical disinfection system, which she has used for several years and has worn the same lens brand for the last 2 years.

SOLUTION: Upon examination with the biomicroscope, mild diffuse punctate staining is noted OU. The patient reports using "Visine" drops during the day if her lenses feel dry and look red. The patient is given a new pair of lenses and contact lens rewetting drops. She is advised to continue the use of her current MPS care regimen. She is asked to not use any rewetting solutions except the one prescribed to her. When the patient returns for her follow-up examination, she reports good comfort with her lenses. No corneal staining is evident with the biomicroscope. The patient is educated on using only solutions that are specified for contact lens use, and that if she is unsure to call the office to verify that, she may alter her care regimen. Eye drops that are not recommended for soft contact lenses may have incompatible preservatives or buildup preservatives within the matrix, resulting in corneal staining.

CASE 11

A 50-year-old woman with a history of dry eyes complains of her soft lenses tearing in her eye.

SOLUTION: This patient has exhibited a low TBUT; however, she was fit in a lens material that has been found to be more successful in dry-eye patients. In addition, this has happened over a period of time, so a defective lot of lenses is not likely. A material change may be warranted to find a lens material that works better for this patient; however, other recommendations may be needed to keep this patient successfull in lens wear. First, this patient should instill a drop of rewetting solution prior to lens removal to make sure the lens is hydrated and moving on the eye prior to removal. She should be using a deep-welled case or a lens vial, and make sure that the lenses are not being caught in the lid when the lid is placed on the case. Her lenses should be inspected prior to insertion to make sure the lenses are in good condition with no tears prior to placing them in the eye. The most likely reasons for the lens tearing is that she is tearing the lens upon removal due to lens dehydration, she is damaging it with her fingernails, damaging it upon handling, or in her lens case. It is highly unusual for a lens to tear in the eye unless it has previous damage. It would be suspected that the lens has been damaged via one of the aforementioned methods and after insertion, the damaged lens tears more between handling the lens and the blink process. Careful education and recommendation of good lens care should correct this patient's problem.

CLINICAL PROFICIENCY CHECKLIST

- Chemical disinfection (MPSs) generally provides one-bottle systems that encourage patient compliance; however, rubbing and rinsing the lenses prior to disinfection is still the best method to fight bacteria, fungi, *Acanthamoeba,* and lens cleanliness.
- Oxidative disinfection (hydrogen peroxide) is an effective method of disinfection and is especially beneficial for patients prone to preservative sensitivities.
- Thorough cleaning and rinsing should be performed prior to lens disinfection.
- The value of patient education should not be underestimated. Patients should be taught insertion, removal, lens care and handling, and risks of noncompliance.
- Patients should be told to contact their eye-care practitioner with any questions.
- The best type of in-office disinfection of diagnostic lenses is disposable diagnostic lenses.
- Patients should be taught simple hygiene; they should wash their hands with soap and water, and dry them prior to handling lenses.
- Frequent case replacement will aid in the prevention of biofilm and case contamination.
- Frequent lens replacement prevents soft lens deposits such as jelly bumps, lipid and mucoprotein deposits, and the complications that may result.
- Tap water should never be used on soft lenses because of the risk of *Acanthamoeba* keratitis.
- Many complications with soft lenses are a result of noncompliance, which for prevention require thorough patient education and a good example demonstrated in the practitioner's office.

REFERENCES

1. Gromacki S. Hydrogel and Silicone Hydrogel Lens Care. Available at: www.visioncareeducation.com/no-feece/course1.asp. Accessed December 2011.
2. Campbell R, Caroline P. Multipurpose non-keratitis. *Contact Lens Spectrum*. 1997;12(3):56.
3. Soni PS, Horner DG, Ross J. Ocular response to lens care systems in adolescent soft contact lens wearers. *Optom Vis Sci*. 1996;73:70–85.
4. Carnt N, Evans V, Holden BA, et al. IER matrix update: adding another silicone hydrogel. *Contact Lens Spectrum*. 2008;23(3):40–43.
5. Andrasko G. Andrasko corneal staining grid. http://www.staininggrid.com. Updated August 19, 2011. Accessed June 4, 2012.
6. Epstein AB. How products fail: déjà vu solution and lens material incompatibilities once again appear on the radar, but this time with more serious consequences. *Rev Optom*. 2007;144(10)(suppl):11–14.
7. Chang DC, Grant GB, O'Donnell K, et al; Fusarium Keratitis Investigation Team. Multistate outbreak of Fusarium Keratitis associated with use of a contact lens solution. *JAMA*. 2006;296(8):953–963.
8. Ward MA. Mycotic keratitis and lens care. *Contact Lens Spectrum*. 2006;21(7):27.
9. Joslin CE, Tu EY, McMahon TT, et al. Epidemiological characteristics of a Chicago-area Acanthamoeba Keratitis outbreak. *Am J Ophthalmol*. 2006;142(2):212–217.
10. Gutman C. Acanthamoeba Keratitis increasing at alarming rate. *Ophthalmology Times* January 1, 2006.
11. Weisbarth RE, Henderson BA. Hydrogel lens care regimens and patient education. In: Bennett ES, Weissman BA, eds. *Clinical Contact Lens Practice*. Philadelphia, PA: Lippincott, Williams & Wilkins; 2005:381–419.
12. Penley CA, Willis SW, Sickler SG. Comparative antimicrobial efficacy of soft and rigid gas permeable contact lens solutions against *Acanthamoeba*. *CLAO J*. 1989;15(4):257–260.
13. Liedel KK, Begley CG. The effectiveness of soft contact lens disinfection systems against Acanthamoeba on the lens surface. *J Am Optom Assoc*. 1996;67:135–142.
14. Zadnik K. *Acanthamoeba* and bacterial keratitis in hydrogel lens wearers. Presented at: Twenty-ninth Annual Contact Lens and Primary Care Congress of the Heart of America Contact Lens Society; Febrauary 1990; Kansas City, MO.
15. Bennett ES. *Acanthamoeba* keratitis in 2007: stay informed but calm. *Contact Lens Spectrum*. 2007;22(7):50–52.

16. Gromacki SJ. An update on regulatory changes for lens care systems. *Contact Lens Spectrum.* 2011;26(2):21.
17. Shovlin JP, Kislan TP, Papas E, et al. Build your practice with next-generation contact lens care. *Contact Lens Spectrum.* 2012;27(2)(suppl):3–8.
18. Klein P, Solomon J, Snyder RP. Cleaning: the key to contact lens care. *Rev Optom.* 1990;127(4):42–44.
19. FDA. Ensuring safe use of contact lens solution. 2009. Available at: www.fda.gov/forconsumers/consumerupdates/ucm164197.htm. Accessed December 2011.
20. Sakuma S. Reeh B, Dang D, et al. Comparative efficacies of four soft contact lens disinfection solutions. *Int Cont Lens Clin.* 1996;23:234–239.
21. http://www.menicon.com/ Accessed June 14, 2012.
22. Watanabe RK. Contact Lens Solution Update 2006. *Contact Lens Spectrum.* 2006;21(8):26–31.
23. Thompson TT. Tyler's Quarterly Soft Contact Lens Parameter Guide. 2012;29(3):65–66.
24. White P. 2011 Contact Lenses & Solutions Summary Supplement to Contact Lens Spectrum. 2011; 26(7)(Suppl):26–28.
25. Eiden B. Does One Contact Lens Solution Fit All? *Rev Cornea Contact Lenses.* 2011; Available at: http://www.reviewofcontactlenses.com/content/d/specialty_lenses/c/28321/. Accessed December 2011.
26. Gromacki SJ. Taking a closer look at hydrogen peroxide products. *Contact Lens Spectrum.* 2007;22(2):26.
27. Gromacki SJ. Hydrogen peroxide disinfection. *Contact Lens Spectrum.* 2006;21(12):19.
28. Gromacki SJ. Hydrogen peroxide contact lens disinfection. *Contact Lens Spectrum.* 2012;27(5, pt 1):23.
29. Connor CG, Presley L, Finchum SM, et al. The effectiveness of several current soft contact lens care regimens against Aspergillus. *CLAO J.* 1998;24:82–84.
30. Ward M. Revisiting hydrogen peroxide disinfection. *Contact Lens Spectrum.* 2006;21(5):23.
31. Sibley MJ. Hydrogen peroxide residues: a comparison between chemical and osmotic extraction. *Contact Lens Spectrum.* 1988;3(8):39–43.
32. Melton JW, Phillips JH. Patient comfort comparison of hydrogen peroxide systems. *Contact Lens Spectrum.* 1988;3(9):48–51.
33. Anger CB, Ambrus K, Stoecker J, et al. Antimicrobial efficacy of hydrogen peroxide for contact lens disinfection. *Contact Lens Spectrum.* 1990;5(11):46–51.
34. Key JE, Monnat K. Comparative disinfectant efficacy of two disinfecting solutions against *Pseudomonas aeruginosa*. *CLAO J.* 1996;22:118–121.
35. Hughes R, Kilvington S. Comparison of hydrogen peroxide contact lens disinfection systems and solutions against *Acanthamoeba polyphaga*. *Antimicrob Agents Chemother.* 2001;45(7):2038–2043.
36. Mowrey-McKee M, George M. Contact lens solution efficacy against *Acanthamoeba castellani*. *Eye Contact Lens.* 2007;33(5):211–215.
37. Simmons PA, Edrington TB, Lao KF, et al. The efficacy of disinfection systems for in-office storage of hydrogel contact lenses. *Int Cont Lens Clin.* 1996;23:94–97.
38. Mandell RB. Symptomatology and aftercare. In: Mandell RB, ed. *Contact Lens Practice.* 4th ed. Springfield, IL: Charles C. Thomas; 1988:598–643.
39. Friedberg DN, Stenson SM. AIDS and your eye exam. CLAO Patient information pamphlet 1994–2004.
40. Ward M. In-office hydrogel contact lens disinfection. *Contact Lens Spectrum.* 2005;20(7):27.
41. Kleist FD. Appearance and nature of hydrophilic contact lens deposits. I. Protein and other organic deposits. *Int Cont Lens Clin.* 1979;6(3):49–58.
42. Kleist FD. Appearance and nature of hydrophilic contact lens deposits. II. Inorganic deposits. *Int Cont Lens Clin.* 1979;6(4):177–186.
43. Begley CG, Waggoner PJ. An analysis of nodular deposits on soft contact lenses. *J Am Optom Assoc.* 1991;62(3):208–214.
44. Caroline PJ, Robin JB, Gindi JJ. Microscopic and elemental analysis of deposits on extended wear soft contact lenses. *CLAO J.* 1985;11(4):311–316.
45. Ward M. Soft lens daily cleaners: what's available. *Contact Lens Spectrum.* 2006;21(11):21.
46. 510(k) Summary of safety and effectiveness. Available at: www.accessdata.fda.gov/cdrh_docs/pdf7/K071203.pdf. Accessed December 2011.
47. Thomas E, Stein H, Cox D, et al. A new standard in lens hygiene. *Contact Lens Spectrum.* 1996;11:32–36.
48. Szczotka-Flynn LB. Chemical properties of contact lens rewetters: a review of hyaluronic acid as a contemporary ingredient in contact lens rewetters. *Contact Lens Spectrum.* 2006;21(4):40–45.
49. Harris MG. Lens care systems—pros and cons. Presented at: Twenty-eighth Annual Contact Lens and Primary Care Congress of the Heart of America Contact Lens Society; February 1989; Kansas City, MO.
50. Schafer J. Improving compliance with patient education. *Contact Lens Spectrum.* 2007;22(10):50.
51. Lens-care systems: what they cost. Consumer Reports 1989; June:416–420.
52. O'Connor M (A. C. Nielson, Inc.). The "real" cost of soft contact lens care: a Nielson report. Presented at: Eighteenth Annual National Research Symposium to the AOCLE; August 1991; Toronto, Canada.
53. Schornack JA, Watanabe R, Dillehay SM, et al. Annual soft contact lens solution usage and costs. *Contact Lens Spectrum.* 1998;13:43–48.
54. Dumbleton KA, Woods CA, Jones LW, et al. Relationship between compliance with lens replacement and contact lens-related problems in silicone hydrogel wearers. *Cont Lens Anterior Eye.* 2011;34(5):216–222.

55. Hickson-Curran S, Chalmers R, Sencer S. Making the case for daily disposable contact lenses: patient non-compliance with storage case hygiene and replacement. Presented at: American Academy of Optometry meeting; November 2010; San Francisco.
56. Woods C, Dumbleton K, Richter D. Compliance with lens care and contact lens case care and replacement. Presented at: American Academy of Optometry meeting; 2010; San Francisco.
57. Gromacki SJ. New research on compliance. *Contact Lens Spectrum*. 2010;25(12):21.
58. Thimons JJ. A new-generation multipurpose disinfecting solution. *Contact Lens Spectrum*. 2011;26(12):36–39.
59. Nichols JJ. Contact lenses 2011. *Contact Lens Spectrum*. 2012;27(1):20–25.
60. Ward MA. How private-label solutions affect your practice. *Contact Lens Spectrum*. 2006;21(3):25.
61. Forister JF, Forister EF, Yeung KK, et al. Prevalence of contact lens-related complications: UCLA contact lens study. *Eye Contact Lens*. 2009;35(4):176–180.
62. Lowther GE. Patient compliance. *Int Cont Lens Clin*. 1988;15(5):142.
63. "Horror stories" fail to stir compliance. *Rev Optom*. 1987;124(11):10.
64. Willcox MDP, Power KN, Stapleton F, et al. Potential sources of bacteria that are isolated from contact lenses during wear. *Optom Vis Sci*. 1997;74:1030–1038.
65. Velasco J, Bermudez J. Comparitive study of the microbial flora on contact lenses, in lens cases and in maintenance liquids. *Int Cont Lens Clin*. 1996;23:55–58.
66. Lakkis C, Harding AS, Brennan NA. Case contamination with hydrogel lens wear. *Clin Exp Optom*. May–June 1997:111.
67. Snyder C. Planned replacement of contact lens cases: rationale and practical approaches. Presented at: Eighteenth Annual National Research Symposium; August 1991; Toronto, Canada.
68. Gromacki S. Make case care a priority in your practice. *Contact Lens Spectrum*. 2010;25(8):23.
69. Hickson-Curran SB. Compliance before, during and after contact lens wear. *Contact Lens Spectrum*. 2012;27(1):38–43.
70. Smythe JL. The forgotten lens care step. *Contact Lens Spectrum*. 2003;18(9):21.
71. Gromacki SJ. Making a case for clean cases. *Contact Lens Spectrum*. 2006;(special edition):12–13.
72. Tlachac CA. Cosmetics for contact lens wearers. *Contact Lens Spectrum*. 1988;3(8):65–70.
73. Ghormley NR. Contact lens solutions and materials: cosmetics and contact lenses. *Int Eyecare*. 1986;1(3):218.
74. Coopersmith L, Weinstock FJ. Current recommendations and practice regarding soft lens replacement and disinfection. *CLAO J*. 1997;23:172–176.

Chapter 13

Soft Lens Problem Solving

J. Bart Campbell, Vinita Allee Henry, and Stephanie Woo

Two significant developments in the field of soft lenses have enormously enhanced the clinician's available tools for soft lens problem solving: the development of modern disposable lenses (particularly daily disposable lenses) and the development of silicone hydrogel lenses. During the 1990s, disposable contact lenses rapidly became the modality of choice for most wearers being fitted for the first time or being refitted with hydrogel lenses. This resulted in changes in the way contact lenses are perceived and cared for by the public, and in the way practitioners manage fittings and many complications.

However, many disposable contact lenses are manufactured with the same hydrogel materials initially used for conventional replacement lenses. Consequently, there is no inherent difference in the interaction between the eye and the lens. That said, hydrogel disposable contact lenses do provide substantial benefits in managing deposition-related complications. In fact, such complications should be eliminated when disposable lenses are used properly. The recent introduction of daily disposable lenses in silicone hydrogel materials will offer the benefits of daily disposable lenses with the benefits of higher oxygen transmission.

Disposable lenses have also encouraged manufacturers to develop a generation of care systems that emphasize convenience through the utilization of multipurpose solutions (MPSs). Although these systems should enhance compliance, they may not accomplish the task of disinfection and cleaning when patients do not follow instructions.[1,2]

The emergence of silicone hydrogel lenses in the late 1990s addressed a major problem not solved by the initial generation of hydrogel disposable lenses: oxygen transmissibility (Dk/t). Lenses manufactured from silicone hydrogel materials have vastly improved Dk/t values compared to conventional hydrogel materials. This characteristic, combined with the existing disposable modality, has enabled the clinician to address two of the biggest causes of soft lens problems: lens deposition and corneal hypoxia. However, patient compliance remains a key issue in avoiding complications. This fact, combined with a demand for 30-day continuous wear (CW) of silicone hydrogel lenses, has resulted in the conclusion that even these lenses are not without complications.[3]

Although rare, conventional replacement contact lens wearers exist in small numbers. Most commonly, such patients have extremely high refractive errors, high amounts of astigmatism, and other special conditions because there are fewer lenses available in the required parameters. More often, patients who wear lenses longer than 1 to 3 months without replacement are noncompliant patients who are not replacing their disposable lenses as recommended. These patients, who experience non–deposition-related complications, continue to provide the practitioner with ample justification to be concerned with soft lens problem solving.

TERMINOLOGY

Most lenses that practitioners refer to as "disposable" do not actually meet the criteria for disposable lenses that have been defined by the US Food and Drug Administration (FDA). To meet the FDA criteria, a device must be used only once and then discarded. Only the so-called 1-day or daily disposable lenses are routinely used in this fashion. Typically, practitioners prescribe "disposable" lenses to be replaced every 7 to 14 days. Further complicating the terminology issue are lenses prescribed as "planned-replacement," "frequent-replacement," or "programmed-replacement" lenses. In this replacement schedule, the lenses are usually replaced every 1 to 3 months.

SYMPTOMS

Reduced Vision

Visual reduction as a result of contact lens wear may be attributed to a number of causes (Fig. 13.1). A problem-oriented case history is often invaluable in disclosing the factor(s) instrumental in contact lens-induced reduction of visual acuity. The clinician should determine onset and duration, and whether the reduced visual acuity is present when spectacles are worn. Reasons for contact lens-related visual acuity reduction may include lens contamination, uncorrected refractive error, defective lens material, improper lens-to-cornea fitting relationship, lens dehydration, and excessive tearing. The use of pinhole visual acuity measurement may assist in determining if the cause of decreased visual acuity is uncorrected refractive error. Visual acuity reduction, noted with both contact lens and spectacle correction, may be attributed to corneal abnormalities, including edema, abrasions, punctate keratitis, and infectious keratitis. The presence of intraocular abnormalities as a source of visual acuity reduction must also be recognized, and all contact lens wearers should undergo regularly scheduled comprehensive eye examinations.

Lens Deposits

Surface deposits are most often attributed to inadequate lens hygiene. A mucoproteinaceous film, primarily composed of lysozyme, is frequently the major factor in causing reduced vision.[4] Complaints of "foggy" or "hazy" vision with distortion, especially when bright lights are viewed, are often expressed by affected patients. This symptom will not be noted after the lens is removed. If it is, the possibility of corneal edema must be considered. Lipid deposits and calcium–lipid complexes (e.g., "jelly bumps"), in addition to other organic and inorganic debris, may cause visual reduction, but their principal effect is on lens comfort.[5] Diagnosis is achieved by examining the lens in vivo with the biomicroscope; excessive deposition may be noted without the use of magnification.

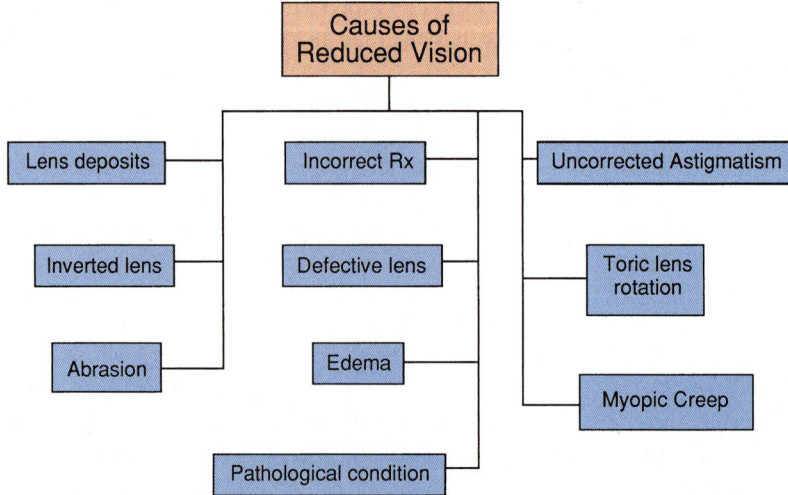

FIGURE 13.1 Summary of causes of reduced vision.

Treatment of lens deposition often depends on the type of deposit. Protein coatings, if observed before extensive accumulation is present, may be removed with enzymatic cleaning because of their superficial nature. If the lens is moderately coated, a series of two or three successive enzymatic cleanings may be necessary to remove the protein adequately; a weekly enzymatic cleaning should be sufficient for most patients. Use of a daily protein remover, either one incorporated into a MPS or a separate solution like SupraClens (Alcon Laboratories), may be helpful. Rubbing of the lens following enzyme soaking with a MPS or saline solution or cleaner in addition to the recommended daily cleaning, may be beneficial in removing any remaining protein. The presence of jelly bumps on the lens surface necessitates replacement of the lens because of their penetrating nature into the lens matrix. Removal of the jelly bumps results in subsequent holes or pits, rendering the lens inadequate for continued wear. Nevertheless, the current practice is to refit the patient in disposable contact lenses if possible. This precludes the need for "heroic" measures to save a contaminated lens. Disposing of the soft lens on a regular basis (either daily, 2 weeks, or 1 month) has virtually eliminated the problems associated with deposits and reduced the need for extra surfactant and enzymatic cleaners.

Incorrect Prescription

Reduction in Snellen visual acuity will be observed if the patient is wearing an incorrect lens prescription. Verification of soft lens power is difficult to perform because of the nature of the material, but may be necessary if inadequate visual acuity is noted. If possible, it is desirable to evaluate new lenses on the patient's eyes at the time of dispensing. This can easily detect incorrect prescriptions, visible lens defects, and uncomfortable lenses. Unfortunately, such evaluations may not be possible in every case and are never possible with every disposable lens. In these situations, patients must be thoroughly educated to be aware of symptoms that indicate defective lenses and to discontinue wear of the affected lens. In addition to manufacturer error, the possibility of such problems as lens reversal or an incorrect refraction must be considered. An expedient method of determining whether the reduction in visual acuity is refractive or possibly pathologic in nature is a pinhole visual acuity measurement. An overrefraction is also definitive in indicating whether the patient is wearing an incorrect prescription or whether the lenses may be switched. If the difference in the refractive error between the two eyes is relatively equal, the patient may not notice that the lenses are switched. New lenses must be ordered with the correct prescription or, if switched, each lens should be placed in the appropriate eye.

Uncorrected Refractive Astigmatism

Another source of reduced visual acuity in soft lens wearers is uncorrected refractive astigmatism. The inherent flexibility of these lenses limits their ability to correct effectively for astigmatism generated by the corneal surface. Approximately 16% of the refractive astigmatism is compensated for by the lens–cornea interface, reflecting the inability of the soft lens to conform totally to the corneal surface.[6] Patients with 0.75 D to 1.00 D of refractive astigmatism may begin to experience symptoms of decreased visual acuity while wearing spherical soft lenses.[7] Aspheric soft contact lens designs have been found to provide good vision in some patients with small amounts of astigmatism (i.e., 0.50–1.00 D). Aspheric soft contact lens designs do not correct astigmatism, but enhance the optics by reducing the spherical aberration; thus, the patient may perceive enhanced vision.[8,9] The ability to tolerate small amounts of blur depends primarily on the visual awareness and activities performed by the contact lens wearer. Persons who perform extensive near tasks involving small detail may require a toric lens correction. Overrefraction with placement of the appropriate cylinder in the phoropter will improve visual acuity, allowing the patient to determine the acceptability of the compromised vision. Astigmatic correction may be obtained with the use of either a soft toric or rigid gas-permeable (GP) contact lens.

Toric Lens Rotation

Soft toric lens rotation, either subsequent to each blink or as a result of persistent mislocation, is a principal cause of reduced visual acuity in astigmatic patients. Patients who exhibit astigmatism on an oblique axis are more prone to lens rotation than are those exhibiting with-the-rule and against-the-rule astigmatism. An oblique cross-cylinder effect, generated as a result of misalignment between the refractive cylinder axis and the toric lens, results in disturbances in visual acuity. Near tasks may be compromised by toric lens rotation with eye convergence, resulting from encyclorotation of the globe. A nasal and upward rotation of soft lenses has been noted and may need to be compensated for in axis selection, especially for presbyopic and esotropic patients.[7] This problem is even more pronounced for presbyopic patients wearing toric contact lenses with one eye corrected for distance vision and the other corrected for near vision (i.e., monovision). Slit-lamp examination of the toric lens will determine whether the lens is stable with adequate centration and movement or whether excessive "rocking" occurs after each blink. Refraction performed over the patient's current contact lenses or diagnostic lenses may be beneficial in determining the appropriate power and axis to order for the patient. This is especially apparent in persons with refractive astigmatism >3.00 D, in whom small amounts of rotation that can have a significant impact on visual acuity may be difficult to assess.[10] Excessive lens movement may require a steeper base curve to reduce rotation, increase stability, and improve visual acuity. Changing to a different design (e.g., slab off, thin zone designs) may also be beneficial. The option of refitting into spherical GP lenses may also be considered in a challenging case, especially when corneal toricity accounts for most of the patient's refractive astigmatism.

Defective Lenses

Characteristics of a defective lens include either abrasions in the lens (scratches, tears, nicks, holes) or poor optics. Both may contribute to irritation, discomfort, and reduced visual acuity. During initial wear, lenses with abrasions are the most common cause of lens replacement. Although the actual defect may not always cause reduced vision, deposit accumulation in the area of a scratch or tear may affect visual acuity. Poor lens manufacturing may result in inadequate optics, resulting in the need for lens exchange. Increased tearing and mucous production secondary to irritation of the palpebral conjunctiva from an elevated lens defect may also degrade vision. Biomicroscopy will elicit the source of the problem if a lens abrasion exists. Careful examination of the lens edge may be necessary to locate a nick or small tear, many of which may not be detected by the practitioner. The absence of improvement in visual acuity with an overrefraction may be indicative of poor optics, necessitating lens replacement. A small peripheral tear, if not irritating to the patient, may be clinically tolerable but will undoubtedly increase in size with continued lens manipulation. Lens replacement is undoubtedly the most effective method of handling defective lenses.

Patients may report discomfort or heightened lens awareness when there are no observable lens defects. If the symptoms are present in only one eye, briefly switching the lenses can determine if the discomfort follows the lens or remains in the initially affected eye. If it follows the lens, then the most expedient solution is simply to replace the lens. If the discomfort remains only in the initially affected eye, closer examination of the eye itself is warranted. Replacement of the lens may still be the only way to alleviate the patient's concerns, even when no clinically observable cause for the discomfort is present.

Manufacturing errors occasionally occur with soft contact lenses. Two lenses may be found together in the blister package. At times, due to the thin lens design, it may appear as a single lens and both lenses be inserted into the eye. Patients will likely complain of blurry vision or decreased comfort. The contact lens wearer should be educated to remove the contact lens for rinsing and rubbing if vision or comfort is decreased. If the issue still exists, replace the lens with a new lens. If this does not address the problem, the patient will need to be examined.

Lens Inversion

A common complaint, especially with new soft lens wearers, is difficulty with lens inversion. Patients wearing thin lenses often exhibit frustration in determining whether the lens is properly oriented before insertion (i.e., "right side out"). Mild irritation may be observed as a result of increased movement of the lens. An inverted spherical lens may or may not cause reduced visual acuity. Examination of the lens edge with the biomicroscope will reveal standoff from the bulbar conjunctiva and excessive movement. Some lens manufacturers print their name or a symbol at the periphery of the lens to facilitate determining the presence of lens inversion. Familiarity with each design is essential, as there is no consistency between manufacturers. The "taco test" may assist patients in placing the lens correctly on the eye (Chapter 12). Removal of the lens, accompanied by correct orientation, will resolve any decrease in visual acuity or irritation noted by the patient. Patients should be counseled that an inverted lens will not damage their eye and that if they are unsure whether the lens is inverted, it is acceptable simply to remove it and try wearing it with the other side toward the eye.

Reduction of Visual Acuity with Contact Lenses and Spectacles

A reduction in visual acuity, apparent with both contact lens and spectacle correction, may be indicative of a more serious complication. Removal of the contact lenses and inspection of the cornea and conjunctiva are imperative in determining the cause of the decreased visual acuity. Some physiologic factors that may influence vision with soft contact lens wear include the following:

1. An abrasion secondary to insertion and removal, poor lens fit, surface defects, or a foreign body.
2. Edema related to the physical fit, water content or prescription.
3. Central punctate staining secondary to poor lens fit, solution sensitivity, surface defects, inadequate wetting, poor tear exchange, or trapped debris.
4. Increased mucous production as a result of giant papillary conjunctivitis (GPC).
5. "Myopic creep" resulting from corneal edema.
6. Irregular astigmatism or corneal distortion secondary to keratoconus or other causes.
7. A pathologic condition affecting the anterior or posterior segment that is unrelated to contact lens wear.

Discomfort

When a soft contact lens wearer experiences discomfort, the lens should be removed immediately. If the discomfort persists, the patient should be educated to contact the practitioner immediately. A comprehensive case history will be very important in determining the cause of the pain (Fig. 13.2). A differential diagnosis is possible by classifying the discomfort into one of four categories. It is important to determine if the discomfort occurs on insertion or after lens removal and if the onset is immediate or delayed. Duration of the discomfort (e.g., transient, constant, or intermittent) should be determined. Further biomicroscopic evaluation of the cornea, both with lens wear and on removal, will aid in determination of the source of the discomfort. In addition, evaluation of corneal staining with fluorescein application is important.

Discomfort on Lens Insertion

If discomfort occurs on insertion, the source is most likely either a torn lens, a sensitivity to the solutions used, debris on lens, or (if applicable) the prism ballast of a toric lens. A torn lens can be detected by carefully examining both the entire lens surface and the lens edge with the biomicroscope. The upper lid should be raised to evaluate the superior lens edge. Lens tears may be difficult to observe. The lens should be carefully observed on the blink, which will make the

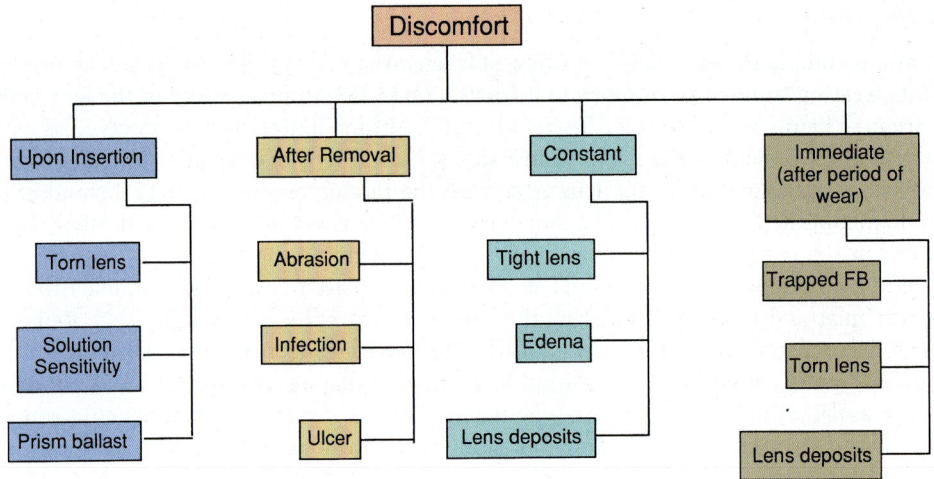

FIGURE 13.2 Summary of causes of discomfort.

tear more evident. The tear may actually be a hole or nick in the lens or have the appearance of a scratch or adhered debris. Apparent trapped debris that cannot be cleaned off and remains on the lens with a blink is most likely a lens defect. A torn lens should be replaced immediately.

If a patient uses an improper solution in the eye or on the soft lens (i.e., hydrogen peroxide or a GP lens solution) or has acquired a sensitivity to the preservative in a solution, an immediate burning and stinging sensation will be experienced. Lens removal should improve the discomfort; however, a mild-to-moderate superficial punctate keratitis will remain; thus, mild discomfort and injection may still be present. By questioning the patient about the solutions used with the lenses and evaluating the cornea and conjunctiva with a biomicroscope, the practitioner will be able to determine if the source of the discomfort is preservative sensitivity. Typically, preservative sensitivity will result in a diffuse superficial punctate keratitis staining pattern.[11] If the practitioner is still unsure, another care system can be prescribed for the patient. Replacing the lens with a fresh, sterile lens and using a fresh case is optimal prior to prescribing a new care system. This will prevent any contamination of the previous solution with the new solution. If the discomfort is eliminated by a change in the solution system, sensitivity to the solution was most likely the cause. In severe cases, lens wear may have to be discontinued until the subjective discomfort has been alleviated. This may occur after a few hours or take up to several days. Artificial tears are recommended to aid patient comfort.

A rare cause of discomfort is the prism ballast of a toric lens. Occasionally, a patient will complain of lens sensation caused by the thickness of the lens in the area of the prism ballast. If no other source of discomfort is found, a change in the type of toric lens design (i.e., use of eccentric lenticulation, double thin zones) may alleviate the lens sensation.

Discomfort with a previously unworn lens versus discomfort with a worn but previously comfortable lens may be approached differently. If the lens is new and the patient experiences discomfort from a design that has previously been satisfactory, the cause may be debris trapped under the lens on insertion. Debris on the lens before insertion is a common cause of discomfort. Possibilities include particles from a tissue or hand towel, a small strand of hair, or other small pieces of debris that are not observable by the naked eye. Simply removing the lens and rinsing it may provide relief from the discomfort. If the discomfort persists and the cause is not visible, the lens itself may be defective in a way that is not visible with conventional inspection techniques. The most expedient course of action is to replace the lens. If the discomfort occurs with a lens that has been previously worn with no discomfort, the most likely cause is a damaged lens. The lens should be removed and inspected. If no damage is found, the lens may be rinsed and inserted again to determine if the discomfort persists.

Discomfort after Lens Removal

When pain or discomfort is present after lens removal, the origin of the problem is typically the cornea. Pain that continues after lens removal is an ocular emergency, and the patient should be evaluated in the office as soon as possible. Corneal abrasions, ocular infections, corneal ulcers, or other ocular problems may be causing the pain. Fluorescein evaluation is important in determining the extent of the corneal disturbance. Discomfort and pain that remain after the removal of soft lenses should be taken seriously until a differential diagnosis is made.

Constant Discomfort during Lens Wear

When the discomfort of soft lenses is constant, the source of the discomfort may be a poorly fitting lens, corneal edema and edema-related symptoms (i.e., microcysts), or lens deposits. Biomicroscopy and fluorescein evaluation will aid in determination of the cause. A compression ring around the limbal area after lens removal is indicative of a tight lens. Higher-modulus silicone hydrogel lenses that are fitted too flat may exhibit edge lift and cause discomfort. After alteration of the lens parameters, either by changing the base curve radius (BCR) or the lens diameter, the symptoms should disappear. For a patient experiencing edema-related symptoms, a change to a higher-Dk/t silicone hydrogel lens will be beneficial.

Another cause of constant discomfort with a soft lens is a deposited lens. These deposits will be evident when the lens is viewed with the biomicroscope. The deposits may be a result of poor lens care, old lenses, or lenses that have been contaminated with substances such as hair spray or lotion. Silicone hydrogel lenses are more prone to lipid deposits than hydrogel lenses. Despite the claims of "no rub" solutions, silicone hydrogel lenses should be rubbed upon removal to aid in the removal of lipid deposits. The authors recommend educating all soft lens patients to rub and rinse their lenses to provide the cleanest and most comfortable lenses. Replacing the deposited lens with a clean, new lens will alleviate the symptoms.

Sudden Discomfort after a Period of Lens Wear

Patients may experience sudden discomfort after the lens has been worn for several hours. The most frequent cause of sudden discomfort is a trapped foreign body, such as dust or cosmetic particles. Removing the lens and rinsing it with solution should eliminate this discomfort. A large foreign body may cause a corneal abrasion; therefore, if the pain continues, it is important for the patient to be evaluated in the office. A deposited lens, especially one with jelly bumps, or a contaminated lens may result in discomfort that increases as the period of lens wear increases. Finally, a torn lens may also cause immediate discomfort; however, typically, the discomfort is noticed on lens insertion. Obviously, the treatment for a foreign body is its removal. If the lens is not damaged, deposited, or torn, the lens may be worn again. Conversely, a damaged lens will require replacement. In the case of a foreign body, the cornea, conjunctiva, and lids should be examined to make sure the foreign body has not become embedded.

Burning or Stinging Sensation

Burning and stinging are most often related to contact lens solution sensitivity (i.e., preservative sensitivity or improper use of solution). Reinforcement of appropriate lens hygiene at each visit is beneficial in maintaining patient compliance and avoiding unnecessary irritation. Irritation with continued use of a chemical disinfecting system may indicate a possible hypersensitivity or toxic reaction to the preservative or an added surfactant. Discomfort noted by patients is typically minimal because of the low concentration of preservatives in the solution. The symptom may be a feeling of dryness, rather than burning. A generalized stippling is indicative of a toxic or hypersensitivity reaction and, if severe enough, may elicit tearing and photophobia as well as decreased visual acuity. Patients who exhibit this problem may achieve success with the use of a preservative-free hydrogen peroxide disinfecting system or of a daily disposable lens that requires no care regimen.

Incomplete neutralization of hydrogen peroxide or use of an old catalytic disc (beyond 90 days or 100 uses) can result in symptoms of burning and stinging. A low pH (4.0) after disinfection and the buffer system to control pH may also contribute to irritation. Although most patients no longer use a separate daily cleaner or enzyme cleaner with their soft lenses, the use of a daily cleaner before insertion or inadequate rinsing of the lens after cleaning may elicit a burning sensation. Any residual cleaner remaining on the lens after enzyme cleaning may also cause discomfort. A comprehensive case history may be extremely beneficial in determining the cause of the ocular irritation. Reviewing cleaning and disinfection procedures at each visit can assist in alleviating solution-related discomfort associated with the use of inappropriate technique. Instructions and diagrams may help in maintaining patient compliance with acceptable cleaning and disinfecting procedures. The emergence of MPSs may make it difficult to determine the offending component, as many of these products contain surfactants and other compounds in the disinfecting solution (Fig. 13.3).

Photophobia

Definition

The term *photophobia* is often used loosely in describing irritation and discomfort as a result of contact lens wear. When the term is used appropriately, photophobia is typically considered a pathologic condition that occurs when light entering the eye causes pain. Photophobia may be contrasted with dazzle, a sensation of discomfort as a result of excessive light that is usually not associated with pain. A temporary sensation of dazzle is experienced with inadequate adaptation of the eye from dark to lighted conditions. Also, dazzle, unlike photophobia, is not accompanied by blepharospasm and lacrimation. Pathologic conditions affecting the anterior segment of the eye are often accompanied by photophobia. Typically, the more superficial the corneal defect, the more severe the photophobia because of the arrangement of the innervation of the epithelium.[12] It is important to remember that photophobia is a *symptom* of an ocular

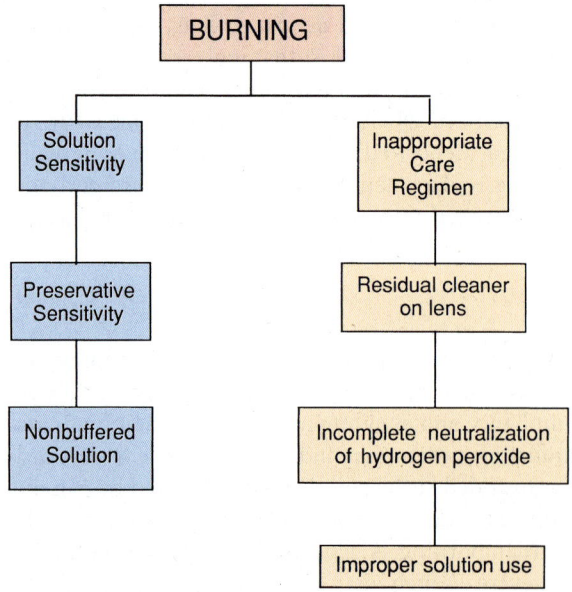

FIGURE 13.3 Summary of causes of burning.

problem and that the logical method to address this symptom is to determine and then treat the condition causing the photophobia.

Causes

Epithelial abrasions may be observed in contact lens wearers and, in severe cases, may induce photophobia. Superficial corneal abrasions may occur as a result of contact lens defects (including tears and nicks), moderate lens "overwear," mild trauma, trapped debris, and an uneven surface. Often, superficial defects go unnoticed by the patient but may result in mild discomfort and irritation. Deeper abrasions typically result in more severe pain, including lacrimation, blepharospasm, and photophobia. Removal of the entire thickness of the epithelium occurs most commonly as a result of blunt trauma (e.g., hand, thumb, or ball in the eye), improper insertion or removal of the contact lens, or a foreign body under the lens.[13]

In addition to abrasions, photophobia has been attributed to other factors.[5,12,14] Initial adaptation to contact lens wear may initiate photophobia, and this is considered normal unless the symptom continues longer than a few weeks. Uncorrected refractive error and residual astigmatism may also contribute to a photophobic response.[12]

Determining the Cause of Photophobia

A thorough case history may be extremely beneficial in eliciting the cause of photophobia. Biomicroscopic examination of both the contact lens and the cornea will eliminate any gross defects contributing to the symptoms. The presence of discharge, in conjunction with lacrimation and blepharospasm, may indicate the possibility of infection. The type of discharge (e.g., mucopurulent, watery, stringy) should be elicited in determining the possible etiology. Fluorescein staining is beneficial in determining the presence, location, and depth of an abrasion. The configuration of the staining pattern may allude to a causative factor (e.g., tear, nick, foreign body, deposited lens). Examination of the lens under magnification may further assist in locating any lens defects.

Treatment of the Causes of Photophobia

Conservative treatment of superficial abrasions includes contact lens removal to ensure proper healing. Epithelial cell coverage of the abrasion usually is complete within 24 hours. Although antibiotic therapy is typically not warranted, consideration may be necessary in patients exhibiting poor lid hygiene, coated lenses, or poor compliance. Deeper corneal abrasions require more aggressive therapy, including lens removal and antibiotic use if the threat of infection is present; however, preservatives found in medications may slow down the healing process.[13] Because of the increased risk of developing a *Pseudomonas* infection, a bandage contact lens is not appropriate for a contact lens wearer with a corneal abrasion. In a non-contact lens patient, a corneal abrasion may be treated with a bandage contact lens.[15]

Infections require discontinuation of contact lens wear and appropriate antibiotic treatment (see Chapter 23). Microbial keratitis (MK) is a serious infection found primarily in overnight wear of contact lenses. More information on MK is provided in Chapter 16. Lens wear should not be resumed until the clinician is comfortable that the infection has resolved.

Dryness

Dry-eye symptoms are very common among soft contact lens wearers.[16–19] This may be a result of the patient's poor tear quality or quantity or of the effect of the contact lens itself on the tear film.[20] Historically, the tear film was described as composed of three layers: aqueous, lipid, and mucin. More recent theories have described the tear film as a gel-like structure with several layers derived from these components.[21] If a deficit occurs in any component, contact lens wear may be affected.

Applying a contact lens to the cornea changes and disrupts the precorneal tear film thickness by displacing a portion of the tear volume. The normal precorneal tear thickness decreases to about half the thickness after the contact lens is applied.[22–24] In addition, the tear breakup time (TBUT) occurs more rapidly in contact lens wear than in non-contact lens wearing normal individuals.[25] A complete blink approximately every 5 seconds is required to spread the tear film over the cornea. Incomplete or partial blinks will result in dryness of the inferior region of the cornea. Blinking exercises may alleviate dryness in these cases. Other factors that can contribute to dry-eye symptoms with soft contact lenses are the environment, medications, computer use, and pregnancy.

Patient and Environmental Factors

A thorough case history will be important to elicit possible causes of dryness. Additionally, the patient should be questioned about any medical conditions, such as Stevens–Johnson syndrome (mucin deficiency), pregnancy (increase in tear viscosity), or Sjogren's syndrome (aqueous deficiency). Medications that can alter the tear film are antihistamines, anticholinergics, antianxiety agents, phenothiazines, and oral contraceptives.[26]

The occupational environment (e.g., working near heating and air conditioning vents) may exacerbate dryness symptoms. Circulating air from automobile vents may also cause discomfort. The use of vent covers to redirect the air away from the wearer or changing the angle of the automobile vents should relieve dryness. Long-term computer use may cause a decreased blink rate, resulting in symptoms of dryness. This may be alleviated by having the wearer take blink breaks, such as at the end of each page of material. The same technique may be useful for others, such as students, who spend significant amounts of time reading. Airline passengers may also experience dryness, particularly on long trips, because of the low relative humidity in airplane cabins at high altitude (Fig. 13.4).

Refitting the patient into a different material may be beneficial in reducing symptoms of dryness. Lenses containing phosphorylcholine have been reported to provide improved comfort.[27,28] Additionally, some manufacturers incorporate compounds such as polyvinylpyrrolidone and polyvinyl alcohol into lenses during the manufacturing process in an effort to provide comfort and lens hydration.[29–31]

Silicone hydrogel lenses have also been reported to provide increased comfort.[32] This may be due in part to the low water content of silicone hydrogel lenses, which results in less lens dehydration. There is additional evidence that the increased oxygen provided by silicone hydrogel materials may decrease the ocular inflammatory response that may be found in hydrogel materials with low oxygen permeability (Dk). This inflammatory response may be responsible for ocular surface and lacrimal gland damage, which may cause ocular dryness; therefore, silicone hydrogel materials eliminate this damage and the dryness that results.[33] Additional treatment for ocular dryness can be found in Chapter 23.

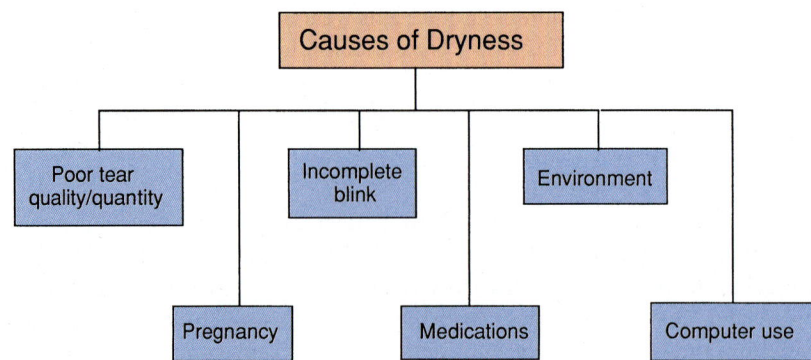

FIGURE 13.4 Summary of causes of dryness.

Excessive Lens Movement

Deposited Lens

Surface deposits have been found to occur less frequently on disposable contact lenses than on conventional replacement lenses.[34] Conventional replacement soft lenses or those that are used beyond their recommended replacement schedule may become very deposited and exhibit excessive movement. The patient may present with symptoms of decentration of the lens during eye movement or with complaints that the lens is easily dislodged from the eye. On observation with the biomicroscope, it will be apparent that the soft lens has become deposited. These deposits may be filmy coatings or elevated deposits. The most common and effective treatment for lens deposition is to fit the patient in disposable lenses. If the patient is already wearing disposable lenses, then education on compliance with replacement instructions is recommended.[35]

In addition, a patient exhibiting signs and symptoms of a dry eye may also experience lens decentration or lenses that dislodge as a result of dehydration of the lens. Use of a soft lens that is recommended for dry eyes or the use of lens lubricants may alleviate dryness.

Inverted Lens

Another cause of a lens moving excessively or dislodging from the eye easily is an inverted lens. Patients should be educated on how to determine lens inversion at the dispensing visit; however, this is more difficult to distinguish with certain types of lenses and some patients. Methods of determining lens inversion by visual inspection have been described previously (see Chapter 12). Repeated demonstration of these two methods may aid the patient in determining lens inversion. Graphics and photographs demonstrating lens inversion may be of additional help. When the lens is observed with the biomicroscope, it may exhibit excessive movement and edge lift. In addition, visual acuity may be reduced. If the patient finds visual inspection of lens inversion difficult and is experiencing decreased visual acuity, excessive lens movement, minor discomfort, or a lens that dislodges, the patient should suspect lens inversion and attempt to insert the lens in the other direction.

Flat Lens

Excessive lens movement is also observed in soft lenses with a BCR that is too flat. Biomicroscopic evaluation of a soft lens that is too flat may reveal any of the following signs or combination of signs: inferior lens decentration with the patient gazing straight ahead, corneal exposure on lens movement, edge lift, superior decentration on downward gaze, or lens movement >1.5 mm with the blink. A change to a steeper base curve or larger lens diameter should improve the soft lens-to-cornea fitting relationship (Fig. 13.5).

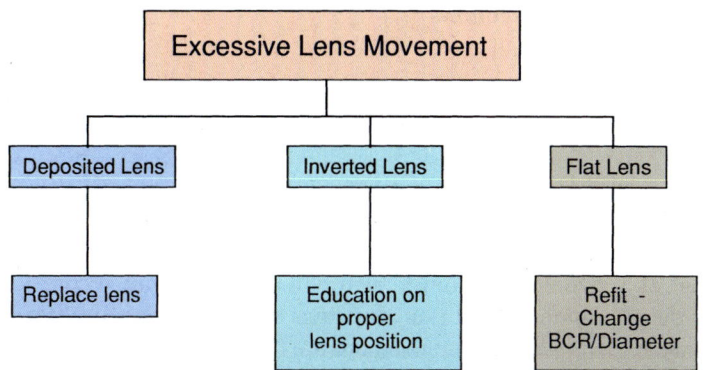

FIGURE 13.5 Summary of causes and management of excessive lens movement.

Foggy/Hazy Vision

Diagnosis

Foggy or hazy vision through a soft contact lens may result from a coated lens, corneal edema, or dry eye. A common symptom elicited from patients may be the appearance of halos around or distortion of bright point sources of light. Clinical signs of either a contaminated lens or corneal edema may be observed with a biomicroscope. To assist in determining the cause of the reduced vision, the patient may be questioned about the frequency of cleaning, method of disinfection (chemical, hydrogen peroxide), use of a daily cleaner and weekly enzyme, cleanliness of hands before lens handling, use of hand lotions or soaps containing moisturizers, and age of lenses. Patients in whom corneal edema is suspected should be questioned about their wearing time. The presence of epithelial edema as a result of "overwear" is infrequently noted in soft lens wearers but may be observed in wearers of thick, low-water-content hydrogel lenses.[13] Symptoms may be more prevalent after long periods of lens wear. Patients experiencing foggy vision as a result of dryness may experience improved vision with the use of preservative-free artificial tears as needed.

Treatment

In cases of a contaminated or coated lens, visual acuity will improve with the placement of a new lens on the eye. If the patient's lens modality is only available in a conventional lens, they may need to use surfactants or enzymatic cleaners, replace the contact lenses more frequently, or switch to a GP material. Patient education on proper cleaning and disinfecting techniques will help prolong the viability of the contact lens.

Removal of the contact lens and exposure of the cornea to air will result in a reduction of epithelial edema.[13] Hypertonic solutions may be beneficial in severe cases of edema, although their use may be unnecessary with the level of epithelial edema found in hydrogel contact lens wearers.[36] Switching patients to a lens material with a higher Dk/t (e.g., silicone hydrogel) and maintaining the patient on a daily-wear (DW) schedule will help reduce or eliminate the edema.[13] Likewise, those patients who were fitted in lower-water-content lenses for comfort (e.g., dry-eye patients) may be refitted in silicone hydrogel lenses to alleviate epithelial edema.

CLINICAL SIGNS

The practitioner will detect clinical signs during biomicroscopic evaluation of the patient's anterior segment. The use of grading scales and diagrams is beneficial to monitor and evaluate changes in the various conditions discussed in this section. The individual practitioner may develop the grading scale, or a currently published scale may be used. Regardless, the scale is typically based on numeric grades, as follows[5]:

0 = not present
1 = minimal
2 = mild
3 = moderate
4 = severe

This scale may be more descriptive when applied to a specific clinical sign (e.g., edema, injection). Assignment of a grade to the clinical sign will aid in accurate record keeping and further evaluation of the condition. In addition, drawings of the findings (infiltrates, staining, vessel growth) will enable the practitioner to compare the findings at each visit to determine if any changes have occurred.

Staining

The use of fluorescein can be an effective method of monitoring alterations in corneal integrity secondary to contact lens wear. Practitioners often choose not to use fluorescein during routine examination because of its inconvenience for patients wearing hydrogel lenses (e.g., discoloring the lens). Following the application of fluorescein, either the eye should be rinsed with saline solution or the patient should be instructed not to reinsert the lenses for approximately 2 hours after insertion of the dye. A hand-held ultraviolet lamp is useful in checking for the presence of residual fluorescein. The introduction of high-molecular-weight fluorescein (fluorexon) and its ability to be used with the soft lens in the eye have helped to increase the use of fluorescein as a diagnostic tool in the evaluation of the corneal response to hydrogel contact lens wear; however, it should be noted that this type of fluorescein exhibits reduced fluorescence in comparison with fluorescein strips. In the authors' experience, silicone hydrogel lenses are less likely to be stained by fluorescein dye (see Chapter 10).

The configuration of corneal punctate staining may be used to identify its cause (Fig. 13.6). Infection, mechanical trauma, trapped debris, desiccation, oxygen deprivation, inappropriate corneal bearing, and solution hypersensitivity are some of the more common causes of decreased corneal integrity.[13] Because of its serious nature, the presence of infectious keratitis must be considered in patients presenting with corneal staining. A comprehensive case history and evaluation of patient symptoms may be beneficial in determining the possibility of infection.

Mechanical trauma can arise from excessive pressure on the cornea from the contact lens. The center and edge of the lens represent the most common areas of bearing. A ring-shaped pattern of staining may result from contact between the peripheral edge of the central bearing area of the lens and the cornea.[5] More isolated areas of staining can occur as a result of lens tears or nicks. Evaluation of the lens for damage is often easiest with the use of the biomicroscope while the lens is on the eye. Fluorescein pooling will be evident within the epithelial break and may mimic the pattern of damage to the contact lens.

Lifting the upper lid may reveal an arc-shaped pattern of staining secondary to epithelial splitting, also known as superior epithelial arcuate lesions (SEALs). The cause of this phenomenon is thought to be mechanical in nature. Patients are typically asymptomatic; therefore, appropriate evaluation of the superior cornea is necessary to detect this condition. Treatment consists of removal of the lenses until healing occurs. Higher-modulus silicone hydrogel lenses have been associated with this finding.[37] Switching to a different design usually alleviates the problem (Chapter 16).[38–40]

Linear corneal staining may be secondary to a foreign body trapped under the lens. The appearance of "tracking" may occur as a result of lens movement during the blink. Removal of the lens in combination with appropriate cleaning of the lens and flushing of the eye will

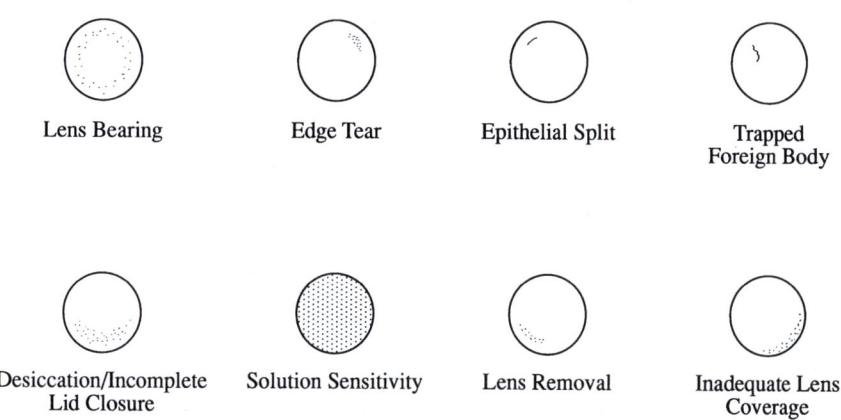

FIGURE 13.6 Diagram representing staining patterns found with soft lenses.

assist in removing any foreign particles. Lens deposits, as well as trapped epithelial debris, may result in scattered punctate staining. Appropriate lid and lens hygiene may help in alleviating this source of staining, in addition to use of a disposable or planned-replacement contact lens.

Lens dehydration may also be a source of punctate staining in hydrogel lens patients. Silicone hydrogel lenses have a lower water content, so are not as prone to dehydration. Typically, drying occurs in the region of the cornea where the lids meet as a result of minimal wiping of the cornea with tears in this area. Incomplete lid closure on blinking may also result in inferior punctate staining. Patients who have a tendency to this type of staining and are wearing thin, high-water-content hydrogel lenses may benefit from switching to a lower-water-content, thicker hydrogel or a silicone hydrogel lens. Frequent use of rewetting drops may also help alleviate corneal desiccation.

A generalized form of superficial punctate staining may develop following a solution hypersensitivity to a chemical preservative. This condition is most often bilateral and disappears following removal of the offending substance. The patient may also experience a foreign-body sensation and photophobia in severe cases. Replacing the lens and the case, in combination with switching the patient to a different preservative or to preservative-free solution will help prevent further reaction. Cold compresses may help alleviate discomfort in severe cases.

Diffuse punctate staining has been found in silicone hydrogel lens materials in combination with a multipurpose care system.[41] Treatment of this type of staining requires switching to a different MPS or a hydrogen peroxide care system, or changing the silicone hydrogel material.

Trauma to the cornea secondary to lens removal may be found in soft lens wearers who remove the lens directly from the cornea rather than sliding the lens down onto the bulbar conjunctiva before removal. The use of the fingernails, instead of the pads of the fingers, will result in a midperipheral staining pattern at the area corresponding to the pinching of the lens. This area of staining is typically arcuate or V-shaped. If the area of staining arouses suspicion, the practitioner may observe the patient's lens removal technique to confirm the cause.

Inadequate soft lens coverage or lens decentration may result in fluorescein staining near the corneal–scleral junction. Typically, this area will also be injected. Refitting with a larger-diameter lens or one that achieves better centration and coverage will alleviate this problem.

Corneal Edema

Clinical Evaluation

Fortunately, the introduction of silicone hydrogel lens materials have reduced the amount of corneal edema and the symptoms and signs associated with it. Clinical signs of corneal edema secondary to conventional hydrogel lens wear are typically apparent only in severe cases (Table 13.1). Alterations in the corneal structure may be clinically apparent initially with

TABLE 13.1 Signs and Symptoms of Corneal Edema
Reduced visual acuity
Foggy/hazy vision
Increase in myopia
Generalized loss of corneal transparency
Striae
Microcysts
Folds of Descemet membrane
Endothelial changes
Possible steepening of keratometry readings

the presence of approximately 6% edema.[5] The absence of significant changes in the radius of curvature and spectacle blur in hydrogel lens wearers can be attributed to the symmetry of the edema throughout the epithelium.[42,43] The presence of a generalized epithelial edema is noted in hydrogel lens wearers and may be partially responsible for a progressive increase in myopia (myopic "creep" or myopic shift).[44] Silicone hydrogel lens materials have increased the oxygen transmission to the cornea by as much as eight times the amount of transmission of conventional hydrogel lenses.[45]

In evaluating corneal structural changes as a result of edema, the biomicroscope and pachometer are both acceptable clinical instruments, although the biomicroscope is used far more frequently in clinical practice. Striae and epithelial edema may initially be visible with 4% to 6% corneal thickening. Mild folds of Descemet membrane become apparent with approximately 7% edema, whereas major folds become apparent with swelling in excess of 15%.[44]

Primary changes are typically apparent within the epithelium and may be observed with the microscope focused on the corneal surface and the illumination source directed toward the limbus. Magnification of, at minimum, 25× must be used to visualize these changes. Vertical striae may also be present in conjunction with epithelial edema and are typically much easier to identify. They may be observed within the deep stroma and are detected by using a narrow parallelepiped. During assessment of the presence of striae, a differentiation must be made from corneal nerves. Striae appear as white lines and usually occur within the pupillary region of the cornea. They are typically 1 to 6 mm in length and rarely bifurcate. Corneal nerves bifurcate and extend to the peripheral limbus. When striae do bifurcate, the angle formed is much smaller than the angle observed with corneal nerves.[5]

Corneal Swelling

Placement of a contact lens on the eye results in a decrease in the amount of oxygen available to the cornea. Lid closure further decreases the oxygen tension at the anterior surface of the contact lens in comparison with the open-eye condition. Indirect endothelial function studies of the corneal swelling response to the overnight use of conventional hydrogel contact lenses confirm corneal swelling between 8% and 15% after overnight wear, in comparison with a swelling rate of 4% in a control, non–lens-wearing group.[46] Variation in the level of swelling is evident as a result of differences in individual responses to decreased oxygen availability.[47] The presence of clinically observable edema secondary to hydrogel lens wear indicates a significant level of swelling, necessitating appropriate alterations in current contact lens management.

In contrast to conventional hydrogels, silicone hydrogels have been found to demonstrate overnight corneal swelling similar to that of a closed eye with no contact lens.[48] The use of silicone hydrogel lenses for DW or overnight wear has virtually eliminated corneal hypoxia in most patients.[49]

Epithelial Edema

A principal cause of epithelial edema may be exposure of the cornea to a hypotonic solution. Intercellular penetration of fluid results in an increase in the fragility of the cornea caused by the increased separation between the epithelial cells and loosening of the junctional complexes. As a result of the vulnerability of the cornea in this state, there is a dramatic increase in its susceptibility to an abrasion.[50] Removal of the corneal barriers to fluid penetration may also be compromised by trauma. A "roughening" of the epithelial surface will allow pooling of tears within the abraded area, as well as edema of the surrounding cells.[13]

The use of fluorescein will significantly enhance the appearance of edema adjacent to the abrasion. A central area of green will appear as a result of pooling of tears within the abraded area, and the edges will appear gray as a result of "heaping" of the epithelium surrounding the lesion. Therefore, a green haze will demarcate the surrounding edema. Generalized edema may best be viewed by retroillumination, whereas the addition of fluorescein may elicit a green, mottled appearance. Because of the difference in refractive indices between the epithelium and water, epithelial edema will also generate a "sparkly" appearance when viewed with white light.[13]

Microcysts

Epithelial microcysts, a complication found with both DW and extended wear (EW) of hydrogel lenses, can be observed biomicroscopically. Microcysts typically are found in the midperipheral cornea, are characterized by reverse illumination and become apparent between 3 weeks and 6 months after EW is initiated with conventional hydrogel lenses.[51] They may vary from 15 to 50 μm in diameter and appear as spheres scattered throughout all layers of the epithelium. These cysts, thought to be composed of disorganized epithelial growths rather than fluid, result from abnormal metabolism during conditions of corneal hypoxia. Reduction of wearing time has not been found successful in reducing the number of microcysts.[47] Lens removal will often result in an increase in the number of microcysts during the first week, but a gradual reduction will occur within a 5- to 10-week period.[52,53] Surfacing of the microcysts will produce punctate staining with fluorescein. Hydrogel contact lens wear should be discontinued and the patient refitted in a silicone hydrogel lens.

Management

The current standard of care for managing patients in this situation is to refit them in a silicone hydrogel lens. For those patients for whom this is not an option, thin, higher-water-content lenses will maximize the level of oxygen reaching the cornea. In hydrogel lenses, a combination of both water content and lens thickness determines the level of Dk/t to the cornea. Average lens thickness is a more accurate determinant of central corneal edema than is center thickness. Higher-power lenses with the same center thickness as lower-power lenses of the same material cause a higher degree of central corneal swelling.[46]

"Tight-Lens" Syndrome

Corneal edema may or may not arise secondary to a lens that is clinically deemed to be "too tight." A soft lens that exhibits no movement under magnification is typically considered to be a "tight lens." The significant exchange of new tears under a soft lens is minimal compared with that under a GP contact lens. Therefore, a variation in the lens-to-cornea fitting relationship has little to do with preventing corneal edematous changes by altering the flow of tears under the lens. The thickness of a hydrogel lens appears to be the parameter that determines the amount of corneal edema.[54] Silicone hydrogel lenses have a high Dk value. Even when the thickness is taken into consideration, the Dk/t (where t is the thickness and Dk/t is oxygen transmissibility) is high, allowing, in most of the materials, for the oxygen transmission to exceed the recommended Dk/t of 125×10^{-9} (cm $\times$ mL O_2)/(sec $\times$ mL $\times$ mm Hg)[45] (see Chapters 10 and 16).

The presence of minimal or no lens movement on the cornea may result in conjunctival injection caused by impingement of the limbal vasculature. Limbal vascular compression results from a "suctioning" of the lens to the eye subsequent to a steep fitting relationship. Biomicroscopic examination of the limbus may reveal congestion of the limbal blood flow posterior to the lens edge with blanching of the vessels just anterior to the lens edge. Conjunctival movement with the blink may also be observed; this is termed *conjunctival drag*. If conjunctival compression occurs with an inadequately fit lens, either the base curve should be flattened or the diameter reduced to provide better movement. The presence of corneal edema may or may not accompany this condition. Its resolution may be accomplished by changing to a silicone hydrogel lens material. Additional edema-related conditions found primarily in EW or CW are addressed in Chapter 16.

Injection

Generalized Injection

A symptom and clinical sign found with both soft and GP lens wear is conjunctival injection (typically expressed as "redness" by patients). There are many causes of generalized injection found in soft contact lens wearers that may or may not be related to contact lens wear (Table 13.2). Typically, if the soft lens is the cause, the injection results from corneal hypoxia, a tight lens, solution sensitivity, trapped foreign body, deposits, lens defects, inflammatory reaction to overnight wear (i.e., Contact Lens Acute Red Eye [CLARE]), or ocular complications of these conditions. The injection may also be a result of conditions not related to the lens, such as allergic, viral, or bacterial conjunctivitis or other ocular and systemic conditions. To identify the cause of injection, a thorough case history should include questions such as the following: When was the injection initially observed? Does it continue after the lenses are removed? Is the injection of recent onset or is it chronic? Are the eyes irritated, burning, or itching? Is there any discharge and, if so, of what type—mucous, watery, or stringy? Was there an occurrence that preceded the injection, such as change in solutions, swimming, lack of sleep, illness, traumatic injury, or foreign body? Based on the case history, the elimination of causative factors, and a thorough evaluation with the biomicroscope, the diagnosis can be made.

Lens-Related Generalized Injection: Narrowing a diagnosis of injection to contact lens-related causes is based on symptoms, lens-to-cornea fitting relationship, lens condition, and wearing time. Moderate-to-severe injection of the eye at any time should be treated as an ocular emergency because of the risk of corneal ulcers and infection. It is not unusual for some patients to present with mild injection caused by a variety of factors (e.g., environment, dryness); however, if the injection is acute with no known cause, a thorough evaluation is necessary to rule out serious conditions.

Symptoms: Lens-related injection will typically occur upon insertion or after lens wear and will improve as lens wear is discontinued. Immediate injection with burning on insertion will most likely be related to solution sensitivity. The use of preservatives such as thimerosal, chlorhexidine, and benzalkonium chloride in increased concentrations or for a prolonged period of time have resulted in patient sensitivity.[55] Newer preservatives found in MPS regimens are more subtle in sensitivity symptoms. Symptoms may be dryness, loss of wearing time, or minor discomfort. Immediate discomfort and injection may also be the result of improper

TABLE 13.2 Factors Resulting in Injection

RELATED TO CONTACT LENSES	NOT NECESSARILY RELATED TO CONTACT LENS WEAR
Damaged lens	Foreign body
Edema	Conjunctivitis
Solution sensitivity	Ocular pathology
Tight lens	Trauma
Deposited lens	Cigarette smoke
Contaminated lens	Swimming in chlorinated pools
Trapped foreign body	Lack of sleep
Poor-fitting lens	Excessive alcoholic beverages
Improper use of solutions	Allergies
CLARE	Dryness

CLARE-contact lens acute red eye.

use of the soft lens solutions, which includes use of a daily cleaner before insertion without a thorough rinsing, inadequate neutralization of hydrogen peroxide disinfecting solutions, and use of incompatible solutions. Management of injection resulting from preservatives requires changing to a care regimen with a different preservative, to a nonpreserved system (such as hydrogen peroxide disinfection with nonpreserved solutions), or to a solution-free lens (i.e., daily disposable contact lenses).

As the wearing time increases over the period of a day with DW or over a period of days with EW, corneal hypoxia, a tight lens, or a deposited or damaged lens may result in a generalized injection. By evaluating the lens and eye with the biomicroscope, the cause of the injection may be determined. Eliminating the injection requires either replacing the lens with a new lens or refitting to improve the fitting relationship or Dk/t of the lens.

Lens Fitting Relationship: As noted previously, a tight-fitting lens may impinge on the limbal vasculature, resulting in injection. When the lens movement is evaluated, no movement will be observed, even with the use of the "push-up test," which consists of manipulating the soft lens with the lower lid in an attempt to push the lens upward. A tightly fitting lens will resist movement when pushed up with the lower lid, whereas a lens that is not adherent will exhibit movement with this test. In addition, the lens should adequately cover the cornea and extend onto the sclera. A lens that is too small may result in injection in the area not adequately covered or in the area of the limbus on which the lens impinges. Altering the soft lens parameters to achieve better movement and coverage will eliminate this form of injection.

Lens Condition: An old, deposited, contaminated, or damaged soft lens may result in a generalized injection. When the lens is removed from the eye, the injection should resolve unless further corneal insult has occurred. Evaluation with the biomicroscope will reveal the condition of the lens. The cornea should be evaluated after lens removal to ensure that the cornea is not affected. Simple replacement of the soft lens with a fresh, clean lens will alleviate the symptoms. In addition, reeducating the patient on the proper care and handling and recommended replacement schedule for the lens may be necessary. Refitting the patient in a more frequently replaced lens, if possible, may preclude recurrence of the problem.

Wearing Time: An acute red eye associated with excessive or overnight wear should be treated with extreme caution. One large-scale study found that conventional hydrogel EW patients who wore their lenses overnight had a 10 to 15 times greater risk of ulcerative keratitis than did DW patients who did not wear their lenses overnight.[56] Fortunately, the use of conventional hydrogel materials for EW has been primarily replaced with silicone hydrogel materials, which provide more oxygen to the cornea for overnight wear.

CLARE, characterized by an EW patient awakening with a red, watery eye, is an inflammatory reaction that occurs with overnight wear of soft contact lenses. This inflammatory reaction is observed in both hydrogel and silicone hydrogel lenses. More information on CLARE and other complications (i.e., contact lens peripheral ulcer, infiltrates) found primarily in overnight wear are discussed in Chapter 16.

For the acute red eye, the cornea should be examined with and without fluorescein for signs of edema, ulceration, or other compromise. If the corneal epithelium is intact, discontinuing lens wear, use of an ocular lubricant, and frequent monitoring until the injection disappears may be all that is necessary. Returning to overnight wear depends largely on the patient's compliance with wearing instructions. Wearing contact lenses for longer than the recommended wearing schedule is likely to result in corneal compromise. A compliant patient may be fitted into a silicone hydrogel lens with a higher Dk/t. The wearing time may be reduced as needed. A CW or EW soft lens worn on a flexible wear (FW) or DW basis or a GP lens may also improve the patient's success at lens wear. In any case, the patient should be educated about why the injection is occurring and about the importance of following directions pertaining to wearing schedule.

Injection Not Related to Contact Lens Wear: It may be difficult for the practitioner to determine if the injection is not lens related. If the soft lens is fitting properly, nonpreserved solutions are used, the lens is clean and new, and the injection continues after lens wear is discontinued, the assumption would be to evaluate the eye for other causative factors. A simple case history may elicit the cause, such as allergies, dryness, lack of sleep, trauma, or cigarette smoke. Further evaluation with the biomicroscope with and without fluorescein will aid in diagnosing the problem. Some patients present with mild injection on a consistent basis, which may be improved with the use of lens lubricants to rinse the lens off, to rinse and relieve the eye exposed to chlorine in swimming pools and cigarette smoke, and to rewet the lens and relieve dry eye.

Sectorial Injection

Injection located in a specific area of the eye typically signals an irritation in that specific area. With soft contact lenses, this is generally the result of a lens tear or deposit that is located in the same area as the injection. Any damaged lens should be replaced, and the injection will disappear.

Another form of sectorial injection sometimes occurs when a lens impinges on a pinguecula. If the lens is observed to be irritating a pinguecula, the lens should be refitted with a larger or smaller diameter that either covers the pinguecula to a greater extent or does not contact the pinguecula. A GP lens may need to be fitted to eliminate contact between the contact lens and the pinguecula.

Episcleritis, a condition that is not contact lens related, often presents as a form of sectorial injection. It is usually unilateral and recurrent, and it may be accompanied by variable levels of discomfort. It is a self-limiting disease that can be treated with topical steroids or topical NSAIDs.[57,58]

Corneal Vascularization

Introduction

Vascularization of the normally avascular cornea is a serious complication of hydrogel contact lens wear. Severe cases involving visual reduction and corneal translucency typically occur after surgery or as a result of a pathologic incident. The presence of a vascular response to contact lens wear, whether involving limbal capillary filling or "true" corneal vascularization, is indicative of contact lens intolerance. This intolerance is generally a result of a tight-lens fit, limbal compression, corneal edema, or excessive wear by the patient.[59] Corneal vascularization occurs more commonly in EW than in DW hydrogel patients. Filling of preexisting limbal capillaries is a common vascular response noted in daily wearers of hydrogel lenses, with the possibility of prolonged engorgement leading to new vessel growth. Silicone hydrogel materials have been shown to reduce limbal hyperemia and corneal vascularization for previous lens wearers in DW or overnight wear, and not to cause vascularization in new wearers.[60] A dramatic reduction in corneal vascularization and limbal hyperemia can be observed in a short period of time after refitting a symptomatic hydrogel patient in a silicone hydrogel lens.

Normal versus Abnormal

Variation in the anatomic configuration of the corneo–limbal junction can lead to difficulty in defining actual new vessel growth from capillary engorgement. Difficulty may arise in defining an anatomic reference point at the limbus to be used to measure the vascular response.[50] A vascularized translucent overlay, composed of conjunctival and subconjunctival tissue, may extend onto the cornea and varies in width depending on the peripheral limit of the Bowman membrane.[61,62] The extension of the overlay is greatest at the superior limbus (up to 2.5 mm) and is least nasally and temporally.[61] The vascular nature of this region may be misleading when an attempt is made to determine the presence of abnormal vessel growth or looping.

Penetration of the limbal vasculature beyond the leading edge of the overlay should be considered indicative of contact lens intolerance, but it may be difficult to assess because of leakage of exudate into the surrounding tissue, causing translucency of the normally transparent cornea.[59] The narrow separation between stromal collagen fibrils normally inhibits the advancement of vessels beyond 1 mm from the limbus. Edematous changes to the stroma may result in an increase in the separation between the collagen fibrils, facilitating extension of the limbal vasculature into the visual axis and resulting in reduced vision.[63]

Appearance

The appearance of the vascular response will vary depending on the duration of corneal irritation and type of pathology. Decompensation of the highly organized architecture of the corneal stroma will result in tortuosity of the penetrating vasculature, whereas maintenance of stromal uniformity and compactness will render a straighter course.[64] Peripheral corneal edema secondary to hydrogel contact lens wear may predispose the tissue to vascular penetration.[65] High minus and prism-ballast lenses (e.g., soft toric lenses) that have thick edges are more likely to cause such a response. Superficial vascularization is typically nonuniform and irregular and may consist of individual "spikes" that on greater resolution may be connected to a venous return. The loop formed between the vessels is much narrower than the anastomoses seen in normal limbal arcades.[59]

Initiating Factors

A variety of factors may be necessary for the initiation of a corneal vascular response. It is apparent that a single mechanism is not entirely responsible for the initiation of this event. Predisposing factors most important in promoting contact lens-induced vascularization include anaerobic metabolism, inflammatory cells within the cornea, and damaged or disturbed epithelial cells. Hypoxic conditions resulting in the buildup of lactic acid, the inability to remove metabolic waste and debris caused by impingement of the conjunctival venous return, and irritation or damage to the corneal epithelium may all initiate the release of vasostimulator substances, resulting in vascularization.[59] Inflammatory cells that migrate to the cornea in response to an inadequate contact lens fit may also elicit a vascular response.[66,67]

Stages

Three stages occur in the process of corneal vascularization secondary to contact lens wear. The first stage encompasses the filling of a preexisting limbal capillary plexus. The second stage involves new vessel growth in the form of endothelial "spikes" or "sprouts" that extend from limbal arcades toward the central cornea. Thirdly, these sprouts form canaliculi and then "true" vessels that may be at any depth within the cornea. This network of abnormal vessel growth may form new arcades.[63] Removal of the contact lens from the eye will result in the emptying of blood from the patent vessels. Actual vascular regression may occur but appears to depend on the length of time the vessels are present, resulting in a critical period of growth beyond which regression may not occur. Remaining empty blood vessels, or "ghost vessels," appear as fine white lines extending in a nonbranching linear pattern toward the central cornea.[59]

Management and Treatment

The management of corneal vascularization is initiated by removal of the causative source of ocular irritation. Isolation of any obvious source of vascularization may be easily addressed, but often the presence of a variety of contributing factors may hinder successful management. It is necessary in each situation to identify the most prominent causative factors in an attempt to eliminate any potential source for vascular growth. Other pathologic conditions, including dry eye, blepharitis, acne rosacea, seasonal allergies, and sensitivity to a solution preservative, may contribute to the vascular response and must be eliminated. Detection of vascularization while the vessels are in their immature state may allow for total regression of the capillary "spikes" and emptying of the filled limbal vascular arcades.[59]

A tight lens-to-cornea fitting relationship, causing a constriction in venous return, may need to be loosened. Peripheral constriction, appearing as a distinct ring circumscribing the limbus on lens removal, may be observed with the use of fluorescein.

One of the most effective means of controlling vascularization is through refitting the patient in a silicone hydrogel lens material, which, as previously noted, provides up to eight times more oxygen to the cornea than hydrogel lens materials.[45] If this is not effective, a reduction of wearing time, such as reducing the number of nights the lens is worn overnight or wearing the lens DW only, should manage vascularization with a silicone hydrogel lens material. In situations in which contact lens wear must be discontinued, a pair of current spectacles is essential. The patient may be more likely to wear spectacles if they are attractive and the prescription is current.

Silicone hydrogel lenses are becoming increasingly available in toric, multifocal, daily disposable, and custom designs to meet the needs of all patients. This availability provides high oxygen transmission to patients who require high minus, high plus, or prism-ballast toric lenses, which in the past might have contributed to corneal vascularization.

The presence of corneal vascularization is often considered innocuous by the patient but can be a primary indicator to the practitioner of contact lens intolerance. Typically, changing a patient's wearing schedule or lens design to afford more adequate lens tolerance will help to diminish the vascular response and allow the patient to maintain successful contact lens wear. This is an excellent opportunity to educate the patient on the advantages of a silicone hydrogel over a hydrogel lens and make the switch to a healthier modality.

Giant Papillary Conjunctivitis (Contact Lens-Induced Papillary Conjunctivitis)

Clinical Signs and Symptoms

GPC, also termed contact lens-induced papillary conjunctivitis (CLPC), is a complication affecting both soft and rigid contact lens wearers. The condition, first described in 1974 by Spring[68] in an attempt to differentiate the entity from other forms of allergic conjunctival disease, was further described by Allansmith et al.[69]

GPC is most often associated with contact lens wear, although irritation from ocular prosthetics and exposed suture ends after penetrating keratoplasty and cataract extraction have also contributed to its development.[68–72] Clinical signs commonly accompanying this condition include conjunctival hyperemia, excess mucus, giant papillae on the upper tarsal conjunctiva, and increased contact lens movement. The development of GPC has been noted in both rigid and soft contact lens wearers, with earlier initiation occurring in soft lens wearers.[69] This is a complication in which the symptoms do not appear to be improved via refitting into silicone hydrogel lens materials. Silicone is naturally hydrophobic and prone to deposits; in addition, silicone hydrogel materials tend to have an increased lens modulus, all of which may contribute to GPC (see Chapter 16). Newer designs with a lower modulus appear to be decreasing the mechanical irritation that may increase the risk of GPC.

Because of size and material differences, the papillary appearance may vary between soft and rigid lens wearers. In documenting papillary response location, the upper tarsal conjunctiva may be divided into three zones: zone 1 represents the superior one-third of the tarsus, zone 2 the middle one-third, and zone 3 the lower one-third near the lid margin. Papillae in soft lens wearers are typically noted to occur in zone 1 initially, progressing inferiorly with advancement of the condition (Fig. 13.7).

Mild hyperemia of the upper tarsal conjunctiva is often the initial clinical sign observed in GPC and may be accompanied by small strands of mucus.[73] Lid eversion, accompanied by fluorescein staining, is essential in the early diagnosis of GPC and should be performed on all contact lens patients before fitting and at each subsequent visit. Initial signs of mild lens

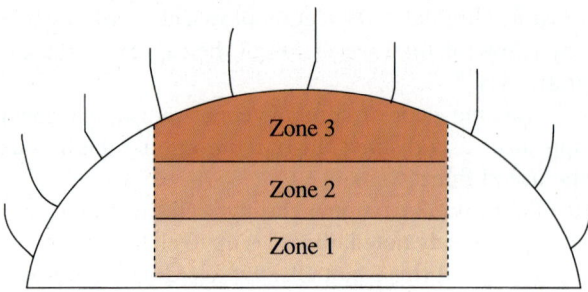

FIGURE 13.7 Diagram representing zones of upper tarsal conjunctiva.

coating, formation of giant papillae, and increased mucus production (stage 1) may progress to the formation of excessive mucus, the presence of giant papillae and erythema, and heavy lens coating (stage 4)[69] (Table 13.3). A distinction has been made between the papillae found in persons who do not wear contact lenses and those in patients with GPC. To assist in this distinction, the appearance of the upper tarsal conjunctiva has been divided into four types: a satin-textured conjunctiva with a smooth surface devoid of papillae, a uniform papillary response (4–8/mm), a nonuniform papillary response (approximately 0.4–0.8 mm in size), and a giant papillary appearance with papillae, at minimum, 1 mm in diameter.

Although papillae are the most common inflammatory sign in GPC, follicles may also be observed with active inflammation of the conjunctiva. The practitioner often experiences confusion in differentiating these two signs. Follicles, or lymphoid elevations, are typically located

TABLE 13.3 Stages of Giant Papillary Conjunctivitis

SYMPTOMS	SIGNS
Stage 1	
Few strands of mucus	None
Mild itching	
Stage 2	
Minimal mucus	Mild lens coating
Moderate itching	Elevation of normal papillae
Slight lens awareness	Beginning of underlying giant papillae
Slight decrease in vision through lens	Mild hyperemia
Mild sheets over papillae	
Stage 3	
Moderate-to-severe mucus	Moderate-to-severe lens coating
Moderate-to-severe itching	Increase in the number, size, and elevation of papillae
Increased blinking with intermittent blurring of vision	Variable hyperemia and edema
Slight lens movement	Heavy mucus
Stage 4	
Severe mucus with adhesion of eyelids	Excessive mucus
Moderate-to-severe itching	Giant papillae with flat apices
Extreme lens awareness, pain	Marked hyperemia and edema
Blurring of vision	Heavy lens coating
Excessive lens movement	

in the inferior conjunctiva and fornix. They appear translucent and exhibit a superficial vascular pattern. Papillae are composed of a central vascular tuft or stalk of vessels and may in later stages exhibit white "tops" as a result of collagen scarring. They are more commonly noted to occur in the upper tarsal conjunctiva.[73]

Patient symptoms often precede objective signs in GPC. The presence of mucus in the nasal corners of the eye in the morning and itching following lens removal (stage 1) may often be noted in lieu of objective signs, including giant papillae, conjunctival thickening, and erythema. Symptoms may progress in later stages (stage 4) to extreme contact lens intolerance, marked hyperemia, moderate-to-severe itching, and excessive mucus production leading to eyelid adherence on awakening. With the progression of the papillary response, contact lens movement becomes more excessive, resulting in discomfort to the patient and a reduction in wearing time. Pseudoptosis has also been reported in some patients.[73]

The papillary reaction of the upper tarsal conjunctiva in GPC has been most often attributed to both an immunologic response to and a mechanical irritation from surface deposits on the contact lens. A cutaneous basophil hypersensitivity reaction (including both a type 1, IgE-mediated reaction and a variety of type 4 delayed reactions) has been implicated.[73] The allergic reaction results from the presence of antigens (e.g., proteins, lipids) on the surface of the lens. Omission of proper and frequent cleaning and infrequent replacement of the contact lens contribute to the initiation and exacerbation of the disease process.

Treatment

Many cases of GPC can be alleviated by early intervention. Contact lens removal will cause the disease process to subside and eventually cease. Most patients, however, are dissatisfied with discontinuing lens wear for long periods. The goal of therapy is to control the clinical signs and symptoms of GPC while allowing contact lens wear to continue with minimal disturbance to the patient.

Patients presenting with GPC should be replacing lenses on a recommended replacement schedule, ideally daily disposable or not greater than monthly replacement. Altering the replacement schedule to a more frequent replacement will aid in eliminating the symptoms of GPC. Most refractive errors can now be corrected, at maximum, with a monthly replacement lens. The patient should be educated about the necessity of replacing the lenses on schedule. The emergence of disposable lenses as the primary choice for fitting soft lens wearers has accomplished more than anything else to decrease the incidence of GPC in contact lens wearers.

The following recommendations are provided for those patients whose refractive errors can only be corrected with a conventional replacement (6–12 months) lens material. In the early stages of GPC, regular surfactant and enzymatic cleaning should alleviate most symptoms. Surfactant cleaning is essential for the removal of deposits, especially lipids, and should be performed daily or after every lens removal. If symptoms persist with daily cleaning, an abrasive cleaner or more frequent cleanings are recommended. Weekly enzymatic cleaning to remove denatured proteins (predominantly lysozyme) is essential in maintaining a relatively deposit-free surface; the possibility of biweekly or even more frequent cleaning may be beneficial in cases of GPC. The use of hydrogen peroxide disinfection systems, accompanied by preservative-free saline solution if needed will assist in reducing the number of possible antigens exposed to the ocular surface.[55]

Replacement of conventional replacement lenses on a more frequent basis, 3 or 6 months, will minimize the incidence of GPC. Low-water-content, nonionic materials are advantageous in these cases because of their greater resistance to deposits in comparison with high-water-content, ionic materials. Changing the lens material or lens design or switching to a GP lens are all alternatives that may increase the likelihood of continued lens wear.

Discontinuing lens wear, exclusive of the severity of the condition, will result in the disappearance of symptoms within approximately 5 days following lens removal. In patients with severe GPC (stages 3 or 4), discontinuing lens wear is usually necessary to terminate progression of the condition.[74] Lenses may be reinserted following the resolution of hyperemia, excessive mucous production, and itching, although the presence of giant papillae may persist for several months to years.[55]

The most effective way to treat moderate-to-severe GPC is the use of a combination antihistamine/mast cell stabilizer once or twice a day before lens insertion and after lens removal, depending on the dosage (see Chapter 23). This, in combination with clean, new lenses, will be effective in most cases. Severe cases of GPC may warrant discontinuing lens wear and use of topical steroids. The use of short-term applications of 0.10% fluorometholone or 0.5% lotoprednol (one drop in each eye four times daily for 1 week, tapered by one drop each week for 3 weeks) is effective in reducing both clinical signs and symptoms of the condition.[55,75] Once the patient is stabilized, the use of an antihistamine/mast cell stabilizer while tapering the steroid can be used. A conservative approach to topical steroid use is necessary in avoiding complications, including glaucoma and cataracts. The use of disposable lenses and mast cell stabilizers has been reported as successful treatment of 93% of patients presenting with GPC.[76]

SUMMARY

Thorough, ongoing patient care may prevent future complications associated with soft contact lens wear. Symptoms elicited from the patient during the case history and clinical signs observed with the biomicroscope signal contact lens-related conditions that should be eliminated or monitored before severe complications develop. Disposable/frequent-replacement soft lenses and silicone hydrogel lens materials are beneficial to the patient and have played a role in the reduction of soft contact lens complications. Frequent follow-up evaluations, every 6 months for DW patients and every 3 months for EW/CW patients, are recommended for monitoring. Contact lenses are not a cosmetic device but a medical device and therefore require evaluation by an eye care practitioner to ensure successful wear.

CLINICAL CASES

CASE 1

A first-time lens wearer presents with the inability to wear soft lenses because of poor comfort and dryness. He has discontinued lenses fitted at another office after not being able to achieve any substantial wearing time and having "dry eyes." During the case history, the patient reported wearing 2-week replacement contact lenses for about 2 to 3 months with wear time not greater than 8 hours per day because of dryness and slight burning. He reports to being compliant with the care regimen and replacement schedule. The patient had previously used two MPS care regimens. His TBUT is 10 seconds and all findings appear normal.

SOLUTION: Preservative sensitivity is suspected. The patient is fit with daily disposable lenses and is instructed to use nonpreserved saline solution if necessary. The patient is able to achieve all-day wear and has good comfort.

CASE 2

A patient presents with reduced vision and a mild burning sensation in the left eye only. She is a long-term soft lens wearer. She reports that she had something "stuck" behind her left lens that morning and that she was not able to remove the lens for a period of time. She notices that her vision is still reduced with spectacles after the contact lenses are removed. On examination, best-corrected visual acuity is OD 20/20 and OS 20/80. Evaluation with the biomicroscope reveals a central coalesced area of staining.

SOLUTION: This patient has a central corneal abrasion. Treatment of the abrasion depends on its severity. The current lens wear should be discontinued until the abraded area has healed.

A mild abrasion might be monitored only. In more severe cases, a broad-spectrum antibiotic may be used prophylactically. In addition, a cycloplegic agent might be administered. Patching or placing a bandage contact lens on a contact lens-induced abrasion is *contraindicated* because the lens may have introduced bacteria to the eye that will thrive in the warm, moist environment that results from patching. The patient should be monitored frequently (e.g., 24 hours, 3 days, and 1 week after the abrasion) until the area has healed completely. The cause of the abrasion should be confirmed so the condition will not occur again. For example, the abrasion might be the result of a damaged lens, a tight lens, solution misuse, removal with the fingernails, or a foreign body. This may require that the lens be refitted or the patient reeducated regarding care and handling.

CASE 3

A patient has EW hydrogel lenses. He wears the lenses for 5 days before removal. He complains of hazy vision. What should you think of and look for?

SOLUTION: The cornea should be evaluated for signs of edema (striae, microcysts). Keratometry and subjective refraction should also be performed to detect changes resulting from edema (e.g., steepening of the keratometric readings, increase in myopia). If the presence of edema is verified, the patient should be fitted into a lens with a higher Dk/t (e.g., silicone hydrogel). If refitting is not an option, EW should be discontinued.

CASE 4

A contact lens patient is fitted in daily disposable contact lenses. The patient remarks that at times, one or both lenses are mildly uncomfortable and can become annoying as the day progresses. What is the probable cause?

SOLUTION: This lens is most likely inverted. Soft lenses have become very thin, and it may be quite difficult to determine if the lens is inverted. At times, an inverted lens may result in less comfort, reduced vision, and more movement than a lens that is not inverted, but with newer designs, vision can be good despite lens inversion. By removing the lens, checking to see if it is in the proper position, and reinserting it, the patient should notice that the symptoms have disappeared.

CASE 5

The patient has been refitted with silicone hydrogel lenses for 30-day CW. The patient has been wearing hydrogel lenses for 7 days and 6 nights for about 2 years. When the patient returns at the 1-week follow-up visit, she has discontinued the silicone hydrogel lenses as she thinks they are not as comfortable as her previous lenses.

SOLUTION: Most likely, this patient has had corneal edema with her previous hydrogel contact lenses. As her cornea rehabilitated with the silicone hydrogel lenses, it has become more sensitive (or less numb). The higher modulus of the 30-day lens, in addition to the healthier cornea, has resulted in more lens sensation. Typically, if the patient is educated on this and asked to wear the silicone hydrogel lenses, at minimum, for 2 weeks (DW or CW), she will be comfortable in the new lenses. If this does not improve the lens comfort, fitting with a lower modulus silicone hydrogel lens material can be attempted. Most patients will adapt well to the silicone hydrogel lenses with education and patience with the adaptation process.

CASE 6

A patient comes to the office complaining of reduced vision in the right eye. Overrefraction is OD −0.50 D and OS +0.50 D. The patient was dispensed the following parameters:

OD: BCR 8.6 mm, overall diameter 14.5 mm, Rx − 3.75 D
OS: BCR 8.6 mm, overall diameter 14.5 mm, Rx − 3.00 D

What is the problem?

SOLUTION: This patient has switched the lenses. The lenses should be switched back to the proper eye and the patient reeducated about removing the right lens first and the left lens second to avoid confusing the two lenses. Patients will typically refuse to believe, sometimes adamantly, that they have switched their lenses until it is demonstrated to them.

CASE 7

A patient has corneal vascularization of 2 mm superiorly and 1.5 mm inferiorly. He has not returned for follow-up evaluation for more than a year. What might be the cause of the vascularization?

SOLUTION: This patient should be questioned about his wearing schedule. He is very likely overwearing his contact lenses or, less likely, the patient's corneal oxygen requirement may be greater than what the current lenses provide. The patient should be educated about the importance of both a proper wearing schedule and routine follow-up evaluations. A refit into a silicone hydrogel lens material that provides more oxygen to the cornea would be beneficial.

CASE 8

A long-term soft lens wearer comes to your office for her annual examination. She sleeps in her hydrogel lenses about two times a week. The fit of the lenses is good and the patient is content with her current lens brand but, upon slit-lamp examination, limbal hyperemia and neovascularization inferiorly are noted.

SOLUTION: The patient is refitted into a silicone hydrogel lens material that can be worn for 7 days and 6 nights EW. The patient intends to continue her current wearing schedule of about 2 nights per week of overnight wear. At the 2-week follow-up examination, the limbal region is white and clear, and the neovascularization has regressed. The new lenses provide more oxygen to the cornea, thus improving ocular health.

CASE 9

A patient has been wearing her current lenses for 3 weeks. She complains of discomfort immediately on insertion. Fluorescein evaluation with the lenses off reveals a superficial staining pattern in the nasal periphery. What might be wrong?

SOLUTION: When the lens is evaluated on the eye, it is likely that there will be damage to the lens. The lens should be replaced and the patient educated about the care and handling of soft lenses. The patient should be reminded not to wear lenses that cause discomfort. Depending on the severity of the staining, the patient may have to discontinue lens wear until the cornea heals.

CASE 10

A patient complains of dry eyes and increased lens intolerance. She received her lenses in April, and it is now November. Her solution regimen has remained the same. She finds the symptoms to be worse at work. What might be the problem?

SOLUTION: The two most likely causes are a dry environment at work, caused by the heating system or antihistamine use. Seasonal allergies and sinus conditions often occur in the spring and fall, and antihistamines are taken. The heat may have recently been turned on at the patient's workplace, creating a dry environment. She should check vents in her work area to prevent air from being directed toward her, especially her head. The use of lens lubricants or perhaps even discontinuation of lens wear while on antihistamines may be helpful. Another factor with a female patient is pregnancy. If the patient has recently become pregnant, this may result in dryness of the eyes not noticed previously. In addition, this patient might benefit from a lens material better suited for dry eyes (i.e., Proclear, Proclear 1 Day, Biofinity-CooperVision, 1 Day Acuvue Moist, Acuvue TruEye, Acuvue Oasys-Vistakon, Dailies Aquacomfort Plus, Dailies Total 1, Air Optix Aqua-Alcon, PureVision 2, Biotrue Oneday-Bausch + Lomb or other silicone hydrogel lens not listed).

CASE 11

A patient has worn soft lenses for 1 year. He admits failing to replace his disposable lenses as scheduled and cannot remember the last time he did so. He experiences mild itching and increased mucus discharge on awakening. Biomicroscopic evaluation reveals grade 2 papillae, and the lenses are moderately coated.

SOLUTION: This patient has GPC. His lenses should be replaced and the patient reeducated about the proper care of the soft lenses. If the GPC does not resolve with new lenses and increased cleaning, the patient may need to discontinue lens wear until the GPC improves. Daily disposable lenses would be beneficial for this patient.

CLINICAL PROFICIENCY CHECKLIST

- Daily disposable, disposable, and frequent-replacement lenses may aid in providing the patient with relatively problem-free wear.
- Two of the most valuable tools used to diagnose complications associated with soft contact lens wear are the case history and the biomicroscope.
- Frequent evaluations, every 6 months for DW patients and every 3 months for EW patients, will aid in reducing serious complications that may result from soft lens wear.
- Reduced vision with contact lenses *and* spectacles may be attributed to corneal abnormalities that require immediate attention.
- Discomfort with a soft lens is not normal and requires evaluation of the patient and the lens. Generally, the lens is found to be damaged or deposited; however, abnormalities of the cornea such as abrasions or ulcers may be observed.
- A recent onset of dryness with lens wear is often found to be the result of antihistamine use, a dry environment, solution sensitivity, or pregnancy.
- The symptom of burning is often related to solution sensitivity or improper solution use.
- Fluorescein evaluation of the cornea after lens removal should be a routine part of any soft lens evaluation.
- Striae and epithelial edema may be visible with 4% to 6% corneal thickening.
- A tight lens may be associated with conjunctival "drag," in which the conjunctiva is seen to move with the soft lens on the blink.
- Silicone hydrogel lenses have reduced complications due to hypoxia by providing greater oxygen transmission to the cornea.
- GPC may be prevented by compliance with disposable lens replacement schedules and rubbing the lens with solution upon removal. For the treatment of GPC, the use of disposable soft lenses and an antihistamine/mast cell stabilizer are beneficial.

REFERENCES

1. Connor CG, Presley L, Finchum SM, et al. The effectiveness of several current soft contact lens care systems against *Aspergillus*. *CLAO J*. 1998;24:82–84.
2. Sakuma S, Reeh B, Dang D, et al. Comparative efficacies of four soft contact lens disinfection solutions. *Int Cont Lens Clin*. 1996;23:234–239.
3. Szczotka-Flynn L, Diaz M. Risk of corneal inflammatory events with silicone hydrogel and low Dk hydrogel extended contact lens wear: a meta-analysis. *Optom Vis Sci*. 2007;84:247–256.

4. Benjamin WJ, Hill RM. Surface coating: the fatal facade. *Contact Lens Forum.* 1979;4:107–109.
5. Mandell RB. Symptomatology and aftercare. In: Mandell RB, ed. *Contact Lens Practice.* 4th ed. Springfield, IL: Charles C Thomas; 1988:598–643.
6. Sarver MD. Vision with hydrophilic contact lenses. *J Am Optom Assoc.* 1972;43:316–320.
7. Mandell RB. Hydrogel lenses for astigmatism. In: Mandell RB, ed. *Contact Lens Practice.* 4th ed. Springfield, IL: Charles C Thomas; 1988:659–680.
8. Snyder C. Aspheric hydrogels "correct" minimal astigmatism? *Contact Lens Spectrum.* 2000;15(12):15.
9. Edrington TB, Barr JT. Creating better locus of focus. *Contact Lens Spectrum.* 2002;17(6):44.
10. Blaze P. Refining toric soft lens correction. *Contact Lens Forum.* 1988;13:53–58.
11. Jones L. Understanding incompatibilities. *Contact Lens Spectrum.* 2004;19(7):S4–S8.
12. Mandell RB. Symptomatology and refitting. In: Mandell RB, ed. *Contact Lens Practice.* 4th ed. Springfield, IL: Charles C Thomas; 1988:388–439.
13. Bergmanson JPG. Contact lens-induced epithelial pathology. In: Bennett ES, Weissman BA, eds. *Clinical Contact Lens Practice.* Philadelphia, PA: JB Lippincott Co; 1991:60-1–60-16.
14. Mandell RB. Clinical procedures. In: Mandell RB, ed. *Contact Lens Practice.* 4th ed. Springfield, IL: Charles C Thomas; 1988:310–325.
15. Clemons CS, Cohen EJ, Arentsen JJ, et al. Pseudomonas ulcers following patching of corneal abrasions associated with contact lens wear. *CLAO J.* 1987;13(16):1–4.
16. Doughty MJ, Fonn D, Richter D, et al. A patient questionnaire approach to estimating the prevalence of dry-eye symptoms in patients presenting to optometric practices across Canada. *Optom Vis Sci.* 1997;74:624–631.
17. Chalmers RL, Begley CG, Edrington T, et al. The agreement between self-assessment and clinician assessment of dry-eye severity. *Cornea.* 2005;24:804–810.
18. Nichols JJ, Mitchell GL, Nichols KK, et al. The performance of the contact lens dry eye questionnaire as a screening survey for contact lens-related dry eye. *Cornea.* 2002;21:469–475.
19. Nichols JJ, Ziegler C, Mitchell GL, et al. Self-reported dry eye disease across refractive modalities. *Invest Ophthalmol Vis Sci.* 2005;46:1911–1914.
20. Nichols JJ, Sinnott LT. Tear film, contact lens, and patient-related factors associated with contact lens-related dry eye. *Invest Ophthalmol Vis Sci.* 2006;47:1319–1328.
21. Lorentz H, Jones, L. Lipid deposition on hydrogel contact lenses: how history can help us today. *Optom Vis Sci.* 2007;84:286–295.
22. Nichols JJ, Mitchell GL, King-Smith, PE. Thinning rate of the precorneal and prelens tear films. *Invest Ophthalmol Vis Sci.* 2005;46:2353–2361.
23. Sindt CW, Longmuir RA. Contact lens strategies for the patient with dry eye. *Ocul Surf.* 2007;5:294–307.
24. Grant R. Developments in contact len surfaces. *Contact Lens Spectrum.* 2010;25(12):30–35.
25. Epstein AB, Stone R. Surface and polymer chemistry: the quest for comfort. *Rev Cornea Cont Lens.* April 2010. http://www.reviewofcontactlenses.com. Accessed February 29, 2012.
26. Bennett ES, Gordon JM. The borderline dry-eye patient and contact lens wear. *Contact Lens Forum.* 1989;14:52–74.
27. Young G, Bowers R, Hall B, et al. Clinical comparison of Omafilcon A with four control materials. *CLAO J.* 1997;23:249–258.
28. Lemp MA, Caffery B, Lebow K, et al. Omafilcon A (Proclear) soft contact lenses in a dry eye population. *CLAO J.* 1999;25:40–47.
29. Peterson RC, Wolffsohn JS, Nick J, et al. Clinical performance of daily disposable soft contact lenses using sustained release technology. *Cont Lens Anterior Eye.* 2006;29:127–134.
30. Nick J, Winterton L, Lally J. Enhancing comfort with a lubricating daily disposable. *Optician.* 2005;229:30–32.
31. Osborn K, Veys J. A new silicone hydrogel lens for contact lens-related dryness. Part 1: material properties. *Optician.* 2005;229:39–41.
32. Dumbleton K, Keir N, Moezzi A, et al. Objective and subjective responses in patients refitted to daily-wear silicone hydrogel contact lenses. *Optom Vis Sci.* 2006;83:758–768.
33. Dillehay SM. Does the level of available oxygen impact comfort in contact lens wear?: review of literature. *Eye Contact Lens.* 2007;33(3):148–155.
34. Ilhan B, Irkec M, Orhan M, et al. Surface deposits on frequent replacement and conventional daily wear soft contact lenses. *CLAO J.* 1998;24:232–235.
35. Coopersmith L, Weinstock FJ. Current recommendations and practice regarding soft lens replacement and disinfection. *CLAO J.* 1997;23:172–176.
36. Luxenberg MN, Green K. Reduction of corneal edema with topical hypertonic agents. *Am J Ophthalmol.* 1971;71:847–853.
37. Jalbert I, Sweeney DF, Holden BA. Epithelial split associated with wear of a silicone hydrogel contact lens *CLAO J.* 2001;27(4):231–233.
38. Pole JJ, Malinovsky VE, Pence NA, et al. Epithelial splits of the superior cornea in hydrogel contact lens patients. *Int Cont Lens Clin.* 1989;16:252–255.
39. Dumbleton K. Noninflammatory silicone hydrogel contact lens complications. *Eye Contact Lens.* 2003;29(suppl 1): S186–S189; discussion S190–S191, S192–S194.

40. Dumbleton K. Adverse events with silicone hydrogel continuous wear. *Cont Lens Anterior Eye.* 2002;25:137–146.
41. Carnt N, Willcox MDP, Evans V, et al. Corneal staining: the IER matrix study 2007;22(9):38–43.
42. Benjamin WJ, Hill RM. Ultra-thins: the case for continuous care. *J Am Optom Assoc.* 1980;51:277–279.
43. Hill JF. Changes in corneal curvature and refractive error upon refitting with flatter hydrophilic contact lenses. *J Am Optom Assoc.* 1976;47:1214–1216.
44. Kame RT, Hayashida JK. Lens evaluation procedures and problem solving. In: Bennett ES, Weissman BA, eds. *Clinical Contact Lens Practice.* Vol. 38. Philadelphia, PA: JB Lippincott Co; 1991:1–10.
45. Sweeney D, Fonn D, Evans K. Silicone hydrogels: the evolution of a revolution. *Contact Lens Spectrum.* 2006;(special edition):14–19.
46. Holden BA, Mertz GW, McNally JJ. Corneal swelling response to contact lenses worn under extended wear conditions. *Invest Ophthalmol Vis Sci.* 1983;24:218–226.
47. Mandell RB. Extended wear. In: Mandell RB, ed. *Contact Lens Practice.* 4th ed. Springfield, IL: Charles C Thomas; 1988:683–717.
48. Steffen RB, Schnider CM. The impact of silicone hydrogel materials on overnight corneal swelling. *Eye Contact Lens.* 2007;33(3):115–120.
49. Fonn D, Dumbleton K, Jalbert I, et al. Benefits of silicone hydrogel lenses. *Contact Lens Spectrum.* 2006;(special edition):38–44.
50. Bergmanson JPG. Histopathological analysis of the corneal epithelium after contact lens wear. *J Am Optom Assoc.* 1987;58:812–818.
51. Zantos SG. Cystic formations in the corneal epithelium during extended wear of contact lenses. *Int Cont Lens Clin.* 1983;10:128–143.
52. Madigan MC, Holden BA, Kwok LS. Extended wear of hydrogel contact lenses can compromise the corneal epithelium. *Invest Ophthalmol Vis Sci.* 1986;27(suppl):140.
53. Humphreys JA, Larke JR, Parrish ST. Microepithelial cysts observed in extended contact lens-wearing subjects. *Br J Ophthalmol.* 1980;64:888–895.
54. Mandell RB. The "tight" soft contact lens. *Contact Lens Forum.* 1979;4:21–32.
55. Silbert JA. Contact lens-related inflammatory reactions. In: Bennett ES, Weissman BA, eds. *Clinical Contact Lens Practice.* Philadelphia, PA: JB Lippincott Co; 1991:65-1–65-9.
56. Schein OD, Glynn RJ, Poggio EC, et al. The relative risk of ulcerative keratitis between extended and daily wear soft contact lens wearers: a case-control study. *N Engl J Med.* 1989;321:773–778.
57. Jones WL. Diseases of the sclera. In: Bartlett JD, Jaanus SD, eds. *Clinical Ocular Pharmacology.* Boston: Butterworth-Heinemann; 1995:763–765.
58. Darcy F, Kirwan C, O'Keefe. Episcleritis following keratorefractive surgery. *Br J Ophthalmol.* 2009;93(11):1554.
59. McMonnies CW. Corneal vascularization. In: Bennett ES, Weissman BA, eds. *Clinical Contact Lens Practice.* Philadelphia, PA: JB Lippincott Co; 1991:61-1–61-9.
60. Papas E, Willcox M. Reducing the consequences of hypoxia: the ocular redness response. *Contact Lens Spectrum.* 2006;(special edition):32–37.
61. Wolff E. *The Anatomy of the Eye and Orbit.* London: HK Lewis; 1958:30–180.
62. Duke-Elder S, Leigh AG. Diseases of the outer eye. In: *System of Ophthalmology.* Vol. 8. London: Henry Kimpton; 1977:676.
63. Allansmith MR. Palpebral conjunctiva: factors associated with papillary response and contact lens wear. *J Am Optom Assoc.* 1984;55:199–200.
64. McMonnies CW. Contact lens-induced corneal vascularization. *Int Cont Lens Clin.* 1983;10:12–21.
65. Larke JR, Humphreys JA, Holmes R. Apparent corneal neovascularization in soft lens wearers. *J Br Contact Lens Assoc.* 1981;4:105.
66. McMonnies CW. Risk factors in the aetiology of contact lens-induced corneal vascularization. *Int Cont Lens Clin.* 1984;11:286–293.
67. Arentsen JJ. Corneal neovascularization in contact lens wearers. In: Cohen EJ, ed. *International Ophthalmology Clinics.* Vol. 26. Boston: Little Brown; 1986:15–23.
68. Spring TF. Reaction to hydrophilic lenses. *Med J Aust.* 1974;1:499–503.
69. Allansmith MR, Korb DR, Greiner JV, et al. Giant papillary conjunctivitis in contact lens wearers. *Am J Ophthalmol.* 1977;83:697–708.
70. Sugar A, Meyer RF. Giant papillary conjunctivitis after keratoplasty. *Am J Ophthalmol.* 1981;91:239–242.
71. Srinivasan BD, Jakobiec FD, Iwamoto T, et al. Giant papillary conjunctivitis with ocular prosthesis. *Arch Ophthalmol.* 1979;97:892–895.
72. Donshik PC, Ballow M, Luistro A, et al. Treatment of contact lens-induced giant papillary conjunctivitis. *CLAO J.* 1984;10:346–350.
73. Allansmith MR. Giant papillary conjunctivitis. *J Am Optom Assoc.* 1990;61(Suppl):S42–S46.
74. Stenson S. Superior limbic keratoconjunctivitis associated with soft contact lens wear. *Arch Ophthalmol.* 1983;101:402–404.
75. Karpecki P. Contact lens wear and ocular allergy. *Contact Lens Spectrum.* 2012;27(3):26–32.
76. Ehlers WH, Donshik PC. Allergic diseases of the lids, conjunctiva, and cornea. *Curr Opin Ophthalmol.* 1994;5:31–38.

Section IV

Challenging Cases

Chapter 14

Correction of Astigmatism

Edward S. Bennett, Kimberly A. Layfield, Dawn Lam, and Vinita Allee Henry

The purpose of this chapter is to discuss methods of managing the astigmatic contact lens patient. These patients can often be challenging to the eye care practitioner; however, it is the ability to fit these people successfully that makes practice both enjoyable and profitable. The principles of residual and high astigmatic correction with gas-permeable (GP) lenses and astigmatic correction with soft toric lenses are reviewed.

GAS-PERMEABLE CONTACT LENS APPLICATIONS

Residual Astigmatism

Residual astigmatism can be defined as the astigmatic refractive error present when a contact lens is placed on the eye to correct an existing ametropia. When a spherical lens is applied, the residual astigmatism is approximately equal to the difference between the corneal astigmatism and the refractive or total astigmatic error of the eye.

Residual astigmatism can be classified as either induced or physiologic. *Induced* residual astigmatism is associated with lens application and can be caused by lens warpage, flexure, decentration, or a toric anterior or posterior lens surface. This section of the chapter primarily addresses *physiologic* residual astigmatism, which commonly results from curvature refractive index differences of the posterior cornea and crystalline lens.

Calculated and Actual Residual Astigmatism

The calculated (or predicted) residual astigmatism (CRA) can be defined as the amount of astigmatism one would predict to result when a spherical GP lens is placed on the eye. It can be obtained directly by subtracting the patient's central anterior corneal toricity (as measured by keratometry) from the total astigmatism of the eye at the plane of the cornea. The following examples illustrate the determination of CRA. In these examples, TRA refers to the total refractive astigmatism and ΔK refers to the difference between the keratometric readings of the two corneal meridians.

EXAMPLE 1

Given: Spectacle Rx = $-1.00 - 2.00 \times 090$

Keratometry = 42.00 @ 090; 43.00 @ 180

Then: CRA = TRA − ΔK
 = $-2.00 \times 090 - (-1.00 \times 090)$
 = -1.00×090

EXAMPLE 2

Given: Spectacle Rx = $-2.00 - 1.50 \times 180$

Keratometry = 41.00 @ 180; 44.00 @ 090

Then: CRA = TRA − ΔK

$= -1.50 \times 180 - (-3.00 \times 180)$

$= +1.50 \times 180$ or transposed:

$= +1.50 - 1.50 \times 090$

$= -1.50 \times 090$

EXAMPLE 3

Given: Spectacle Rx = $+3.00 - 3.50 \times 180$

Keratometry = 40.00 @ 180; 43.00 @ 090

Then: CRA = TRA − ΔK

$= -3.50 \times 180 - (-3.00 \times 180)$

$= -0.50 \times 180$

EXAMPLE 4

Given: Spectacle Rx = $-8.00 - 2.50 \times 180$

Keratometry = 42.50 @ 180; 45.00 @ 090

$$F90 \text{ (12 mm vertex distance)} = \frac{-10.50}{1-0.012\,(-10.50)} = 9.33 \text{ D}$$

$$F180 \text{ (12 mm vertex distance)} = \frac{-8.00}{1-0.012\,(-8.00)} = 7.30 \text{ D}$$

Spectacle Rx (at corneal plane) = $-7.25 - 2.00 \times 180$

Then: CRA = TRA − ΔK

$= -2.00 \times 180 - (-2.50 \times 180)$

$= +0.50 \times 180$ or transposed to:

$= +0.50 - 0.50 \times 090$

$= -0.50 \times 090$

EXAMPLE 5

Given: Spectacle Rx = $+13.50 - 3.00 \times 010$

Keratometry = 41.00 @ 010; 44.00 @ 100

$$F010 \text{ (12 mm vertex distance)} = \frac{+13.50}{1-0.012\,(+13.50)} = +16.11 \text{ D}$$

$$F100 \text{ (12 mm vertex distance)} = \frac{+10.50}{1-0.012\,(+10.50)} = +12.01 \text{ D}$$

Spectacle Rx (at corneal plane) = $+16.00 - 4.00 \times 010$

Then: CRA = TRA − ΔK

$$= -4.00 \times 010 - (-3.00 \times 010)$$

$$= -1.00 \times 010$$

In Examples 4 and 5, the importance of vertexing the patient's refraction to the corneal plane is quite apparent. In both cases, if vertex distance was ignored, the CRA would equal zero.

If a GP spherical lens of standard thickness (to minimize or eliminate the effects of flexure) is selected for a diagnostic fitting, the predicted sphero–cylindrical overrefraction (OR) can be calculated by using the following guidelines[1]:

1. List the spectacle correction (Rx) and keratometric readings.
2. The effective power should be determined at the corneal plane (if indicated).
3. Determine the lacrimal lens power (LLP) induced by the base curve radius (BCR) of the lens.
4. Add together the powers of the contact lens, lacrimal lens, and the difference between the keratometric readings of the principal corneal meridians.
5. With the following formula, subtract the value obtained in step 4 from the spectacle Rx to obtain the OR:

$$\text{Overrefraction (OR)} = \text{Spectacle Rx} - (\text{Contact Lens Power [CLP]} + \text{LLP} + \Delta K)$$

The following example illustrates this principle:

EXAMPLE 6

1. Spectacle Rx $= -2.00 - 2.50 \times 180$

   Keratometry $= 43.00 @ 180; 45.00 @ 090$

   Diagnostic Lens $= -3.00 \text{ D}; 43.25 \text{ D BCR}$

2. At Corneal plane, spectacle Rx $= -2.00 - 2.25 \times 180$

3. LLP $= 43.25 - 43.00 = +0.25$

4. CLP + LLP + ΔK $= \text{LLP} + \Delta K = [-3.00 + (+)0.25] + (-)2.00 \times 180$

   $= -2.75 - 2.00 \times 180$

5. OR $= \text{Spectacle Rx} - (\text{CLP} + \text{LLP} + \Delta K)$

   $= -2.00 - 2.25 \times 180 - (-2.75 - 2.00 \times 180)$

   $= +0.75 - 0.25 \times 180$

Does the CRA correlate well with the residual astigmatism actually obtained after diagnostic lens application (i.e., actual residual astigmatism, or ARA)? There does appear to be some correlation, although often the ARA will be slightly less.[2-5] In one study of over 400 eyes fitted with spherical GP lenses, the mean CRA was found to be $-0.51 \text{ D} \times 090$, whereas the mean ARA was equal to $-0.23 \text{ D} \times 090$.[3] The difference between the CRA and ARA values could be caused by many factors, including inaccuracy of the keratometer for determining anterior corneal curvature (i.e., it evaluates only a few points on the paracentral cornea). In addition, examiner error in performing both refraction and keratometry could produce a difference between these two astigmatic values.

When a patient has refractive and keratometric cylinder axes that differ by >15 degrees, it can be assumed that the axes are unequal and the use of conventional crossed-cylinder equations are necessary to determine the CRA. Because of the time involved, unless the appropriate tables or a computer-assisted contact lens design program is available, the use of a GP, spherical diagnostic lens for OR to determine the residual astigmatism is advisable.

Methods of Correcting Residual Astigmatism

A GP contact lens may cause a reduction in visual acuity (VA) that is unacceptable to a patient because of the amount of residual astigmatism. This depends on the amount of residual astigmatism, the patient's refractive error, and whether critical vision demands are common. Highly ametropic patients may be able to tolerate a higher amount of residual cylinder than low ametropes. Therefore, individual variance is determined by the amount of residual astigmatism necessary to contraindicate the use of a spherical GP lens; however, patients exhibiting >0.75 D often experience subjectively compromised vision. Methods of correcting residual astigmatism include spherical GP lenses, spherical soft lenses, soft toric lenses, and front surface toric GP lenses.

Spherical Gas-Permeable Lenses: Spherical GP lenses can be successfully fitted to patients exhibiting residual astigmatism if any one of the following conditions exists:

1. ARA differs in amount from CRA. For example, you may predict a CRA of -1.00×090, but your OR results in a value of -0.50×090. Rechecking keratometry or the subjective refraction may determine where the error was made. However, the most important factor is to never allow the CRA to prevent spherical GP lens application because of the possibility of obtaining a lower ARA value.
2. The lens can flex on the eye to reduce residual astigmatism. In most cases, flexure or bending of a GP lens on the eye will increase the existent residual astigmatism. However, there is one case in which flexure will actually reduce or totally correct residual astigmatism. It has been found that when the corneal toricity is with-the-rule and the residual astigmatism is against-the-rule, a thin spherical GP lens will flex and reduce the amount of residual astigmatism.[6] This is illustrated in the following example:

EXAMPLE 7

Given: Spectacle Rx = $-2.00 - 1.00 \times 180$

Keratometry = 41.00 @ 180; 43.00 @ 090

Then: CRA = TRA $-$ ΔK

$= -1.00 \times 180 - (-)2.00 \times 180$

$= +1.00 \times 180$ transposed to:

$= +1.00 - 1.00 \times 090$

A thin lens can flex between 0.25 and 0.50 D to correct some of this residual astigmatic error.[6,7] The use of a GP lens with high oxygen permeability (high-Dk) in a thin, large-diameter design fitted "steeper than K" (e.g., the Menicon Z thin design) should, in theory, correct even a greater amount of residual astigmatism.
3. The demand on critical vision is low.
4. The patient's VA is not decreased to an unacceptable level.

Spherical Soft Lenses: There is one situation in which a spherical soft lens would definitely be indicated. If very little or no refractive astigmatism is present in the patient's spectacle correction, a spherical soft lens should provide acceptable VA. This is demonstrated in Example 8.

EXAMPLE 8

Given: Spectacle Rx = $-4.00 - 0.25 \times 180$

Keratometry = 43.00 @ 180; 44.50 @ 090

Then: CRA = $-0.25 \times 180 - (-)1.50 \times 180$

$= +1.25 \times 180$ or transposed to:

$= +1.25 - 1.25 \times 090$

The other advantage of spherical soft lens use is the avoidance of a more complicated and expensive lens design.

Soft Toric Lenses: The most common reason for the rapid decline in front surface toric GP lenses for correction of residual astigmatism is the optical quality, parameter availability, and disposability of soft toric lenses. With few exceptions, patients with >0.75 D of ARA can be fitted successfully into soft torics. The availability of large diagnostic sets incorporating numerous astigmatic corrections has also made this an easy option for fitting patients. The following examples illustrate representative applications for soft toric lenses in patients with a high amount of residual astigmatism:

EXAMPLE 9

Given: Spectacle Rx = $-2.50 - 1.25 \times 180$

Keratometry = 43.00 DS

Then: CRA = TRA $- \Delta K$

$= -1.25 \times 180 - 0$

$= -1.25 \times 180$

EXAMPLE 10

Given: Spectacle Rx = $-2.50 - 1.25 \times 180$

Keratometry = 43.00 @ 180; 45.50 @ 090

Then: CRA = TRA $- \Delta K$

$= -1.25 \times 180 - (-)2.50 \times 180$

$= +1.25 \times 180$ or

$= +1.25 - 1.25 \times 090$

In Examples 9 and 10, these patients exhibited no and high corneal astigmatism, respectively; however, they were both good candidates for soft toric lenses. Soft toric lenses are most successful when the refractive cylinder is between -0.75 and -2.00 D and the cylinder axis is not oblique. The reasons for this are fourfold:

1. Most soft toric lenses are available in these parameters; higher-cylinder-power custom lenses are available at slightly more—to much greater—expense.
2. Most diagnostic sets and inventories are in these parameters.
3. In high refractive astigmatism, rotation of the lens with the blink may reduce VA.
4. Oblique cylinder axes tend to result in greater lid effect on the lens edge; therefore, rotational instability is possible.

Front Surface Toric Gas-Permeable Lenses: Application of the patient's residual astigmatic correction onto the front of the GP lens surface was, until the introduction of soft toric lenses, the most common method of correcting this problem. It is still a recommended option in some cases, including patients who desire or benefit visually from a GP lens and those who have experienced soft lens-induced complications (i.e., edema, giant papillary conjunctivitis [GPC]). Three stabilization methods have been used: (a) prism ballast, (b) prism ballast and truncation, and (c) periballast.

Prism ballast: Prism ballast can be incorporated into a GP lens to allow the patient's residual cylinder to be ground onto the front surface of the lens. The purpose of the prism is to stabilize the lens from possible rotational movement induced by the action of the lids. It is recommended when patients have lower lids at or below the lower limbus, when large palpebral apertures with loose lids are present, and whenever discomfort is experienced with truncated, prism-ballasted lens designs.[8]

The amount of prism to be incorporated into the lens design is the minimum amount that produces stabilization and is dependent on lens power. An amount equal to 0.75 to 1 Δ for moderate and high minus lenses and 1.25 to 1.5 Δ for low minus and plus lenses has been recommended.[9] A greater amount of prism is indicated with plus power lenses because of the thinner edge present in these designs.

Because of the greater center thickness (CT) of these lenses in comparison to spherical designs, a high-Dk lens material (>50) is recommended. A minimum overall diameter (OAD) of 8.8 mm is recommended, both to incorporate the prism effectively and help offset the possible effects of flare from a heavier, potentially inferiorly decentering lens design. To estimate the CT of a prism-ballasted lens, the following equation can be used[9]:

$$CT \times 100 = \text{Prismatic power} \times OAD$$

Therefore, if 1 Δ were used for stabilizing a 9.0-mm OAD, 0.09 mm would need to be added to a conventional spherical lens design of the same power (more plus meridian) to obtain an estimate of the CT in prism-ballasted form. If the conventional spherical CT for the lens power in the most plus meridian is 0.15 mm, in prism-ballasted form the CT would equal 0.15 + 0.09, or 0.24 mm.

The most accurate method of ultimately determining the exact powers and axis would be to order a spherical power prism-ballasted lens and have the laboratory mark the base-apex line.[10] If a diagnostic fitting set is present, a slightly "steeper than K" lens should be selected. As the center of gravity tends to be more anterior and the mass of these lenses tends to defy gravity somewhat, a plus tear film centrally should assist with centration. If the lens is riding inferiorly with little or no movement after the blink, a minus carrier should be indicated in the final order. A well-fitted lens will move slightly superiorly with the blink but with little or no rotation (i.e., a direct vertical movement).[11] Evaluating the amount of lens rotation with the blink is very important. This effect will vary as a result of such factors as the lid configuration, location, tightness, and forcefulness of the blink. As a result of the natural alignment or symmetry of the superior lid, there is a tendency for the lid to rotate nasally or excyclorotate. Therefore, the presence of tight lids or a forceful blink may contraindicate a front surface toric design. Assuming the base of the prism is dotted on the diagnostic lens, the amount of rotation can be evaluated in several ways, including the following:

(a) **Trial frame.** The patient can also wear a trial frame in combination with a low-power cylinder trial lens having hash marks for judgment of rotation (Fig. 14.1). The marks on the spectacle trial lens can be aligned with both the prism base and the optical section beam, and the degree reading can be read directly from the trial frame.
(b) **Slit-lamp beam rotation.** Many of the slit lamps in use today allow the practitioner to rotate the optical section to align with the position of the prism base. The amount of rotation can be read directly from a scale on the slit lamp.
(c) **"Guesstimate."** The most commonly used (and convenient) method is simply to estimate the amount of rotation with the blink. Because it is very easy to underestimate the amount of rotation, always think of the lens as a clock, with each hour equivalent to 30 degrees. If the prism base appears to be at approximately 6:30 (not 6 o'clock), the prism base has

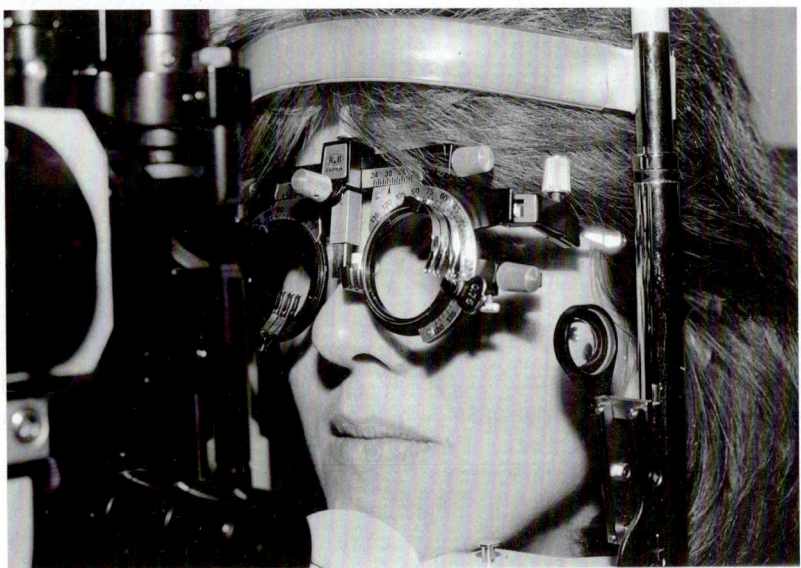

FIGURE 14.1 Trial frame use with trial lens and hash marks to estimate toric lens rotation.

rotated 15 degrees. The importance of proper evaluation of rotational amount and stability is discussed further in the section of this chapter on soft toric lenses.

After the amount of rotation has been determined by one of the aforementioned methods, the CLPs must be adjusted accordingly. If, as you observe the lens, the right lens rotates 15 degrees nasally (to the observer's right) and the left lens rotates 15 degrees nasally (to the observer's left), then the LARS (left add, right subtract) principle is used (Fig. 14.2). In this case, the axis of the final cylinder power of the right lens is decreased by 15 degrees, while the cylinder axis of the left lens is increased 15 degrees. On the average, prism-ballasted lenses tend to rotate 10 to 15 degrees nasally.

When a desirable lens-to-cornea fitting relationship has been achieved and an OR performed through the ballasted sphere, the lenses can be ordered. If a diagnostic fitting set is not available (as is often the case), an OR over the best-fitting spherical lenses will assist in determining the

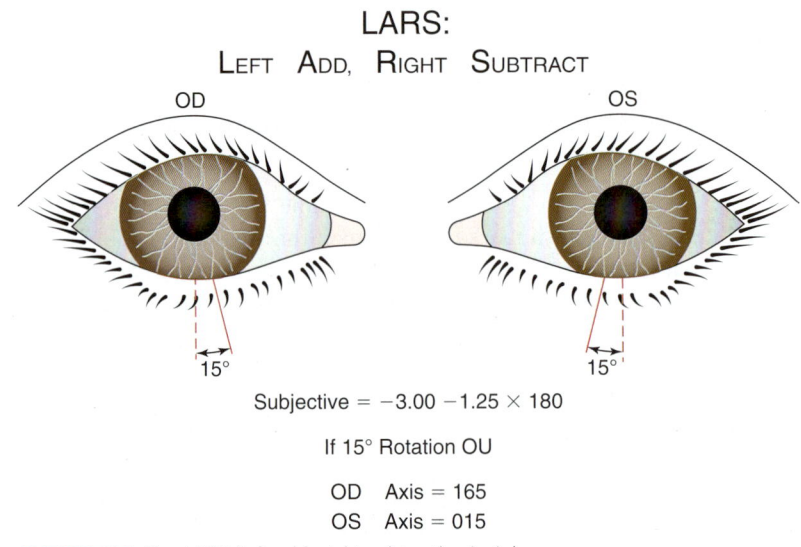

FIGURE 14.2 The LARS (left add, right subtract) principle.

final lens powers. The calculations required to arrive at the final parameters are illustrated in the following example[1]:

EXAMPLE 11

	OD	OS
Spectacle Rx	$-1.50 - 1.00 \times 090$	$-2.50 - 1.25 \times 090$
Keratometry	43.25 DS	43.00 @ 090; 43.25 @ 180
Diagnostic lens	43.50 DS, -3.00 D	43.25 DS, -3.00 D
SLE	Good centration OU	
OR	$+1.25 - 1.50 \times 090$	$+0.25 - 1.00 \times 090$
Final power	$-1.75 - 1.50 \times 090$	$-2.75 - 1.00 \times 090$

The LLP can be obtained by subtracting the combined powers of the contact lens and the OR from the spectacle Rx.

The values obtained in the ORs above actually equal the predicted values. These can be obtained by performing the following calculations:

OD

LLP = Spectacle Rx − (CLP + OR)
 = $[-1.50 - 1.00 \times 090]$
 $- [(-3.00) + (+)1.25 - 1.50 \times 090]$
 = $[-1.50 - 1.00 \times 090]$
 $- [(-)1.75 - 1.50 \times 090]$
 = $+0.25 + 0.50 \times 090$

OS

$[-2.50 - 1.25 \times 090]$
$- [(-3.00) + (+)0.25 - 1.00 \times 090]$
$[-2.50 - 1.25 \times 090]$
$- [(-)2.75 - 1.00 \times 090]$
$+0.25 - 0.25 + 090$

The CLP can be derived simply by subtracting the LLP from the spectacle Rx:

OD

CLP = Spectacle Rx − LLP
 = $[-1.50 - 1.00 \times 090]$
 $[+ 0.25 + 0.50 \times 090]$
 = $-1.75 - 1.50 \times 090$

OS

$[-2.50 - 1.25 \times 090]$
$-(+)0.25 - 0.25 \times 090$
$-2.75 - 1.00 \times 090$

As the cylinder will be grounded on the front surface of the lens in plus cylinder form, the CLPs are transposed to

OD	OS
$-3.25 + 1.50 \times 180$	$-3.75 + 1.00 \times 180$

As compensation for lens rotation is often desired, this could become

OD	OS
$-3.25 + 1.50 \times 165$	$-3.75 + 1.00 \times 015$

The contact lens order could be written as follows:

Parameter	OD	OS
BCR	43.50 (7.76)	43.50 (7.76)
CLP	−3.25 + 1.50 × 165	−3.75 + 1.00 × 015
OAD	9.0	9.0
Optical zone diameter (OZD)	7.8	7.8
Secondary curve radius/width (SCR/W) (=BCR + 1 mm)	8.8/.3	8.8/.3
Peripheral curve radius/width (PCR/W) (= SCR + 2 mm)	10.8/.3	10.8/.3
CT	0.26	0.25
Prism	1 Δ, double dot base	1 Δ, dot base
Material	Fluoroperm 60	Fluoroperm 60
Add. information	Minus carrier	Minus carrier

Prism ballast and truncation: In most cases in which a front toric GP lens is desirable, the lens of choice is a prism-ballasted truncated design. The addition of truncation assists in providing good rotational stability.

Most of the design and fitting information provided for prism ballast-only designs also pertains to lenses that incorporate prism ballast. The primary differences pertain to OAD, prism, and the shape of the inferior edge. Typically, vertical diameters are 8.7 to 9.2 mm, with horizontal diameters usually 0.4 to 0.5 mm larger.[8] Truncating a prism-ballasted lens reduces the ballast for minus lenses and increases it for plus lenses. Therefore, especially in high minus powers, the need for more prism ballast is imperative to maintain the truncation in contact with the lower lid; an amount equal to 1.25 to 1.5 Δ would be recommended, whereas a smaller amount is indicated for low minus and plus power lenses. Finally, the shape of the truncation is quite important. As the truncation should rest evenly against the lower lid, the edge should be flat to increase the distribution of lens pressure across as much of the lid as possible.[8] Anterior tapering of the lens edge may result in the truncation slipping under the lower lid; posterior edge tapering may result in subjective discomfort. Because of the typical nasal rotation of the base, ordering the truncation at approximately 15 degrees temporal to the base-apex line would be recommended. Referring back to Example 11, the order of a prism-ballasted truncated design might be similar to the following:

Parameter	OD	OS
BCR	43.50 (7.76)	43.50 (7.76)
CLP	−3.25 + 1.50 × 165	−3.75 + 1.00 × 015
OAD	9.4/8.9	9.4/8.9
OZD	7.8 (decentered 0.5 mm) UP	7.8 (same as OD)
SCR/W	8.8/0.3	8.8/0.3
PCR/W	10.8/0.3	10.8/0.3
CT	0.26	0.25

Prism	1.25 Δ	1.25 Δ
Material	Fluoroperm 60	Fluoroperm 60
Add. information	Double dot base	Dot base
	Truncation 15° temp OU	

The above examples assumed that diagnostic lenses were unavailable. Obviously, the success rate would be higher if diagnostic lenses were used. A recommended diagnostic set is provided in Table 14.1.

Prism-ballasted, front surface toric lens designs, both truncated and nontruncated, are associated with some problems that limit their use. These include the following[1]:

1. Vision is blurred.
2. Discomfort results from prism, truncation, or both.
3. Quality control is poor.
4. Inferior decentration causes flare and possibly corneal desiccation.
5. It is not possible to modify the front surface.
6. If unilateral, asthenopia can result from a vertical imbalance, although low amounts of prism (i.e., 0.75 − 1 Δ) can usually be tolerated.
7. Edema can develop if a low-Dk GP lens material is used.

Verification of front surface toric lenses is straightforward. The back surface of the lens is placed against the lens stop of the lensometer and is rotated until the position of the target image indicates prism base down (axis = 90 degrees). If, for example, the left lens cylinder was ordered at axis 105 degrees, the base of the prism should be rotated nasally 15 degrees to obtain the power in that meridian. The lens is then rotated 90 degrees to obtain the power in the other meridian. The cylinder power of the lens is the same on the eye as in air when measured with the lensometer, as the cylinder is on the front surface only. If the lens was ordered with the power $-3.25 + 1.25 \times 075$, this should be the power read with the lensometer.

Periballast: A periballasted lens design is cut in lenticular form with a high minus carrier. Two forms of this lens design are available. In one form, the final lens is cut with no flange at the top and with the entire 1.0 to 1.3 mm of flange left at the bottom to achieve the ballast. In the

TABLE 14.1 Circular Prism-Ballasted Trial Lens Set (10 Lenses)

BASE CURVE	OAD/OZD	CLP	SCR/W	PCR/W
1. 40.50 (8.33)	9.2/8.0	−3.00	9.30/0.3	11.30/0.3
2. 41.50 (8.13)	9.2/8.0	−3.00	9.10/0.3	11.10/0.3
3. 42.00 (8.04)	9.2/8.0	−3.00	9.00/0.3	11.00/0.3
4. 42.50 (7.94)	9.0/7.8	−3.00	8.90/0.3	10.90/0.3
5. 43.00 (7.85)	9.0/7.8	−3.00	8.90/0.3	10.90/0.3
6. 43.50 (7.76)	9.0/7.8	−3.00	8.80/0.3	10.80/0.3
7. 44.00 (7.67)	9.0/7.8	−3.00	8.70/0.3	10.70/0.3
8. 44.50 (7.58)	8.8/7.8	−3.00	8.60/0.3	10.60/0.3
9. 45.00 (7.50)	8.8/7.8	−3.00	8.50/0.3	10.50/0.3
10. 46.00 (7.34)	8.8/7.8	−3.00	8.30/0.3	10.30/0.3

CLP, contact lens power; OAD, overall diameter; OZD, optical zone diameter; PCR/W, peripheral curve radius/width; SCR/W, secondary curve radius/width.

other form, the lens is manufactured such that a small amount of flange remains at the top to provide a minus carrier effect.

A periballast does reduce some of the prism ballast-induced problems. The advantages include better optical quality, a thinner design, and no vertical imbalance. However, it is rarely used because of the rotational instability and flange-induced discomfort.

High Astigmatism

The correction of high astigmatic error, defined as ≥2.50 D of corneal astigmatism, is quite different from correction of residual astigmatic error. In most cases, the selection of a carefully designed spherical or bitoric design will be successful with these patients. The latter design alternative is most often recommended, and these designs are easy to fit and evaluate. Other alternatives include aspheric designs, soft toric lenses, and back surface toric GP lenses.

Spherical Gas-Permeable Lenses

Although the benefits of a spherical design in high astigmatism include the use of an uncomplicated lens design and less expense, the selection of this alternative will, in most cases, eventually result in failure because of such problems as decentration-induced symptoms of visual flare, corneal desiccation resulting from excessive peripheral clearance, flexure-induced fluctuation in VA, and lens rocking resulting in corneal staining.[11,12] In addition, although good centration is possible to achieve regardless of the amount of corneal astigmatism, these lenses will, as a result of poor corneal alignment, apply excessive pressure (i.e., bearing zones) against the cornea, possibly resulting in corneal distortion.[12,13] This condition is accelerated if poor centration is present.[14] However, a borderline candidate (i.e., 2.0–2.5 D of corneal cylinder) with their corneal cylinder localized centrally (i.e., not limbus-to-limbus), a spherical lens can be successful.[15]

In many cases, it is not a bad idea to use a spherical lens as the initial diagnostic lens and evaluate vision, corneal alignment, and centration. A relatively low-Dk material (i.e., 25–50) should be selected to minimize flexure and facilitate manufacture. The BCR should be about one-third of the difference "steeper than K" to achieve a well-centered intrapalpebral lens-to-cornea fitting relationship. The CT in minus lens powers should be 0.02 to 0.04 mm thicker than with low astigmatic patients to minimize flexure. Overkeratometry should also be performed to rule out flexure. If toricity >0.50 D exists with overkeratometry, either a flatter BCR or a bitoric lens design should be considered.

Aspheric Designs

An aspheric design may provide better centration and a more uniform fluorescein pattern than a spherical lens design. In particular, designs with an elliptic back surface (i.e., the progressive and the so-called biaspheric designs) have been shown to exhibit good centration in patients having 2 to 3 D of corneal astigmatism (Fig. 14.3).[16] However, to minimize symptoms of visual flare, good centration is imperative with these designs.

Soft Toric

Improvements in quality control, enhanced quality of vision, and greater oxygen transmissibility currently make this modality an option to consider when a high astigmatic patient with no evidence of corneal distortion is strongly motivated toward soft lens wear.[17] In addition, numerous companies manufacture custom soft toric lenses in practically any axis and power, and improvements in edge designs have resulted in better subjective comfort than was attained with previous-generation designs. Finally, computer-assisted lens design programs are available that are especially beneficial in cross-cylinder situations and currently are being used by both practitioners and manufacturers.[18] This type of program is capable of providing a recommended cylinder axis and power based on the patient's refractive data, the diagnostic lens parameters, and the amount of rotation on the eye.

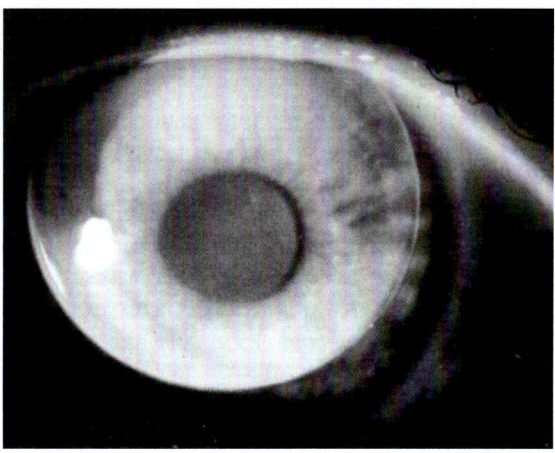

FIGURE 14.3 An aspheric lens (Boston Envision) providing good centration and a less obvious "dumbbell-shaped" fluorescein pattern than present with a spherical design.

Excellent quality control is imperative with these lenses, and they should also be stable on the eye; rotation of only a few degrees can significantly affect visual performance, especially with patients having more than 3 D of corneal astigmatism. If corneal distortion or irregular astigmatism is present, a much better visual result can be attained with the selection of a GP lens. Manufacturers' claims of success and accuracy may also be erroneous; therefore, it is important to consider soft toric lenses when the patient is motivated, astigmatism is regular, and the need for critical distance vision is not great.

Back Surface Toric

A back surface toric lens design has the advantage of providing greater alignment of the posterior lens surface to the cornea; therefore, better centration is present. In addition, problems such as flexure, lens rocking, and flare are minimized.

There are numerous philosophies on how to determine the BCRs for any posterior surface (i.e., back surface or bitoric designs). The Mandell-Moore philosophy for determining the BCRs is provided in Table 14.2.[19] To assist in achieving alignment between lens and cornea, toric peripheral curves may be beneficial.[20] To determine the specific PCRs to select, the following philosophy can be used:

Secondary curve radii (SCRs) = 1.0 mm flatter than the BCRs (e.g., if the BCRs are 41 D [8.23 mm] and 44 D [7.67 mm], the SCRs would be 9.23/8.67 mm or rounded off to 9.2/8.7 mm].

PCRs = 3.0 mm flatter than the BCRs; in the above case, they would be equal to 11.2/10.7 mm.

If a spherical periphery is desired, simply add 1.0 mm to the average BCR to determine the SCR and add 3.0 mm to determine the PCR. In the above example, the average between

TABLE 14.2 Mandell-Moore Fit Factor

CORNEAL CYL (D)	FIT FLAT MERIDIAN	FIT STEEP MERIDIAN
2.0	On K	0.50 D Flatter
2.5	0.25 D Flatter	0.50 D Flatter
3.0	0.25 D Flatter	0.75 D Flatter
3.5	0.25 D Flatter	0.75 D Flatter
4.0	0.25 D Flatter	0.75 D Flatter
5.0	0.25 D Flatter	0.75 D Flatter

Reprinted with permission from Mandell RB, Moore CF. A bitoric lens guide that really is simple. *Contact Lens Spectrum*. 1988;3(11):83–85.

41 D and 44 D equals 42.50 D (7.94 mm); the SCR would equal (approximately) 8.9 mm and the PCR would equal 10.9 mm.

When determining the BCRs, the tear layer power will result in a change in power. To determine these values, Sarver's formula can be used[21]:

$$Fs = Ff + Kf - Ks$$

where

    Fs = the back vertex power of the contact lens in the steeper principal meridian (in air)
    Ff = the back vertex power of the contact lens in the flatter principal meridian (in air)
    Ks = the BCR of the contact lens in the steeper principal meridian
    Kf = the BCR of the contact lens in the flatter principal meridian

All of this information can be incorporated into the following example:

EXAMPLE 12

Spectacle Rx: $+0.50 - 4.00 \times 180$
Keratometry: 40.50 @ 180; 44.50 @ 090

A spherical diagnostic lens with a BCR of 41.50 D was attempted. However, this lens resulted in inferior decentration and some flexure-induced uncorrected corneal astigmatism confirmed by toric readings by keratometry performed over the lenses. A back surface toric lens design, using the Mandell-Moore base curve philosophy, is then ordered. The parameters can be obtained from the following:

$$Kf = 40.50 + (-)0.25 = 40.25 \text{ D}$$
$$Ks = 44.50 - 0.75 = 43.75 \text{ D}$$
$$Ff = +0.50 + (0.25) \text{ (LLP)} = +0.75 \text{ D}$$
$$Fs = +0.75 + (40.25 - 43.75) = -2.75 \text{ D}$$

The peripheral curves can be determined as follows:

$$\text{Average BCR} = \frac{40.25 + 43.75}{2} = 42.00 \text{ D (8.04 mm)}$$

$$\text{SCR} = 8.00 \text{ mm (rounded off from 8.04)} + 1.00 = 9.00 \text{ mm}$$

$$\text{PCR} = 8.00 + 3.00 = 11.00 \text{ mm}$$

Final order (empirical):

BCR (mm)	Power (D)	SCR/W (mm)	PCR/W (mm)	OAD (mm)
40.25/43.75 (8.38)(7.71)	+0.75	9.00/.3	11.00/.3	9.2

Unfortunately, the great majority of high astigmatic patients would not be able to achieve optimum VA from a back surface toric design because of the problem of induced cylinder. A back surface toric GP contact lens in situ induces a cylinder in the optical system (contact lens–fluid lens) designed to correct the ametropia. The minus cylinder is the result of the difference between the refractive index of the contact lens (n = 1.47 –1.49 in most cases; 1.49 will be used here) and the index of the tear lens (n = 1.336). The exact amount would be 0.456 times the back surface toricity. The minus cylinder axis will lie along the flatter principal meridian of the toric back surface of the contact lens. This induced cylinder rarely corrects and sometimes compounds the residual astigmatism.

The following contact lens conversion factors are important when determining the changes in power induced by a toric back surface contact lens.

1. From back surface lens toricity (measured with the radiuscope) to contact lens cylinder power in air (measured with the lensometer)—multiply by 1.452 (or approximately 1.5).
2. From back surface lens toricity (measured with the radiuscope) to the contact lens cylinder power measured in fluid (on the eye or induced)—multiply by 0.456 (or approximately one-half).
3. From contact lens cylinder power in air (measured with the lensometer) to the contact lens cylinder power in fluid (on the eye or induced)—multiply by 0.314 (or approximately one-third).
4. From the contact lens cylinder power in fluid (on the eye or induced) to the contact lens cylinder power in air (measured with the lensometer)—multiply by 3.19 (or approximately 3).

Essentially, this concept can be simplified to a 1:2:3 principle (Fig. 14.4). This would represent a fractional component by which if one component is known, the other two can be easily determined. If "2" equals the amount of base curve toricity verified with the radiuscope, "1" equals 1 divided by 2 or one-half the base curve toricity, "3" equals both three times the "1" value or 3/2 times the base curve toricity. If the base curve toricity equals 3 D, the induced cylinder predicted with lens wear is one-half this value or 1.5 D; the value verified with a lensometer is 4.5 D or 3/2 times the radiuscope value.

Referring back to Example 12, the amount of induced astigmatism would equal approximately $0.5 \times \Delta K$ (back surface or -3.50×180) = -1.75×180. A plus correcting cylinder of the same amount and axis is applied to the front surface; therefore, in this case, $+1.75$ D $\times$ 180 is the front surface cylinder power. This will result in a power of -3.50×180 while creating a spherical power effect (SPE; i.e., the lens can rotate on the eye without affecting vision); this will be discussed later in this section of the chapter.

The other factor to consider when verifying a back surface toric lens is that because the induced astigmatism is not corrected, when the cylinder power is verified with a lensometer,

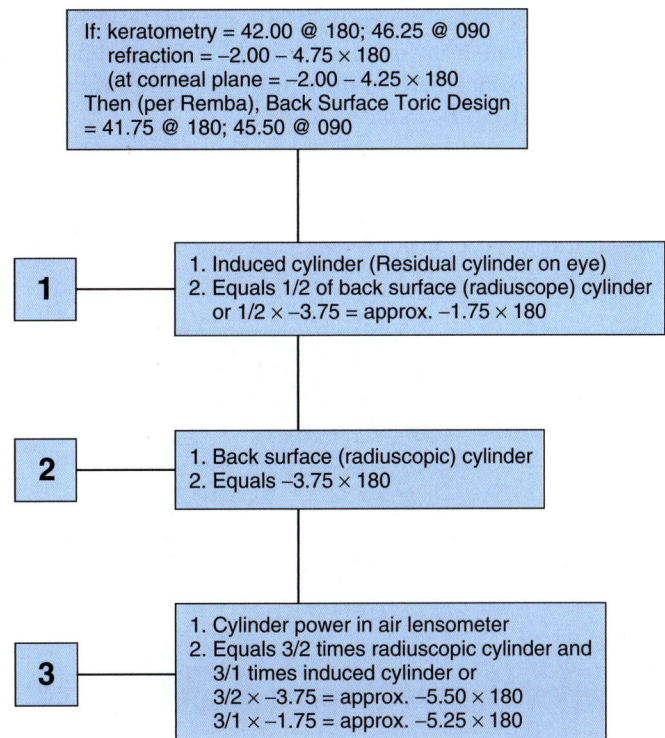

FIGURE 14.4 The 1:2:3 principle.

a value equal to approximately 1.5 times the back surface toricity (radiuscope cylinder) will be read. In the previous example, the amount of cylinder power recorded with a lensometer is $-3.50 \times 1.5 = -5.25$ D $\times$ 180. This is a key factor when a back surface toric is differentiated from a bitoric lens because a bitoric design with the induced cylinder corrected on the front surface (unless a significant residual astigmatism is also being incorporated into the lens) will verify with a similar cylinder for both the radiuscope and the lensometer.

It is also important to emphasize the fact that it is often not a true "1-2-3" relationship, particularly if the patient is fit into a low-refractive-index material. For example, if the patient is fit into a lens having 2 D of base curve material and a material refractive index of 1.485, the lensometer cylinder will equal -2.87 D (i.e., $1.485 - 1.00/1.3375 - 1.00 \times 2$). If they are fit into a lens material with a refractive index of 1.415, using the same equation, the lensometer cylinder will only equal -2.45 D.[22]

To summarize this discussion, it is apparent that to obtain both good centration and good VA, a bitoric lens is indicated. There is one situation in which a back surface toric design would provide the preferable vision correction. This design is the lens of choice when the corneal toricity is against-the-rule and the residual astigmatism is approximately 0.5 times the amount of back surface toricity of the lens (as measured with the radiuscope).

Bitoric Design

In most cases of high corneal astigmatism, a bitoric lens design should be used. Typically, they are indicated for ≥2.50 D of corneal toricity; however, they can be fit to individuals with as low as 1.50 D if limbus-to-limbus astigmatism is present. The benefits of centration (Fig. 14.5) and, if the lenses are well designed and manufactured, satisfactory VA are present with this option.

It was mentioned earlier that if the induced astigmatism that was created as a result of the toric anterior tear layer is corrected, a SPE is created. In other words, if this front surface correction is ground onto the lens in the correct meridian relative to the principal meridian of the base curve, lens rotation will not alter the correction and the bitoric lens will provide a spherical effect when correcting only for the induced astigmatism.[23,24] This is shown in Figure 14.6 in which the extreme case of 90-degree rotation is provided. It is shown that the tear layer will compensate, and the front surface cylinder correction will still equal the new cylinder and axis of the induced cylinder.

Fitting Methods: A misperception of bitoric lenses is that they are very challenging to fit. However, this has not been substantiated by recent research.[25,26] In a survey of the Diplomates of the Cornea and Contact Lens Section of the American Academy of Optometry (AAO),

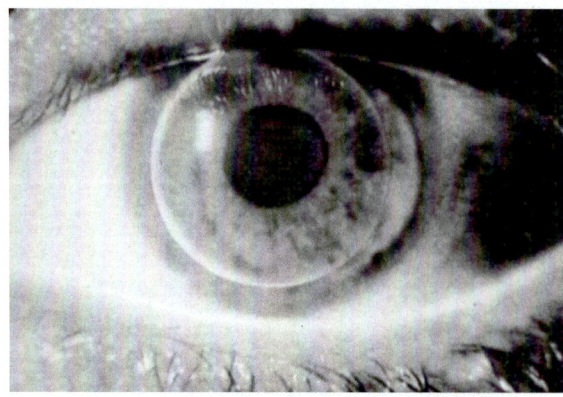

FIGURE 14.5 A well-centered bitoric lens on a highly astigmatic cornea.

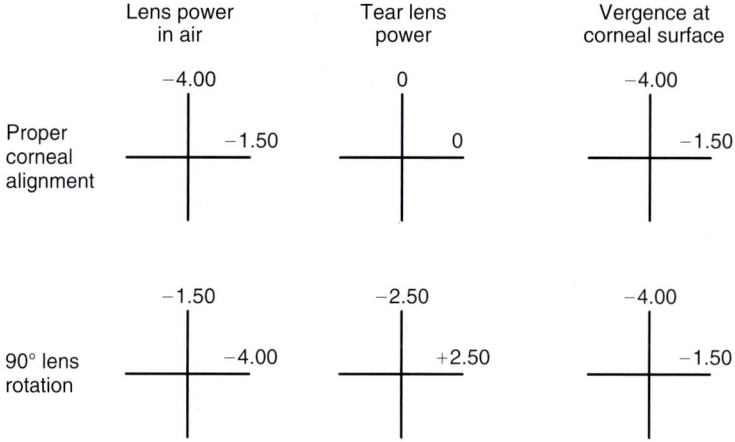

FIGURE 14.6 The principle of spherical power effect.

approximately 90% responded that bitoric GP lenses varied from acceptable to very easy to fit.[26] These lenses are fitted either empirically or via a bitoric diagnostic set.

Empirical Methods: Fitting toric back surface lenses empirically has become very popular due to the benefits of efficiency of fit as well as first-fit success due to the quality of manufacturing of these designs today.[27,28] In a recent study, 19 subjects wore empirically designed bitoric lenses for 1 month and soft toric lenses for 1 month.[28] Ten of these subjects were soft toric lens wearers entering study while seven were spectacle wearers (i.e., contact lens dropouts), and two were GP toric wearers. They had an average of −3.62 D of refractive cylinder. However, at the conclusion of the study, 14/19 preferred the vision of the GP lenses and 11/19 elected to stay in this modality.

The lens powers and BCRs of any back surface or bitoric lens design can be determined by several methods, including the previously demonstrated computational method.[11,29,30] Example 13 shows how these values can be determined for a bitoric design using both computational and optical cross methods:

EXAMPLE 13

Keratometry: 42.50 @180; 45.50 @90

Refraction (at corneal plane): −6.00 − 3.00 × 180

1. *Computational method*
   (a) Calculate residual cylinder:

   Spectacle cylinder corneal cylinder = −3.00 × 180 − (−)3.00 × 180 = 0

   (b) Select BCRs via Mandell-Moore:

   $$K_f = 42.50 - (+)0.25 = 42.25 \text{ D or } 7.99 \text{ mm}$$
   $$K_s = 45.50 - (+)0.75 = 44.75 \text{ D or } 7.54 \text{ mm}$$

   (c) Calculate back vertex powers:

   $$F_f = -6.00 + (+)0.25 = -5.75 \text{ D}$$
   $$F_s = F_f + (K_f - K_s) = -5.75 + (42.25 - 44.75) = -8.25 \text{ D}$$

   Power of lens in air = −5.75 − 2.50 × 180

2. *Optical cross method*

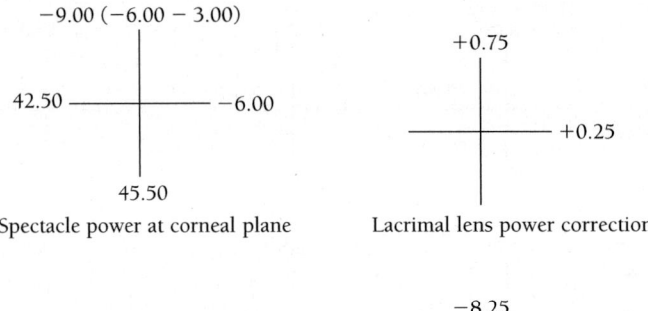

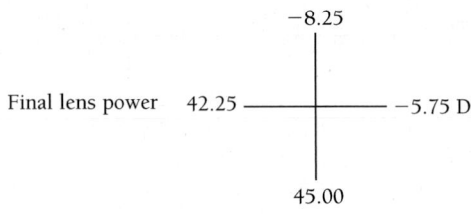

Bitoric lens correction: −5.75/−8.25 42.25(7.99 mm)/44.75(7.46 mm)

It is important for the laboratory to understand that these are the values that should be verified with the lensometer. Therefore, the powers should represent compensated values with the induced cylinder correction on the front surface. In this case, approximately 0.50 ×−2.50 (back surface cylinder) = −1.25 D × 180. + 1.25 D × 180 will need to be added to the front surface to arrive at the final lens powers of −5.75/−8.25.

As the optical cross method illustrates, it is not necessary to use a formula to determine the final lens powers. Essentially, a bitoric design can be considered as two spherical designs when tear lens power calculations are performed. In this example, a BCR was selected that was 0.25 D "flatter than K" in the horizontal meridian. Using the SAM–FAP philosophy (i.e., steep add minus/flat add plus), the power in the meridian becomes 0.25 D more plus or −5.75 D. In the steep meridian, a BCR was selected that was 0.75 D "flatter than K" in the steep meridian; therefore, the final lens power becomes 0.75 D more plus or −8.25 D.

It is important to emphasize that most philosophies recommend a flat BCR that is either "On K" or 0.25 D flatter than "K" and a steep BCR approximately 0.75 D flatter than steep "K." This designs results in a slight amount of with-the-rule toricity, which promotes vertical movement in the with-the-rule astigmatic patients.[29]

3. *Mandell-Moore Bitoric Lens Guide*

Another computational method for determining the bitoric lens specifications is the Mandell-Moore bitoric lens guide.[16] This is a simple reference guide in which the keratometric and refraction information is entered and the final values are derived using the recommended BCRs. This is an excellent empirical method for determining powers and BCRs in which it is not necessary to compute lacrimal lens effects. It has also been found to result in a comparable success rate when compared with diagnostic fitting of bitoric lenses.[31] An example of this method is provided in Figure 14.7. The form is downloadable from the GP Lens Institute website (www.gpli.info). There is also a calculator to perform the calculations on this website.

4. *GPLI Toric and Spherical Lens Calculator.*

A calculator to determine, not only BCRs but the other parameters for back surface and bitoric lens designs is available from the GP Lens Institute on their website: www.gpli.info.[30] Once the refraction and keratometry values are inputted, the calculator will recommend a particular design (i.e., spherical, back surface toric, or bitoric). The toric program was developed by Dr. Tom Quinn.[29] It dynamically shows the tear lens powers and shows the recommended BCRs and powers on the "lens." (Fig. 14.8) In addition, it will provide other lens parameters as well as any recommendations or precautions resulting from this design.

GP CLINICAL EDUCATION:
Mandell-Moore bitoric lens guide
Click here for a blank guide which you can then print for your office.

Mandell-Moore bitoric lens guide - per eye

	Flattest K	Sphere power	Steepest K	SPH + CYL power
1. Keratometry	43.00 @ 180		46.50 @ 090	
2. Spectacle Rx (Minus cyl form)		−40.00 − 4.00 x 180		
3. Enter K	43.00		46.50	
4. Enter spectacle power		−4.00		−8.00
5. Vertex adjust line 4		−3.75		−7.25
6. Insert fit factor	(−) 0.25	(+) 0.25	(−) 0.75	(+) 0.75
Add lines	3&8	5&8	3&8	5&8
7. Final CL Rx	42.75	−3.50	45.75	−6.50
	Base curve	Power	Base curve	Power

Bitoric lens fit factor

Corneal cyl (D)	Fit flat meridian	Fit steep meridian
2.0	On K (0 D)	0.50 D Flatter
2.5	0.25 D Flatter	0.50 D Flatter
3.0	0.25 D Flatter	0.75 D Flatter
3.5	0.25 D Flatter	0.75 D Flatter
4.0	0.25 D Flatter	0.75 D Flatter
5.0	0.25 D Flatter	0.75 D Flatter

FIGURE 14.7 Mandell-Moore bitoric lens guide.

5. *Newman's GP Toric Guide.*

    This empirical guide, developed by Dr. Clarke Newman, is also available at www.gpli.info. It is a downloadable form that has all of the base curve selection, BCR-mm conversion, vertex conversion, and lens design selection information for the practitioner to design a bitoric lens.

Spherical Power Effect Bitoric Diagnostic Lenses: The use of bitoric diagnostic lenses is the preferable method of fitting these patients. Most Contact Lens Manufacturers Association (CLMA) member laboratories have bitoric diagnostic fitting sets available for loaner use as well as for purchase. Excellent success rates have been reported by fitting high astigmatic patients by using the Polycon II SPE bitoric diagnostic lenses (formerly available from Ciba Vision Corp.).[32–34] In fact, in the aforementioned survey of AAO Diplomates, the Mandell-Moore Empirical Fitting Guide was the most commonly used empirical fitting method and the Polycon II SPE design was the most commonly used bitoric diagnostic fitting set.[25] This concept makes fitting bitoric designs as simple as fitting spherical lens designs, and many patients obtain VA equal to or better than that achieved with their optimum spectacle correction.

As this lens design is no longer available, a similar fitting set can be provided by your laboratory. A set with 3 D of back surface toricity is recommended. Such a set is shown in Table 14.3. It can consist of a ten lens set with the BCRs ranging from 40.50/43.50 to 45.00/48.00 in 0.50 D steps, all with powers of pl/−3.00 D. The induced cylinder correction is already incorporated into the lens.

I. Residual Astigmatic Correction

Front Toric GP
1. Rarely indicated; used when soft lenses contraindicated
2. Example: keratometry = 42.00 @ 180; 43.25 @ 090
   refraction = −1.00 − 2.75 x 180

Spherical GP
1. Can flex to reduce induced cylinder
2. Example: keratometry = 41 @ 180; 43 @ 090
   refraction = −2.00 − 1.00 x 180

Spherical Soft
1. Indicated when refractive cylinder is low and corneal cylinder is moderate or high
2. Example: keratometry = 42.00 @; 43.50 @ 090
   refraction = −5.00 − 0.25 x 180

Soft Toric
1. Indicated when refractive astigmatism is between 1–2 diopters and significant residual astigmatism is present
2. Example: keratometry = 43.00 DS
   refraction = −3.00 − 1.50 x 090

II. High Astigmatic Correction

Spherical GP
1. <3D corneal cylinder or when oblique astigmatism-especially in ATR cylinder
   Example: keratometry = 42.00 @ 145; 46.00 @ 055
   refraction = −2.50 − 4.50 x 162
2. Consider aspheric design with 2–3 diopters of corneal astigmatism-especially in ATR cylinder

Soft Toric
1. Any refractive astimatic patient with regular astigmatism and motivated for soft lens wear

Back Surface Toric
1. Indicated when corneal toricity is ATR and residual astigmatism = 0.5 x radiuscopic toricity; otherwise, BS torics are contraindicated
2. Example: keratometry = 42.25 @ 090; 45.00 @ 180
   refraction = −1.00 − 4.50 x 090
   back surface −41.50 @ 090; 44.50 @ 180

Bitoric
1. Indicated in all regular astimatic cases with ≥ 3D of corneal toricity
2. Example: keratometry = 41.00 @ 180; 45.00 @ 090
   refraction = −3.00 − 4.75 x 180
   (at corneal plane) −3.00 − 4.00 x 180
Two methods can be used:
a. Empirical power: order BCR :40.75/44.25, powers −2.75/−6.25
b. spherical power effect:
   select: 40.50/43.50 base curve radius pl/−3.00 powers
   predicted OR = −2.50 DS
Final predicted lens design = 40.50/43.50   −2.50/−5.50

FIGURE 14.8 Gas-permeable toric fitting guide.

TABLE 14.3 10 Lens Bitoric SPE Set		
BCR (mm)	POWER (D)	DIAMETER (mm)
8.33/7.76	pl/−3.00	9.0
8.23/7.67	pl/−3.00	9.0
8.13/7.58	pl/−3.00	9.0
8.04/7.50	pl/−3.00	9.0
7.95/7.42	pl/−3.00	9.0
7.85/7.34	pl/−3.00	9.0
7.76/7.26	pl/−3.00	9.0
7.67/7.18	pl/−3.00	9.0
7.59/7.11	pl/−3.00	9.0
7.50/7.03	pl/−3.00	9.0

The initial SPE diagnostic lens flat meridian BCR should be 0.12 to 0.50 D flatter than the flat K reading. As the diagnostic lenses are designed in 0.50 D steps, there should only be one lens to meet this criterion. The determination of the final lens powers is a two-step procedure:

1. Perform a spherical refraction over the selected SPE diagnostic lens.
2. Add the OR to the powers in the flat and steep meridians of the diagnostic lens.

Example 14 shows how the SPE concept is used in the diagnostic fitting process:

EXAMPLE 14

Spectacle Rx: +2.00 − 3.00 × 180

Keratometry: 41.50 @ 180; 44.50 @ 090

Diagnostic lens parameters:

BCR = 41.00/44.00

Power: pl/−3.00

SLE: good centration; alignment fluorescein pattern

OR: +2.50 DS (VA = 20/20)

Final order: BCR = 41.00 (8.23 mm)/44.00 (7.67 mm)

Power = +2.50/−0.50

Boston ES bitoric

In the above example, a higher-Dk lens material (>50) would be recommended because of the powers necessary. As there was no predicted residual astigmatism and assuming the VA was acceptable with a spherical-only OR, it can be concluded that it was negligible. In most cases, if there is <0.75 D of residual astigmatism, it is not necessary to incorporate it into the lens correcting power. However, if the patient's VA is reduced significantly (typically, at minimum, one line worse than the optimum correction) with a spherical-only OR but is optimally corrected with the residual cylinder present, a cylinder power effect (CPE) bitoric lens design is indicated. This design incorporates both the induced and the residual cylindrical error (as determined with a SPE bitoric diagnostic lens). The following steps summarize the CPE fitting process:

1. Select the recommended SPE diagnostic lens.
2. Perform a spherical OR; if the VA is reduced, perform a sphero–cylindrical OR.
3. Use Silbert's rule[8] to determine the final lens powers: "If the axes are at or near the principal corneal meridians, add the appropriate power in the refraction to the air power of the corresponding meridian in the diagnostic lens, and order."

Examples 15 and 16 are representative examples of CPE bitoric fitting.

EXAMPLE 15

Keratometry: 41.50 @ 180; 44.50 @ 090

Spectacle Rx: $-0.75 - 4.00 \times 180$

Diagnostic SPE lens: 41.00/44.00

Power: pl/−3.00

OR (sphere): −0.25 DS 20/30 + 2

OR (sphere–cyl): $-0.25 - 1.00 \times 180$ 20/20

Add the OR to the corresponding power in the diagnostic lens to obtain the final lens powers:

180 meridian: $-0.25 + \text{pl} = -0.25$ D

090 meridian: $(-0.25 + -1.00) + (-)3.00 = -4.25$ D

Final order: 41.00 (8.23 mm)/44.00 (7.67 mm) −0.25/−4.25

Fluoroperm 30 bitoric

EXAMPLE 16A

Keratometry: 41.50 @ 180; 44.50 @ 090

Spectacle Rx: $-0.75 - 2.00 \times 180$

Diagnostic SPE lens: 41.00/44.00

Power: pl/−3.00

OR (sphere): −0.25 DS 20/25 − 2

OR (sphere–cyl): $+0.75 - 1.00 \times 090$ 20/20

Add the OR to the corresponding power in the diagnostic lens to obtain the final lens powers:

180 meridian: $-0.25 + \text{pl} = -0.25$ D

090 meridian: $+0.75 + (-)3.00 = -2.25$ D

Final order: 41.00 (8.23 mm)/44.00 (7.67 mm) −0.25/−2.25

Fluoroperm 30 bitoric

As the Polycon II lens has such a low-Dk value, a higher-Dk material, as shown in the two examples, should be ordered. In addition, it is important to mention that the incorporation of the residual astigmatic correction negates the benefit of an SPE lens. Therefore, rotation of a CPE bitoric lens could compromise vision. However, on high astigmatic corneas, bitoric lens designs typically orient properly on the eye and satisfactory vision is achieved.

To verify the BCRs of a bitoric (or back surface toric) lens design, rotate the lens mount until one mire image comes into focus and record that value. Then turn the focusing knob until the image 90 degrees away comes into focus and record this value. Essentially, a bitoric lens will have the same radiuscopic appearance as a warped lens. Verifying the power is straightforward when the lensometer is used. For both SPE and CPE bitoric lenses, the air powers should equal what was ordered (i.e., with SPE lenses, the cylinder power amount should equal the toricity measured with the radiuscope). If a back surface toric lens was ordered, the air power cylinder should be approximately 1.5 times the radiuscopic cylinder.

Other Considerations: Other factors to consider when fitting bitoric GP lenses include the CT, peripheral curve design, very high astigmatic corneas, and irregular astigmatism.

1. Center thickness. Bitoric lenses are thin lens designs. The CT for a bitoric lens is equal to the CT of a spherical in the most plus bitoric lens power. For example, in Example 16A, if the recommended CT for a Fluoroperm 30 lens material in −0.25 D power is 0.19 mm, that would be the recommended CT for this bitoric lens design.
2. Peripheral curve design. Either spherical or toric peripheral curves can be ordered. However, as a result of improvements in manufacturing technology such that automated numeric lathes can create accurate toric peripheral curves without crimping the lens as was performed in the past.[15,35] The primary author's philosophy is to select toric PCRs such that the toric SCR are 1 mm flatter than the toric BCR and the toric PCR are 2 mm flatter than the toric SCR.[36] In Example 16A, the BCRs are 41.00 (8.23 mm)/44.00 (7.67 mm). The SCR would be (rounding off the values): 9.2/8.7 mm and the PCR would equal 11.2/10.7 mm. The final order would be the following:

EXAMPLE 16B

BCR: 41.00 (8.23 mm)/44.00 (7.67 mm)

Powers: −0.25/−2.25

OAD/OZD: 9.4/8.2 mm

CT: 0.19 mm

SCR/W: 9.2/8.7 mm @ 0.3 mm

PCR/W: 11.2/10.7 mm @ 0.3 mm

Fluoroperm 30 bitoric

3. Very high astigmatic corneas. It is not unusual to have a very highly astigmatic patient fitted with a bitoric diagnostic lens of much lesser toricity. The resulting fluorescein pattern is not alignment but actually somewhat astigmatic in appearance. When this is the case, the fit should proceed as in Examples 14 through 16. An OR is performed and added to the diagnostic lens powers to achieve the lens powers. Next, the steeper BCR can be steepened to improve the fitting relationship and the power in that meridian increased in minus by the same amount. This is demonstrated in Example 17.

EXAMPLE 17

Spectacle Rx: +2.00 − 5.50 × 180

Keratometry: 41.00 @ 180; 46.50 @ 090

Diagnostic lens parameters: BCR = 40.50/43.50

Power: pl/−3.00

SLE: good centration; mild bearing horizontally; excessive clearance vertically

OR: +2.50 DS (equal to predicted; VA = 20/20)

Tentative order: 41.00 (8.23 mm) + 2.50 D/44.00 (7.67 mm) −0.50 D

Steepen vertical meridian 1.5 D to improve fitting relationship and add −1.50 D to power in that meridian

Final order: 41.00 (8.23 mm) +2.50 D/45.50 (7.42 mm) −2.00 D

Toric peripheral curves: SCR = BCR + 1 mm; PCR = SCR + 2 mm

$$SCR = 8.2/7.4 + 1\ mm = 9.2/8.4\ mm$$

$$PCR = 9.2/8.4 + 2\ mm = 11.2/10.4\ mm$$

Fluorex 700 bitoric

4. Irregular astigmatism. There are some situations in which a bitoric lens would exhibit limited success. These are cases in which the keratometric axis differs significantly (usually 15 degrees or more) from the spectacle cylinder axis as a result of hypoxia, trauma, surgery, or other factors. In this situation, it may be preferable to use a spherical GP lens design. Bitoric lenses are most successful from both a fitting and a vision standpoint when the steep and flat meridians of the cornea are 90 degrees apart. The decision about whether to use a bitoric lens will depend on corneal topography. If the topography map exhibits a symmetric pattern and, in particular, the astigmatism is limbus-to-limbus (termed "global" astigmatism), a bitoric lens design should be successful.[37]

In summary, a recommended toric fitting guide is presented in Figure 14.8.

It would be appropriate to mention that the most important problem with any toric lens design is hesitancy on the part of the practitioner to use it. Comments pertaining to the complexity of the design, the difficulty in fitting, expense (especially if numerous refittings occur), and the time involved are not uncommon. Even many practitioners who pride themselves on their ability to fit GP lenses rarely fit toric designs, often indicating that a spherical design will work just as well, if not better. Certainly, the selection of a laboratory that can fabricate a toric lens with good optical quality is paramount to success. Fortunately, the quality of bitoric lenses today is quite good and very consistent as a result of improvements in manufacturing technology. Numerous educational resources on bitoric design and fitting are available from the GP Lens Institute and are listed in Table 14.4.

SOFT (HYDROGEL AND SILICONE HYDROGEL) CONTACT LENS APPLICATIONS

It has been estimated that about 45% of a contact lens-seeking population have an astigmatic correction ≥0.75 D,[38] and 35% require ≥1.00 D.[39] If the criterion for significant astigmatism is taken at the 0.75 D level, then approximately 40% of the spectacle-wearing population are

TABLE 14.4 Bitoric Educational Resources Available From the Gas-Permeable (GP) Lens Institute (www.gpli.info)

1. Mandell-Moore Bitoric Lens Calculator and Guide
2. GP Lens Management Guide
3. GP Lens Grand Rounds Troubleshooting Guide
4. GP Online webinars
5. GPLI Toric and Spherical Lens Calculator
6. Newman's GP Toric Guide

potential candidates for astigmatic-correcting soft lenses. Obviously, there is a considerable need for contact lenses that correct astigmatism, especially when a soft lens is the lens of choice. This need is currently being met in the United States as manufacturers continue to develop and improve toric lenses. This section of the chapter will present an overview and update of toric lens technology and its clinical application, and will discuss the techniques necessary to fit these lenses successfully.

Patient Selection and Indications

Clinical success with soft toric lenses is based on the standard criteria of good physical and physiologic performance, along with other visual considerations, which include the following:

1. Good vision in all directions of gaze.
2. Stable vision, minimally affected by lid actions.
3. Sustained vision (i.e., minimal effects from dehydration or base curve change that may affect meridional orientation).

One of the most important benefits of soft toric lenses pertains to the -0.75 to -1.00 D astigmatic patient. Clinical studies have concluded that vision is significantly better with soft toric lens wear than with spherical soft lenses.[40–42] Although the percent of individuals with greater than or equal to 0.75 D of refractive astigmatism is much greater than the current 23% of soft lens wearers with a soft toric correction, the percent of soft toric lens wear is increasing.[43] Careful patient selection and proper selection of lens type or brand maximize the probability of success. A good idea of showing the individuals with ≥0.75 D, but wearing a spherical soft correction, the benefits of a toric correction is simply showing them in the phoropter the difference in vision between a spherical and sphero–cylindrical correction.[44] The following patient characteristics should be considered:

Patient History

First, patients must be good candidates for fitting with soft contact lenses. The usual contraindications for soft lens wear also apply to soft toric lens wear. Patients who have failed to adapt to GP lenses because of discomfort or edge awareness are often motivated by the comfort of soft lenses. Patients with astigmatism who wear GP lenses and demonstrate chronic 3- and 9 o'clock staining, glare from optic zone and peripheral curve junctions, flare, excessive or insufficient lens movement, or poor wetting characteristics are often good candidates for soft lenses.[41] For first-time contact lens wearers, clinician and patient preference will determine if GP or soft lenses are selected. Both can correct all types of astigmatism effectively. Diagnostic evaluation of the lenses on the eyes is still the best method of evaluating lens fit, and it also aids in designing the lens specifications.

Amount of Astigmatism

Uncorrected refractive astigmatism that is ≥0.75 D is usually unacceptable to patients with low spherical refractive errors. In these cases, best corrected spectacle vision is usually quite good, and patients are less tolerant of any compromise that might occur with the use of spherical soft lenses. In contrast, patients having corrections with larger spherical refractive errors often tolerate an uncorrected cylinder better. It has been suggested that in patients whose astigmatic correction is <25% of their spherical correction, a spherical soft lens first should be tried first.[45] Studies that have measured the effect of masking the astigmatism with spherical soft lenses have found little or no clinically significant amounts to occur.[46–50] Lenses with aspheric surfaces have been said to improve VA in some astigmatic patients, although no evidence exists demonstrating actual cylinder masking or correction.[51] Moderate refractive astigmatism of 1.25 to 2.25 D is now easily managed with most disposable soft toric lenses. Some disposable hydrogel toric lens designs are available in high cylinder powers (>2.25 D), which would be beneficial to high astigmatic patients, but they may still be sensitive to axis rotation or mislocation and may require custom toric lenses. Custom toric lenses are available in a wide range of cylinder powers, and their use should be considered a viable option in high astigmatism of any axis.[17,52–54]

The Axis of the Refractive Astigmatism

It has been speculated that the axis of the correcting cylinder could affect rotational position of the toric lens because of the resulting thickness profiles.[55] Individuals with oblique cylinder axes, in particular, are more prone to experience lens rotation.[12] Other studies showed that no correlation exists between refractive cylinder power and axis to rotational position.[56] Perhaps lens stabilization mechanisms offsets the variation in lens thickness profiles with the idea that the lids interact with the different edge thicknesses influencing the rotational position of the lens. However, modern soft toric lenses with uniform edge thickness around the full circumference of the lens minimize the potential for this problem.[52,57,58]

Types of Astigmatism

Whenever the use of a toric lens is indicated, a quantitative comparison of the relative amount of corneal toricity and refractive astigmatism is helpful. Refractive or total astigmatism is the sum of corneal and lenticular astigmatism. Corneal astigmatism, or better yet, corneal toricity is the difference in curvature between the two principle meridians of the corneas. When a spherical GP lens is placed on the eye, corneal astigmatism is masked and residual astigmatism may result in the sphero–cylinder OR. If the residual astigmatism is significant, a soft toric lens is preferred. It corrects the internal cylinder that would remain if a spherical GP lens were fitted and eliminates the need for a more complex prism ballast, front toric, or bitoric GP lens design. Internal astigmatism is found most commonly in conjunction with spherical corneas or moderately against-the-rule corneas and is usually in the range of −0.75 to −1.50 D at axes of 90 ± 15 degrees.

As a general rule, if the refractive astigmatism is less than the corneal toricity, a GP lens would be the least complex option. If the refractive astigmatism is greater than the corneal toricity, a soft toric is usually the lens of choice.

If the axes of the primary corneal meridians and the spectacle cylinder do not coincide, a GP lens is preferable.[58] The masking ability of a GP lens avoids the crossed-cylinder result that occurs with a soft toric lens because of its tendency to align with the primary corneal meridians and not with the refraction axis.

When the cylinder power in a soft toric lens is prescribed, only the total refractive cylinder needs to be considered. The relationship of the ocular lens surface and the cornea does not create a significant tear lens, as in the case of GP lenses. However, rotational effects of soft lenses may affect the final prescription and require lens power or axis compensations. Irregular astigmatism and keratoconus patients require GP lens correction for best vision, although soft toric lenses can be attempted when GP lenses cannot be tolerated. In keratoconus, soft lenses should be considered as a last resort because visual performance of GP lenses are far superior and soft contact lens visual performance is comparable to that measured in spectacles.[59]

Lid Configuration and Anatomy

Because the dynamics of lid action are one of the principal causes of lens mislocation and undesired rotation, eyelid anatomy and function can be taken into consideration when toric lenses are fitted.[60] Lid anatomy, lid tension, palpebral aperture size, lid closure dynamics, refractive corrections, and lens parameters play a role in lens stabilization.[61] The ideal eye has a relatively wide aperture, normal lid tension, complete closure, a lower lid at the inferior limbus, and no raised conjunctival tissue. Lids that are unusually tight or eyes that have small palpebral apertures often produce excessive force on the lens and result in unpredictable orientation. However, one study found eyes of small palpebral fissures tend to have better lens stability.[56] This may have been related to lens design (prism-ballasted, back surface soft toric contact lens). When the lower lid is positioned higher than 2 mm above the limbus or is sharply angled from the horizontal plane, undesired axis mislocations often result. An incomplete blinking pattern adversely affects toric lenses because of localized dehydration and build up of surface deposits at the inferior region of the lens. Reduced tear volume or an unstable tear film may also cause unwanted lens rotation as a result of dehydration of the lens during wear, with subsequent changes in lens adherence to the cornea.

Occupational Considerations

Soft toric lenses may be unacceptable for patients with intolerance to slight prescription changes or for people who have critical vision requirements at work. Patients with early presbyopia require special consideration because lens axis shifts in the downward gaze position can affect VA and add stress to an already fatigued accommodative system. Use of soft toric lenses in presbyopic monovision can be successful, but several lenses may be required to optimize the correction. For patients needing only slight astigmatic corrections and for whom comfort is a factor, a soft toric lens may be the best option because the immediate comfort with these lenses is equal to that found with spherical soft lenses, and the attainable vision is often comparable as well. Several hydrogel toric multifocal designs are available and have provided an additional contact lens option for these patients (Table 14.5).[54]

TABLE 14.5 Soft Toric Multifocal Lenses

LENS	MANUFACTURER
Clearion Progressive Toric	Acuity One
Intelliwave Multifocal Toric	Art Optical
Essential Soft Toric Multifocal	Blanchard Contact Lens
CO Soft 55 Custom Bifocal Toric	California Optics
Proclear Multifocal Toric	CooperVision
Triton Translating Bifocal Toric	Gelflex USA
Synergy Translating Bifocal Toric	Gelflex USA
Metrofocal Toric	Definitive Metro Optics
Metrofocal Toric	Metro Optics
Satureyes Multifocal Toric	Metro Optics
OCU-FLEX 55 Toric Multifocal	Ocu-Ease/Optech
Aqua-Ease Toric Multifocal	Ocu-Ease/Optech
HDX-Toric Progressive	PolyVue Distribution
SpecialEyes 54 Multifocal Toric	SpecialEyes
C-VUE Advanced Toric Multifocal	Unilens Corporation
C-VUE HydraVue Toric Multifocal	Unilens Corporation
C-VUE 55 Toric Multifocal	Unilens Corporation
MVT Multifocal Toric	Unilens Corporation
UCL Multifocal Toric	United Contact Lens
UCL Sonic View Toric	United Contact Lens
Horizon 55 Bi-Con Toric	Westcon Contact Lens

Lens Design and Stabilizing Techniques

The various methods of providing specific lens orientation include prism ballasting, truncation, dynamic stabilization with double-thin zones, periballasting, eccentric lenticulation, back surface toricity, and combinations of all of the above. No matter what method of stabilization is selected, orientation is achieved as a result of a thickness differential along the superior, central, and inferior portions of the lens. These techniques are described below.

Prism Ballasting

Incorporating 0.75 to 2 D of base-down prism can stabilize a soft lens and allow it to resist rotational forces. The general principle behind prism ballasting is to balance the various forces acting on the lens to obtain stabilization. Some have suggested that the prism stabilizes the lens by lowering the center of gravity on the lens.[12,62] Others have shown that increasing the amount of prism does not increase rotational stability.[63] Prism stability has been explained more accurately by the *watermelon seed principle*.[64] Essentially, if a moist wedge is squeezed, the resultant action is for the wedge to be expelled by the pressure in a direction away from the wedge apex. Thus, lid pressure squeezes the lens into the base-down direction.[55] This principle works in a similar way with both prism and nonprism toric lenses. The nonprism torics have thinner regions in the superior and inferior portions (double-thin zones) and a greater thickness in the center, thereby creating a biprism effect with bases joined along the horizontal plane at the center of the lens. It has been found that prism-ballasted lenses rotate significantly away from their base position when wearers rotate their heads perpendicular (90 degrees) to vertical.[65]

Truncation

Prism ballasting is occasionally combined with truncation and has been found to be reasonably successful, particularly when utilized on lenses with thicker edges.[12] Truncated soft lenses result by removing an area of lens material 0.4 to 1.5 mm from the lower edge of the lens, with larger truncations used with larger OADs. Truncation is successful via assisting the inferior lens to position adjacent to the lower lid margin, which provides a shelf for stability. Although truncation raises the center of gravity on a lens, the stability of orientation is not reduced because of the minor role of gravity. Truncated lenses had some success in creating lens stability, but it resulted in corneal exposure and consequently, patient discomfort. Soft toric lenses today are being designed as round, nontruncated lenses without loss of stable meridional orientation and with greater comfort as a result.[48]

Dynamic Stabilization and Double-Thin Zones

Thinning the upper and lower sections of a lens results in the thickest portion of the lens being in the center of the lens. The thin zones at the top and bottom are covered by the lids, and because of the *watermelon seed principle* described previously, the thicker center of the lens positions horizontally between the lids. These stabilization zones are beveled equally or are double slab-off in form, and the lens is nonprismatic. This design is often referred to as "double slab-off," "thin zone," or "reverse prism" and is one of the most commonly used methods of soft toric lens stabilization.[12] This thin-zone design is most successful when the thickness differential of the horizontal and vertical profiles is greatest, as in higher myopic or against-the-rule cylinder corrections, because the wedge effect is maximized. With lower amounts of lens power, rotational stability is not as good with this design.[66,67] Plus lenses in this design were less stable at first; however, design changes have incorporated a minus carrier before the thin zones are added, which allows the increased thickness differential to work in much the same way as it does for minus toric lenses. The thin-zone design usually provides good comfort, good optics, sometimes unpredictable axis location, but reasonably good stability.[68] In cases in which fitting a toric lens on one eye might produce a vertical imbalance from a prism-ballasted toric lens, the double thin-zone design, which contains no prism, is especially beneficial. It is interesting to note that in practice, vertical imbalance, secondary to prism ballasting a soft toric lens, is seldom a problem, even if one eye is fit with a toric prism lens.[69,70] The effective prism of a contact lens on the eye is related to the position of the visual axis relative to its geometric center and to its refractive power.[71] Thus, the effective prism power of a prism contact lens varies along its vertical meridian. The effectiveness of the prism will depend on the refractive index of the surrounding media. In addition, one design in particular has been designed with an independent optic zone to minimize stability inconsistency with different lens powers.[72]

Accelerated Stabilization

This design utilizes four zones with a thicker profile placed at the midperiphery of the lens to minimize lens rotation.[73] The thinner portions of the lens rest under the open lids. The "active" portions of the lens with the accelerated thickness slope orient within the interpalpebral fissure to work with the lid dynamics to quickly reorient the lens when it becomes misaligned.[73,74]

Periballasting

The periballasted design differs from prism-ballasted lenses in that it has no prism in the optical portion of the lens, only in the periphery. The lens is fabricated by thinning or removing the superior portion of a high minus lenticular carrier, which reduces lid–lens edge interaction and produces a peripheral ballast in the inferior portion of the lens. Eliminating prism in the optical zone may reduce the CT, and improved optical quality is achieved.[75]

Eccentric Lenticulation

This is a front surface, off-center (eccentric), lenticular cut in the direction of the prism apex that is similar to periballasting. The removal of excess material on the anterior surface provides several benefits, which include a reduced differential in edge thickness that increases both stability and comfort, a reduced mass of the lens so that it behaves similarly to a spherical soft lens, better limbal–scleral draping, and minimized compression on the scleral conjunctiva.

The eccentric lenticulation feature is especially important in front toric lens construction, in which edge thickness can vary significantly. The increased stability is particularly evident in oblique cylinder corrections in which the lid margin closure first meets the thicker part of the lens at an oblique angle, often resulting in torsional mislocation.[76] The eccentric lenticulation creates superior and inferior thin portions and nearly equal thicknesses around the entire lens periphery. The prism remains only in the central two-thirds of the lens. Many of the laboratories making soft toric contact lenses incorporate eccentric lenticulation into their lenses.

Back Surface Toricity

Some clinicians using toric lenses have presumed that back cylinder construction may aid in lens stability, especially on eyes with a corneal toricity >3.00 D.[45,77] It seems logical to expect that an effect similar to that observed with back surface toric GP lenses is present and may enhance the stability of soft toric lens orientation. However, back surface toricity alone is insufficient to stabilize rotation.[78,79] It is usually used in conjunction with another lens stability design. Many second-generation toric lenses and most custom soft toric lenses are made with back toricity and with the toric zone limited to the central optic area. Toric curves that are confined to the central optic zone reduce differential edge thickness, which minimizes lid blink-related torsional effects. Whether by design or by manufacturing preference, back surface toric construction functions very well in terms of predictable location and nonrotation, but only when combined with prism ballasting. There is no difference or advantage in front or back toric construction in terms of optical performance of soft toric lenses, as there is in GP toric lenses.

Fitting Principles and Problem Solving

Lens Selection

Toric contact lenses are available in a variety of replacement modalities including daily disposable, 2-week, 1-month, and 3-month, and yearly replacement schedules. The increasing availability of frequent-replacement and disposable soft toric lenses has allowed practitioners to fit common lens parameters from inventory. Many manufacturers produce stock lenses in cylinder powers of −0.75 to −2.25 D with axes in 5- or 10-degree steps, often ranging from 0 to 180 degrees. Extended power ranges are also available in frequent-replacement modalities for higher cylinder corrections, often with 1-degree axis increments from 0 to 180 degrees.[53] Additionally, the advent of silicone hydrogel lens materials has allowed astigmatic patients the option of overnight wear due to the increased oxygen transmissibility of the material. All of the available silicone hydrogel toric lenses meet the cornea's oxygen needs under open-eye conditions.[80] In the closed-eye environment, there can be regions of corneal swelling corresponding to the thick areas of the lens; however, this is much less than with hydrogel lenses and the thicker areas are less in area[44,81] (Fig. 14.9).

The availability of disposable lenses has also allowed patients to have spare lenses readily available, and deposit-related problems, such as GPC, are minimized.[82,83] Daily disposable lenses, in particular, offer many benefits, especially for young active people who may desire part-time wear or may, in some cases, be more prone to noncompliance.[29,84] In addition, the parameter range is expanding for these designs.[29,54,84]

As materials and parameters of soft toric lenses continue to expand, the need for custom lenses on a conventional replacement basis is decreasing, although there will always be patients requiring corrections beyond these ranges.[12] The recent introduction of the Definitive material (Contamac) provides the practitioner with a latheable, custom silicone hydrogel material, which can be successful with high astigmatic patients. It is available from Art Optical, Metro Optics, Unilens, and X-Cel.[54]

Axis Location and Orientation

A major influence on lens orientation is the torsion forces of the lids during a blink. The temporal-to-nasal motion created by the upper lid during the blink process creates a tendency for nasal rotation upward (encyclorotation) of a contact lens, commonly observed with GP lenses. Other patient factors that have been found to influence lens orientation include the intercanthal angle, degree of myopia, and palpebral fissure size.[56] Lids with a higher outer canthus tend to create inferior-temporal rotation, whereas lids with a higher inner canthus tend to create inferior-nasal rotation.[56,61,85,86] Most toric lenses will stabilize within 5 and 10 degrees of the zero position and most will stabilize within 10 minutes of insertion. However, as different designs interact with the lids in unique ways, not all designs will orient in the same position on a given eye.[85,86] A number of physical and physiologic variables noted below can make predicting orientation difficult, especially in the case of soft toric lenses.

Lens rotation resulting in mislocation of axis is another factor responsible for inadequate soft toric lens performance and can result in reduced VA.[87] Lens rotation in and of itself is not an issue, but lens stability and consistency of that mislocation is important.[88] Blink-initiated rotation,

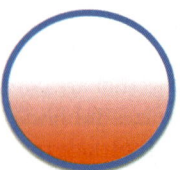

Traditional Prism Ballast

Air Optix for Astigmatism

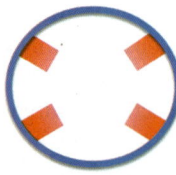

Oasys for Astigmatism

FIGURE 14.9 Compared with traditional prism ballasting, some newer designs modify the regions of greater thickness. (Reprinted with permission from Jackson JM. Back to basics: soft lenses for astigmatism. *Contact Lens Spectrum.* 2012;27(6):28–32.)

or rocking, is usually caused by a loose fit or insufficient lens stabilization features or forces. The amount of visual disruption resulting from a nonstable lens depends on the power of the cylinder, the degree of rocking, and the speed of recovery as the lens regains its resting position following a blink or change of gaze. Selecting a steeper BCR, if available, or another soft toric lens design often solves the problem of the unstable, or rocking, soft toric lens.[89] Fortunately, recently introduced soft toric designs appear to be more stable than their hydrogel predecessors.[90–93]

Diagnostic Lens Procedures

Although clinical studies have found empirical fitting (i.e., without diagnostic lens application) to be quite successful, diagnostic lens evaluation is strongly recommended when the use of soft toric lenses is being considered, especially with the availability of frequent replacement and disposable soft toric contact lenses.[94–96] Toric lens thickness profiles, power, cylinder axis, and patient head position can affect lens orientation. The following suggestions will help minimize any unpredictable orientation or mislocation of an ordered toric lens.

First, diagnostic lenses should be relatively close to the spherical and cylinder powers and axis (± 20 degrees and ± 1.00 D) of the manifest refraction of the eye to be fitted. Second, 10 to 15 minutes should be allowed for trial lens equilibration. Third, axis location on the eye should be accurately determined. Only a well-centered, freely moving lens that is accurately labeled can provide a basis for reliable axis correction on the next lens. As discussed in the section on front toric GP lenses, if the base-down position rotates to the left of the center line (clockwise), the amount of axis deviation to compensate for the mislocation in the ordered lens must be added to the spectacle axis. Conversely, if the rotation is to the right of the center line (counterclockwise), subtraction is needed (i.e., LARS). Once the axis mislocation has been compensated, the new lens is expected to mislocate to the same position, otherwise the compensation would have been for naught (Fig. 14.2).

The amount of axis mislocation can be estimated by using one of the following methods. It is beneficial that most slit lamps allow the examiner to rotate the beam to align with the axis identification mark(s) on the lens and be able to read the amount of rotation directly off the protractor on the slit lamp. If this is not available, it is not uncommon to use a gross estimate method, in which a clock dial is visualized on the lens, with each deviation of an hour (e.g., from 5 o'clock to 6 o'clock, 6 o'clock to 7 o'clock) being equivalent to a 30-degree arc. Obviously, this "guesstimate" method is limited and should be applied carefully to cylinder evaluations of ≥ 2.00 D, which are meridionally very sensitive. This is especially important in higher-cylinder-power lenses as the more the lens rotates (without compensation), the greater the residual astigmatism that results[81] (Table 14.6).

The importance of an accurate sphero–cylindrical OR when determining the powers to be ordered cannot be overemphasized.[97] When small amounts of lens rotation in high cylinder cases are being considered, sphero–cylindrical OR data can be combined with the in-air lens powers in

TABLE 14.6 Effect of Lens Rotation on Residual Astigmatism

LENS CYLINDER POWER (DC)	10° OF AXIS MISALIGNMENT GIVES RESIDUAL ASTIGMATISM OF (DC)..
−0.75	−0.25
−1.25	−0.42
−1.75	−0.58
−2.25	−0.75
−2.75	−0.92

Reprinted with permission from Jackson JM. Back to basics: soft lenses for astigmatism. *Contact Lens Spectrum*. 2012;27(6):28–32.

TABLE 14.7 Soft Toric Lens Calculators

http://ecp.acuvue.com/en_US/practice-resources-fitting.jsp
http://coopervision.com/practitioner/fitting-tips-and-tools/toric-support/toritrack-calculator
http://virtualconsultant.cibavision.com/toric_lens.jsp
http://www.aoa.org/x4783.xml
http://www.eyedock.com
Opticalc (iPhone app)

a crossed-cylinder calculation to determine the next (and corrected) lens specifications.[98,99] Some manufacturers offer desktop or personal digital assistant-based crossed-cylinder calculators. These programs typically apply a simple sphero–cylinder OR formula for a precise determination of the corrected lens power and axis specifications. Online sources of crossed-cylinder calculator programs are provided in Table 14.7.[100] While sphero–cylindrical OR is a useful tool, a clear OR endpoint and lens stability are important to ensure clinical success with this technique.[101]

Markings on soft toric lenses are used as reference points for assessing lens rotation and do not represent the cylinder axis of the lens. A useful guide is shown in Figure 14.10.

Other Useful Suggestions for Evaluating Toric Lens Performance

Any mislocation caused by a tightly fitting lens should be determined. Steeply fitting lenses tend to lock at unpredictable and incorrect orientations. Lenses that move freely will respond properly to the orientation forces that stabilize them. In contrast, loosely fitting lenses often result in blink-initiated variable rotation by not allowing the lens-stabilizing forces to work.

Rotational velocity should be checked on the edge. This is the speed with which a poorly oriented toric lens will rotate in its effort to recover and to reorient.[66,88,102] After deliberate mislocation of about 45 degrees and then release, it should take no more than 15 seconds (with normal blinking) for the lens to return to its initial stable orientation. A tightly fitting lens will

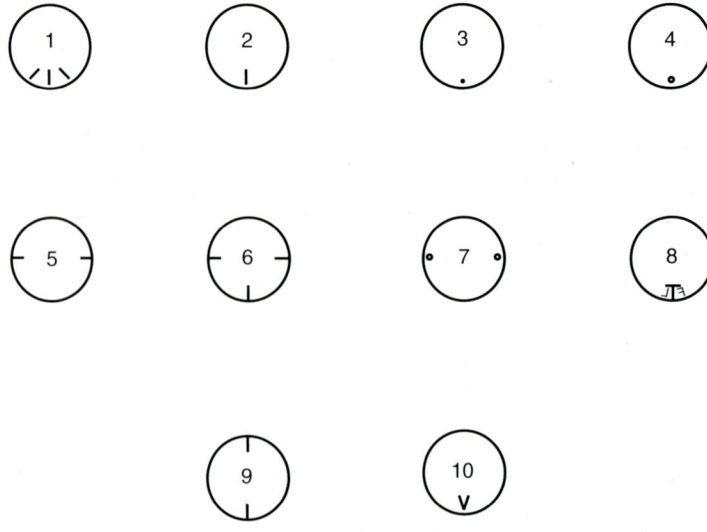

FIGURE 14.10 Soft toric lens identification guide.

demonstrate stable lens orientation with a slow return to correct axis orientation. A loosely fitting lens will demonstrate unstable and inconsistent orientation.[12] A rapid return is desired and is particularly important for those patients who engage in demanding sports or occupations that require accurate vision.

Equilibration or a settling time of 20 minutes for most lens types should be adequate for reliable assessment of fit, with lower-water-content lenses requiring less time. If after equilibration, a lens shows unpredictable rotation or a mislocation >30 degrees, a base curve change, a larger diameter, or a different type of toric lens should be considered. Small degrees of mislocation or rocking (0–5 degrees) are visually acceptable to most patients, especially in cylinder powers ≤2.00 D.[103]

Amounts of mislocation must be corrected using axis compensation. The result of cylinder mislocation is a sphero–cylinder OR with the amount of the resultant cylinder equal to twice the power of the spherical component but of opposite sign.[76] Some clinicians have suggested undercorrecting the cylinder, as the patient is less sensitive to shifts of axis and the variable vision from crossed-cylinder effects.[104] In addition, remembering to vertex the manifest

Soft Toric Identification Guide

1.
   - Purevision Toric (Bausch + Lomb) marks at 5,6,7 o'clock
   - Optima Toric (Bausch + Lomb) marks at 5,6,7 o'clock
   - Soflens Toric (Bausch + Lomb) marks at 5,6,7 o'clock
   - Proclear Toic (Coopervision) 3 laser marks
   - Metrofocal Toric Definitive (Metro Optics) 3 lines 6 o'clock
   - Revitaleyes Toric Definitive (Metro Optics) 3 lines 6 o'clock
   - Metrosoft Toric (Metro Optics) 3 lines 6 o'clock & 10° both sides
   - Satureyes Lite Toric (Metro Optics) 3 lines 6 o'clock & 10° both sides
   - Extreme H2O Toric LC & MC (Hydrogel Vision) marks at 6 o'clock & 20° either side
   - HD-T Toric (PolyVue) 3 scribe lines: 5,6,7 o'clock

2.
   - Biocurve Toric (Biocurve)
   - Biofinity Toric (CooperVision)
   - Avaira Toric (CooperVision)
   - Biomedics Toric (CooperVision)
   - Frequency 55 Toric and XR(CooperVision)
   - Hydrasoft Toric (CooperVision)
   - Preference Toric and XR (CooperVision)
   - Proclear Toric XR (CooperVision)
   - Vertex Toric and XR (CooperVision)
   - PureVision 2 for Astigmatism (Bausch + Lomb)
   - Clearsight 1 Day Toric (Coopervision)
   - Preferred T (Preferred Vision Group)
   - C-Vue 55 Custom Toric (Unilens)
   - C-Vue Advanced Custom Toric (Unilens)
   - C-Vue HydraVUE Custom Toric (Unilens)
   - Eyedia Precise (clearLab)
   - Ocu-Ease Elite Toric (OcuEase)
   - Tresoft Toric (United Contact Lens)
   - UCL Toric (United Contact Lens)
   - Alden Classic 38 Toric (Alden Optical)
   - Alden Classic 55 Toric (Alden Optical)

3.
   - Synergy (Gelflex) OD: 1 dot 6 o'clock, OS: 2 dots 6 o'clock

4.
   - CO Soft 55 Toric (California Optics)

5.
   - Focus Dailies Toric (Alcon)
   - Fresh Look Toric (Alcon)
   - Alden HP49 Toric (Alden Optical)
   - Alden HP54 Toric (Alden Optical)
   - Alden HP59 Toric (Alden Optical)
   - Proclear Multifocal Toric (CooperVision)

6.
   - Air Optix for Astigmatism (Alcon Vision Care)

7.
   - SpecialEyes 59 & 54 Toric (SpecialEyes, LLC)

8.
   - Freshlook Color Blends Toric (Alcon)

9.
   - Acuvue Advance for Astigmatism (Vistakon)
   - Acuvue Oasys for Astigmatism (Vistakon)
   - 1 Day Acuvue Moist for Astigmatism (Vistakon)

10.
    - Flexlens Toric (X-Cel Contacts)

FIGURE 14.10 *(Continued)*

refraction will aid in choosing the correct contact lens sphere and cylinder power. Performing a sphero–cylindrical OR is an important and accurate method of predicting success with soft toric fitting and gives the clinician an accurate means to evaluate whether poor VA is caused by the fit of the lens or by poor optical quality.[103]

An interesting method of predicting soft toric success is the so-called "Becherer twist."[104] This is performed after the patient's best subjective refraction is in the phoropter. The cylinder knob is twisted, and when the patient observes a blurring or degrading of the sharpness of the image on the VA chart, this value is recorded. If the twisting is >20 degrees in each direction, regardless of where the axis is located or the amount of cylinder, success will be achieved ≥90% of the time or greater with the first lens. If the twist is 15 degrees, then the success achieved will be about 90% with two lenses. If the twist is 10 degrees, then the success achieved will be 70% with three lenses necessary. If the twist is <5 degrees, any success will depend on how much decrease in contrast the patient is willing to accept. This method is simply determining the patient's tolerance to blur when cylinder axis is shifted.

Managing Poor Visual Response

Soft toric lenses, even when optimally fitted, may result in visual quality and acuity that is "softer" than that attained with spectacles. This must be explained to the patient in advance, or expectations will be unrealistic. The lenses available today should correct the patient's sight to a consistent 20/20 acuity, and most unexpected visual responses can be managed. Common reasons for poor visual performance during the early fitting phase include axis mislocation, incorrect sphere or cylinder power, poor centration, poor lens stability, lens dehydration, and optically poor (defective) lenses (Fig. 14.11).

Several simple diagnostic tests may be used to isolate the factors causing the reduced vision. First, the correct axis location should be verified by relocating or dialing the contact lens base to either side of its stabilized position. The effect on vision should be noted as the lens is moved off axis and then allowed to return to its original position. If a slight off-axis movement reduces VA significantly and equally on either side of the shift, then the axis is correctly positioned. If axis location is correct and consistent, a sphero–cylinder OR should be performed. If the equivalent dioptric sphere is plano, then the powers of the toric lens are correct. If the axis of the OR matches the axis of the toric lens, then the patient is accepting the cylinder power of the soft toric lens. If the axis is 90 degrees away, then the patient is rejecting the amount of cylinder power and indicating that there is too much cylinder power in the soft toric lens. If the OR axis is at an oblique angle, then there may be an axis mislocation of the lens. The amount of cylinder power from the OR can also predict the amount of mislocation of the lens. If 100% of the toric lens cylinder power manifests in the OR, then it would be predicted that the lens is rotated 30° either to the left or the right.[105]

Historically, verification of suspect or poorly performing soft toric lenses by standard lensometry was advisable to identify the offending element in a soft toric lens failure. To do this, the lens is prepared by lightly "blot"-drying it with a lint-free cloth. The lens should then be geometrically centered over the lensometer stop, convex side up, with the prism base or lens marking positioned in the base-down (90 degrees) position. The use of a smaller aperture (3–4 mm) stop attachment to the vertically mounted lensometer is beneficial and eliminates peripheral aberrations, thus allowing more accurate power and axis measurements. These inexpensive plastic mounts are available for most lensometers. Measuring with the lens ocular surface down (back vertex) will determine the true axis, cylinder, and sphere. If the lens is placed convex side down on the aperture stop, the measured axis will be complementary or mirror reversed from the true axis (i.e., axis 80 degrees will be read as axis 100 degrees). Currently, contact lens technology results in more replicable lenses and if a lens is suspected of being anomalous, a second diagnostic lens can usually be found from the diagnostic fitting set. Current diagnostic lenses are most often disposed of; therefore, the risk of misfiling/mislabelling a lens is much less likely.

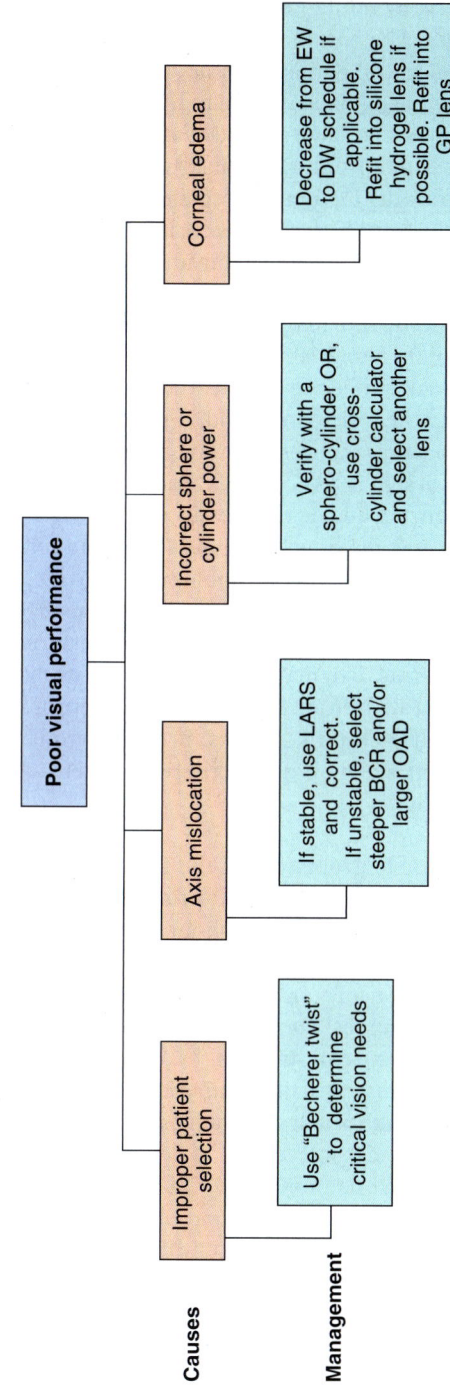

FIGURE 14.11 Soft toric lens problem solving.

The use of the retinoscopic reflex will help assess the optical quality of a toric lens on the eye. A distorted retinoscopic reflex also can indicate an incorrect base curve relationship (usually too steep) or irregular wrapping of the back surface around the central cornea. Improperly draping lenses distort vision, which varies during the blink. This phenomenon may also be observed using overkeratometry, by noting the change in the shape and the clarity of the mires immediately following the blink. The best fit is the flattest lens that allows good centration and regular lens wrapping over the central cornea with no edge buckling.

In general, eyes with refractive astigmatism equal to the corneal toricity may be best corrected with a back toric design, and eyes that have refractive astigmatism with minimal or no corneal toricity may be best corrected with a front toric construction. However, the improved stability of soft toric lens designs blurs this distinction.[101] Soft lens flexure transfers toricity to either surface, from the back surface to the front surface, thus creating a bitoric form on the eye. Theoretically, a well-draping toric lens induces no significant unexpected optical power effects in situ.

Front Versus Back Toricity: Current soft toric lenses are thinner in design and are available in the common cylinder powers of 0.75 to 2.50 D (usually in 0.50 D steps). There appear to be no advantages to either front or back surface toric construction. Soft toric lenses assume a bitoric configuration when draped over the toric cornea and, if properly prescribed, will result in a SPE on the eye.[45] Soft lens toricity in situ is transferred from one surface to the other. From a manufacturing standpoint, a front toric design is less complex. Back toric fabrication requires more steps, but lenses can be made with higher cylinders more easily and probably more accurately. However, modern toric-generator lathes and molding techniques have simplified the manufacturing of back toric lenses.[101] Trends in lens fabrication technology are moving toward back toric designs.

It has been suggested that a back toric lens may provide better wrap and stability in highly toric corneas, and conversely, front toric construction may perform better on nearly spherical corneas with significant internal astigmatism.[106] It seems reasonable, then, to assume that spherical corneas may work best with front toric designs, and corneas with significant toricity (2.00 D) may be best fitted with back toric designs. If neither front nor back soft toric lenses yield acceptable quality of vision when all other criteria are met, then it is advisable to use a GP lens to achieve the best vision.

Physiologic Problems: A soft toric lens must fulfill the same physiologic criteria as a spherical soft lens. Because of the addition of cylinder and prism ballasting, the toric lens thickness is increased both centrally and regionally throughout most of the lens profile. While these lenses are thicker than spherical soft lenses, improvements in lens design have allowed for decreased overall thickness in most soft toric lenses.[12] The averaging of oxygen transmission throughout the entire lens determines the oxygen available to the cornea and the physiologic changes that may occur because of hypoxia.[107] An increased corneal swelling response induced by prism has been demonstrated in comparison to nonprism lenses.[108] The added thickness and increased mass of soft toric lenses suggest that they may impair normal corneal metabolism more often than spherical soft lenses.[109] Because of this, physiologic changes detected by the biomicroscope should be monitored. The availability of silicone hydrogel toric lenses has resulted in a reduction in physiologic problems associated with soft toric lenses. This material allows increased oxygen transmission throughout the entire lens and results in overall better eye health.[110]

Superficial punctate keratitis (SPK), if present with soft toric lenses, is usually observed in the inferior cornea. Edema, if present, is also observed more often at the lower hemisphere, often associated with areas of lens thickness.[111] A probable cause of SPK, in addition to localized hypoxic edema, is localized dehydration of toric lenses.[112] With toric (nonrotating) lenses, dehydration is more common in the inferior region as evidenced by a tendency for surface deposits to form in this area.[111] This problem is more common in patients with partial blinking patterns.

Conjunctival or scleral indentation from the pressure of lens edges is observed with larger lenses, bulky edges, tight fits, and base curve steepening caused by lens aging. If not resolved, this mechanical compression can lead to perilimbal congestion, limbal swelling, or an acute red-eye response.

Superior epithelial arcuate lesions (SEALs) are typically observed near the superior limbus and can result from mechanical pressure or rubbing of the lens at the superior peripheral cornea. While these lesions can occur with any type of soft lens, there is increased incidence with higher-Dk or silicone hydrogel materials.[113] A SEAL will typically resolve after discontinuing lens wear for a short period of time or by changing the base curve of the lens.

Corneal epithelial edema is a concern because of the increased thickness of toric lenses. This is especially true in lenses with a lower-water-content or thicker profiles. Studies have shown that corneal swelling of between 2.6% and 4.9% occurs after 3 hours of lens wear with some currently available soft toric lenses.[66] Although most patients wearing toric hydrogel lenses on a daily-wear (DW) basis tolerate their lenses well when they follow a reasonable wearing schedule, there is a trend to refit patients into a higher-Dk silicone hydrogel soft toric lens.

Neovascularization can be a response to a variety of factors, such as hypoxia, mechanical irritation, infections, allergies, or a toxin-mediated condition. The decreased oxygen supply that occurs with thicker toric lens designs increases the risk of neovascularization. Inferior corneal vascularization has been reported with extended-wear (EW) hydrogel toric lenses[114] and may be related to mechanical, as well as hypoxic causes. When corneal hypoxia secondary to soft toric contact lens wear is suspected, better oxygenation can be achieved with a silicone hydrogel material, a thinner lens design, or GP lenses.[12,51]

Higher-water-content hydrogel materials (55%) were once the best soft lens option available for patients who wear their lenses overnight and for patients whose corneas need increased oxygenation. With the introduction of EW silicone hydrogel toric lenses, hydrogel lenses should be considered for a flexible-wear schedule at best. While the water content of silicone hydrogel lenses is lower than that of hydrogel lenses, the Dk value is higher.[78] This allows for much higher oxygenation and has resulted in improved patient tolerance and safety of EW regimens.

SUMMARY

The ability to fit toric contact lenses successfully separates the expert from the novice contact lens clinician. The successful fitting of toric lenses requires clinical skills pertaining to contact lens evaluation and fit assessment; a familiarity with simple optical principles, product design, and availability; and eventually a feel for lens behavior on the eye. All these skills can be developed quickly by the clinician who resolves to practice full-scope contact lens care.

CLINICAL CASES

CASE 1

A patient enters your office with a strong desire to be refitted into GP contact lenses. His previous doctor fitted him with soft lenses 1 year ago, and he has experienced both blurred vision and frequent lens replacements because of lens surface deposits and fingernail tears.

Your examination results in the following refractive data:

	OD	OS
Keratometry	42.25 @ 180; 44.25 @ 090	42.50 @ 180; 44.25 @ 090
Refraction	$-2.00 - 0.75 \times 180$	$-1.50 - 0.75 \times 180$
CRA	-1.25×090	-1.00×090

What lens material should this patient be fitted with?

SOLUTION: As the corneal astigmatism is with-the-rule and the residual astigmatism is against-the-rule, a high-Dk GP lens material should flex to reduce the residual astigmatism sufficiently. For example, the Menicon Z is a hyper-Dk material that is manufactured in a thin lens design. In addition, if it is fitted slightly "steeper than K" (i.e., 0.25 D), the flexure may be such that almost all the residual astigmatism will be compensated for by the flexing of the lens.

CASE 2

Your patient is being evaluated for possible contact lens wear. She has never worn contact lenses before and has no lens material preference. Your examination results in the following refractive data:

	OD	OS
Keratometry	44.00 @ 180; 44.25 @ 090	43.50 @ 180; 44.00 @ 090
Refraction	−3.25 − 1.25 × 180	−3.00 − 1.25 × 180
CRA	−1.00 × 180	−0.75 × 180

Assuming (based on all other examination findings) that she is a good contact lens candidate, into what lens material would you fit her?

SOLUTION: As the patient does not have a preference for lens material and the residual astigmatism may be of sufficient magnitude to compromise vision with GP lens wear, soft toric lenses are recommended. This patient has an excellent probability of success based on the refraction (i.e., low cylinder amount, regular astigmatism, and the availability of lens parameters).

CASE 3

Your patient has been a spherical GP lens wearer for 2 years after previously being a soft lens failure because of GPC. Although he enjoys the wettability, ease of care, comfort, and durability of these lenses, he thinks his vision has never been "crisp." Your examination results in the following information:

	OD	OS
Keratometry	43.25 @ 010; 44.25 @ 100	43.75 @ 170; 44.25 @ 080
Refraction	+2.00 − 2.25 × 010	+1.25 − 1.75 × 170
CRA	−1.25 × 010	−1.25 × 170

Evaluation of current contact lenses:

	OD	OS
VA	20/25 − 2	20/25 − 1
OR	pl − 1.25 × 010 20/20 + 2	+0.25 − 1.00 × 170 20/20 + 1
SLE	Good centration and lag	Good centration and lag
Lens parameters		
BCR	43.50 D (7.76 mm)	43.75 D (7.71 mm)
Power	+2.00	+1.00
OAD	9.4 mm	9.4 mm
CT	0.24 mm	0.22 mm
Edge	Minus lenticular	Minus lenticular

Into what material would you fit this patient?

SOLUTION: As a result of this patient's motivation to continue GP lens wear, a front surface toric lens design is recommended. If this is to be empirically designed, the following parameters can be ordered:

	OD	OS
BCR	43.50 D (7.76 mm)	43.75 D (7.71 mm)
Power	+2.00 − 1.25 × 175	+1.25 − 1.00 × 005
	or	or
	+0.75 + 1.25 × 085	+0.25 + 1.00 × 095

These values were determined by adding OR of spherical lens to lens power and compensating 15 degrees for possible rotational effects.

OAD	9.4/9.0 mm	9.4/9.0 mm
CT	0.24 + 0.11 (1.25 × 9.0)	0.22 + 0.11
	= 0.35 mm	= 0.33 mm
Edge	Minus lenticular	Minus lenticular
Prism	1.25 Δ	1.25 Δ

A higher amount of prism is not indicated as truncation will actually increase ballast effect.

Lens: As a result of the CT, a minimum 50-Dk lens material is recommended.

CASE 4

This patient is a previous GP lens failure as a result of discomfort and is highly motivated for soft lenses. Your refraction reveals the following:

OD: −4.00 − 3.00 × 175   OS: −4.25 − 3.25 × 005

Assuming the ocular health is normal and all other tests indicate that contact lens wear is recommended, would you fit this patient into soft lenses?

SOLUTION: With the increase in optical quality accompanied by the availability of numerous custom soft toric lens designs, it would be worthwhile to attempt to fit this patient with soft lenses. If lens rotation is not excessive or unstable, soft toric lenses should be successful in this case. Likewise, if the patient is very motivated and does not have very critical vision demands, the probability of success is very high. However, if critical vision demands are accompanied by unstable lens rotation, a bitoric GP lens material should be recommended.

CASE 5

A patient who has recently moved to your town enters your office with a desire to have his current contact lenses evaluated and possibly refitted. He was fitted 6 months ago by an eye doctor who told him these lenses were "hard astigmatism contacts." Until today he had not worn the lenses for 2 months as a result of poor VA. Your evaluation of these lenses reveals the following:

	OD	OS
VA	20/30 + 1	20/25 − 2
OR	pl − 1.50 × 180 20/20	pl − 1.25 × 180 20/20
SLE	Good centration/alignment	Good centration/alignment
	Fluorescein pattern	Fluorescein pattern

Lens parameters		
BCR	41.50 (8.13 mm)/44.50 (7.58 mm)	42.00 (8.04 mm)/44.50 (7.58 mm)
Power	−1.50/−6.00	−2.00/−5.75

What type of lens design is this and how should you manage this patient?

SOLUTION: It is very apparent that these are back surface toric lens designs. This information matches the 1:2:3 principle exactly. The residual astigmatism equals one-half of the back surface toricity as verified with the radiuscope and equals one-third of the lensometry cylinder. This patient would benefit from application of a bitoric lens design. In this particular case, as the induced cylinder equals −1.50 × 180 OD and −1.25 × 180 OS, it would be compensated for by adding +1.50 × 180 OD and +1.25 × 180 OS to these respective lenses to create SPE bitoric lenses. The final powers (as determined in the absence of a bitoric diagnostic set and assuming the back surface toric lenses provided a good lens-to-cornea fitting relationship) would be obtained by simply adding the induced cylinder correction to the corresponding meridian of the back toric lens (i.e., the vertical meridian). The final lens powers would equal the following:

OD: −1.50/−4.50   OS: −2.00/−4.50

These values should be verified with the lensometer.

CASE 6A

A patient wants to wear contact lenses for the first time and exhibits no preference for lens material. Good motivation and normal ocular health are present. The refractive findings are the following:

	OD	OS
Keratometry	41.50 @ 180; 45.75 @ 090	41.00 @ 180; 44.50 @ 090
Refraction	−4.25 − 4.75 × 180	−3.50 − 4.00 × 180
Vertexed	−4.00 − 4.25 × 180	−3.50 − 3.50 × 180

What material/lens design would you fit this patient with?

SOLUTION: This appears to be an excellent candidate for a bitoric lens design, especially as the patient exhibits no preference for lens material. In addition, a back surface toric design should result in a significant amount of induced cylinder. If a bitoric diagnostic fitting set is not available, spherical lenses can be fit initially to evaluate both the patient's reaction to contact lens wear and the lens-to-cornea fitting relationship. An initial BCR approximately one-fourth the difference "steeper than K" can be selected (i.e., 42.50 D OD; 41.75 D OS). However, even if good centration is present, the fluorescein pattern will most likely exhibit areas of harsh bearing adjacent to regions of excessive clearance, which could ultimately result in excessive corneal curvature changes and possible distortion. Therefore, a bitoric lens design is recommended to provide an improved alignment relationship with the cornea. Two methods will be shown to arrive at the lens powers:

Method 1: Computational

BCR (Mandell-Moore):

OD
41.25 (8.18 mm)/45.00 (7.50 mm)
$F_f = -4.00 +$ (tear lens correction)
$-4.00 + (+)0.25$
$= -3.75$ D
$F_s = F_f + K_f - K_s$
$= -3.75 + (41.25 - 45.00)$
$= -7.50$ D

OS
40.75 (8.28 mm)/43.75 (7.71 mm)
$F_f = -3.50 +$ (tear lens correction)
$-3.50 + (+)0.25$
$= -3.25$ D
$F_s = F_f + K_f - K_s$
$= -3.25 + (40.75 - 43.75)$
$= -6.25$ D

Method 2: Consider as two spherical lens designs

BCR (Mandell-Moore):

OD
41.25 (8.18 mm)/45.00 (7.50 mm)

Using "SAM-FAP," the powers become 0.25 D more plus in the horizontal meridian and 0.75 D more plus in the vertical meridian:
$-4.00 + (+)0.25 = -3.75$ D
$-8.25 + (+)0.75 = -7.50$ D

OS
40.75 (8.28 mm)/43.75 (7.71 mm)

Using "SAM-FAP," the powers become 0.25 D more plus in the horizontal meridian and 0.75 D more plus in the vertical meridian:
$-3.50 + (+)0.25 = -3.25$ D
$-7.00 + (+)0.75 = -6.25$ D

Because no residual astigmatism is predicted with this design, addition of the induced cylinder correction on the front surface should result in an SPE bitoric design. The induced cylinder equals one-half of the back surface (radiuscope) toricity.

	OD	OS
	IC = 0.5 × −3.75 × 180 = (approx.) −1.75 D × 180 + 1.75 D × 180 should be added to front surface	IC = 0.5 × − 3.00 × 180 = −1.50 D × 180 +1.50 D × 180 should be added to the front surface

Final Design

	OD	OS
BCR	41.25 (8.18 mm)/45.00 (7.50 mm)	40.75 (8.28 mm)/43.75 (7.71 mm)
Power	−3.75 D/−7.50 D	−3.25 D/−6.25 D
OAD	9.2 mm	9.2 mm
SCR	9.20/8.50 mm	9.30/8.70 mm
PCR	11.20/10.50 mm	11.30/10.70 mm
CT	0.14 mm	0.15 mm

Material Boston ES bitoric

CASE 6B

What would you predict the final bitoric lens design to be if an SPE bitoric diagnostic fitting set is used in the above case?

	OD	OS
Keratometry	41.50 @ 180; 45.75 @ 090	41.00 @ 180; 44.50 @ 090
Refraction (vertexed)	−4.00 − 4.25 × 180	−3.50 − 3.50 × 180

Select BCR 0.12 − 0.50 D flatter than flat K value:

	41.00 (8.23 mm)/44.00 (7.67 mm)	40.50 (8.33 mm)/43.50 (7.76 mm)
	pl/−3.00	pl/−3.00
Power (horizontal meridian)		
	−4.00 + (+)0.50 D = −3.50 D	−3.50 + (+)0.50 D −3.00 D

SOLUTION: Because the diagnostic lens has a plano power in the horizontal meridian and residual astigmatism is not a factor in this case, the predicted OR is spherical and equals the predicted lens power.

	OD	OS
Predicted OR	−3.50 DS	−3.00 DS

Final predicted lens powers = Diagnostic lens powers + OR

	= pl + (−)3.50 = −3.50	= pl + (−)3.00 = −3.00
	= −3.00 + (−)3.50 = −6.50	= −3.00 + (−)3.00 = −6.00

Final order (if good fitting relationship is obtained and lens powers equal predicted values):

BCR:	41.00 (8.23 mm)/44.00 (7.67 mm)	40.50 (8.33 mm)/43.50 (7.76 mm)
Power	−3.50 D/−6.50 D	−3.00 D/−6.00 D
CT	0.14 mm	0.14 mm
SCR/W	9.20/8.70 @ 0.3mm	9.30/8.80 @ 0.3mm
PCR/W	11.20/10.70 @ 0.3mm	11.30/10.80 @ 0.3mm
Material	Paragon HDS bitoric	

CASE 7

This patient enters your office with a situation identical to that of the patient in Case 6 except for refraction. Your findings reveal the following:

	OD	OS
Keratometry	41.50 @ 180; 45.75 @ 090	41.00 @ 180; 44.50 @ 090
Refraction	−4.25 − 5.75 × 180	−3.50 − 5.00 × 180
Refraction (vertexed)	−4.00 − 5.00 × 180	−3.50 − 4.25 × 180

With what lens material/design would you fit this patient?

SOLUTION: As with Case 6, you may want to fit a spherical GP lens design; however, if an SPE diagnostic fitting set is available, this would be the lens of choice in this case. To arrive at the predicted final lens parameters, the same diagnostic lenses as used in Case 6B should be used:

	OD	OS
BCR	41.00 (8.23 mm)/44.00 (7.67 mm)	40.50 (8.33 mm)/43.50 (7.76 mm)
	pl/−3.00	pl/−3.00

To arrive at the final predicted lens powers, perform the tear lens calculations:

Power (horizontal meridian) = −4.00 + (+)0.50 = −3.50 D (i.e., this meridian was 0.50 D flatter than flat K)

= −3.50 + (+)0.50
= −3.00 D (i.e., this meridian was 0.50 D flatter than flat K)

Power (vertical meridian) = −9.00 + (+)1.75 = −7.25 D (i.e., this meridian was 1.75 D flatter than steep K)

= −7.75 + (+)1.00
= −6.75 D (i.e., this meridian was 0.50 D flatter than K)

or
−3.50 − 3.75 × 180

or
−3.00 − 3.75 × 180

Final predicted lens power = Diagnostic lens powers + OR; therefore, predicted OR = Final predicted lens power − Diagnostic lens powers

= (−3.50 − 3.75 × 180) − (pl − 3.00 × 180)
= −3.50 − 0.75 × 180

= (−3.00 − 3.75 × 180) − (pl − 3.00 × 180)
= −3.00 − 0.75 × 180

If these are the actual ORs found with these lenses, Silbert's rule can be used to determine the final lens powers:

Horizontal meridian: Add −3.50 D to pl = −3.50 D
Vertical meridian: Add −4.25 D to −3.00 D = −7.25 D

Add −3.00 D to pl = −3.00 D
Add −3.75 D to −3.00 D = −6.75 D

As can be observed, this is simply another method of obtaining the same values derived earlier. Final order (if good fitting relationship exists and final powers equal predicted values):

	OD	OS
BCR	41.00 (8.23 mm)/44.00 (7.67 mm)	40.50 (8.33 mm)/43.50 (7.76 mm)
Power	−3.50/−7.25	−3.00/−6.75

Fluoroperm 30 bitoric

It should also be mentioned that 0.75 D residual astigmatism is borderline for determining whether a CPE design would be indicated. Obviously, this would be dictated by such factors as the patient's vision demands and the vision obtained with the best spherical OR (not spherocylindrical) over an SPE bitoric diagnostic lens.

CASE 8

Your patient is deemed a viable candidate for bitoric GP lenses. The following refractive information has been obtained:

	OD	OS
Spectacle Rx:	−2.00 −6.00 × 180	−1.50 − 5.00 × 180

Spectacle plane:	$-2.00 - 5.25 \times 180$	$-1.50 - 4.50 \times 180$
Keratometry	42.00 @ 180; 47.25 @ 090	41.50 @ 180; 46.00 @ 090

With what bitoric lens design and material would you fit this patient?

SOLUTION: If, in fact, a 3 D SPE fitting set is the only option, the following lenses can be fitted and the vertical meridian compensated to achieve an improved fitting relationship. Likewise, toric peripheral curves would be recommended.

	OD	OS
Dx Lenses:	BCR = 41.50/44.50	41.00/44.00
	Power: pl/−3.00	Power: pl/−3.00

SLE: Good centration; mild bearing horizontally; excessive clearance vertically OU

OR:	-1.50 DS (20/20)	-1.00 DS (20/20)
Tent. order:	41.50 (8.13 mm) − 1.50 D/	41.00 (8.23 mm) − 1.00 D/
	44.50 (7.58 mm) − 4.50 D	44.00 (7.67 mm) − 4.00 D

Steepen vertical meridian 1.5 D and add −1.50 D to power in that meridian

Steepen vertical meridian by 1 D and add −1 D to power in that meridian

Final order: 41.50 (8.13 mm) − 1.50 D/ 46.00 (7.34 mm) − 6.00 D

41.00 (8.23 mm) − 1.00 D/ 45.00 (7.50 mm) − 5.00 D

Toric peripheral curves: SCR = BCR + 1 mm; PCR = SCR + 2 mm

SCR = 8.1/7.3 + 1 mm = 9.1/8.3
PCR = 11.1/10.3 mm

8.2/7.5 + 1 mm = 9.2/8.5
11.2/10.5 mm

Material: Optimum Classic bitoric

CASE 9A

Your patient is a good candidate for soft toric lenses. The following refractive data has been obtained:

	OD	OS
Keratometry	42.25 @ 180; 43.50 @ 090	42.50 @ 180; 43.25 @ 090
Refraction	$-2.50 - 1.25 \times 180$	$-2.75 - 0.75 \times 180$

You apply the following soft toric diagnostic lenses:

BCR	8.6 mm	8.6 mm
Power	$-3.00 - 1.25 \times 180$	$-3.00 - 0.75 \times 180$

With slit-lamp evaluation, you estimate that the middle laser mark on the right lens has shifted 10 degrees to the right and 20 degrees to the left on the left eye.

What axis change would be indicated for the new diagnostic lenses? If a good, stable fit is achieved, what would be the predicted OR and final lens powers?

SOLUTION: Using the LARS principle, you would subtract 10 degrees from the spectacle axis for the right lens axis and add 20 degrees for the left lens axis. The new diagnostic lenses would be

OD: $-3.00 - 1.25 \times 170$ OS: $-3.00 - 1.25 \times 020$

If both a good fitting relationship and rotation stability exists with these lenses, the predicted OR would simply equal the difference between the refraction and the diagnostic lens power:

OD: $(-2.50 - 1.25) - (-3.00 - 1.25) = +0.50$ DS
OS: $(-2.75 - 0.75) - (-3.00 - 1.25) = +0.25$ DS

Final predicted lens order:

OD: BCR = 8.6 mm Power = $-2.50 - 1.25 \times 170$
OS: BCR = 8.6 mm Power = $-2.75 - 0.75 \times 020$

CASE 9B

In the above case, what changes would you make if the right lens exhibited poor rotational stability—in other words, if it rotated excessively and periodically failed to return to its original position.

SOLUTION: The selection of a steeper BCR would be recommended (i.e., 8.3 mm, if available). Other possible options would be to select a lens with either a larger OAD or a greater amount of prism (if appropriate). As this problem is only present with one lens, it is quite probable that one of these options will result in a successful fit. However, if both lenses are exhibiting unstable rotation, these changes may not solve the problem. If this is the case, a different type of soft toric lens can be attempted (i.e., prism ballast if the previous lens was nonprism ballasted and vice versa). If this fails, a GP lens material is recommended.

CASE 10

You have recently fit a patient having the following refractive information with soft toric lenses:

	OD	OS
Refraction	$-2.50 - 2.75 \times 170$	$-2.00 - 2.25 \times 010$
Keratometry	42.50 @ 170; 45.50 @ 080	42.75 @ 010; 45.25 @ 100

Current lens parameters

BCR	8.6 mm	8.6 mm
Power	$-2.50 - 2.25 \times 160$	$-2.00 - 2.00 \times 020$
Design	Front toric	Front toric

At the dispensing visit, the patient complained of intermittent blurry vision, and SLE revealed poor rotational stability. Nevertheless, the patient was instructed to adapt to lens wear and return to the office in 1 week. At this visit, the same symptoms and clinical signs were present. How would you handle this situation?

SOLUTION: Because of the high amount of corneal astigmatism, it is possible that a back toric lens design might provide better stability. It is recommended that a back toric design be diagnostically fit to determine if better stability exists. If this design fails also, either a spherical or bitoric GP lens design can be used.

CASE 11

You have recently fit a patient with the following refractive information with soft toric lenses:

	OD	OS
Refraction	$-5.50 - 1.75 \times 180$	$-6.00 - 1.75 \times 180$
Keratometry	43.00 @ 180; 44.50 @ 090	42.50 @ 180; 44.00 @ 090

As appropriate diagnostic lenses were not available, the following lenses were ordered after empirical determination:

BCR	8.6 mm	8.6 mm
Power	$-5.25 - 2.00 \times 180$	$-5.75 - 2.00 \times 180$

At the 1-week follow-up evaluation, this patient complained of poor vision in the right eye. What is the likely cause of this problem assuming good rotational stability is present?

SOLUTION: The solution should reside in the OR. As this lens material was only available in cylinder powers of -1.25 and -2.00 D, this practitioner ordered the -2.00 D power because this was closer to the -1.75 D refractive astigmatism value. In addition, the sphere was compensated for by reducing the minus by -0.25 D. However, vertex distance was ignored. Once vertexed, the cylinder power should be -1.25×180 for the right eye. One would expect an OR with a cylinder axis 90 degrees away from the cylinder power.

CASE 12*

A 26-year-old male patient presents wearing disposable spherical soft lenses, and is satisfied with the clarity of his vision. His lenses are worn on a DW basis with occasional overnight wear.
VA with contact lenses:

    OD   20/25−   OR: +0.25 − 0.75 × 180 20/20 +
    OS   20/25−   OR: +0.25 − 0.75 × 180 20/20 +

Biomicroscopy with contact lenses:
OU Good centration and lens lag with the blink
Manifest refraction:

    OD   −3.00 − 0.75 × 180 20/20 +
    OS   −3.50 − 0.75 × 180 20/20 +

Keratometry:

    OD   44.00 @ 180; 44.75 @ 090
    OS   44.00 @ 180; 44.75 @ 090

SOLUTION: The uncorrected astigmatism would best be corrected by a soft toric lens. It was considered best to select a lens that would correct the refractive cylinder and could also be worn on a flexible-wear schedule.
He was fit with the following lenses:

    OD   BCR: 8.6   Power: −3.00 − 0.75 × 180 20/20 +
                           Air Optix for Astigmatism (Alcon)

    OS   BCR: 8.6   Power: −3.50 − 0.75 × 180 20/20 +
                           Air Optix for Astigmatism (Ciba Vision)

Biomicroscopy with contact lens wear:
OU good centration and lens lag with the blink
These lenses were prescribed for DW with occasional overnight wear.

CASE 13*

A 23-year-old female patient presented desiring contact lenses. She had been told by several previous doctors that she was a poor candidate for contact lenses. Several years earlier, she had attempted GP lens wear and was unsuccessful.

Manifest refraction:

    OD   +4.50 − 6.00 × 010 20/30+
    OS   +3.75 − 5.50 × 180 20/25−

Keratometry:

    OD   46.00 @ 010; 50.00 @ 100
    OS   46.00 @ 180; 51.00 @ 090

SOLUTION: Custom soft toric lenses were designed using a company desktop or personal digital assistant-based crossed-cylinder programmed calculator. The spectacle Rx conversion for vertex distance was entered and resulted in the following Custom Hydrasoft Toric EW (CooperVision) lenses:

    OD   BCR 8.6 mm   OAD 15.0 mm   Rx +6.00 − 6.00 × 010
    OS   BCR 8.6 mm   OAD 15.0 mm   Rx +4.75 − 5.50 × 180

These lenses were dispensed and reevaluated at 1 week and then at 3 weeks. Although the patient was asymptomatic and was satisfied with her vision, at the 3-week follow-up evaluation,

---

* Cases 12 through 15 are modified from Bennett et al.[98]

the right lens was rotated 6 degrees counterclockwise (i.e., the 6 o'clock mark shifted to the right) and the left lens was rotated about 5 degrees clockwise (i.e., the 6 o'clock mark was shifted to the left).

VA with contact lenses:

    OD   20/50 (stable) OR $-0.50 - 0.50 \times 127$ 20/25+

    OS   20/30 (stable) OR $-0.25 - 0.75 \times 043$ 20/25+

Biomicroscopy with contact lenses:

OU   Both lenses resulted in good centration and movement with the blink.

According to the LARS rule, the axis should be reordered at about 5 degrees for the right lens and 175 degrees for the left lens. However, a more accurate method would be to insert the OR into a desktop or personal digital assistant-based crossed-cylinder calculator, which is quite simple and quick. Using the cross-cylinder equations programmed into the calculator, the resultant powers were ordered. The following lenses were dispensed with the corresponding visual acuities:

    OD $+5.00 - 5.50 \times 007$ 20/25

    OS $+4.25 - 5.50 \times 003$ 20/25

It should be noted that Proclear XR Toric, also manufactured by CooperVision, is available in the above plus powers and cylinder powers up to -5.75 D in 0.50 D steps and 5 degree steps from 0 to 180 degrees. If the patient could successfully wear -5.25×005, these lenses would be available in a 6 pack for monthly replacement at a lower cost to the patient.

CASE 14*

A 50-year-old female gemologist wearing soft toric lenses for 16 years has become disillusioned with contact lens wear because of vision limitations. At work, she more often had to use a jeweler's loop to look at jewelry. Monovision was acceptable, although she was unwilling to compromise distance or near vision anymore. She required accurate distance, intermediate, and near vision for tasks at work and at home. A spectacle prescription was not an option for cosmetic reasons and because of the aberrations her present prescription provided. She was replacing her contact lenses every 18 months because of deposit buildup. This patient was on a DW schedule using the Clear Care (Alcon) disinfection regimen to clean and disinfect her lenses. She was not currently taking any medications. Her primary reason for requesting an eye examination was to investigate the possibility of improving her distance and near vision with soft toric DW lenses.

Biomicroscopy:
Lid eversion revealed a slightly hyperemic appearance of the tarsal conjunctiva without papillae or follicles, a result of the present contact lens surface characteristics. When pressure was applied to the meibomian glands on the lid margin, normal contents were expressed. Lid appearance was slightly flaccid, typical for a 50-year-old woman. The inferior tear meniscus was adequate in height to support contact lens wear. Fluorescein staining revealed intact corneas without defects. Neither eye exhibited any signs of neovascularization or edema. Grade 1 bulbar conjunctival injection was present.

Manifest refraction:

    OD $+1.75 - 2.50 \times 100$ 20/20   Add $+1.50$ 20/20 Dominant eye

    OS $+1.75 - 2.00 \times 70$ 20/20   Add $+1.50$ 20/20

Keratometry:

    OD   42.87 @ 180; 44.62 @ 090

    OS   42.62 @ 180; 44.37 @ 090

Schirmer I without anesthetic:

    OD   26 mm in 5 min

    OS   24 mm in 5 min

Tear breakup time OD 10 seconds; OS 10 seconds

SOLUTION: The patient was determined to continue wearing soft lenses. She was not motivated to try GP lenses. An aspheric multifocal soft toric lens modality was an option that was available in her prescription. The commitment of office time and possible multiple lens orders were discussed to make the patient aware of the difficulties in achieving the visual requirement. The aspheric multifocal toric bifocal lens was fitted and ordered empirically because of the multiple visual demands at work and at home.
The contact lens specifications from CooperVision were as follows:

Proclear Multifocal Toric

Base curve: 8.8 mm (OD); 8.8 mm (OS)

Diameter: 14.4 mm (OD); 14.4 mm (OS)

| Power: $+1.75 - 2.00 \times 100$ | Add $+1.50$ (OD) distance lens |
| $+1.75 - 2.00 \times 70$ | Add $+1.50$ (OS) near lens |

The patient was dispensed the soft toric multifocal contact lenses and educated about deposit buildup. VA and OR exhibited the following:

| OD | 20/25 − (distance and near) plano -0.50×100 |
| OS | 20/20 (distance and near) $-0.25 - 0.25 \times 70$ |

Biomicroscopy with contact lenses:
The lenses centered well and revealed a 0.5-mm lag with the blink. The toric markings on both eyes were positioned at 3 and 9 o'clock and exhibited slight temporal rotation with the blink, although recovery was rapid. The lens surface appeared to be clean and wet evenly. A 1-week follow-up appointment was scheduled to discuss the acceptability of this lens design. The right lens was reordered to achieve better acuity.

CASE 15*

A 32-year-old man who is part owner of a very busy 24-hour restaurant was evaluated. His sleep habits were very erratic. He came into the office as a previously unsuccessful GP lens wearer because of intolerance; therefore, he was asking for soft contact lenses. He mentioned that eyeglasses were very troublesome, especially during warm weather. His primary reason for requesting an eye examination was to investigate the possibility of wearing soft EW lenses.

Biomicroscopy:
Lid eversion revealed a normal satin appearance of the tarsal conjunctiva without papillae or follicles. Fluorescein staining revealed intact corneas without defects. Neither eye exhibited any signs of neovascularization or edema. Conjunctiva and sclera exhibited no inflammation or congestion. The tear meniscus was normal.

Retinoscopy:

| OD | $-3.00 - 1.50 \times 180$ 20/20 − 2 |
| OS | $-2.50 - 1.00 \times 180$ 20/20 |

Manifest refraction:

| OD | $-3.25 - 1.75 \times 165$ 20/20 |
| OS | $-2.50 - 1.25 \times 180$ 20/20 |

Keratometry:

| OD | 40.00 @ 180; 41.75 @ 090 |
| OS | 40.00 @ 180; 41.50 @ 090 |

Tear breakup time OD 12 seconds; OS 11 seconds

SOLUTION: He required a correction for his compound myopic astigmatism. Because of his visual demands, erratic work habits, and EW criteria, monthly replacement PureVision Toric

(Bausch + Lomb) contact lenses were prescribed. It was suggested that this patient be fitted with a monthly frequent-replacement toric EW lens.

Lens specifications	OD	OS
Base curve	8.7	8.7
Diameter	14.0	14.0
Power	−3.00 − 1.75 × 180	−2.50 − 1.00 × 180

With dispensing, the following visual acuities were obtained:

	OD	OS
VA (distance)	20/20	20/20
VA (near)	J1	J1

The OR was plano OU.

Biomicroscopy with contact lenses:
Good centration and lens movement with the blink were present OU. The toric markings at 6 o'clock on each lens showed slight nasal rotation with rapid recovery.

CLINICAL PROFICIENCY CHECKLIST

- CRA can be obtained by subtracting the patient's keratometric astigmatism from the refractive astigmatism. This value equals the predicted amount of astigmatism when a GP lens is placed on the eye.
- Because the ARA sometimes differs from the calculated, it is advisable to first use a spherical GP lens for diagnostic purposes.
- In certain cases, soft lenses are recommended when a high amount of residual astigmatism is present. If very little or no refractive cylinder is present, a spherical lens is often successful; if between −1.00 and −2.00 D of nonoblique refractive astigmatism is present, a soft toric lens is recommended.
- When a prism-ballasted, front surface toric design is used, use a high-Dk (>45) lens material, a minimum 8.8 mm OAD, slightly "steeper than K" BCR, and 0.75 to 1 Δ for moderate and high minus lenses and 1.25 to 1.50 Δ for low minus and plus power lenses (for prism-ballasted *and* truncated lenses, the prism amounts are reversed).
- A spherical lens design is rarely indicated in cases of high astigmatism (defined as ≥2.50 D) even if good centration is present. Poor alignment with the cornea can result in staining, corneal distortion, and flexure-related reduced VA.
- Selecting the BCRs for a back surface or bitoric lens can be performed easily using an available philosophy such as Remba's. Determining the power in each meridian can be performed by calculating the tear lens power in each meridian (i.e., as if two spherical lenses were present).
- The primary problem with using a back surface-only GP toric lens is that this design will induce a cylinder amount equal to approximately one-half of the back surface toricity (as measured with a radiuscope); the lensometer (i.e., power in air) will measure a value equal to 3/2 times the radiuscope value and 3 times the induced amount, hence the term *1:2:3 principle*.
- Correction of the induced cylinder requires adding the same amount of cylinder (but opposite in sign) to the front surface of the lens. If, for example, the induced cylinder equals −1.75 × 180 (i.e., the radiuscopic toricity was approximately −3.50 × 180), +1.75 × 180 would need to be added to the front surface. With this plus cylinder addition, an SPE bitoric lens is created; this lens can rotate in any direction without having an effect on vision.

- The use of a SPE bitoric diagnostic set is recommended. When the appropriate lens has been selected, a spherical OR is performed and this value is then added to the diagnostic lens powers to derive the final powers. If less than optimum vision is obtained, a sphero–cylindrical OR should be performed and the use of Silbert's rule is beneficial in deriving the final powers (i.e., add the OR power to the power in the same meridian of the diagnostic lens).
- Patients with astigmatism who are good contact lens candidates and are either first-time wearers motivated for soft lens wear or have failed with GP lenses because of such factors as discomfort, chronic 3 and 9 o'clock staining, or a poor fitting relationship are good candidates for soft toric lenses.
- Several methods of stabilizing soft toric lenses are used. Whereas truncation, prism ballast, and periballast have often been used in the past, dynamic stabilization (i.e., thinning the top and the bottom of the lens) and eccentric lenticulation (i.e., use of a front surface, off-center lenticular cut in the direction of the prism apex similar to periballast) are becoming popular.
- When fitting a soft toric lens, it is important to use diagnostic lenses close to the patient's refractive sphere power, cylinder power, and axis values (i.e., ±1.00 D and ±20 degrees). If the lens rotates on the eye, the LARS principle should be used. For example, if the lens moves 10 degrees to the right and the cylinder axis of the manifest refraction is 180 degrees, a lens with an axis equal to (180 − 10) or 170 degrees should be ordered.
- One method of predicting soft toric success is to place the subjective refraction in the phoropter and have the patient twist the cylinder knob in both directions. If a blurring or degrading of the VA chart occurs with <5 degrees of a twist, the chance for success is low.
- Physiologic problems that can be induced by a soft toric lens include SPK, edema, scleral indentation, and neovascularization. For the more sensitive or oxygen-demanding cornea patients, a silicone hydrogel toric lens or GP lens should be considered.

REFERENCES

1. Bennett ES. Astigmatic correction. In: Bennett ES, Grohe RM, eds. *Rigid Gas Permeable Contact Lenses*. New York, NY: Professional Press; 1986:345–380.
2. Dellande WD. A comparison of predicted and measured residual astigmatism in corneal contact lens wearers. *Am J Optom Arch Am Acad Optom*. 1970;47(6):459–463.
3. Sarver MD. A study of residual astigmatism. *Am J Optom*. 1969;46(8):578–582.
4. Kratz JD. A modification on Javal's rule for the correction of astigmatism. *Am J Optom*. 1949;26(7):295–306.
5. Carter JH. Residual astigmatism of the human eye. *Optom Weekly*. 1963;54(27):1271–1272.
6. Harris MG, Chu CS. The effect of contact lens thickness and corneal toricity on flexure and residual astigmatism. *Am J Optom*. 1972;49(4):304–307.
7. Harris MG. Contact lens flexure and residual astigmatism on toric corneas. *J Am Optom Assoc*. 1970;41(3):247–248.
8. Silbert JA. Rigid lens correction of astigmatism. In: Bennett ES, Weissman BA, eds. *Clinical Contact Lens Practice*. Philadelphia, PA: JB Lippincott; 1991:1–24.
9. Borish IM. Vision correction with contact lenses. *Clinical Refraction*. 3rd ed. Chicago: Professional Press; 1970:971–1005.
10. Laurenzi A. Fitting front-surface toric GPs. *Contact Lens Spectrum*. 2009;24(11):17.
11. Henry VA, Bennett ES. Contact lenses for the difficult-to-fit patient. *Contact Lens Forum*. 1989;14(10):49–68.
12. Lindsay RG. Toric contact lens fitting. In: Phillips AJ, Speedwell L, eds. *Contact Lenses*. Edinburgh: Elsevier; 2007:255–270.
13. Wilson SE, Lin DTC, Klyce SD, et al. Topographical changes in contact lens-induced corneal warpage. *Ophthalmology*. 1990;97:734–744.
14. Wilson SE, Lin DTC, Klyce SD, et al. RGP decentration: a risk factor for corneal warpage. *CLAO J*. 1990;16(3):177–183.

15. Bennett ES, Newman CD. GP toric technology and applications. *Contact Lens Spectrum.* 2008;23(12):17.
16. Seibel DB, Bennett ES, Henry VA, et al. Clinical evaluation of the Boston Equacurve. *Contact Lens Forum.* 1988;13(5):39.
17. Snyder C. Evaluation of "High-Cylinder" soft toric contact lenses. *Int Cont Lens Clin.* 1997;24(5):160–165.
18. Budd J. Using your computer to design and evaluate lenses. *Contact Lens Spectrum.* 1988;3(7):53–60.
19. Mandell RB, Moore CF. A bitoric lens guide that really is simple. *Contact Lens Spectrum.* 1988;3(11):83–85.
20. Lowther GE. RGP bitoric lenses. *Int Cont Lens Clin.* 1988;15(2):44.
21. Sarver MD, Mandell RB. Toric lenses. In: Mandell RB, ed. *Contact Lens Practice.* Springfield, IL: Charles C. Thomas; 1988:284–309.
22. Rinehart JM. Torics decoded. *Rev Cornea Contact Lenses.* April, 2010.
23. Grosvenor TP. Optical principles of toric contact lenses. *Optom Weekly.* 1976;67(2):37–39.
24. Bergenske PD. A recipe for SPE. *Contact Lens Spectrum.* 2001;16(2):15.
25. Blackmore K, Bachand N, Bennett ES, et al. Gas permeable toric use and applications: survey of Section on Cornea and Contact Lens Diplomates of the American Academy of Optometry. *Optometry.* 2006;77(1):17–22.
26. Kajita M, Ito S, Yamada A, et al. Diagnostic bitoric rigid gas permeable contact lens. *CLAO J.* 1999;25(3):163–166.
27. Bennett ES. Counterpoint: when correcting astigmatism, vote yes to GP lenses. *Contact Lens Spectrum.* 26(10):16–18.
28. Michaud L, Barriault C, Dionne A, et al. Empirical fitting of soft or rigid gas-permeable contact lenses for the correction of moderate to severe refractive astigmatism: a comparative study. *Optometry.* 2009;80:373–383.
29. Quinn TG. Choosing the right toric option. *Contact Lens Spectrum.* 2010;25(9):24–29.
30. http://www.gpli.info
31. Pitts K, Pack L, Edmondson W, et al. Putting a bitoric RGP lens fitting guide to the test. *Contact Lens Spectrum.* 2001;16(10):34–40.
32. Sarver MD, Kame RT, Williams CT. A bitoric rigid gas permeable contact lens with spherical power effect. *J Am Optom Assoc.* 1985;56(3):184–189.
33. Kame RT, Hayashida JK. A simplified approach to bitoric gas permeable lens fitting. *Int Con Lens Clin.* 1988;15(2):53–58.
34. Weissman BA, Chun MW. The use of spherical power effect bitoric rigid contact lenses in hospital practice. *J Am Optom Assoc.* 1987;58(8):626–630.
35. Edrington TB. When to correct astigmatism with soft and GP lenses. *Contact Lens Spectrum.* 2010;25(10):17.
36. Bennett ES. Astigmatic correction. In Bennett ES, Hom MM, eds. *Manual of Gas Permeable Contact Lenses.* 2nd ed. St. Louis, MO: Elsevier; 2004:286–323.
37. McMahon TT, Szczotka-Flynn LB. Contact lens applications for ocular trauma, disease and surgery. In: Bennett ES, Weissman BA, eds. *Clinical Contact Lens Practice.* Philadelphia, PA: Lippincott Williams & Wilkins; 2005; 549–576.
38. Dabkowski JA, Roach MP, Begley CG. Soft toric versus spherical contact lenses in myopes with low astigmatism. *Int Cont Lens Clin.* 1992;19(11–12):252–256.
39. Kruse A, Lofstrom T. How much visual benefit does an astigmat achieve being corrected with a toric correction? *Int Cont Lens Clin.* 1996;23(3–4):59–65.
40. Richdale K, Bernsten DA, Mack CJ, et al. Visual acuity with spherical and soft toric contact lenses in low- to moderate-astigmatic eyes. *Optom Vis Sci.* 2007;84(10):969–975.
41. Snyder C, Wiggins NP, Daum KM. Visual performance in the correction of astigmatism with contact lenses: spherical RGPs versus toric hydrogels. *Int Cont Lens Clin.* 1994;21(7–8):127–131.
42. Bayer S, Young G. Fitting low astigmats with soft toric contact lenses—what are the benefits and how easily is it achieved? Poster presented at: Annual Meeting of the American Academy of Optometry; December, 2005.
43. Morgan PB, Woods CA, Tranoudis IG, et al. International contact lens prescribing in 2011. *Contact Lens Spectrum.* 2012;27(1):26–32.
44. Quinn TG. Soft toric advances and fitting trends. *Contact Lens Spectrum.* 2009;24(3):48.
45. Remba MB. Part II. Clinical evaluation of toric hydrophilic contact lenses. *J Am Optom Assoc.* 1981;52(3):211–221.
46. Snyder C, Talley DK. Masking of astigmatism with selected spherical soft contact lenses. *J Am Optom Assoc.* 1989;60(10):728–731.
47. Morgan PB, Efron SE, Efron N, et al. Inefficacy of aspheric soft contact lenses for the correction of low levels of astigmatism. *Optom Vis Sci.* 2005;82(9):823–828.
48. Edmondson L, Edmondson W, Price R. Masking astigmatism: CIBA Focus Night & Day vs Focus Monthly. *Optom Vis Sci.*2003;80(12):184.
49. Harris MG, Lau S, Ma H, et al. Do disposable contact lenses mask astigmatism? *Contact Lens Spectrum.* 1995;10:21–28.
50. Cho P, Woo GC. Vision of low astigmats through thick and thin lathe-cut soft contact lenses. *Cont Lens Anterior Eye.* 2001;24(4):153–160.
51. Bergenske PD. Prescribing soft toric contact lenses. *Contact Lens Spectrum.* 2005;20(2):33–39.
52. Blaze P, Downs S. Fitting soft toric lenses in high astigmatics. *J Am Optom Assoc.* 1984;55:12.
53. Thompson TT. Tyler's quarterly soft contact lens paramenter guide. *TQ.* 2012;29(3):6–56.

54. Brujic M, Miller J. Taking stock in your astigmatic options. *Rev Cornea Contact Lenses.* April 2012.
55. Hanks A. The watermelon seed principle. *Contact Lens Forum.* 1983;8(9):31.
56. Young G, Hunt C, Covey M. Clinical evaluation of factors influencing soft toric contact lens fit. *Optom Vis Sci.* 2002;79(1):11–19.
57. Gasson A. Correction of astigmatism and hydroflex soft toric lenses. *Contact Lens J.* 1979;8(2):3.
58. Dain SJ. Over-refraction and axis mislocation of toric lenses. *Int Cont Lens Clin.* 1979;6(2):57.
59. Jinabhai A, Radhakrishnan H, Tromans C, et al. Visual performance and optical quality with soft lenses in keratoconus patients. *Ophthalmic Physiol Opt.* 2012;32(2):100–116.
60. Tomlinson A, Bibby MM. Lid interation and soft toric lens axis location. *Am J Optom Physiol Opt.* 1982;59(4):60.
61. Epstein AB, Remba MJ. Hydrogel toric contact lens correction. In: Bennett ES, Weissman BA, eds. *Clinical Contact Lens Practice.* Philadelphia, PA: Lippincott Williams and Wilkins; 2005:515–529.
62. Ott W. Soft toric contact lenses. *Optician.* 1978;45(34):29.
63. Harris MG, Decker MR, Funnell JW. Rotation of spherical nonprism and prism-ballast hydrogel contact lenses on toric corneas. *Am J Optom Physiol opt.* 1977;54(4):149–152.
64. Knoll HA. The stability of the shape of the human cornea. *Am J Optom Physiol Opt.* 1976;53(7):360.
65. Young G, McIlraith R, Hunt C. Clinical evaluation of factors affecting soft toric lens orientation. *Optom Vis Sci.* 2009;11:E1259–E1266.
66. Snyder C. Overcoming soft toric lens challenges. *Contact Lens Spectrum.* 1998;13(6):2s–4s.
67. Castellano CF, Myers RI, Becherer PD, et al. Rotational characteristics and stability of soft toric lenses. *J Am Optom Assoc.* 1990;61(3):167–170.
68. Hanks AJ, Weisbarth RE, McNally JJ. Clinical performance comparisons of soft toric contact lens designs. *Int Cont Lens Clin.* 1987;14(1):16.
69. Cons S, Ng J, Carter D, et al. Solution to the contact lens prism paradox. *Contact Lens Spectrum.* 1992;7:52–54.
70. Nilsson M, Stevenson SB, Leach N, et al. Vertical imbalance induced by prism-ballasted soft toric contact lenses fitted unilaterally. *Ophthalmic Physiol Opt.* 2008;28(2):157–162.
71. Mandell RB. Contact lens optics. In: Mandell RB, ed. *Contact Lens Practice.* Vol 14. Springfield, IL: Charles C. Thomas; 1988:16:954–980.
72. Hickson-Curran S, Veys J, Dalton L. A new dual-thin zone disposable toric lens. *Optician.* 2000;219:18–26.
73. Ficco CW. A model for fitting success. *Contact Lens Spectrum.* 2006;21(7):s2–s4.
74. Edrington TB. Toric torque. *Contact Lens Spectrum.* 2006;21(8):17.
75. Braff SM. A new corneal contact lens design for the correction of residual astigmatism. *Optom Weekly.* 1970;61(1):24.
76. Holden BA. The principles and practice of correcting astigmatism with soft contact lenses. *Aust J Optom.* 1975;58:279.
77. Strachan JPF. Further comments on the fitting of spherical hydrophilic lenses and the correction of astigmatism with toric lenses. *Contacto.* 1971;20(5):22.
78. Harris MG, Laconic M, Ward J. Stability of back-toric prism-ballast hydrogel contact lenses. *Am J Optom Physiol Opt.* 1978;55(1):15–18.
79. Remba M. Soft toric lenses: a clinical review. *Optom Monthly.* 1983;74:77–80.
80. Brennan NA. Corneal oxygenation during toric contact lens wear. Poster presented at: Annual Meeting of the American Academy of Optometry; October 2008.
81. Jackson JM. Back to basics: soft lenses for astigmatism. *Contact Lens Spectrum.* 2012;27(6):27–32.
82. Choate W, Shaw R, West W, et al. A clinical evaluation of a custom toric lens for planned replacement. *Contact Lens Spectrum.* 1997;12(9):s2–s4.
83. Cabrera JV, Rodriguez JB. Vision with disposable toric contact lenses and daily-wear toric contact lenses. *Ophthalmic Physiol Opt.* 1998;18(1):66–74.
84. Miller JR. Don't forget daily disposables when fitting astigmats. *Contact Lens Spectrum.* 2011;26(8):19.
85. Voyles S, Henry VA, DeKinder JO, et al. Determining the most likely rotational direction of soft toric contact lenses. Presented at: Annual meeting of the American Academy of Optometry; 2006; Denver, CO.
86. Young G, Hickson-Curran S. Reassessing soft toric lens fitting. *Contact Lens Spectrum.* 2005;20(1):42–45.
87. McMonnies C, Parker D. Predicting the rotational performance of soft toric lenses. *Aust J Optom.* 1977;60(4):130–138.
88. Tan J, Papas E, Carnt N, et al. Performance standards for soft toric contact lenses. *Optom Vis Sci.* 2007;84:422–428.
89. Andrzejewski T, Pence N. Design, materials, and fitting of toric silicone hydrogel lenses. *Contact Lens Spectrum.* 2011;26(9):32–37,43.
90. Pence N, Doke-Borden C, Sellars S, et al. Rotational characteristics of Acuvue Oasys for Astigmatism contact lenses. Poster presented at: Annual Meeting of the American Academy of Optometry; 2009; Orlando, FL.
91. Pence N, Sera N, Kovacich S. Rotational characteristics of Air Optix for Astigmatism contact lenses. Poster presented at: Annual Meeting of the American Academy of Optometry; 2008; Anaheim, CA.
92. Pence N, Howard D, et al. Rotational characteristics of Acuvue Advance for Astigmatism contact lenses. Poster presented at: Annual Meeting of the American Academy of Optometry; 2008; Anaheim, CA.
93. Pence N, Kovacich S, et al. Rotational characteristics of purevision toric contact lens. Poster presented at: Annual Meeting of the American Academy of Optometry; 2007; Tampa, FL.
94. Lieblein JS. To trial fit torics or not. *Contact Lens Spectrum.* 1991;6(4):35–38.

95. Snyder AC, Bowling E. Diagnostic versus empirical fitting with the eclipse soft toric contact lens. *Contact Lens Spectrum.* 1990;5(12):29–36.
96. Hallak J. Standard soft toric lenses: a problem of orientation. *Int Cont Lens Clin.* 1982;9(4):250.
97. Lindsay RD, Bruce AS, Brennan NA, et al. Determining axis misalignment and powers of soft toric lenses. *Int Cont Lens Clin.* 1997;24(3):101–106.
98. Bennett ES, Davis RL. Toric Grand Rounds. In: Bennett ES, Weissman BA, eds. *Clinical Contact Lens Practice.* Philadelphia, PA: Lippincott, Williams & Wilkins; 2005:969–995.
99. Blaze P. Refining soft toric contact lens correction. *Contact Lens Forum.* 1988;13(11):52.
100. Jackson JM. A closer look at soft toric contact lens calculators. *Contact Lens Spectrum.* 2012;27(3):46.
101. Hom MM. Soft contact lenses for astigmatism. In: Hom MM, ed. *Manual of Contact Lens Prescribing and Fitting with CD-Rom.* Edinburgh: Butterworth Heinemann; 2000:219–230.
102. Covey M. A clinical evaluation of Frequency 55 toric. *Optician.* 2000;219:24–28.
103. Myers RI, Jones DH, Meinell P. Using overrefraction for problem solving in soft toric fitting. *Int Cont Lens Clin.* 1990;17(9–10):232–235.
104. Becherer PD. Soft torics: a viable modality. *Contact Lens Update.* 1990;9(2):17–21.
105. Snyder C. A review and discussion of crossed cylinder effects and over-refractions with soft toric contact lenses. *Int cont lens clin* (New York, NY). 1989;16:113–117.
106. Maltzman B, Rengel A. Soft toric lenses: an update. *CLAO J.* 1985;11(4):335.
107. White P, Miller D. Corneal edema. *Complications of Contact Lenses.* Boston: Little, Brown; 1981.
108. Soni PS, Borish IM, Keech P. Ballasted contact lenses: topographical comparative changes in corneal thickness. Fifth National Research Symposium on Contact Lenses; 1978; Boston.
109. Hallak J, Cohen H. Localized edema with soft toric contact lenses. *J Am Optom Assoc.* 1985;56:12.
110. Hom MM. Ten reasons to prescribe silicone hydrogel soft torics. *Optom Manag.* 2006;41(11):53–56.
111. Maltzmann BA. Lipid protein precipitates in soft toric lenses. *Contact Lens Forum.* 1988;13(1):74.
112. Clompus R. Custom correction for astigmats and soft torics. *Rev Optom.* 1986;23(4):1986.
113. Bowling E, Shovlin JP, Russell GE, et al. The corneal atlas. *Rev Optom.* 2007;144(1):19–20.
114. Westin E, Benjamin WJ. Inferior corneal neovascularization associated with extended wear of prism-ballasted soft toric lenses. Poster presented at: Annual Meeting of the American Academy of Optometry; 1988; Columbus, Ohio.

Chapter 15

Bifocal Contact Lenses

Edward S. Bennett and Vinita Allee Henry

INTRODUCTION

There is very little doubt that tremendous potential exists for expanding your contact lens practice in the ever-increasing presbyopic marketplace. It is rapidly growing and is currently the largest segment of the population as well as the largest relatively untapped segment of the contact lens market.[1-4] An international survey concluded that there is significant underprescribing of contact lenses for presbyopia.[5] With 78 million baby boomers (i.e., those born in the United States between 1946 and 1964) now entering presbyopia, a large group of potential bifocal contact lens wearers exist.[1] It is certainly evident that a contact lens that provides more natural vision will appeal to them as would any product or service that claims to be all natural. More than 90% of contact lens wearers in the 35 to 55 age category have worn contact lenses for a large period of their life, and they are committed to continuing contact lens wear.[6] In the next decade, a large opportunity exists for eye care practitioners to fit presbyopes with contact lenses as individuals in the over-50 age group as this age group should be around 28% of all contact lens wearers.[7] This older cohort—consisting of those in the 45-to-54 age range—is in its peak earning period. They are willing to pay extra for features and benefits they perceive to be of value or that enhance the quality or services being provided.[1] Therefore, with the natural vision, binocularity, and cosmesis provided by bifocal contact lenses to a population in which vanity is important, the bifocal market has much potential in the coming decade.[1,8,9] Although this chapter will refer to this form of contact lens as "bifocals," most of these designs provide correction for more than two distances and would best be described as "multifocals." Other forms of presbyopic contact lens correction include single-vision distance-correcting contact lenses in combination with reading glasses, and monovision in which one eye is optimally corrected for distance and the other eye is optimally corrected for near.

The primary question is: will practitioners fit them? Although only 18% of soft lenses in the United States are prescribed for presbyopia, 45% of those are fit with multifocals and 25% are fit with monovision. Worldwide, the values are slightly smaller with 11% of soft lenses prescribed for presbyopia; 41% wearing multifocals and 12% wearing monovision.[10]

The numbers are steadily increasing and bifocals have become the standard of care for presbyopic contact lens wearers. The question is why are the numbers not greater? Certainly, the reasons are multifold and include practitioner apprehension. Common comments from patients have indicated that when asked about bifocal contact lenses, it is not uncommon to hear such responses as: "I never knew bifocal contact lenses existed" or "I've heard of them but my previous doctor said they don't work." Actually the latter is a true comment. Bifocal contact lenses are not successful until they are diagnostically fit to the patient. This is confirmed via a study by Jones et al.[11] who divided subjects into "reactive" (i.e., contact lenses were not presented them initially as an option) and "proactive" (i.e., contact lenses were actively discussed as a viable option). The results showed that, whereas 9 of 80 subjects were fit into contact lenses in the reactive group, 46 of 80 subjects, including 21 of 33 presbyopic patients, were fit into contact lenses from the proactive group.

Bifocal contact lens patients not only receive the binocular vision advantages and more natural vision, but they also can represent the most enthusiastic patients in the practice who can refer others and allow practitioners to build their contact lens practice. Patients being told either that there is no such option, bifocal lenses are not successful, or automatically being fit into monovision (one eye optimally corrected for distance, the other eye for near) are not being properly managed. Instead these patients should be referred to a practitioner who is fitting bifocal contact lenses. There are numerous stories in the literature of how fitting presbyopic patients into bifocal contact lenses had a significant impact on their lives.[12,13]

Some explanations for the limited bifocal contact lens applications do have merit. Although translating GP bifocal designs can claim as good or better vision at distance and near versus progressive addition spectacle lenses (PALs), most contact lens bifocal/multifocal designs do represent some compromise. Most designs have multiple vision corrections in front of the pupil at the same time, termed "simultaneous vision" designs. Although the compromise in vision may only be mild with some designs, it must be considered with patients having critical vision demands. In addition, the spectacle lens market is enjoying considerable success as a result of the enormous amount of publicity aimed at showing the glamour and beauty of today's fashion frames. Presbyopic spectacle sales also benefit practice income.

Nevertheless, presbyopic patients deserve the opportunity to be educated and, if interested, to be fit with bifocal contact lenses. These specialty contact lenses are not for everyone, as will be discussed later in this chapter. However, consumer interest is increasing—and will continue to increase—as a result of several recent advancements with these designs, including the following: (a) Soft disposable multifocal and bifocal designs allowing both the ability of the presbyope to minimize lens deposit-related problems, not to mention have replacement lenses readily available while allowing the practitioner the ability to trial a pair of lenses for a short-time period (typically 1 week) and make any indicated changes; (b) silicone hydrogel materials in presbyopic soft and hybrid designs have allowed a cohort of contact lens wearers who require high oxygen transmission to achieve this goal; (c) high add aspheric multifocal GP designs have resulted in allowing the more mature presbyope to see at all distances via an aspheric design; and (d) GP-segmented, translating designs with intermediate vision capabilities to allow the advanced presbyope with critical vision needs at all distances to meet these needs. In addition, this population is more active than their predecessors, making spectacle correction a less desirable option for visual freedom. As PALs often require numerous head movements to find the optimum position for computer use and other intermediate tasks, due to the varying corrective powers present during any eye movement, they can also represent compromise.[14-17] Also, as will be emphasized in this chapter as well, the fitting and problem solving of these designs are not nearly as complicated as one might perceive them to be. With the baby boomers becoming presbyopic, it makes good sense to present this option to all presbyopic patients in your office.

PATIENT SELECTION AND EVALUATION

Practice Promotion

The first important step toward achieving success with a potential bifocal contact lens patient is practice promotion of this contact lens option. Patient brochures can be displayed in the reception area as well as the examination rooms. This gives the patient every opportunity to review this material prior to the examination and introduce them to the possibility of wearing bifocal contact lenses. Obviously practice newsletters, websites, facebook pages, and other social media can be used to inform both current and potential future patients about bifocal contact lenses. The idea should be given to the patient before they become a presbyope and emphasized again when they reach presbyopia.

Comprehensive Preliminary Evaluation

Aging Changes

To determine if the patient is a good candidate, an understanding of normal changes occurring over time is important.[18,19] Aqueous tear production and stability of the tear film both decrease with age, making the patient more susceptible to dry eye, which can affect the wetting and comfort of contact lenses. In fact it has been found that, whereas 28% of presbyopic patients reported dryness prior to contact lens wear, 68% reported dryness after 6 months of lens wear.[20] Older eyes are also more likely to have developed pingueculae and pterygia, which can further disrupt the tear film and decrease contact lens comfort. Loss of endothelial cells throughout the lifespan makes the cornea more susceptible to edema, and since most bifocal contact lenses are thicker by nature, materials must be chosen with oxygen transmission in mind. As a result of crystalline lens changes, reduction in light transmission, a decrease in retinal sensitivity, and reduced contrast sensitivity occur as well. Loss of eyelid tonicity occurs with age and can present problems with translating bifocals.

Tests to Perform

Fitting a patient who is not a good candidate for bifocal contact lenses will almost always result in failure and with the high cost of chair time and patience, it is advisable to rule these patients out before any fitting begins (Table 15.1).

1. Case history. A comprehensive case history should be performed to determine the patient's goals, motivation (to be discussed), history of medications, history of surgery (notably cosmetic surgery), visual requirements, and occupational requirements. It is important to ask if the patient is currently taking any medications and record all medications being used. Numerous medications—including antihistamines, ibuprofen, estrogen, tricyclic antidepressants, anticholinergics, and scopolamine patch—can reduce tear volume.[20] It is important to ask about previous surgeries. With cosmetic lid surgery becoming increasingly popular, this may affect GP bifocal and multifocal lens positioning by exerting excessive lifting with the blink.
2. Visual requirements. The patient's visual requirements need to be carefully evaluated. Open discussions between the doctor and the patient about life- and work-styles are mandatory if success is to be obtained. This will be further discussed in the forthcoming section on consultation.
3. Anatomical measurements. Performing anatomical measurements such as vertical fissure size, horizontal visible iris diameter, and pupil diameter is beneficial. Pupillary size determination should be obtained both in normal room illumination and with the lights

TABLE 15.1 Preliminary Evaluation Tests for the Potential Presbyopic Contact Lens Patient

1. Case history
    Medications
    History of surgery
    Visual requirements
    Occupational environment
    Goals

2. External findings
    Vertical fissure size
    Lid position and tonicity
    Pupil size (normal room illumination; dim illumination)
    Blink rate/quality

3. Tear volume and quality
4. Corneal integrity
5. Refraction: BVA at distance and near; add power
6. Keratometry/corneal topography
7. Dominant eye

BVA, best corrected visual acuity.

dimmed. Patients wearing simultaneous vision designs will be impacted by the variance in pupil diameter with changes in illumination. In particular, patients with a large pupil sizes (>5 mm in normal room illumination), although relatively uncommon in the presbyopic population, would be contraindicated for a GP aspheric lens design due to the glare and ghosting of images that would occur during low illumination conditions.[17] In addition, patients with a "low" lower lid (i.e., over 1 mm inferior to lower limbus) will not be good candidates for GP translating bifocals because of poor or no alignment of truncation to lid. Likewise, patients exhibiting poor (i.e., loose) lid tonicity/elasticity would be poor candidates for translating designs.

4. Tear film evaluation. The patient should blink completely and frequently (at minimum, every 5 seconds). The tear meniscus should be evaluated, and the customary tests for tear quality (tear breakup time or TBUT.) and quantity (i.e., Zone-Quick or Schirmer) should be performed. Patients exhibiting a 10-second TBUT or greater should experience successful all-day wear,[21] whereas those with less than this value should be advised that they will not typically achieve an all-day wearing period.[22] In particular, if the TBUT is between 6 and 9 seconds, patients should be informed that all-day wear may not be possible and extended wear is not recommended.[23] These individuals tend to optimize their wearing period via the use of either silicone hydrogel disposable lenses or GP lenses. They also benefit from regular cleaning of their lenses as well as frequent rewetting drop use. A 5 second or less TBUT typically contraindicates contact lens wear, especially if the measurement is repeatable.[24]

5. Biomicroscopy. A careful biomicroscopic evaluation is important to rule out corneal dry spots or other causes of staining. Lid eversion is important to ensure that significant papillary hypertrophy is not present.

6. Refraction. A refraction assists in determining motivation. The best candidates for bifocal contact lenses should have more than 1 D of hyperopia or more than 1.25 D of myopia.[25] Low hyperopic patients typically expect better vision through the contact lenses since spectacles were not necessary prior to presbyopia. Low myopic and emmetropic patients entering presbyopia are also difficult to please since they can typically see quite well at near without any correction. However, they should not be excluded if, in fact, they are motivated. These individuals may appreciate wearing one distance lens only (if exhibiting low myopia) or a soft bifocal lens on one eye if emmetropic. If the patient is amblyopic, unless an optimum translating bifocal fitting relationship can be achieved, a bifocal lens is often contraindicated due to possible further compromise in vision.

7. Corneal topography. Finally, corneal topography evaluation assists in both determining whether the patient is a good candidate for bifocal lenses and what specific lens design would be indicated. Although corneal topography evaluation is not essential when fitting the presbyopic patient into contact lenses, it is beneficial to determine the size and location of the apex, the eccentricity of the cornea and, in some cases, assisting with the design parameters.[17] In particular, when GP lenses are the preferred option, a centrally positioned apex lends itself to an aspheric design whereas an inferior positioned apex would be desirable for segmented, translating designs. Patients having keratoconus or other forms of irregular cornea are often poor candidates due to some compromise in distance acuity that may result with bifocal contact lenses.

Good and poor candidates for bifocal contact lens wear are given in Table 15.2.

Patient Consultation

This is perhaps the most important factor when considering bifocal contact lens success. Good bifocal contact lens patients need to be sufficiently motivated to give their lenses appropriate care and should be made thoroughly aware of the level of visual quality to be expected well before the initial fitting. A comprehensive education program is extremely valuable as it will

TABLE 15.2 Good and Poor Candidates for Bifocal Contact Lens Wear

GOOD CANDIDATES	POOR CANDIDATES
Motivated presbyopes (do not want to wear spectacles)	Unmotivated presbyopes
Normal lid tonicity	Critical vision demands
Good ocular health	Amblyopia
Good tear quality (>10 s TBUT) and volume	Poor tear quality (≤5 s) and volume
	Irregular cornea

help to develop the correct amount of optimism and realism concerning bifocal contact lens wear. A well-informed patient is your best patient.

What are the patient's expectations? Is poor cosmesis with spectacles present? If the patient spends most of the time performing critical near tasks, failure with bifocal contact lenses is probable. The questions about lifestyle/visual demand presented in Table 15.3 have been recommended for potential presbyopic bifocal contact lens wearers.[26]

The process begins by always asking the patients if they are interested in contact lenses. They may not be aware that you fit contact lenses, not to mention bifocal contact lenses. They may be assuming that bifocal spectacle wear is their only option. This simple invitation to try bifocal contact lenses may significantly change a patient's quality of life; nevertheless, it has been found that practitioners ask <20% of their spectacle-wearing patients if they would be interested in wearing contact lenses.[13] If the patients show interest and appear to be qualified, it can be communicated to them that about all of the patients experience an enhanced quality

TABLE 15.3 Determining Potential Bifocal Contact Lens Patient Success

	GOOD CANDIDATE	QUESTIONABLE
1. Time spent in public eye?		
a. A lot	X	
b. Very little		X
2. Are spectacles undesirable when in the public eye?		
a. Yes	X	
b. No		X
3. How much time do you spend doing precise work like accounting?		
a. Very little	X	
b. A lot		X
4. How much time do you spend doing intense reading during the day?		
a. Very little	X	
b. A lot		X
5. Are spectacles bothersome in your sports and leisure activities?		
a. Yes	X	
b. No		X
6. Do you dislike spectacles?		
a. Yes	X	
b. No		X

From Friant RJ. When bifocal lenses are most likely to succeed. *Contact Lens Spectrum*. 1986;1(6):14–23.

of life through bifocal contact lenses as they are free from spectacle lens wear. The availability of disposable bifocal lenses allows the practitioner the opportunity to prescribe them on a trial basis for those patients deemed good soft lens candidates.

It is important to determine what their goals from contact lens wear are and, specifically, to determine which distances are most important to them. How do they spend their time during the day and what visual tasks are especially important and time-consuming (i.e., computer use, driving, reading, etc.) should be asked. The goal should be to satisfy their primary visual demands. Patients should not be guaranteed that spectacles will not be necessary if they are fit into a presbyopic contact lens correction. Not only should they have a spectacle correction to use as a backup to contact lenses—perhaps for morning or evening wear or to have available if lens loss or an eye infection occurs—but monovision wearers should be encouraged to wear overspectacles for critical distance tasks—especially driving—and some aspheric multifocal wearers appreciate additional plus power when reading fine print (especially in dim illumination) or perhaps some additional minus power when driving at night.

A positive, optimistic but realistic approach is best. It is particularly important to "under-promise and overdeliver" with presbyopic patients being fit into contact lenses. They need to be aware of possible compromises, including the fact that they do not have the focusing ability of a teenager. Even with the best technology available, bifocal contact lenses will not meet all of their visual demands. They need to appreciate that bifocal contact lenses are different from spectacles. Patients should be told that they may not experience the same quality of vision as with spectacles. Contact lenses are dynamic devices that sit directly on the eye unlike spectacles in which good near vision can be obtained via simply dropping the eyes to view through the bifocal segment. If the patients appear to be quite satisfied with spectacle wear or are extremely concerned about any possible compromise in vision, they can be told that bifocal lenses may not be the best option for them. In that way, their motivation can be assessed. Conversely, there are patients who will accept reasonable visual compromise to experience the benefits of contact lens wear. "20/Happy" is a phrase in common use today to describe patients who experience a slight decrement in acuity chart vision (often 20/25–20/30) but are extremely satisfied with their bifocal contact lenses.

Finally, it is important to review all of the contact lens corrective options with the patient. Single-vision contact lenses, supplemented by reading glasses, can be mentioned first. Patients can be told that this option should provide them with their best vision at near and distance. They should also be informed that some patients do not like to put the spectacles on and take them off frequently (not to mention the wearing of spectacles in general). The second option to explain would be monovision. A surprising number of patients have already heard of this option but it should be defined to patients nevertheless as an option in which one eye sees optimally at distance whereas the other eye will see well at near. The fact that the opposite eye will be somewhat blurred for any visual task and the need for supplemental vision correction (i.e., a second distance contact lens or "driving" glasses) for critical vision tasks should be explained. Finally, bifocal contact lenses can be presented. This option allows the patient the aforementioned benefits of visual freedom and binocularity. Although the higher cost should be mentioned (often 1 1/2–2 times the cost of conventional designs) as well as the possibility of a lens exchange or two to fine tune the fit (although the patient rarely needs to discontinue lens wear during this period), the patient can be told that if he/she remains patient and motivated, there is a good likelihood for success.

The authors having reached the stage of presbyopia and enjoying the benefits of multifocal contact lenses (one GP and one soft) have gained a new appreciation for the benefits of the lenses and the education involved with fitting the lenses. Being presbyopic is an advantage when describing the benefits. Patients react well to the fact that their practitioner is promoting a contact lens design that they are successfully wearing. Success stories and testimonials help the new wearer feel that they can achieve success too and it increases their patience with the process. That said, younger practitioners can relate patient success stories to encourage their new fits to stay the course and experience the newfound benefits.

SOFT BIFOCAL AND MULTIFOCAL LENSES

Soft contact lenses for presbyopia were introduced in the 1980s. The first lenses were expensive to manufacture and custom-made; therefore, the cost to the patient was high. This compounded with the inherent nature of soft lenses to deposit and tear, in addition to lack of success of the designs and product discontinuation, made this a less than desirable modality for practitioners and patients. Translating designs in GP lenses are beneficial for providing increased near vision; however, translating designs have not been very successful in soft contact lenses. Most soft contact lenses for use with presbyopia are a simultaneous vision design. This may result in slightly compromised vision, as this design does not provide the same clarity as spectacles, but many patients are satisfied with the vision. The simultaneous existence of a focused image and an out-of-focus image on the retina results in a reduction in retinal image quality.[9,27] Despite this, many patients experience satisfactory vision and success when wearing these lenses.

The introduction of disposable/frequent-replacement soft hydrogel lenses and silicone hydrogel lenses have increased the popularity and success of soft bifocal and multifocal contact lenses. As the baby boomer population increases and their desire to remain lifelong contact lens wearers has increased, bifocal contact lens use is on the rise.[28,29] In addition to the disposable lenses and the increased oxygen transmission, material changes that aid dry-eye patients and the ease in fitting and dispensing trial lenses have been a large part of this upward trend in bifocal/multifocal use.

Patient Selection

Motivation is a key factor for these patients. Planting the seed in single-vision soft lens wearers prior to them requiring a presbyopic correction is beneficial to them remaining lifelong contact lens wearers. Although the process of fitting is easier than in the past, enthusiasm on the part of the practitioner and patient will affect patient motivation.[30]

Patient education is another key factor for success. This requires a thorough explanation for what is occurring in presbyopia, and methods of correcting for it, including reading glasses over contact lenses, monovision, and bifocal contact lenses. The patient needs to know that these lenses are a little more complicated and may require some compromise, but with motivation and patience, success is obtainable. Thorough education makes the patient feel a part of the fitting and makes the process more understandable. Their input is vital in arriving at a successful endpoint.

Normal age-related changes may affect the patient's ability to wear soft multifocals successfully. Ocular dryness may be an issue and may be managed by lens materials and solutions. More complicated age-related changes, like cataracts and macular degeneration, may result in unacceptable vision.

Good candidates for soft multifocals include successful single-vision soft lens wearers, dissatisfied monovision patients, low amounts of astigmatism (unless fit in a toric multifocal), moderate myopes and hyperopes, and those with a healthy cornea and tears. The patient may have to accept some compromise, usually in one area, either distance, intermediate, or near (Table 15.4).

TABLE 15.4 Soft Multifocal Patient Selection

- Motivated
- Successful soft lens patient
- Computer users (can provide intermediate vision)
- Dissatisfied monovision wearer
- Healthy cornea, lids, and tear film
- Low astigmats (unless fitting a toric multifocal)
- Moderate myopes and hyperopes
- Healthy cornea and tears

TABLE 15.5 Disposable/Frequent-Replacement Presbyopic Soft Contact Lenses (Center-Near Designs)

NAME	MANUFACTURER
Focus Dailies Progressive, Air Optix Aqua Multifocal	Alcon
Soflens Multi-Focal, PureVision Multi-Focal, PV2 for Presbyopia	Bausch + Lomb
Quattro	Blanchard
Proclear 1 day multifocal, Proclear, Proclear XR, Biofinity and Proclear Toric Multifocal (N lenses)	CooperVision
C-Vue 55 & Toric Multifocal, C-Vue Hydravue & Toric Multifocal, C-Vue Advanced and Toric Multifocal	Unilens
EMA Multifocal, Unilens 38, Softsite	Unilens
SpecialEyes and SpecialEyes Toric Multifocals	SpecialEyes

Lens Designs

Center-Near

Many of the soft multifocal lenses are aspheric with a center-near correction. Disposable/frequent-replacement center-near multifocals can be found in Table 15.5. These center-near designs are discussed in this section.

The Air Optix Aqua Multifocal (Alcon) is a center-near design, which compensates for patient loss of accommodation by extending the depth of focus to provide clear vision at distance and near (Fig. 15.1). It delivers smooth transitions between near, intermediate, and distance powers. It is a silicone hydrogel monthly replacement lens, which is available in three add powers (Lo, Med, and Hi) and one base curve radius (BCR) (8.6 mm). This lens material provides high oxygen permeability combined with the wettability from the Aqua Moisture System.[31]

When fitting Air Optix Aqua Multifocal lenses, select a Lo add for spectacle add powers up to +1.25 D, a Med add for spectacle add powers between +1.50 and +2.00 D, and a Hi add for spectacle add powers of +2.25 to +2.50 D (Table 15.6). It is important to follow the fitting guide when fitting this lens design for good success.

The Soflens Multi-Focal and the PureVision Multi-Focal (Bausch + Lomb) are aspheric, center-near designs. The anterior surface is aspheric and the back surface is a spherical bicurve. The Soflens Multi-Focal is available in two BCRs (8.5 and 8.8 mm) and is a 2-week replacement lens. The PureVision Multi-Focal is a silicone hydrogel lens and is available in one BCR (8.6 mm), and is a monthly replacement lens.

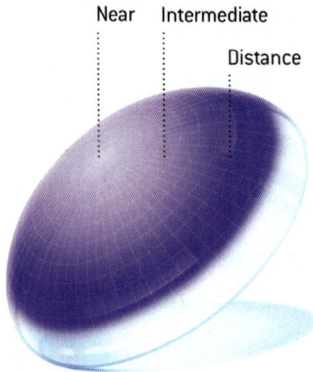

FIGURE 15.1 Air Optix Aqua Multifocal. (Courtesy of Alcon.)

TABLE 15.6 Add Selection for Air Optix Aqua Multifocal

INITIAL CONTACT LENS ADD	SPECTACLE ADD
Lo	Up to +1.25
Med	+1.50 to +2.00
Hi	+2.25 to +2.50

When fitting the PureVision Multi-Focal lens, the 8.6 mm BCR is used. The lenses come with two add powers, Low and High add. If the patient has a spectacle add ≤+1.25 D, the Low add is recommended OU. For an add power between +1.50 and +1.75 D, High adds OU (with −0.25 to −0.50 D over the distance Rx) or mixed adds (Low add on the dominant eye and High add on the nondominant eye) are recommended. For spectacle add powers >+1.75 D, High add powers on both eyes are recommended (Table 15.7).

The PureVision 2 (PV2) for Presbyopia (Bausch + Lomb) is a monthly replacement silicone hydrogel multifocal lens designed to provide near, intermediate, and distance vision with a unique aspheric power profile. The lenses come with two add powers, Low and High add.

Shack–Hartmann analyses by Bausch + Lomb of current aspheric multifocal lenses can demonstrate inconsistencies in the power available for near, intermediate, and distance. PV2 for Presbyopia was designed to have consistent add powers for the near and intermediate zones and accurate distance powers for all labeled lens powers. Additionally, the design provides a higher available add power (Low and High) and a broader intermediate zone compared to PureVision Multi-Focal (Fig. 15.2). Bausch + Lomb reports that this lens provides better near and intermediate vision with good distance vision as compared to the PureVision Multi-Focal and other popular soft multifocal lenses and improved predictability of fitting. (Merchea M. Personal communication October 26, 2012.)

C-Vue 55 and EMA Multifocals (Unilens Corp.) are aspheric center-near designs with two adds, Low and High, similar to the Bausch + Lomb lens designs. Quattro (Blanchard) is an aspheric center-near design, which is available in two BCRs (8.4 and 8.8 mm). It is available in an add power that corrects up to +2.50 D. When fitting this lens, the spherical power is based on the distance spherical equivalent power corrected for the required add (Table 15.8). If the patient has an add <+1.25 D, it is recommended that the dominant eye be fit in a spherical distance lens and the nondominant eye be fit with a lens of a power equal to the distance power (spherical equivalent, vertexed) with +1.25 D added. For example, a patient with a −2.50 D OU and +1.00 D Add right eye dominant, would wear a spherical −2.50 D lens on the OD and a −1.25 D Quattro lens on the OS. BCR selection is 8.4 mm with a 14.2 mm diameter for keratometry readings ≥44.50 D, and 8.8 mm with a 14.5 mm diameter for keratometry readings ≤44.25 D.

Focus Dailies Progressive lenses (Alcon) are an aspheric, center-near design with an add power that corrects up to +3.00 D. A formula is used to determine the distance prescription to select. The formula is based on adding half the patient's add power to his or her spherical

TABLE 15.7 Add Selection for PureVision Multi-Focal

INITIAL CONTACT LENS ADD	SPECTACLE ADD
Low	Up to +1.25
High (Add −0.25 or −0.50 to distance Rx)	+1.50 to +1.75
High	>+1.75

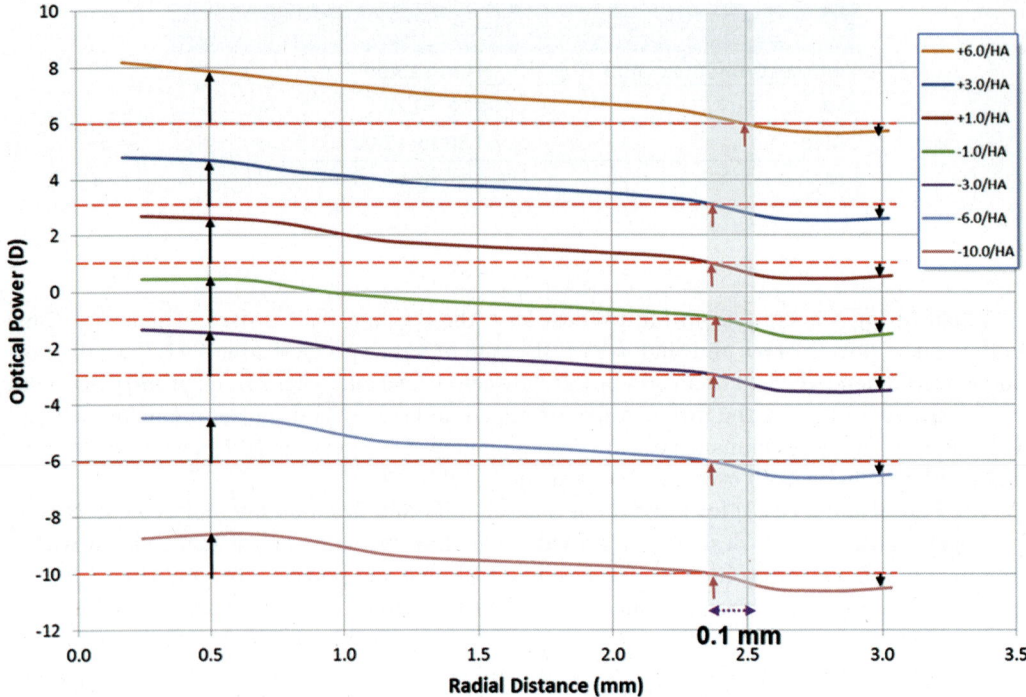

FIGURE 15.2 Power profiles for PureVision 2 for Presbyopia High Add (+6.00 D to −10.00 D) demonstrating consistency of near add power (see *arrow* at 0.5 mm radius) above the labeled distance power (*dashed line*) for each distance lens power, and a broad intermediate zone, and accurate distance labeled power. (Courtesy of Bausch + Lomb.)

equivalent, vertex-corrected distance prescription. For example, a patient with 3.00 D spectacle prescription and a +1.00 D add would require the following:

$$-3.00 + (0.50) = -2.50 \text{ D}.$$

The lenses are labeled with only the distance prescription. This simplifies the fitting process, but limits the available choices for the patient. If the patient's distance vision is not acceptable, decreasing the amount of the plus power added to the distance prescription of, at minimum, the distance eye, may be beneficial.[32] A recent addition to the daily disposable multifocal market is the Proclear 1 day Multifocal lens (CooperVision). It is made from the Proclear material, which is quite successful with dry-eye patients. It is an aspheric center-near design

TABLE 15.8 Quattro Power Selection

ADD* (PATIENT AGE)	DOMINANT EYE RX	NONDOMINANT EYE RX
+1.25 (46 or less)	1.00	1.25
+1.50 (47–48)	1.00	1.25
+1.75 (49–50)	1.25	1.50
+2.00 (51–52)	1.50	1.75
+2.25 (53–54)	1.75	2.00
+2.50 (55 & older)	1.75	2.25

*Added to distance Rx-spherical equivalent, vertexed.

TABLE 15.9 Power Selection for Proclear 1 Day Multifocal

DISTANCE CONTACT LENS RX	SPECTACLE ADD POWER
SE of distance Rx	+1.00 to +1.25
SE of distance Rx on dominant eye/add +0.75 to nondominant eye distance Rx	+1.50 to +1.75
SE of distance Rx on dominant eye/add +0.75 to +1.00 to nondominant eye distance Rx	+2.00 to +2.25

SE, spherical equivalent.

with a gradual transition and comes in one add power and one BCR (8.7 mm). Both eyes are fit with the spherical equivalent of the patient's distance prescription when the add power is +1.00 to +1.25 D. For higher add powers, the dominant eye power remains the same and the nondominant eye is fit with a "near boost" by adding plus to the lens for the nondominant eye (i.e, if the add power is +1.50 to +1.75 D, add +0.75 D to the nondominant eye power and for add powers of +2.00 to +2.25 D, add +0.75 to +1.00 D to the nondominant lens power) (Table 15.9). Daily disposable multifocal lenses are convenient and can be advantageous for occasional wearers, frequent travelers, and those with allergies.[33]

Flexlens Multifocal (X-Cel Contacts) is an aspheric front surface design providing near and distance vision. It is fit only on the nondominant eye and a spherical Flexlens is fit on the dominant eye.[34]

There are very few laboratories that make lenses in high sphere values (≤20 D) and toric lenses with high cylinder values for presbyopic patients. One lens design that meets this need is Intelliwave lenses (Art Optical), which are available as quarterly replacement multifocal lenses in a center-near design. They are manufactured from the Definitive silicone hydrogel material (Contamac). Intelliwave uses wavefront technology to control aberrations.[35–37] Alden Optical makes the Astera Multifocal Toric in a center-near design. It is available in multiple base curves and diameters. It is a quarterly replacement hydrogel lens.

There are conventional replacement (6–12 months) center-near lenses available, which are fit similar to these lenses. Due to the number of conventional center-near lenses, they will not be discussed individually in this chapter.

Center-Distance

Currently available disposable/frequent-replacement center-distance lenses can be found in Table 15.10.

The Acuvue Bifocal (Vistakon) is a 2-week replacement concentric bifocal with five alternating concentric rings and four add powers (+1.00, +1.50, +2.00, and +2.50 D). The central

TABLE 15.10 Disposable/Frequent-Replacement Presbyopic Soft Contact Lenses (Center-Distance Designs)

NAME	MANUFACTURER
Proclear EP	CooperVision
Proclear, Proclear XR, Biofinity and Proclear toric Multifocals (D lens)	CooperVision
Acuvue Bifocal, Acuvue Oasys for Presbyopia	Vistakon
UCL Multifocal	United Contact Lens
SaturEyes and SaturEyes Toric Multifocals, Metrofocal and Metrofocal Toric and Metrofocal and Metrofocal Toric Definitive	Metro Optics
SpecialEyes and SpecialEyes Toric Multifocals	SpecialEyes

distance zone is 2 mm wide surrounded by a near zone, alternating distance and near for a total width of 8 mm. The add power selection is based on the patient's age.

This lens is less dependent on pupil size than aspheric designs due to the alternating zones within the pupil, which aid in providing an equal area of distance and near over a range of pupil sizes.[38] One study found that the Acuvue Bifocal, when compared with progressive addition spectacles at varying illuminations, resulted in similar near performance.[39]

The Acuvue Oasys for Presbyopia (Vistakon) improves on the Acuvue Bifocal by providing a 2-week replacement silicone hydrogel material to increase oxygen and providing an aspheric zonal design (Stereo Precision Technology; Fig. 15.3). This technology combines the concentric zones (less pupil size dependence) with aspheric technology, which provides clear, balanced vision.[31]

The Acuvue Oasys for Presbyopia lens is available in three add powers (Low, Mid, and High) with an 8.4 mm-BCR. When fitting this lens, select the Low add for patient add powers ≤+1.25 D and Mid add for +1.50 to +1.75 D add powers. For patient add powers of +2.00 to +2.50 D, try the Mid add on the dominant eye and the High add on the nondominant eye. For early presbyopes, fitting the dominant eye in an Acuvue Oasys sphere and the nondominant eye in a Low add may be preferable (Table 15.11).

Proclear EP (CooperVision) has a center spherical distance zone with a progressive aspheric zone that provides intermediate and near vision for emerging presbyopes (Fig. 15.4). The design is similar to the D lens of other CooperVision multifocals. This lens is easy to fit as there is only one BCR and the lens power is selected based on the patient's distance spectacle prescription. This lens can provide an effective add power of, at maximum, +1.50 D. No add power is recorded on the lens pack as it is the same for all lenses. This lens is made of omafilcon A (Proclear material); therefore, it is recommended for dry-eye patients. This is beneficial for those presbyopic patients who experience dryness.

Proclear and Biofinity Multifocals (CooperVision) have a unique design that allow creativity in fitting patient's visual needs. These lenses are available in one BCR and four add powers (+1.00, +1.50, +2.00, and +2.50 D). The Proclear XR Multifocal has expanded parameters for distance powers of ±20 D and add powers from +0.75 to +4.00 D in 0.50 D steps. This creates a wide range of multifocal lenses for almost every patient, regardless of his or her spectacle power. The Biofinity Multifocal is a monthly replacement silicone hydrogel material with an increased Dk/t.

These multifocals have a D lens, which may be fit on the dominant eye and has a center-distance spherical zone, surrounded by an aspheric progressive intermediate zone and then an outer spherical near zone. The N lens, fit on the nondominant eye, has a center-near spherical

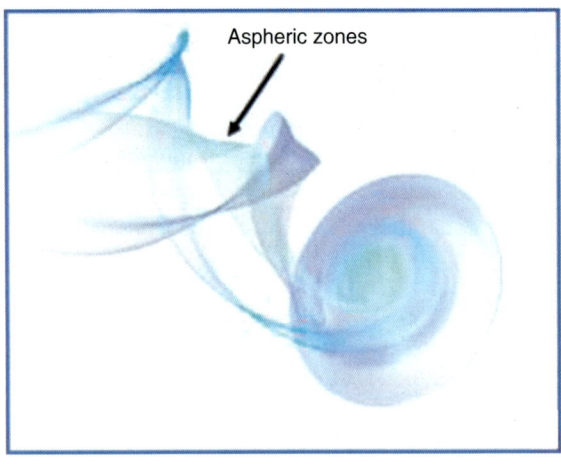

FIGURE 15.3 Acuvue Oasys for Presbyopia. (Courtesy of Vistakon.)

TABLE 15.11 Add Selection for Acuvue Oasys for Presbyopia

INITIAL CONTACT LENS ADD	SPECTACLE ADD
Low (May consider an Acuvue Oasys Sphere for dominant eye)	≤+1.25
Mid	+1.50 to +1.75
Mid for dominant eye & high for nondominant eye	+2.00 to +2.50

zone, surrounded by the aspheric intermediate progressive zone and a distance spherical zone. This design is termed Balanced Progressive Technology (Fig. 15.5). This lens design has been very successful.

When fitting this design, the initial power is based on the spherical equivalent of the current refraction, vertexed back to the cornea. The add should be equivalent to the add for spectacles unless it is between add powers; if this occurs, the lower add should be selected. For add powers of +1.00 to +1.50 D, it is recommended that the patient be first fit in two D lenses. If poor near vision occurs after wear, the nondominant eye should be switched to an N lens. For spectacle add powers of +2.00 or +2.50 D, the D lens should be used on the dominant eye and the N lens on the nondominant eye.[40] The manufacturer recommends that 20/20 vision be obtained binocularly at distance and near. Monocular visual acuities with the D lens should be 20/20 at distance and 20/40 or better at near. The reverse is true of the N lens, where distance visual acuity (VA) should be 20/40 or better and near VA 20/20. If the VA does not meet these criteria, then an overrefraction should be performed monocularly to improve the vision[41] (Table 15.12).

Other center-distance designs that are available for quarterly replacement are Satureyes Multifocal and Metrofocal (Metro Optics). In addition, there is the Metrofocal Definitive material, which is a silicone hydrogel material available from Metro Optics. SpecialEyes 54 Multifocal sphere (SpecialEyes) is available in a concentric design with D and N lenses. Conventional lens replacement materials, available in this center-distance design, include 4Vue and XTRA (Unilens Corp.).

Translating

The only soft lens currently available in a translating design is the Triton Translating Bifocal (Gelflex). Translation is more challenging with a soft lens bifocal than a GP bifocal, but can provide better vision than simultaneous designs. The thicker inferior edge may cause more lens awareness.[42] The Triton lens is available in sphere and toric conventional replacement lenses. It

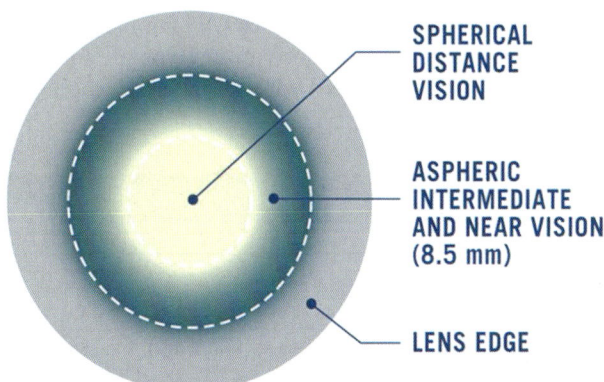

FIGURE 15.4 Proclear EP. (Courtesy of CooperVision.)

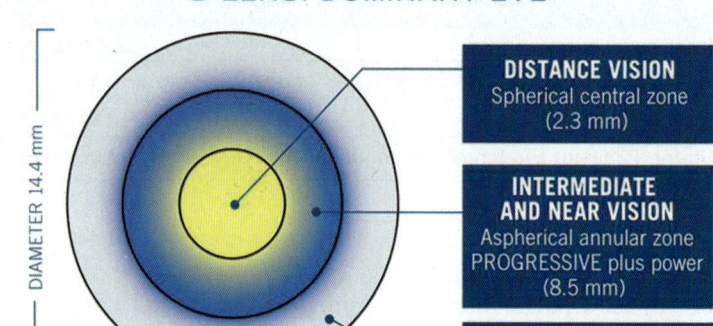

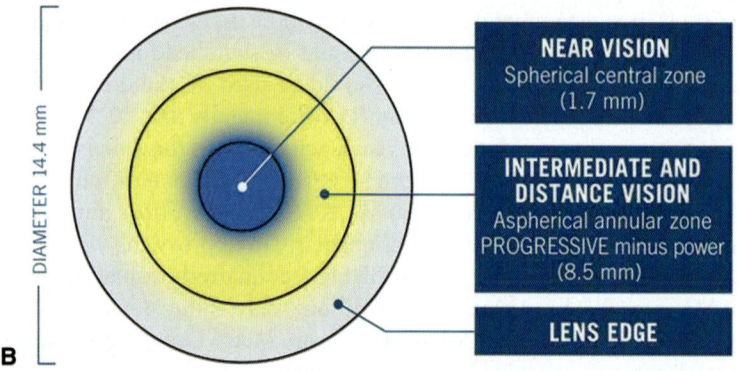

FIGURE 15.5 (A,B) The Proclear and Biofinity Multifocals Multifocals utilize a distance center ("D" in **A**) and near center ("N" in **B**). (Courtesy of CooperVision.)

is a back surface design with biprism and truncation for stability and position.[43] The horizontal diameters are 14.5 and 15.0 mm with vertical diameters of 11.4 to 13.9 mm. The near segment is located 1 mm below the geometric center. Marker dots on the lens at the 3- and 9 o'clock positions mark the geometric center of the lens and aid the practitioner in adjusting the vertical size to affect the fit and segment position.[44]

Soft Toric Multifocals

Several manufacturers make soft toric multifocal lenses, which increases the range of refractive errors that can be corrected. Until there are more of this type of lens available in disposable/frequent-replacement modalities and silicone hydrogel materials, the lenses will be limited in

TABLE 15.12 Add Selection for Biofinity Multifocal

INITIAL CONTACT LENS ADD	SPECTACLE ADD
D Lenses OU	+1.00 and +1.50
D lens dominant eye and N lens nondominant eye	+2.00 and +2.50
D lens +2.00 add on dominant eye and N Lens +2.50 add on nondominant eye	+2.25

use, but each year there is expansion in this lens category. Soft toric multifocals that are available in multipacks for frequent replacement are the Proclear Multifocal Toric (CooperVision), replaced monthly, and the C-Vue 55 Toric Multifocal (Unilens Corp.), Intelliwave Definitive Toric Multifocal (Art Optical), SaturEyes, Metrofocal, Metrofocal Definitive toric multifocals (Metro Optics), and SpecialEyes 54 Toric Multifocal (SpecialEyes), replaced quarterly. These designs are similar to their spherical counterparts. Proclear XR, C-Vue, and Intelliwave are available in a prescription of ± 20 D and a large range of cylinder powers and full axis range. In addition, there are additional conventional replacement soft toric multifocals, which are not mentioned here by name.

Fitting

Preliminary Testing

The fitting process is important to the success of the bifocal contact lens fitting. Examination procedures that should be performed before lenses are placed on the eye include current refraction, add determination, keratometry readings, determination of dominant eye, pupil size, TBUT, and a discussion pertaining to the patient's visual needs. Initiating the process with a current refraction and add power aids in the selection of the initial diagnostic lenses. In cases where the lenses must be ordered empirically, errors in the refraction contribute to patient and practitioner frustration and increase chair time. Keratometry may not be crucial with every lens design, as many of the lenses are only available in one BCR; however, it is beneficial if the cornea is exceptionally steep or flat, or if the lenses are available in more than one BCR.

There are several methods of determining the dominant eye. One of the most common methods is to have the patient view a 20/30 or 20/40 letter on the VA chart with both eyes open. The patients are instructed to sight through their hands, and upon closing their right eye, asked whether the letter is still visible. This is repeated with the left eye. The eye in which the letter disappears upon closure is the dominant eye. This can be confirmed by having the practitioner observe which eye the patient is using. Another common method is the use of a plus lens over each eye monocularly while viewing the VA chart binocularly. This can be performed with the patient behind the phoropter or by simply placing a trial lens ($+1.00 - +2.00$ D) in front of each eye individually and asking the patient which eye has greater blur. The eye that observes greater blur is the dominant eye.[45] A final method is to hand the patients a camera and ask them to hold the camera's viewfinder to their eye as they would if they were going to take a photograph. Typically, they will sight the camera with their dominant eye. This method can be used to confirm the prior methods.

Pupil size may play a critical role in the resulting vision in simultaneous designs. A small pupil size may affect distance vision when wearing a center-near design or near vision for a center-distance design. A large pupil may lead to glare and poor image quality. A lens that is successful during the day, may not be satisfactory at night. If pupil size appears to be affecting vision, a different lens design should be attempted.[46]

Successful soft contact lens wearers should be able to be refit into a multifocal design that is a similar material or replacement modality as their current lenses. Those who have not worn contact lenses before or who have been unsuccessful, may have similar challenges with the multifocal lenses. As with any contact lens patient, a healthy ocular surface and good tear quality aids in successful lens wear. As age-related changes may result in a dry eye, eliminating environmental issues, encouraging the patient to drink more water, and managing blepharitis or meibomian gland dysfunction can be beneficial. The use of either hydrogen peroxide solutions or multipurpose solutions, especially formulated to increase wettability should be used. In addition, using a lens material, such as omafilcon or a silicone hydrogel, may add to patient comfort. Rewetting drops and blinking exercises should also be encouraged.[46]

The patients should be asked about their daily visual needs at work and for hobbies. Do they primarily have distance, near, or intermediate tasks? How much time do they spend performing these tasks? Someone who works all day on a computer has different needs than a truck driver or an accountant. Practitioners strive for 20/20 VA at distance and near, but a computer user may not desire or require 20/20 VA at near. Near-point VA charts that simulate everyday reading tasks (i.e., newsprint, phone book, map, music, menu, etc.) are helpful (Fig. 15.6). If the patients have a specific near task that they need to be able to see, they should be encouraged to bring it along to use for testing. The patients can evaluate their intermediate vision at a computer in the office if this is important to them. All the handheld electronic devices today make it easy for the patients to test their vision with "real-world" visual tasks. The patients should be encouraged to use good lighting and adjust their working distance to provide optimum clarity.[47] The benefit of disposable soft multifocals is the ability to send the patients out into their everyday environment for a few days to try the lenses. Wearers who participate in sporting activities may desire one or two distance-vision-only lenses for occasional wear.

Diagnostic Lenses

When selecting diagnostic lenses, the current refraction should be converted to the spherical equivalent for spherical lenses and vertexed back to the cornea for both spherical and toric lenses. Distance powers should represent the "least minus" "most plus" power accepted by the patient. Add powers should be selected as prescribed unless the add falls between available add powers; in that case, the lower add power should be used. Typically, if there are two BCRs available, the steeper BCR should be selected first, unless the manufacturer's fitting guide specifies differently. Fitting guides and manufacturer calculators can be helpful for selecting the initial diagnostic lenses and for troubleshooting. Table 15.13 contains information regarding online fitting guides and contact lens calculators.

It is important to note that there are many different designs for the soft multifocal lenses. The diagnostic lens should be the identical design as the lens that will be ordered. In most cases, these lens designs are not interchangeable, so the practitioner is doing the patient a disservice if he or she believes he or she can overrefract over one design to try to order a different design. If the desired diagnostic lens is not in stock, it would be better to use a fitting guide,

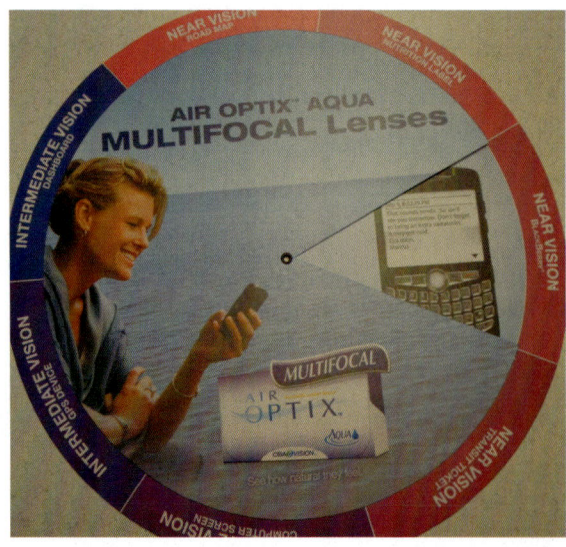

FIGURE 15.6 Example of near vision chart for use with multifocals.

TABLE 15.13 Online Contact Lens Fitting Guides and Calculators

Blanchard: www.blanchardlab.com/products/essential_soft/home.html
Bausch + Lomb: http://www.bausch.com
Alcon: www.virtualconsultant.cibavision.com
CooperVision: www.coopervision.com
Vistakon: www.ecp.acuvue.com

contact a laboratory consultant or use a laboratory calculator to select a lens to be ordered empirically, rather than trying to use a different design.

Another important tip is to use the fitting guide for the particular lens design selected. The fitting guide has been based by the manufacturer on numerous patient encounters to determine how the lens design reacts on the eye. So in a sense, the fitting guide is similar to having hundreds of previous patient encounters to assist in the fit. Even if this is the first patient that a practitioner has fit in this lens design, the practitioner can know that the fitting guide is supported by previous experience, so how it can assist in obtaining a successful fit should not be underestimated.

Once the diagnostic lenses are selected, they should be inserted and allowed to sit for 10 to 20 minutes prior to evaluating VA at near and distance. During this period of time, the patients should be cautioned not to judge their vision as the lenses are settling. The patients may want to take a walk around the office or outside the office to initially evaluate their lenses. If the patients choose to read during this period of time, they may become discouraged by their near vision and feel the lenses will not be successful before allowing the lenses to settle. The authors like to encourage the patients to try the lenses over a period of a few weeks as typically the vision improves as the patients adapt to their new vision. The patient should be encouraged not to give up too early. Thorough education and encouragement helps the patient to become successful.

The fit of the lenses should be evaluated before checking the VA. The lenses should fit like an acceptable soft spherical lens. The lenses should center, move with the blink, or have a positive push-up test. If the fit is not satisfactory and the BCR cannot be changed, then the lens should be removed and another design should be used.

Testing of the lenses should be performed under normal illumination and with trial lenses or flippers (± 0.25 and ± 0.50 D flippers). When overrefracting, 0.25 D steps can be significant to vision; therefore, the practitioner should be cautious about making large changes in power. Monocular overrefraction with the patient viewing binocularly is encouraged. Any overrefraction should be checked at distance and near so as not to compromise near vision to obtain good distance vision or poor distance to achieve good near vision. Vision should be checked binocularly at distance and near. If vision is reduced, monocular visual acuities and overrefraction should be checked to see if a change needs to be made. The patient should be encouraged to assess vision binocularly, not monocularly. Charts for testing near VA should include paragraphs to be read, not individual letters, and should have examples of news print, music, maps, telephone books, and other everyday reading material.[47] Many of the manufacturers make near cards like this but, if not, the practitioner can keep a sample of different reading materials for multifocal fittings.

Modified Monovision

Some patients will benefit from creative combinations of lenses. This could include enhancing the distance vision or near vision in one eye depending on if it is the dominant or nondominant eye (this will be discussed in more detail in the next section), using unequal add powers, combining two different bifocal lens designs, or fitting a spherical or toric distance lens in the dominant eye and a multifocal lens in the nondominant eye.

Although all of the aforementioned combinations may be a form of enhanced bifocal fitting, the use of a spherical lens in the dominant eye and a multifocal in the nondominant eye is an example of modified monovision. This is often successful for persons who require good distance vision and have few near visual tasks or patients who need little to no correction for distance. The disposable/frequent-replacement multifocals make this an easier alternative as the patient can wear the same material and replacement schedule on both eyes, but have one lens which is a distance-only lens and one that is a multifocal. As noted, typically the full distance prescription is provided in the contact lens to be placed on the dominant eye and the multifocal lens is placed on the nondominant eye. The multifocal lens should be adjusted so that distance and near VA is good, priority being given to near vision.

Follow-Up and Care/Problem Solving

If, upon fitting the initial diagnostic lenses, the patient has slightly reduced distance vision, monocular visual acuities should be checked to make sure that the distance correction is at least 20/40 or better in both eyes. If not, then an overrefraction should be performed over the lens that has reduced VA. If both eyes have better than 20/40 distance VA, then trial lenses or flippers should be used in an attempt to increase the power on the dominant eye by -0.25 D. It the overrefraction is >-0.50 D, reducing the add in the dominant eye may be the best alternative. Typically, the order for making alterations in the lens power for distance blur is

1. to add -0.25 D steps to dominant eye distance prescription
2. to decrease the add power in the dominant eye
3. increasing minus in the distance prescription of both lenses

An example of this is

OD lens -3.00 D, Add $+1.50$ D Dominant eye
OS lens -3.00 D, Add $+1.50$ D

If this patient has poor distance vision, the first step would be to add -0.25 D to the OD lens resulting in -3.25 D. If it requires >-0.50 D to improve the distance vision, then the add in the OD lens should be reduced to $+1.00$ D, rather than increasing the minus power.

When the patient is experiencing near vision blur, this is often solved by adding plus ($+0.25$ D) to the nondominant distance prescription. If the overrefraction at near is $+0.50$ D or greater, then the add power in the nondominant eye should be increased. The order of making changes is

1. add $+0.25$ D to the nondominant eye distance prescription
2. increase the add in the nondominant eye

An example of this is

OD lens -3.00 D, Add $+1.50$ D Dominant eye
OS lens -3.00 D, Add $+1.50$ D

If this patient has poor near vision, the first step would be to add $+0.25$ D to the left lens resulting in -2.75 D. If it requires $>+0.50$ D to improve the near vision, then the add power in the left lens should be increased to $+2.00$ D, rather than increasing the plus power.

If there is blur at distance and near, the distance vision should be corrected first. If several lens changes have been made and the VA is still not satisfactory, then another design should be used. When 20/20 vision is achieved or when vision is satisfactory, the patient should be sent home with the lenses to try them in their natural environment. The patient should make a mental note of any visual concerns experienced with the lenses, so that at the follow-up visit (typically in 7–14 days) the patient can tell the practitioner what visual tasks are satisfactory and which ones are not satisfactory. Changes in the power, fit, or design can be made at this visit.

Care and handling of these lenses is no different than any other soft contact lens (see Chapter 12). If the patient is a new wearer, he or she may experience more difficulty handling the lens—notably inserting the lens—due to difficulty in seeing the lens at near and loss of manual dexterity. Care regimens that improve wettability or are preservative-free may be helpful for patients with dry eye. A summary of fitting pearls can be found in Table 15.14.

GP LENS DESIGNS

Traditionally, GP multifocal and bifocal designs enjoyed greater success than their soft lens counterparts. The optical quality achieved with a rigid lens as well as the ability to achieve translation is important in obtaining success. These designs can be divided into aspheric multifocal and translating designs.

Types of Designs

Aspheric Multifocal

Aspheric lens designs have a gradual change in curvature along one of their surfaces (anterior or posterior) based upon the geometry of conic sections. The eccentricity or rate of flattening of the lens surface is greater than with single-vision lens designs; therefore, an increase in plus power is generated toward the periphery of the lens. Although often available in a back surface aspheric, several front surface designs have been introduced. Aspheric multifocal GP lenses, unlike soft lens designs, often have very good optical quality and, like soft lenses, are relatively easy to fit. These are thin lens designs, fit steeper than K, in an effort to achieve optimum centration with very little (usually about 1 mm) of movement with the blink. High success rates have been reported with these lenses, often >75%.[48–52]

TABLE 15.14 Fitting Pearls for Soft Multifocal Contact Lenses

- Use the manufacturer fitting guide for selecting the diagnostic lens and for problem solving
- If there is more than one BCR, start with the steeper BCR
- Start with current refraction and add power
- Remind patients to have good light and adjust their working distance to the optimal distance
- If the patient has slightly reduced distance and near vision, fix the distance vision before working with near vision
- Use normal room illumination
- Let lenses settle for 10–20 min prior to evaluating
- Assess vision binocularly
- Use handheld trial lenses or flippers to overrefract
- Overrefract in 0.25 D steps
- Overrefract monocularly with both eyes open and recheck any overrefraction at near and distance
- Use everyday reading material when evaluating patient's near vision
- Test vision at the distances required by the patient's visual needs (e.g., a computer user needs good intermediate vision and may accept reduced near vision)
- Round add powers down
- It is acceptable to use unequal add powers

BCR, base curve radius.

Patient Selection: As aspheric designs utilize the simultaneous vision principle with near and distance power corrections in front of the pupil at the same time, the best candidates are early-to-moderate presbyopes. Some of the newer designs have been able to incorporate a higher add power into the lens via modification of the front surface; therefore, high add patients should not be excluded. GP aspheric multifocals are a good option for individuals with a high intermediate distance demand including accountants, electricians, plumbers, and those with mechanical responsibilities.[53] Most important is the individual who devotes much of his or her time to computer use. GP aspheric multifocals have been recommended for individuals spending, at minimum, one-third of their waking hours at a computer.[54] Early presbyopes who are current GP wearers also tend to prefer the ease of transition from a thin spherical design into a relatively thin aspheric design. It is important to select patients with a small-to-medium pupil size (i.e., <5 mm in room illumination) as glare and ghosting of images is possible at night with individuals having large pupil diameters due to the effect created by paracentral and midperipheral plus powers.[17] Patients with critical distance or near demands may obtain greater benefit from a translating design, although the vision achieved with the early presbyope having an optimum fit is often quite satisfactory. Part of this may be the result of a slight amount of shift, or translation, with downward gaze. Individuals who are still quite active athletically are good candidates for aspheric lenses due to their low risk of displacement. Individuals who are not good candidates for translating multifocals due to an inferior positioned or a flaccid lower lid are typically good aspheric candidates. Good candidates for aspheric multifocal lenses are summarized in Table 15.15.

Lens Design/Fitting: Until recently, most aspheric designs were of such high eccentricity, that the manufacturer recommended a BCR selection of as much as 3 D steeper than "K." The VFL 3 lens from Conforma is an example of such a design. However, most lens designs in common use—whereas higher in eccentricity than single-vision lenses—are typically fit approximately 1 D steeper than "K."

Low-Eccentricity Back-Surface Designs: There are a large and increasing number of lens designs that have a lower posterior rate of flattening and are fit in a more conventional (i.e., not as steep) as higher-eccentricity designs. As with previously discussed lens designs, these lenses need to position centrally (or slightly superiorly) with limited lens movement with the blink. Approximately 1 mm lag is optimum with these designs. Although they are fit approximately 1 D steeper than "K," the fluorescein pattern should exhibit an alignment or near-alignment pattern due to the back surface geometry (Fig. 15.7). There are numerous such designs on the market and the specific manufacturers with their designs can be located at www.gpli.info.

A representative example of a lower-eccentricity, posterior aspheric lens design is the ESSentials multifocal from Blanchard. This design has three Series of add powers, with the increase in add resulting from an effective decrease in the central distance power zone.[55] Series I is for the beginning presbyope; Series II is for the early-moderate presbyope, and Series III is for the moderate-high presbyope. However, it is not uncommon for the advanced presbyopes, especially if they have small pupils, to require additional add power. The introduction of the ESSential CSA design allows for more add power to be placed on a concentric ring surrounding the central

TABLE 15.15 Good Candidates for GP Aspheric Multifocal Lenses

- Early-to-moderate presbyopes
- Computer users
- Present single-vision GP wearers
- Small-to-medium pupil size
- Low or flaccid lower lid

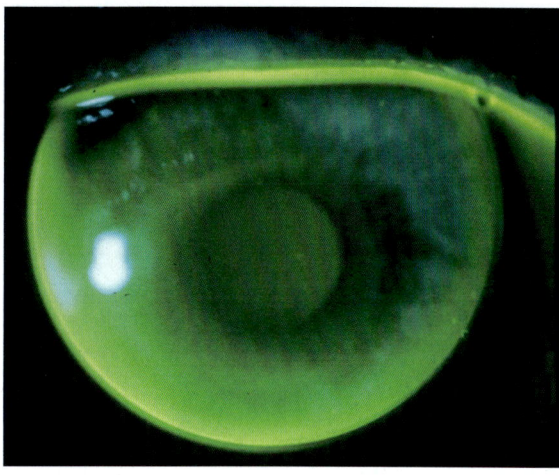

FIGURE 15.7 A well-fitting aspheric GP multifocal lens.

distance zone—which is 4.0 to 4.6 mm in diameter—on the front surface of the lens (Fig. 15.8). If the patient, for example, is wearing the Series II design but requires an additional +0.75 D add power, this lens can be ordered with the identical parameters but specified with a +0.75 D CSA. This is one of several aspheric multifocal designs that can provide higher add powers.

Optimum HR (Contamac) and Paragon HDS HI (Paragon Vision Sciences) are high-refractive-index materials, which incorporate a higher add power on the front surface. Centration is optimized with these materials because they have less lens mass than conventional materials.[37]

High-Eccentricity Back-Surface Designs: Although not as popular as the lower-eccentricity designs, very high-eccentricity designs such as the VFL 3 Lens (Conforma) are available. This high-eccentricity, posterior aspheric lens design is available in the Fluoroperm 30 and Boston ES lens materials and incorporates aberration control. The high-definition, advance presbyopia (HD–AP) lens design, incorporating a slightly higher add power, is available in the Paragon HDS material. It is typically fit several diopters steeper than "K." In addition, its best application is in the early-to-moderate presbyopic patient, although a high add is obtained by fitting a steeper BCR, the "distance" zone is reduced, and distance VA can be compromised. Typically, good centration (which is essential) is obtained because of the steep BCR and the absence of prism ballast. A mild apical clearance fluorescein pattern will be observed (Fig. 15.9). The lens should not move more than 1.0 to 1.5 mm with the blink and, therefore, it often fails on flat corneas because of excessive lens lag with the blink.

Front Surface Aspheric Designs: Several laboratories have available front surface aspheric lens designs including the Naturalens Progressive (Advanced Vision Technologies) and the Renovation Multifocal (Art Optical). Although the amount of add generated with these designs can be limited, this is a viable option in cases in which the back surface design decenters and causes flattening and possibly distortion of the cornea. This is likely if the lens decenters superiorly and either adheres

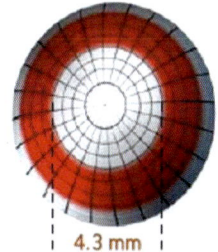

4.3 mm

FIGURE 15.8 The ESSential CSA lens design from Blanchard Contact Lens. The red region represents the area on the front surface in which additional add power is placed.

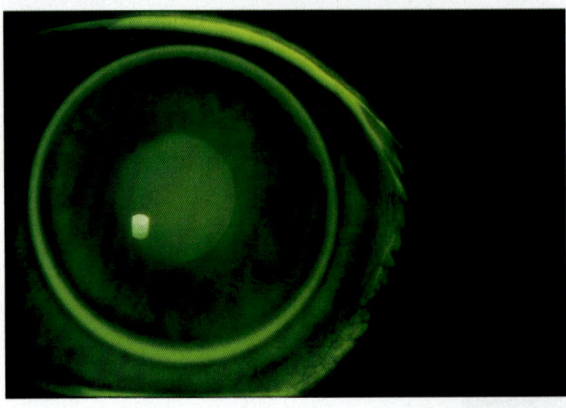

FIGURE 15.9 An optimum fitting VFL 3 aspheric multifocal lens.

or moves very minimally. The front surface of the Renovation Multifocal has the additional benefit of being designed to reduce spherical aberration.

Problem Solving: Possible problems with these designs include decentration and blur at near due to insufficient near add power. If the lens moves excessively with the blink and decenters inferiorly, the BCR should be steepened, typically by 0.50 D.[24] Superior decentration, if excessive and resulting in undesirable corneal topography changes, should be solved by changing to a front surface aspheric design. A steeper BCR may be beneficial as well in this case. If lateral decentration is present, a larger-diameter lens can be attempted, although if the decentration is due to a decentered corneal apex, the use of another lens design or material is recommended.

In some cases, patients experience blur at near due to insufficient add power being provided from these designs. As indicated previously, there are higher add designs available for the management of this problem. In addition, either via the use of unequal adds or a "modified bifocal approach" in which one lens is overplussed by a small amount (i.e., 0.25–0.50 D), this problem can be easily solved.

Summary: Aspheric multifocal fitting and problem solving is actually quite simple and straightforward. After proper patient selection, a good fitting relationship with minimal movement with the blink is required. It is recommended to have, at minimum, one of these designs and the manufacturer can provide assistance with the management of patients wearing these designs.

Translating Bifocals

Translating or alternating vision bifocals are prism-ballasted, and sometimes truncated, lens designs that utilize the lower lid as a stop gap such that when the patients drop their eyes inferiorly to read, the lens is pushed superiorly such that they are viewing through the inferior near portion of the lens. With this method, when properly fit, excellent vision can be obtained at distance and near. The segments represent many of the common types of spectacle segments including executive, crescent, and D shaped. In addition, a few annular or concentric translating bifocal designs with a superiorly decentered distance zone are available as well. Some representative examples include executive (Tangent Streak, Fused Kontacts of Missouri; Solitaire, Truform, Euless, TX), crescent (Solutions, X-Cel, Duluth, GA; Metro-Seg, Metro Optics, Austin, TX), and concentric (Mandell Seamless, ABB-Concise, Alameda, CA).

Whereas these lenses may take more initial chair time to fit, they are not as difficult as a novice practitioner may perceive them to be. In fact, they often represent the bifocal lens of choice in many contact lens practices as a result of the excellent vision obtained.[56–58] The BiExpert (Art Optical and Essilor) is a segmented, translating lens, which can be designed empirically by providing the refraction, horizontal visible iris diameter, pupil size, lower lid to lower pupil distance, palpebral aperture width, lower lid to limbus position, and lid tension.[37] Initial comfort is actually quite good with these designs as a result of the thin edge and limited movement with the blink desired with these lenses. In fact, due to the fact that both aspheric multifocal and segmented translating designs should move little with the blink, the initial comfort of these designs has been comparable to, if not slightly better than, spherical single-vision GP designs.[59] The fitting and problem-solving guidelines outlined in this chapter will be important for patient success.

Patient Selection: As mentioned previously, patients desiring excellent vision, or having critical vision demands, are good candidates for this form of bifocal lens. In addition, the ability to incorporate any add power makes this a good option for moderate-to-advanced presbyopes who have unsatisfactory vision at near with an aspheric lens design. Although there are an increasing number of segmented translating designs that provide intermediate vision, one limitation of translating bifocals is the inability to provide intermediate vision, limiting their use in patients needing vision at this distance (or requiring them to have over spectacles for either reading or intermediate work). When good centration and limited movement is not possible with an aspheric design or the patient has large pupils, a translating design will often be successful. These patients should, however, have a lower lid within 1 mm of the lower limbus. Conversely, if the palpebral fissure size is too small, the lens may position too superiorly and the segment may position in front of the pupil on straightahead gaze. Specifically, if the lower lid is positioned >1.5 mm above the lower limbus, it may be difficult to provide a sufficient segment height for acceptable near vision.[24] To allow translation to occur, lid tension should be moderate-to-tight. GP translating bifocal patient selection is summarized in Table 15.16.

Fitting: These lens materials are customarily available in either a high- or hyper-Dk material due to the thickness of the prism-ballasted design. Most laboratories have warranty programs, which allow you to exchange lenses for a higher overall fee and this is recommended, especially for the novice fitter. Diagnostic fitting is extremely important for successful fitting of GP translating bifocals. Regardless of the lens design to be used, the manufacturer's fitting guide is typically not complicated and straightforward in regard to BCR selection and lens evaluation. It is important to have in office, at minimum, one diagnostic fitting set of these lenses. When in doubt as to which set to use, contact your local Contact Lens Manufacturer's Association (CLMA) member laboratory.

These lenses typically incorporate 1 to 3Δ in an effort to position on or close to the lower lid. Likewise, they are fit slightly flatter than K to increase the likelihood that the lenses will fall quickly to the lower lid and move not more than 1 mm with the blink. It is important to evaluate the position of the segment line to the pupil in normal room illumination with straightahead gaze. With few exceptions, the segment line should position at or near the lower pupil margin. If the patient is viewing even slightly superior or inferior, this will shift the position of the segment line to the pupil and could result in ordering an incorrect segment height. Patients with a slightly low lower lid (i.e., 0.5–1 mm below the limbus) would benefit from both a larger overall diameter and segment height and vice versa for patient exhibiting a lower lid 1 to 1.5 mm above the limbus.

TABLE 15.16 Good Candidates for GP Translating Bifocal Lenses

- All presbyopic add powers
- Critical vision demands
- Any pupil size
- Lower lid positioned near to or above lower limbus
- Moderare-to-tight lid tension
- Inferior corneal apex

Translation should also be evaluated. While in the biomicroscope the patient should view inferiorly and, with the upper lid held back, the lens should push up or translate such that, at minimum, one-half of the pupil is covered by the segment as the practitioner views it in straightahead gaze. Alternatively, the ophthalmoscope can be used from an inferior position to simulate reading; in which case, the segment should appear to be predominantly in front of the pupil. As with aspheric designs, the use of loose trial lenses or flipper bars is important when performing the overrefraction.

Representative Examples

Prism Ballasted/Truncated (Tangent Streak): This is a prism-ballasted, often truncated, one-piece translating bifocal lens design. It is available in almost any lens material. It has an executive style segment line, which should be positioned at or slightly below the lower pupil margin (Fig. 15.10).

The 20-lens diagnostic set has BCRs in 0.50 D steps for both +2.00 D and −2.00 D distance lens powers. Any segment is available; the segment power in the fitting set is +2.00 D. The overall diameter is 9.4 (horizontally)/9.0 mm (vertically) with a 4.2 mm segment height and 2 Δ base down. Any diameter, segment height, and prism can be ordered based upon the diagnostic fitting relationship. For spherical corneas, a BCR 1 D flatter than K is recommended; for 0.50 D of corneal cylinder, a 0.50 D flatter-than-K base curve should be fit; for >1 D of corneal toricity, an "On K" to slightly steeper BCR can be selected.

Prism-Ballasted Only (Solutions): This is a crescent design that utilizes diagnostic fitting set parameters as well as base curve fitting philosophy, which are similar to the Tangent Streak lens (Fig. 15.11). The lens is available in low, medium, and high prism as well as 5 segment heights, in 0.5 mm increment differences. The benefit to the fitter is the ease of fitting due to the limited choices available including the absence of prism.

Concentric (Annular) Alternating Designs: These are also prism-ballasted designs with a central distance zone of approximately 4 mm in diameter, which is decentered slightly superior in an effort to be positioned directly in front of the pupil during distance gaze but in close proximity to the lower lid such that translation can occur with inferior gaze.[17,60] This is surrounded by a near-concentric periphery. Increasing the central distance zone can result in improved distance vision but degraded near vision and vice versa. These designs—like segmented designs—are often fit slightly flatter than "K."

Segmented, Translating Designs with Intermediate Correction: There are several designs available including executive trifocal designs such as the Tangent Streak Trifocal (Fused Kontacts), and Llevations (Truform), an aspheric intermediate zone such as Presbylite (Lens Dynamics) to an aspheric back surface and segmented front surface such as ESSential Solutions (X-Cel) and

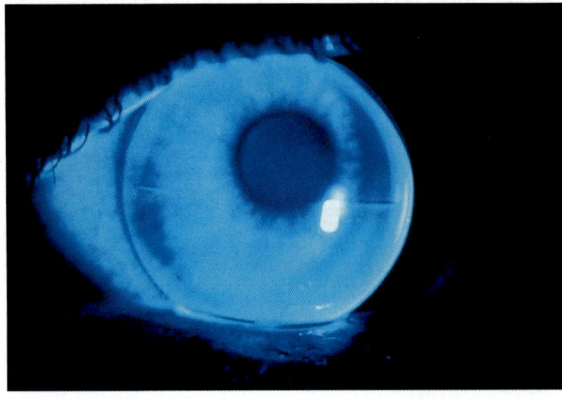

FIGURE 15.10 An optimum fitting Tangent Streak translating design GP bifocal lens.

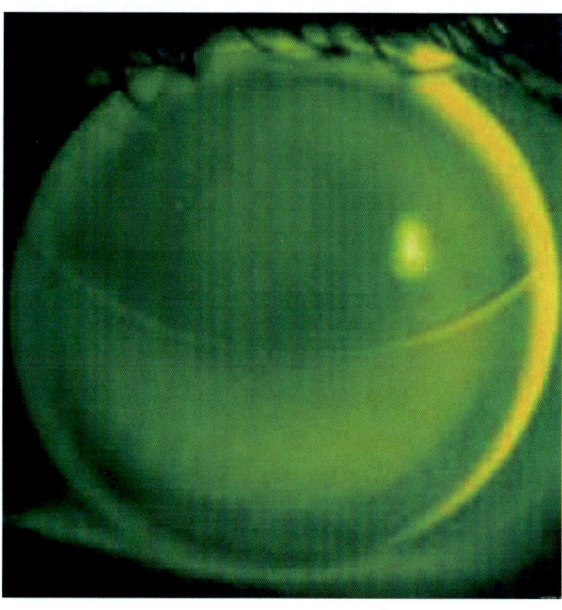

FIGURE 15.11 An optimum position and fluorescein pattern for the Solutions Bifocal (X-Cel).

EZEyes Multifocal (Essilor). Truform Optics has a multitude of such designs and, in fact, have more types of segmented, translating designs than any other laboratory in the country. For patients who desire critical distance or near vision but spend much time every day at a computer, this type of design represents a preferable alternative to wearing a bifocal design accompanied by overspectacles for computer work.

Problem Solving: Problem-solving translating lens designs can be divided into five categories: (a) excessive lens rotation with the blink; (b) lens is positioned too superiorly; (c) poor lens translation; (d) poor distance vision; and (e) poor near vision.[61]

Excessive rotation with the blink is often the result of a base curve that is too steep. The apical clearance fitting relationship results in a lens that will attempt to position more centrally as opposed to fall inferiorly (Fig. 15.12). Therefore, the lens will be impacted more by the upper lid. Selecting a lens that is 0.50 D flatter in BCR should reduce or eliminate this problem. Another cause of excessive rotation is the presence of an upswept lower-lid contour (Fig. 15.13).

When this is present, if the lenses can be truncated, the RALS (right add left subtract) acronym can be used to determine the axis. For example, if both lenses rotate 15 degree toward the nose due to the shape of the lower lid, the prism can be ordered at 105 degrees OD and 75 degrees OS.

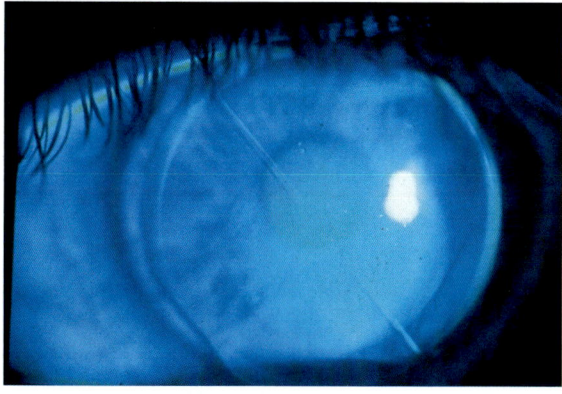

FIGURE 15.12 Excessive rotation of a Tangent Streak bifocal lens fit 1 D steeper than K.

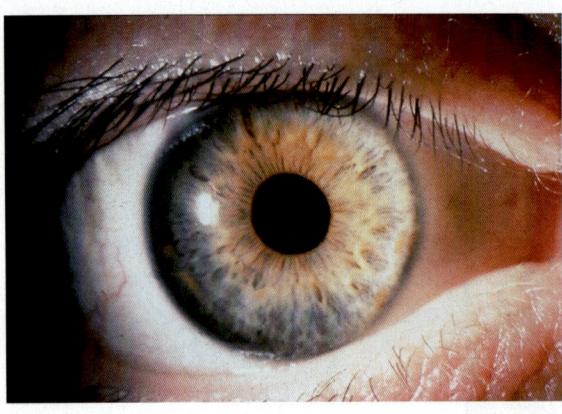

FIGURE 15.13 An upswept lower-lid contour.

When the lens is being lifted too superior with the blink such that the segment is in front of the pupil with distance gaze, increasing the prism ballast (again by 0.50 Δ) should bring the lens down (Fig. 15.14). In addition, flattening the peripheral curve radius can be beneficial.

When the lens exhibits intermittent or no translation with the blink, the edge clearance of the lens should be increased (Fig. 15.15). This can be accomplished easily in-office by selecting a flatter BCR. Likewise, the peripheral curve could be made flatter and wider. Another option would be to increase prism or truncation. If the lens continues to not translate, an aspheric design is indicated.

If poor distance vision is present, it is often the result of one of the following causes: (a) Lens is too high/moves excessively (increase prism); (b) Lens is not adequately covering the pupil with straightahead gaze (increase overall diameter); (c) Segment height is too high (reorder with smaller segment height). If poor near vision is present, it is often the result of one of the following causes: (a) Segment height is too low (increase segment); (b) Lens is not translating (increase edge clearance); (c) Excessive rotation is present (flatten BCR); (d) Patient is dropping head—not eyes—when reading (reeducate patient).

GP translating bifocal problem solving is summarized in Table 15.17.

Irregular Cornea Designs

In the past, highly astigmatic, keratoconic, and postrefractive surgery patients were at a loss for a design to fit their cornea. Several labs are producing lenses to meet these needs. Reclaim HD (Blanchard) has front surface multifocal optics. It can be manufactured with a toric back surface on all Rose K designs for keratoconic individuals and on the RSS lens (Refractive Surgery Specific) for postrefractive individuals. Another company that provides reverse geometry back surface lenses with a front surface multifocal for refractive surgery patients is LasikNear (Valley Contax).[37]

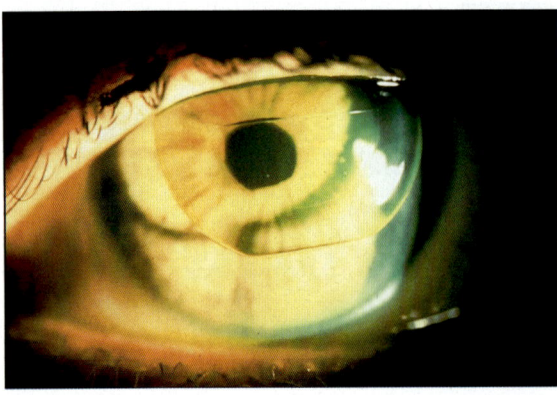

FIGURE 15.14 A superiorly decentered translating bifocal.

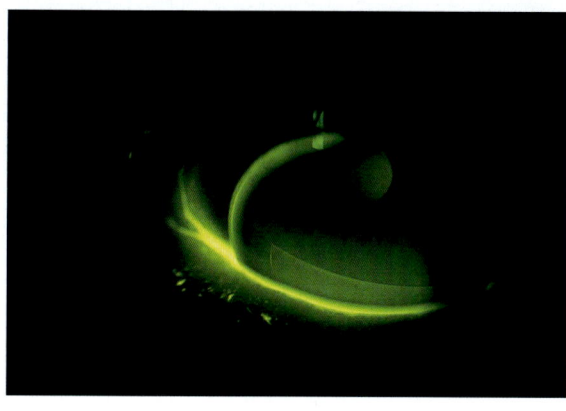

FIGURE 15.15 Absence of translation in a segmented bifocal lens design.

Scleral Designs

Scleral lens designs are offering new opportunities for patients. The combination of initial comfort with a multifocal design may aid in the success of some individuals. The So$_2$Clear Progressive (Dakota Sciences/Art Optical/Metro Optics) can be fit using the standard So$_2$Clear design and the lens is ordered in a center-near presbyopic version. Both the Digiform and Digiform 18 lenses (Truform Optics) are available in an adjustable center-near design with various add powers or a center-distance design surrounded by a near zone. The Dyna Semi Scleral (13.5–16 mm diameter) and Dyna Scleral (17–19 mm diameter) (Lens Dynamics) have a front aspheric design. If needed, the Quad Sym edge design or front aspheric can be added. Other designs that will be forthcoming are a front aspheric center-near design by Blanchard and a back surface aspheric, center-distance design with reverse curves by Advanced Vision Technologies.[62]

Hybrid Designs

SynergEyes has a hybrid option for presbyopic patients, the Duette Multifocal. The Duette Multifocal has a GP 8.4 mm center made of a 130 Dk material and an 84 Dk silicone hydrogel skirt. The total diameter of the lens is 14.5. The lens is a center-near design and has two sizes of add zones. It is fit the same as a Duette with the additional step of selecting the add zone, which provides the best vision at distance, intermediate, and near.[37]

TABLE 15.17 GP Translating Bifocal Problem Solving

PROBLEM	MANAGEMENT
Excessive rotation	1. Flatten BCR 0.50 D 2. Change prism axis
Lens positions too superiorly	1. Increase prism 0.50 Δ
Poor lens translation	1. Increase Edge Clearance (flatten BCR or PCR) 2. Increase prism or truncation
Blur at distance	1. Increase prism (if too high) 2. Increase OAD if too little pupil coverage 3. Lower seg height (if high)
Blur at near	1. Higher seg (if low) 2. Increase edge clearance (if poor translation) 3. Reeducate patient (if drops head not eyes to read 4. Flatten BCR (if excessive rotation)

BCR, base curve radius; PCR, peripheral curve radius; OAD, overall diameter; seg, segment.

GP Multifocal and Bifocal Educational Resources

The most important educational resource to the practitioner who desires to fit GP presbyopic lens designs is the laboratory consultant. These individuals can provide useful information on lens designs, provide diagnostic fitting sets, and assist in the lens design, fitting, and troubleshooting process. In addition, many useful resources have been developed by the GP Lens Institute, the educational division of the CLMA. These include a comprehensive resource on GP presbyopic contact lens education for practitioner, staff, and patient, entitled "Rx for Success," in addition to other GP resources. These resources can be found at http://www.gpli.info.

OTHER FORMS OF PRESBYOPIC CONTACT LENS CORRECTION

Other contact lens options available for presbyopic patients include single-vision lenses in combination with reading glasses and monovision.

Single-Vision Contact Lenses/Reading Glasses

The use of single-vision lenses (soft or GP) in combination with reading glasses affords the benefits of ease of fit, optimum vision at distance and near, and limited expense. However, patients with varied near and distance tasks will complain of the inconvenience of frequently applying and removing their spectacles. In addition, many patients desire contact lenses to eliminate the need for spectacle wear. Nevertheless, it is important for this option to be presented to all potential presbyopic contact lens patients. Some patients will prefer to begin with this option; however, at a later date, they will change to one of the other presbyopic contact lens options mentioned to them at the original fitting/consultation visit.

Monovision

Monovision was first reported as a form of presbyopic contact lens correction in the 1960s.[63] For many years, it was the most popular form of contact lens correction for presbyopia; however, it has been surpassed by soft multifocals in the last few years and today multifocals are considered the new standard of care for presbyopes.[64]

In the past year, soft multifocals topped the list of contact lens correction for presbyopia at 37%, with soft monovision at 30%, spectacles worn over soft lenses at 19%, GP bifocals/multifocals at 5%, GP monovision at 4%, and hybrid/scleral multifocals around 1%. Although practitioners prefer multifocals 67% of the time compared to 23% for monovision, in actual fits, the difference is only 42% multifocal to 37% monovision.[65] This is most likely due to patient perception that multifocals do not work, are more expensive, or the concept that if it is not broken do not fix it. Newer lens designs are changing those perceptions. Internationally, multifocal fits are increasing and monovision fits are decreasing.[10]

Several studies directly comparing monovision to soft or GP multifocal contact lenses have found that 68% to 76% of wearers prefer multifocals over monovision.[66–69] A separate study compared high- and low-contrast acuity and contrast sensitivity of four different presbyopic corrections; progressive addition spectacles, a GP multifocal lens, a soft bifocal lens, and monovision. The monovision lenses performed poorest in all categories tested.[70] The reason multifocals are preferred by wearers over monovision appears to be related to "real-world" viewing. It has been found that although monovision contact lenses perform better in an examination room setting, soft multifocals wearers appreciate the multifocal contact lenses not only for clinical testing, but even more in their everyday tasks (i.e., daytime and nighttime driving, intermediate vision, watching television, reading detail on television).[71]

All this said, the success rate for monovision has been between 70% and 76%[72,73]; however, it is evident that for monovision to be successful, the brain must suppress blur from the defocused eye.[74] There has been much heightened consumer awareness about monovision resulting from a report of an aviation accident in which three passengers were injured in a plane in which the pilot was wearing a monovision correction.[75]

The advantages of monovision include[4,17,76] (a) ease of fitting; (b) uninterrupted vision out of each eye separately; (c) changing one lens only for present lens wearers; (d) less expense to patient and practitioner; and (e) avoidance of some of the problems present in multifocal contact lenses, including ghost images and fluctuating vision due to pupil size change.

Disadvantages/Problems

A major problem with monovision is a decrease in stereopsis. A decrease of anywhere from 37 to 150 seconds of arc has resulted when subjects have been refit from monovision into multifocal contact lenses.[73,77,78] Several studies have demonstrated that stereoacuity loss increases with increasing monocular add powers.[79,80] Some monocular suppression of blur also occurs as the add increases.[81] Subjects with monovision correction have demonstrated contrast sensitivity loss and sometimes compromise on critical distance vision tasks.[82,83,70] In addition, an increase in anisometropia of ≥ 0.50 D and as much as 1.25 D has been found in 29% of monovision wearers.[84]

Driving with monovision wear is also a concern and should, in fact, add to the problems presbyopes already experience with night driving.[85] As many as 80% of monovision patients have reported problems with night driving.[86] This would especially be true with glare.[87] It has also been found that monovision wearers have a very difficult time suppressing headlights while driving at night with one-third of the subjects experiencing glare while night driving.[88] Interestingly, when evaluating habitual monovision wearers on several simulated driving tasks under daytime conditions, no difference was found in driving performance between monovision and their habitual distance correction.[89] Nevertheless, it has been advised for monovision patients to avoid driving or operating dangerous machinery during the first 2 to 3 weeks of adaptation.[90]

Patient Selection

The authors feel that multifocals should be the first and primary option provided for presbyopes. In those patients where multifocals may not be a viable option, the following information may be helpful for fitting monovision.

The age and add powers of the patient are predictive of success with lower add power patients (+1.25 to +2.00 D) being more successful than higher add power patients.[73,91] The visual needs as well as the lifestyle of the patient must be evaluated when considering monovision. If prolonged and critical distance vision is desirable, monovision is not a good option. Likewise, if depth perception is important to a given occupation, for example, with construction workers, monovision would not be recommended.[92] Individuals in occupations like teaching, performing arts, public speaking, and sales who desire the benefit of being able to constantly change viewing distances and still remain focused could benefit from monovision lens wear.

Due to an esophoric shift in eye posture, esophoria at distance and a reduction in nearpoint visual acuity and stereopsis have also been shown to indicate a poor prognosis for success with monovision.[91,93] A patient's personality has also been found to be important for monovision success.[94] A significant correlation between initial negative response and unsuccessful monovision wear has been found.[95] In addition, it has been found that introverted males tend to reject monovision most frequently whereas the most successful patients were laid-back and optimistic.[96]

Lens Selection and Fitting Considerations

Both GP lenses and silicone/hydrogel lens materials lend themselves well to monovision due to their resultant visual performance, oxygen permeability, and wettability. As a result of the greater tendency for dryness and surface deposition, if soft lenses are deemed preferable, a disposable (daily to monthly) lens is essential for long-term success.

The eye to be selected for near point depends upon several factors. It has been found that in 95% of the cases it has been the nondominant eye.[73] A "swinging plus" test in which the patient simply walks around the room holding a plus power trial lens equal to their required add over one eye—repeating the procedure over the other eye—has been advocated.[97] This is also beneficial in simulating the impact monovision will potentially have on their quality of vision. The eye

TABLE 15.18	Important Factors for Monovision Fitting and Prescribing
1.	Binocular vision testing should be performed to determine the effect of monovision on stereopsis.
2.	The proper eye for near vision should be selected. This often is the nondominant eye and/or the eye in which vision is reduced relative to the other eye.
3.	The indicated add power should be demonstrated to the patient such that they can obtain a realistic impression of the resulting blur.
4.	It is recommended to prescribe the full amount of correction and avoid the temptation of prescribing less plus power in the near-corrected eye and/or prescribing more plus power in the distance-corrected contact lens.
5.	Patients should be strongly encouraged—if not required—to obtain a pair of driving spectacles (i.e., minus correction in the lens over the near-corrected eye) to wear for driving or any other critical distance tasks.
6.	Although most individuals adapt within 2 wk, patients should be instructed that it could take up to 6 wk to fully adapt to monovision.

Modified from Bennett ES, Jurkus JM. Presbyopic correction. In: Bennett ES, Weissman BA, eds. *Clinical Contact Lens Practice*. 2nd ed. Philadelphia, PA: Lippincott Williams and Wilkins; 2005; 531–548.

that the patients deem more comfortable with the overplus correction will be the eye corrected for nearpoint. The full distance and near powers are typically prescribed. It is possible that by overplussing the power of the distance lens and/or underplussing the power of the near lens, not only is the patient's vision compromised at one or both distances, but it may also reduce the interocular suppression of blur that is important for monovision to be successful.[4] It is recommended to perform binocular vision testing to determine the effect of monovision on stereopsis. As indicated previously, it is important to strongly encourage—if not require—the patient to have over spectacles for use while driving and for any other critical distance-vision tasks. Although full adaptation to monovision may take up to 2 to 3 weeks,[73] patients should be told that it may take as long as 4 to 6 weeks. If they experience difficulty in adapting (i.e., experience headaches, eyestrain, blurred vision), switching the near and distance-corrected eyes should be considered. Important factors for successful monovision lens wear are provided in Table 15.18.

Problem Solving

Several problems induced by monovision and their clinical management have been reported[98]:

Asthenopia: If the patient reports frequent or prolonged asthenopic symptoms, the optics and power of the lenses should be verified and an overrefraction performed. Often poor optics, inappropriate powers, or uncorrected cylinder are to blame. It is often necessary to fit a toric soft lens for a monovision wearer with astigmatism of 0.75 D.

Blur at Distance: If the patient's complaint is poor distance vision, it is first important to evaluate for optical problems. It may be necessary to completely correct the astigmatism in the distance eye or, in the case of a low add, the patient may not be suppressing at distance.

Blur at Intermediate Distances: Demand for intermediate vision will be best provided by multifocals; however, another option may require the use of a modified monovision system by fitting a simultaneous multifocal lens on the near eye and a distance lens on the other eye. The multifocal alone may provide adequate intermediate vision or the distance zone of the multifocal lens may be fit to provide intermediate power with the add providing near vision.

Blur at Near: It is important to determine if the blur is constant or task-specific. If the blur is constant, the add should be adjusted. You should then overrefract, adding plus to the near eye until clear vision is achieved. If clear vision is not achieved, the optics of the near lens should be evaluated. If the blur is task-specific (e.g., most noticeable at work in near-intensive demands), a pair of over spectacles may be required.

Fatigue and Flare: A frequent complaint of monovision patients is eye strain or fatigue when performing an intensive amount of near work. Prescribing a pair of single-vision glasses with plus over the distance eye and plano over the near will often alleviate the symptoms.

As for flare caused by a cosmetic fit, the cause of flare in monovision is too small of an optical zone for scotopic conditions. To verify the condition, it is important to examine the patient under both dim and normal room illumination. The pupil size should be measured under dim illumination, with 2 mm added to determine the minimum optical zone size.

Headaches: Some early presbyopes who have a reasonable amount of accommodation remaining only need a very low add and may be fighting excess plus prescribed for near. They try to accommodate to clear their distance eye at near and, as a result, are overplussed on their near eye. If increasing the add to 1.25 or 1.50 D does not alleviate the symptoms, the fitting should be deferred until a higher add is required. Hyperopic patients find being fit with single-vision contact lenses optically provides them with an advantage, and monovision may not be necessary during the first year of lens wear.

Involuntary Eye Switching: Often patients will observe that, especially under visual stress, they momentarily switch eyes. An example of this is the executive fit with the distance eye dominant, who is reviewing annual budgets; as she concentrates on the budget, the dominant eye attempts to see the text. These are usually transient episodes of very short duration during adaptation. If eye switching continues after the first week of lens wear, the eyes are inappropriately fit and the near eye should be refit for distance, and vice versa.

Persistent Blur or Haze: If blurring and haze unrelated to the fit of the contact lens persist after 2 weeks of monovision wear, an adjustment is necessary. The practitioner must first ensure that the blur is not caused by edema as a result of a poorly fitting lens. If the lens is suspect, it should be adjusted before any other step is taken. If the fit of the lens is not the cause, the duration of the blur or haze should next be determined.

If the blur is constant, the optics of the lenses should be evaluated and an overrefraction should be performed. If the problem is optically induced, a new lens should correct the problem. If the blur is not related to the optics of the lens or refraction, the amount of add should be examined next.

In cases of low adds (>1.00 D), there may not be enough stimulus for the patient to learn to selectively suppress. In these cases, increasing the amount of the add by 0.50 D has been successful in alleviating the symptom.

If the add is over 2.00 D, the patient may not be a suitable candidate for monovision. In some cases, reducing the add by 0.50 D has been successful, but most patients will not accept the near blur this creates. The best solution is to abandon the monovision fitting for multifocal corrections. If the add is between 1.00 and 2.00 D and blur persists, the lenses should be switched. Often, this symptom reflects an inappropriate eye being fit for distance.

Slight or Intermittent Blur/Haze: This normal symptom of adaptation is encountered by most monovision patients at some time in their initial weeks of wear. It is generally found to be most common in circumstances requiring visual concentration under scotopic conditions; for example, viewing television in a dim room. If the blur or haze is slight, intermittent, and transient, the patient should be instructed that no correction is necessary. If possible, they should try to avoid these conditions in the first week of monovision wear. The practitioner should be alert for blur or haze caused by a poor contact lens fit and take action if necessary. If blurring or haze is persistent, an office visit is required.

Vague complaints of discomfort: Most nonspecific complaints can be alleviated by switching eyes: the dominant eye has not been fit for the dominant task. This is more common in cases in which a clear eye dominance cannot be established during in-office testing. In the vast majority of cases, simply switching eye function between the eyes alleviates all symptoms, and the patient becomes successful.

SUMMARY

This chapter presented an overview of important fitting and problem-solving considerations of bifocal contact lens designs. It is hoped that this information will be of value in determining who is a good candidate and what lens material(s) would be most beneficial. Bifocal contact lenses represent potentially the biggest contact lens market. The new and improved designs and materials make bifocal contact lenses a viable option for every interested and eligible presbyopic patient.

CLINICAL CASES

CASE 1

A 56-year-old patient is undergoing an eye examination in your office. During the course of the examination, this patient "inquires" about contact lenses, showing mild interest. Her refractive findings are as follows:

$$OD + 0.50 - 0.25 \times 180 \; 20/20$$
$$OS + 0.25 - 0.25 \times 180 \; 20/20$$
$$Add +2.25 \; D$$

Her TBUT is 4 seconds OU.

SOLUTION: Contact lens wear appears to be contraindicated for this patient. The ambivalent motivation, in combination with poor tear quality and small distance error, would most likely result in failure. After thorough education on fees, lens design and care, and ocular dryness, if the patient's motivation appears to be good, the patient might be fit in a bifocal lens on the nondominant eye only. A material like the Proclear or a silicone hydrogel material would be recommended due to her low TBUT.

CASE 2

A 46-year-old patient is strongly motivated for bifocal contact lenses. She is a first-time wearer who is especially interested in soft contact lenses. Her refraction is as follows:

$$OD -3.75 - 0.25 \times 180 \; 20/20$$
$$OS -3.50 - 0.25 \times 180 \; 20/20$$
$$Add +1.00 \; D$$

Keratometry readings:

$$OD \; 42.00 \; @ \; 180; \; 42.50 \; @ \; 090$$
$$OS \; 42.25 \; @ \; 180; \; 42.50 \; @ \; 090$$

Dominant eye: OD

The preliminary evaluation shows the presence of an inferiorly positioned lower lid (i.e., 1 mm below the limbus). All other findings indicate she is a good bifocal contact lens candidate.

SOLUTION: This patient appears to be a good candidate for any of the available soft bifocal lens designs. All the options should be explained, and if she is still interested, one of these designs can be diagnostically fitted.

If Acuvue Oasys for Presbyopia was selected, the trial lenses would be

$$OD \; BCR \; 8.4 \; mm, \; Rx \; -3.75 \; D \; Add \; Low$$
$$OS \; BCR \; 8.4 \; mm, \; Rx \; -3.50 \; D \; Add \; Low$$

The patient sees 20/25 OU at distance and 20/20 OU at near. A −0.25 D overrefraction OD improves distance acuity to 20/20 OU and does not affect near vision. The patient is sent home for 1 to 2 weeks with the following trial lenses:

OD BCR 8.4 mm, Rx −4.00 D, Add Low
OS BCR 8.4 mm, Rx −3.50 D Add Low

Another option might be the Proclear EP.

If Proclear EP lenses were chosen, the initial diagnostic lenses would be

OD BCR 8.7 mm, Rx −3.75 D
OS BCR 8.7 mm, Rx −3.50 D

CASE 3

A 53-year-old patient is strongly motivated for soft bifocal contact lens wear. She has worn spherical soft lenses before presbyopia developed. She then attempted monovision and failed because she did not like the loss of stereoacuity. She is currently wearing reading glasses over her distance vision soft lenses but desires to be spectacle-free. Her refraction is as follows:

OD $-3.00 - 0.25 \times 090$ 20/20
OS -2.75 DS 20/20
Add $+2.00$ D

Keratometry readings:

OD 43.00 @ 180; 43.25 @ 090
OS 43.50 DS

Dominant eye: OD

Her TBUT is 10 seconds.

Her lower lid is positioned slightly above (0.5 mm) the limbus. All other findings indicate that she is a good bifocal contact lens candidate.

SOLUTION: This patient would be a good candidate for any soft bifocal lens design that can provide a +2.00 D add. If this patient is fit with the Biofinity Multifocal, the following trial lenses would be selected:

OD BCR 8.6 mm, Rx −3.00 D Add +2.00 D lens
OS BCR 8.6 mm, Rx −2.75 D Add +2.00 N lens

With these lenses, her distance vision was 20/30 OU and her near vision 20/20 OU. Monocular acuities should then be checked. Monocular acuities were OD 20/30 at distance and 20/25 at near, and OS 20/30 at distance and 20/20 at near. A −0.25 D trial lens over the OD improves monocular distance acuity to 20/20. The patient is sent home with the following lenses:

OD BCR 8.6 mm, Rx −3.25 D Add +2.00 D lens
OS BCR 8.6 mm, Rx −2.75 D Add +2.00 N lens

Distance and near acuities are 20/20 OU. The patient is to return for a follow-up visit in 1 to 2 weeks.

CASE 4

Your 48-year-old patient is a long-term soft lens wearer. He has recently noticed that his near vision is not as good as it used to be. He is currently wearing Air Optix Night and Day. His examination reveals the following:

OD −4.50 D 20/20
OS −5.00 D 20/20
Add +1.50 D

Keratometry readings:

OD 42.00 @ 180; 42.25 @ 090
OS 42.50 DS

Dominant eye: OS

His TBUT is 10 seconds.

SOLUTION: This patient is a good candidate for bifocal contact lens wear. This patient is fit with Air Optix Aqua Multifocal. The diagnostic lenses selected for this patient would be

OD BCR 8.6 mm, Rx −4.25 D Add Med
OS BCR 8.6 mm, Rx −4.75 D Add Med

Vision is good with the trial lenses.

The patient can go home wearing the trial lenses and return for follow-up in 1 to 2 weeks. The authors would recommend 2 weeks.

CASE 5

A long-term soft toric patient, who has worn monovision for about 3 years, wants to try bifocal contact lenses. He replaces his current contact lenses on a monthly basis. His spectacle Rx is

OD −2.50 − 1.25 × 180 VA 20/20
OS −2.00 − 1.75 × 180 VA 20/20
Add +1.50 D

Dominant eye: OD
Keratometry readings:

OD 43.00 @ 180; 44.00 @ 090
OS 43.00 @ 180; 44.25 @ 090

His TBUT is 9 seconds.

SOLUTION: This patient would be a good candidate for the Proclear Multifocal Toric lens. Diagnostic lenses can be ordered for the patient. For this patient, as no vertexing back to the cornea is necessary, contact lenses matching the spectacle prescription can be ordered and the identical add used. Based on the more recent fitting guidelines, both eyes would start with a D lens. At the dispensing visit, acceptable vision is 20/20 at distance and near OU with 20/40 or better at near with the OD and 20/40 or better distance acuity with the OS. This lens is a monthly replacement lens and is good for less than ideal tear quality. Ideally, the patient would have a TBUT $\geq$10 seconds for good tear quality. If the vision falls within the acceptable range at the dispensing, the patient should wear the lenses on a trial basis and return for follow-up in 1 to 2 weeks.

CASE 6

A 46-year-old woman has been wearing soft contact lenses since she was 15 years old. She has been tolerating her current soft lenses for the past few years by wearing some discount store readers over the top for near work. She is currently wearing PureVision lenses. She would like to try bifocal contact lenses. She would like to not have to rely on the readers all the time and they tend to break often.
Her current refraction is

OD −3.50 DS Add +1.50 D Dominant eye
OS −3.25 DS Add +1.50 D

Keratometry readings:

42.00 @ 180; 42.50 @ 90 OU

SOLUTION: The patient is fit with PureVision Multi-Focals. Her diagnostic lenses are

OD BCR 8.6 mm −3.75 D Add High
OS BCR 8.6 mm −3.50 D Add High

The patient has 20/20 vision at distance and 20/30 at near. Increased plus over the left eye affects her distance vision slightly and she prefers to try the diagnostic lenses. At a 2-week follow-up visit, she is reasonably happy with her new lenses. She finds that probably 90% of the time she can see well for driving, computer, and near work. Occasionally, when she is sewing or reading smaller print materials, she has difficulty seeing optimally. The dispensary has a selection of premade readers in high-quality frames and lenses. The patient purchases a pair of +1.00 D readers to carry in her purse for those occasional times she needs a little more help and has a pair of discount readers from a dollar store tucked in her sewing bag. Even though she still could use some reading glasses occasionally, the majority of the time she can get along without them.

CASE 7

This 45-year-old patient is a current GP lens wearer who is beginning to be symptomatic at near. He enjoys playing squash and basketball. His refraction shows the following:

$$OD: +4.00 - 1.00 \times 180 \; 20/20$$
$$OS: +4.50 - 1.25 \times 005 \; 20/20$$
$$Add \; +1.00 \; D$$

The pupil size is normal (4.5 mm), and the lower lid is positioned 1 mm below the limbus. All other findings indicate that this patient is a good bifocal contact lens candidate.

SOLUTION: All presbyopic contact lens options should be explained to this patient. If this patient is receptive to a bifocal design, an aspheric design can be considered, especially since this patient is an early presbyope. The position of the lower lid and possibly the refractive error may contraindicate an alternating design. Likewise, he is very active and these lenses would be much less likely to dislodge than a translating design.

CASE 8

A 44-year-old male patient had been a long-term spherical GP wearer and was recently refit into a back surface aspheric GP lens design. The patient was pleased with both vision at all distances and comfort with these lenses. However, despite changes in both BCR and diameter, the lenses positioned superiorly and exhibited very little (if any) movement with the blink. Corneal topography revealed superior flattening (approximately 2.25 D change 2.5 mm superior from center and 3 D of steepening 3 mm inferior from center immediately) after lens removal. In addition, there was mild distortion evident superiorly OU.

SOLUTION: This is a good case for the use of a front surface aspheric GP design. The lens should position more centrally and the spherical back surface should minimize the topography changes that resulted with the back surface aspheric design.

CASE 9

A 50-year-old female patient has been a 7-year wearer of the ESSential Multifocal lens design (Blanchard). She has recently been experiencing blurred vision when performing critical near work, especially reading. Her refraction information is as follows:
Refraction:

$$OD: -6.50 - 1.50 \times 172 \; 20/20$$
$$OS: -6.25 - 1.50 \times 006 \; 20/20$$
$$Add \; +2.00 \; D$$

Keratometry readings:

$$OD: 43.00 \; @ \; 180; \; 44.25 \; @ \; 090$$
$$OS: 43.25 \; @ \; 180; \; 44.50 \; @ \; 090$$

Her anatomical measurements are the following:
Lower-lid position: 1 mm below the limbus
Pupil size: 3.5 mm
She is wearing the following lenses in a "modified bifocal approach."
OD: ESSentials Series II: BCR: 7.67 mm OAD: 9.5 mm Power: −7.00 D
OS: ESSentials Series III: BCR: 7.63 mm OAD: 9.5 mm Power: −6.50 D
VA: 20/20 OD, OS and OU at distance; 20/40 OD, 20/30+2 at near. A +1.00 D overrefraction over OD and +0.75 D over OS resulted in 20/20 at near.
Both lenses exhibited good centration and about 1 mm lag with the blink.

SOLUTION: Reorder the lenses in a Series II OU with the same lens parameters but order with a +1.00 D CSA on the front surface OU. With a small pupil diameter, it is apparent that this patient required a higher add earlier than with most presbyopic patients. A 4.0 mm central distance zone is also recommended to optimize near vision via mild translation of the lens with downward gaze.

CASE 10

This 49-year-old patient is a former spherical GP lens wearer who discontinued contact lens wear 2 years ago after failing to achieve adequate vision at distance and near with monovision. Currently, he is wearing progressive addition spectacles, but as a result of his prescription, he is very motivated to return to contact lens wear. His refraction and keratometric measurements are as follows:

Refraction:

OD: −5.00 − 1.00 × 005 20/20
OS: −4.50 − 1.50 × 175 20/20
Add +1.75 D

Keratometry readings:

OD: 42.00 @ 180; 43.00 @ 090
OS: 42.50 @ 180; 44.00 @ 090

His anatomical measurements are the following:

Lower-lid position: 0.5 mm above the limbus

Pupil size: 5.5 mm

All other findings indicate that this patient is a good bifocal contact lens candidate.

SOLUTION: Once all of the options have been explained to this patient, it is very likely he will be fit with a translating design such as the Tangent Streak. Using the fitting guide, the following diagnostic lenses can be selected:

	OD	OS
BCR	8.08 mm	7.94 mm
OAD	9.4/9.0 mm	9.4/9.0 mm
Power	−2.00/+2.00 D Add	−2.00/+2.00 D Add

If the lens fits as predicted, the overrefraction is equal to the predicted value, and the segment position is at or near the lower pupil margin, the following lens design could be ordered:

	OD	OS
BCR	8.08 mm	7.94 mm
OAD	9.4/9.0 (11−2) mm	9.4/9.0 (11−2) mm
Power	−4.50/+1.75 D Add (the −4.50 results from vertexing the −5.00 D sphere to −4.75 and adding the +0.25 D tear lens power compensation)	−4.25/+1.75 D Add (the −4.25 results from vertexing the −4.50 D sphere to −4.25)
Seg height	4.2 mm	4.2 mm
Prism	2.00 PD	2.00 PD

CASE 11

Solitaire lens (Truform Optics) diagnostically fit to a motivated and qualified candidate both moves and rotates excessively after the blink on the right eye. The patient's refractive, keratometric, and lens design information is provided below:

Refraction: −2.00 −0.75 ×170 20/20
Add +2.00 D

Keratometry: 43.00 @ 180; 43.75 @ 090

Lens design:
>
> BCR: 7.85 mm (43.00 D)
> Power: −2.00/+2.00 D Add
> Prism: Standard

SOLUTION: A flatter BCR lens should be selected; for example, 42.50 D (remember: make the design change a *significant* one). If excessive rotation is still present, increasing the prism should be considered.

CASE 12

A 53-year-old wearer of the Solutions Bifocal (X-Cel) inquired if there was any way she could achieve better vision from her contact lenses when she is working at her computer. She spends several hours every day at her computer and for the past 2 years has been wearing a pair of +1.00 D reading glasses she bought at a pharmacy.

SOLUTION: With the increasing number of translating designs with an intermediate correction, this patient would benefit from any one of these designs. As she is already wearing the Solutions Bifocal, it would be recommended to refit her into the Essential Solutions. The aspheric back surface will assist in providing an intermediate correction while the segmented crescent front surface design will continue to provide her with both distance and near correction.

CASE 13

A monovision wearer has symptoms of fatigue when performing prolonged near work. These symptoms initiated after she changed to a job that required long periods of intense near work.

SOLUTION: Prescribing a pair of "overspectacles" is recommended. Plus is prescribed over the distance eye and plano over the near eye to relieve the visual fatigue caused by a monovision correction.

A better option would be to refit this patient in multifocal soft lenses for a trial period to see if she might be happier. There are some indications that it may take longer for her to adapt to multifocals since she is an adapted monovision wearer. At minimum, a discussion of her options should take place.

CLINICAL PROFICIENCY CHECKLIST

- Bifocal contact lenses are increasing in popularity, and new technology has resulted in better lens designs and successful fitting. Bifocal contact lenses are preferred over monovision fitting.
- The best candidates for bifocal contact lens correction include those who are very motivated, have good tear quality, and have >1 D of refractive error. Patients with poor tear quality, eye disease, amblyopia, or poor motivation should be ruled out.
- There are numerous simultaneous vision (i.e., the patient views through the distance and near zones at the same time) soft bifocal designs, including center-near and center-distance designs, either aspheric or concentric, and a translating design.
- The increased popularity of soft bifocal designs can be contributed to disposable/frequent-replacement lenses, silicone hydrogel materials, and toric multifocal lenses. Disposable/frequent-replacement lenses allow the practitioner to fit lenses from inventory and have the patient wear the lenses on a trial basis. In addition, deposit-related problems and torn lenses are less of an issue because of the regular replacement schedule and spare lenses.

(continued)

- There are several available simultaneous vision GP bifocal lens designs, including aspheric and center-distance and center-near concentric designs. The primary benefit of the aspheric designs is good vision for early presbyopes and persons requiring good intermediate vision. The primary limitations include the need for good lens centration, achieving high add powers for advanced presbyopes, and reduced vision at distance if pupil size is large.
- Alternating vision bifocal designs include one-piece "no image jump" segmented designs, a fuse segmented design, and an alternating distance-center concentric design.
- The segmented, translating designs have a good probability of success, especially with advanced presbyopic patients. This is true because if the lenses are fitting and translating properly, the patient will be viewing through the distance zone when viewing at a distance and the near zone when viewing at near. Patients who have a low lower-lid position (i.e., 1 mm or more below the lower limbus), very loose lower-lid tension, or tight lids (creating excessive lens rotation) are not good candidates for these lenses.
- When fitting a segmented GP bifocal design, it is extremely important to take careful measurements of the patient's pupil size, corneal diameter, and distance from the lower lid to the center of the pupil.
- For monovision patients, it is important to select a wettable contact lens material, perform binocular function testing to determine the effect of loss of stereopsis, select the proper eye for near (often the nondominant eye, although it should be the eye with reduced vision or with higher myopia if anisometropia is present), and encourage either "driving" spectacles or a second distance contact lens.
- Another contact lens option for presbyopic patients is the use of reading glasses over a spherical (distance-only) contact lens prescription. Although this option provides the benefits of ease of fit, optimum vision at distance and near, and limited expense, most patients will be unhappy with the frequent application and removal of spectacles.

REFERENCES

1. Schwartz CA. Portrait of a presbyope in 1999. *Optom Today.* 1999;(Suppl):5–7.
2. Meyler J, Veys J. A new pupil-intelligent design for presbyopic correction. *Optician.* 1999;217:18–23.
3. Edwards K. Contact lens problem-solving: bifocal contact lenses. *Optician.* 1999;218:26–32.
4. Bennett ES, Jurkus JM. Presbyopic correction. In: Bennett ES, Weissman BA, eds. *Clinical Contact Lens Practice.* 2nd ed. Philadelphia, PA: Lippincott Williams and Wilkins; 2005; 531–548.
5. Morgan PB, Efron N, Woods CA. International contact lens prescribing survey consortium. *Clin Exp Optom.* 2011;94(1):87–92.
6. Edmonds F, Reindel W. As cited in Tan J: "Contact Lens Options for Presbyopia" http://www.siliconehydrogels.org/editorial_jackie_tan.asp. Accessed January 2012.
7. Studebaker J. Soft multifocals: practice growth opportunity. *Contact lens Spectrum.* 2009;24(6):40–43.
8. Bennett ES. Bifocal and multifocal contact lenses. In: Phillips AJ, Speedwell L, eds. *Contact Lens Practice.* 5th ed. Oxford, UK: Butterworth-Heinemann; 2006;311–331.
9. Pujol J, Gispets J, Arjona M. Optical performance in eyes wearing two multifocal contact lens designs. *Ophthalmol Physiol Opt.* 2003;23:347–360.
10. Morgan PB, Woods CA, Tranoudis IG, et al. International contact lens prescribing in 2011. *Contact Lens Spectrum.* 2012;27(1):26–31.
11. Jones L, Jones D, Langley C, et al. Reactive or proactive contact lens fitting – does it make a difference? *J Br Contact Lens Assoc.* 1996;19(2):41–43.
12. Schwartz C, Bennett ES. How RGPs changed my life *Optom Manag.* 1997;32(4):51–56.
13. Bennett ES. Bifocal contact lenses changed my life. *Contact Lens Spectrum.* 1999;14(10):19.
14. Fisher K, Bauman E, Schwallie J. Evaluation of two new soft contact lenses for correction of presbyopia: the Focus Progressives Multifocal and the Acuvue Bifocal. *Int Cont lens Clin.* 1999;26:92–103.
15. Martin DK, Dain SJ. Postural modifications of VDU operators wearing bifocal spectacles. *Appl Ergonom.* 1988;19:293–300.
16. Afanador AJ, Aitsebaomo P, Gertzman DR. Eye and head contribution to gaze at near through multifocals: the useable field of view. *Am J Optom Physiol Opt.* 1986;63:187–192.

17. Bennett ES. Contact lens correction of presbyopia. *Clin Exp Optom.* 2008;91:265–278.
18. Jurkus JM, Nichols S. Contact lenses and the aging eye. *Optom Today.* 1999;7(3) (suppl):53–60.
19. Bennett ES, Weissman BA, Remba MR. Contact lenses and the older adult. In: *Rosenbloom & Morgan's Vision and Aging.* St. Louis, MO: Elsevier; 2007;215–240.
20. du Toit, Situ P, Simpson T, et al. The effects of six months of contact lens wear on the tear film, ocular surfaces, and symptoms of presbyopes. *Optom Vis Sci.* 2001;78:455–462.
21. Hansen DW. Current concepts of RGP multifocal contact lenses. *Practical Optom.* 1992;3(2):70–78.
22. Andres S, Henriques A, Garcia ML, et al. Factors of the precorneal fluid breakup time (BUT) and tolerance of contact lenses. *Int Cont Lens Clin.* 1987;4:81–120.
23. Bennett ES, Jurkus JM, Schwartz CA. Bifocal contact lenses. In: Bennett ES, Henry VA, eds. *Clinical Manual of Contact Lenses.* 2nd ed. Philadelphia, PA: Lippincott Williams & Wilkins; 2000:410–449.
24. Bennett ES, Hansen D. Presbyopia: gas permeable bifocal fitting and problem-solving. In: Bennett ES, Hom MM, eds. *Manual of Gas-Permeable Contact Lenses.* 2nd ed. St. Louis, MO: Elsevier Science; 2004:324–356.
25. Josephson J, Caffery B. Hydrogel bifocal lenses. In: Bennett ES, Weissman BA, eds. *Clinical Contact Lens Practice.* Philadelphia, PA: JB Lippincott; 1991:43.1–43.12.
26. Friant RJ. When bifocal lenses are most likely to succeed. *Contact Lens Spectrum.* 1986;1(6):14–23.
27. Gispets J, Arjona M, Pujol J. Image quality in wearers of a center-distance concentric design bifocal contact lens. *Ophthalmic Physiol Opt.* 2002;22:221–223.
28. Mack CJ. Contact lenses 2007. *Contact Lens Spectrum.* 2008;23(1):26–34.
29. Kirby J. 2007 Annual contact lens update. *Optom Manag.* 2007;42(4):26–28.
30. Norman CW. Communicate and demonstrate soft multifocal benefits. *Contact Lens Spectrum.* 2003;18(9):15.
31. Watanabe RK. Design characteristics of two new soft multifocals. *Contact Lens Spectrum.* 2010;25(2):18.
32. Davis RL. Contact lens options for presbyopes. *Optom Manag.* 2004;39(4):37–43.
33. Andre M. Proclear 1 day multifocal. Presented at: Annual Workshop of the Association of Optometric Contact Lens Educators; June 2012; Bloomington, IN.
34. Flexlens product information. http://www.xcelcontacts.com/our-lenses/flexlens-multi. Accessed July 2012.
35. Product Spectrum: line of custom soft lenses now available. *Contact Lens Spectrum.* 2008;23(9):52.
36. Pence NA. Can I get that in a silicone hydrogel? *Contact Lens Spectrum.* 2010;25(11):23.
37. Bennett ES, Henry VA. Contemporary multifocal primer. *Contact Lens Spectrum.* 2012;27(2):24–32.
38. Bergenske PD. The presbyopic fitting process. *Contact Lens Spectrum.* 2001;16(8):34.
39. Jimenez JR, Durban JJ, Anera RG. Maximum disparity with Acuvue bifocal contact lenses with changes in illumination. *Optom Vis Sci.* 2002;79:170–174.
40. Pence NA. Two new SiHy options. *Contact Lens Spectrum.* 2011;26(11):21.
41. Henry VA. Soft multifocals – fitting and case presentations. Presented at: 47th Annual Meeting of the Heart of America Contact Lens and Primary Care Congress; February 2008; Kansas City, MO.
42. Gasson A, Morris J. Lenses for presbyopia. In: Gasset A, Morris J, eds. *The Contact Lens Manual.* 3rd ed. London: Butterworth-Heinemann; 2003:298–317.
43. Ezekial DF, Ezekial DJ. A soft bifocal lens that does not compromise vision. *Contact Lens Spectrum.* 2002;17(6):40–42.
44. http://www.gelflex.com/pdf/triton_. Last accessed February 28, 2008.
45. Quinn TG. The role of ocular dominance in presbyopic lens correction. *Contact Lens Spectrum.* 2007;22(1):48.
46. Gromacki SJ. Preventing contact lens challenges for presbyopes. *Contact Lens Spectrum.* 2004;19(8):S1–S8.
47. Richdale K. Presbyopic soft lens design options. *Contact Lens Spectrum.* 2008;23(3):34.
48. Lieblein JS. Finding success with multifocal contact lenses. *Contact Lens Spectrum.* 2000;14(3):50–51.
49. Byrnes SP, Cannella A. An in-office evaluation of a multifocal RGP lens design. *Contact Lens Spectrum.* 1999;14(11):29–33.
50. Anderson G. A GP bifocal for active presbyopes. *Optom Manag.* 2003;38(6):74.
51. Smith VM, Koffler BH, Litteral G. Evaluation of the ZEBRA 2000 (Z10) Breger Vision bifocal contact lens. *CLAO J.* 2000;26(4):214–220.
52. Bierman A. Beyond monovision. *Optom Manag.* 2003;38(4):70.
53. Hansen DW. RGP bifocals and computer users—the real world. *Contact Lens Spectrum.* 1996;11(2):15.
54. Ames K. Fitting the presbyope with gas permeable contact lenses. *Contact Lens Spectrum.* 2001;16(10):42–45.
55. Businger U, Byrnes S, Baker R. An RGP multifocal for moderate to high presbyopes. *Contact Lens Spectrum.* 2000;15(10). Available at www.clspectrum.com/articleviewer.aspx?articleid=12035. Accessed April 2013.
56. Kirman St, Kirman GS. The Tangent Streak bifocal contact lens. *Contact Lens Forum.* 1988;13(6):38–40.
57. Remba MJ. The Tangent Streak rigid gas permeable bifocal contact lens. *J Am Optom Assoc.* 1988;59(3):212–216.
58. Bennett ES. The RGP bifocal patient: how to optimize success. *Optom Today.* 1996;4(1):16–17.
59. Bennett ES. Researching GP multifocals. *Contact Lens Spectrum.* 2005;20(2):21.
60. Hansen DW. Multifocal contact lenses – the next generation. *Contact Lens Spectrum.* 2002;17(11):42–48.
61. Bennett ES, Luk B. Rigid gas permeable bifocal contact lenses: an update. *Optom Today.* 2001;15:34–36.
62. Bennett ES. Sclerals for dry-eyed presbyopes. *Contact Lens Spectrum.* 2012;27(7):19.
63. Fonda G. *Trans Ophthalmol Soc Australia.* 1966;25:46–50.
64. Schachet JL, Kading D, Lowinger S, et al. Multifocals: the new standard of care. *Contact Lens Spectrum.* 2012;27(6)(suppl):3–5.

65. Nichols JJ. Market and survey data suggest 2011 was a year of rebuilding for many. *Contact Lens Spectrum.* 2012;27(1):20.
66. Benjamin W. Comparing multifocals and monovision. *Contact Lens Spectrum.* 2007;22:35–39.
67. Richdale K, Mitchell GL, Zadnik K. Comparison of multifocal and monovision soft contact lens corrections in patients with low astigmatic presbyopia. *Optom Vis Sci.* 2006;83:266–273.
68. Situ P, Du Toit R, Fonn D, et al. Successful monovision contact lens wearers refitted with bifocal contact lenses. *Eye Contact Lens.* 2003;29:181–184.
69. Johnson J, Bennett ES, Henry VA. Multivision™ versus monovision: a comparative study. Presented at: Annual Meeting of the Contact Lens Association of Ophthalmologists; Febrauary 2000; Las Vegas, NV.
70. Rajagopalan AS, Bennett ES, Lakshminarayanan V. Visual performance of subjects wearing presbyopic contact lenses. *Optom Vis Sci.* 2006;83(8):611–615.
71. Woods J, Woods CA, Fonn D. Early symptomatic presbyopes—what correction modality works best? *Eye Contact Lens.* 2009;35(5):221–226.
72. Westin E, Wick B, Harrist RB. Factors influencing success of monovision contact lens fitting: survey of contact lens diplomates. *Optometry.* 2000;71(12):757–763.
73. Jain S, Arora I, Azar DT. Success of monovision in presbyopes: review of the literature and potential applications to refractive surgery. *Surv Ophthalmol.* 1996;40:491–499.
74. Collins MJ, Goode A. Interocular blur suppression and monovision. *Acta Ophthalmol.* 1994;72(3):376–380.
75. Nakagawara VB, Veronneau SJH. Monovision contact lens use in the aviation environment: a report of a contact lens-related aircraft accident. *Optometry.* 2000;71:390–395.
76. Gasson A, Morris J. Lenses for presbyopia. In: Gasset A, Morris J, eds. *The Contact Lens Manual.* 3rd ed. London: Butterworth-Heinemann; 2003:298–317.
77. Kirschen DG, Hung CC, Nakano TR. Comparison of suppression, stereoacuity and interocular differences in visual acuity in monovision, and Acuvue Bifocal contact lenses. *Optom Vis Sci.* 1999;76:832–837.
78. Richdale K, Mitchell GL, Zadnik K. Comparison of multifocal and monovision soft contact lens corrections in patients with low-astigmatic presbyopia. *Optom Vis Sci.* 2006;83(5):266–273.
79. Heath DA, Hines C, Schwartz F. Suppression behavior analyzed as a function of monovision addition power. *Am J Optom Physiol Opt.* 1986;63:198–201.
80. Larsen WL, Lachance A. Stereoscopic acuity with induced refractive errors. *Am J Optom Physiol Opt.* 1983;60:509–513.
81. Collins MJ, Goode A, Brown B. Distance visual acuity and monovision. *Optom Vis Sci.* 1993;70:723–728.
82. Loshin DS, Loshin MS, Comer G. Binocular summation with monovision contact lens correction for presbyopia. *Int Cont Lens Clin.* 1982;9:161–165.
83. Collins MJ, Brown B, Bowman KJ. Contrast sensitivity with contact lens correction for presbyopia. *Ophthalmic Physiol Opt.* 1989;9:133–138.
84. Wick B, Westin E. Change in refractive anisometropia in presbyopic adults wearing monovision contact lens correction. *Optom Vis Sci.* 1999;76:33–39.
85. Wood JM. Aging, driving and vision. *Clin Exp Optom.* 2002;85(4):214–220.
86. Josephson JE, Caffery BE. Monovision versus aspheric bifocal contact lenses: a crossover study. *J Am Optom Assoc.* 1987;58:652–654.
87. Johannsdottir KR, Stelmach LB. Monovision: a review of the scientific literature. *Optom Vis Sci.* 2001;78:646–651.
88. Hansen DW. It's time to minimize monovision. *Contact Lens Spectrum.* 2001:16(1):15.
89. Wood JM, Wick K, Shuley V, et al. The effect of monovision contact lens wear on driving performance. *Clin Exp Optom.* 1998;81(3):100–103.
90. Harris MG, Classe JG. Clinicolegal considerations of monovision. *J Am Optom Assoc.* 1988;59:491–495.
91. Erickson P, McGill EC. Role of visual acuity, stereoacuity and ocular dominance in monovision patient success. *Optom Vis Sci.* 1992;69:761–764.
92. Davis RL. Pinpoint success with GP multifocal lenses. *Contact Lens Spectrum.* 2003;18(10):25–38.
93. McGill EC, Erickson P. Sighting dominance and monovision distance binocular fusional ranges. *J Am Optom Assoc.* 1991;62(10):738–742.
94. MacAlister GO, Woods CA. Monovision versus RGP translating bifocals. *J Br Contact Lens Assoc.* 1991;14:173–178.
95. du Toit R, Ferreira JT, Nel ZJ. Visual and nonvisual variables implicated in monovision wear. *Optom Vis Sci.* 1998;75(2):119–125.
96. Erickson DB, Erickson P. Psychological factors and sex differences in acceptance of monovision. *Percept Mot Skills.* 2000;91(3, pt 2):1113–1119.
97. Hom MM. Monovision and bifocals. In Hom MM, ed. *Manual of Contact Lens Fitting and Prescribing with CD-ROM.* 2nd ed. Boston: Butterworth-Heinemann; 2000;327–354.
98. Schwartz CA, Jurkus JM. Troubleshooting the monovision fit. *Contact Lens Forum.* 1991;16(4):24–26.

Chapter 16

Overnight Contact Lens Wear

Kathy Dumbleton and Lyndon Jones

INTRODUCTION

While most patients choose to wear their lenses on a daily basis, removing them at the end of each day before going to sleep, this modality does not offer the convenience of permanent vision correction sought by many contact lens wearers. The opportunity for day and night lens wear has therefore been attractive to contact lens wearers since their very inception. This modality of contact lens wear is referred to as extended (up to 6 consecutive nights) wear (EW) or continuous (up to 30 consecutive nights) wear (CW).[1] Overnight lens wear first became a reality some 35 years ago,[2–4] but its popularity and success have been extremely turbulent over this time.

Overnight contact lens wear has historically been associated with a high rate of complications[5–7] and, as a result, practitioners and patients alike have become concerned about the potential safety issues associated with EW. Hypoxic complications, resulting from poor oxygen supply to the cornea, were common with low-oxygen permeability (Dk) materials.[8,9] Fortunately, with the widespread use of silicone hydrogel materials and high-Dk rigid gas-permeable (GP) materials, these complications are now relatively rare.[1,10–12] Unfortunately, the major concern with overnight lens wear, corneal infection, still remains.[13–21]

For overnight lens wear to be successful, contact lenses must not only be convenient, they must also be safe and comfortable. While the risk of microbial keratitis (MK) remains the major source of anxiety associated with overnight lens wear, comfort and dryness are also major limiting factors for patients desiring the convenience of this modality of lens wear.

HISTORY OF EXTENDED WEAR

Throughout the 1970s and early 1980s, manufacturers released a variety of materials that were intended for overnight wear. These early materials were often worn for up to a month at a time without being removed and achieved great commercial success, with John de Carle reporting success with over 2,000 patients in the early 1970s and other authors reporting similarly high levels of clinical success up to the mid-1980s.[22–26] As a result of such positive data, EW for cosmetic use for up to 30 days was approved by the US Food and Drug Administration (FDA) in 1981, sparking an explosion in the number of patients being fitted with lenses for overnight wear. However, very soon afterward, reports of corneal ulceration with significant vision loss began appearing in journals,[27,28] and the safety of overnight wear was questioned in both peer-reviewed journals and the lay media. The Contact Lens Institute in the United States sponsored studies to investigate the relative risk and incidence of infectious keratitis. The results from these studies were published in 1989[5,6] and clearly demonstrated that overnight wear of lenses carried with it a significantly increased risk of corneal infection. As a result, the FDA immediately reduced the approved length of time for overnight wear without removal from 30 to 7 days.

In the mid-1980s, it was believed that the corneal infections seen with overnight wear were probably due to poor hygiene and compliance and that the principal factor driving such infection rates was because of patients reinserting poorly disinfected lenses. It was hypothesized that using lenses on a disposable or frequent-replacement basis, in which the lenses were inserted once only and then discarded upon removal, would likely have an impact on the infection rates reported. Such a concept became a clinical reality with the introduction of disposable EW lenses to the United States in 1987. The first published large-scale study appeared to support such a concept,[29] but soon thereafter, reports of infectious keratitis started to appear.[30] The final proof that disposability had no impact on the rate of ulceration with conventional hydrogel materials worn overnight came with the publication of a paper in 1999,[7] which showed that the rate of ulcerative keratitis was exactly that found 10 years previously in the United States,[5,6] before disposability was commonplace. This publication clearly showed that overnight wear with conventional soft lens materials should be discouraged due to the increased risk that such a modality had on the development of sight-threatening keratitis.

Despite this, patients still seek methods to liberate them of spectacles, with refractive surgery being extremely popular, despite the known risks.[31–37] Patients still sleep in lenses overnight even when told not to do so, with an estimated 32% of patients in the United States reporting that they sleep in their lenses occasionally, frequently, or almost every night.[38] Clearly, some patients continue to desire a lens that can be worn overnight and will undertake this procedure whether their practitioner sanctions it or not and regardless of the fact that they acknowledge that "infection" is a potential consequence if they sleep in lenses.[39] To determine the potential safety of materials to be worn overnight, at least from the perspective of hypoxia, requires a detailed knowledge of the oxygen requirements of the cornea.

CORNEAL OXYGEN REQUIREMENTS AND OXYGEN TRANSMISSIBILITY

The cornea is avascular and derives most of its oxygen supply from the atmosphere. Any contact lens acts as a potential barrier to oxygen transport and the ability of a material to transport oxygen through the lens is a major factor in determining the clinical success of that material.

Oxygen delivery to the cornea through the lens depends upon both the Dk of the material and the thickness (t) of the lens in question. The Dk of conventional hydrogels is directly related to the amount of water that a polymer can hold, as the oxygen dissolves into the water phase of the material and diffuses through the lens from the anterior to the posterior lens surface. The Dk increases logarithmically with increasing water content of the material,[40] and can be determined from the water content using either the nonedge corrected Fatt formula ($Dk = 2.0 \times 10^{-11} e^{0.0411 WC}$)[41] or boundary and edge-corrected Morgan and Efron formula ($Dk = 1.67 \times 10^{-11} e^{0.0397 WC}$),[42] in which "WC" is the quoted water content of the material concerned. The units of Dk are 10^{-11} (cm^2/sec) (mL O$_2$/mL $\times$ mm Hg) or "barrer". The term Dk/t describes the oxygen transmissibility of a lens and gives a quantitative indication of the amount of oxygen that a lens-wearing eye will receive through the lens and is a more clinically useful number than Dk, which gives no indication of the effect of lens thickness or lens design.[43] The units of Dk/t are 10^{-9} (cm/sec) (mL O$_2$/mL $\times$ mm Hg).

The minimum acceptable oxygen level to prevent edema is a critical factor in determining the clinical success of a particular lens for a particular patient. Studies using Dk/t values to determine minimum oxygen levels for overnight wear calculate the Dk/t of a lens type, place lenses of varying oxygen transmissibilities on the cornea of individuals, and then use a physiological marker of some description to determine the response of the cornea to that level of oxygen. The marker most commonly used is corneal swelling. In a landmark study, Holden and Mertz[44] determined that a lens with a Dk/t of 87×10^{-9} units would limit overnight corneal swelling to 4%, which is a similar level of corneal swelling seen without lens wear. However, at that time no hydrogel lens could meet this criterion for EW. Therefore, based on the relationship between corneal swelling and Dk/t from their study, Holden and Mertz[44] suggested that a Dk/t of 34 units would be a suitable compromise for EW, since this Dk/t would induce an average of 8% overnight swelling and allow full recovery soon after eye opening. However, it must be reiterated that these values are "averages" and patients exhibit widely different corneal metabolic requirements.[45,46]

A different method of determining minimum oxygen requirements uses a modelling approach, in which a computational model of the cornea is developed to calculate a theoretical value. Fatt pioneered corneal oxygen distribution studies[47,48] and provided an early model of corneal oxygen profile underneath a lens, by considering the cornea as a single layer.[49] Later, Harvitt and Bonanno[50] updated Fatt's model to a five-layer mathematical model of distribution of oxygen tension across the cornea under a lens and included the effect of increasing acidification from contact lens wear on the corneal oxygen consumption model. They determined that a Dk/t of 125 units was the average required to prevent anoxia throughout the entire corneal thickness. Brennan[51] described several shortfalls of the Harvitt and Bonanno diffusion model, including an inherent problem with allowing theoretical consumption of oxygen when zero oxygen tension is predicted, as well as underestimating the average corneal thickness and overestimating average tear layer thickness, leading to overestimation of the required lens transmissibility to avoid corneal anoxia. Brennan[51] proposed an eight-layer model of corneal oxygenation during contact lens wear, in which the shortfalls of Harvitt and Bonanno's model were corrected. Using this model, he devised a mathematical method based on the total oxygen consumption of the cornea and estimated that lenses with a Dk/t of only 50 units for EW should suffice.[52]

Once the Dk/t of the lens in question is known and it is appreciated that such a lens material and design would provide the cornea with suitable levels of oxygenation, then the issue becomes more related to the suitability of the patient to safely adapt to overnight wear.

PATIENT SELECTION FOR OVERNIGHT LENS WEAR

Patient selection is crucial for success when prescribing contact lenses for any wearing modality, but is particularly important for EW and CW. Practitioners are fortunate to have a wide array of contact lens designs and materials available, allowing almost every patient to be successfully fitted. However, care must still be taken to select only those patients suitable for overnight lens wear and then to prescribe the most appropriate lens type for their individual optical, physiological, vocational, and environmental needs.

A thorough history is essential, not only to assess the patient's motivation and reasons for an overnight wearing modality, but also to evaluate their general and ocular health. Systemic disease, medications, allergies, dry eyes, and previous inflammation or infection may contraindicate how contact lenses are worn and information about the patient's occupation, work environment, and leisure pursuits may also be crucial.

Suitable Candidates

While this appraisal is not intended to serve as an exhaustive list, there are a number of good reasons for considering an overnight wear modality. A group of obvious candidates for CW are patients with high refractive errors who are vulnerable as a result of their unaided visual performance. These patients benefit enormously from being able to see clearly at all times, particularly when waking during the night. Other prospective patients include those who have an active lifestyle or occupation in which spectacle wear is hazardous or impractical. These groups may include members of the emergency workforce, who often undertake shift work with unpredictable hours and schedules. EW or CW may also be beneficial for parents of young children who demand functional vision within seconds of waking, day and night. There may also be situations where hygiene is a concern and patients are unable to disinfect or handle their contact lenses each day in a sanitary manner because of location. Examples include outdoor enthusiasts and military personnel. It is noteworthy that males are overrepresented in those patients who use lenses overnight, potentially reflecting their preference for the convenience afforded by an overnight wear modality.[53]

An overnight wear modality may also be used for a number of therapeutic, drug delivery, and bandage applications,[54–60] and in certain binocular conditions, where the chances of improving corrected visual acuity (VA) in the amblyopic eye are much greater with continuous visual correction. A group of potential candidates for EW or CW also worthy of mention is those individuals who are considering refractive surgery. These modalities of lens wear can be offered either in the short term, such that patients can experience 24-hour visual correction, or as a permanent alternative to irreversible surgical procedures. In addition, as mentioned earlier, many current contact lens wearers admit to occasionally or regularly sleeping while wearing their lenses and those individuals who report doing this should be proactively counseled on the options of EW and CW, when appropriate. For reasons such as these, practitioners continue to fit soft EW lenses to approximately 9% of their patients.[61]

Unsuitable Candidates

Unfortunately, not all prospective EW and CW candidates are suitable, due to their lifestyle, general health, or ocular appearance. Patients who have a history of noncompliance with instructions for wearing time, replacement frequency, and lens care should probably be avoided, since the consequences of being noncompliant when wearing lenses overnight are potentially higher than in a daily wear (DW) mode and these individuals have also been reported to be at a greater risk of infection, inflammation, and other complications with lens wear.[18,20,21,62–67] A number of studies have also reported a higher prevalence of infiltrative complications in smokers,[6,20,67–70] and while smoking is not strictly a contraindication to overnight wear, these patients should be counseled with respect to this factor. Another activity that has been reported to be associated with a higher risk of complications among lens wearers is swimming,[71–74] and for this reason, EW and CW modalities should be avoided for regular swimmers. General health is also a consideration and individuals with systemic conditions associated with increased inflammation or a slower healing response may be better suited to a DW modality.[75]

There are also a number of ocular conditions that can preclude overnight wear with contact lenses. Patients with chronic blepharitis or meibomian gland dysfunction typically have a higher bacterial load (especially gram-positive organisms) on the ocular adnexa,[76–78] increasing their risk for developing corneal infection or inflammation. Severely symptomatic dry-eye patients should also be avoided, since their chance of successful wear is unlikely and patients with chronic desiccation staining may also be better with a DW modality, as breaks in the epithelial barrier may lead to corneal infection.[79] The decision to fit patients with a history of inflammation will be dependent upon the most likely cause of the infiltrates. Corneal scars should be regarded with great suspicion, particularly if they have the typical circular appearance indicative of a resolved contact lens peripheral ulcer or CLPU (Fig. 16.1). Once there has been one corneal inflammatory response event, there is a much higher risk of the patient developing a further inflammatory event,[69,80–82] and overnight wear should either be avoided or the patient monitored extremely closely.

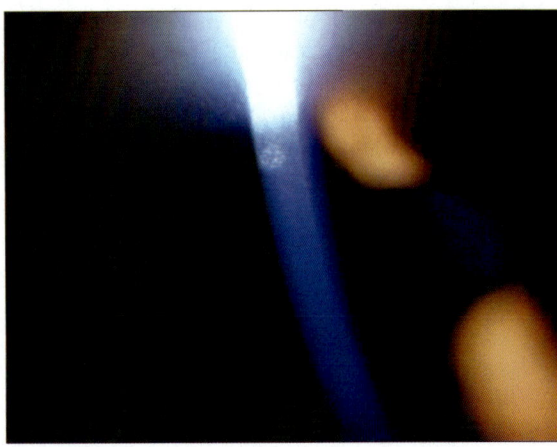

FIGURE 16.1 Scar remaining from a resolved contact lens peripheral ulcer (CLPU).

Once a decision has been made to fit lenses on an overnight basis, then the choice of contact lens material becomes the next important issue.

MATERIAL SELECTION FOR EXTENDED AND CONTINUOUS WEAR

Currently, practitioners have four options for fitting patients who desire overnight wear. They are as follows.

Conventional Hydrogel Materials

As described above, oxygen diffuses through conventional hydrogel materials through the water phase. Unfortunately, this reliance on water to maximize Dk has been a severely limiting factor for the development of hydrogels for overnight wear, since water has a Dk value of only 80 barrer,[83] and thus the oxygen diffusion through the lens is limited. Using the Morgan and Efron formula[42] it can be seen that the most basic of soft lens polymers, poly hydroxyethylmethacrylate (HEMA), has a Dk of only 9 to 10 barrers. In order to increase the Dk of a conventional hydrogel contact lens material beyond that of poly HEMA, it is necessary to incorporate monomers that will bind more water into the polymer.[43,84,85] These higher-water-content materials typically use HEMA or methyl methacrylate (MMA) as the "backbone" monomers, with more hydrophilic monomers such as N-vinyl pyrrolidone (NVP) or methacrylic acid (MA) increasing the water content to 60% to 70%, providing Dk values of close to 30 barrers.[43,84–86] Table 16.1 reports the Dk/t values for a number of commonly prescribed conventional hydrogel lenses, using the Morgan and Efron formula[42] to derive the Dk values from the published water content and center thickness of -3.00 D lenses. It must be remembered that these Dk/t values will be lower for positively powered lenses and high minus lenses, due to the increased lens thickness inherent in such lens designs.

Inspection of Table 16.1 clearly shows that conventional hydrogel lens materials provide very inadequate oxygen transmissibilities for safe, edema-free overnight wear, given the required Dk/t values reported above for overnight wear. This awareness of the short-comings of conventional hydrogel materials resulted in the development of novel materials that would provide increased amounts of oxygen to the corneal surface.

Silicone Elastomers

The first group of materials to provide significantly enhanced oxygen transmission was based on silicone rubber, and these "silicone elastomers" became clinically available in the early 1970s.[87,88] These lenses provided sufficient oxygen transport to the ocular surface for overnight

TABLE 16.1 Common Conventional Hydrogel Contact Lens Materials

COMMERCIAL NAME	MANUFACTURER	WATER CONTENT	Dk (EDGE & BOUNDARY CORRECTED)	CT	Dk/t
Frequency 38 (polymacon)	CooperVision	38.0	8	0.07	11
SofLens 38 (polymacon)	Bausch + Lomb	38.0	8	0.035	22
Preference Sphere (tetrafilcon A)	CooperVision	42.5	9	0.07	13
Biomedics 55 (ocufilcon D)	CooperVision	55.0	15	0.07	21
Acuvue 2 (etafilcon A)	Vistakon	58.0	17	0.084	20
SofLens daily disposable (hilafilcon B)	Bausch + Lomb	59.0	17	0.09	19
Proclear (omafilcon A)	CooperVision	62.0	20	0.065	30
Focus Dailies (nelfilcon A)	Alcon	69.0	26	0.10	26

Dk, oxygen permeability; CT, center thickness; Dk/t, oxygen transmissibility wear, with Dk values >300 barrers,[89] and they were used for both therapeutic and pediatric applications for over 20 years.[90] However, despite their exceptional oxygen transmission and durability, a number of major limitations were associated with their use in clinical practice. Fluid is unable to flow through these materials, resulting in frequent lens binding to the ocular surface,[91] and the lens surfaces are extremely hydrophobic, resulting in marked lipid and mucous deposition.[92,93] A silicone elastomer lens is still available (Silsoft, Bausch + Lomb), but its clinical usage is very low due to high cost, limited parameter availability, and poor surface wettability.

Rigid Gas-Permeable Materials

In the 1960s and early 1970s, the only rigid lens material available was polymethyl methacrylate (PMMA). Despite their low cost and excellent biocompatibility, PMMA lenses gradually lost their popularity due to their lack of Dk, and in 1978 the first truly GP lens material (Boston 1) was introduced, which incorporated a silicon-containing monomer commonly called TRIS, which resulted in a marked increase in Dk.[84,94] Over the next decade, polymer chemists started to increase the silicone content of rigid GP lenses, in an attempt to increase Dk.[95] This strategy worked well, until a Dk value in the mid-50s was reached, at which point the silicone content was so high that the surface acquired a small but significant electrostatic charge.[95,96] This negative charge attracted positively charged lysozyme from the patients tear film and, after a few months of lens wear, tenacious protein deposits bound to the lens surface, preventing the surface from wetting properly and inducing inflammatory changes in some patients. In addition, such materials often displayed poor dimensional stability,[97] were relatively brittle,[98] easily scratched[99] and occasionally exhibited lens "crazing", due to poor or variable polymerization procedures.[100–103]

In an attempt to reduce surface deposition but maintain gas permeability, manufacturers started to produce fluoro-silicone/acrylates (F-S/A) in the late 1980s, in which fluorine was added to enhance wettability and Dk to levels above that previously available in silicone/acrylates (S/A).[89,104] Studies have demonstrated that F-S/A deposit less protein than S/A,[105] while maintaining high levels of oxygen transmission.

S/A GP materials for overnight wear were initially fitted in the early 1980s and proved relatively successful.[106–108] However, some patients still showed hypoxic complications when lenses were worn for extended periods of time.[109] Improved manufacturing methods have now resulted in the development of a number of sophisticated GP lens materials that have Dk values over 100 barrer (Table 16.2), which provide adequate oxygenation for overnight wear in the majority of patients.[110–112] Of these, the Menicon Z material is the only GP material that is FDA approved for up to 30 nights CW and has proven to be successful when worn in this way.[113–117]

Despite the fact that GP lenses have been successful from a physiological perspective, issues relating to lens binding,[109,118,119] acquired ptosis,[120] and peripheral corneal staining[109,121] have limited their clinical usage, although GP materials are widely used on an overnight basis for orthokeratology, which is described in detail in Chapter 22.

Silicone Hydrogel Materials

Since the development of S/A GP and silicone elastomeric soft lens materials, the advantages of incorporating siloxane groups into contact lens materials, from an oxygen transmission perspective, have been well known. Since the late 1970s, manufacturers have tried to incorporate silicone into conventional HEMA-based hydrogel materials to develop high-Dk hydrogels. However, the chemistry required to successfully achieve this is very complex and it was not until the late 1990s that this became commercially possible.

Several silicone hydrogel lenses approved for overnight wear (for both EW and CW) are currently available, with their major features being summarized in Table 16.3. As described

TABLE 16.2 Common Rigid Lens Materials

NAME	MATERIAL TYPE	MANUFACTURER QUOTED Dk	Dk/t
Boston II	S/A	12	8
Boston IV	S/A	19	13
Boston Equalens	F-S/A	47	31
Boston EO	F-S/A	58	39
Boston Equalens II	F-S/A	85	57
Boston XO	F-S/A	100	67
Boston XO$_2$	F-S/A	141	94
Fluoroperm 30	F-S/A	30	20
Fluoroperm 60	F-S/A	60	40
Fluoroperm 92	F-S/A	92	61
Fluoroperm 151	F-S/A	151	101
Menicon Z	Siloxanylstyrene-based fluoromethacrylate	163	125*
Paragon HDS	F-S/A	58	39
Paragon HDS 100	F-S/A	100	67

Dk\t, oxygen transmissibility at a "standardized" center thickness of 0.15 mm
* = manufacturers quoted Dk/t for −3.00 D lens

above, the incorporation of siloxane groups into hydrogel materials is complex, as silicone is inherently hydrophobic and a huge impediment to the development of silicone hydrogel lenses related to the decreased surface wettability, increased lipid interaction, and accentuated lens binding previously seen in silicone elastomers. In order to make the surfaces of silicone hydrogel lens materials hydrophilic and more wettable, techniques incorporating plasma into the surface processing of the lens have been developed.[94,122–124] More recent techniques have involved incorporating hydrophilic monomers into the lens material that assist with surface wetting.[125,126] The purpose of these surface modifications is to mask the hydrophobic silicone from the tear film, increasing the surface wettability of the materials and reducing lipid deposition. In addition to complications induced by poor surface wettability, the incorporation of siloxane results in an increase in the modulus or "stiffness" of the lens materials, resulting in silicone hydrogel materials being significantly "stiffer" than their conventional hydrogel counterparts.

Space limitations prevent an extensive review of the technology behind these materials and fuller reviews can be found elsewhere.[1,85,86,94,127] However, the differences that do exist are fairly closely related to the company that manufactures them, and thus a brief overview of the lenses will be provided by dividing them into the companies who currently have commercially available lenses approved for overnight wear.

Bausch + Lomb

Bausch and Lomb's PureVision material, balafilcon A, is a homogeneous combination of the silicone-containing monomer polydimethylsiloxane (a vinyl carbamate derivative of trimethylsiloxy silane [TRIS]) copolymerized with the hydrophilic hydrogel monomer NVP.[128–131] PureVision lenses are surface treated in a reactive gas plasma chamber, which transforms the silicone components on the surface of the lenses into hydrophilic silicate compounds.[94,122,129,132] Glassy, discontinuous silicate "islands" result,[129,133,134] and the hydrophilicity of the transformed surface areas "bridges" over the underlying balafilcon A material. PureVision is one of only two

TABLE 16.3 Silicone Hydrogel Materials Approved for Overnight Wear

PROPRIETARY NAME	AIR OPTIX NIGHT & DAY AQUA	O_2 OPTIX OR AIR OPTIX AQUA	PUREVISION	ACUVUE OASYS	BIOFINITY	MENICON PREMIO
United States adopted name	lotrafilcon A	lotrafilcon B	balafilcon A	senofilcon A	comfilcon A	asmofilcon A
Manufacturer	Alcon	Alcon	Bausch + Lomb	Vistakon	CooperVision	Menicon
CT (@ −3.00 D) mm	0.08	0.08	0.09	0.07	0.08	0.08
Water content (%)	24	33	36	38	48	40
Dk ($\times 10^{-11}$)	140	110	91	103	128	129
Dk/t ($\times 10^{-9}$)	175	138	101	147	160	161
Modulus (MPa)	1.4	1.0	1.1	0.72	0.75	0.9
Surface treatment	25 nm plasma coating with high refractive index	25 nm plasma coating with high refractive index	Plasma oxidation process	No surface treatment. Internal wetting agent (PVP)	None	Plasma oxidation
Principal monomers	DMA + TRIS + siloxane macromer	DMA + TRIS + siloxane macromer	NVP + TPVC + NVA + PBVC	mPDMS + DMA + HEMA + siloxane macromer + TEGDMA + PVP	FM0411M; HOB; IBM; M3U; NVP; TAIC; VMA	undisclosed

DMA, (N,N-dimethylacrylamide); FM0411M, (α-Methacryloyloxyethyl iminocarboxyethyloxypropyl-poly(dimethylsiloxy)-butyldimethylsilane); HEMA, (poly-2-hydroxyethyl methacrylate); HOB, (2-Hydroxybutyl methacrylate); IBM, (Isobornyl methacrylate); M3U, (α-Bis(methacryloyloxyethyl iminocarboxy ethyloxypropyl)-poly(dimethylsiloxane)-poly(trifluoropropylmethylsiloxane)-poly (ω−methoxy-poly(ethyleneglycol)propyl methylsiloxane); mPDMS, (monofunctional polydimethylsiloxane); NVA, N-vinyl aminobutyric acid; NVP, (N-vinyl pyrrolidone); PBVC, (poly[dimethysiloxy] di [silylbutanol] bis[vinyl carbamate]); PVP, (polyvinyl pyrrolidone); TAIC, (1,3,5-Triallyl-1,3,5-triazine-2,4,6(1H,3H,5H)-trione); TEGDMA, (tetraethyleneglycol dimethacrylate); TPVC, (tris-(trimethylsiloxysilyl) propylvinyl carbamate); TRIS, (trimethylsiloxy silane); VMA, (N-Vinyl-N-methylacetamide).

soft lenses approved for up to 30 days of CW and clinical trials have shown the lens to be effective when used in this way.[135–137] It is also approved for use as a therapeutic bandage lens and several studies have demonstrated its value when used in this manner.[54,138,139]

Alcon

Alcon has two silicone hydrogel materials that are approved for overnight use. The lotrafilcon A material (AIR OPTIX Night & Day AQUA), employs a co-continuous biphasic or two-channel molecular structure, in which two phases persist from the front to the back surface of the lens[123]; lotrafilcon B (O_2OPTIX / Air Optix AQUA) is based upon very similar technology. The surfaces of both materials are permanently modified in a gas plasma chamber using a mixture of trimethylsilane, oxygen, and methane to create a permanent, ultrathin (25 nm), high refractive index, continuous hydrophilic surface.[123,129,133,134,140–142] The lotrafilcon A material is approved for up to 30 nights of CW and successful results have been reported with the lens used in this manner,[81,137,143–148] and it is also approved for use as a therapeutic lens.[55–58,138,149,150] On a DW basis, both lotrafilcon materials have proven to be clinically successful.[151–155]

CooperVision

CooperVision offers two silicone hydrogel materials, comfilcon A (Biofinity) and enfilcon A (Avaira), of which the latter is only approved for DW. Both materials reportedly have a higher Dk than would be predicted from their water content,[127,156] implying that the chemistry upon which they are based is different to that employed in other silicone hydrogels. Comfilcon A is approved for EW and enfilcon A contains a ultraviolet (UV) blocker.[157–159] To date, little clinical data is published on either lens, but the performance of comfilcon A appears comparable on overnight wear to other silicone hydrogels.[160,161]

Vistakon

Vistakon has two silicone hydrogel materials approved for reusable wear. The Acuvue Advance material, galyfilcon A has a relatively high water content compared with other silicone hydrogel materials (47%) and thus a relatively low Dk and is only approved for DW. It has an (UV) blocker, with a reported Class 1 UV protection, blocking >90% of UVA and >99% of UVB rays.[162–164] The Acuvue OASYS material (senofilcon A) also has Class 1 UV blocking capabilities.[164–167] The Acuvue Advance lens material was the first non–surface-treated silicone hydrogel to become a commercial reality, closely followed by Acuvue OASYS. The senofilcon A material used to manufacture the Acuvue OASYS lens is based upon similar chemistry to that of the galyfilcon A material in Acuvue Advance. Both materials incorporate a long-chain high-molecular-weight internal wetting agent based on polyvinylpyrolidone (PVP), which reduces the degree of hydrophobicity typically seen at the surface of siloxane-hydrogels.[162,163] The Advance lens internal wetting agent is termed Hydraclear and that used for the OASYS lens is "HydraClear Plus," implying that more PVP is probably incorporated. The OASYS lens has been particularly successful in studies investigating subjects with symptoms of contact lens-induced dryness.[168–171]

Menicon

Menicon has a silicone hydrogel material, asmofilcon A (PremiO), which is only available in a limited number of markets[172] and has limited published data on its clinical performance.[173] The lens uses a patented polymerization system to combine the siloxane and hydrophilic monomers (Menisilk) and uses a novel plasma surface treatment which, according to Menicon, combines the benefits of both plasma coating (as exemplified in the lotrafilcon A and lotrafilcon B materials from Alcon)[124,133,174] and plasma oxidation (as seen in the surface treatment process used with the Bausch + Lomb balafilcon A material).[124,130,133]

CLINICAL PERFORMANCE OF SOFT CONTACT LENS MATERIALS WORN OVERNIGHT

Hypoxia and acidosis are perhaps the greatest challenges for any soft lens worn on an overnight basis. Acidosis results from hypercapnia (increase of carbon dioxide) and is often associated with hypoxia.[175,176] In addition, oxygen flow and the release of carbon dioxide waste products are impeded by the contact lens and all these factors result in significant stresses on the cornea.

Recent data would suggest that while highly oxygen permeable silicone hydrogels now dominate EW fits, almost 25% of all EW fits still occur with hydrogel lenses, despite their lower Dk/t.[61] Recent data published on almost 7,500 EW fits over a 5-year period (2006–2010) from 39 countries represents the most up-to-date information on the materials fitted to EW patients globally.[53] It demonstrated that 28% of all new fits and refits into an EW modality were undertaken with hydrogel materials. However, a large range was observed, with some countries (such as China and Egypt) using hydrogels for almost 90% of their EW fits and other more mature markets (such as Australia and Canada) only using hydrogels for 5% of their EW patients.

The potential complications associated with the overnight wear of these two broad categories of materials are summarized in Table 16.4 and detailed below.

Potential Complications Associated with Conventional Hydrogel Materials

The major complications induced by overnight wear of HEMA-based materials are due to the fact that they provide insufficient oxygen to the cornea.

Striae and Folds

Hypoxia within the corneal stroma results in the accumulation of lactic acid and a subsequent influx of fluid from the anterior chamber, resulting in "edema" and a physical increase in corneal thickness.[177] This is an acute response to hypoxia and very often there are no symptoms associated with mild edema but, in extreme cases, decreased vision, glare, halos, and photophobia can occur. With overnight wear of low-Dk conventional hydrogel lens materials, corneal swelling is typically in the order of 1% to 5% during the day, increasing to approximately 10% overnight.[178–181] Measurements of corneal thickness are made using a pachometer. Clinically, the presence of corneal swelling may be observed as the appearance of striae and folds, which occur as a direct result of corneal swelling.[182–186] Striae are vertical, grayish-white, wispy lines in the stroma seen with a parallelepiped and appear when edema exceeds 5%.[186] Folds appear

TABLE 16.4 Potential Complications for HEMA-Based and Silicone Hydrogel Materials Worn Overnight

HEMA-BASED HYDROGEL	SILICONE HYDROGEL	EITHER HYDROGEL
Stromal striae	Mucin balls	Contact lens acute red eye
Stromal folds	Superior epithelial arcuate lesions	Contact lens peripheral ulcer
Epithelial microcysts	Conjunctival flaps	Infiltrative keratitis
Endothelial polymegethism	Corneal erosions	Microbial keratitis
Limbal hyperemia	Papillary conjunctivitis	
Stromal neovascularization		
Reduced corneal sensitivity		
Reduced epithelial thickness		
Stromal thinning		

as a physical "buckling" in Descemet's membrane and are seen as black, deep grooves with direct focal illumination and are observed when edema of 10% or more occurs.[186] These acute responses are reversible on eye opening, but repeated overnight wear with conventional hydrogel lenses have been shown to result in many detrimental effects on corneal structure and function. The amount of oxygen required to eliminate edematous complications is a matter for some conjecture, with estimates suggesting that during overnight wear, 87 to 125 Dk/t units are necessary.[44,51,187–189] Conventional lenses clearly fall drastically short of these requirements (see Table 16.1) and edema can therefore be expected to occur for the vast majority of patients who wear these materials overnight. The same cannot be said for highly oxygen-transmissible GP and silicone hydrogel lenses (see Tables 16.2 and 16.3), and striae and folds would be expected to rarely, if ever, be observed in these patients.

Epithelial Microcysts

In addition to acute responses to hypoxia, the cornea also responds to chronic hypoxia. A common chronic response is the development of epithelial microcysts, which present as small (5–30 μm) inclusions or dots located in the epithelium.[190–192] Low numbers of microcysts can occur without lens wear, but their prevalence increases when conventional hydrogel lenses are worn overnight,[193] and they are rarely seen in patients wearing silicone hydrogel lenses.[194,195] They are comprised of necrotic cellular tissue or debris, which has a relatively high refractive index and results in the characteristic reversed illumination observed when viewed using marginal retroillumination.[192,193,196] Patients with microcysts are usually asymptomatic. Microcysts typically occur after approximately 2 months of chronic hypoxia and increase in number over the next 2 to 4 months, after which their numbers level off. Microcysts originate in the deeper layers of the epithelium and migrate anteriorly. If they reach the surface, they break through the epithelium, causing staining and occasionally a mild interference in vision. Treatment is discontinuation of lens wear or refitting with a contact lens of greater Dk/t. Recovery typically takes 4 to 6 weeks, and an initial increase in the numbers of microcysts usually occurs, as the cornea suddenly becomes reoxygenated.[197] The numbers of microcysts then gradually reduce over a 2- to 3-month period, to the point where they are eliminated.[192]

Endothelial Polymegethism

The endothelium has also been shown to demonstrate changes in morphology due to chronic hypoxia. Polymegethism was first reported 30 years ago[198] and describes a change in size of the endothelial cells that occurs when low-Dk/t lenses are worn.[199–204] While this condition is initially asymptomatic, patients may eventually exhibit intolerance to contact lens wear.[205] Polymegethism does not occur in wearers of silicone hydrogel lens materials[194] or when hyperpermeable GP lenses are worn overnight.[206]

Limbal Hyperemia

Overnight lens wear with conventional hydrogels frequently results in limbal hyperemia.[207] Increases in limbal redness are seen rapidly when conventional lens materials are worn, even on a DW basis, with detectable differences being seen within just a few hours of lens insertion.[188] Hypoxia has been shown to be a major contributing factor to limbal hyperemia, particularly in studies comparing the limbal response between silicone hydrogel lenses and conventional hydrogel lenses, where changes can be seen over both short- and long-term periods of time.[154,188,208–210] Further, extremely good evidence now exists to support the theory that limbal hyperemia is directly related to lens material Dk/t.[211] A rapid reduction in limbal redness is observed when patients are refitted into silicone hydrogel lenses, even when they are worn on an overnight basis (Fig. 16.2).[11,208–210]

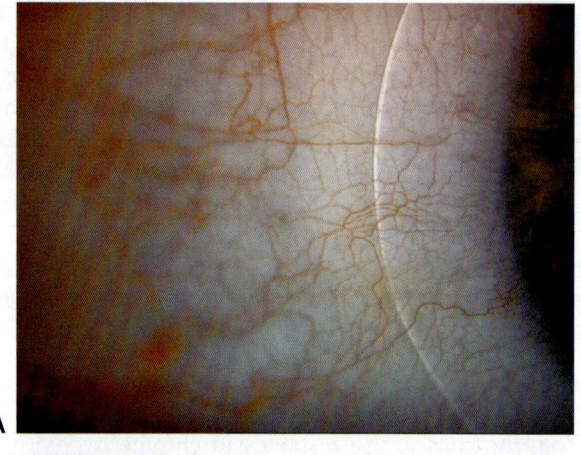

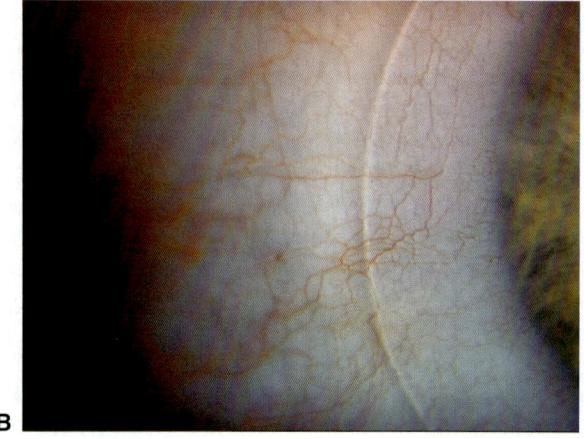

FIGURE 16.2 **(A)** Limbal hyperemia subsequent to conventional hydrogel lens wear on an extended wear basis. **(B)** Reduction in limbal hyperemia in the same eye as **A** when refitted with a silicone hydrogel lens for extended wear.

Neovascularization

In addition to limbal hyperemia associated with EW of conventional hydrogel lenses, chronic new vessel formation also frequently occurs. This "neovascularization" is defined as the formation and extension of capillaries into a previously avascular corneal area.[212] Studies have indicated that up to 65% of patients using conventional hydrogel lenses on an EW basis exhibit some level of neovascularization.[178] This is in comparison with no evidence of neovascularization in patients using silicone hydrogel lens materials.[137,178,208] Patients who do exhibit neovascularization demonstrate regression of the vessel response following refitting with silicone hydrogels in as little as 1 month (Fig. 16.3).[80,154] The new vessels do not simply disappear, but "ghost vessels" remain,[213] and these ghost vessels can fill rapidly if adversely stimulated again.

Other Chronic Corneal Changes

Several other changes to the cornea frequently occur as a result of EW-induced hypoxia, but these may not be so apparent to the eye care practitioner. They include reduced corneal sensitivity,[214,215] reduced oxygen uptake by the epithelium,[200] decreased epithelial thickness[200] and, perhaps of greatest concern, greater bacterial adherence.[216–219] In addition, although acute hypoxia is known to result in corneal swelling, chronic hypoxia can result in long-term stromal thinning.[200,220,221]

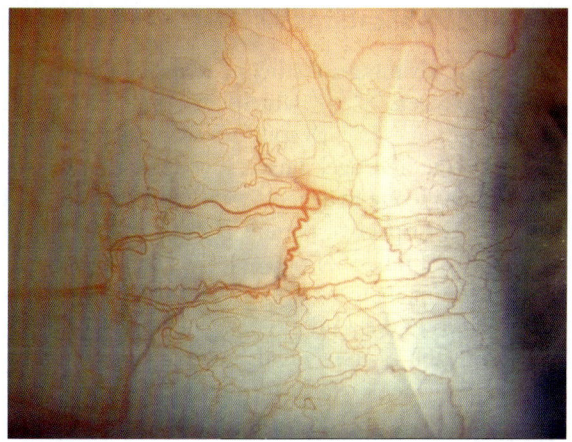

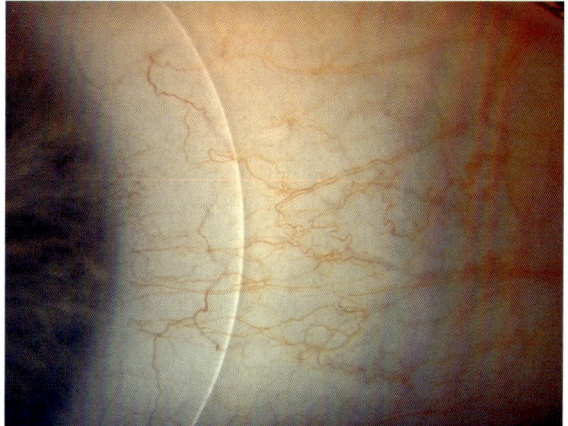

FIGURE 16.3 **(A)** Neovascularization subsequent to extended wear with a conventional low oxygen permeability lens. **(B)** Regression of neovascularization in the same eye as **A** following refitting with a silicone hydrogel lens worn on an extended wear basis for 1 month.

Myopic Shift

Chronic hypoxia is also the presumed cause of a myopic prescription shift, which can occur in some patients who wear conventional hydrogel lenses on an EW basis.[26,222,223] Similar to the reversal of other chronic responses to hypoxia, patients may show a hyperopic shift when refitted with silicone hydrogel lenses.[144,222,223] This can be clinically significant if a refitting occurs in a patient who is on the verge of presbyopia. Approximately 1-month post refitting, all patients should be carefully overrefracted, as the patient may be wearing a lens that is overminused or underplussed, possibly resulting in near vision problems.

Corneal Staining

A common complication observed with EW of conventional hydrogel lenses is corneal staining, also called superficial punctate staining (SPS) or superficial punctate keratitis (SPK). This can take on the appearance of small punctate spots to large, dense, confluent patches.[224] One of the possible causes of staining is hypoxia, and it is particularly important to monitor staining in EW and CW wearers because it represents a break in the epithelial barrier, which may act as a subsequent portal for the entry of bacteria.

The disadvantages of overnight wear with these HEMA-based materials relate to both the very low levels of oxygen provided by these lenses compared with silicone hydrogels[225,226] and to the increased rates of complications reported when such lenses are worn overnight.[5–7]

Potential Complications Associated with Silicone Hydrogel Materials

The principal advantage of silicone hydrogel lenses for overnight wear is their excellent ability to transmit oxygen,[94,187,226] which has resulted in the elimination of the hypoxic complications described earlier.[12,81,194] Despite these higher levels of oxygen available to the cornea when wearing silicone hydrogel lenses, mechanical, inflammatory, and infectious complications still occur. When silicone hydrogels were first introduced, limitations in parameter availability prevented every prospective patient from being able to realize their benefits for overnight wear, but with current ranges of powers, base curves and lens designs, there are very few individuals who are now unable to be fitted with these lenses, if desired.

As discussed in the section on silicone hydrogel materials, the major disadvantages with these materials are their relatively hydrophobic surfaces and higher modulus of elasticity. The first two silicone hydrogel lenses to be introduced (lotrafilcon A and balafilcon A) had very high modulus values compared with HEMA-based hydrogels, as they were primarily intended for overnight wear and thus oxygen transport was critical. This resulted in the lenses having high siloxane contents (providing very high-Dk values), but correspondingly very high modulus values.[1,85,127] While this increased rigidity was beneficial for lens handling, it was certainly implicated in a variety of mechanical complications, which were initially seen with these lenses, particularly when they were worn on a CW basis.[10,12,80,81,227] The silicone hydrogels that were subsequently introduced into the market were aimed more for the DW market, could thus have lower-Dk/t values with lower siloxane amounts, and therefore tended to have lower-modulus values[1,85,127] (Fig. 16.4). As a result, clinicians tended to see fewer mechanical complications with newer materials. In addition, companies became more accustomed to designing silicone hydrogel lenses in these higher moduli and quickly redesigned the first-generation materials to reduce their thickness profile, offered more base-curve options and redesigned the back surface, which resulted in reduced mechanical complications with even these original high modulus materials.

Inflammatory and infectious complications remain a concern with overnight wear of silicone hydrogel lenses and appear to be more patient than material dependent. The following section will briefly review the complications that tend to occur with silicone hydrogel materials.

Mucin Balls

Posttear lens debris often occurs with overnight lens wear, particularly with silicone hydrogel lenses. The most commonly reported debris is referred to as "mucin balls."[228–232] These are pearly, translucent, 20 to 100 μm spherical particles observed between the back surface of

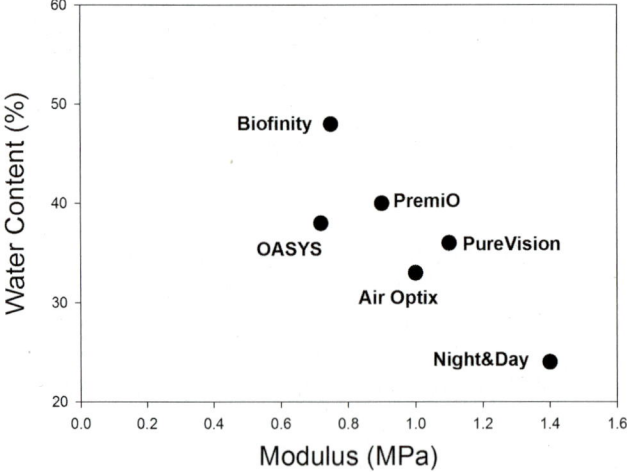

FIGURE 16.4 A graph of water content (%) versus modulus for silicone hydrogel lens materials.

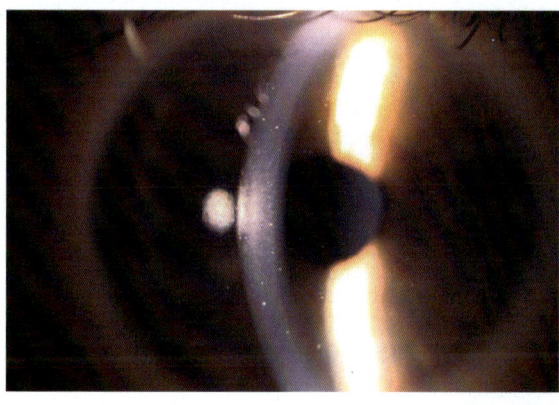

FIGURE 16.5 Mucin balls observed between the back surface of a silicone hydrogel lens and the cornea.

a contact lens and the cornea[10] (Fig. 16.5), which have been shown to consist of mucin and lipid.[232] They are believed to occur when relatively stiff lens materials "shear" the tear film and roll up small balls of mucin and lipid from the tear film. When the lenses are removed, transient depressions are left in the epithelium,[230,233,234] which pool with fluorescein.[10,228] In most cases, patients are asymptomatic and there is complete resolution within a few hours. Mucin balls have not been directly linked with any clinical complications, although two studies have shown the presence of mucin balls to be associated with a decreased incidence of corneal inflammatory events.[235,236] It has been hypothesized that mucin ball presence implicates a more concentrated or viscous mucus layer on the surface of the cornea, which prevents upregulation of the immune response against bacterial ligands.[236]

Superior Epithelial Arcuate Lesions

Another mechanical complication that can occur with all hydrogel lenses, but which is more common with stiffer materials, is superior epithelial arcuate lesions (SEALs).[10,80,224,237–243] These typically present as an arcuate break in the epithelium approximately 1 mm from the limbus; however, in some silicone hydrogel wearers, the lesion may be closer to the central cornea.[238,241,244] The edges may be irregular, roughened or thickened, particularly if the SEAL is associated with diffuse or focal infiltration. SEALs are frequently asymptomatic, but may be associated with a mild foreign body sensation following lens removal.[10,81] SEALs can occur for a number of reasons, but are most likely the result of the stiff nature of silicone hydrogel materials or their inflexibility to conform to the limbus, causing increased mechanical pressure.[238,242] Management requires temporary discontinuation of lens wear for 1 to 2 days. Patients should be warned that their symptoms may increase initially and ocular lubricants can be dispensed to relieve discomfort. In cases of recurrence, refitting with a different design or material may be indicated.[10,80] An example of SEAL occurring in a silicone hydrogel lens wearer is described in Case 1 at the end of this chapter.

Bulbar Conjunctival Disruptions

Indentation and mild staining of the conjunctival tissue can occur with all soft lenses and is generally not too concerning, if there is no subjective discomfort and associated adverse effects do not occur. A relatively new clinical finding affecting the bulbar conjunctiva associated with silicone hydrogel lenses, particularly when worn on an EW or CW basis, has been reported, referred to as "lens-induced epithelial flaps" or "conjunctival epithelial flaps" (CEF).[245–251] These terms are used to describe areas of conjunctival epithelium that separate from the underlying tissue. They can be best appreciated with the use of fluorescein and a yellow barrier filter.[252] The "flaps" are usually observed up to 1 mm away from the lens edge superiorly or inferiorly and have a roughened or jagged appearance (Fig. 16.6). Recent impression cytology studies have shown that CEFs appear to be formed by healthy epithelial and goblet cells that have been

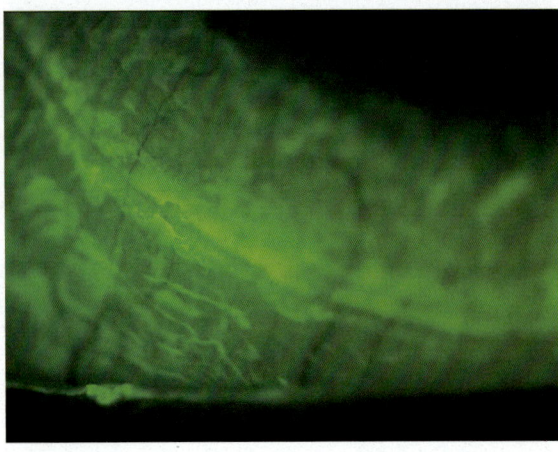

FIGURE 16.6 Conjunctival disruption, as shown with fluorescein staining, subsequent to continuous wear with a silicone hydrogel lens ("epithelial flap").

dislocated from their normal location along the conjunctival surface by the lens edge.[250] There does not appear to be any sign of associated inflammation in the area,[251] and lens wearers are asymptomatic. While the condition appears benign, clinicians may choose to refit patients with alternative lens designs or materials if the presentation persists.

Corneal Abrasions and Erosions

Corneal abrasions and erosions can occur with all lens types. The etiology for these conditions is trauma from either a foreign body getting under the lens and abrading the superficial epithelial cells or the contact lens becoming "bound" to the epithelium and disturbing the cells when it regains mobility. This is more likely with overnight lens wear than daily lens wear,[80,227,253] and the severity of symptoms associated with these conditions varies considerably. The epithelium is disrupted (Fig. 16.7) and the affected area stains with fluorescein. In almost all cases, simply removing the lens allows rapid resolution. Ocular lubricants may be used, but in most cases no medication is required. Severe cases may benefit from a prophylactic topical antibiotic, analgesics, or mydriatics.[227]

Contact Lens Papillary Conjunctivitis

Contact lens papillary conjunctivitis (CLPC; also referred to as giant papillary conjunctivitis or GPC) is believed to be both mechanical and immunological in nature.[10,80,227,254–256] CLPC had become a relatively rare complication with conventional hydrogel EW since the introduction

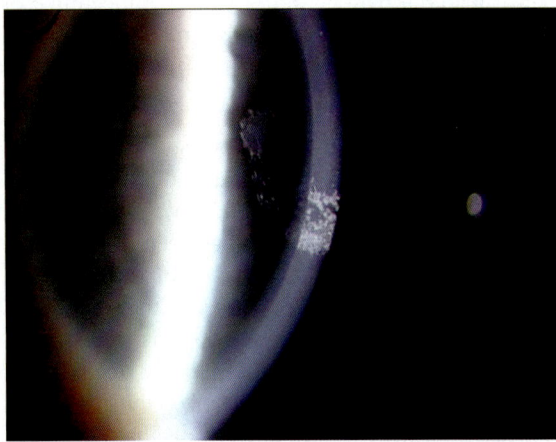

FIGURE 16.7 Corneal erosion in a patient wearing silicone hydrogel lenses on a continuous-wear basis.

of frequent-replacement lenses,[146,254,257–260] but the introduction of CW silicone hydrogels initially saw a resurgence of this condition.[10,227,243,261–264] A combination of the increased stiffness and edge designs of some of these lenses was implicated,[10,227,264] but newer designs and lower-modulus silicone hydrogel materials appear to have diminished the prevalence once again. CLPC presents with changes to the palpebral conjunctiva, consisting of increased hyperemia and papillary excrescences. The papillae present either diffusely across the entire palpebral conjunctiva or may be in a localized area.[146,227,261,262] The symptoms associated with this condition in silicone hydrogel wearers are generally rapid in onset and include foreign body sensation or discomfort, itching, stringy or ropy mucous discharge and, in some cases, lens mislocation, particularly during sleep.[10,227,264] Cases of CLPC that are mechanical in origin generally resolve very quickly, simply by ceasing lens wear and either wearing spectacles or daily disposable lenses for a period of approximately 2 weeks.[264] A topical antihistamine/mast cell stabilizer may also be used to manage CLPC. Changes to wearing schedule, lens design, and material may then be required to prevent recurrence. An example of CLPC occurring in a silicone hydrogel lens wearer is described in Case 2 at the end of this chapter.

Potential Complications Associated with all Hydrogel Materials

While the previous two sections have concentrated on the complications associated with conventional hydrogel or silicone hydrogel lenses, it is important to emphasize that there are many complications that can occur with EW and CW of all soft, hydrogel lenses and these are covered in the following section.

Contact Lens Acute Red Eye

Contact lens acute red eye (CLARE) is a unilateral, acute inflammatory condition that occurs with EW and CW in response to gram-negative organisms (e.g., *Pseudomonas* spp.) colonizing the lens and releasing endotoxins.[265–270] A higher incidence of CLARE occurs in patients with upper respiratory infection, and these cases may be due to the presence of other gram-negative organisms including *Haemophilus influenzae*.[267,270] Patients with CLARE typically awaken in the early morning by a moderately painful (foreign body sensation) red eye, with associated epiphora and photophobia. Focal or diffuse subepithelial infiltrates are usually observed in the midperiphery of the cornea close to the limbus. The infiltrates rarely stain and rapidly resolve.[227] CLARE is self-limiting on removal of contact lenses. It is therefore generally managed with temporary discontinuation of lens wear and ocular lubricants during the acute stage.

Contact Lens Peripheral Ulcer

CLPU is an inflammatory response that results in lesions often termed "sterile ulcers".[271,272] The etiology of this condition is a hypersensitive reaction to the (usually gram positive) exotoxins released by pathogenic bacteria.[270,273,274] Clinical signs include a single, small, circular, peripheral or midperipheral grayish-white, grey lesion in the anterior stroma.[227,272] Symptoms include mild to moderate pain (foreign body sensation), mild lacrimation, and mild photophobia.[80,227,272] Following the acute presentation, the epithelium regenerates within a few days. Diffuse infiltration surrounding the lesion may develop. A very well-defined circular "scar" remains, gradually fading with time, but still present several months after the event.[80,227,272] Differential diagnosis from MK is extremely important.[80,275] An example of CLPU occurring in a silicone hydrogel lens wearer is described in Case 3 at the end of this chapter.

Infiltrative Keratitis

Infiltrative keratitis (IK) is a general term used to describe inflammatory events within the cornea. All cases of IK exhibit the presence of infiltrates within the cornea, which can be located anywhere but are usually peripherally situated in the limbal area, often with associated limbal hyperemia.[80,227,276] Many IK cases are due to the presence of gram-positive exotoxins found on the lid margin.[268,276] Symptoms include mild to moderate irritation (often a foreign body discomfort), mild redness, lacrimation, photophobia, and occasional mild discharge.[80,227,276] There is a large degree of variability in the severity of symptoms associated with IK and in some cases there are no symptoms that are associated with the infiltrates. This condition is termed asymptomatic infiltrative keratitis (AIK) and its cause is frequently unknown.[227] Temporary discontinuation of lens wear results in full resolution of clinical signs and symptoms, normally within a few days. In most cases, no additional treatment is required; however, ocular lubricants may be dispensed to alleviate symptoms.[80]

Incidence of Inflammatory Complications

It is extremely difficult to accurately report the incidence rates for inflammatory conditions, as the percentages reported for corneal infiltrates vary significantly, depending upon the study design and the criteria used for reporting infiltrates, which can vary widely.[277]

It is recognized that overnight wear, in addition to increasing the risk of MK, also increases the risk of inflammation in contact lens wearers,[68,277,278] with more recent estimates suggesting that EW increases the risk for corneal infiltrates 2–8×.[21,279,280] When silicone hydrogel lenses initially became available in the late 1990s, they were prescribed predominately for overnight lens wear, for periods of up to 1 month. Most of the clinical trials conducted to investigate the incidence of inflammatory events with silicone hydrogel lenses therefore report primarily on an overnight wearing modality.[16,21,135,136,243,280–282] These studies report incidence rates for sterile keratitis ranging from 1.3 to 5.5 per 100 patient years for conventional hydrogel lenses and from 2.9 to 6.7 per 100 patient years for silicone hydrogel lenses. Szczotka-Flynn and Diaz performed a metaanalysis to evaluate the risks of corneal inflammatory events in users of silicone hydrogel and low-Dk/t hydrogel EW lenses.[283] They reported rates of 14.4 per 100 eye years for silicone hydrogel wearers and 7.7 per 100 eye years for conventional hydrogel wearers. This represents an approximately two times higher risk of developing corneal infiltrates in patients wearing silicone hydrogel lenses on an EW basis for up to 30 days as compared with low-Dk/t lenses worn for 7 days EW. It is not clear from this finding, however, whether the material or the length of overnight wear, or a combination of the two, was responsible for this apparent increase in risk. Three other studies also support this 2× increased risk of IK with the wearing of silicone hydrogels.[21,279,284] The reason for this remains unknown, but factors such as solution interactions, modulus, deposition with tear film components, and reduced wettability have all been proposed as potentially being relevant.[21,279,284] There also appears to be a patient predisposition for inflammatory events[270] and approximately 10% to 25% of EW and CW patients in clinical trials have been reported to experience repeat episodes.[80,82,285] It may be advisable for those who do experience repeated events to switch to a flexible wear schedule, with only occasional overnight lens wear.

Microbial Keratitis

MK is the most serious complication associated with contact lens wear and was the greatest concern with EW of conventional hydrogel lenses. Fortunately, the prevalence of MK within the general population is extremely low, due in part to the exceptional defense mechanisms that protect the ocular surface.[286–288] The microorganisms most commonly associated with MK in contact lens wearers are the *Pseudomonas* spp. (principally *aeruginosa*),[289–292] but many different microorganisms have been cultured from cases of MK in contact lens patients.[293] The major risk factors for MK include overnight wear, poor compliance with lens and case hygiene, epithelial trauma, smoking, male gender, and swimming in lenses.[18,20,294–296] The generally accepted figure for the annualized incidence of MK in conventional hydrogel DW patients is 4 per 10,000 wearers,[5,7,277] and EW has been reported to increase this risk by approximately five times.[5–7,277] Although it was initially hoped that the risks would be lower with CW of silicone hydrogels, study results now indicate that the risk level is similar to that found with conventional HEMA-based materials.[16,18,20,277,295]

Patients with MK usually experience severe pain, lacrimation, hyperemia, and photophobia.[80,227,275] Any area of the cornea may be affected and the clinical appearance is usually of a single irregular infiltrative lesion with excavation of the epithelium, Bowman's layer, and the stroma. An anterior chamber reaction and lid edema are also common and VA may be reduced.[80,227,275] An example of MK occurring in a conventional hydrogel lens wearer is described in Case 4 at the end of this chapter.

MK is considered an ocular emergency and treatment must be instigated immediately in order to achieve the best possible outcome.[294,297–300] As most cases of MK in contact lens wearers are bacterial, treatment is with antibiotic agents unless other prognostic signs exist. Initial treatment is generally with fluoroquinolone monotherapy, and supplemental cycloplegics and analgesics are given as required.[292,301–304] In severe cases, fortified antibiotics may also be prescribed.[292,305,306] Prognosis for most patients is good and most cases resolve without visual loss,[16] even though a scar remains, but this does depend upon the causative organism. The cases of fusarium keratitis[307–311] and acanthamoeba keratitis[312–314] associated with lens wear are typically much more severe and have frequently resulted in significant loss of best-corrected vision and, in many cases, corneal transplantation is required.[310,315]

PATIENT EDUCATION

Prescribing contact lenses for overnight wear represents some unique challenges and certain adaptations to the contact lens fitting routine and management of patients using these lenses require discussion. In an increasingly litigious society, clinicians should exercise caution when fitting contact lenses that may result in an increased risk of complications. The most likely legal claim is one of negligence, and the most common causes of liability are inappropriate patient selection, providing inadequate instructions, prescribing improper wearing schedules, inadequate monitoring of ocular health, and incorrect management of contact lens-related complications. Appropriate patient education plays a key role in the success of overnight wearing modalities and reduces the likelihood of possible litigation.[316]

Informed Consent or Patient Agreement

It is highly recommended that practitioners develop documents that give clear information about the contact lenses to be worn, the overnight wearing modality (EW or CW), the risks and benefits for this modality, instructions on how to avoid complications, and what steps to take if a complication is suspected.[317–322] A number of separate documents can be utilized or the information can be amalgamated into one. An important element is either an informed consent or a patient–practitioner agreement and examples of such documents have been previously described.[323]

Comfort and Adaptation

Properly fitted lenses are vital in order to provide optimum patient comfort and minimize the risk of mechanically induced adverse responses. Trial lens fitting should always be undertaken before the commencement of overnight contact lens wear and, if any problem with fit is observed or if significant discomfort is reported, an alternative design or product should be tried. Initial comfort during trial fitting greatly influences the patient's perception of contact lenses,[324] and may have an effect on their ultimate success.

Lenses that decenter or do not provide complete corneal coverage should be avoided since they may result in corneal desiccation or limbal chafing. As discussed previously, the higher modulus of some silicone hydrogel lenses renders them stiffer and therefore the physical lens-to-cornea curvature relationship is more critical to successful fitting. A phenomenon that is consequently observed more often with silicone hydrogel lenses than conventional soft lenses is lens "fluting,"[325] which usually causes a foreign-body-like discomfort to the patient. Unfortunately, fluting does not reduce with increased wear and, if observed, an alternate base curve or design must be evaluated.

Adaptation to well-fitted lenses for overnight wear should be rapid. However, there is justification for recommending that patients who are new to contact lenses should adapt to DW for a period of at least 1 week, mainly to ensure that they are capable of wearing, handling, and looking after contact lenses before initiating EW or CW. When prescribing EW or CW for adapted wearers, these individuals should be instructed to commence overnight wear immediately. With highly permeable silicone hydrogel materials, a follow-up visit after the first night of lens wear is unnecessary since the only reason for this visit would be to assess any possible acute hypoxic responses. It is more appropriate to see patients after approximately a week when they have had an opportunity to adapt to an overnight wearing modality. It is, however, very important to discuss how the patient is likely to feel upon waking in their lenses. Changes in the tear film overnight may result in mild dryness and blurring of vision, which generally resolve with blinking but may also be alleviated with rewetting drops. Patients must also be instructed to contact their eye care practitioner if they experience any problems before their first follow-up visit is scheduled.

All wearers should be seen for an initial follow-up visit after the first week, to ensure that lenses are comfortable and patients are able to tolerate overnight wear. Subsequent follow-up visits should occur after a further 2 to 3 weeks and then 3 months after commencing EW or CW. It is particularly important to assess patients who have been refitted into silicone hydrogel lenses from conventional hydrogel materials within the first weeks of wear, especially if they have been worn on an EW basis. Changes relating to recovery from chronic hypoxia may occur within the first month or so of lens wear, including a possible reversal of a previous myopic shift[222] and a transient appearance of microcysts.[195] Assessments of VA and overrefraction and a careful slit-lamp biomicroscope examination are therefore recommended at each visit. Changes in lens parameters can be made before a supply of lenses is ordered for the patient. Subsequent follow-up visits should be scheduled at 3 to 6 monthly intervals thereafter.

Wearing Schedule

The wearing schedule is determined by a number of factors. These include the current approvals of wearing time by the regulatory authorities (e.g., FDA, CE, etc.). Some lenses are only approved for up to 6 nights of overnight wear (EW) and others for up to 30 nights (CW). Even then, these approvals are the maximum recommended wearing schedule. The optimal number of consecutive nights should be considered for each patient on an individual basis and it should be emphasized that patients can always remove their lenses after a shorter time period if they wish to. Flexibility in wearing schedule must be emphasized. If lenses are worn for shorter periods, they must be cleaned and disinfected with an appropriate care system before reinsertion. Regardless of wearing schedule, patients should be advised that they must NEVER continue to wear an uncomfortable lens or wear a lens when they have a painful or red eye.

Every 6 or 30 nights of overnight wear should be followed by one night with no lenses and lenses should either be discarded, or in the case of lenses approved for 6 nights, they may be cleaned and disinfected and then reworn for a further 6-night period if this is indicated by the manufacturers. It is important that all patients replace their lenses according to the recommended schedule. Some practitioners suggest replacing monthly replacement lenses at the beginning or end of a month to improve compliance. Text messaging systems and e-mails are also being used by some companies and practices to remind patients when they should be replacing their lenses.

Solutions and Rewetting Drops

Patients must be dispensed with a care regimen, which they can use in the event of either a scheduled or unscheduled lens removal. Typically, multipurpose care regimens are prescribed due to their ease of use and relatively low cost, but care should be taken to ensure that there is compatibility between the lens material and the system. The use of a rub and rinse cycle is highly recommended, even with "no-rub" regimens, particularly for patients who are prone to lipid deposition.[326,327] Hydrogen peroxide systems can also be used if the practitioner prefers these systems. It is important to also provide rewetting drops to all EW and CW patients. These are very useful for the alleviation of dryness on eye waking and during their normal wear. They can also be used at night if desired and should be recommended for patients exhibiting high numbers of mucin balls, as their regular use prior to sleep has been reported to decrease their frequency of observation.[228] Ideally, these drops should be of relatively low viscosity, to prevent blurring following their insertion. Rewetting drops with surface-active agents have been shown to improve the clinical performance of silicone hydrogel contact lenses[328] and patients experiencing lipid deposition may also find them helpful. Periodic lens removal with a rub and rinse with a care regimen containing a surfactant may also be helpful for some patients experiencing lipid buildup.[326]

Emergencies

Patients should be advised to remove their EW or CW lenses if they feel physically unwell, as they are often prone to adverse events during these times. Most importantly, they should be advised that they must NEVER sleep in an uncomfortable lens or when they have a painful or red eye and that they must check their eyes on waking each morning to ensure that they look "good," feel "good," and that they can see well, a three-point safety check they should perform every morning.[329] If they are at all concerned, they must remove the lenses and contact their practitioner urgently, as delayed treatment in cases of MK has a significant impact on eventual prognosis and recovery.[294,296,297,300] To facilitate this, they should be supplied with emergency contact details, which must include a 24-hour emergency contact number (via either a pager or practitioner home contact number). It may be possible for practitioners in a locality to arrange an on-call system, where practitioners rotate this duty.

Office staff play a vital role in the management of potential emergency situations for EW and CW patients. This is only possible with some degree of in-office training being undertaken and such training is well worthwhile, from both a clinical and legal standpoint. It is particularly important that staff schedule patients with potential adverse responses quickly or arrange referral for an emergency appointment externally if necessary. Suitable in-office protocols should be developed and reviewed regularly.

Follow-Up Care

Contact lens follow-up is extremely important for EW and CW patients and is the best method of avoiding complications or identifying the cause of problems when they occur. It is important to emphasize the importance of follow-up visits to patients whether they are experiencing problems or not. They should be made aware of symptoms that may indicate a problem, but it is also crucial to explain that some complications may occur without any associated symptoms, in the initial stages.

The visit should begin with a thorough history, preferably in the form of a patient discussion and the use of "open" rather than "closed" questions is recommended. For example, "how would you describe your contact lens wear" or "what seems to be the main problem with your contact lenses/eyes/vision?" Once the chief complaint is established, further questioning can follow. The measurement of VA is extremely important, particularly if a complication is suspected or observed and recording the best level of corrected acuity with or without the lenses in place is crucial both to establish whether any temporary or permanent loss of VA has occurred and for the requirements of complete record keeping.

A thorough slit-lamp examination should be performed at all follow-up visits. It is particularly important that lens surface characteristics and wettability be evaluated. After lens removal, the eyelids, lashes, margins, conjunctiva, and cornea should be examined using the appropriate illumination techniques. Lid eversion and fluorescein staining (with the use of an additional yellow barrier filter)[252] must be performed at all visits. The eye can be irrigated with saline prior to reinsertion of the lenses and as with all lens removals, patients should be advised to disinfect their lenses prior to wearing them again overnight. Evaluation of the anterior chamber for flare or cells may also be necessary for the differential diagnosis of certain complications.

Comprehensive record keeping is crucial for EW and CW patients. A record of all findings, verbal communication, and instructions must be clearly recorded in the patient's record.[319,320,330] The use of grading scales to rate the severity of ocular findings is strongly recommended.[322,331-333] Increasingly, photography and video recording are also being utilized as an accurate means of documenting findings.

SUMMARY

Overnight wear of contact lenses is certainly not for everyone, but does offer many advantages over DW for many patients. When discussing the opportunity for EW or CW with patients, it is important to provide a carefully balanced point of view. Patients appreciate learning about the potential disadvantages, as well as being informed of the positive aspects. Thorough follow-up examinations are crucial for patient success with overnight lens wear. While newer GP and silicone hydrogel materials appear to have solved hypoxia problems for the majority of patients choosing to wear lenses overnight, some patients will experience inflammation and mechanical complications and practitioners must be equipped to handle these complications when they occur. A number of strategies have been suggested to reduce a patient's risk of complications. The initiation of lid hygiene measures is also recommended for patients predisposed to inflammatory responses. Even though these new materials are an enormous improvement over older generation materials, further modifications to lens designs and surface treatments are vital to the continuing success of overnight wear modalities.

CLINICAL CASES

CASE 1

The patient is a 23-year-old Asian woman wearing AIR OPTIX Night & Day AQUA (Alcon) lenses (−3.00 D OU) on a CW basis, with monthly replacement for 3 months. She came in for a routine follow-up visit with no symptoms. Visual acuities were 20/20 OD and OS. Slit-lamp examination revealed an arcuate lesion superiorly OS extending from 12 o'clock to 1 o'clock (Fig. 16.8A). Following lens removal, she reported mild discomfort under her eyelid OS. The lesion stained with fluorescein (Fig. 16.8B).

SOLUTION: A diagnosis of SEAL was made. Ocular lubricants were dispensed q1h OS and contact lens wear was temporarily discontinued. The patient was seen for follow-up the next day, at which time she was asymptomatic and the epithelium was intact in the affected area. She was refitted with AIR OPTIX AQUA lenses OU for EW with weekly removal without further complications. This case emphasizes the importance of reviewing all EW and CW patients at regular intervals, even when they do not report any problems.

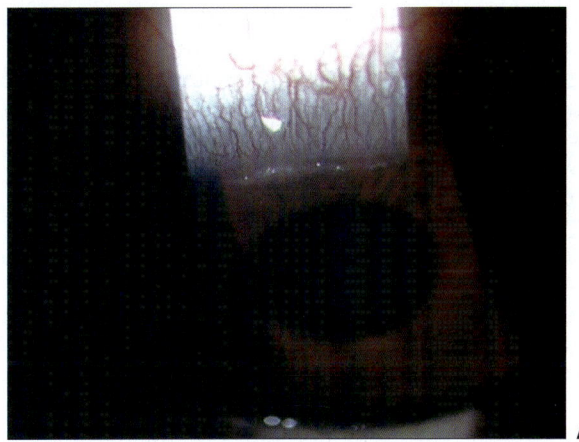
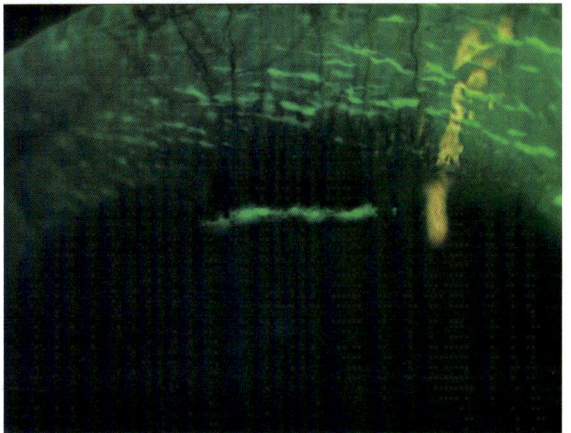

FIGURE 16.8 **(A)** Superior epithelial arcuate lesion (SEAL) subsequent to silicone hydrogel continuous wear. **(B)** Same lesion as observed with fluorescein staining.

CASE 2

The patient is a 27-year-old Caucasian man wearing PureVision (Bausch + Lomb) lenses (−4.00 D OU) on a CW basis for 1 month. He reported discomfort, mucus, and itchiness, and suspected seasonal allergies. Visual acuities were 20/15 OD and OS. Slit-lamp examination of the cornea and bulbar conjunctiva showed no abnormalities. Lid eversion revealed hyperemia and an area of large, papillary excrescences in the central area, adjacent to the lid margin OU (Fig. 16.9).

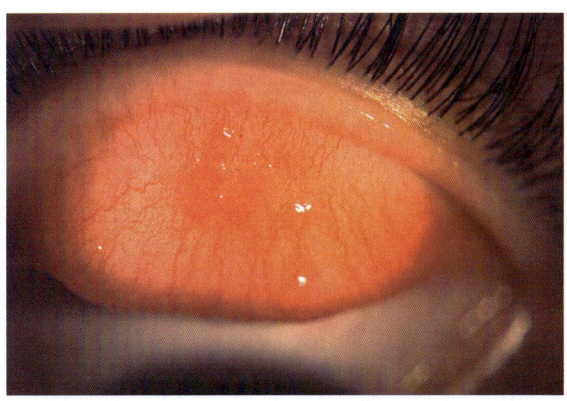

FIGURE 16.9 Localized contact lens-associated papillary conjunctivitis (CLPC) subsequent to silicone hydrogel continuous wear.

SOLUTION: A diagnosis of CLPC was made. PureVision CW lenses were discontinued, and a supply of daily disposables was dispensed for sporting activities only. At the follow-up visit 2 weeks later, the tarsal conjunctiva was smooth and no symptoms were reported. The patient appreciated the convenience of daily disposable lenses and elected to remain in this modality.

CASE 3

The patient is a 31-year-old Caucasian woman wearing PureVision (Bausch + Lomb) lenses (OD −2.75 D, OS −3.50 D) on a CW basis for 3 years. She called to report pain, photophobia, and lacrimation OS, and a foreign body sensation that had started the previous day. She was instructed to immediately schedule an appointment. Visual acuities were 20/15 OD and OS. Slit-lamp examination revealed a small (0.3-mm) circular lesion in the paracentral cornea at 10 o'clock OS and sectoral bulbar and limbal hyperemia superior nasally (Fig. 16.10A). The epithelium in this region stained with fluorescein (Fig. 16.10B).

SOLUTION: A tentative diagnosis of CLPU was made. The patient was directed to wear her spectacles and given current-generation fluoroquinolone drops q.i.d. prophylactically and ocular lubricants prn. Later that evening, she reported a marked improvement in her symptoms and at a follow-up visit the next day, she was asymptomatic and only showed mild epithelial disturbance in the area of the lesion. She continued the antibiotic therapy for a further 3 days, and at the next follow-up visit, the epithelium was intact and treatment was ceased. At the 3-week follow-up visit, the patient was anxious to resume lens wear and was recommended to commence with DW only. Six months later, she had reverted to CW and experienced a second CLPU event. CW was discontinued and a daily/flexible wear recommended.

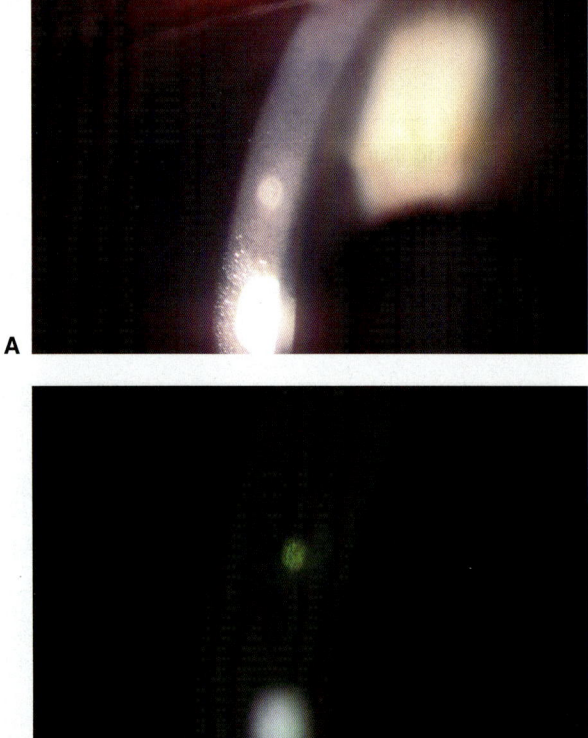

FIGURE 16.10 (A) Contact lens peripheral ulcer (CLPU) subsequent to 30-night silicone hydrogel lens wear. **(B)** The same ulcer as observed with fluorescein staining.

CASE 4

The patient is a 19-year-old Caucasian man wearing Acuvue 2 (Vistakon) lenses (−2.50 D OU) on a DW basis with monthly replacement. He reported napping in his lenses the previous evening but removing them overnight and waking on the day of presentation with marked pain, photophobia, and redness in his right eye (Fig. 16.11A). Visual acuities were 20/20 OD and 20/15 OS. Slit-lamp examination revealed a small irregular oval lesion in the midperiphery at 7 o'clock (Fig. 16.11B). The epithelium stained with fluorescein and there was rapid stromal leakage. Anterior chamber examination showed grade 3 cells and flare.

SOLUTION: A diagnosis was made of probable MK, and the patient was treated with moxifloxacin HCL (0.5%). There was complete resolution of symptoms within 4 days and the epithelium was intact by day 5. A small scar remained, but the VA returned to 20/15 OD. This case demonstrates that even DW patients do occasionally nap while wearing their lenses and can experience serious complications as a result. Careful counseling is crucial.

CASE 5

The patient is a 38-year-old Caucasian man wearing AIR OPTIX Night & Day AQUA (Alcon) lenses (OD −6.00 D, OS −6.50 D) on a CW basis for 2 years. He is a volunteer firefighter, father of young children, and outdoor enthusiast.

SOLUTION: The patient initially started CW in a clinical trial and has subsequently continued in this modality with his own eye care practitioner. What he appreciates most about the lenses is that when he has to get up in the night for an emergency call or for one of his children, he immediately

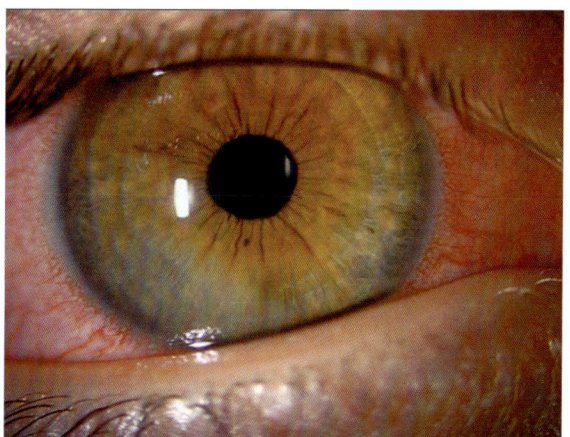

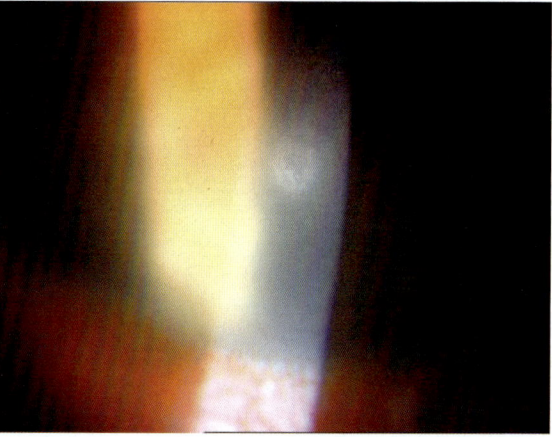

FIGURE 16.11 (A) Bulbar and limbal hyperemia associated with microbial keratitis. (B) Ulceration associated with microbial keratitis following napping in contact lenses.

has functional vision without having to find spectacles or insert contact lenses. What he dislikes most about his lenses is that he has to take 1 night away from lens wear each month when he replaces his lenses and it is "Murphy's law" that this is always a night where he is called out!

CASE 6

The patient is a 22-year-old Caucasian man who was successfully wearing FDA group IV Acuvue (Vistakon) lenses on a DW basis while using ReNu MultiPlus (Bausch + Lomb), but showed signs of limbal hyperemia. He was refitted into PureVision (Bausch + Lomb) lenses and wished to wear them on a CW basis for up to 30 days. However, after 7 to 8 days, the lenses continually appeared to be "greasy" and his comfort and vision was reduced. He also complained of burning sensation and mild crusting on lashes. Examination of the lid margins revealed the presence of plugged meibomian glands with translucent secretions.

SOLUTION: The patient has meibomian gland dysfunction. He was advised to remove the lenses every 5 days, rub and rinse them with his ReNu MultiPlus, soak them overnight, and insert them the next day for up to another 5 to 6 nights. In addition, he was given artificial lubricants and lid scrubs and advised to use warm compresses and lid massages for his lid margin disease (when not wearing his lenses). This solved the problem, and he now successfully wears the lenses on an EW basis with no complaints. This case is fairly typical of what occurs with patients who have marginal tear film quality because of lid disease and wish to use their lenses on a CW basis. Figure 16.12A shows mild meibomian gland dropout in the lower lid, and Figure 16.12B shows no meibomian gland dropout in the upper eye lid. Acuvue lenses attract very little lipid deposition compared with silicone hydrogel lenses,[334,335] and switching a patient may result in symptoms because of deposition of the silicone hydrogel material.

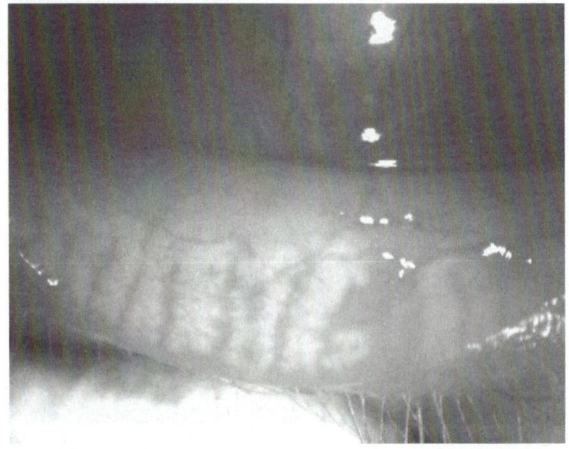

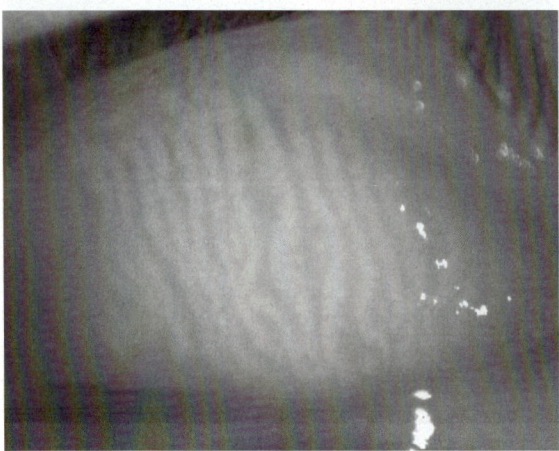

FIGURE 16.12 The upper and lower eyelids were everted and images of the meibomian glands were captured using the Keratograph 4, OCULUS (Wetzlar, Germany). **(A)** Meibography of the lower lid showing mild meibomian gland dropout. **(B)** Meibography of the upper lid showing no meibomian gland loss. (Dr. Sruthi Srinivasan, CCLR, University of Waterloo.)

Reverting to a shorter period of wear without removal and using a rub and rinse process will help to control the lens deposition. It also demonstrates that not all patients who wish to wear their lenses for 30 nights can do so.

CASE 7

The patient is a 54-year-old woman who presented having worn soft contact lenses for more than 30 years. She wore her lenses 7 days a week, 17 hours per day, with the last 5 to 6 hours being somewhat uncomfortable because of symptoms of dryness. She also admitted to regularly napping in her lenses during the day. On presentation, she was wearing Acuvue 2 (Vistakon) lenses in a monovision format (OD for near), with visual acuities of 20/40− and 0.8 M binocularly. Her spectacle prescription was OD −17.50−2.00 × 130 (20/40−) and OS −10.25 −2.25 × 010 (20/40) with a +1.50 D reading add. Keratometry readings were OD 45.75 D × 47.50 D and OS 46.25 D × 48.25 D, and her horizontal visible iris diameter was 12 mm. Slit-lamp examination revealed extensive limbal hyperemia, obvious neovascularization, stromal striae, and endothelial polymegethism (OD > OS) because of chronic hypoxia.

SOLUTION: The patient was fitted with the C-Vue HydraVue Toric Multifocal (Unilens). The lens is a completely custom-designed lens lathed from the Definitive silicone hydrogel material supplied by Contamac, and is replaced on a monthly replacement schedule. Based on the corneal curvatures and spectacle prescriptions, she was initially fit in a multifocal toric with:

OD −14.50 − 1.25 × 130 +1.50 D ADD, BC 8.3 mm, DIA 14.5 mm
OS −9.00 − 1.75 × 010 +1.50 D ADD, BC 8.3 mm, DIA 14.5 mm

The initial fit was beset by a few challenges, as both binocular distance and near vision proved unacceptable to the patient at 20/40− and 1.0 M. Examination of both lenses showed both to be well centered and to have adequate movement; however, the OS lens was rotated by 20 degrees counterclockwise after settling. Binocular loose lens overrefraction with +0.25 held over the right eye improved near vision considerably. The patient remained highly motivated to continue with the lens fitting process and thus a new lens pair was ordered:

OD −14.25 − 1.25 × 130 +1.50 D ADD, BC 8.3 mm, DIA 14.5 mm
OS − 9.00 − 1.75 × 170 +1.50 D ADD, BC 8.3 mm, DIA 14.5 mm

The new pair was much better received, with binocular distance and near VA being 20/30+2 and 0.8M.

At her 1-week follow-up visit, the patient's distance VA was 20/20, and she managed 0.63 M with ease. There were no striae present and her limbal vessels appeared dramatically different, with an obvious reduction in both limbal hyperemia and neovascularization. Her wearing time was still 17 hours and, despite being advised that the material is only approved for DW, she still reported napping in her lenses while taking public transit home each day! She also reported a marked improvement in end-of-day dryness symptoms. The improvement in her ocular appearance continued over the next 3 weeks and at her 1-month visit all signs of chronic hypoxia (with the exception of endothelial polymegethism, which is not expected to recover substantially) were absent.

CLINICAL PROFICIENCY CHECKLIST

- EW and CW are not recommended for all contact lens patients, but these modalities can offer incredible convenience for many wearers.
- Complications will occur with overnight wear as with DW, but the chances of them occurring can be reduced and, in the case of hypoxic complications, can be eliminated with current contact lens materials.
- Only high-Dk/t GP and silicone hydrogel materials should be prescribed for overnight wear unless no other alternatives exist.

(continued)

- Optimal lens fitting characteristics are vital for success with high-Dk/t GP and silicone hydrogel materials.
- Appropriate patient selection is crucial for overnight wear. Patients with a history of poor compliance and a prior history of complications should be avoided or meticulously counseled.
- Certain changes can be expected when refitting low-Dk/t wearers with high-Dk/t materials for EW or CW. These include a transient microcyst response and rebound hyperopic prescription changes.
- Mechanical complications can generally be reduced by changing lens designs or materials.
- Inflammatory complications tend to be patient dependent. If they occur, pay close attention to the prospect of lid margin disease such as blepharitis or meibomian gland disease.
- Differential diagnosis of inflammatory and infectious complications is crucial. If in doubt, the patient should be treated as if the case were infectious. If resolution is rapid, inflammation is the most likely etiology.
- Inflammation can be prevented by suspending overnight wear during periods of ill health or stress.
- Even if lenses are "approved" for wear for up to 6 or 30 consecutive nights, a flexible wearing schedule is recommended.
- The risk of inflammation and infection can be reduced by avoiding swimming in contact lenses or at least cleaning and disinfecting the lenses before wearing them overnight after swimming and hot tub use.
- Inflammation and infection can be reduced by careful and appropriate use of contact lens care products and following instructions for wearing schedules and lens replacement.
- Thorough record keeping is essential.
- All patients should be told that if they are "in doubt," they should "take their lens(es) out."

ACKNOWLEDGMENTS

The authors thank Dr. Sruthi Srinivasan and Dr. Alex Hui for their assistance with Cases 6 and 7.

REFERENCES

1. Jones L, Dumbleton K. Soft lens extended wear and complications. In: Hom MM, Bruce A, eds. *Manual of Contact Lens Prescribing and Fitting*. Oxford: Butterworth-Heinemann; 2006; 393–441.
2. Fatt I. Water flow conductivity and pore diameter in extended-wear gel lens materials. *Am J Optom Physiol Opt.* 1978;55:43–47.
3. Kersley HJ. Contact lens in aphakia. *Trans Ophthalmol Soc U K.* 1977;97:142–144.
4. Nesburn AB. Prolonged-wear contact lenses in aphakia. *Ophthalmology.* 1978;85:73–79.
5. Poggio EC, Glynn RJ, Schein OD, et al. The incidence of ulcerative keratitis among users of daily-wear and extended-wear soft contact lenses. *N Engl J Med.* 1989;321:779–783.
6. Schein OD, Glynn RJ, Poggio EC, et al. The relative risk of ulcerative keratitis among users of daily-wear and extended-wear soft contact lenses. A case-control study. Microbial Keratitis Study Group. *N Engl J Med.* 1989;321:773–778.
7. Cheng KH, Leung SL, Hoekman HW, et al. Incidence of contact-lens-associated microbial keratitis and its related morbidity. *Lancet.* 1999;354:181–185.
8. Brennan N, Coles M. Extended wear in perspective. *Optom Vis Sci.* 1997;74:609–623.
9. Donshik PC. Extended wear contact lenses. *Ophthalmol Clin North Am.* 2003;16:305–309.
10. Dumbleton K. Noninflammatory silicone hydrogel contact lens complications. *Eye Contact Lens.* 2003;29:S186–S189.

11. Sweeney DF. Clinical signs of hypoxia with high-Dk soft lens extended wear: is the cornea convinced? *Eye Contact Lens.* 2003;29:S22–S25.
12. Stapleton F, Stretton S, Papas E, et al. Silicone hydrogel contact lenses and the ocular surface. *Ocul Surf.* 2006;4:24–43.
13. Lim L, Loughnan MS, Sullivan LJ. Microbial keratitis associated with extended wear of silicone hydrogel contact lenses. *Br J Ophthalmol.* 2002;86:355–357.
14. Lee KY, Lim L. Pseudomonas keratitis associated with continuous wear silicone-hydrogel soft contact lens: a case report. *Eye Contact Lens.* 2003;29:255–257.
15. Syam P, Hussain B, Hutchinson C. Mixed infection (Pseudomonas and coagulase negative staphylococci) microbial keratitis associated with extended wear silicone hydrogel contact lens. *Br J Ophthalmol.* 2004;88:579.
16. Schein OD, McNally JJ, Katz J, et al. The incidence of microbial keratitis among wearers of a 30-day silicone hydrogel extended-wear contact lens. *Ophthalmology.* 2005;112:2172–2179.
17. Landers JA, Crompton JL. Microbial keratitis associated with overnight wear of silicone hydrogel contact lenses. *Med J Aust.* 2006;185:177–178.
18. Dart JK, Radford CF, Minassian D, et al. Risk factors for microbial keratitis with contemporary contact lenses: a case-control study. *Ophthalmology.* 2008;115:1647–1654, 1654 e1–1654 e3.
19. Keay L, Stapleton F. Development and evaluation of evidence-based guidelines on contact lens-related microbial keratitis. *Cont Lens Anterior Eye.* 2008;31:3–12.
20. Stapleton F, Keay L, Edwards K, et al. The incidence of contact lens-related microbial keratitis in Australia. *Ophthalmology.* 2008; 115:1655–1662.
21. Radford CF, Minassian D, Dart JK, et al. Risk factors for nonulcerative contact lens complications in an ophthalmic accident and emergency department: a case-control study. *Ophthalmology.* 2009;116:385–392.
22. Leibowitz HM, Laing RA, Sandstrom M. Continuous wear of hydrophilic contact lenses. *Arch Ophthalmol.* 1973;89:306–310.
23. Ezekiel D. High water content hydrophilic contact lenses. *Aust J Optom.* 1974;57:317–324.
24. Benson C. Continuous use of contact lenses. *Trans Ophthalmol Soc N Z.* 1976;28:71–74.
25. Stark WJ, Martin NF. Extended-wear contact lenses for myopic correction. *Arch Ophthalmol.* 1981;99:1963–1966.
26. Binder PS. Myopic extended wear with the Hydrocurve II soft contact lens. *Ophthalmology.* 1983;90:623–626.
27. Hassman G, Sugar J. Pseudomonas corneal ulcer with extended-wear soft contact lenses for myopia. *Arch Ophthalmol.* 1983;101:1549–1550.
28. Weissman BA, Mondino BJ, Pettit TH, et al. Corneal ulcers associated with extended-wear soft contact lenses. *Am J Ophthalmol.* 1984;97:476–481.
29. Donshik P, Weinstock FJ, Wechsler S, et al. Disposable hydrogel contact lenses for extended wear. *CLAO J.* 1988; 14:191–194.
30. Killingsworth DW, Stern GA. Pseudomonas keratitis associated with the use of disposable soft contact lenses. Case report. *Arch Ophthalmol.* 1989;107:795–796.
31. Gritz DC. LASIK interface keratitis: epidemiology, diagnosis and care. *Curr Opin Ophthalmol.* 2011; 22:251–255.
32. Kim HJ, Silverman CM. Traumatic dislocation of LASIK flaps 4 and 9 years after surgery. *J Refract Surg.* 2010;26:447–452.
33. Jain V, Mhatre K, Shome D. Flap buttonhole in thin-flap laser in situ keratomileusis: case series and review. *Cornea.* 2010;29:655–658.
34. Al-Mezaine HS, Al-Amro SA, Al-Obeidan S. Incidence, management, and visual outcomes of buttonholed laser in situ keratomileusis flaps. *J Cataract Refract Surg.* 2009; 35:839–845.
35. Ambrosio R, Jr., Tervo T, Wilson SE. LASIK-associated dry eye and neurotrophic epitheliopathy: pathophysiology and strategies for prevention and treatment. *J Refract Surg.* 2008;24:396–407.
36. Schallhorn SC, Amesbury EC, Tanzer DJ. Avoidance, recognition, and management of LASIK complications. *Am J Ophthalmol.* 2006;141:733–739.
37. Mozayan A, Madu A, Channa P. Laser in-situ keratomileusis infection: review and update of current practices. *Curr Opin Ophthalmol.* 2011;22:233–237.
38. Dumbleton K, Richter D, Woods C, et al. Compliance with contact lens replacement in Canada and the United States. *Optom Vis Sci.* 2010;87:131–139.
39. Bui TH, Cavanagh HD, Robertson DM. Patient compliance during contact lens wear: perceptions, awareness, and behavior. *Eye Contact Lens.* 2010;36:334–339.
40. Ng C, Tighe B. Polymers in contact lens applications VI. The 'dissolved' oxygen permeability of hydrogel and the design of materials for use in continuous wear lenses. *Br Polymer J.* 1976;8:118–123.
41. Fatt I, Chaston J. Measurement of oxygen transmissibility and permeability of hydrogel lenses and materials. *Int Cont Lens Clin.* 1982;9:76–88.
42. Morgan PB, Efron N. The oxygen performance of contemporary hydrogel contact lenses. *Cont Lens Anterior Eye.* 1998;21:3–6.
43. Jones L. Modern contact lens materials: a clinical performance update. *Contact Lens Spectrum.* 2002;17:24–35.
44. Holden BA, Mertz GW. Critical oxygen levels to avoid corneal edema for daily and extended wear contact lenses. *Invest Ophthalmol Vis Sci.* 1984;25:1161–1167.

45. Larke JR, Parrish ST, Wigham CG. Apparent human corneal oxygen uptake rate. *Am J Optom Physiol Opt.* 1981;58:803–805.
46. Efron N. Intersubject variability in corneal swelling response to anoxia. *Acta Ophthalmol (Copenh).* 1986;64:302–305.
47. Fatt I, St Helen R. Oxygen tension under an oxygen-permeable contact lens. *Am J Optom Arch Am Acad Optom.* 1971;48:545–555.
48. Fatt I, Freeman RD, Lin D. Oxygen tension distributions in the cornea: a re-examination. *Exp Eye Res.* 1974;18:357–365.
49. Fatt I, Ruben C. A new oxygen transmissibility concept for hydrogel contact lenses. *J Br Contact Lens Assoc.* 1993;16:141–149.
50. Harvitt DM, Bonanno JA. Re-evaluation of the oxygen diffusion model for predicting minimum contact lens Dk/t values needed to avoid corneal anoxia. *Optom Vis Sci.* 1999; 76:712–719.
51. Brennan NA. Corneal oxygenation during contact lens wear: comparison of diffusion and EOP-based flux models. *Clin Exp Optom.* 2005;88:103–108.
52. Brennan NA. Beyond flux: total corneal oxygen consumption as an index of corneal oxygenation during contact lens wear. *Optom Vis Sci.* 2005;82:467–472.
53. Efron N, Morgan PB, Woods CA. The International Contact Lens Prescribing Survey C: International survey of contact lens prescribing for extended wear. *Optom Vis Sci.* 2012; 89(2):122–129.
54. Lim L, Tan DT, Chan WK. Therapeutic use of Bausch & Lomb PureVision contact lenses. *CLAO J.* 2001;27:179–185.
55. Montero J, Sparholt J, Mely R. Retrospective case series of therapeutic applications of a lotrafilcon A silicone hydrogel soft contact lens. *Eye Contact Lens.* 2003;29:S54–S56; discussion S57–S59, S192–S194.
56. Ambroziak AM, Szaflik JP, Szaflik J. Therapeutic use of a silicone hydrogel contact lens in selected clinical cases. *Eye Contact Lens.* 2004;30:63–67.
57. Szaflik JP, Ambroziak AM, Szaflik J. Therapeutic use of a lotrafilcon A silicone hydrogel soft contact lens as a bandage after LASEK surgery. *Eye Contact Lens.* 2004;30:59–62.
58. Ozkurt Y, Rodop O, Oral Y, et al. Therapeutic applications of lotrafilcon a silicone hydrogel soft contact lenses. *Eye Contact Lens.* 2005;31:268–269.
59. Xu J, Li X, Sun F. In vitro and in vivo evaluation of ketotifen fumarate-loaded silicone hydrogel contact lenses for ocular drug delivery. *Drug Deliv.* 2011;18:150–158.
60. Boone A, Hui A, Jones L. Uptake and release of dexamethasone phosphate from silicone hydrogel and group I, II, and IV hydrogel contact lenses. *Eye Contact Lens.* 2009;35:260–267.
61. Morgan PB, Woods C, Tranoudis I, et al. International contact lens prescribing in 2011. *Contact Lens Spectrum.* 2012;27:26–31.
62. Dart JK, Stapleton F, Minassian D. Contact lenses and other risk factors in microbial keratitis. *Lancet.* 1991;338:650–653.
63. Dart J. Predisposing factors in microbial keratitis: the significance of contact lens wear. *Br J Ophthalmol.* 1988;72:926–930.
64. Cheung J, Slomovic AR. Microbial etiology and predisposing factors among patients hospitalized for corneal ulceration. *Can J Ophthalmol.* 1995;30:251–255.
65. Dumbleton KA, Woods CA, Jones LW, et al. The relationship between compliance with lens replacement and contact lens-related problems in silicone hydrogel wearers. *Cont Lens Anterior Eye.* 2011;34:216–222.
66. Yeung KK, Forister JF, Forister EF, et al. Compliance with soft contact lens replacement schedules and associated contact lens-related ocular complications: the UCLA Contact Lens Study. *Optometry.* 2010;81:598–607.
67. Stapleton F, Edwards K, Keay L, et al. Risk factors for moderate and severe microbial keratitis in daily wear contact lens users. *Ophthalmology.* 2012;119:1516–1521.
68. Cutter GR, Chalmers RL, Roseman M. The clinical presentation, prevalence, and risk factors of focal corneal infiltrates in soft contact lens wearers. *CLAO J.* 1996;22:30–37.
69. McNally JJ, Chalmers RL, McKenney CD, et al. Risk factors for corneal infiltrative events with 30-night continuous wear of silicone hydrogel lenses. *Eye Contact Lens.* 2003;29:S153–S156; discussion S166, S192–S194.
70. Lam DS, Houang E, Fan DS, et al. Incidence and risk factors for microbial keratitis in Hong Kong: comparison with Europe and North America. *Eye.* 2002;16:608–618.
71. Radford CF, Minassian DC, Dart JK. Acanthamoeba keratitis in England and Wales: incidence, outcome, and risk factors. *Br J Ophthalmol.* 2002;86:536–542.
72. Stehr-Green JK, Bailey TM, Brandt FH, et al. Acanthamoeba keratitis in soft contact lens wearers. A case-control study. *JAMA.* 1987;258:57–60.
73. Mena KD, Gerba CP. Risk assessment of Pseudomonas aeruginosa in water. *Rev Environ Contam Toxicol.* 2009;201:71–115.
74. Stapleton F, Ozkan J, Jalbert I, et al. Contact lens-related acanthamoeba keratitis. *Optom Vis Sci.* 2009;86:E1196–E1201.
75. O'Donnell C, Efron N. Diabetes and contact lens wear. *Clin Exp Optom.* 2012;95:328–337.
76. Dougherty JM, McCulley JP. Comparative bacteriology of chronic blepharitis. *Br J Ophthalmol.* 1984;68:524–528.

77. Groden LR, Murphy B, Rodnite J, et al. Lid flora in blepharitis. *Cornea.* 1991;10:50–53.
78. van der Meulen IJ, van Rooij J, et al. Age-related risk factors, culture outcomes, and prognosis in patients admitted with infectious keratitis to two Dutch tertiary referral centers. *Cornea.* 2008;27:539–544.
79. Fleiszig SM, Glenn A. Fry award lecture 2005. The pathogenesis of contact lens-related keratitis. *Optom Vis Sci.* 2006;83:866–873.
80. Dumbleton K. Adverse events with silicone hydrogel continuous wear. *Cont Lens Anterior Eye.* 2002;25:137–146.
81. Sweeney D, du Toit R, Keay L, et al. Clinical performance of silicone hydrogel lenses. In: Sweeney D, ed. *Silicone Hydrogels: Continuous Wear Contact Lenses.* Oxford: Butterworth-Heinemann; 2004;164–216.
82. Sweeney DF, Stern J, Naduvilath T, et al. Inflammatory adverse event rates over 3 years with silicone hydrogel lenses. *Invest Ophthalmol Vis Sci.* 2002;43:40.
83. Fatt I. Now do we need 'effective permeability'? *Contax.* 1986:6–23.
84. Tighe B. Soft lens materials. In: Efron N, ed. *Contact Lens Practice.* Oxford: Butterworth-Heinemann; 2002; 71–84.
85. Tighe B. Contact Lens Materials. In: Phillips A, Speedwell L, eds. *Contact Lenses.* Edinburgh: Butterworth-Heinemann; 2006;59–78.
86. Maldonado-Codina C. Soft lens materials. In: Efron N, ed. *Contact Lens Practice.* Oxford: Butterworth-Heinemann; 2010;67–85.
87. Zekman TN, Sarnat LA. Clinical evaluation of the silicone corneal contact lens. *Am J Ophthalmol.* 1972;74:534–537.
88. Refojo MF. Contact lens materials. *Int Ophthalmol Clin.* 1973;13:263–277.
89. Refojo MF. Mechanism of gas transport through contact lenses. *J Am Optom Assoc.* 1979;50:285–287.
90. Gurland JE. Use of silicone lenses in infants and children. *Ophthalmology.* 1979;86:1599–1604.
91. Rae ST, Huff JW. Studies on initiation of silicone elastomer lens adhesion in vitro: binding before the indentation ring. *CLAO J.* 1991;17:181–186.
92. Huth S, Wagner H. Identification and removal of deposits on polydimethylsiloxane silicone elastomer lenses. *Int Cont Lens Clin.* 1981;8:19–26.
93. Dahl AA, Brocks ER. The use of continuous-wear silicone contact lenses in the optical correction of aphakia. *Am J Ophthalmol.* 1978;85:454–461.
94. Tighe B. Silicone hydrogels: Structure, properties and behaviour. In: Sweeney D, ed. *Silicone Hydrogels: Continuous Wear Contact Lenses.* Oxford: Butterworth-Heinemann; 2004;1–27.
95. Loveridge R. Dk 30, 60, 90 and 120—can the cornea tell the difference? *Optom Today.* 1997:36.
96. Walker J. High Dk RGPs: the lens of first choice. *Optician.* 1992;203:18–25.
97. Schwartz C. Radical flattening and RGP lenses. *Contact Lens Forum.* 1986;11:49–52.
98. Yokota M, Goshima T, Itoh S. The effect of polymer structure on durability of high Dk gas permeable materials. *J Br Contact Lens Assoc.* 1992;15:125–129.
99. Tranoudis I, Efron N. Scratch resistance of rigid contact lens materials. *Ophthal Physiol Opt.* 1996;16:303–309.
100. Walker J. Handling high DK lenses. *Optician.* 1989;197:30–39.
101. Walker J. Cracking and crazing - a practitioner's viewpoint. *Optician.* 1990;199:19–21.
102. Lembach RG, McLaughlin R, Barr JT. Crazing in a rigid gas permeable contact lens. *CLAO J.* 1988;14:38–41.
103. Arnestad J. Cracking of Persecon CE contact lenses. *Contact Lens J.* 1989;17:86–87.
104. Bark M, Hanson D, Grant R. A guide to rigid gas-permeable contact lens materials. *Optician.* 1994;207:17–20.
105. Walker J. A clinical and laboratory comparison of the deposition characteristics of both silicone/acrylate and fluoro-silicone/acrylate lenses. *J Br Contact Lens Assoc.* 1988;11:83–86.
106. Levy B. The use of a gas permeable hard lens for extended wear. *Am J Optom Physiol Opt.* 1983;60:408–409.
107. Ichikawa H, Kozai A, MacKeen DL, et al. Corneal swelling responses with extended wear in naive and adapted subjects with menicon RGP contact lenses. *CLAO J.* 1989;15:192–194.
108. Koetting RA, Castellano CF, Nelson DW. A hard lens with extended wear possibilities. *J Am Optom Assoc.* 1985;56:208–211.
109. Fonn D, Holden BA. Rigid gas-permeable vs. hydrogel contact lenses for extended wear. *Am J Optom Physiol Opt.* 1988;65:536–544.
110. Ichijima H, Imayasu M, Tanaka H, et al. Effects of RGP lens extended wear on glucose-lactate metabolism and stromal swelling in the rabbit cornea. *CLAO J.* 2000;26:30–36.
111. Ichijima H, Cavanagh HD. How rigid gas-permeable lenses supply more oxygen to the cornea than silicone hydrogels: a new model. *Eye Contact Lens.* 2007;33:216–223.
112. Gardner HP, Fink BA, Mitchell LG, et al. The effects of high-Dk rigid contact lens center thickness, material permeability, and blinking on the oxygen uptake of the human cornea. *Optom Vis Sci.* 2005;82:459–466.
113. Ladage PM, Yamamoto K, Ren DH, et al. Effects of rigid and soft contact lens daily wear on corneal epithelium, tear lactate dehydrogenase, and bacterial binding to exfoliated epithelial cells. *Ophthalmology.* 2001;108:1279–1288.
114. Ren DH, Yamamoto K, Ladage PM, et al. Adaptive effects of 30-night wear of hyper-O_2 transmissible contact lenses on bacterial binding and corneal epithelium: a 1-year clinical trial. *Ophthalmology.* 2002;109:27–39.
115. Gleason W, Albright RA. Menicon Z 30-day continuous wear lenses: a clinical comparison to Acuvue 7-day extended wear lenses. *Eye Contact Lens.* 2003;29:S149–S152; discussion S166, S192–S194.
116. Maldonado-Codina C, Morgan PB, Efron N, et al. Comparative clinical performance of rigid versus soft hyper Dk contact lenses used for continuous wear. *Optom Vis Sci.* 2005;82:536–548.

117. Albright RA, Venuti BD, Ichijima H, et al. Postmarket surveillance of Menicon Z rigid gas-permeable contact lenses for up to 30 days continuous wear in the United States. *Eye Contact Lens.* 2010;36:241–244.
118. Swarbrick HA, Holden BA. Ocular characteristics associated with rigid gas-permeable lens adherence. *Optom Vis Sci.* 1996;73:473–481.
119. Swarbrick HA, Holden BA. Effects of lens parameter variation on rigid gas-permeable lens adherence. *Optom Vis Sci.* 1996;73:144–155.
120. Fonn D, Holden BA. Extended wear of hard gas permeable contact lenses can induce ptosis. *CLAO J.* 1986;12:93–94.
121. Key JE, Mobley CL. Paraperm EW lens for extended wear. *CLAO J.* 1989;15:134–137.
122. Grobe G, Kunzler J, Seelye D, et al. Silicone hydrogels for contact lens applications. *PMSE.* 1999;80:108–109.
123. Nicolson PC, Vogt J. Soft contact lens polymers: an evolution. *Biomaterials.* 2001;22:3273–3283.
124. Nicolson PC. Continuous wear contact lens surface chemistry and wearability. *Eye Contact Lens.* 2003;29:S30–S32; discussion S57–S59, S192–S194.
125. Maiden A, Vanderlaan D, Turner D, et al. Hydrogel with internal wetting agent. US Patent 6,367,929. 2002.
126. McCabe K, Molock F, Hill G,et al. Biomedical devices containing internal wetting agents. US Patent 7,052,131. 2006.
127. Jones L, Subbaraman LN, Rogers R, et al. Surface treatment, wetting and modulus of silicone hydrogels. *Optician.* 2006;232:28–34.
128. Bambury R, Seelye D. Vinyl carbonate and vinyl carbamate contact lens materials. US Patent 5,610,252. 1997.
129. Lopez-Alemany A, Compan V, Refojo MF. Porous structure of Purevision versus Focus Night & Day and conventional hydrogel contact lenses. *J Biomed Mater Res (Appl Biomat).* 2002; 63:319–325.
130. Kunzler J. Silicone-based hydrogels for contact lens applications. *Contact Lens Spectrum.* 1999;14:9–11.
131. Grobe G. Surface engineering aspects of silicone-hydrogel lenses. *Contact Lens Spectrum.* 1999;14:14–17.
132. Valint PL Jr, Grobe GL III, Ammon DM Jr, et al. Plasma surface treatment of silicone hydrogel contact lenses. US Patent 6,193,369. 2001.
133. Gonzalez-Meijome JM, Lopez-Alemany A, Almeida JB,et al. Microscopic observation of unworn siloxane-hydrogel soft contact lenses by atomic force microscopy. *J Biomed Mater Res B Appl Biomater.* 2006;76:412–418.
134. Teichroeb JH, Forrest JA, Ngai V, et al. Imaging protein deposits on contact lens materials. *Optom Vis Sci.* 2008;85:1151–1164.
135. Nilsson SE. Seven-day extended wear and 30-day continuous wear of high oxygen transmissibility soft silicone hydrogel contact lenses: a randomized 1-year study of 504 patients. *CLAO J.* 2001;27:125–136.
136. Brennan NA, Coles ML, Comstock TL, et al. A 1-year prospective clinical trial of balafilcon a (PureVision) silicone-hydrogel contact lenses used on a 30-day continuous wear schedule. *Ophthalmology.* 2002;109:1172–1177.
137. Morgan PB, Efron N. Comparative clinical performance of two silicone hydrogel contact lenses for continuous wear. *Clin Exp Optom.* 2002;85:183–192.
138. Foulks GN, Harvey T, Raj CV. Therapeutic contact lenses: the role of high-Dk lenses. *Ophthalmol Clin North Am.* 2003;16:455–461.
139. Arora R, Jain S, Monga S, et al. Efficacy of continuous wear PureVision contact lenses for therapeutic use. *Cont Lens Anterior Eye.* 2004;27:39–43.
140. Nicolson P, Baron R, Chabrecek P, et al. Extended wear ophthalmic lens. US Patent 5,760,100. 1998.
141. Weikart CM, Matsuzawa Y, Winterton L, et al. Evaluation of plasma polymer-coated contact lenses by electrochemical impedance spectroscopy. *J Biomed Mater Res.* 2001;54:597–607.
142. Gonzalez-Meijome JM, Lopez-Alemany A, Almeida JB, et al. Microscopic observations of superficial ultrastructure of unworn siloxane-hydrogel contact lenses by cryo-scanning electron microscopy. *J Biomed Mater Res B Appl Biomater.* 2006;76:419–423.
143. Montero Iruzubieta J, Nebot Ripoll JR, Chiva J, et al. Practical experience with a high Dk lotrafilcon A fluorosilicone hydrogel extended wear contact lens in Spain. *CLAO J.* 2001;27:41–46.
144. McNally J, McKenney CD. A clinical look at a silicone hydrogel extended wear lens. *Contact Lens Spectrum.* 2002;17:38–41.
145. Malet F, Pagot R, Peyre C, et al. Clinical results comparing high-oxygen and low-oxygen permeable soft contact lenses in France. *Eye Contact Lens.* 2003;29:50–54.
146. Stern J, Wong R, Naduvilath TJ, et al. Comparison of the performance of 6- or 30-night extended wear schedules with silicone hydrogel lenses over 3 years. *Optom Vis Sci.* 2004;81:398–406.
147. Chalmers RL, Dillehay S, Long B, et al. Impact of previous extended and daily wear schedules on signs and symptoms with high Dk lotrafilcon A lenses. *Optom Vis Sci.* 2005;82:549–554.
148. Bergenske P, Long B, Dillehay S, et al. Long-term clinical results: 3 years of up to 30-night continuous wear of lotrafilcon A silicone hydrogel and daily wear of low-Dk/t hydrogel lenses. *Eye Contact Lens.* 2007;33:74–80.
149. Kanpolat A, Ucakhan OO. Therapeutic use of Focus Night & Day contact lenses. *Cornea.* 2003;22:726–734.
150. Bendoriene J, Vogt U. Therapeutic use of silicone hydrogel contact lenses in children. *Eye Contact Lens.* 2006;32:104–108.
151. Schafer J, Mitchell GL, Chalmers RL, et al. The stability of dryness symptoms after refitting with silicone hydrogel contact lenses over 3 years. *Eye Contact Lens.* 2007;33:247–252.

152. Dillehay SM, Miller MB. Performance of Lotrafilcon B silicone hydrogel contact lenses in experienced low-Dk/t daily lens wearers. *Eye Contact Lens.* 2007;33:272–277.
153. Long B, McNally J. The clinical performance of a silicone hydrogel lens for daily wear in an Asian population. *Eye Contact Lens.* 2006;32:65–71.
154. Dumbleton K, Keir N, Moezzi A, et al. Objective and subjective responses in patients refitted to daily-wear silicone hydrogel contact lenses. *Optom Vis Sci.* 2006;83:758–768.
155. Long B, Schweizer H, Bleshoy H, et al. Expanding your use of silicone hydrogel contact lenses: using lotrafilcon A for daily wear. *Eye Contact Lens.* 2009;35:59–64.
156. Jones L. Comfilcon A: a new silicone hydrogel material. *Contact Lens Spectrum.* 2007;22:21.
157. DeLoss KS, Walsh JE, Bergmanson JP. Current silicone hydrogel UVR blocking lenses and their associated protection factors. *Cont Lens Anterior Eye.* 2010;33:136–140.
158. Szczotka-Flynn L. Looking at silicone hydrogels across generations. *Optom Manag.* 2008:68–71.
159. Chou B. The evolution of silicone hydrogel lenses. *Contact Lens Spectrum.* 2008;22:37–39.
160. Moezzi AM, Fonn D, Simpson TL. Overnight corneal swelling with silicone hydrogel contact lenses with high oxygen transmissibility. *Eye Contact Lens.* 2006;32:277–280.
161. Brennan NA, Coles ML, Connor HR, et al. A 12-month prospective clinical trial of comfilcon A silicone-hydrogel contact lenses worn on a 30-day continuous wear basis. *Cont Lens Anterior Eye.* 2007;30:108–118.
162. Steffen R, Schnider C. A next generation silicone hydrogel lens for daily wear. Part 1 - Material properties. *Optician.* 2004;227:23–25.
163. Schnider C, Steffen R. A next generation silicone hydrogel lens for daily wear. Part 2 - clinical performance. *Optician.* 2004;228:20–24.
164. Moore L, Ferreira JT. Ultraviolet (UV) transmittance characteristics of daily disposable and silicone hydrogel contact lenses. *Cont Lens Anterior Eye.* 2006;29:115–122.
165. Chandler HL, Reuter KS, Sinnott LT, et al. Prevention of UV-induced damage to the anterior segment using class I UV-absorbing hydrogel contact lenses. *Invest Ophthalmol Vis Sci.* 2010;51:172–178.
166. Andley UP, Malone JP, Townsend RR. Inhibition of lens photodamage by UV-absorbing contact lenses. *Invest Ophthalmol Vis Sci.* 2011;52:8330–8341.
167. Giblin FJ, Lin LR, Leverenz VR, et al. A class I (Senofilcon A) soft contact lens prevents UVB-induced ocular effects, including cataract, in the rabbit in vivo. *Invest Ophthalmol Vis Sci.* 2011;52:3667–3675.
168. Sulley A. Practitioner and patient acceptance of a new silicone hydrogel contact lens. *Optician.* 2005;230:15–17.
169. Riley C, Young G, Chalmers R. Prevalence of ocular surface symptoms, signs, and uncomfortable hours of wear in contact lens wearers: the effect of refitting with daily-wear silicone hydrogel lenses (senofilcon a). *Eye Contact Lens.* 2006;32:281–286.
170. Young G, Riley CM, Chalmers RL, et al. Hydrogel lens comfort in challenging environments and the effect of refitting with silicone hydrogel lenses. *Optom Vis Sci.* 2007;84:302–308.
171. Ousler GW III, Anderson RT, Osborn KE. The effect of senofilcon A contact lenses compared to habitual contact lenses on ocular discomfort during exposure to a controlled adverse environment. *Curr Med Res Opin.* 2008;24:335–341.
172. Jones L. A new silicone hydrogel lens comes to market. *Contact Lens Spectrum.* 2007;22:23.
173. Lakkis C, Vincent S. Clinical investigation of asmofilcon a silicone hydrogel lenses. *Optom Vis Sci.* 2009;86:350–356.
174. Weikart CM, Miyama M, Yasuda HK. Surface modification of conventional polymers by depositing plasma polymers of trimethylsilane and of trimethylsilane + O_2. *J Colloid Interface Sci.* 1999;211:18–27.
175. Ang J, Efron N. Carbon dioxide permeability of contact lens materials. *Int Cont Lens Clin.* 1989;16:48–57.
176. Ang JH, Efron N. Corneal hypoxia and hypercapnia during contact lens wear. *Optom Vis Sci.* 1990;67:512–521.
177. Klyce S. Stromal lactate accumulation can account for corneal edema osmotically following epithelial hypoxia in the rabbit. *J Physiol.* 1981;321:49–64.
178. Fonn D, MacDonald KE, Richter D, et al. The ocular response to extended wear of a high Dk silicone hydrogel contact lens. *Clin Exp Optom.* 2002;85:176–182.
179. Holden BA, Mertz GW, McNally JJ. Corneal swelling response to contact lenses worn under extended wear conditions. *Invest Ophthalmol Vis Sci.* 1983;24:218–226.
180. Fonn D, du Toit R, Simpson TL, et al. Sympathetic swelling response of the control eye to soft lenses in the other eye. *Invest Ophthalmol Vis Sci.* 1999;40:3116–3121.
181. Fonn D, Bruce AS. A review of the Holden-Mertz criteria for critical oxygen transmission. *Eye Contact Lens.* 2005;31:247–251.
182. Polse KA, Mandell RB. Etiology of corneal striae accompanying hydrogel lens wear. *Invest Ophthalmol.* 1976;15:553–556.
183. Polse KA, Sarver MD, Harris MG. Corneal edema and vertical striae accompanying the wearing of hydrogel lenses. *Am J Optom Physiol Opt.* 1975;52:185–191.
184. Kerns RL. A study of striae observed in the cornea from contact lens wear. *Am J Optom Physiol Opt.* 1974;51:998–1004.

185. La Hood D. Daytime edema levels with plus powered low and high water content hydrogel contact lenses. *Optom Vis Sci.* 1991;68:877–880.
186. Efron N. Stromal oedema. In: Efron N, ed. *Contact Lens Complications.* London: Elsevier; 2012; 185–197.
187. Alvord L, Court J, Davis T, et al. Oxygen permeability of a new type of high Dk soft contact lens material. *Optom Vis Sci.* 1998;75:30–36.
188. Papas EB, Vajdic CM, Austen R, et al. High-oxygen-transmissibility soft contact lenses do not induce limbal hyperaemia. *Curr Eye Res.* 1997;16:942–948.
189. Holden BA, Sweeney DF, Sanderson G. The minimum precorneal oxygen tension to avoid corneal edema. *Invest Ophthalmol Vis Sci.* 1984;25:476–480.
190. Ruben M, Brown N, Lobascher D, et al. Clinical manifestations secondary to soft contact lens wear. *Br J Ophthalmol.* 1976;60:529–531.
191. Zantos S, Holden B. Ocular changes associated with continuous wear of contact lenses. *Aust J Optom.* 1978;61:418–426.
192. Efron N. Epithelial microcysts. In: Efron N, ed. *Contact Lens Complications.* London: Elsevier;2012;167–173.
193. Holden BA, Sweeney DF. The significance of the microcyst response: a review. *Optom Vis Sci.* 1991;68:703–707.
194. Covey M, Sweeney DF, Terry R, et al. Hypoxic effects on the anterior eye of high-Dk soft contact lens wearers are negligible. *Optom Vis Sci.* 2001;78:95–99.
195. Keay L, Sweeney DF, Jalbert I, et al. Microcyst response to high Dk/t silicone hydrogel contact lenses. *Optom Vis Sci.* 2000;77:582–585.
196. Zantos S. Cystic formations in the corneal epithelium during extended wear of contact lenses. *Int Cont Lens Clin.*1983;10:128–146.
197. Keay L, Jalbert I, Sweeney DF, et al. Microcysts: clinical significance and differential diagnosis. *Optometry.* 2001;72:452–460.
198. Schoessler J. Corneal endothelial polymegethism associated with extended wear. *Int Cont Lens Clin.* 1983;10:148–155.
199. Efron N. Endothelial polymegethism. In: Efron N, ed. *Contact Lens Complications.* London: Elsevier;2012; 291–298.
200. Holden BA, Sweeney DF, Vannas A, et al. Effects of long-term extended contact lens wear on the human cornea. *Invest Ophthalmol Vis Sci.* 1985;26:1489–1501.
201. Carlson KH, Bourne WM. Endothelial morphologic features and function after long-term extended wear of contact lenses. *Arch Ophthalmol.* 1988;106:1677–1679.
202. Dutt RM, Stocker EG, Wolff CH, et al. A morphologic and fluorophotometric analysis of the corneal endothelium in long-term extended wear soft contact lens wearers. *CLAO J.* 1989;15:121–123.
203. Polse KA, Brand RJ, Cohen SR, et al. Hypoxic effects on corneal morphology and function. *Invest Ophthalmol Vis Sci.* 1990;31:1542–1554.
204. Yagmur M, Okay O, Sizmaz S, et al. In vivo confocal microscopy: corneal changes of hydrogel contact lens wearers. *Int Ophthalmol.* 2011;31:377–383.
205. Sweeney DF. Corneal exhaustion syndrome with long-term wear of contact lenses. *Optom Vis Sci.* 1992;69: 601–608.
206. Barr JT, Pall B, Szczotka LB, et al. Corneal endothelial morphology results in the Menicon Z 30-day continuous-wear contact lens clinical trial. *Eye Contact Lens.* 2003;29:14–16.
207. Efron N. Limbal redness. In: Efron N, ed. *Contact Lens Complications.* London: Elsevier;2012; 133–139.
208. Dumbleton KA, Chalmers RL, Richter DB, et al. Vascular response to extended wear of hydrogel lenses with high and low oxygen permeability. *Optom Vis Sci.* 2001;78:147–151.
209. du Toit R, Simpson TL, Fonn D, et al. Recovery from hyperemia after overnight wear of low and high transmissibility hydrogel lenses. *Curr Eye Res.* 2001;22:68–73.
210. Woods J, Jones L, Woods C, et al. Use of a photographic manipulation tool to assess corneal vascular response. *Optom Vis Sci.* 2012;89(2):215–220.
211. Papas E. On the relationship between soft contact lens oxygen transmissibility and induced limbal hyperaemia. *Exp Eye Res.* 1998;67:125–131.
212. Efron N. Corneal neovascularization. In: Efron N, ed. *Contact Lens Complications.* London: Elsevier;2012; 214–224.
213. McMonnies C. Contact lens induced corneal vascularisation. *Int Cont Lens Clin.* 1983;10:12–21.
214. Millodot M, O'Leary DJ. Effect of oxygen deprivation on corneal sensitivity. *Acta Ophthalmol (Copenh).* 1980;58:434–439.
215. Millodot M. A review of research on the sensitivity of the cornea. *Ophthal Physiol Opt.* 1984;4:305–318.
216. Fleiszig S, Efron N, Pier G. Extended contact lens wear enhances *Pseudomonas aeruginosa* adherence to human corneal epithelium. *Invest Ophthalmol Vis Sci.* 1992;33:2908–2916.
217. Latkovic S, Nilsson SE. The effect of high and low Dk/L soft contact lenses on the glycocalyx layer of the corneal epithelium and on the membrane associated receptors for lectins. *CLAO J.* 1997;23:185–191.
218. Ren H, Petroll WM, Jester JV, et al. Adherence of Pseudomonas aeruginosa to shed rabbit corneal epithelial cells after overnight wear of contact lenses. *CLAO J.* 1997;23:63–68.

219. Ren DH, Petroll WM, Jester JV, et al. The relationship between contact lens oxygen permeability and binding of Pseudomonas aeruginosa to human corneal epithelial cells after overnight and extended wear. *CLAO J.* 1999;25:80–100.
220. Holden B. The ocular response to contact lens wear. *Optom Vis Sci.* 1989;66:717–733.
221. Liesegang TJ. Physiologic changes of the cornea with contact lens wear. *CLAO J.* 2002;28:12–27.
222. Dumbleton KA, Chalmers RL, Richter DB, et al. Changes in myopic refractive error with nine months' extended wear of hydrogel lenses with high and low oxygen permeability. *Optom Vis Sci.* 1999;76:845–849.
223. Jalbert I, Stretton S, Naduvilath T, et al. Changes in myopia with low-Dk hydrogel and high-Dk silicone hydrogel extended wear. *Optom Vis Sci.* 2004;81:591–596.
224. Efron N. Corneal staining. In: Efron N, ed. *Contact Lens Complications.* London: Elsevier; 2012;155–166.
225. Bruce A. Local oxygen transmissibility of disposable contact lenses. *Cont Lens Anterior Eye.* 2003;26:189–196.
226. Efron N, Morgan PB, Cameron ID, et al. Oxygen permeability and water content of silicone hydrogel contact lens materials. *Optom Vis Sci.* 2007;84:328–337.
227. Sankaridurg P, Holden B, Jalbert I. Adverse events and infections: which ones and how many? In: Sweeney D, ed. *Silicone Hydrogels: Continuous Wear Contact Lenses.* Oxford: Butterworth-Heinemann; 2004; 217–274.
228. Dumbleton K, Jones L, Chalmers R, et al. Clinical characterization of spherical post-lens debris associated with lotrafilcon high-Dk silicone lenses. *CLAO J.* 2000;26:186–192.
229. Craig JP, Sherwin T, Grupcheva CN, et al. An evaluation of mucin balls associated with high-DK silicone-hydrogel contact lens wear. *Adv Exp Med Biol.* 2002;506:917–923.
230. Ladage PM, Petroll WM, Jester JV, et al. Spherical indentations of human and rabbit corneal epithelium following extended contact lens wear. *CLAO J.* 2002;28:177–180.
231. Tan J, Keay L, Jalbert I, Naduvilath TJ, et al. Mucin balls with wear of conventional and silicone hydrogel contact lenses. *Optom Vis Sci.* 2003;80:291–297.
232. Millar TJ, Papas EB, Ozkan J, et al. Clinical appearance and microscopic analysis of mucin balls associated with contact lens wear. *Cornea.* 2003;22:740–745.
233. Jalbert I, Stapleton F, Papas E, et al. In vivo confocal microscopy of the human cornea. *Br J Ophthalmol.* 2003;87:225–236.
234. Efron N. Contact lens-induced changes in the anterior eye as observed in vivo with the confocal microscope. *Prog Retin Eye Res.* 2007;26:398–436.
235. Evans V, Carnt N, Naduvilath T, et al. Risk factors associated with corneal inflammation in soft contact lens daily wear. *Contact Lens Ant Eye.* 2007;30:302.
236. Szczotka-Flynn L, Benetz BA, Lass J, et al. The association between mucin balls and corneal infiltrative events during extended contact lens wear. *Cornea.* 2011;30:535–542.
237. Hine N, Back A, Holden B. Aetiology of arcuate epithelial lesions induced by hydrogels. *J Br Contact Lens Assoc.* 1987:48–50.
238. Holden BA, Stephenson A, Stretton S, et al. Superior epithelial arcuate lesions with soft contact lens wear. *Optom Vis Sci.* 2001;78:9–12.
239. Jalbert I, Sweeney DF, Holden BA. Epithelial split associated with wear of a silicone hydrogel contact lens. *CLAO J.* 2001;27:231–233.
240. Malinovsky V, Pole J, Pence N, et al. Epithelial splits of the superior cornea in hydrogel contact lens patients. *Int Cont Lens Clin.* 1989;16:252–254.
241. O'Hare N, Stapleton F, Naduvilath T, et al. Interaction between the contact lens and the ocular surface in the etiology of superior epithelial arcuate lesions. *Adv Exp Med Biol.* 2002;506:973–980.
242. Young G, Mirejovsky D. A hypothesis for the aetiology of soft contact lens-induced superior arcuate keratopathy. *Int Cont Lens Clin.* 1993;20:177–179.
243. Donshik P, Long B, Dillehay SM, et al. Inflammatory and mechanical complications associated with 3 years of up to 30 nights of continuous wear of lotrafilcon A silicone hydrogel lenses. *Eye Contact Lens.* 2007;33:191–195.
244. O'Hare N, Naduvilath T, Sweeney D, et al. A clinical comparison of limbal and paralimbal superior epithelial arcuate lesions (SEALs) in high Dk EW. *Invest Ophthalmol Vis Sci.* 2001;42:s595.
245. Lofstrom T, Kruse A. A conjunctival response to silicone hydrogel lens wear. *Contact Lens Spectrum.* 2005;20:42–44.
246. Carnt N, Keir N. A conjunctival response to silicone hydrogel lens wear. http://www.siliconehydrogels.org/featured_review/may_06.asp 2006.
247. Lin M. Conjunctival epithelial flaps: what are they and do we need to worry? http://www.siliconehydrogels.org/editorials/may_06.asp 2006.
248. Santodomingo-Rubido J, Wolffsohn J, Gilmartin B. Conjunctival epithelial flaps with 18 months of silicone hydrogel contact lens wear. *Eye Contact Lens.* 2008;34:35–38.
249. Graham AD, Truong TN, Lin MC. Conjunctival epithelial flap in continuous contact lens wear. *Optom Vis Sci.* 2009;86:e324–e331.
250. Bergmanson JP, Tukler J, Leach NE, et al. Morphology of contact lens-induced conjunctival epithelial flaps: a pilot study. *Cont Lens Anterior Eye.* 2012;35:185–188.

251. Markoulli M, Francis IC, Yong J, et al. A histopathological study of bulbar conjunctival flaps occurring in 2 contact lens wearers. *Cornea.* 2011;30:1037–1041.
252. Cox I, Fonn D. Interference filters to eliminate the surface reflex and improve contrast during fluorescein photography. *Int Cont Lens Clin.* 1991;18:178–181.
253. Markoulli M, Papas E, Cole N, et al. Corneal erosions in contact lens wear. *Cont Lens Anterior Eye.* 2012;35:2–8.
254. Katelaris CH. Giant papillary conjunctivitis—a review. *Acta Ophthalmol Scand.* 1999;77(suppl):17–20.
255. Donshik PC. Contact lens chemistry and giant papillary conjunctivitis. *Eye Contact Lens.* 2003;29:S37–S39; discussion S57–S59, S192–S194.
256. Stapleton F, Stretton S, Sankaridurg PR, et al. Hypersensitivity responses and contact lens wear. *Cont Lens Anterior Eye.* 2003;26:57–69.
257. Nilsson SE. Ten years of disposable contact lenses—a review of benefits and risks. *Cont Lens Anterior Eye.* 1997;20:119–128.
258. Porazinski AD, Donshik PC. Giant papillary conjunctivitis in frequent replacement contact lens wearers: a retrospective study. *CLAO J.* 1999;25:142–147.
259. Marshall E, Begley C, Nguyen C. Frequency of complications among wearers of disposable and conventional soft contact lenses. *Int Cont Lens Clin.* 1992;19:55–59.
260. Poggio EC, Abelson M. Complications and symptoms in disposable extended wear lenses compared with conventional soft daily wear and soft extended wear lenses. *CLAO J.* 1993;19:31–39.
261. Skotnitsky C, Sankaridurg PR, Sweeney DF, et al. General and local contact lens induced papillary conjunctivitis (CLPC). *Clin Exp Optom.* 2002;85:193–197.
262. Skotnitsky CC, Naduvilath TJ, Sweeney DF, et al. Two presentations of contact lens-induced papillary conjunctivitis (CLPC) in hydrogel lens wear: local and general. *Optom Vis Sci.* 2006;83:27–36.
263. Santodomingo-Rubido J, Wolffsohn JS, Gilmartin B. Adverse events and discontinuations during 18 months of silicone hydrogel contact lens wear. *Eye Contact Lens.* 2007;33:288–292.
264. Sorbara L, Jones L, Williams-Lyn D. Contact lens induced papillary conjunctivitis with silicone hydrogel lenses. *Cont Lens Anterior Eye.* 2009;32:93–96.
265. Holden BA, La Hood D, Grant T, et al. Gram-negative bacteria can induce contact lens related acute red eye (CLARE) responses. *CLAO J.* 1996;22:47–52.
266. Sankaridurg PR, Vuppala N, Sreedharan A, et al. Gram negative bacteria and contact lens induced acute red eye. *Indian J Ophthalmol.* 1996;44:29–32.
267. Sankaridurg PR, Willcox MD, Sharma S, et al. Haemophilus influenzae adherent to contact lenses associated with production of acute ocular inflammation. *J Clin Microbiol.* 1996;34:2426–2431.
268. Sankaridurg PR, Sharma S, Willcox M, et al. Bacterial colonization of disposable soft contact lenses is greater during corneal infiltrative events than during asymptomatic extended lens wear. *J Clin Microbiol.* 2000;38:4420–4424.
269. Hume EB, Willcox MD. Adhesion and growth of Serratia marcescens on artificial closed eye tears soaked hydrogel contact lenses. *Aust N Z J Ophthalmol.* 1997;25(suppl):S39–S41.
270. Willcox M, Sharma S, Naduvilath TJ, et al. External ocular surface and lens microbiota in contact lens wearers with corneal infiltrates during extended wear of hydrogel lenses. *Eye Contact Lens.* 2011;37:90–95.
271. Grant T, Chong MS, Vajdic C, et al. Contact lens induced peripheral ulcers during hydrogel contact lens wear. *CLAO J.* 1998;24:145–151.
272. Holden BA, Reddy MK, Sankaridurg PR, et al. Contact lens-induced peripheral ulcers with extended wear of disposable hydrogel lenses: histopathologic observations on the nature and type of corneal infiltrate. *Cornea.* 1999;18:538–543.
273. Hume E, Wu P, Thakur A, et al. Contact lens induced peripheral ulcers (CLPU) are produced by an alpha-toxin deficient mutant of Staphylococcus aureus. *Invest Ophthalmol Vis Sci.* 2001;42:s593.
274. Wu P, Stapleton F, Willcox MD. The causes of and cures for contact lens-induced peripheral ulcer. *Eye Contact Lens.* 2003;29:S63–S66; discussion S83–S84, S192–S194.
275. Aasuri MK, Venkata N, Kumar VM. Differential diagnosis of microbial keratitis and contact lens-induced peripheral ulcer. *Eye Contact Lens.* 2003;29:S60–S62; discussion S83–S84, S192–S194.
276. Willcox M, Sankaridurg P, Zhu H, et al. Inflammation and infection and the effects of the closed eye. In: Sweeney D, ed. *Silicone hydrogels: Continuous Wear Contact Lenses.* Oxford: Butterworth-Heinemann; 2004; 90–125.
277. Keay L, Stapleton F, Schein O. Epidemiology of contact lens-related inflammation and microbial keratitis: a 20-year perspective. *Eye Contact Lens.* 2007;33:346–353, discussion 362–363.
278. Stapleton F, Dart JK, Minassian D. Risk factors with contact lens related suppurative keratitis. *CLAO J.* 1993;19:204–210.
279. Chalmers RL, Wagner H, Mitchell GL, et al. Age and other risk factors for corneal infiltrative and inflammatory events in young soft contact lens wearers from the Contact Lens Assessment in Youth (CLAY) study. *Invest Ophthalmol Vis Sci.* 2011;52:6690–6696.
280. Efron N, Morgan PB, Hill EA, Raynor MK, Tullo AB. Incidence and morbidity of hospital-presenting corneal infiltrative events associated with contact lens wear. *Clin Exp Optom.* 2005;88:232–239.
281. Chalmers RL, Keay L, Long B, et al. Risk factors for contact lens complications in US clinical practices. *Optom Vis Sci.* 2010;87:725–735.

282. Morgan PB, Efron N, Hill EA, et al. Incidence of keratitis of varying severity among contact lens wearers. *Br J Ophthalmol.* 2005;89:430–436.
283. Szczotka-Flynn L, Diaz M. Risk of corneal inflammatory events with silicone hydrogel and low dk hydrogel extended contact lens wear: a meta-analysis. *Optom Vis Sci.* 2007;84:247–256.
284. Chalmers RL, Keay L, McNally J, et al. Multicenter case-control study of the role of lens materials and care products on the development of corneal infiltrates. *Optom Vis Sci.* 2012;89:316–325.
285. Dumbleton K, Fonn D, Jones L, et al. Severity and management of contact lens related complications with continuous wear of high Dk silicone hydrogel lenses. *Optom Vis Sci.* 2000;77:216.
286. Smolin G. The defence mechanism of the outer eye. *Trans Ophthalmol Soc U K.* 1985;104(pt 4):363–366.
287. Knop E, Knop N. The role of eye-associated lymphoid tissue in corneal immune protection. *J Anat.* 2005;206:271–285.
288. Meek B, Speijer D, de Jong PT, et al. The ocular humoral immune response in health and disease. *Prog Retin Eye Res.* 2003;22:391–415.
289. Willcox MD. Which is more important to the initiation of contact lens related microbial keratitis, trauma to the ocular surface or bacterial pathogenic factors? *Clin Exp Optom.* 2006;89:277–279.
290. Willcox MD. New strategies to prevent Pseudomonas keratitis. *Eye Contact Lens.* 2007;33:401–403; discussion 410–411.
291. Willcox MD. Pseudomonas aeruginosa infection and inflammation during contact lens wear: a review. *Optom Vis Sci.* 2007;84:273–278.
292. Willcox MD. Management and treatment of contact lens-related Pseudomonas keratitis. *Clin Ophthalmol.* 2012;6:919–924.
293. Willcox MD, Holden BA. Contact lens related corneal infections. *Biosci Rep.* 2001;21:445–461.
294. Keay L, Edwards K, Naduvilath T, et al. Factors affecting the morbidity of contact lens-related microbial keratitis: a population study. *Invest Ophthalmol Vis Sci.* 2006;47:4302–4308.
295. Keay L, Edwards K, Stapleton F. An early assessment of silicone hydrogel safety: pearls and pitfalls, and current status. *Eye Contact Lens.* 2007;33:358–361.
296. Edwards K, Keay L, Naduvilath T, et al. Characteristics of and risk factors for contact lens-related microbial keratitis in a tertiary referral hospital. *Eye.* 2009;23:153–160.
297. Miedziak AI, Miller MR, Rapuano CJ, et al. Risk factors in microbial keratitis leading to penetrating keratoplasty. *Ophthalmology.* 1999;106:1166–1170; discussion 1171.
298. Laspina F, Samudio M, Cibils D, et al. Epidemiological characteristics of microbiological results on patients with infectious corneal ulcers: a 13-year survey in Paraguay. *Graefes Arch Clin Exp Ophthalmol.* 2004;242:204–209.
299. Butler TK, Males JJ, Robinson LP, et al. Six-year review of Acanthamoeba keratitis in New South Wales, Australia: 1997–2002. *Clin Experiment Ophthalmol.* 2005;33:41–46.
300. Titiyal JS, Negi S, Anand A, et al. Risk factors for perforation in microbial corneal ulcers in north India. *Br J Ophthalmol.* 2006;90:686–689.
301. Smith A, Pennefather PM, Kaye SB, et al. Fluoroquinolones: place in ocular therapy. *Drugs.* 2001;61:747–761.
302. Mather R, Karenchak LM, Romanowski EG, et al. Fourth generation fluoroquinolones: new weapons in the arsenal of ophthalmic antibiotics. *Am J Ophthalmol.* 2002;133:463–466.
303. Pachigolla G, Blomquist P, Cavanagh HD. Microbial keratitis pathogens and antibiotic susceptibilities: a 5-year review of cases at an urban county hospital in north Texas. *Eye Contact Lens.* 2007;33:45–49.
304. Parmar P, Salman A, Kalavathy CM, et al. Comparison of topical gatifloxacin 0.3% and ciprofloxacin 0.3% for the treatment of bacterial keratitis. *Am J Ophthalmol.* 2006;141:282–286.
305. Rattanatam T, Heng WJ, Rapuano CJ, et al. Trends in contact lens-related corneal ulcers. *Cornea.* 2001;20:290–294.
306. Leeming JP. Treatment of ocular infections with topical antibacterials. *Clin Pharmacokinet.* 1999;37:351–360.
307. Yu DK, Ng AS, Lau WW, et al. Recent pattern of contact lens-related keratitis in Hong Kong. *Eye Contact Lens.* 2007;33:284–287.
308. Saw SM, Ooi PL, Tan DT, et al. Risk factors for contact lens-related fusarium keratitis: a case-control study in Singapore. *Arch Ophthalmol.* 2007;125:611–617.
309. Iyer SA, Tuli SS, Wagoner RC. Fungal keratitis: emerging trends and treatment outcomes. *Eye Contact Lens.* 2006;32:267–271.
310. Chang DC, Grant GB, O'Donnell K, et al. Multistate outbreak of Fusarium keratitis associated with use of a contact lens solution. *JAMA.* 2006;296:953–963.
311. Alfonso EC, Cantu-Dibildox J, Munir WM, et al. Insurgence of Fusarium keratitis associated with contact lens wear. *Arch Ophthalmol.* 2006;124:941–947.
312. Thebpatiphat N, Hammersmith KM, Rocha FN, et al. Acanthamoeba keratitis: a parasite on the rise. *Cornea.* 2007;26:701–706.
313. Joslin CE, Tu EY, Shoff ME, et al. The association of contact lens solution use and Acanthamoeba keratitis. *Am J Ophthalmol.* 2007;144:169–180.
314. Foulks GN. Acanthamoeba keratitis and contact lens wear: static or increasing problem? *Eye Contact Lens.* 2007;33:412–414; discussion 424–425.

315. Khor WB, Aung T, Saw SM, et al. An outbreak of Fusarium keratitis associated with contact lens wear in Singapore. *JAMA.* 2006;295:2867–2873.
316. Foulks GN. Prolonging contact lens wear and making contact lens wear safer. *Am J Ophthalmol.* 2006;141:369–373.
317. Classe JG. Liability for extended-wear contact lenses. *Optom Clin.* 1991;1:51–62.
318. Harris MG, Dister RE. Informed consent for extended-wear patients. *Optom Clin.* 1991;1:33–50.
319. Classe JG. Avoiding liability in contact lens practice. *Optom Clin.* 1994;4:1–12.
320. Harris M. Informed consent for contact lens patients. *J Br Contact Lens Assoc.* 1994;17:119–134.
321. Classe JG. Informed consent and contact lens practice. *J Am Optom Assoc.* 1996;67:132–134.
322. Brennan NA, Coles C, Jaworski A, et al. Proposed practice guidelines for continuous contact lens wear. *Clin Exp Optom.* 2001;84:71–77.
323. Brennan N, Coles C, Dahl A. Where do silicone hydrogels fit into everyday practice? In: Sweeney D, ed. *Silicone Hydrogels: Continuous Wear Contact Lenses.* Oxford: Butterworth-Heinemann; 2004;275–308.
324. Efron N, Brennan NA, Currie JM, et al. Determinants of the initial comfort of hydrogel contact lenses. *Am J Optom Physiol Opt.* 1986;63:819–823.
325. Dumbleton KA, Chalmers RL, McNally J, et al. Effect of lens base curve on subjective comfort and assessment of fit with silicone hydrogel continuous wear contact lenses. *Optom Vis Sci.* 2002;79:633–637.
326. Ghormley N, Jones L. Managing lipid deposition on silicone hydrogel lenses. *Contact Lens Spectrum.* 2006;21:21.
327. Nichols JJ. Deposition rates and lens care influence on galyfilcon A silicone hydrogel lenses. *Optom Vis Sci.* 2006;83:751–757.
328. Subbaraman LN, Bayer S, Glasier MA, et al. Rewetting drops containing surface active agents improve the clinical performance of silicone hydrogel contact lenses. *Optom Vis Sci.* 2006;83:143–151.
329. Yamane S, Paragina S. Patient education. In: Bennett ES, Weissman, BA, eds.*Clinical Contact Lens Practice.* Philadelphia, PA: Lippincott; 1991;1–9.
330. Miller PJ. Liability issues in contact lens practice. *J Am Optom Assoc.* 1986;57:227–229.
331. Efron N. Grading scales for contact lens complications. *Ophthal Physiol Opt.* 1998;18:182–186.
332. Efron N, Morgan PB, Katsara SS. Validation of grading scales for contact lens complications. *Ophthalmic Physiol Opt.* 2001;21:17–29.
333. IER. IER Grading Scales. In: Phillips A, Speedwell L, eds. *Contact Lenses.* Edinburgh: Butterworth-Heinemann; 2006;628–631.
334. Jones L, Senchyna M, Glasier MA, et al. Lysozyme and lipid deposition on silicone hydrogel contact lens materials. *Eye Contact Lens.* 2003;29:S75–S79.
335. Carney FP, Nash WL, Sentell KB. The adsorption of major tear film lipids in vitro to various silicone hydrogels over time. *Invest Ophthalmol Vis Sci.* 2008;49:120–124.

Chapter 17

Aphakia

Dennis Burger and Larry J. Davis

INTRODUCTION

While the number of patients undergoing cataract surgery continues to increase, the number that remains aphakic following surgery has been declining rapidly since the mid-1980s. The quality of intraocular lenses (IOLs), the improved surgical techniques, and the safety of IOLs have combined to be a driving force in reducing the number of aphakic patients. Although IOLs have resulted in greatly reducing the number of new aphakic patients, they have not eliminated aphakia for all patients requiring removal of the crystalline lens. The use of IOLs is considered risky for some patients following trauma or complicated intraocular surgery and for relatively young patients, especially infants.

Perhaps no single population has experienced the benefits of contact lenses more than those who are aphakic. The thick spectacle lenses necessary for the aphakic eye (usually +12.00–+16.00 D) induce a magnification of at least 30%.[1] Restrictions of the peripheral visual field are also found while wearing spectacle lenses for the correction of aphakia. Prismatic effect is found to increase toward the edge of the lens, resulting in a ring scotoma. Although lenticular designs reduce the thickness and mass of these lenses, they may reduce the "optical" size of the lens, further restricting the visual field. Patients attempt to compensate for these effects by turning their head to scan the visual field. Contact lenses offer reduced magnification and better visual performance by eliminating visual field restrictions, and eliminate the use of the thick spectacle lenses, which are heavy, cosmetically unattractive, and optically inferior to contact lenses[2,3] (Appendix A).

ADULT APHAKIC PATIENTS

Patient Selection

All contact lens wearers must perform routine lens care to maintain a lens with clear optical quality that is free from contamination. Once the decision is made to proceed with a contact lens correction, the patient, or in the case of extremely young or old patients, the guardian, should be advised of the required lens maintenance. Some factors to consider include specific visual requirements, best potential visual acuity (VA), manual dexterity, willingness or ability to participate in lens care, and if indicated, social support system.

Ideally, the corneal astigmatism should be 2 D or less to maintain a well-fitting contact lens. In most cases (with the exception of infantile aphakia), this would mean fitting approximately 4 to 6 weeks following the primary surgical procedure. Against-the-rule corneal cylinder, which may occur from loose sutures or wound gape, can complicate the fitting of a contact lens. Therefore, while an attempt should be made to reduce the corneal cylinder as much as possible, having a moderate amount of with-the-rule cylinder is better than leaving the patient with even a small amount of against-the-rule corneal cylinder. Patients who have become aphakic as a result of blunt or penetrating trauma should be allowed sufficient time to reduce any intraocular inflammation. While a period of 4 to 6 weeks is also usually adequate in this group of patients, some may require a longer amount of time. This is usually of no consequence if the patient is beyond the critical period and without risk of refractive amblyopia and if good VA is maintained in the paired eye. Correction of the pediatric aphakic patient should be performed as soon as possible. Most often this can be achieved within 5 days following the primary surgical procedure. This is especially true if small-incision techniques are used, which allow for a short healing period and reduced postoperative astigmatism.

Fitting Principles

Because of the large vertex powers and frequent unpredictability of lens dynamics on the eye, diagnostic lens application is essential. During the prefitting evaluation, in addition to the usual evaluation of corneal curvature, refractive status, VA, tear quality, and external disease, any results of undercorrecting the refractive cylinder should be evaluated. As the BCVA in many of these patients is 20/40 or worse, residual cylinder may have no effect on their optimum VA. Diagnostic fitting, using high-powered plus lenses, will improve the accuracy of the initial prescription by reducing any errors in compensating for vertex distance. It is also essential to evaluate lens movement and centration while performing a diagnostic fitting. When fitting gas-permeable (GP) lenses, they will frequently be found to decenter and a careful fluorescein pattern evaluation is indicated. The use of a soft lens requires careful evaluation of lens fit as well. Adequate lens movement is essential to reduce complications resulting from tight-fitting lenses.

Lens Materials

Gas-Permeable Lenses

When to Use: Once the decision is made to proceed with contact lenses, practitioners are presented with an initial decision of whether to use a soft or GP contact lens design. Patients having no contact lens experience are usually fit with a rigid lens. This is especially true if the corneal curvatures are 43.00 D or flatter, with 2.00 D or less with-the-rule corneal cylinder, and if the upper lid is positioned at or below the superior limbus. Any amount of against-the-rule astigmatism can negatively influence centration of a rigid lens design. GP contact lenses offer several distinct advantages over their soft lens counterparts (Fig. 17.1). Often, patients most

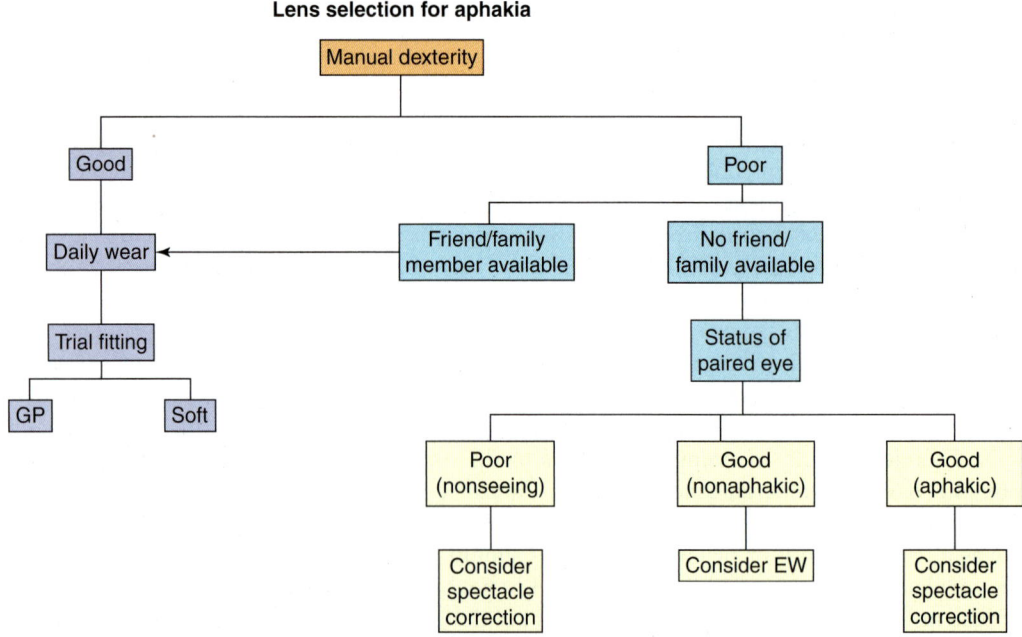

FIGURE 17.1 Factors influencing the initial lens of choice for contact lens correction of aphakia.

likely to reject GP contact lens wear are those having previous experience wearing a soft contact lens. If, after proceeding with the fitting and evaluation of GP lenses, it is determined that an adequate fitting relationship or comfort cannot be achieved, refitting with a soft lens design is usually well accepted by the patient. Patients who have experienced serious adverse reactions (e.g., tight lens syndrome, keratitis, severe giant papillary conjunctivitis [GPC]) while using a soft contact lens are more likely to successfully adapt to GP lenses than those wearing soft lenses without apparent adverse effects. These patients must possess the motivation to accept the change in lid sensation, movement, and handling required for a GP lens design.

Lens Designs: Because of the high plus powers of aphakic lenses resulting in a large center thickness (CT), those attempting to fit rigid lenses must be familiar with various design characteristics that may improve the fitting relationship and enhance patient comfort. In most cases, a minus lenticular type of design is indicated. This results in both reducing lens mass by decreasing CT and creating a more posteriorly positioned center of gravity, thus enhancing lens centration. Lenticulation also produces a thicker lens edge profile and creates greater lens-to-lid interaction. This enhances lens movement and improves centration of the optical zone diameter over the pupil. Because of intralaboratory variability in the manufacture of lenticular lens designs, it is advisable to specify a specific lenticular design for better consistency and performance. This is achieved, in part, by requesting a particular flange radius (lenticular curve) and optic cap (front optical zone) to be used during lens manufacture (Fig. 17.2). While a flatter flange radius will usually assist in maintaining a superior lens-to-cornea fitting relationship, this may also result in increased lens awareness. An approximate, desired flange radius between 1.0 and 2.0 mm flatter than the base curve radius (BCR) in millimeters is recommended.[4] For example, if a lens is ordered with a 45.00 D (7.50 mm) BCR, one would expect to order a flange radius of 8.5 to 9.5 mm. With few exceptions, the optic cap should be equal to the back optic zone diameter. A recommended diagnostic fitting set for lenticular lenses is found in Table 17.1.[5] Effective Power and Vertex Power optical considerations are provided in Appendix A and B, respectively, at the end of this chapter.

Occasionally, patients having corneas >45.00 D may be fitted using a small-diameter, single-cut lens design. These lenses will require fitting at least 1 D steeper than K to improve lens centration. A recommended diagnostic fitting set for single-cut aphakic lenses is provided in Table 17.2.[5] Because of the large CT of these lenses, it is recommended to order aphakic designs in a lens material with medium to high oxygen permeability (Dk). These lenses demonstrate

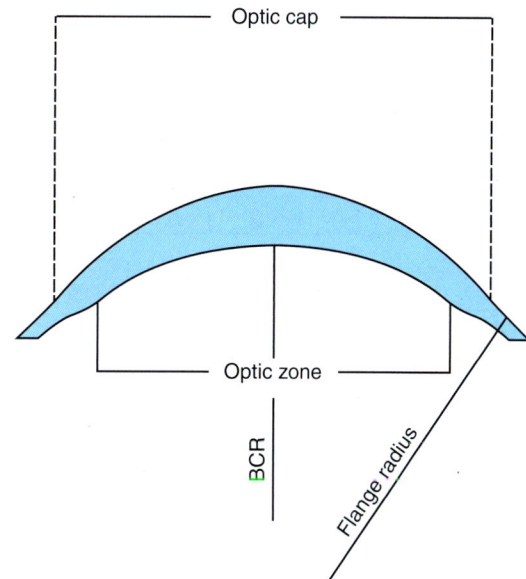

FIGURE 17.2 Design of a minus carrier aphakic contact lens.

TABLE 17.1 Suggested Lenticular Aphakia Trial Lens Set (Recommended Material is PMMA or a Low-Dk Gas-Permeable Material)

BASE CURVE	OAD	OZD	BACK VERTEX POWER	SCR/W	PCR/W	CT	FLANGE RADIUS
39.00	9.50	8.0	+13.00	BCR + 1.0 mm/.4	SCR + 1.5/.35	0.44	BCR + 1.50 mm
40.00	9.50	8.0	+13.00	BCR + 1.0 mm/.4	SCR + 1.5/.35	0.44	BCR + 1.50 mm
40.50	9.50	8.0	+13.00	BCR + 1.0 mm/.4	SCR + 1.5/.35	0.44	BCR + 1.50 mm
41.00	9.50	8.0	+13.00	BCR + 1.0 mm/.4	SCR + 1.5/.35	0.44	BCR + 1.50 mm
41.50	9.50	8.0	+13.00	BCR + 1.0 mm/.4	SCR + 1.5/.35	0.44	BCR + 1.50 mm
42.00	9.50	8.0	+13.00	BCR + 1.0 mm/.4	SCR + 1.5/.35	0.44	BCR + 1.50 mm
42.50	9.50	8.0	+13.00	BCR + 1.0 mm/.4	SCR + 1.5/.35	0.44	BCR + 1.50 mm
43.00	9.30	7.8	+13.00	BCR + 1.0 mm/.4	SCR + 1.5/.35	0.42	BCR + 1.50 mm
43.50	9.30	7.8	+13.00	BCR + 1.0 mm/.4	SCR + 1.5/.35	0.42	BCR + 1.50 mm
44.00	9.30	7.8	+13.00	BCR + 1.0 mm/.4	SCR + 1.5/.35	0.42	BCR + 1.50 mm
44.50	9.30	7.8	+13.00	BCR + 1.0 mm/.4	SCR + 1.5/.35	0.42	BCR + 1.50 mm
45.00	9.00	7.6	+13.00	BCR + 1.0 mm/.4	SCR + 1.5/.3	0.40	BCR + 1.50 mm
45.50	9.00	7.6	+13.00	BCR + 1.0 mm/.4	SCR + 1.5/.3	0.40	BCR + 1.50 mm
46.00	9.00	7.6	+13.00	BCR + 1.0 mm/.4	SCR + 1.5/.3	0.40	BCR + 1.50 mm
47.00	9.00	7.6	+13.00	BCR + 1.0 mm/.4	SCR + 1.5/.3	0.40	BCR + 1.50 mm
48.00	9.00	7.6	+13.00	BCR + 1.0 mm/.4	SCR + 1.5/.3	0.40	BCR + 1.50 mm

BCR, base curve radius; CT, center thickness; Dk, oxygen permeability; PCR/W, peripheral curve radius/width; PMMA, polymethylmethacrylate; OAD, overall diameter; OZD, optical zone diameter; SCR/W, secondary curve radius/width.
From Davis LJ, Bergin C, Bennett ES. Aphakia. In: Bennett ES, Weissman BA, eds. *Clinical Contact Lens Practice*. Philadelphia, PA: Lippincott Williams & Wilkins; 2005:595–604.

good stability even when materials having Dk values above 100 are used. Most lens designs are now available including spherical, front toric, bitoric, bifocal, and multifocal powers.

Soft (Hydrogel and Silicone Hydrogel) Lenses

When to Use: Soft contact lenses offer potential advantages over their GP counterparts. Perhaps the most important advantage is immediate patient comfort. Second, a well-fitting contact lens is almost always obtainable. Therefore, one indication for using a soft aphakic contact lens is

TABLE 17.2 Suggested Single-Cut Aphakia Trial Lens Set

BASE CURVE	OAD	OZD	BACK VERTEX POWER	SCR/W	PCR/W	CT
45.00	9.00	7.6	+13.00	BCR + 1.0 mm/.4	SCR + 1.5/.3	0.40
45.50	9.00	7.6	+13.00	BCR + 1.0 mm/.4	SCR + 1.5/.3	0.40
46.00	9.00	7.6	+13.00	BCR + 1.0 mm/.4	SCR + 1.5/.3	0.40
46.50	9.00	7.6	+13.00	BCR + 1.0 mm/.4	SCR + 1.5/.3	0.40
47.00	9.00	7.6	+13.00	BCR + 1.0 mm/.4	SCR + 1.5/.3	0.40
48.00	9.00	7.6	+13.00	BCR + 1.0 mm/.4	SCR + 1.5/.3	0.40

BCR, base curve radius; CT, center thickness; PCR/W, peripheral curve radius/width; OAD, overall diameter; OZD, optical zone diameter; SCR/W, secondary curve radius/width.
From Davis LJ, Bergin C, Bennett ES. Aphakia. In: Bennett ES, Weissman BA, eds. *Clinical Contact Lens Practice*. Philadelphia, PA: Lippincott Williams & Wilkins; 2005:595–604.

when an inadequate fit occurs while using a GP lens design. In cases of low refractive astigmatism, soft contact lenses usually perform quite well. If residual astigmatism reduces VA, the appropriate cylindrical error can be incorporated into spectacles and worn over the contact lens. Finally, the ability to inventory most lens parameters provides immediate correction in cases of high refractive error without interruption of lens wear in the event of lens loss or damage. Patients who have become aphakic secondary to trauma may also have iris defects resulting in large or ectopic pupils. These patients may benefit from a dark-tinted, hydrogel contact lens creating an artificial pupil and iris, which attenuates bright light. Hydrogel lens designs are more suitable for this application, as they more readily accept tint and encompass more of the corneal surface while providing better centration with decreased movement.

Lens Designs: Several soft lens designs are available for aphakic contact lens fitting. As many aphakic patients are elderly and benefit from using an extended-wear (EW) contact lens material, various aphakic contact lenses have been designed for use on an EW schedule. An attempt is made to increase oxygen transmission by reducing lens thickness using lenticulation, increasing the water content of the material, or both. It has been several years since any new hydrogel contact lens materials or designs have been investigated for use in aphakia on an EW basis. Most recently, silicone hydrogel lenses and numerous spherical, toric, and bifocal planned-replacement lenses in aphakic powers have been introduced. A list of these lens designs is provided in Table 17.3.[6]

TABLE 17.3 Hydrogel and Silicone Hydrogel Planned-Replacement Lenses in Aphakic Powers

COMPANY	NAME	AVAILABILITY
I. Silicone Hydrogel		
ABB Optical	Concise Definitive & toric	4-pack
Gelflex USA	Synergy SiHy & toric	1+3-pack
Metro Optics	Metrosoft Definitive	4-pack
Unilens	C VUE HydraVUE[a]	6-pack
II. Hydrogel		
A. Spherical		
Alden Optical	Alden HP49	4- or 6-pack
Alden Optical	Alden HP54	4- or 6-pack
Alden Optical	Alden HP59	4- or 6-pack
Alden Optical	Alden Classic 38 or 55	4- or 6-pack
CooperVision	Proclear/Hydrasoft	4- or 6-pack
Gelflex USA	Synergy	1+3-pack
Metro Optics	Metrosoft II	4-pack
Metro Optics	Metrolite	4-pack
Metro Optics	Metrotint	4-pack
Ocu-Ease	Ocu-Flex 55	4-pack
SpecialEyes	SpecialEyes 54 & 59 Sphere	4- or 6-pack
United Contact Lens	UCL-55	4-pack
United Contact Lens	Tresoft	4-pack
X-Cel Contacts	Flexlens	1+3-pack
X-Cel Contacts	Adult Aphakic	1+3-pack

(continued)

TABLE 17.3 Hydrogel and Silicone Hydrogel Planned-Replacement Lenses in Aphakic Powers *(Continued)*

COMPANY	NAME	AVAILABILITY
B. Toric		
Advanced Ultra Vision	CO Soft 55 Toric	6-pack
Alden Optical	Alden HP49,54, & 59 Toric	4- or 6-pack
Alden Optical	Alden Classic 38 & 55 Toric	4- or 6-pack
California Optics	CO Soft 55 Toric	4-pack
Gelflex USA	Synergy Quarterly Replacement Toric	1+3-pack
United Contact Lens	UCL Toric	4-pack
X-Cel Contacts	Flexlens Toric	1+3-pack
C. Multifocal and Multifocal Toric		
ABB Optical	Concise MF & MF Toric	4-pack
CooperVision	Proclear Multifocal XR	6-pack
CooperVision	Proclear Multifocal Toric	6-pack
Gelflex USA	Synergy Translating Bifocal	1+3-pack
Gelflex USA	Synergy Bifocal Toric	1+3-pack
SpecialEyes	SpecialEyes 54 Multifocal	4-pack
SpecialEyes	SpecialEyes Multifocal Toric	4-pack
United Contact Lens	UCL Sonic View Multifocal	4-pack
United Contact Lens	UCL Sonic View MF Toric	4-pack

[a]Available in toric, multifocal, and multifocal toric.
From Thompson TT. *Tyler's Quarterly.* 2012;29(2):28–56.

Complications

The thick lens designs necessary for aphakia create a hypoxic environment for the cornea. It is thought that many contact lens-related complications such as corneal infiltrates, neovascularization, corneal edema, and more serious complication of infectious corneal ulceration are caused in part by the relative hypoxia that occurs while wearing contact lenses. Contributing factors in the elderly population are reduced aqueous tear secretion, meibomian gland dysfunction, blepharitis, and possibly decreased activity of the immune system. Periodic evaluation of proper lens fit should be performed, at minimum, every 6 months. Occasionally, a hydrogel lens is found to fit tighter with age. Routine annual or semiannual lens replacement may be beneficial in reducing acute tight lens syndrome. It has been demonstrated that lens removal before sleep is an important factor reducing the frequency of serious lens-related complications. Therefore, it is advisable to discourage the use of EW for most aphakic patients.

Occasionally, patients are unable or reluctant to perform lens care. Many patients lack the necessary manual dexterity to insert and remove contact lenses. Others may have a psychological reluctance to be actively involved in the required lens manipulation and care. Routine removal and cleanings may then be performed by a friend or a family member, or as a last resort in the office.

PEDIATRIC APHAKIC PATIENTS

One of the most challenging and rewarding uses of contact lenses is for the pediatric aphakic. Pediatric aphakia, although rare, is a condition that is made for the use of contact lenses. Cataracts can be either congenital or acquired and either monocular or binocular.

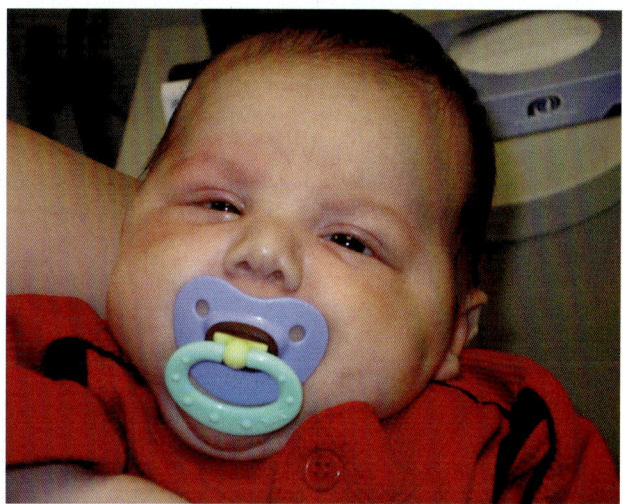

FIGURE 17.3 Two-week-old aphakic.

Congenital cataracts are estimated to occur in approximately 1.4 to 2.3 per 10,000 births and can be unilateral or bilateral.[7-11] Although the incidence is rare, the visual implications are severe if the cataract is not removed early and the child is not properly treated (Fig. 17.3).

Treatment for congenital cataracts consists of early cataract extraction, contact lens correction, and amblyopia treatment before age 4 months to have reasonable expectation of good VA in the affected eye.[12]

Treatment Options

Treatment options for the pediatric aphakics include glasses, IOLs, and contact lenses. Glasses can be a viable option for the bilateral aphakic. Glasses allow both eyes to be corrected; however, there are significant limitations. Patients will experience reduced visual fields, magnification distortion (30% increase), and problems with achieving properly fitted frames, especially for infants (Fig. 17.4).

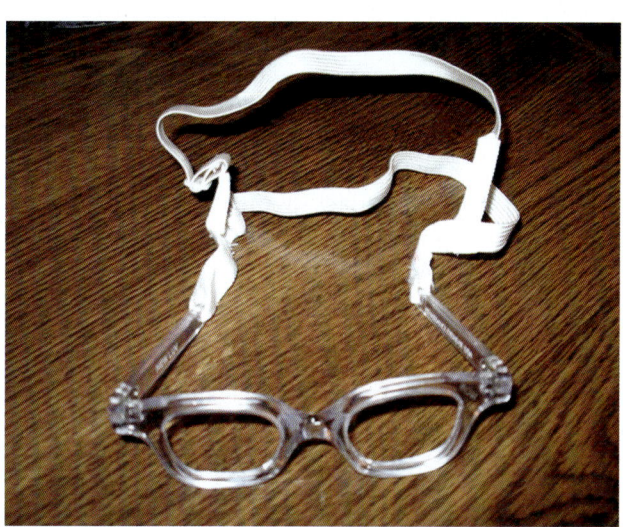

FIGURE 17.4 Headband frame.

Unilateral aphakics have the additional problem of anisometropia and, as a result, cannot be effectively corrected in spectacles. The development of amblyopia is a major concern in unilateral aphakics since it is unlikely that the patient is using both eyes. Bilateral aphakics are more successful as both eyes have similar refractive errors; the problem of anisometropia is eliminated.[13]

IOLs have been suggested for pediatric aphakics, but this is controversial.[14–19] Problems exist with this treatment modality in that the eye changes rapidly during the first 4 years of life because of axial length.[20] The average refractive error at the corneal plane for a 1-month-old infant is +31 D, while at age 4 it is +16 D.[21] Because of this change in refractive power, the IOL would either have to be changed multiple times or additional vision correction would be needed to properly correct the child's vision. IOLs would be best served in the aphakic population that is over the age of 4.

Currently, contact lenses are the best option for the pediatric aphakic. The power and fit of the lens can be easily changed as the eye grows.[17,18,22,23] The problem of anisometropia for the unilateral aphakic is significantly reduced to allow for binocular correction. There are multiple contact lens options for the pediatric patient. These options include soft lenses, rigid GP lenses, and silicone lenses.

Soft lenses are commonly used in the adult population or in the nonaphakic pediatric population. New materials, including silicone hydrogels, allow for long-term wear of lenses with minimal complications. Additionally, the disposable modality has allowed for ease of replacement for lost lenses with these patients. However, soft lenses are not extensively used in the pediatric population. The powers required for the pediatric aphakic are generally >+20 D. Many of these soft lenses need to be custom-made (Table 17.4). Infants under the age of 1 year often have lenses in the +25 to +32 D range. These lenses are extremely thick. Aphakic lenses in this power range are generally ≥1 mm thick. Additionally, the Dk of the soft lens material is low, in the range of 15 to 24. Therefore, these lenses are very thick with very low Dk. This creates a lens that has low oxygen transmissibility (Dk/t) and can result in problems with acute red-eye response. If soft aphakic lenses are used, they must be used as a daily wear (DW) option and should never be used in an EW modality. Other problems associated with aphakic soft lenses are increased difficulty for insertion by the parents and some compromise in vision versus GP lenses.

GP lenses are another option for the pediatric aphakic patient. Advantages of GP lenses versus soft include that they are easier for the parents to handle, have higher Dk/t, offer better vision, can be obtained in any power, are the least costly contact lens alternative, and have good durability. There are several disadvantages, namely, problems with comfort, ease of displacement of the lens, need for custom lenses, and difficulty in fitting the lens. It is difficult to fit a rigid lens; keratometry readings may not be possible, diagnostic lenses have to be used, and the fitting on noncooperative children may need to be performed under general anesthesia in the operating room.

The last option is a flexible silicone elastomer, the Silsoft lens. Advantages of the Silsoft lens are that they have the highest Dk (Dk = 340), they can be used as EW, they provide good comfort, there is availability of stock parameters, they stay in the eye better than a rigid lens, they are easier to handle for parents than soft lenses, and fluorescein can be used with the lens. Disadvantages are that they are the most expensive lens option, there is limited power availability (3 D steps), they attract lipid deposits and have to be replaced, and they can adhere to the eye and become excessively tight. Despite all these disadvantages, the Silsoft lens remains the workhorse lens for the pediatric aphakic. This lens has high Dk/t, good comfort, and the ability to stay in the eye, thus allowing it to be used as an EW lens with fewer complications than soft lenses. Silsoft lenses also cause less irritation and, with the ability to be used in an EW modality, are more convenient for the parents than GP lenses.

TABLE 17.4 Pediatric Aphakic Lenses

MANUFACTURER	LENS	BASE CURVE	DIAMETER	POWER	DK
Acuity One	Clearion Custom	5.8–11.0	8.0–16.0	Pl–+ 50 D	15
Advanced Vision Tech	AVT	8.3–8.9	14.5	+10.25 D & above	15
Alden Optical	HP49, HP54, HP59, Classic 38, Classic 55	6.5–9.7	10–16	+10.25–+30 D	15 21 24 8.4 18.8
Bausch + Lomb	Silsoft	7.5–8.3	11.3, 12.5 under +20	+11.50–+32 D	340
Biocurve	Biocurve Aphakic	8.0–9.5	13–15.5	+10.25–+25	18.8
California Optics	CO Soft	8.3–9.2	13.0–15.0	Pl–+30 D	18.8
Continental	Pediatric Aphakic	5.8–10.4	8.5–14.0	Pl–+40 D	18.1
Gelflex USA	Synergy SiHy	8.0–9.2	14.3–15.3	unlimited	60
Ocu-Ease	Pediatric Aphakic	6.0–8.6	8.0–16.0	+10 +40	18.1
SpecialEyes	SpecialEyes 49, 54, 59	6.9–9.5	12.5–16.0	Pl–+25 D	15 23 24
Visionary Optics	XP	3.5–35	6.0–17.0	Pl–+50 D	21
Westcon Contact Lens	Horizon 55 Custom	6.0–11.0	10–18	Pl–+50 D	18.8
X-Cel	Pediatric Aphakic	5.0–11.0	8.0–16.0	Pl–+50 D	17
Various	Rigid Gas-Permeable	Any	Any	Any	Up to 163

Anatomic Considerations

There are many differences between pediatric and adult eyes that the practitioner must be aware of: axial length, corneal diameter, corneal curvature, palpebral aperture, and pupil size.[21,24,25] All of these are important features to recognize when fitting a contact lens to a child.

The axial length is one of the key features, as it contributes so much to refractive error. In newborns, the axial length is typically 17 mm, whereas the adult eye's length is 24 mm. This short eye results in very high refractive errors. The typical aphakic power in an infant at 1 month is 31 D, but by the time the child is age 4, it has decreased to 17 D.[21] The average corneal diameter in infants is much smaller than adults. In infants, the average diameter is 9.8 mm, whereas in the adult eye it is between 11.5 and 12.5 mm.[21] The cornea also undergoes significant change during the first year of life. In premature infants, the average curvature is 49.50 D; in 1- to 2-month-old infants it is 47 D, and in 4-year-old it is 43 to 44 D.[21] Also, the palpebral aperture in infants is smaller than that of the adult and the tension of the lids tighter than that of the adult. This makes it a challenge to insert a contact lens onto the eye. The pupil diameter of the infant is also much smaller than the adult eye, with the average pupil size of an infant being 2 mm. With all these factors, the contact lens fit becomes critical. The contact lens has to fit these characteristics: relatively small in diameter to be inserted on the eye, steep in corneal curvature so the lens will stay centered, and high power because the refractive error is very high. Any contact lens that is used for the pediatric aphakic should also have exceptional Dk, as this lens may be used in an EW modality.

Contact Lens Fitting

Determining Lens Parameters

Fitting a contact lens to an infant is one of the most challenging techniques that the contact lens practitioner must perform. Different age groups require different methods for successful contact lens fitting. Different strategies need to be employed for the infant, the toddler, and the young child. In general, it may not be possible to obtain corneal curvature measurements on children under the age of 4 to 5 years.[26,27] The practitioner will also not be able to obtain subjective responses. The use of an autorefractor may be limited to older children. Therefore, the practitioner needs to be skilled in performing retinoscopy. This will be the determining factor in deciding on the power of the contact lens. When determining an aphakic correction, it should be noted that the infant is going to have a very high refractive error and that the younger the child, the higher the refractive error.

Determining the initial power can be frustrating because of the lack of cooperation of the child. Retinoscopy can be performed in several ways: using loose lenses, using retinoscopic lens bars, or using a single high plus lens. In using loose lenses, the practitioner places a lens in front of the child's eye and determines motion and then attempts a different lens depending on what was initially elicited. The problem is that the child often loses interest and the practitioner is constantly exchanging lenses. The use of a lens bar eliminates this, but typically the child will attempt to grab the bar. A simple way to determine the power is to take a high plus lens (e.g., +20 D) and move it away from the eye until neutralization is obtained (Fig. 17.5). If the distance is measured from where the lens is to the corneal plane, the power can be calculated for the lens using the following formula: $P_C = P_S/1 - dP_S$, where P_C is the power at the corneal plane and P_S is the power at the spectacle plane. This will yield an initial power for the contact lens. The practitioner should always keep in mind that the power of the eye will continue to change as the child gets older and it is not unusual for a newborn to have a lens with the power of +32 D while a 4-year-old may be only +17 D. In all cases, the first lens is a sophisticated diagnostic lens and retinoscopy needs to be performed over the lens to determine, with accuracy, the power needed for the patient.

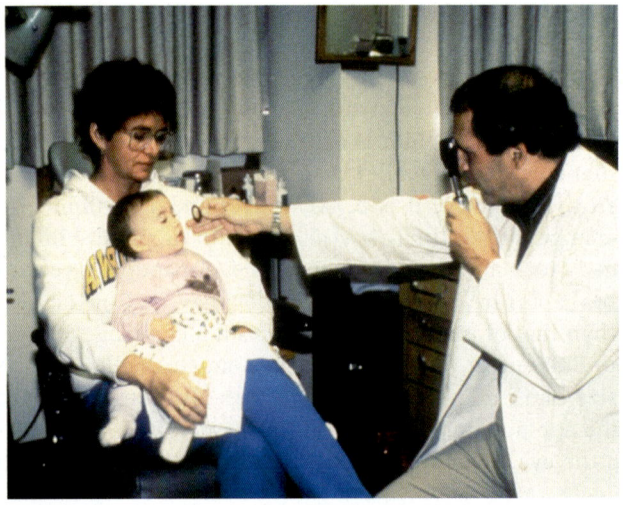

FIGURE 17.5 Vertex lens technique.

Assessing the Lens-to-Cornea Fitting Relationship

All contact lenses should be assessed after they are placed in the eye. Determination of the power of the lens needs to be performed. Retinoscopy will yield how close the correction is. Typically, infants and toddlers are overplussed by 3 D. The reason for this is the fact that young infants and toddlers work in a near world, often holding things very close to their eyes. As the child ages, the correction changes until he or she is properly corrected for distance and uses reading overglasses, typically in the form of bifocals.

The fit of the lens needs to be evaluated. The primary author does not use soft lenses for pediatric aphakics who are under the age of 5. The use of GP contact lenses and Silsoft lenses allows the practitioner to use fluorescein to determine the fitting relationship. Both types of lenses should center well and move easily. The fluorescein patterns should be of minimal apical clearance. Rigid lenses will need to be fit a little larger than normal to help keep the lens centered. Whenever possible, the use of the slit lamp to access the lens-to-cornea fitting relationship is preferable. Even young children can be placed in the slit lamp for observation (Fig. 17.6).

Care should be taken to look for staining or lens binding. If these conditions are found, steps must be taken to eliminate them. The surface of the lens should also be evaluated. The Silsoft lens is a hydrophobic material that is coated to allow tears to cover the lens. A side effect of the coating is that it has an affinity for lipids and the lens will get deposited and have to be replaced.

Lens Handling and Care

Handling

Insertion for an Infant: Fitting a contact lens to an infant under the age of 1 year can be both frustrating and rewarding. The type of contact lens, the power, the overall diameter (OAD), and the BCR have to be selected. Once the lens has been selected, the lens must be inserted onto the eye. For the infant group, the most successful technique is to have the mother cradle the child against her breast and use her arms to secure the child so he or she cannot move (Fig. 17.7).

The lids are then separated and the lens is placed on the eye. Problems inserting the lens may exist if the child has very tight lids and the practitioner cannot get the lids sufficiently separated to get the lens in the eye. In situations like this, the use of a speculum to separate the lids will allow the practitioner to insert the lens onto the eye (Fig. 17.8).

Care should be taken not to express the contact lens when the speculum is removed. Although the technique with the speculum appears awkward and uncomfortable, it allows for fast insertion on an infant, in whom it is challenging to apply a lens.

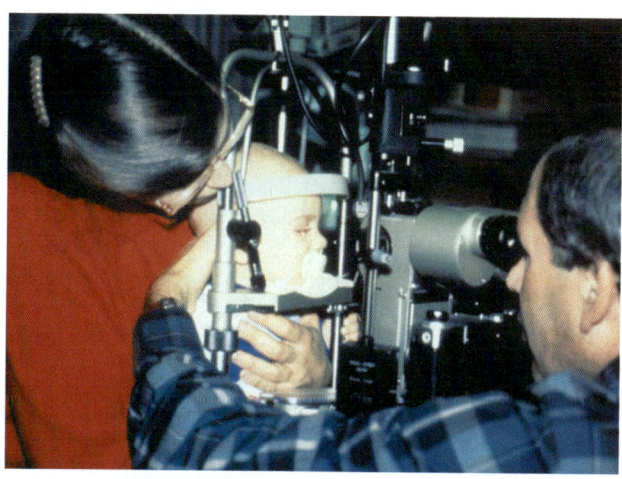

FIGURE 17.6 Infant in slit lamp.

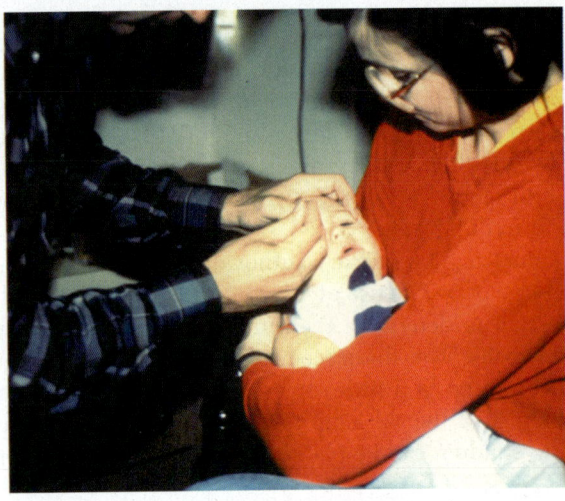

FIGURE 17.7 Infant insertion.

Insertion for a Toddler: Insertion for the toddler age group between $1^1/_2$ and 4 years of age is the most difficult group in which to insert a lens. These children are very active and know what they want and what they do not want. The contact lens insertion is extremely difficult on an uncooperative child in this age group. They will turn their heads, squeeze their eyes shut, physically fight, and often generally resist. Many practitioners will use some form of restraint to aid in the insertion of the lens. The restraints will keep the child moderately immobile to allow lens insertion. Commercial restraints, such as the papoose board, have Velcro strips to hold the child still (Fig. 17.9).

The use of blankets or sheets will often be equally successful. When using a blanket, it is important to lay the child on the ground and then either roll the child in the blanket or wrap the blanket around the child, making sure that the arms and legs are securely within the blanket (Fig. 17.10). This then allows the practitioner to insert the lens onto the eye with minimal movement of the child. Additionally, it frees the practitioner's hands to make lens insertion easier. In some of these cases, the practitioner may have to use the speculum as an aid to separate the lids to allow insertion. This technique is not as traumatic to the child as is a protracted lens insertion battle. Inserting the aphakic lens can be cumbersome. The lens is thick and heavy and will not stay on a finger. It is best to "pinch" the lens between two fingers to insert it. The lens should either be placed directly on center or, if not possible, the lens should be slid underneath the upper lid to allow the lens to adhere to the eye. These techniques should be used for all age groups. The practitioner should always remember that the goal is to place the contact lens on the eye because the child is aphakic and that this lens is therapeutically indicated.

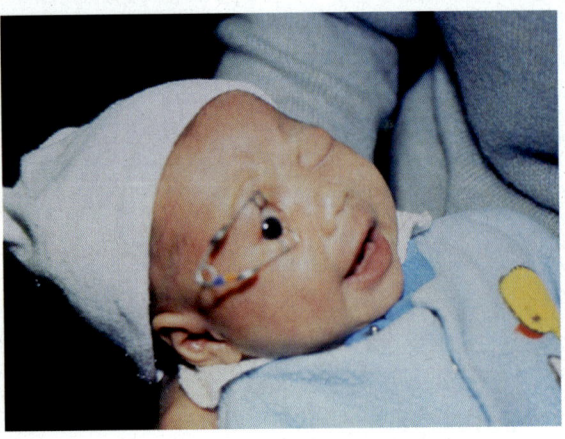

FIGURE 17.8 Speculum on infant.

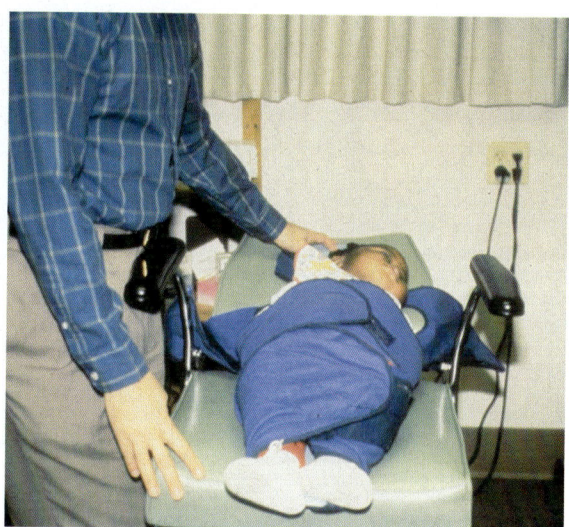

FIGURE 17.9 Infant on papoose board.

Insertion for a Child: Children who are older (>5 years) are generally more cooperative; thus, determining the necessary contact lens is easier. Children of this age group can have keratometry performed, can use the autorefractor, and can tell you what they see and may be able to participate in a subjective refraction. This age group is the one that can be reasoned with. The technique that the first author uses is the following. A discussion of the contact lens is provided. A lens is then shown to the child (Fig. 17.11). The child can touch the lens and see how it feels (Fig. 17.12). The lens is then placed on different parts of the child such as the cheek, the nose, or the hand. At this point, the author then places a lens on his eye so the child can see that it is okay. The child then is allowed to handle the lens and the lens is placed on the child's eye (Fig. 17.13). The child is often rewarded for his or her effort after the lens is in place. Suitable rewards can be the stickers, the surprise goody box, or, as we often use, some jelly beans.

Removal of the Lens: The technique for lens removal is the same for all age groups. The technique is the two-hand method using both lids to expel the lens (Fig. 17.14). To remove the lens, fingers from each hand should be placed at the lid margin of both the top and bottom lids. Pressure should be placed on the lids so the margin presses against the globe. The lids should then be pushed toward each other. Care should be taken not to evert the lids. When performed properly, the lens will be expressed from the eye. This technique will work for Silsoft, rigid, and even soft lenses. Soft lens solutions are used for Silsoft and soft lenses. GP solutions are used for GP lenses.

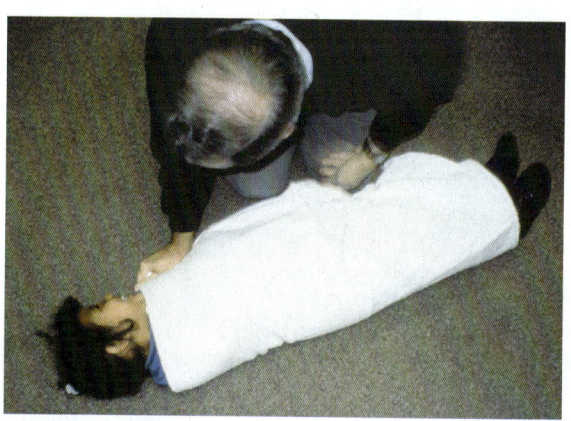

FIGURE 17.10 Blanket technique.

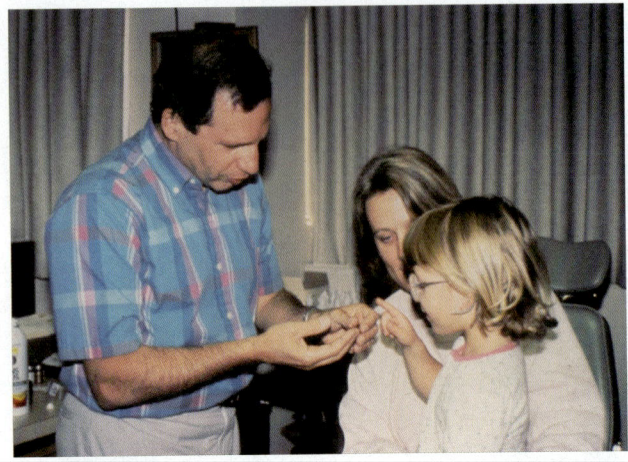

FIGURE 17.11 Initial presentation of lens to child.

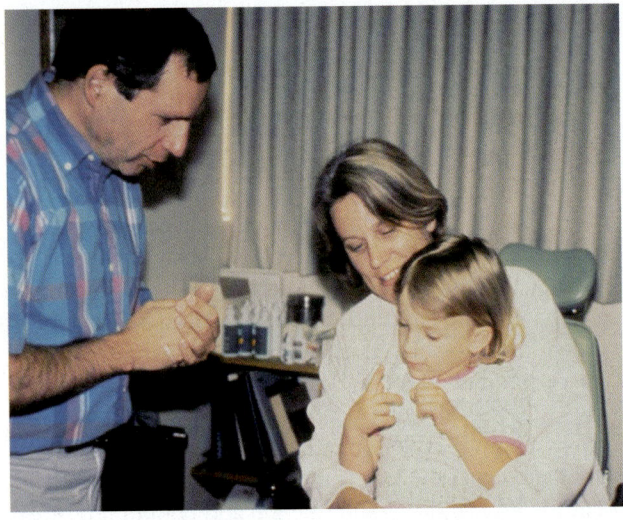

FIGURE 17.12 Child handling lens.

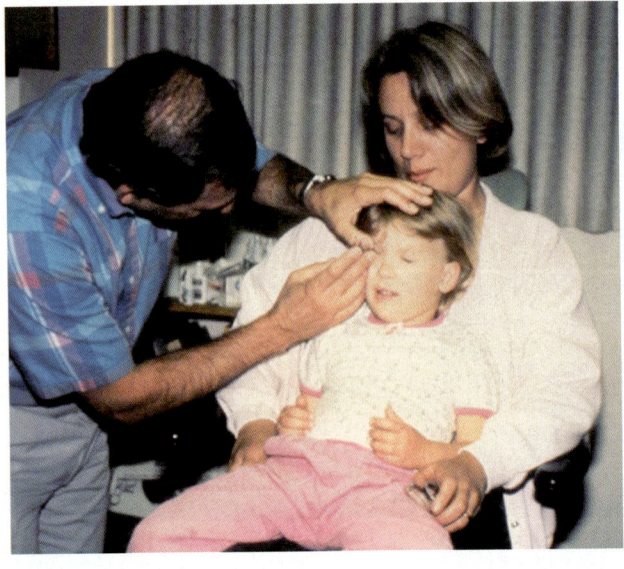

FIGURE 17.13 Insertion on child.

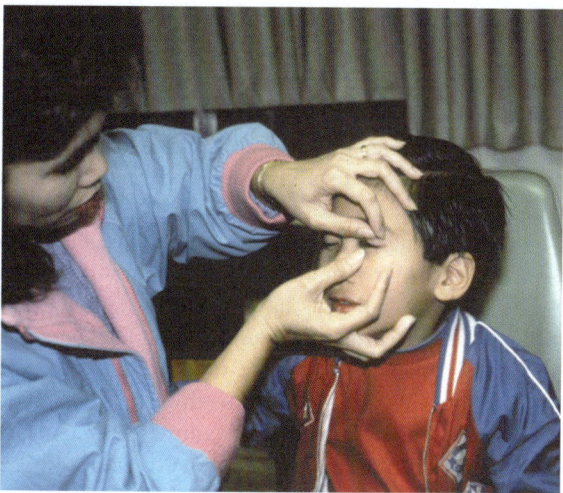

FIGURE 17.14 Two-hand removal.

Care

Wearing Schedule: The wearing schedule for a pediatric aphakic will vary depending on the age of the child and the contact lens modality used. If a soft aphakic lens is used, this lens must be removed on a daily basis. The low Dk and thick lens does not lend itself to an EW modality. Rigid lenses have more flexibility. These lenses have higher Dk. This allows the child to sleep with a lens in place. The authors recommend removal of the rigid lens at night, but leaving the lens in during daytime naps. The Silsoft lens, with its high permeability, is the most flexible. These lenses can be worn either as DW or as EW. The lens is durable enough to be removed every day if the practitioner chooses, or oxygen permeable enough that the lenses can stay in the eye for 1 week or more at a time. The practitioner will decide how long the lens should be used before removal. When the lens is removed, it is advised that the lens be cleaned and sterilized.

Follow-Up Appointments: Pediatric patients will be evaluated very frequently by the contact lens practitioner. The patient should be seen the day after dispensing to evaluate how the lens is being tolerated, especially if the lens is being worn in an EW modality. Follow-up visits should be scheduled at 1 week and again in 1 month. The child should then be evaluated every 2 to 3 months to monitor the fitting relationship of the lens and the resulting vision.

Potential Problems

With any type of contact lens there is a potential for problems. Pediatric patients are often more difficult to assess. In many cases, they cannot verbalize the problem. The practitioner's first encounter of a problem may be a red eye. Parents should be made aware of signs of a normal and an abnormal response. Red eyes are the biggest concern. This can be secondary to erosion, an infection, or a tight lens. Parents should immediately have the child examined by a practitioner to determine the underlying cause. Once the cause is found, the practitioner should proceed with the proper treatment. Other less significant problems that will most likely be encountered include lens loss and lens degradation. Pediatric patients will lose lenses; this is always expected. A spare lens should always be available so the patient is not without a lens. Silsoft lenses will also degrade with use because of the film on the lens. Frequent removal and cleaning will help prevent this problem.

What Parents Need to Know

Successful contact lens wear for the pediatric aphakic patient is going to be directly related to the success achieved with the parents. Parents need to be informed of the child's condition, treatment, prognosis, and follow-up care. They need to be aware that they will be involved in all aspects of the child's lens care including insertion, removal, and cleaning. It is important that the parents are educated about the child's condition, are properly motivated, and have the ability and desire to make the contact lens work. They must be able to observe the eye for any potential complications secondary to lens use and need to recognize an adverse event. They need to be aware of the costs involved with the treatment. In the primary author's experience, the average pediatric aphakic uses six lenses per eye per year. Replacement of lenses can be because of loss, damage, or prescription change. Parents should also be aware that the contact lens is a long-term treatment and not a short-term management option. Parents need to be aware that not only will they have a contact lens to be responsible for, but, in all likelihood, the child will need treatment for amblyopia. They need to know that patching may be required to achieve the child's best possible vision. Once the parents are educated, it is important for them to comply. This will pertain to exhibiting proficiency with inserting, removing, cleaning, and recentering of the contact lens. Failure to perform these functions will cause failure of the patient to successfully wear the lens. Finally, it would be ideal to have a cooperative child, but, in many cases, this will not be the result. Lenses have to be inserted and cared for by whatever means necessary and, especially if the child is not cooperative, perseverance is important. Although these patients are difficult to care for, the rewards can be extremely satisfying.

SUMMARY

Aphakic patients are motivated by a strong desire to enhance their quality of vision. Despite this strong will to proceed with the indicated treatment of contact lenses, they often face disappointment from high expectations regarding convenience and best visual performance. This is especially true if the paired eye is phakic with excellent VA or if the affected eye experiences glare. Reluctance to perform lens care or insertion/removal and persistent lens awareness may also result in dissatisfaction with contact lens wear. It is advisable to inform each potential contact lens candidate of the necessary lens care and handling before proceeding with fitting. This should be followed by fitting a lens that provides the best and most comfortable VA and the best fit with the least lens awareness possible.

ACKNOWLEDGEMENTS

The authors would like to thank Amy Langford, OD, for her contribution to this chapter.

CLINICAL CASES

CASE 1

A 46-year-old man developed a cataract of the right eye following penetrating trauma. This has left him with aphakia and a small area of corneal scarring outside of the visual axis. Manifest refraction:

$$OD: +12.50 - 0.75 \times 145 \; 20/25$$
$$OS: -4.00 - 0.75 \times 180 \; 20/20$$

Keratometry:

$$OD: 41.75 @ 150; 43.00 @ 60$$
$$OS: 41.00 @ 180; 42.00 @ 90$$

SOLUTION: Because of the relatively flat corneal curvatures and young age, this patient would be expected to perform well with a rigid contact lens. It is recommended to begin with a relatively large lens of about 9.50 mm in diameter with a BCR "on K." It would be expected that a lenticular edge design would be necessary to provide for adequate lens centration. The predicted lens design would be as follows:

BCR	41.75 D (8.08 mm)
Power +14.75 D (vertex distance = 12 mm)	
Diameter	9.50 mm
Optic zone	8.0 mm
Flange radius/optic cap	9.50 mm/8.0 mm
Peripheral curve radii/widths	9.0/0.4 mm, 12.0/0.35 mm

Another important consideration is the myopic refractive error of the paired eye. Aphakic contact lenses result in 3% to 5% image magnification. This, combined with the relative minification from the left spectacle lens, may result in aniseikonia-related asthenopia or diplopia (Appendix C). Therefore, overcorrecting the aphakic eye by 3 to 4 D will allow for a balanced spectacle prescription. Fitting both eyes with contact lenses would be an alternative method to reduce these magnification effects. If the keratometry readings were steeper (e.g., 45.00 @ 150; 46.00 @ 60), a smaller-diameter lens would be indicated. It is recommended to fit an initial lens that is approximately 0.50 D steeper than K using a 9.0-mm diameter lens. A lenticular design will usually be indicated provided the upper eyelid is at or below the superior limbus. The predicted lens would therefore be as follows:

BCR	45.50 (7.42 mm)
Power +14.25 D (vertex distance = 12 mm)	
Diameter	9.0 mm
Optic zone	7.6 mm
Flange radius/optic cap	9.0 mm/7.6 mm
Peripheral curve radii/widths	8.5/0.4 mm, 11.0/0.3 mm

CASE 2

A 73-year-old aphakic patient has worn a hydrogel contact lens in her left eye with weekly removals for 5 years. She reports a 1-day history of discomfort in the eye with no discharge. The VA in the affected eye is reduced to 20/50 but improved to 20/30 with a +2.00 D overrefraction. The best VA 3 months previously was 20/30 using a plano overrefraction. Slit-lamp examination demonstrates a nonmoving hydrogel lens that is well centered. The conjunctiva is injected, and the cornea demonstrates stromal edema by the presence of several large striae. No corneal inflammatory cells are present. A diffuse, epithelial, punctate stain is apparent on instillation of fluorescein.

SOLUTION: These findings are consistent with acute tight lens syndrome. On dehydration, hydrogel lenses undergo parameter changes that result in a tighter fitting relationship. This, combined with corneal flattening from overnight corneal edema, may result in a lens adhering to the eye. Since aphakic hydrogel lenses with a medium to high water content can develop a large amount of dehydration, sufficient lens lag of at least 1.0 to 1.5 mm is indicated. Possible solutions would be to remove the lens more frequently, replace the lens more frequently (at minimum every 6 months), or loosen the fit by selecting a flatter BCR or smaller diameter. Another alternative would be to use a GP lens design.

CASE 3

A 36-year-old man with a history of penetrating trauma is aphakic with a large iris defect in the affected eye. This results in a subjective complaint of glare. A corneal scar exists somewhat outside the visual axis. The best refraction of the right eye using a +14.00 D sphere provides a VA of 20/40. There is no improvement with pinhole. The paired eye is emmetropic with a VA of 20/20.

SOLUTION: In addition to correction of the aphakic refractive error, one must consider the large iris defect. Two options are available. First, the use of dark sunglasses while outdoors may improve the subjective comfort. If glare continues to be a problem while indoors, a tinted aphakic hydrogel lens with an artificial pupil would be indicated. The patient has excellent VA with a spherical spectacle refraction. Therefore, a hydrogel lens design would also be expected to provide good VA. It is recommended to begin with a hydrogel lens having a dark-tinted, opaque iris that also has a central clear pupil of about 3 mm. This design would allow for clear central VA while reducing glare by simulating the natural iris.

CASE 4

A 65-year-old aphakic man wears a GP lens for aphakia in the right eye. He reports lens intolerance for the past 3 to 4 days while wearing the lens. Upon examination, two to three areas of lens edge chipping are observed. Inspection of the lens demonstrates a very thin-lens edge profile.

SOLUTION: The thin-lens edge design has developed several chips that create lens awareness. A new lens must be ordered incorporating a thicker edge. This may be accomplished simply by increasing the lens CT. However, additional modifications may also be desirable since increasing lens CT may also produce a heavy lens that positions inferiorly. As this patient's lens had a very thin lens edge, it is likely that it did not have a lenticular design. Reordering a lenticular design would increase the lens edge thickness profile while reducing the lens CT. This is probably preferred in most cases as lens centration may also be improved.

CASE 5

A 73-year-old aphakic patient presents after 3 months of extended hydrogel contact lens wear. Her care regimen includes weekly lens removal, last removing the lenses 5 days previously. During the examination, her best VA is 20/30 with an overrefraction of +1.50 D. A corresponding flattening of both corneal meridians is also found by keratometry after lens removal. Slit-lamp examination demonstrates two to three large Descemet folds in the central cornea. Consistent with previous examinations, the cornea also exhibits dot/fingerprint, epithelial basement membrane changes. The contact lens provides an excellent fitting relationship with approximately 1 to 2 mm of lens lag with the blink.

SOLUTION: This patient demonstrates corneal edema secondary to a high corneal oxygen demand. Despite a well-fitting contact lens, corneal hypoxia has resulted in corneal curvature and refractive power changes. If this patient continues with the present lens design and wearing schedule, more serious complications may result. Patients having vitreous prolapse touching the corneal endothelium may also demonstrate corneal edema with hydrogel lenses even when removed daily. The quality of vision may vary throughout the day because of fluctuating refractive error and corneal curvature changes. A reduction in wearing time is indicated. Alternatively, a silicone hydrogel contact lens material (see Table 17.3) would provide much better oxygen transmission and, therefore, minimize the risk of serious lens-related complications. A hyper-DK GP lens material is another option and should provide a more stable vision correction. She may also be considered for a secondary intraocular lens.

CASE 6

A 65-year-old aphakic patient wearing a hydrogel contact lens has experienced for the past 12 months recurrent episodes of GPC, soiled lenses, and lens awareness. He is unable to care for the lens himself because of a tremor related to Parkinson disease. Lens maintenance includes weekly lens removal by his wife, followed by cleaning and disinfection overnight.

SOLUTION: This patient is found to have GPC along with poor tear layer and blepharitis. He is fortunate to have someone who can participate in lens care. However, weekly removals of a hydrogel lens have resulted in recurrent episodes of GPC. Therefore, more frequent lens removal is indicated. The patient also appears to have a tear layer that is incompatible with comfortable hydrogel lens wear.

The use of a GP lens may be advantageous in these cases. As the deposits are more easily removed with cleaning, lens soilage is reduced. These lenses can be worn overnight provided a good fit is obtainable and one of the new materials having a Dk of at least 70×10^{-11} is used. Another consideration is the patient's blepharitis and poor tear layer. Medical treatment in the form of hot packs or antibiotic/steroid drops is indicated for the lid disease. Tear supplements may be necessary to reduce lens deposits. GP contact lenses tend to become more comfortable following 1 or 2 days of overnight wear. If the patient is very motivated toward continuing soft lens wear, a planned-replacement lens—preferably silicone hydrogel—would be recommended. Alternative therapy may include the use of a secondary intraocular lens.

CASE 7

An aphakic patient reports wearing a GP contact lens without complaints. The lens is observed to position inferiorly without movement on blinking. Coalesced 3- and 9 o'clock staining is present along with distorted keratometer mires following lens removal.

SOLUTION: A low-riding aphakic rigid lens may result from a steep lens-to-cornea fitting relationship, a thin-lens edge design, thick heavy lenses, or a loose upper eyelid. A recommended solution includes a lenticular design that will reduce the CT while increasing the edge thickness to maintain a superior lens fit. If the lens is already of lenticular design, flattening the flange radius or increasing the OAD may enhance the interaction between the lens and the upper eyelid, creating a higher lens fit (Fig. 17.15). In the event that a lens continues to drop with no improvement in corneal stain and distortion, hydrogel lenses should be considered. When indicated, the appropriate astigmatic correction is placed into a spectacle lens to be worn while wearing the soft lens.

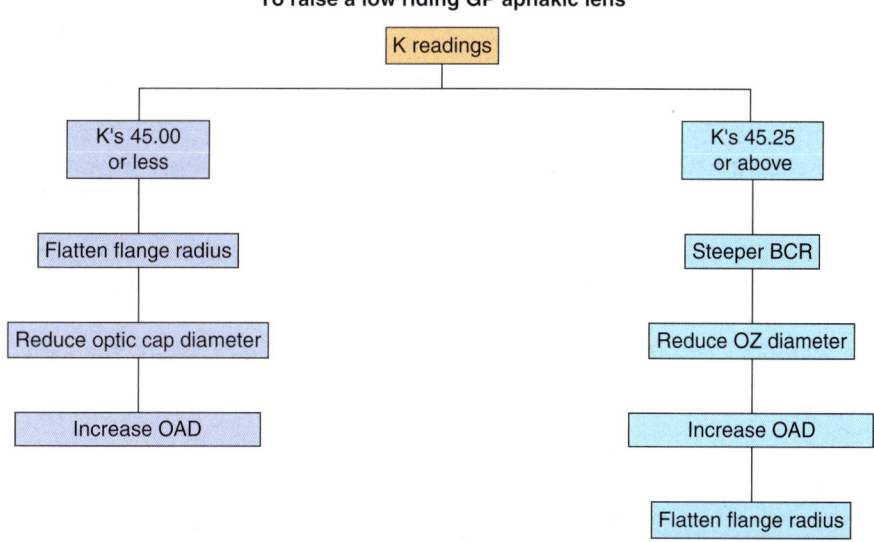

FIGURE 17.15 Raising a low-riding gas-permeable aphakic lens.

CASE 8

A 9-year-old aphakic patient had cataract extraction because of lens subluxation secondary to Marfan syndrome. She presents for a contact lens follow-up. She wears her lenses daily and reports no problems. She is currently wearing the following:

OD BCR 8.3 mm   Dia. 13.8 mm Rx +15.00 D   VA: 20/80
OS BCR 8.3 mm   Dia. 13.8 mm Rx +14.50 D   VA: 20/60 − 1

FlexLens, ReNu care system keratometry:

OD: 42.50 @ 090; 42.75 @ 180
OS: 40.00 @ 090; 42.75 @ 180

Horizontal visible iris diameter (HVID): 11.5 mm
Manifest refraction:

OD: +12.75 − 2.75 × 0.25 VA: 20/25
OS: +12.50 − 2.00 × 150 VA: 20/30

Slit-lamp examination revealed neovascularization, microcystic edema, and superficial punctate keratitis. The lenses were heavily deposited.

SOLUTION: Because of the anterior segment findings, the patient was refit into a silicone hydrogel lens to provide greater oxygen transmission. The initial trial lenses ordered were:

OD BCR: 8.3 mm, OAD: 14.0 mm, Rx +15.00 − 2.75 × 25   Distance VA 20/25
                                                          Near VA 20/50

OS BCR: 8.3 mm, OAD: 14.0 mm, Rx +14.50 − 2.00 × 150   Distance VA 20/30
                                                          Near VA 20/50

Overrefraction:

OD: +1.25 − 2.25 × 15 Distance VA 20/25, near VA 20/50
OS: +0.50 − 2.00 × 165 Distance VA 20/30, near VA 20/50

A spherical overrefraction of +1.00 D OU gave the patient no blur at distance and 20/30 near vision. The patient was given a spectacle prescription to wear over the contact lenses at near.

CASE 9

A 4-year-old patient had a history of congenital cataract in the left eye that was removed in the first year of life. She was initially fit with Silsoft contact lenses. At the age of 3, she became intolerant to the Silsoft lenses. She was successfully fit with a hydrogel lenses (BCR 8.3 mm, OAD 13.0 mm, Rx +20.00 D). Four months after dispensing the hydrogel lens, the patient began to experience discomfort and the lens was decentering. The mother expressed interest in trying a different lens.

SOLUTION: Silicone hydrogel (see Table 17.3) trial lenses are to be ordered. The patient's pertinent information is as follows:

Refraction:

OD: plano BCVA 20/20
OS: +15.00 BCVA 20/60

HVID: 10 mm

Keratometry values: unable to obtain because of the patient's age and cooperation. In young aphakic patients, keratometry readings cannot be taken with accuracy; therefore, it is best to perform a diagnostic fit with a trial lens. The laboratory should be able to provide consultation as to an initial trial lens to order.

The following lens was ordered for her OS: BCR 8.3 mm, OAD: 13.0 mm, Rx: +20.00 D. (The power was chosen to make the patient artificially myopic to allow for clear vision at near because of lack of accommodation in the aphakic eye.) At her follow-up visit, the results of testing were:
VA

OD: 20/20
OS: 20/100 with an overrefraction of ×4.00 + 1.00 × 180; VA was still 20/100.

The lenses centered well. The patient was to continue patching for amblyopia. After 3 months of amblyopia treatment, her VA with contact lenses was OS 20/40. Her overrefraction was −0.50 + 2.00 × 135 for 20/30 acuity. A new lens was ordered with the same parameters, except the power was changed to +16.00 D. The lens centers well and provides a good fit.

CLINICAL PROFICIENCY CHECKLIST

- Diagnostic fitting using aphakic lenses is essential to provide for an accurate prescription and to evaluate fitting dynamics of these thick lens designs.
- Ideally, new wearers should be fit into a hyper-Dk GP or silicone hydrogel lens material, provided a good fit can be achieved.
- Altering lens edge profile by using lenticular designs is essential to providing thin, well-fitting, GP aphakic contact lenses.
- When indicated in unilateral aphakic patients, consider the refractive error of the paired eye to provide for a balanced spectacle prescription. Consider fitting both eyes with contact lenses, or if bifocal spectacles are to be worn, fit the aphakic eye and adjust the contact lens power to balance the spectacle prescription.
- Planned replacement of soft aphakic lenses reduces the effects of parameter changes and complications associated with soiled lenses.
- Hydrogel aphakic lenses having a water content of >45% require sufficient lens lag (1.5–2.0 mm) at the fitting visit to reduce complications resulting from tight lenses.
- Front vertex versus back vertex power specification may influence the accuracy of final lens power.
- Hydrogel aphakic lenses may produce significant corneal edema, especially in patients having a prolapsed vitreous making contact with the corneal endothelium. Methods of reducing edema include reduction in wearing time, the use of silicone hydrogel lenses, or using a hyper-Dk GP contact lens material.
- Soft, large GP, and silicone elastomer lenses are recommended for the pediatric aphakic patient, with the latter two options recommended for patients under the age of 5.
- The younger the child, the higher the refractive error; a newborn can have a refractive error of +32 D, which may be reduced to +17 D at age 4.
- A simple way to measure the power on a pediatric aphakic patient is to take a +20 D lens and move it away from the eye until stabilization has been achieved.
- For the pediatric infant, it is recommended to have the mother cradle the child for lens insertion; for the toddler, a papoose board can be used.

OPTICAL CONSIDERATIONS FOR APHAKIA

Appendix A: Effective Power

When moving a lens from the spectacle plane toward the cornea, the effective vergence of light rays is altered. Therefore, the same aphakic eye will require a different power in a spectacle lens placed 12 mm in front of the cornea than in a contact lens placed on the cornea. It is necessary to increase power in the positive direction when moving close to the cornea.

The following equation is used to determine the effective power:

$$Fe = \frac{F}{1 - dF}$$

where

Fe = effective power (diopters)
F = back vertex power of lens (diopters)
d = vertex distance, or distance lens is moved in meters; $(+)$ if lens is moved toward cornea, $(-)$ if lens is moved away from the cornea

For example, what would be the power of a lens placed on the cornea that would be equivalent to a $+12.00$ D lens placed at a distance of 12 mm in front of the cornea (vertex distance = 12 mm)?

$$Fe = \frac{+12}{1 - .012(12)} = +14.02 \text{ D}$$

Therefore, a contact lens having a power of $+14.00$ D would have an effective power equal to a $+12.00$ D lens placed in the spectacle plane.

Note: The magnitude of astigmatism increases at the corneal plane.

Appendix B: Vertex Power

The power of a spectacle and contact lens is measured from the surface along the visual axis. It is the dioptric power from this point that influences the plane of focus for light passing through these thick lenses. Since the lens shape is of meniscus form (front surface has $[+]$ positive power, back surface has $[-]$ negative power), the vertex power is different when measuring from a reference point on the front of the lens compared to one on the back of a lens. These values are dependent on the lens CT, according to the following equations:

$$\text{Front Vertex Power } (Fv) = \frac{F_2}{1 - t/n\, F_2} + F_1$$

$$\text{Back Vertex Power } (Fv') = \frac{F_1}{1 - t/n\, F_1} + F_2$$

where

F_1 = power of front surface
F_2 = power of back surface
t = lens thickness (meters)
n = lens index of refraction

For example, determine the front and back vertex powers of an aphakic contact lens that has the following parameters:

$$F_1(\text{air}) = +76.00 \ (r_1 = 6.32 \text{ mm})$$
$$F_2(\text{air}) = -64.00 \text{ D} \ (r_1 = 7.50 \text{ mm})$$
$$n(\text{air}) = 1.48$$
$$CT = .50 \text{ mm } (.0005 \text{ m})$$

$$Fv' = \frac{+76.00}{1 - \frac{.0005}{1.48}(+76.00)} + -64.00 = +14.00 \text{ D}$$

$$Fv = \frac{+76.00 + -64.00}{1 - \frac{.0005}{1.48}(-64.00)} = +13.35 \text{ D}$$

In this example, there is a difference of 0.65 D between back vertex power and front vertex power. These differences increase in magnitude for lenses having higher vertex powers and increased CT.

Appendix C: Magnification

The spectacle-corrected aphakic eye is found to experience an image magnification of approximately 30%. These effects may be calculated from the following equations:

$$SM = \frac{1}{1 - t/n \, F_1} \times \frac{1}{1 - dFv'}$$

where

F_1 = power of front surface
Fv' = power of back surface
t = lens thickness (meters)
n = lens index of refraction
d = distance from back of lens to eye's entrance pupil (meters)

Using our example of an eye that requires a spectacle lens with a power of +12.00 D and a contact lens having a power of +14.00 D gives the following result (vertex = 12 mm):

Magnification: spectacle lens $\dfrac{1}{1 - \frac{.007}{1.49}(+15.00)} \times \dfrac{1}{1 - .015(12)}$

$F_1 = +15.00$
$Fv' = +12.00$
$t = 7.0$ mm
$n = 1.49$ (plastic) $1.076 \times 1.219 = 1.31$
$d = 12 + 3 = 15$ mm   or 31% magnification

Magnification: contact lens $\dfrac{1}{1 - \frac{.0005}{1.48}(+76.00)} \times \dfrac{1}{1 - .003(14)}$

$F_1 = +76.00$
$Fv' = +14.00$
$t = .50$ mm
$n = 1.48$ $(1.026) \times 1.043 = 1.07$
$d = 3$ mm   or 7% magnification

The above example demonstrates that contact lenses decrease magnification to at least one-fourth of that produced using an aphakic spectacle lens. It can be shown that an IOL further reduces this magnification to one-half of that found with contact lenses.

REFERENCES

1. Boeder P. Spectacle correction of aphakia. *Arch Ophthalmol.* 1962;68(6):870–874.
2. Davis JK, Torgersen DL. The properties of lenses used for the correction of aphakia. *J Am Optom Assoc.* 1983;54(8):685–693.
3. Borish IM. Aphakia: perceptual and refractive problems of spectacle correction. *J Am Optom Assoc.* 1983;54(8):701–711.
4. Nelson G, Mandell RB. The relationship between minus carrier design and performance. *Int Cont Lens Clin.* 1975;2(2):75–81.
5. Davis LJ, Bergin C, Bennett ES. Aphakia. In: Bennett ES, Weissman BA, eds. *Clinical Contact Lens Practice.* Philadelphia, PA: Lippincott Williams & Wilkins; 2005;595–604.
6. Thompson TT. *Tyler's Quarterly.* 2012;29(2):28–56.
7. Abrahamsson M, Magnusson G, Sjostrom A, et al. The occurrence of congenital cataract in western Sweden. *Acta Opthalmol Scand.* 1999;77(5):578–580.
8. San Giovanni JP, Chew EY, Reed GF, et al. Infantile cataract in the collaborative perinatal project: prevalence and risk factors. *Arch Ophthalmol.* 2002;120:1559–1565.
9. Bhatti TR, Dott M, Yoon PW, et al. Descriptive epidemiology of infantile cataracts in metropolitan Atlanta, GA, 1968–1998. *Arch Pediatr Adolesc Med.* 2003;157(4):341–347.
10. Wirthe MG, Russell-Eggitt IM, Graig JE, et al. Aetiology of congenital and paediatric cataract in an Australian population. *Br J Ophthalmol.* 2002;86(7):782–786.
11. Rahi JS, Dezatraux C. Measuring and interpreting the incidence of congenital ocular anomalies: lessons for a national study of congenital cataracts in the UK. *Invest Opthalmol Vis Sci.* 2001;42:1444–1448.
12. Beller R, Hoyt CS, Marg E, et al. Good visual function after neonatal surgery for congenital monocular cataracts. *Am J Ophthalmol.* 1981;91:559–565.
13. Davis LJ. Complex refractive errors in pediatric patients: cause, management, and criteria for success. *Optom Vis Sci.* 1998;75(7):493–499.
14. Anisworth JR, Cohen S, Levin AV, et al. Pediatric cataract management with variation in surgical technique and aphakic optical correction. *Ophthalmology.* 1997;104:1096–1101.
15. Basti S, Ravishankar U, Gupta S. Results of a prospective evaluation of three methods of management of pediatric cataracts. *Ophthalmology.* 1996;103:713–720.
16. Braverman DE. Pediatric contact lenses. *J Am Optom Assoc.* 1998;69:452.
17. Ozbek Z, Durak I, Berk TA. Contact lenses in the correction of childhood aphakia. *CLAO J.* 2002;28:28–30.
18. Chia A, Johnson K, Marrin F. Use of contact lenses to correct aphakia in children. *Clin Exp Ophthalmol.* 2002;30:252–255.
19. Buckley EG. Scleral fixated (sutured) posterior chamber intraocular lens implantation in children. *J AAPOS.* 1999;3:289–294.
20. McClatchey SK, Parks MM. Myopic shift after cataract removal in childhood. *J Pediatr Ophthalmol Strabismus.* 1997;34:88–95.
21. Moore BD. Changes in the aphakic refraction of children with unilateral congenital cataracts. *J Pediatr Ophthalmol Strabismus.* 1989;26:290–295.
22. Ellis P. Extended wear contact lenses in pediatric ophthalmology. *CLAO J.* 1983;9:317–321.
23. Cutler SI, Nelson LB, Calhoun JH. Extended wear contact lenses in pediatric aphakia. *J Pediatr Ophthalmol Strabismus.* l985;22:86–91.
24. Chase WW, Fronk SJ, Micheals BA. A theoretical infant schematic eye. Presented at: Annual Meeting of the American Academy of Optometry; 1984; St. Louis, MO.
25. Enoch JM. The fitting of hydrophilic (soft) contact lenses to infants and young children. Mensuration data on aphakic eyes of children born with congenital cataracts. *Contact Lens Med Bull.* 1972A:36–40.
26. Pratt-Johnson JA, Tillson G. Hard contact lenses in the management of congenital cataracts. *J Pediatr Ophthalmol Strabismus.* 1985;22:94–96.
27. Saunders RA, Ellis FD. Empirical fitting of hard contact lenses in infants and young children. *Ophthalmology.* 1981;88:127–130.

Chapter 18

Children and Contact Lenses

Jeffrey J. Walline, Marjorie J. Rah, Christine W. Sindt, and Edward S. Bennett

INTRODUCTION

A common question by parents and young people alike is: "What age can someone start wearing contact lenses?" Certainly they are often told that contact lens wear cannot begin until a certain age (often anywhere from 8 to 12 years of age). However, as with many presbyopic, borderline dry eye, and astigmatic individuals, most young people are good candidates for contact lenses if this option is presented to them. The purpose of this chapter is twofold: (a) To answer the question about what age to begin fitting young people as well as how to select qualified wearers, the fitting process, and the follow-up care, and (b) How myopia control is becoming a more available—if not exciting—option for young people. Pediatric aphakia will only be briefly addressed as it is described in great detail in Chapter 17.

Why Fit Contact Lenses to Young People?

There are many benefits, some life-changing, of fitting young people into contact lenses (Table 18.1). Children may require contact lens wear as a result of aphakia,[1–8] amblyopia therapy,[9–11] ocular trauma,[9,12] or refractive error. As the medically necessary applications are discussed elsewhere, the emphasis in this chapter pertains to the elective use of contact lenses for the correction of a young person's refractive error.

Often a young person is motivated to wear contact lenses after experiencing spectacle lens wear. The limitations to spectacles are many and include limitations in peripheral vision, induced aberrations and prism when viewing away from the optical center, and possible problems with excessive magnification and minification.[13] All of these problems are minimized, if not eliminated with contact lens wear. Spectacle wear has been associated with negative attributes, such as disfigurement and less attractiveness,[14,15] not to mention shyness, introversion, and less social forcefulness.[16,17] All children have an active lifestyle and spectacles can compromise their ability, not to mention their motivation, to participate in athletic activities due to the restrictions imposed by both lenses and frames. In addition, young people can become injured while wearing spectacles during athletic activities. For example, if a ball strikes the glasses, it can result in the lenses being pushed into the face, possibly resulting in lacerations and other trauma-induced complications of the eye, orbit, and face.

It is also evident that contact lenses can have benefits pertaining to increased self-esteem and quality of life as compared to spectacles. The Adolescent and Child Health Initiative to Encourage Vision Empowerment (ACHIEVE) Study was a randomized, single-masked trial with 8- to 11-year-old myopic children randomly assigned to wear spectacles or soft contact lenses for a 3-year period.[18] It was concluded that contact lenses significantly improve how children feel about their physical appearance, their ability to play sports, and their acceptance among friends. Their perception of their physical appearance is likely to improve with contact lens wear, even if they do not mind wearing spectacles. Contact lenses even made children more confident about their academic performance if they initially disliked wearing spectacles.

TABLE 18.1 Benefits of Contact Lenses for Young People

1. Minimize or eliminate spectacle-induced problems (i.e., reduced peripheral vision, induced aberrations, and prism)
2. Beneficial in all athletic activities.
3. Increased quality of life; notably, perception of physical appearance, ability to play sports, and social acceptance.
4. The potential to not require a vision correction during the day via OOK.
5. The possibility of myopia control via OOK.
6. Medically beneficial applications such as aphakia, trauma, or amblyopia

Another benefit of contact lenses versus spectacles is the perception of quality of life as it pertains to vision. The Pediatric Refractive Error Profile was administered to the ACHIEVE study subjects at baseline, 1 month, and every 6 months for 3 years.[19] Myopic children younger than 12 years of age reported better vision-related quality of life when fit with contact lenses, versus spectacles. Older children, children who are motivated to wear contact lenses, children involved in recreational activities, and children who did not like their appearance in glasses benefited the most.

Another important benefit of contact lenses, versus spectacles, is the potential for myopia control as provided by overnight orthokeratology (OOK). This application of specially designed lenses only for overnight wear allows qualified young people to see clearly during the day without any vision correction. OOK will be described in more detail later in this chapter.

Why Are Contact Lenses Not Prescribed More Often to Young People?

It is evident that many eye care practitioners (ECPs) are resistant to fitting young people with contact lenses for several reasons, including safety/adverse events, increased chair time, concerns about motivation, maturity, and hygiene.[20,21] However, it has been found that children as young as 8 years old are capable of wearing soft,[18,22–25] rigid gas-permeable (GP) lenses,[22,26–30] and OOK[31–34] contact lenses. In the ACHIEVE study, younger (<10 years of age) contact lens wearers wore their lenses for shorter periods of time than spectacle wearers, but still wore them, on average, about 10 hours per day. Both contact lenses and spectacles can be offered as a primary vision correction option for 8- to 11-year-old myopic children because they are capable of independent contact lens care.[18] As it pertains to chair time, the results of the Contact Lenses in Pediatrics (CLIP) Study found that the total chair time for children 8 to 12 years of age was only 15 minutes more than teens of ages 13 to 17.[35] Most of this difference pertained to a longer instruction time for lens handling, a task that is typically performed by office staff, so it does not impact the productivity of a busy practice.

The perception often held by ECPs is that the risk of infection or severe complications is higher in kids. However, there does not appear to be any scientific evidence indicating a higher risk in children. It is also evident that children as young as 8 years of age are mature enough to independently care for their contact lenses and experience few adverse effects resulting from contact lens wear.[22,24,32,36] It has been found that soft contact lens wear in young people was associated with lower risk of infiltrative events when compared with teens and young adults.[37] Likewise, the incidence of contact lens-induced corneal staining has been found to be less in young people[35,38] than in adults.[39,40] This may be in part due to the overall better ocular health of children compared to adults, including more tear volume, clearer corneas, decreased conjunctival redness, and less lid inflammation.[21] Therefore, provided that proper lens care and compliance are emphasized and reinforced, there is no reason why young people should be more susceptible to contact lens complications than adults.

For contact lenses to be successful in a young person, it depends largely on how proactive the ECP is with both young people and their parents. In a survey conducted by the Good Housekeeping (magazine) Reader Advisory Panel about attitudes and perceptions of parents about children's vision care, 66% believe that their eye doctor's recommendations are the right choice for their child's vision correction.[41] With this in mind, ECPs should routinely consider offering contact lenses as a treatment option, even as young as 8 years old.

PATIENT SELECTION

What Age Can Young People Wear Contact Lenses?

Traditionally, contact lenses were not often prescribed to children and young adults. Anecdotally, they (and their parents) were told that they had to wait until their eyes stopped growing, despite the fact that there are several benefits—as previously described—that could make this modality life-changing to a young person. There is, however, a shift toward contact lenses serving as the primary mode of refractive correction. A research survey, conducted by the AOA Research and Information Center was designed to gauge current trends in prescribing contact lenses in children ranging in age from 8 to 17 years.[42–44] Although responding optometrists most often fit children aged 8 to 9 years (51%) and 10 to 12 years (71%) in spectacles as the primary method of vision correction, a gradual shift was noted, in that 21% indicated they were more likely to fit the 10–12-year-old children into contact lenses than 1 year prior. Nearly half indicated they prescribed contact lenses first for 13- to 14 year olds, and 66% recommended contact lenses as the primary form of correction for 15- to 17 year olds. Factors that influenced the fitting of young people included the availability of daily disposable lenses (cited by 30%), improved contact lens materials (23%), requests from child or parent (19%), and young person's participation in activities and sports (10%).

As mentioned previously, children 8 years and older are often successful with contact lens wear and can both handle lenses and adapt to lens wear.[35] It has also been suggested that if contact lens wear is indicated, parental support is confirmed, and necessary precautions and care taken, there might not be a minimum age for contact lenses.[21]

Other Important Factors for Patient Selection

In addition to age, there are eight important factors for the parent, young person, and practitioner to take into account when considering prescribing contact lenses.[42,45,46] The first seven are ranked in descending order of importance from the results of the AOA study. These include interest and motivation, maturity, ability to take care of lenses independently, personal hygiene habits, sports, prescription requirements, self-esteem, and preexisting medical conditions. These are listed in Table 18.2.

1. Interest and motivation. In the aforementioned AOA survey, almost all of the respondents indicated that the child's interest and motivation to wear contact lenses is the most important factor to consider. However, motivation should be judged after the child has worn contact lenses in the office. Many children are initially apprehensive because they think that anything in the eye feels like the drops that the doctor instills. If the child is still extremely hesitant after experiencing a pair of contact lenses for a short time, then the child may not be a good candidate for contact lens wear until later. Many optometrists and parents believe that the young person who was prescribed spectacles but either fails to wear them or wears them only intermittently is a poor contact lens candidate. However, these individuals may be more compliant with contact lens wear as a refractive correction modality because they dislike spectacle wear, not because they are incapable of the responsibility of wearing vision correction.[47] The other factor to consider is the attitude of the parent(s). It is important to beware of the parents who insist their child needs contact lenses when, in fact, the child exhibits an absence of verbal and nonverbal cues that would confirm such an opinion after experiencing contact lens wear. The parent who is involved but not overbearing is the best indicator for success.[48]

TABLE 18.2 Important Factors for Parent, Child, and Practitioner to Consider Before Prescribing Contact Lenses

1. Interest and motivation
2. Maturity
3. Ability to care for lenses independently
4. Personal hygiene habits
5. Sports
6. Prescription requirements
7. Self-esteem
8. Preexisting medical conditions

It is evident that some young people are resistant to people touching their eyes or instilling drops into their eyes.[21] This may be an indication that the young person is not ready for contact lens wear, but it is not an absolute guarantee that the child will not be successful. Occasionally, children require extra time and patience to learn to handle contact lenses, but they ultimately may be successful. If a child cannot independently remove elective contact lenses after 1 to 2 weeks of wear, and there appears to be little motivation, then contact lens wear should be delayed until the child is comfortable with contact lens care.

2. Maturity. The second most important factor from the AOA study pertaining to when to fit contact lenses with children was their maturity level. This can determined from both input from the parent(s) and also via observation of the young person during the examination.[13] A child who converses easily, appears open to new experiences, and has a good track record in other areas (i.e., schoolwork, activities), should have the maturity to be successful with contact lenses.
3. Ability to take care of lenses independently. Fortunately, it has been shown that children can handle lenses with a slightly longer period for instruction than teenagers.[35] If they are unable to master lens handling during the lens care instruction session, it is likely a sign that they are not ready—and possibly not sufficiently motivated—for elective contact lens wear.
4. Personal hygiene habits. Although input from the parent would be important here, the personal hygiene (hair combed, clean hands, etc.) and how a young person conducts themselves during the examination can speak volumes about their potential to properly care for their contact lenses.
5. Sports. It is important for the practitioner to inquire about the child's activities, including sports. This can serve a twofold purpose: (a) determine if they are a spectacle wearer, how satisfied are they wearing spectacles (if worn) for these activities. (b) this may help in determining what type of contact lens to fit if the young person is deemed a good candidate. As indicated previously, it can be mentioned to parents that contact lenses tend to make young people feel better about their ability to play sports.[18]
6. Prescription requirements. Obviously this can play a very important role in determining whether they are a good contact lens candidate. Both hyperopic (unless the prismatic benefit of spectacles is necessary) and myopic young people can appreciate the benefits of an unobstructed field of view (FOV), not to mention viewing images that are not excessively magnified or minified. Young progressive myopes can also benefit from the potential myopia control provided by OOK or soft bifocal contact lenses.

Where a potential problem can develop is with the emmetropic young person and cosmetically tinted contact lenses. As a result of sight-threatening complications resulting from plano power tinted contact lenses,[49–52] which consumers could often obtain without a prescription, without appropriate instruction, and with the potential to provide to other young people (i.e., "swapping lenses"), in 2005, the United States Food and Drug Administration (FDA) classified all contact lenses, whether they correct vision or are used simply for cosmetic purposes, as medical devices.[53] They cannot be provided without a valid prescription. Nevertheless, despite this fact, contact lenses continue to be purchased over the internet, which places the individual at risk for harmful eye care practices,[54] and has been found to result in four times greater risk for microbial keratitis (MK).[55] This can be the result of such factors as not practicing good hygiene, not cleaning or using the correct care products, sleeping in lenses, not replacing the lenses on a healthy schedule, and sharing the lenses with other people.[56] A recent report of 13 cosmetic lens wearers who all experienced a MK is quite relevant.[52] Seven of these individuals received their lenses from unlicensed optical shops, five shared lenses with friends and relatives, and one found the lenses in the garbage. *Pseudomonas* was the causative organism in seven of the cases and eight eyes had an ulcer ≥5 mm in size with a corresponding visual acuity of worse than or equal to 6/24.

Of course, the increasing introduction of decorative contact lenses (i.e., "Halloween designs," "Circle Lens") has created additional concerns.[57–59] When Lady Gaga wore the larger iris look created by the so-called "Circle Lens," it resulted in a craze in which teenagers began to acquire these lenses directly over the internet from foreign sites. Once again, the fact that these lenses are obtained without the fitting and instruction from ECPs makes it imperative that young people and their parents are informed both that contact lenses are medical devices as well as the potential problems associated with cosmetic tinted lenses.

7. Preexisting medical conditions. As with a potential contact lens wearer of any age, it is important to determine if there are any existing medical conditions that may rule out or delay contact lens fitting. As with adult patients, it is important to treat underlying conditions, such as allergies, blepharitis, and meibomian gland dysfunction prior to fitting contact lenses.[13]

Fortunately, dryness is a rare problem, occurring much less in children than in adults.[60–63] In fact, it has been found that only 4% of pediatric contact lens wearers were classified as dry-eye sufferers, compared to more than half of adult contact lens wearers.[63]

The Discussion with Parents

The decision for their child to wear contact lenses must first be presented to the parents. If the young person is a good candidate and the parents agree, both parents and child must be educated about myopia (if present), how it progresses with age, and how it can impact the child's performance in both school and in sports.[21,64] They should also be informed about the pros and cons of contact lenses, as well as the possible risks. This is especially important with OOK, in which the risk of severe complications is higher than with daily wear (DW) lenses.[55,65,66] That said, it should be emphasized that contact lenses are a very safe modality if the young person complies with the wearing schedule and lens care instructions provided by the ECP.

THE CONTACT LENS EXAMINATION AND FITTING

The Examination

The work-up or prefitting examination assists in determining not only if the patient is a good contact lens candidate but also what type of lenses would be best. The tests are the same as for the adult with particular attention to how the patient reacts to such tests as tonometry, lid eversion, and drop instillation. When the decision has been made to try contact lenses, it is important to radiate confidence in presenting contact lenses as a good option for them. Otherwise young people will reflect the anxiety that is present in the room.[67]

Soft or Gas-Permeable: The Decision-Making Process

The lens to be fit depends upon several factors. For the young athlete, soft lenses—especially daily disposable lenses—are often a desirable option if their prescription is consistent with the available lens parameters. This option eliminates the need for daily lens cleaning and disinfection and provides a clean lens on the eye each day they are worn.[68] As some children may not need to wear them every day (i.e., perhaps just for sports or other extracurricular activities), daily disposable lenses can even be cost-effective. When daily disposable lenses are not an option due to factors such as price or prescription, 2-week or monthly soft lenses are often prescribed. As they may be wearing these lenses for several decades, a 2-week or monthly replacement silicone hydrogel lens material is recommended.

GP lenses are an option for several young patients. Highly astigmatic young people can appreciate the visual benefits of GP lenses and it would beneficial to present this to both the patient and the parents. Obviously, the fact that these lenses are smaller in size and move more on the eye must be mentioned such that they can understand that they will experience some initial awareness that may take up to 2 weeks to go away. However, approximately 80% of children are able to initially adapt to GP contact lens wear, which is similar to adult adaptation rates. [26,69] The increasing introduction of corneoscleral and semi-scleral lens designs for healthy eyes, however, provides an option when vision is a high priority and initial awareness is a concern with conventional GP designs. For the young, progressive myope, it makes sense to present the option of OOK or soft bifocal contact lenses (to be discussed) and with today's internet-educated parents and children, it is not uncommon for them to initially present this potential option to their ECP.

Fitting Soft Lenses

Fitting soft lenses in young people is similar to an adult. As it is understandable for a young person to be apprehensive about the initial application of contact lenses, it can be made easier by having them handle a lens prior to it being applied for initial evaluation of the fit. They can be told it is like a big drop of water touching the eye. They may feel a little "tickling" sensation once it is on the eye, but it will go away fairly soon and they will love the fact they can experience vision (or the blackboard, the baseball, etc.) without having to wear glasses.

Fitting Gas-Permeable Lenses

The first step is to explain to the patient that these are small lenses that are actually quite easy to put on the eye. If the ECP or a staff member could demonstrate by inserting a lens on themselves, that would also help reduce anxiety. They should be told about the initial awareness caused by a small lens that moves on the eye and the upper lid "senses this movement" when the lid touches the lens edge on the blink. However, this sensation reduces over time. The use of a topical anesthetic has been found to result in a better perception of adaptation as well as a higher success rate by reducing the initial awareness.[70] The anesthetic effect should be allowed to dissipate, however, such that the young person can gradually experience a realistic sensation of lens wear. During the time between application and evaluation, the child should be encouraged to view inferiorly to reduce lid awareness. The evaluation of the lens-to-cornea fitting relationship is similar to adults. Such factors as an ultrathin design and the use of a lenticular when indicated (i.e., a minus lenticular for all plus and very low minus power lenses, and a plus lenticular for all high minus power designs) will optimize the initial comfort. Likewise, empirically fitting will allow the young person to experience the primary benefit of GP lenses, good vision, which then may actually reduce their perceptions about awareness.

Fitting an infant is discussed in more detail in the Chapter on aphakia (i.e., Chapter 17). However, the coauthor prefers GP lenses on infants, and there are some important guidelines to consider when fitting the very young patient into this modality.[71,72] When approaching these patients, it is a good idea to know the predicted keratometry values by age, especially if keratometry is impossible to perform.[73] In addition, it is necessary to dilate the pupils of young people to make retinoscopy easier. Cyclopleging nonaphakes will help in obtaining a true power without fear of accommodation. As most eye growth occurs within the first year of life, it is recommended to fit pediatric GP lenses on the large side to provide sufficient movement and to increase comfort. A good rule of thumb is to fit the lens 1 mm smaller than the horizontal visible iris diameter. If it is impossible to use a manual keratometer or a topographer, there is no better substitute than applying a lens using the aforementioned keratometry guide and allowing the fluorescein pattern to dictate what changes (if any) to make. The five-LED cobalt blue flashlight from Inova (Emmisive Energy Corp.) provides the brightest illumination—brighter than the slit lamp—and it is portable, which can make infant GP contact lens fitting much easier.[72] An alignment fitting relationship is desired. The lens may begin dislocating or popping off of the eye as the eye grows. This could be due to the fact that the lens may start exhibiting a steep fitting relationship, and a flatter base curve radius, possibly accompanied by a larger diameter. Changes in the fit are expected at 6 to 8 weeks, 4 to 6 months, 1 year, and 2 to 3 years of age.

PATIENT EDUCATION AND FOLLOW-UP CARE

There are actually many similarities in educating children and adults. As mentioned before, the time period for education is only slightly longer for children than for teenagers.[35] Although, like adults, young people can become complacent with lens care, they are actually easier to influence and educate than adults because they are more willing to listen, learn, and to please.[21] Proper instructions on lens handling, which results in mastery of insertion and removal, supplemented by reinforcing care procedures with the young person and parent at every follow-up visit should result in successful contact lens wear.

Lens Handling

1. When can young people independently handle their lenses? Children may be able to assume the responsibility of lens removal at as early an age as 4 to 5 years, insertion at 6 to 8 years of age, and cleaning and lens care at 10 to 12 years old.[74] However, this is dependent upon such factors as dexterity and maturity. Certainly children under the age of 11 often require parents to partner in the care and handling process. For a first-time contact lens wearer, it is more important to prove the ability to remove a contact lens than it is to prove the ability to insert a contact lens. If a child cannot insert the contact lens, then he or she will not hurt their eye. However, the inability to remove a lens can be devastating. Prior to dispensing of an elective contact lens, children should prove that they can remove their own lenses at least two times.
2. Lens handling instructions. It can be beneficial to both have the young person handle a contact lens simply to see how it feels on the finger as well as have a staff person demonstrate how easy it is to handle the lenses and the fact that they can feel comfortable on the eye. Then it is important to demonstrate proper hand washing to the young person and parent, drying the hands with a clean towel or tissue after washing and before handling the lenses. For insertion, as with adults, it is important to pin the lids back with the middle finger of the opposite hand (as eye) under the upper lashes and the middle finger of the same hand (as eye) positioned over the lower lashes. Likewise, for removal, it is important for the lid margins to be pinned against the eye and, as with insertion, for maximum success the lids can be handled similar to insertion (i.e., opposite hand for upper lid; same hand for lower lid) and the lids can be pulled temporally or vertically to eject the lens.

Care and Compliance Instructions

1. Have the young person repeat instructions. Once the patient has exhibited mastery of lens handling, it is important to review the care of the lenses. This includes removal at night, cleaning with recommended solution in the palm of the hand (unless daily disposable),

placed into a clean empty case, which is then filled with the prescribed disinfecting solution. In the morning, the lenses are removed and inserted with the appropriate wetting solution. After insertion, the case should be rinsed out with saline, wiped dry, then allowed to air dry upside down with caps off. Once this has been explained, it is important for the child or, at minimum, for the parent to be able to repeat these instructions. It is also important to ask the child these questions during every biannual visit, to make sure that they continue good contact lens hygiene for life.

2. Reward success. After the young person demonstrates mastery with handling and care instructions, they can be rewarded and a "parent-approved" treat drawer could serve this purpose.[67]

3. Symptoms to be aware of. It is important to emphasize to the patient and parent(s) the importance of removing the lenses if the eyes become red, irritated, or they are unable to see clearly. They should also be advised that if these problems do not clear up after lens removal, they should talk to their parents about calling their ECP.[75]

4. DW if at all possible. There are many reasons why DW is recommended for young people, especially during adaptation.[74] (a) Children work better in a routine; (b) both child and parents become proficient in handling the lenses; and (c) lenses stay cleaner and the eye is not exposed to a greater reduction of oxygen at night, resulting in better comfort, fewer infections, and better vision.

5. Water and contact lens wear/care. Children should be told not to wear their lenses while swimming. Ideally, it would be recommended not to wear them while showering or in the sauna due to possibility of Acanthamoeba keratitis. It can be mentioned to the parents that the FDA has recommended that contact lenses not be exposed to any form of water for this reason.[76] If they do swim in their lenses, it is important to have them instill some saline to help loosen up the lenses, then remove them, and either dispose of or disinfect them. And, of course, they should be advised not to use tap water or have saliva come in contact with their lenses.

6. Wearing schedule and follow-up visit schedule. Both of these schedules depend upon the lens chosen and practitioner preference. One recommended wearing schedule is to wear the lenses 6 to 8 hours the first day, 10 hours the second day, and then all waking hours.[74] The most important follow-up visit is the first one, typically scheduled after 1 week of lens wear. Further visits could be scheduled at 1 month, 3 months, and every 6 months after dispensing. The importance of adhering to the prescribed wearing and follow-up schedules should be emphasized to both patient and parent(s).[77]

7. Backup spectacles. Children who are fitted with contact lenses as the primary vision correction device should also be prescribed a pair of spectacles for backup purposes to minimize the risk of contact lens overwear.[78]

8. Other important factors. Patients should be advised to remove lenses approximately 1 hour before bedtime to minimize the risk of becoming tired and falling asleep with lenses on. In addition, a small bottle of solution in the child's desk or locker is a good idea, especially when they are adapting to lens wear.[75]

9. Contact lens consent/assent forms. To help both the child and parental understanding as well as have them more accountable for any problems that occur, it can be beneficial to explain all potential risks of contact lens wear and how these problems can occur as a result of failure of the patient to comply with the recommended wearing schedule and care instructions. The parent can sign such an informed consent at the time of fitting. Another approach is to partner the young person in the care by having them sign an assent form such as that provided in Table 18.3.[79]

10. Useful websites. There are several consumer-friendly websites that provide contact lens wear and care guidelines, important tips for safe contact lens wear, and videos on how to handle lenses. These are listed in Table 18.4.

TABLE 18.3 Contact Lens Assent

I am going to wear contact lenses. To keep my eyes from being hurt I have to:
- Clean my hands before touching my contact lenses
- Remove my contact lenses from my eyes
- Clean my contact lenses every night
- Rinse my contact lenses only with solutions (never with water)
- Throw away my contact lenses every _____
- Tell my mom or dad if my eyes hurt.

Name of Child: _____

Date: _____

Reprinted from Walline JJ, Rah MJ. Children and informed consent. *Contact Lens Spectrum*. 2008;23(5).

Follow-up Visits

The follow-up visits are an excellent opportunity to review compliance and reinforce important care instructions. The patient should be questioned as to how proficient they feel in their handling of the lenses or if further instruction is indicated. They should also be asked how they clean their lenses upon removal (unless daily disposable) and confirm that the solutions they are using are those originally prescribed. They should also be asked how many hours they are wearing the lenses every day to ensure they are not overwearing them. When they return for their 6-month evaluation, consideration can be given to giving them a compliance test such as that given in Table 18.5.

It is also important to appropriately manage contact lens complications when they occur with young people, using medications that are FDA-approved and appropriate for their specific age. Two commonly used types of medications for the management of complications with young contact lens wearers are antiallergy and antimicrobial agents. FDA-approved medications and their minimum age are provided in Tables 18.6 and 18.7.[80] Only when no option exists with the appropriate age approval should medications, using appropriate off-label guidelines, be prescribed.

MYOPIA CONTROL

A dynamic and exciting area for contact lens applications with young people is the potential use for slowing eye growth and exhibiting myopia control. Several methods are presented with an emphasis on OOK.

A. Myopia development
   It is evident that myopia is becoming more prevalent in the United States as well as worldwide. Researchers have reported that the prevalence of myopia in the United States has increased from 25% in 1971–1972 to 41.5% in 1999–2004.[81]

   The relationship between normal eye growth and the development of myopia in school-age children was first analyzed in the 1989 Orinda Longitudinal Study of Myopia (OLSM).[82,83] It was found that refractive error decreased toward emmetropia from an

TABLE 18.4 Contact Lens Care and Handling Consumer Sites

- All About Vision: http://www.allaboutvision.com/contacts/contact_lenses.htm#wearandcare
- Bausch + Lomb: http://www.bausch.com/en/Eye-concerns/Wearing-Contact-Lenses/Wearing-and-Caring-for-Contact-Lenses
- Contactlenses.org: www.contactlenses.org
- Contactlenssafety.org: www.contactlenssafety.org
- Menicon: http://www.meniconamerica.com/consumer/lens-care-dos-and-donts

TABLE 18.5 Example of a Compliance Test

T	F	1.	You should throw away your contact lenses every 2 wk.
T	F	2.	You should rub your contact lenses every time after taking them out of your eyes
T	F	3.	You should rub your contact lenses for a total of 20 s
T	F	4.	You should continue to wear your lenses if your eyes become red.
T	F	5.	You should pour the solution out of the case when you have put the lenses on your eyes.
T	F	6.	You should rinse your lenses in water from the sink every night.
T	F	7.	You should remove your contact lenses every night.
T	F	8.	You should call your doctor if your eyes continue to hurt after removing your lenses.
T	F	9.	It is okay to put your contact lenses in your mouth to rinse them.

Answers to Quiz: 1(T), 2(T), 3(T), 4(F), 5(T), 6(F), 7(T), 8(T), 9(F)

Reprinted from Walline JJ, Rah MJ. Emphasizing lens care. *Contact Lens Spectrum.* 2008;23(1):51.

average of +0.73 D at age 6 to an average of +0.50 D at age 12. The Collaborative Longitudinal Evaluation of Ethnicity and Refractive Error (CLEERE) study suggested that children who have two parents with myopia are inherently predisposed to have eyes that are shaped like a nearsighted person, and are also likely to become nearsighted over time.[84] Therefore, this study confirmed the presence of a genetic/anatomical relationship in myopia progression. However, there may also be other factors that contribute to myopia development, including near work, urban locale, education level, and less time spent outdoors.[85]

The interest in—and need for—myopia control is longstanding significance and has numerous potential benefits. Myopia is associated with the inconvenience of costs associated with optical corrections, not to mention the possible complications associated with contact lens and surgical correction.[86] The increase in axial length occurring in high myopia can increase the risk of glaucoma, cataract, and both chorioretinal and idiopathic retinal

TABLE 18.6 FDA-Approved Allergy Medications/Minimum Age

BRAND NAME	GENERIC NAME	AGE
Acular	0.5% ketorolac tromethamine	3 yr
Alamast	0.1% pemirolast potassium	3 yr
Alocril	2% nedocromil sodium	3 yr
Alomide	0.1% lodoxamide tromethamine	2 yr
Alrex	0.2% loteprednol etabonate	12 yr
Crolom/Opticrom	4% cromolyn sodium	4 yr
Elestat	0.05% epinastine hydrochloride	3 yr
Emadine	0.05% emedastine difumarate	3 yr
Optivar	0.05% azelastine hydrochloride	3 yr
Pataday	0.2% olopatadine hydrochloride	3 yr
Patanol	0.1% olopatadine hydrochloride	3 yr
Zaditor/Alaway/Refresh	0.025% ketotifen fumarate	3 yr

Reprinted from Walline JJ, Rah MJ. Lens complications: allergy and antibiotic medications. *Contact Lens Spectrum.* 2009;24(5):49.

TABLE 18.7 FDA-Approved Antibiotic Medications/Minimum Age

BRAND NAME	GENERIC NAME	AGE
AK-Tracin	500 units/gram bacitracin	Not established
AzaSite	1% azithromycin	1 yr
Ciloxan	0.3% ciprofloxacin	1 yr
Genoptic	0.3% gentamycin	1 mo
Ilotycin	0.5% erythromycin	2 mo
Iquix	1.5% levofloxacin	6 yr
Neosporin	Polymyxin B/neomycin/gramicidin	Not established
Ocuflox	0.3% ofloxacin	1 yr
Polysporin	Polymyxin B/bacitracin	Not established
Polytrim	Polymyxin B/trimethoprim	2 mo
Quixin	0.5% levofloxacin	1 yr
Tobrex	0.3% tobramycin	2 mo
Vigamox	0.5% moxifloxacin	1 yr
Zymar	0.3% gatifloxacin	1 yr

Reprinted from Walline JJ, Rah MJ. Lens complications: allergy and antibiotic medications. *Contact Lens Spectrum*. 2009;24(5):49.

degeneration.[87–89] High myopia is also a leading cause of permanent visual impairment.[90,91] Furthermore, high myopes experience less predictable refractive surgery results and poorer vision-specific quality of life.[92]

What is clinically meaningful myopia control? The average rate of progression for myopic progression for myopic children in the United States is approximately −0.50 D per year.[93–96] If, for example, a child has a −1.00 D refractive error at age 8 and the refractive error progresses linearly until age 16 and is halted, the child would become a −5.00 D myope (Table 18.8).[97] It is apparent, therefore, that myopia progression should be slowed by, at minimum, 50% in order to be clinically meaningful to the patient.

B. Noncontact lens methods aimed at myopia control

Several methods have been attempted for slowing myopia progression and the results are presented in Table 18.9. If clinically meaningful slowing of myopia progression is defined as 50% or greater, several methods that do not meet this criterion include undercorrection

TABLE 18.8 Myopia Progression

MYOPIA PROGRESSION SLOWED BY (%)	FINAL MYOPIA
0	−5.00
25	−4.00
50	−3.00
75	−2.00
100	−1.00

If a −1.00 D myope progresses exactly −0.50 D per year for 8 years, the child's final refractive error is shown for each category of slowed myopia progression.

Reprinted from Walline JJ. Current and future developments in myopia control. *Contact Lens Spectrum*. 2012;27(10):34.

TABLE 18.9 Controlled Myopia Control Studies, Categorized by Myopia Control Agent, Showing the Percent Reduction of Myopia Progression

MODALITY	AUTHOR (YR)	% REDUCTION[a]	OVERALL AVERAGE[b]
Undercorrection	Adler ('06)	−16	−19
	Chung ('02)	−22	
Alignment GP lenses	Katz ('03)	−5	−7
	Walline ('04)	−8	
Bifocal or multifocal spectacles	Edwards ('02)	3.1	18
	Fulk ('00)	20	
	Gwiazda ('03)	16	
	COMET2 ('11)	24	
	Cheng ('10)	32	
	Yang ('09)	14	
	Hasebe ('05)	18	
Peripheral myopia spectacles	Sankaridurg ('10)	30	30
Pirenzepine	Siatkowski ('08)	30	35
	Tan ('05)	39	
Corneal reshaping	Cho ('05)	44	46
	Kakita ('12)	36	
	Walline ('09)	58	
Soft bifocal lenses	Sankaridurg ('11)	34	51
	Aller ('06)	79	
	Walline ('11)	40	
	Anstice ('11)	50	
Atropine	Chua ('06)	77	81
	Shih ('99)	96	
	Yen ('89)	76	
	Fang ('10)	76	

[a]Negative numbers indicate an increase in myopia progression.
[b]Overall average is a simple mathematical average of each of the studies, not weighted by sample size or any other considerations.
Reprinted from Walline JJ. Current and future developments in myopia control. *Contact Lens Spectrum*. 2012;27(10):34.

of myopia,[98,99] alignment fit GP contact lenses,[22,30] bifocal or multifocal spectacles,[100–102] peripheral myopia spectacles,[103] and pirenzepine.[104,105] Atropine has been shown to be an effective method for slowing myopia progression.[106–109] However, ECPs rarely prescribe atropine for slowing myopia progression, primarily resulting from their belief that the side effects of atropine, mydriasis, and cycloplegia are uncomfortable for children. However, this is debatable as dropout rates from myopia control studies[108–110] are significantly lower than dropout rates from most alignment fit, DW GP contact lens myopia control studies.[28–30,111]

C. Contact lenses and myopia control
1. Conventional daily wear contact lenses. Anecdotally, the belief for many years was that DW of conventional DW GP lenses results in slowing myopia progression. The results of two randomized clinical trials found that GP lenses did not significantly slow the axial growth of the eye, which indicates that these lenses do not have a permanent effect

on myopia progression.[26,29] Conventional soft lens designs, likewise, have not resulted in any effect on myopia progression.[25,26]

2. OOK

(a) Why Orthokeratology? As described in Chapter 22, orthokeratology is defined (in myopia) as a temporary correction of myopia and astigmatism using specially designed, typically GP contact lenses to flatten the central cornea. Also termed "corneal reshaping," "corneal refractive therapy," and "vision shaping treatment," contemporary use of this modality typically pertains to wearing these lenses at night only. Therefore, the benefits of OOK are many.[112] The advantage of freedom from corrective lens wear is very powerful and potentially life-changing for a young person, notably for an active child involved in swimming, sports, and other activities. In addition, many young people are particularly tough on their spectacles, often necessitating replacement due to damage or loss.

Studies with young people have found that it can take, on average, only 1 week for the desired goal of myopia reduction (often resulting in a slight hyperopic refractive error) to be obtained,[113] and a first-fit success rate of over 80%.[34] However, of primary interest—especially to parents—is the effect of OOK on controlling myopia. Several recent studies from three different continents—United States, China, and Australia—have all confirmed the significant effect OOK has on axial length in young people. The Corneal Reshaping and Yearly Observation of Nearsightedness (CRAYON) study compared axial eye growth to a previous study,[26] which evaluated similar outcomes with soft lens and conventional DW GP lens wear.[114] The Longitudinal Orthokeratology Research in Children (LORIC) study compared spectacle lens wear with OOK in young people.[33] Both studies found a significant reduction in axial elongation and vitreous chamber growth with OOK versus the other modalities (Fig. 18.1). In fact, the axial growth was approximately 57% slower than that of soft lenses, conventional GP lenses, and spectacles. Recent data by Swarbrick[115] showed slowed eye growth for eyes wearing orthokeratology contact lenses compared to the contralateral eyes wearing alignment fit GP contact lenses.

(b) How does OOK effect myopia control? With the aforementioned OOK studies resulting in a reduced progression in axial length growth versus other corrective modalities, the next logical question to ask is "Why does OOK appear to exhibit a significant effect in controlling myopia?" The answer may pertain to changes in the peripheral retina. The retina essentially moves to where light is focused through the emmetropization process. The eye grows faster in response to hyperopic blur and

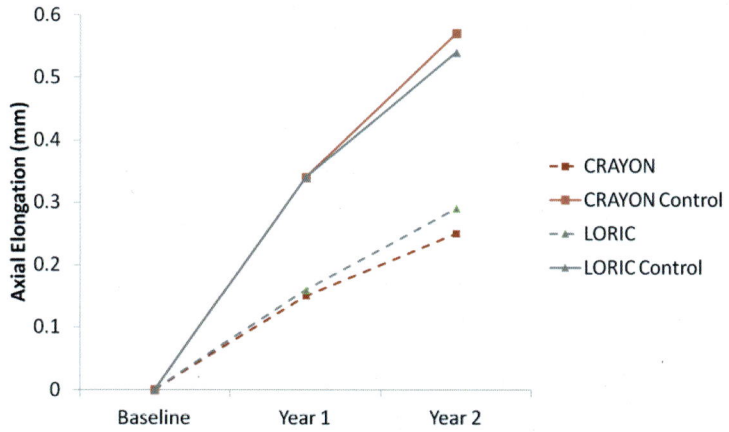

FIGURE 18.1 A comparison of axial length changes in the LORIC versus CRAYON studies.

slower in response to myopic blur to obtain clear vision. Whereas the central retina was once thought to be exclusively responsible for the emmetropization process, recent animal studies indicate that the peripheral retina is more important than originally believed.[116–118] Hyperopic blur presented only to the peripheral retina causes the eye to grow longer, and if the peripheral hyperopic blur is removed, the eye returns to emmetropia, even if the fovea is no longer functioning due to ablation.[118]

Numerous studies have found that myopic eyes typically have a hyperopic peripheral refraction, whereas emmetropes and hyperopes have a relatively myopic peripheral refraction.[119–124] Therefore, it is possible that the peripheral hyperopic defocus could be a cause rather than a result of myopia development and inducing a relatively myopic peripheral defocus in myopic eyes might slow down or stop myopic progression.[125,126] It is apparent that this may be achievable with OOK.[126–129] It has been suggested that the midperipheral ring of steepening in the cornea or the untreated peripheral cornea may cause the peripheral retina to experience a myopic defocus, which in turn may slow down the rate of myopia progression.[114] It has also been proposed that higher-order aberrations induced by orthokeratology lens wear may be a stimulus for the slowing of eye growth.[33] Therefore, although the exact mechanism underlying reduced progression with OOK is unknown at this time, it is apparent that this modality can be used to induce myopic defocus in the periphery in myopic children and thus provide a potential mechanism for myopia control.

(c) What about safety? The greatest concern about OOK in children is the potential for MK. The literature has numerous reports of corneal ulcers in orthokeratology wearers, primarily impacting children.[130–132] The majority of reported cases were from Asian countries, predominantly China, Taiwan, and Hong Kong. This could be representative of the populations most likely to be fitted with OOK lenses as well as poor management and care as represented by the large number of early cases in which Acanthamoeba was the causative organism. Overall, however, it does not appear that the risk of MK or adverse events in general is any higher than any other overnight contact lens modalities,[133–135] and may not be higher in children than in individuals older than 12 years of age.[136]

3. Bifocal soft lenses. Several studies with bifocal soft lens designs have resulted in an average of 50% treatment effect in reducing myopia progression.[137–140] Most recently, a significant reduction in myopia progression resulted from use of a novel lens design to reduce relative peripheral hyperopia in a silicone hydrogel lens material.[140] This design had a central distance vision correction; outside of the central zone, the refractive power of the lens increased progressively with relative plus power of 1 D at 2 mm from center. It appears that soft bifocal/multifocal lenses with a distance center are effective by providing a similar peripheral optical profile as OOK designs; therefore, in theory, they should also slow the growth of the eye (Fig 18.2).[141]

4. Important factors in deciding which option to select. The decision as to whether to fit young people into corneal reshaping or soft bifocal contact lenses to slow myopia progression should be determined after a discussion between the ECP and both the child and the parents. While ECPs cannot unequivocally state that OOK or soft bifocal contact lenses will slow myopia progression, they can discuss the benefits of contact lens wear and include myopia control as a possible beneficial side effect. Important factors to consider include the ECP's comfort level in fitting each modality, the child's perceived ability to handle contact lenses, and the patient's comfort with either type of contact lens. Children who desire only part-time lens wear would benefit from soft lenses (although myopia control effect may be less) as would those who have soft lens-wearing parents. Children who swim regularly or have parents who are uncomfortable with their children wearing contact lenses outside of the home should consider OOK.[97]

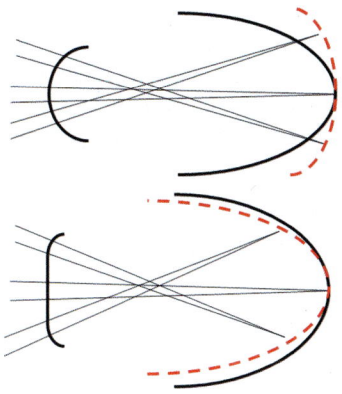

FIGURE 18.2 The impact of corneal reshaping and some bifocal soft designs on peripheral retinal emmetropization (**bottom**) versus peripheral retinal hyperopia induced by standard designs (**top**).

5. The future of myopia control. Future research will include the optimization of OOK and soft bifocal contact lenses to correct peripheral refractive error and the development of testing equipment that can measure a patient's susceptibility to develop myopia based upon peripheral refraction.[142] However, even if researchers confirm the fact that myopic blur presented to the peripheral retina slows myopia progression, they still need to determine what it is that optimizes the signal to slow eye growth and design the lenses accordingly.

SUMMARY

It is evident that most children 8 years of age or above are good candidates for contact lenses and this modality should be offered as a primary vision correction option. There are no large challenges in fitting young people. It is simply important to ask the right questions and perform the appropriate tests to determine if they are qualified and motivated to wear contact lenses. Whether it be with a soft lens, a conventional GP lens, a scleral lens, or an orthokeratology design, the difference you can make in the life of a young person is one that can last a lifetime.

CLINICAL CASES

CASE 1

An 8-year-old girl is interested in contact lenses. She has been a 2-year spectacle wearer and she does not enjoy wearing her spectacles for sports (she plays soccer and softball) and at school. Her refraction is:

$$OD: -2.00 - 0.75 \times 175 \; 20/20 + 2$$
$$OS: -2.25 - 0.50 \times 006 \; 20/20$$

Her parents are highly myopic and they are concerned about the progression of her refractive error.

SOLUTION: It is important to note the child has been a spectacle wearer first and that she—not just her parents—is motivated to wear contact lenses, There are two viable options for this young lady:

1. DW GP lenses. The GP modality may slow down the progression of her myopia. It would also be important to design the lenses such that they would have a large overall diameter (≥10 mm) and low edge clearance to minimize the risk of displacement and loss during sports activities.
2. OOK. She would be an excellent candidate for OOK and this topic will be discussed in Chapter 20.

CASE 2

A 9-year-old myopic girl reported for her annual eye examination. She complained of poor distance vision with gradual onset. She had no other visual or asthenopic complaints. She received her first pair of glasses 2 years prior and needed a new pair of glasses every year. Her vision with the current glasses was:

OD	−2.25 − 0.50 × 175	20/30 − 2
OS	−2.50 − 0.25 × 015	20/40
OU	at 33 cm	20/15

Manifest refraction at this visit was:

OD	−3.25 − 0.25 × 180	20/40
OS	−3.25 − 0.25 × 010	20/30 − 2
OU	at 33 cm	20/15

Her parents, both with significant myopia, asked about ways to keep their child from becoming as nearsighted as themselves. Soft bifocal contact lenses with a distance center design and corneal reshaping contact lenses were discussed. The parents chose to have their daughter fit with corneal reshaping contact lenses.
Keratometry readings were:

OD	43.25/43.87 @ 090 mires clear
OS	43.37/44.12 @ 090 mires clear

SOLUTION: Corneal refractive therapy (CRT) contact lenses with the following parameters were prescribed:

	OD	OS
Base Curve Radius (mm)	8.6	8.6
Return Zone Depth (μm)	550	550
Landing Zone Angle (°)	33	33

One year later, the patient returned, reporting no visual or asthenopic complaints with nightly wear of the same CRT contact lenses she was originally dispensed. Uncorrected visual acuity was 20/20 − 1 OD and 20/15 − 1 OS. Refraction over the contact lenses was −0.25 OD and plano OS to get to 20/15 in each eye. The eyes were healthy, and topographical analysis showed a 3.75 mm treatment zone centered over the pupil in each eye. CRT contact lens wear was continued with the same contact lenses, and the patient was asked to return in 6 months for a contact lens check. The parents were told that new contact lenses may be necessary at the next visit due to advancing myopia, but the changes in nearsightedness experienced over the year were significantly less than the previous 2 years of spectacle wear. Both patient and parents were extremely happy with the outcome following CRT contact lens wear.

While wearing spectacles, this patient experienced greater myopia progression over 1 year (−1.00 D OD and −0.75 D OS) than the expected progression of −0.50 D.[93,94] She also had two parents with significant myopia, increasing the risk of high myopia.[82,143,144] These factors led to a discussion of myopia control, which resulted in the fitting of corneal reshaping contact lenses. This patient experienced only −0.25 D myopia progression in one eye following 1 year of corneal reshaping contact lens wear. Although this patient's myopia progression essentially stopped during the first year of corneal reshaping contact lens wear, corneal reshaping contact lenses slow myopia progression by 43%.[145] Parents should not expect complete cessation of myopia progression over a long period of time. Corneal reshaping contact lenses provide children with clear vision throughout the day[32] and they also slow myopia progression, so they may be presented to patients as an option for myopia control.

CLINICAL PROFICIENCY CHECKLIST

- Benefits of contact lenses versus spectacles in young people include their benefits in an active lifestyle, improved perception of their physical appearance, and their potential for myopia control.
- Several studies have found that children as young as age 8 are capable of wearing soft lenses, rigid GP lenses, and OOK lenses. It has also been found that the amount of time for fitting, education, and follow-up is only slightly longer for a teenager than for a younger child.
- Important factors if considering fitting a young person into contact lenses are (a) interest and motivation, (b) maturity, (c) ability to take care of lenses independently, (d) personal hygiene habits, (e) sports, (f) prescription requirements, and (g) preexisting medical conditions. However, age alone should not be used to determine whether a child is a good contact lens candidate.
- Children and their parents should be advised that all contact lenses—including nonprescription tinted lenses for cosmetic purposes—are medical devices and should not be shared with other individuals or purchased illegally and without the intent for follow-up care.
- Daily disposable lenses are recommended for young people desiring part-time wear, particularly for the young athlete. GP lenses are recommended for highly astigmatic and any other young person desiring the quality of vision benefits, as well as those considering OOK for potential myopia control.
- When fitting GP lenses, it is recommended to fit the lenses empirically as well as use a topical anesthetic immediately before dispensing to optimize the initial experience.
- It is important for both the young children and their parent(s) to know how to handle and care for the lenses and to be able to repeat the care instructions.
- Conventional soft and GP lenses do not exhibit any myopia control effect but both OOK designs and center-distance soft bifocal/multifocal designs have been found to reduce myopia progression.
- Recently, it has been found that contact lens-induced myopia control may be the result of inducing a relatively myopic peripheral defocus in myopic eyes resulting in a slowing of eye growth.
- New orthokeratology and soft bifocal/multifocal designs are being developed in an effort to optimize the focus of light at the peripheral retina and slow eye growth.

REFERENCES

1. Levin AV, Edmonds SA, Nelson LB, et al. Extended-wear contact lenses for the treatment of pediatric aphakia. *Ophthalmology.* 1985;95:1107–1113.
2. Nelson LB, Cutler SI, Calhoun JH, et al. Silsoft extended wear contact lenses in pediatric aphakia. *Ophthalmology.* 1985;92:1529–1531.
3. Cutler SI, Nelson LB, Calhoun JH. Extended wear contact lenses in pediatric aphakia. *J Pediatr Ophthalmol Strabismus.* 1985;22:86–91.
4. Orbek Z, Durak I, Berk TA. Contact lenses in the correction of childhood aphakia. *CLAO J.* 2002;28:28–30.
5. Chia A, Johnson K, Martin F. Use of contact lenses to correct aphakia in children. *Clin Exp Ophthalmol.* 2002;30:252–255.

6. Lightman JM, Marshall D Jr. Clinical evaluation of back optic radius and power determination by age in pediatric aphakia due to congenital cataract fitted with a Silicone elastomer contact lens. *Optom Vis Sci.* 1996;73:22–27.
7. Moore B. The fitting of contact lenses in aphakic infants. *J Am Optom Assoc.* 1985;56:180, 182–183.
8. Weissman BA. Fitting aphakic children with contact lenses. *J Am Optom Assoc.* 1983;54:235–237.
9. Jurkus JM. Contact lenses for children. *Optom Clin.* 1996;5:91–104.
10. Joslin CE, McMahon TT, Kaufman LM. The effectiveness of occluder contact lenses in improving occlusion compliance in patients that have failed traditional occlusion therapy. *Optom Vis Sci.* 2002;79:376–380.
11. Burger DS, London R. Soft opaque contact lenses in binocular vision problems. *J Am Optom Assoc.* 1993;64:176–180.
12. Shaughnessy MP, Ellis FJ, Jeffery AR, et al. Rigid gas-permeable contact lenses are a safe and effective means of treating refractive abnormalities in the pediatric population. *CLAO J.* 2001;27:195–201.
13. Brujic M, Miller J. How young is too young for contact lenses? *Rev Cornea Contact Lenses.* May 2010.
14. Gording EJ, March E. Personality changes of certain contact lens patients. *J Am Optom Assoc.* 1968; 9:266–269.
15. Harris MB. Sex differences in stereotypes of spectacles. *J App Soc Psychol.* 1991;21:1659–1680.
16. Terry RL, Stockton LA. Eyeglasses and children's schemata. *J Social Psychol.* 1993;133:425–438.
17. Terry RL. Eyeglasses and gender stereotypes. *Optom Vis Sci.* 1989;66:694–697.
18. Walline JJ, Jones LA, Sinnott L, et al. Randomized trial of the effect of contact lens wear on self-perception in children. *Optom Vis Sci.* 2009;86(3):222–232.
19. Rah MJ, Walline JJ, Jones-Jordan LA, et al. Vision specific quality of life of pediatric contact lens wearers. *Optom Vis Sci.* 2010;87(8):360–366.
20. Sindt CW. A lifetime of contact lens wear. *Contact Lens Spectrum* (special edition). 2010;25(4):40.
21. Cho P, Cheung SW. Fitting kids with contact lenses. *Contact Lens Spectrum.* 2009;24(8):33–39.
22. Walline JJ, Jones LA, Mutti DO, et al. A randomized trial of the effects of rigid contact lenses on myopia progression. *Arch Ophthalmol.* 2004;122:1760–1766.
23. Walline JJ, Long S, Zadnik K. Daily disposable contact lens wear in myopic children. *Optom Vis Sci.* 2004;81:255–259.
24. Soni PS, Horner DG, Jimenez L, et al. Will young children comply and follow instructions to successfully wear soft contact lenses? *CLAO J.* 1995;21:86–92.
25. Horner DG, Soni PS, Salmon TO, et al. Myopia progression in adolescent wearers of soft contact lenses and spectacles. *Optom Vis Sci.* 1999;76:474–479.
26. Walline JJ, Jones LA, Mutti DO, et al. Use of a run-in period to decrease loss to follow-up in the Contact Lens and Myopia Progression (CLAMP) study. *Control Clin Trials.* 2003;24:711–718.
27. Stone J. The possible influence of contact lenses on myopia. *Br J Physiol Opt.* 1976;31:89–114.
28. Perrigin J, Perrigin D, Quintero S, et al. Silicone-acrylate contact lenses for myopia control: 3-year results. *Optom Vis Sci.* 1990;67:764–769.
29. Khoo CY, Chong J, Rajan U. A 3-year study on the effect of RGP contact lenses on myopic children. *Singapore Med J.* 1999;40:230–237.
30. Katz J, Schein OD, Levy B, et al. A randomized trial of rigid gas permeable contact lenses to reduce progression of children's myopia. *Am J Ophthalmol.* 2003;136:82–90.
31. Fan L, Jun J, Jia Q, et al. Clinical study of orthokeratology in young myopic adolescents. *Int Contact Lens Clin.* 1999;26:113–116.
32. Walline JJ, Rah MJ, Jones LA. The Children's Overnight Orthokeratology Investigation (COOKI) pilot study. *Optom Vis Sci.* 2004;81:407–413.
33. Cho P, Cheung SW, Edwards M. The longitudinal orthokeratology research in children (LORIC) in Hong Kong: a pilot study on refractive changes and myopia control. *Curr Eye Res.* 2005;30:71–80.
34. Eiden SB, Davis RL, Bennett ES, et al. The SMART Study: background, rationale, and baseline results. *Contact Lens Spectrum.* 2009;24(10):24–31.
35. Walline JJ, Jones LA, Rah MJ, et al. Contact Lenses in Pediatrics (CLIP) study: chair time and ocular health. *Optom Vis Sci.* 2007;84(9):896–902.
36. Walline JJ, Jones LA, Mutti DO, et al. Predicting successful RGP contact lens wearers. *Optom Vis Sci.* 2001;78(suppl):27.
37. Chalmers RL, Wagner H, Mitchell GL, et al. Age and other risk factors for corneal infiltrative and inflammatory events in young soft contact lens wearers from the Contact Lens Assessment in Youth (CLAY) study. *Invest Ophthalmol Vis Sci.* 2011;52(9):6690–6696.
38. Li L, Moody K, Tan DTH, et al. Contact lenses in pediatrics study in Singapore. *Eye Contact Lens.* 2009;35(4):188–195.
39. Begley CG, Barr JT, Edrington TB, et al. Characteristics of corneal staining in hydrogel contact lens wearers. *Optom Vis Sci.* 1996;73:193–200.
40. Nichols KK, Mitchell GL, Simon KM, et al. Corneal staining in hydrogel lens wearers. *Optom Vis Sci.* 2002;79:20–30.
41. http://www.jnjvisioncare.com/newsroom-press-releases-parents-barrier.jsp Accessed August 2012.
42. Children & contact lenses. Doctors' attitudes & practices in fitting children in contacts. AOA Research and Information Center, September 2010. Available at www.aoa.org/childrenandcontactlenses.

43. Sindt CW, Riley CM. Practitioner attitudes on children and contact lenses. *Optometry.* 2011(82):44–45.
44. Sindt CW. Pediatric prescribing habits. *Contact Lens Spectrum.* 2010;25(11):48.
45. Sindt CW. Positive opinions about kids in contact lenses. *Contact Lens Spectrum.* 2011;26(1):48.
46. Rah MJ, Walline JJ. Responsibility for contact lens wear is a team effort. *Contact Lens Spectrum.* 2008;23(8).
47. Rah MJ, Walline JJ. Noncompliant eyeglass wearer a good fit for contact lenses. *Contact Lens Spectrum.* 2008;23(12):47.
48. Walline JJ, Rah MJ. Predicting lens wear success. *Contact Lens Spectrum.* 2009;24(11):48.
49. Steinemann TL, Fletcher M, Bonny AE, et al. Over-the-counter decorative contact lenses: cosmetic or medical devices? A case series. *Eye Contact Lens.* 2005;31(5):194–200.
50. Snyder RW, Brenner MB, Wiley L, et al. Microbial keratitis associated with plano tinted contact lenses. *CLAO J.* 1991;17:252–255.
51. Gagnon MR, Walter KA. A case of acanthamoeba keratitis as a result of a cosmetic contact lens. *Eye Contact Lens.* 2006;32(1):37–38.
52. Singh S, Satani D, Patel A, et al. Colored cosmetic contact lenses: an unsafe trend in the younger generation. *Cornea.* 2012;31(7):777–779.
53. "Improper use of decorative contact lenses may haunt you." FDA Consumer Health Information. www.fda.gov/ForConsumers/ConsumerUpdates/ucm164197.htm.
54. Fogel J, Zidile C. Contact lenses purchased over the internet place individuals potentially at risk for harmful eye care practices. *Optometry.* 2008;79(1):23–35.
55. Stapleton F, Keay L, Edwards K, et al. The incidence of contact lens-related microbial keratitis in Australia. *Ophthalmology.* 2008;115:1655–1662.
56. Padilla KL, Harrington TR, Edmondson W. Purchasing lenses from online lens retailers. *Contact Lens Spectrum.* 2004;19(3):38–43.
57. "Why can't decorative contact lenses be purchased on the internet or in drug stores without a current prescription?" Available at: http://www.contactlenssafety.org/lensbuying.html.
58. Joint statement from the American Academy of Optometry Section on Cornea, Contact Lenses and Refractive Technologies and the American Optometric Association Contact Lens and Cornea Section concern regarding cosmetic "Circle" Contact Lenses. Available at: http://www.aoa.org/x16126.xml.
59. Sindt CW. The Circle Lens Craze. *Contact Lens Spectrum.* 2010;25(9):50.
60. Walline JJ, Rah MJ. Dry eyes are less of a problem in young contact lens wearers. *Contact Lens Spectrum.* 2009;24(7):48.
61. Doughty MJ, Fonn D, Richter D, et al. A patient questionnaire approach to estimating the prevalence of dry eye symptoms in patients presenting to optometric practices across Canada. *Optom Vis Sci.* 1997;74:624–631.
62. Hom M, De Land P. Prevalence and severity of symptomatic dry eyes in Hispanics. *Optom Vis Sci.* 2005;82:206–208.
63. Greiner KL, Walline JJ. Dry eye in pediatric contact lens wearers. *Eye Contact Lens.* 2010;36:352–355.
64. Daniels K. Consider Ortho-K for myopia control. *Rev Optom.* 2012;149(7):38–49.
65. Dart JK, Radfort CF, Minassian D, et al. Risk factors for microbial keratitis with contemporary contact lenses: a case-control study. *Ophthalmology.* 2008;115:1647–1654.
66. Morgan PB, Efron N, Brennan NA, et al. Risk factors for the development of corneal infiltrative events associated with contact lens wear. *Invest Ophthalmol Vis Sci.* 2005;46:3136–3143.
67. Sindt CW. Twelve tips to improve your pediatric contact lens fitting. *Contact Lens Spectrum.* 2012;27(6):52.
68. Rah MJ, Walline JJ. Lens selection, follow-up: keys to fitting young lens wearers. *Contact Lens Spectrum.* 2009;24(12):46.
69. Polse KA, Graham AD, Fusaro RE, et al. Predicting RGP daily wear success. *CLAO J.* 1999;25(3):152–158.
70. Bennett ES, Smythe J, Henry VA, et al. The effect of topical anesthetic use on initial patient satisfaction and overall success with rigid gas permeable contact lenses. *Optom Vis Sci.* 1998;75(11):800–805.
71. Sindt CW. Getting started with GP fitting. *Contact Lens Spectrum.* 2011;26(11):47.
72. Sindt CW. Fitting infants and young children with GP lenses. *Contact Lens Spectrum.* 2010;25(1):48.
73. Shin JA, Manny RE, Kleinstein RN, et al. Short-term repeatability of hand-held keratometry measurements. *Optom Vis Sci.* 1999;76:247–253.
74. Sindt CW. Tips for pediatric dispensing. *Contact Lens Spectrum.* 2011;26(9):48.
75. Walline JJ, Rah MJ. Emphasizing lens care. *Contact Lens Spectrum.* 2008;23(1):51.
76. US Food and Drug Administration: http://www.fda.gov/medicaldevices/productsandmedicalprocedures/homehealthandconsumer/consumerproducts/contactlenses/default.htm.
77. Rah MJ, Walline JJ. The most common causes of adverse events in children. *Contact Lens Spectrum.* 2008;23(6):49.
78. Jones-Jordan LA, Chitkara M, Coffey B, et al. A comparison of spectacle and contact lens wearing time in the ACHIEVE study. *Clin Exp Optom.* 2010;93(3):157–163.
79. Walline JJ, Rah MJ. Children and informed consent. *Contact Lens Spectrum.* 2008;23(5).
80. Walline JJ, Rah MJ. Lens complications: Allergy and Antibiotic medications. *Contact Lens Spectrum.* 2009;24(5):49.
81. Vitale S, Sperduto RD, Ferris FL III. Increased prevalence of myopia in the United States between 1971–1972 and 1999–2004. *Arch Ophthalmol.* 127:1632–1639.

82. Zadnik K, Satariano WA, Mutti DO, et al. The effect of parental history of myopia on children's eye size. *JAMA.* 1994;271(17):1323–1327.
83. Zadnik K, Mutti DO, Friedman NE, et al. Initial cross-sectional results from the Orinda Longitudinal Study of Myopia. *Optom Vis Sci.* 1993;70(9):750–758.
84. Zadnik K, Manny RE, Yu JA, et al. Ocular component data in schoolchildren as a function of age and gender. *Optom Vis Sci.* 2003;80(3):226–236.
85. Rose KA, Morgan IG, Ip J, et al. Outdoor activity reduces the prevalence of myopia in children. *Ophthalmology.* 2008;115(8):1279–1285.
86. Sankaridurg P, Holden B, Smith E, et al. Decrease in rate of myopia progression with a contact lens designed to reduce relative peripheral hyperopia: one-year results. *Invest Ophthalmol Vis Sci.* 2011;52(13):9362–9368.
87. Bier C, Kampik A, Gandorfer A, et al. Retinal detachment in pediatrics: etiology and risk factors. *Ophthalmology.* 2010:107:165–174.
88. Praveen MR, Shah GD, Vasavada AR, et al. A study to explore the risk factors for the early onset of cataract in India. *Eye.* 2010;24:686–694.
89. Xu L, Wang Y, Wang S, et al. High myopia and glaucoma susceptibility: the Beijing Eye Study. *Ophthalmology.* 2007;114(2):216–220.
90. Lin LL, Shih YF, Tsai CB, et al. Epidemiologic study of ocular refraction among schoolchildren in Taiwan in 1995. *Optom Vis Sci.* 1999;76:275–281.
91. Xu L, Wang Y, Li Y, et al. Causes of blindness and visual impairment in urban and rural areas in Beijing: the Beijing Eye Study. *Ophthalmology.* 2006;113(7):1134 e1–1134 e11.
92. Rose K, Harper R., Tromans C, et al. Quality of life in myopia. *Br J Ophthalmol.* 2000;84(9):1031–1034.
93. Fulk GW, Cyert LA, Parker DE. A randomized trial of the effect of single-vision vs. bifocal lenses on myopia progression in children with esophoria. *Optom Vis Sci.* 2000;77(8):395–401.
94. Gwiazda J, Hyman L, Hussein M, et al. A randomized clinical trial of progressive addition lenses versus single vision lenses on the progression of myopia in children. *Invest Ophthalmol Vis Sci.* 2003;44(4):1492–1500.
95. Walline JJ, Long S, Zadnik K. Daily disposable contact lens wear in myopic children. *Optom Vis Sci.* 2004;81(4):255–259.
96. Walline JJ, Jones LA, Sinnott L, et al. A randomized trial of the effect of soft contact lenses on myopia progression in children. *Invest Ophthalmol Vis Sci.* 2008;49(11):4702–4706.
97. Walline JJ. Current and future developments in myopia control. *Contact Lens Spectrum.* 2012;27(10):34.
98. Adler D, Millodot M. The possible effect of undercorrection on myopic progression in children. *Clin Exp Optom.* 2006;89:315–321
99. Chung K, Mohidin N, O'Leary DJ. Undercorrection of myopia enhances rather than inhibits myopia progression. *Vision Res.* 2002;42:2555–2559.
100. Berntsen DA, Sinnott LT, Mutti DO, et al. A randomized trial using progressive addition lenses to evaluate theories of myopia progression in children with a high lag of accommodation. *Invest Ophthalmol Vis Sci.* 2012;53(2):640–649.
101. Cheng D, Schmid KL, Woo GC. The effect of positive-lens addition and base-in prism on accommodation accuracy and near horizontal phoria in Chinese myopic children. *Ophthalmic Physiol Opt.* 2008;28(3):225–237.
102. Edwards MH, Li RW, Lam CS, et al. The Hong Kong progressive lens myopia control study: study design and main findings. *Invest Ophthalmol Vis Sci.* 2002;43(9):2852–2858.
103. Sankaridurg P, Donovan L, Varnas S, et al. Spectacle lenses designed to reduce progression of myopia: 12-month results. *Optom Vis Sci.* 2010;87(9):631–641.
104. Siatkowski RM, Cotter SA, Crockett RS, et al. Two-year multicenter, randomized, double-masked, placebo-controlled, parallel safety and efficacy study of 2% pirenzepine ophthalmic gel in children with myopia. *J Aapos.* 2008;12(4):332–339.
105. Tan DT, Lam DS, Chua WH, et al. One-year multicenter, double-masked, placebo-controlled, parallel safety and efficacy study of 2% pirenzepine ophthalmic gel in children with myopia. *Ophthalmology.* 2005;112(1):84–91.
106. Yen MY, Liu JH, Kao SC, et al. Comparison of the effect of atropine and cyclopentolate on myopia. *Ann Ophthalmol.* 1989;21(5):180–182,187.
107. Fang PC, Chung MY, Yu HJ, et al. Prevention of myopia onset with 0.025% atropine in premyopic children. *J Ocul Pharmacol Ther.* 2010;26(4):341–345.
108. Shih YF, Chen CH, Chou AC, et al. Effects of different concentrations of atropine on controlling myopia in myopic children. *J Ocul Pharmacol Ther.* 1999;15(1):85–90.
109. Chua WH, Balakrishnan V, Chan YH, et al. Atropine for the treatment of childhood myopia. *Ophthalmology.* 2006;113(12):2285–2291.
110. Shih YF, Hsiao CK, Chen CJ, et al. An intervention trial on efficacy of atropine and multi-focal glasses in controlling myopic progression. *Acta Ophthalmol Scand.* 2001;79(3):233–236.
111. Baldwin WR, West D, Jolley J, et al. Effects of contact lenses on refractive corneal and axial length changes in young myopes. *Am J Optom Arch Am Acad Optom.* 1969;46(12):903–911.
112. Jedlicka J. Ortho-K and kids: maximize the benefits, minimize the risks. *Rev Cornea Contact Lenses.* May 2012:26–28.

113. Mika R, Morgan B, Cron M, et al. Safety and efficacy of overnight orthokeratology in myopic children. *Optometry*. 2007;78:225–231.
114. Walline JJ, Jones LA, Sinnott LT. Corneal reshaping and myopia progression. *Br J Ophthalmol*. 2009;93:1181–1185.
115. Swarbrick H, Alharbi A, Watt K, et al. Overnight orthokeratology lens wear slows axial eye growth in myopic children [E-abstract 1721]. *Invest Ophthalmol Vis Sci*. 2010;51.
116. Smith EL III, Kee CS, Ramamirtham R, et al. Peripheral vision can influence eye growth and refractive development in infant monkeys. *Invest Ophthalmol Vis Sci*. 2005;46:3965–3972.
117. Smith EL III, Ramamirtham R, Qiao-Grider Y, et al. Effects of foveal ablation on emmetropization and form-deprivation myopia. *Invest Ophthalmol Vis Sci*. 2007;48:3914–3922.
118. Smith EL III, Hung LF, Huang J. Relative peripheral hyperopic defocus alters central refractive development in infant monkeys. *Vision Res*. 2009;49:2386–2392.
119. Mutti DO, Sholtz RI, Friedman NE, et al. Peripheral refraction and ocular shape in children. *Invest Ophthalmol*. 2000;41:1022–1030.
120. Atchison DA, Pritchard N, Schmid KL. Peripheral refraction along the horizontal and vertical visual fields in myopia. *Vision Res*. 2006;46:1450–1458.
121. Chen X, Sankaridurg P, Donovan L, et al. Characteristics of peripheral refractive errors of myopic and non-myopic eyes Chinese eyes. *Vision Res*. 2010;50:31–35.
122. Schmid GF. Variability of retinal steepness at the posterior pole in children 7-15 years of age. *Curr Eye Res*. 2003;27:61–68.
123. Logan NS, Gilmartin B, Wildsoet CF, et al. Posterior retinal contour in adult human anisometropia. *Invest Ophthalmol Vis Sci*. 2004;45:2152–2162.
124. Mutti DO, Hayes JR, Mitchell GL, et al. Refractive error, axial length, and relative peripheral refractive error before and after the onset of myopia. *Invest Ophthalmol Vis Sci*. 2007;48:2510–2519.
125. Charman WN, Radhakrishnan H. Peripheral refraction and the development of refractive error: a review. *Ophthalmic Physiol Opt*. 2010;30:321–338.
126. Charman WN, Mountford J, Atchison DA, et al. Peripheral refraction in orthokeratology patients. *Optom Vis Sci*. 2006;83:641–648.
127. Quieros A, Gonzalez-Meijome JM, Jorge J, et al. Peripheral refraction in myopic patients after orthokeratology. *Optom Vis Sci*. 2010;87:323–329.
128. Kang P, Swarbrick H. Peripheral refraction in myopic children wearing orthokeratology and gas-permeable lenses. *Optom Vis Sci*. 2011;88(4):476–482.
129. Paune-Fabre J. Clinical performance of a new peripheral refraction control GP lens for myopia stabilization. Poster presented at: Global Specialty Lens Symposium; January 2011; Las Vegas, NV.
130. Watt K, Swarbrick HA. Microbial keratitis in overnight orthokeratology: review of the first 50 cases. *Eye Contact Lens*. 2005;31(5):201–208.
131. Watt KG, Boneham GC, Swarbrick HA. Microbial keratitis in orthokeratology: the Australian experience. *Clin Exp Optom*. 2007;90(3):188–189.
132. Young AL, Leung AT, Cheng LL, et al. Orthokeratology lens-related corneal ulcers in children: a case series. *Ophthalmology*. 2004;111(3):590–595.
133. Bullimore MA, Sinnott LT. The risk of microbial keratitis with overnight corneal reshaping lenses [E-abstract 90583]. *Optom Vis Sci*. 2009;86.
134. Swarbrick H. Overnight orthokeratology and the risk of microbial keratitis. *Refractive Eyecare*. June 2012:16.
135. Santodomingo-Rubido J, Villa-Collar C, Gilmartin B, et al. Orthokeratology vs. spectacles: adverse events and discontinuations. *Optom Vis Sci*. 2012;89(8):1133–1139.
136. Lipson MJ. Long-term clinical outcomes for overnight corneal reshaping in children and adults. *Eye Contact Lens*. 2008;34(2):94–99.
137. Walline J, Jones-Jordan LA, Greiner KL, et al. The effects of soft bifocal contact lenses on myopia progression in children [E-Abstract 110642]. *Optom Vis Sci*. 2011;88.
138. Sankaridurg P, Holden B, Smith E III, et al. Decrease in rate of myopia progression with a contact lens designed to reduce relative peripheral hyperopia: one-year results. *Invest Ophthalmol Vis Sci*. 2011;52(13):9362–9367.
139. Aller TA. Results of a one-year prospective clinical trial (CONTROL) of the use of bifocal soft contact lenses to control myopia progression. *Ophthal Physiol Opt*. 2006;26(1):8–9.
140. Anstice NS, Phillips JR. Effect of dual-focus soft contact lens wear on axial myopia progression in children. *Ophthalmology*. 2011;118(6):1152–1161.
141. Walline JJ, Rah MJ. Soft bifocal contact lenses for myopia progression. *Contact Lens Spectrum*. 2009;24(3):52.
142. Herzberg CM. An update on orthokeratology. *Contact Lens Spectrum*. 2010;25(3):22.
143. Jones-Jordan LA, Sinnott LT, Manny RE, et al. Early childhood refractive error and parental history of myopia as predictors of myopia. *Invest Ophthalmol Vis Sci*. 2010;51:115–121.
144. Lam DS, Fan DS, Lam RF, et al. The effect of parental history of myopia on children's eye size and growth: results of a longitudinal study. *Invest Ophthalmol Vis Sci*. 2008;49:873–876.
145. Cho P, Cheung SW. Retardation of myopia in orthokeratology (ROMIO) Study: a 2-year randomized clinical trial. *Invest Ophthalmol Vis Sci*. 2012;53:7077–7085.

Chapter 19

Keratoconus

Edward S. Bennett, Joseph T. Barr, and Loretta Szczotka-Flynn

Keratoconus is a progressive, typically bilateral, asymmetric disease of the cornea that is characterized by steepening and distortion, apical thinning, and corneal ectasia.[1-3] The cause of keratoconus is unknown, although it is most likely a genetic disease. The management of keratoconus is most often in some form of rigid gas-permeable (GP) contact lenses; however, more severe cases require surgery, typically either penetrating keratoplasty (PKP) or deep anterior lamellar keratoplasty (DALK).

The Collaborative Longitudinal Evaluation of Keratoconus (CLEK) Observational Study was the largest multicenter, prospective, observational study designed to describe the course of keratoconus and the associations among its visual and physiological manifestations. The CLEK study characterized the course of keratoconus and identified factors related to vision, progression, and corneal scarring in keratoconus. A total of 1,209 patients were enrolled between 1995 and 1996, at 15 participating clinics, and patients were reexamined annually for 8 years, through mid-2004. The results of the CLEK study will be referenced throughout this chapter.

CHARACTERISTICS

Keratoconus is bilateral in approximately 96% of the cases.[4,5] Typically one eye is diagnosed earlier and progresses more than the fellow eye. It is often diagnosed in the early teens to early 20s.[6,7] It typically stops progressing by the fourth decade, possibly secondary to age-related cross-linking resulting in great rigidity and less likelihood for the ectasia to result.[8-11] For the same reason, keratoconus is unlikely to result after age 40. There does not appear to be a significant difference in the incidence of keratoconus either between left and right eyes or between males and females.

Epidemiology

The prevalence of keratoconus is stated to be 1/2,000 persons. With 270 million Americans, this translates to 135,000 Americans with the diagnosis of keratoconus. However, the only estimate of the incidence and prevalence of keratoconus comes from a study conducted in Olmsted County in Minnesota, which identified 64 incident cases of keratoconus between 1935 and 1982 at Mayo Clinic.[12] Case ascertainment was based solely on medical record review with the diagnosis determined by the "examiner's description of characteristic irregular light reflexes observed during ophthalmoscopy or retinoscopy, or irregular mires detected at keratometry." Kennedy et al.[12] estimated the overall average annual incidence rate at two per 100,000 population with a prevalence of 55 per 100,000. These estimates are most likely low, given current diagnostic techniques such as corneal topography. Other groups have reported the prevalence as high as 86 per 100,000 in Denmark[13] and incidence as high as 25 per 100,000 in populations that have traditions of consanguineous marriages.[14] The higher incidence was suggestive of a genetic factor being significant in the etiology.

ETIOLOGY

The cause of keratoconus is unknown, although metabolic/chemical changes in the corneal tissue have been documented. However, the disease has been associated with atopy,[15-17] connective tissue disorders,[18-22] eye rubbing,[23,24] contact lens wear,[25-28] and inheritance.[29]

Histological Changes

It is still unclear what causes the corneal changes that occur in keratoconus. A triad of classic histopathological changes have been observed, which include[1]

1. Thinning of the corneal stroma
2. Breaks in Bowman layer
3. Iron deposition in the basal layers of the corneal epithelium

Apparently, degeneration of the epithelial cells is followed by breaks in Bowman layer. Specifically, fragmentation of Bowman layer—possibly caused by degradative enzymes and reduced inhibitors in the epithelium—may represent an early change in keratoconus.[30,31] Abnormal enzymes in the corneal epithelium lead to excess collagenase and reduced protease inhibitors in the stroma, most likely resulting in keratocyte death.[32] This increased collagenase activation may be slowly breaking down stromal collagen, resulting in stromal thinning.[33] Biochemical studies have shown the total amount of protein in the cornea to be decreased.[34] The pathology of collagen fibrils has shown abnormally low numbers of collagen lamellae,[35] and it has been suggested that the lamellae are released from their interlamellar attachments or Bowman layer and become free to slide, resulting in thinning without collagenolysis.[36]

Recent research has intimated that the origin of the disease may be epithelial.[37] It was also found that histologically keratoconus is an anterior corneal disease that, in all but severe cases, does not result in compromise of the posterior cornea. It also appears to affect the anterior limiting lamina and the anterior stroma to a greater extent than previously believed. As the anterior limiting lamina provides the foundation that the epithelium requires to remain firmly attached to the cornea,[38,39] if this is compromised, the epithelium becomes irregular and less well organized.

Atopic Relationship

There appears to be a relationship between atopic conditions (i.e., eczema, hay fever, asthma) and keratoconus as approximately 50% of keratoconic patients have some form of atopy.[1,3,4,40,41] As itching is a primary symptom in atopic conditions, it has also been found that most keratoconic patients are vigorous eye rubbers, although a cause-and-effect relationship has not been proven.[23,24,42,43] Korb et al.[44] has found that keratoconus patients use much more force than nonkeratoconic individuals, essentially using their knuckles, when they rub their eyes. It has been proposed that the corneal indentation (fibril buckling) and compensatory curvature transfer, as well as the high intraocular pressure-induced bulging of the cornea immediately adjacent to the indentation, are mechanical responses to eye rubbing that result in high-tissue pressure.[45] Therefore, forceful eye rubbing could play a role in the etiology of keratoconus, and it was recommended that individuals who have atopy, a family history of keratoconus, or have already been diagnosed with this condition, be advised not to rub their eyes.

Genetic and Heredity

Several studies have suggested that keratoconus is genetic[46-60] with possible linkage to various chromosomal regions. There have been reports from single families, and twin studies also reported in earlier literature. Between 6% and 16% of patients with keratoconus have a history of familial disease.[41,61-63] Because the severity of the disease varies from asymptomatic forme fruste conditions to disabling scarring requiring corneal transplantation, the true incidence, prevalence and familial aggregation is difficult to ascertain. However, in asymptomatic conditions, keratoconus may only be detected using sophisticated instrumentation such as videokeratography (VKG). Studies have found that, in fact, 50% to 60% of family members of keratoconic patients will have, at minimum, subtle topographical abnormalities that would be suspicious of keratoconus.[47,64,65] Keratoconus has shown association with rare genetic syndromes, such as Woodhouse Sakati syndrome[66] and Down syndrome,[67] further supporting the genetic hypothesis.

Contact Lenses

It has been suggested, in many reports, that rigid contact lenses may cause keratoconus due to such factors as mechanical pressure and hypoxia.[26,68–70] In one study, 27% of the keratoconic patients were contact lens wearers, all of whom were not diagnosed with keratoconus at the time of fitting.[70] It was found that these individuals were older at the time of diagnosis, had central (vs. decentered) cones, and had a tendency toward flatter corneal curvatures. However, once again, it is difficult to establish a cause-and-effect relationship as the incidence of keratoconus would be expected to be higher with contact lens wearers.[6] This is the age in which keratoconus typically is diagnosed, and these individuals may be corrected for their myopia prior to being diagnosed with keratoconus. A case report of one of the authors supports a hypoxic etiology. A long-term rigid lens wearer lost one of her GP lenses and went back to wearing an older polymethylmethacrylate (PMMA) spare lens for 8 years. Keratoconus developed in the eye wearing the PMMA lens, whereas the GP lens wearing eye was unaffected.[71]

The "Cascade Hypothesis"

Many of the etiological factors mentioned above are linked together via the "Cascade Hypothesis" from Kenney.[9,72–74] According to this theory, a cascade of events occur that ultimately result in keratoconus. It is evident that many different chromosomes have associations with keratoconus and, more likely, keratoconus has multiple genes involved that are related to a final common pathway, which she has termed the "Oxidative Stress Pathway." Young patients have a propensity to produce high levels of reactive oxygen species (ROS or free radicals) in the cornea. These free radicals are typically cleared by superoxide dismutase, ALDH3, and other enzymes that prevent accumulation of these potentially harmful substances. In this theory, apoptosis occurs as a result of buildup of ROS and reactive nitrogen species in susceptible individuals who are unable to produce protective healthy enzymes. This is preceded by damage to the mitochondrial DNA, reducing energy production; therefore, free radicals accumulate, causing damage to the structural integrity of the cornea. This results in a cascade of events in which a compromised cornea weakens, thins, and becomes steeper in curvature. More recently, Mitochondrial complex 1 sequence variations appear to be the main cause of the elevated ROS.[53] Therefore, as exposure to ultraviolet (UV)-B light generates free radicals, it is important for the appropriate eye wear protection to be used. Likewise, mechanical stress such as that caused by a poorly fitted contact lens or via eye rubbing can exaggerate ROS formation. If this is the case, these individuals need to avoid eye rubbing with the appropriate treatment of allergies and atopic conditions also advised. Antioxidative therapy, like those currently used in retinal treatments, could be a possible future option.[73]

Protective Associations

Interestingly, it has been found that a factor that may reduce the likelihood of keratoconus is smoking, perhaps reducing the risk by increasing collagen cross-linking.[75,76] It also appears that diabetic individuals if, in fact, they have keratoconus have a less severe form as diabetic hyperglycemia may also increase collagen cross-linking.[77,78]

DIAGNOSIS AND EVALUATION

The earlier a patient can be diagnosed as having or possibly having keratoconus, the sooner the practitioner can institute the appropriate management and adequately educate the patient. For the condition to be diagnosed, the practitioner must be aware of the symptoms and clinical signs of keratoconus and encourage frequent follow-up care for monitoring progression.

Early Symptoms and Clinical Signs

The diagnosis begins with a thorough case history. The practitioner must ask the right questions and be a good listener, as the symptoms of incipient keratoconus are varied and frequently confused with psychogenic complaints. Quite often the patient has difficulty explaining the actual problem. Monocular diplopia or "ghost" images and blurring of images are common symptoms, but practitioners may fail to ask questions eliciting a description of image blur.[79] Vision may not actually be blurred but distorted; letters may be confused, and parts of letters may be missing or altered. Therefore, the practitioner should ask the patient whether they are experiencing this distortion out of one eye only. In addition, if this condition had been previously undiagnosed, the patient may own several pairs of glasses, none of which are satisfactory. Finally, asthenopic complaints, polyopia, photophobia, and halos around lights may be reported.

A gradual decrease in visual acuity (VA) is often the first clinical sign of keratoconus. The vision of one eye will be affected before the other, and the blur will be present for both near and far distances. The patient may be able to see better by squinting or by holding printed material very close to the eyes. Contrast sensitivity function is reduced as well.[80] In addition, due to the conical distortion, an early clinical sign of keratoconus is a "scissors-like" motion observed during retinoscopy. In the early stages, manifest refraction will often result in satisfactory VA; however, an increase in both myopia and regular or irregular astigmatism may be found.[81] An absence of parallellism of keratometry mires and a localized region of corneal steepening is often observed with VKG (to be discussed). As the condition progresses, it is often necessary to make large changes in both sphere and cylinder power when refracting. In some cases, the Jackson Cross Cylinder (JCC) is not adequate to provide a noticeable difference and the use of a handheld JCC marked with a ±1.00 D and held over the phoropter aperture or trial frame is recommended.[82] In advanced keratoconus, efforts at obtaining a meaningful refraction may be laborious and frustrating. In these cases, the use of a GP diagnostic lens accompanied by an overrefraction will provide more beneficial information as to the patient's potential best-corrected VA.

The early changes in VA and contrast sensitivity is accompanied by an increase in higher-order aberrations.[83-88] Notably, keratoconus patients have an elevated magnitude of the higher-order aberration coma.[84,87,88]

Corneal Topography Change

Keratometry

Keratometry is beneficial in the diagnosis and monitoring of keratoconus. However, the limitations of keratometry, including the measurement of only a few paracentral points on the cornea, can make early diagnosis difficult, especially if the patient has a decentered apex of the cone.

What is often observed in early keratoconus is a lack of parallellism of the keratometric mires. The mires are somewhat distorted, and one may not completely overlap the other. The corneal astigmatism may increase and shift toward an oblique axis. A steepening of the corneal curvature may be observed. If the condition is incipient, the keratometry readings may be in the 43 to 48 D range. Once the condition advances beyond the curvature values of the keratometer, a +1.25 D ophthalmic lens can be mounted over the objective (patient end) to add approximately 8 D to the keratometer reading (Appendix 1). A +2.25 D lens will extend the range approximately 16 D.[82]

Videokeratography

The use of VKG has been an outstanding tool for the diagnosis and monitoring of patients with keratoconus. The location of the apex and the progression of the condition can be observed via evaluation of the color map. The localized area of steepening can easily be observed with a color map (Fig. 19.1).

Although definitive keratoconus cannot be diagnosed in the absence of several slit-lamp or retinoscopy findings, a keratoconus suspect can be determined quite easily via the appearance of the color map. These individuals can then be monitored to determine if further progression and diagnosis of the condition occurs. In addition, a compression of the mires will be present in the affected region via the reflection of the photokeratoscopic rings. In addition, as the unaffected corneal region (typically superior) will not change, an inferior–superior dioptric asymmetry will be present.[1]

The impacted region or "cone" has traditionally been categorized as nipple, oval (i.e., sagging), or globus.[89–91] The nipple cone is smaller and more centralized than the other two types. The oval cone is more inferior, while the globus cone is quite large in diameter. McMahon[92] reported on results from the CLEK study in which the impacted areas were divided into nipple (Fig. 19.2A), oval (Fig. 19.2B), globoid (Fig. 19.2C), and marginal (Fig. 19.1), with the latter group pertaining to a nonround or nonoval cone located in the periphery of the cornea (often inferior). As shown in Table 19.1, most of the cones can be described as nipple or oval. It was also reported that 12.2% have an apex above horizontal with an average location of at 262 degree (inferior-temporal).[93]

Several VKG systems have developed applications for the screening and diagnosis of keratoconus.[79,94–97] This is particularly important as the presence of keratoconus is a contraindication

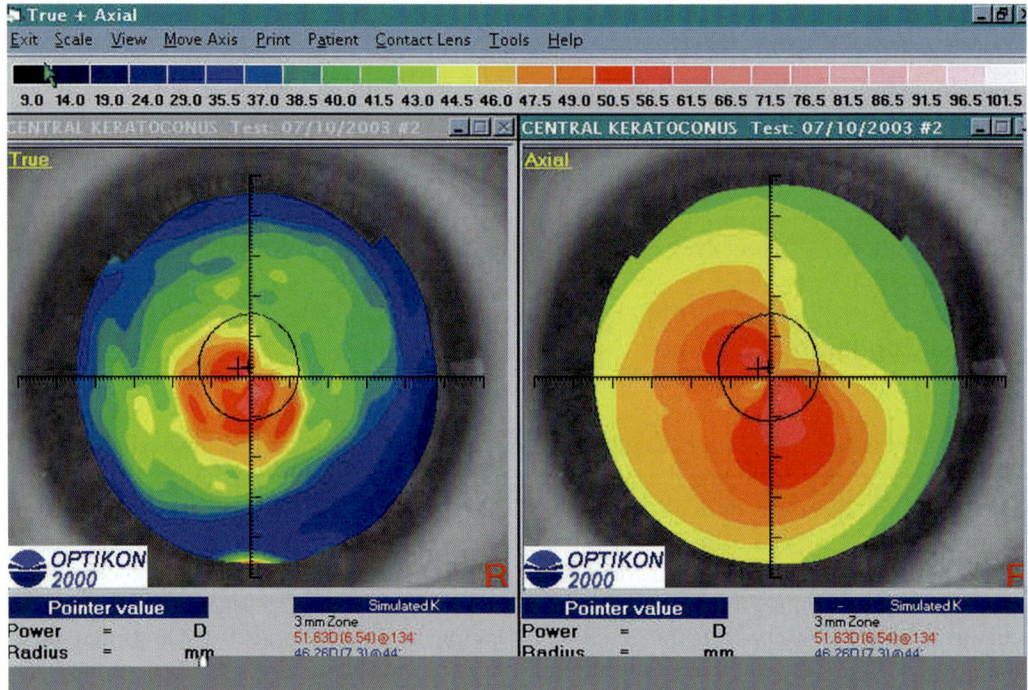

FIGURE 19.1 Representative color map of a keratoconic patient.

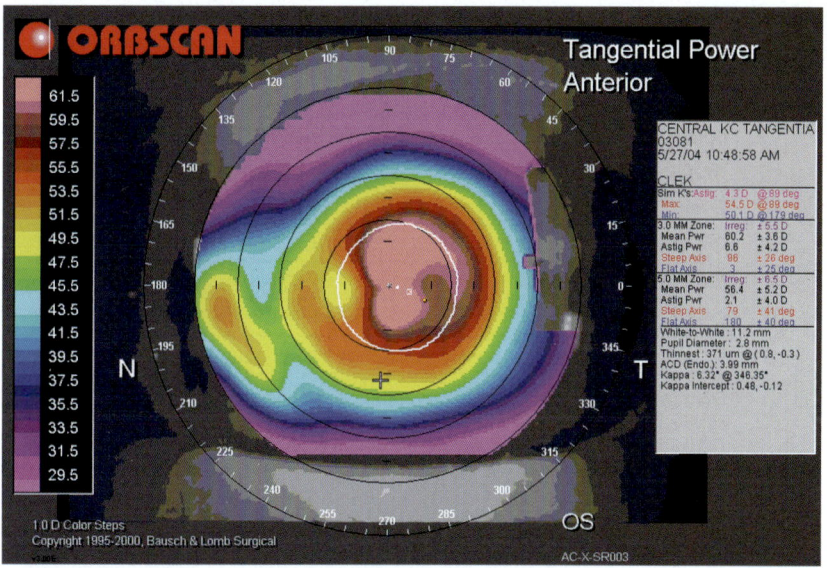
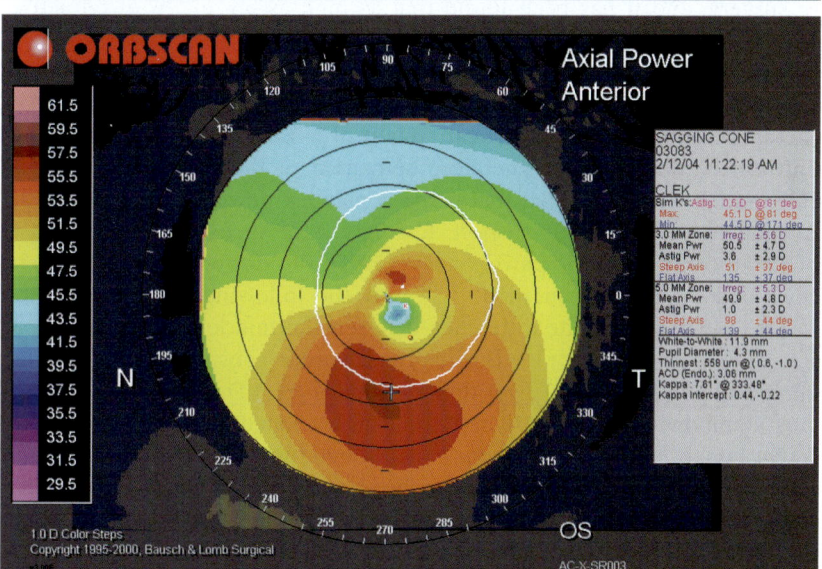
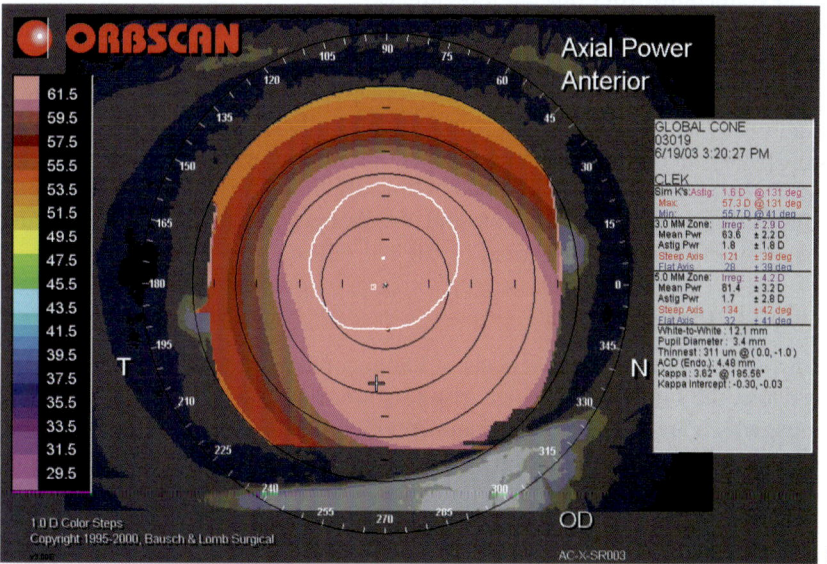

FIGURE 19.2 A nipple cone is shown in **(A)**, an oval or sagging cone in **(B)**, and a globus or globoid cone in **(C)**.

TABLE 19.1 Cone Types and Prevalence

CONE TYPE	PREVALENCE
Nipple	28.7%
Oval	44.3%
Globoid	6.7%
Marginal	5.6%
Other	11.0%
PK	3.7%

From McMahon TT. Collaborative longitudinal evaluation of keratoconus update. Presented at: Annual Meeting of the American Academy of Optometry; December 2006; Denver, CO.

for refractive surgery, and it has been found that as high as 5% to 7% of refractive surgery candidates have subclinical keratoconus.[98,99]

In research clinics, keratoconus has been defined using topographic indices only. VKG readings and differences in corneal shape have been used to diagnose keratoconus. Mandell[6,100], with the cone apex aligned with the optical system of a VKG, determined that a true apex power reading can be obtained and therefore compared to the normal range in the detection of keratoconus. It was concluded that if the cone apex power is 48 to 49 D, the patient should be considered a keratoconus suspect. For powers of 49 to 50 D, there is a very high likelihood of keratoconus, and for powers above 50 D, the diagnosis is almost certain. The modified Rabinowitz–McDonnell method[1,94,101] uses the following guidelines: if the central corneal power is >47.2 D or if the difference between the inferior and superior paracentral corneal regions (i.e., I–S value) is >1.4 D, then the cornea is considered keratoconus suspect. If the central corneal power is >48.7 D or the I–S value is >1.4 D, then the cornea is classified as keratoconus. Rabinowitz and coworkers have also developed an index, the KISA index, to grade the presence or absence of keratoconus.[102] Although this index has the potential to define disease severity, the developers have only described its role in defining normals, keratoconus suspects, and those with the disease. The KISA index has been used to monitor changes in normal eyes of unilateral keratoconus patients[103] and genetic screening where KISA was used to distinguish keratoconus from normal individuals.[47]

The difficulty in using topographic-only methods to define keratoconus is that early forme fruste conditions—which may never progress—can be labeled as keratoconus with unnecessary worry imposed on the patient. Although topographic evidence of keratoconus should be a strong reason to avoid ablative refractive surgery, otherwise asymptomatic patients may not need any special therapeutic treatment other than monitoring. For that reason, a definitive diagnosis of keratoconus is usually made clinically by requiring either a slit-lamp sign of the disease (as discussed below), refractive and VA changes suggestive of keratoconus, or distortion of the anterior cornea as measured by the red reflex.

Slit-Lamp Biomicroscopic Signs

Biomicroscopy is essential for the diagnosis of keratoconus. Only with the biomicroscope can the observer detect the subtle changes occurring within the cornea. The hallmark clinical signs of keratoconus, which are present in the majority of clinically confirmed cases, include Vogt's striae, Fleischer's ring, and scarring. Vogt's striae are a series of vertical or oblique lines located in the posterior stroma or Descemet's membrane (Fig. 19.3). They are most likely the result of the stretching of the corneal lamellae. They temporarily disappear when transient pressure is applied to the globe through the upper lid.[104] Fleischer's ring can be observed in approximately

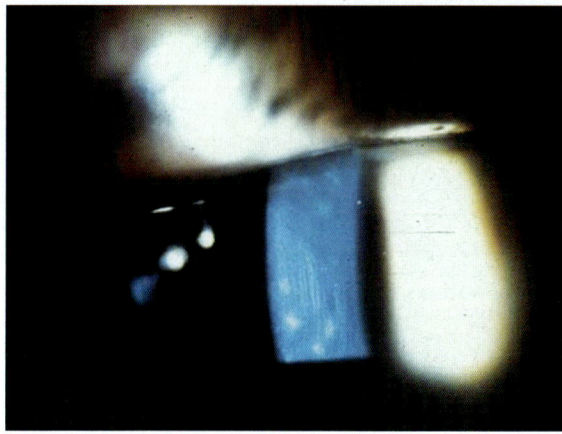

FIGURE 19.3 Vogt's striae.

50% of all diagnosed cases of keratoconus.[41,105] It is a yellow-brown to olive-green discoloration appearing in a broken or interrupted ring encircling the base of the cone (Fig. 19.4). It appears to outline the base of the cone and represents hemosiderin deposits in the deep epithelium near Bowman membrane. Irregular superficial scars can form at the apex of the cone as the condition progresses. They begin as discrete dots in Bowman membrane; fibrillar connective tissue invades the space between the opacities, and they proceed to increase and become opaque (Fig. 19.5).[106,107]

Thinning of the cornea can be observed at the region of the cone via an optic section. Increased visibility of the nerve fibers can be observed at the corneoscleral junction as a result of a change in their density. In severe cases, corneal hydrops can occur secondary to a rupture in Descemet membrane, allowing aqueous humor from the anterior chamber to flow through the damaged endothelium, causing corneal edema and eventually scarring. The results of the CLEK study found that 65% of the patients had Vogt's striae in, at minimum, one eye and 30% in both eyes; 86% had Fleischer's ring in, at minimum, one eye and 56% in both eyes; and 53% had corneal scarring in, at minimum, one eye and 22% in both eyes.[41]

External findings include Munson sign and Rizzuti phenomenon. In advanced cases, the shape of the lid will be altered due to the protrusion of the cone, and Munson sign will be present. This can be confirmed by having the patient look down until the lower lid is at the equator of the cone. According to Rizzuti[108], when illuminating the cornea with a penlight from the temporal side of the cornea, focused anterior to the iris, light is sharply focused on the temporal side of the nasal limbus.

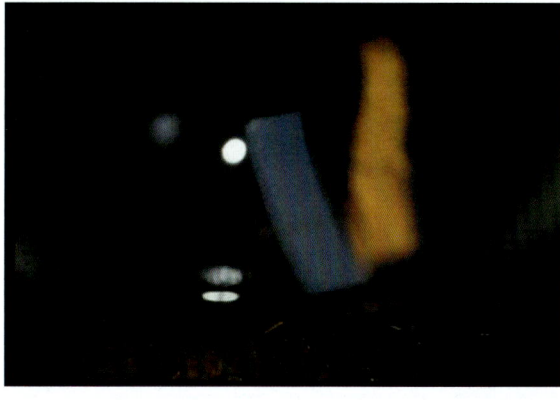

FIGURE 19.4 Fleischer's ring.

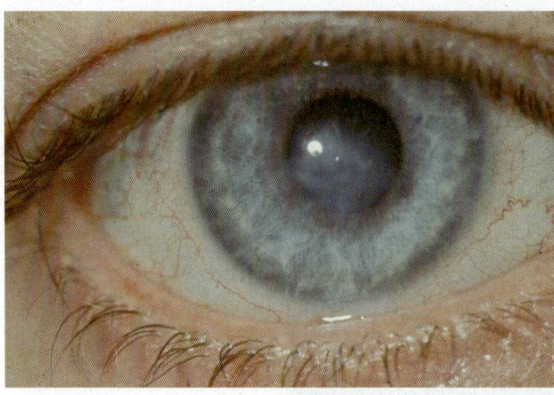

FIGURE 19.5 Corneal scarring.

Ophthalmoscopy

On ophthalmoscopy, a circular, oblong, or dumbbell-shaped shadow may appear that looks like a large indefinite cataract separating the central from the peripheral reflex.[79] On closer evaluation, this phenomenon is observed to be corneal in location. Fundus details are difficult to observe. A technique called photodiagnosis has been useful in diagnosing and monitoring the size, shape, and location of advanced or severe cones. In this technique, the image of the cone is viewed against the red fundus reflex. With the dilated pupil, the examiner views the cornea through the direct ophthalmoscope at a distance of 2 feet. In advanced cases (>50 D), the cone can be easily observed against the red fundus reflex (Fig. 19.6). The image can also be recorded using a fundus camera with a high-plus power condensing lens. The clinical signs of keratoconus are summarized in Table 19.2.

Tomography Applications

Optical coherence tomography (OCT) applications in contact lens practice are greatly increasing. OCT instruments are able to produce two-dimensional cross-section images of the anterior ocular surface. These images are very high resolution and allow for detailed analysis of the corneal layers.[109] This can be beneficial in both diagnosis and monitoring of anterior segment changes. Certainly the benefits of this technology in designing and fitting contact lenses—notably scleral designs—are already evident.

Scheimpflug imaging is based on a rotating camera and a monochromatic slit light source, which rotate together.[110] It pertains to using tomography such that—among other applications—via the measurement of posterior corneal elevation and global pachymetry, and the provision of a series of keratoconic-specific indexes, abnormalities associated with an

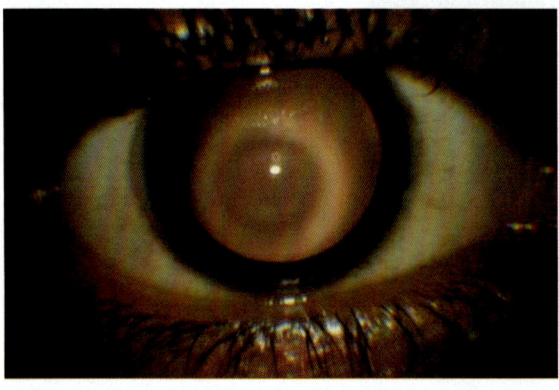

FIGURE 19.6 Photodiagnosis outlining the cone.

TABLE 19.2 Keratoconus Clinical Signs

External signs
    Munson sign
    Rizzuti phenomenon

Refractive signs
    Retinoscopic scissors reflex
    Increased myopia
    Increase in and irregularity of astigmatism

Keratometry signs
    Lack of mire parallelism
    Mire distortion
    Increase in and irregularity of astigmatism

Videokeratoscopy signs
    Compression of mires in affected region
    Color map shows increased power in isolated area of cone
    Inferior–superior dioptric asymmetry

Slit-lamp biomicroscopic signs
    Vogt's striae
    Fleischer's ring
    Scarring
    Increased visibility of nerve fibers
    Corneal thinning
    Hydrops

Ophthalmoscopy

ectatic cornea are detected, quantified, and monitored.[109] The most widely used instrument to provide Scheimpflug imaging is the Pentacam (Oculus).

DIFFERENTIAL DIAGNOSIS

When diagnosing keratoconus, it is important to rule out other mimicking conditions such as corneal warpage syndrome (CWS), corneal molding from a high riding GP lens, keratoglobus, and pellucid marginal degeneration (PMD).

Corneal Warpage Syndrome

Keratoconus and CWS can often be differentiated via a combination of the case history and a comprehensive clinical examination, including videokeratoscopy. CWS patients typically have a long-term history of contact lens wear. This condition occurs as a combination of corneal hypoxia and the mechanical effects induced by the contact lens. It has been most often reported with PMMA lens wear, although soft and GP lenses can induce CWS, the latter via a poor lens-to-cornea fitting relationship. Although corneal distortion and often a scissors-like retinoscopy reflex is present in both conditions, CWS patients typically manifest signs of corneal hypoxia, while rarely exhibiting corneal steepening beyond 50 D.[111] In addition, the degree of mire irregularity or misalignment is typically less with CWS than in keratoconus. Videokeratoscopy will show a localized area of corneal steepening in keratoconus but not necessarily in CWS. Keratoconus can often be differentiated with a comprehensive biomicroscopy examination. Clinical signs such as corneal thinning, Fleischer's ring, Vogt's striae, and in moderate-to-severe cases, corneal scarring are present in keratoconus and not associated with CWS, which is limited to changes in corneal contour.[112] The affected corneal region is limited in keratoconus, often of variable size, encompassing some of (but not limited to) the central and inferior regions. This can be verified via photodiagnosis. Keratoconus, unlike CWS, is a progressive condition,

TABLE 19.3 Corneal Warpage Syndrome versus Keratoconus: Differential Diagnosis		
	CORNEAL WARPAGE SYNDROME	**KERATOCONUS**
Case history	Long-term rigid lens wear: often PMMA or low-Dk GP	Not limited to rigid CL wear Often atopic history
Slit-lamp evaluation	Corneal hypoxia and possibly lens decentration	Corneal thinning in affected region Fleischer's ring Vogt's striae Scarring (in later stages)
Corneal topography	Rarely steeper than 50 D Mire irregularity often mild and improves with either discontinuation of CL wear or refitting into higher-Dk material VKG shows irregularity; not limited in location; if inferior steep region, need to rule out superior decentration	Often steeper than 50 D at apex of cone Continues to progress with increasing mire irregularity and steepening of affected region Location of steepest area is often inferior

CL, contact lens; Dk, oxygen permeability; GP, gas-permeable; PMMA, polymethylmethacrylate; VKG, videokeratography.

typically over a 5- to 10-year period, often resulting in a protruding conical region, easily observable via Munson sign in advanced stages. CWS, conversely, is remediated and often results in a healthy, regular cornea via discontinuation of contact lens wear or refitting into a higher oxygen permeable (Dk) lens material exhibiting a well-centered lens-to-cornea fitting relationship. The differences in keratoconus and CWS are summarized in Table 19.3.

High Riding GP Lens

A pseudo-keratoconic corneal topography can result from wearing a highly positioned GP lens. This fitting relationship induces superior corneal flattening accompanied by inferior steepening, thus simulating a keratoconus color map. As with CWS, none of the classical slit-lamp signs of keratoconus will be present. In addition, once the rigid lens is removed, the inferior cornea will flatten back toward baseline over the course of approximately 7 to 14 days.

Pellucid Marginal Degeneration

As with keratoconus, PMD is a progressive disorder affecting both eyes. However, it is typically characterized by a peripheral band of thinning of the inferior cornea from 4 o' to 8 o'clock with a 1 to 2 mm unaffected area between the region of thinning and the limbus.[1] Slit-lamp evaluation should be beneficial in differentiating the regions of thinning between keratoconus and PMD. In addition, in PMD, the videokeratograph has a classical "butterfly" appearance demonstrating a large amount of against-the-rule astigmatism.[113] Many believe the two conditions are similar and perhaps share the same etiology and pathophysiology, yet different areas of the cornea are affected.

Keratoglobus

Keratoglobus is a condition in which the entire cornea thins, most notably near the limbus as opposed to the localized thinning in keratoconus.[1,2] Although, like keratoconus, a bilateral condition, keratoglobus is typically present from birth and tends to be nonprogressive.

CLASSIFICATION AND PROGRESSION

There are various classification schemes for keratoconus, although no single classification scheme has been universally accepted. One comprehensive classification scheme is presented in Table 19.4, which includes visual symptoms, classical slit-lamp signs, and corneal curvature values as a method to distinguish among different degrees of severity. One classification scheme (Table 19.5) utilizes slit-lamp findings, corneal topography map characteristics, and two easily determined topographic indices, Average Corneal Power (ACP) and higher-order first corneal surface wavefront RMS error (HORMSE).[114]

Apical scarring is included to better delineate moderate-to-severe disease, since corneal scarring is associated with more advanced disease.[115] With the inclusion of higher-order RMS errors, normal from suspect cases are better delineated as coma has been shown to be an excellent differentiator of suspected keratoconus and normal corneas.[116]

Patients first diagnosed with keratoconus want to know the prognosis for progression and loss of vision. Clinicians would like to be able to predict the rate of progression and to identify those patients who will advance to severe keratoconus. However, the rate of progression for a particular patient is impossible to predict. Some patients advance rapidly for 6 months to a year and then stop progressing, with no further change. Often there are periods of several months with significant changes followed by months or years of no change; this may then be followed by another period of rapid change. However, it typically progresses over a time period of 3 to 8 years.[4] In the CLEK study, the slope of the change of flat K was approximately

TABLE 19.4 Keratoconus Classification

STAGE 1
1. Fully correctable with spectacles
2. Slight increase in refractive astigmatism
3. Slight or no keratometric mire distortion
4. Normal keratometry readings
5. Mild area of steepening with videokeratoscopy
6. Mild scissors reflex with retinoscopy
7. Difficult to diagnose
STAGE 2
1. Definite corneal distortion and irregular astigmatism observed with keratometry and videokeratoscopy
2. Further increase in myopia and refractive astigmatism
3. Keratometer values exhibit 1–4 D of steepening
STAGE 3
1. Best-corrected spectacle VA is greatly decreased
2. Accurate keratometry readings are difficult to obtain because of mire distortion
3. Keratometry readings have steepened from 5 to 10 D
4. Increase in irregular astigmatism, commonly ranging from 2 to 8 D
5. Slit-lamp findings, including corneal thinning, increased nerve fiber visibility, Vogt's striae, Fleischer's ring, and possibly scarring, are often present
STAGE 4
1. Intensification of above signs, with the cornea steepening to >55 D
2. Scarring present at apex
3. Munson sign present

TABLE 19.5 Keratoconus Severity Score

Rules: The decision process flows down each grade. For grades 0–1, all of the parameters in a category must be met. For all grades, the italicized features must be met. The worst of the remaining features is then assessed, with the "worst" of the features carrying the greater weight (as long as the italicized features are met).

0	Unaffected—normal topography *Definitely no scar (DNS)* *No slit-lamp signs for keratoconus* Typical axial pattern ACP <47.75 D Higher-order RMS error <0.65

1	Unaffected—atypical topography
	DNS
	No slit-lamp signs for keratoconus
	Atypical axial pattern
	    Irregular pattern
	    Asymmetric superior bowtie
	    Asymmetric inferior bowtie
	    Inferior or superior steepening no more than 3.00 D steeper than ACP
	ACP <48.00
	Higher-order RMS error <1.00

2	Suspect topography
	DNS or probably no scar (PNS)
	No slit-lamp signs for keratoconus
	Axial pattern with isolated area of steepening
	    Inferior steep pattern
	    Superior steep pattern
	    Central steep pattern
	ACP <49.00 D
	or
	Higher-order RMS error >1.00, <1.50

3	Affected—mild disease *Axial pattern consistent with keratoconus* *May have positive slit-lamp signs* *No corneal scarring consistent for keratoconus* ACP <52.00 D or Higher-order RMS error 1.51–3.50
4	Affected—moderate disease *Axial pattern consistent with keratoconus* *Must have positive slit-lamp signs* ACP >52.01 D, <56.00 D or Higher-order RMS error >3.51–5.75 or Corneal scarring grade up to 3.0 overall
5	Affected—severe disease *Axial pattern consistent with keratoconus* *Must have positive slit-lamp signs* ACP >56.01 D or Higher-order RMS error >5.75 or Corneal scarring grade 3.5 or greater overall

ACP, average corneal power; RMS, root-mean-square.

0.20 D per year; over 7 years, this translated into an expected steepening of 1.44 D. Steepening of 3 D or more in either eye had an incidence of 23%.[117]

PATIENT CONSULTATION

As with almost all medical conditions, patients should be informed of the diagnosis (or possible diagnosis) as soon as possible. The progression of the disease can be described and, although most patients will not need a corneal transplant, the possibility of this option should be mentioned. These individuals are often very curious about their condition and desire more information. The Internet is always a good source for information, but patients can also impose undue worry upon themselves if they retrieve faulty information or information not pertaining to them or their specific disease state. One excellent source is the National Keratoconus Foundation site at www.nkcf.org. Keratoconus patients can contact a large number of sources of information here and find answers to commonly asked questions. Likewise, practitioners can utilize this information as well. Additionally, several cities have keratoconus support groups in an effort to allow patients the opportunity to share their experiences with others.

When monitoring these patients, it is important to empathize with the possible changes in their quality of life. Typical keratoconus has an onset early in life, often said to be at puberty.[118] The CLEK study reported a median age of 39 years at enrollment. Thus, keratoconus is a chronic disease with a long duration, affecting people during their prime earning and child rearing years, which may relate to the reported adverse psychological effects reported by some authors.[119–122] Giedd et al.[120] used a standardized questionnaire (Milton Behavioral Health Inventory or MBHI) with subjects recruited through the Internet via the keratoconus-link listserv. The results showed that 96% of respondents indicated that keratoconus had, at minimum, some impact on their lives; 40% indicated the impact was moderate or severe. Keratoconus subjects also scored lower on the respectful coping style scale. This would appear to indicate that keratoconus patients may tend to be less respectful and cooperative with their practitioner, likely resulting in practitioners having a less favorable attitude toward them. In the CLEK study, VA worse than 20/40 was associated with lower quality-of-life scores.[123] A steep keratometric reading >52 D was associated with lower scores on subscales representing mental health, role difficulty, driving, dependency, and ocular pain. Scores for keratoconus patients were between patients with category 3 and 4 age-related macular degeneration (AMD) except general health, which was better than AMD patients, and ocular pain, which was worse than AMD patients.[123] This significantly impaired vision-related quality of life continues to decline over time.[124] Additionally, in those patients with worsening VA and increasing corneal curvature, a significant 10-point decline over 7 years in NEI-VFQ scale scores is found.[124] Therefore, although keratoconus rarely results in blindness, its impact on patients is comparable to that of a person with advanced macular degeneration and, because it affects young adults, the magnitude of its public health impact is disproportionate to its reported prevalence and clinical severity.

Additionally, impact on the quality of life was confirmed by a study in which keratoconus patients were compared to normal controls and to age-matched patients with chronic, nonkeratoconic eye disease via use of a personality questionnaire.[63] Abnormal results were found on the same psychological scales (passive-aggressive, paranoid, hypomanic, disorganized thinking patterns, and substance abuse) in both the keratoconic and chronic eye disease patients. The fact that it has been reported that keratoconus has been associated with both a higher incidence of sleep apnea syndrome[125,126] and floppy eyelid syndrome[127] may be notable to mention to keratoconus patients as well.

SPECTACLE MANAGEMENT

Spectacle correction is an uncommon form of correction in keratoconus. The CLEK study found an incidence of 16% of patients diagnosed with keratoconus wore spectacles as their primary form of distance correction.[41] As a result of the gradual progression of corneal irregularity, spectacles appear to have their best application early in the disease prior to contact lens use. Spectacles do not impact the irregular nature of the corneal curvature. In addition, the refractive error can change quite rapidly and, as the condition progresses, anisometropia may exist due to one eye being more often affected than the other eye.[105]

CONTACT LENS MANAGEMENT

Rigid Lens Fitting

Keratoconus is best corrected with rigid GP contact lenses. Even in the early stages of the disease when spectacle correction may still be an option, rigid contact lenses do the best job at correcting the irregular astigmatism and secondary aberrations that are induced from the irregular cornea as compared to conventional soft toric lenses.[128] In the process of rigid lens fitting, the practitioner may be presented with a difficult fit as a result of an extremely decentered apex of the cone. This is particularly true in cases in which the apex is decentered several millimeters inferiorly as the lens tends to position at the steepest region of the cornea.

In the CLEK study, 65% of patients were best corrected bilaterally with rigid lenses; 8% unilaterally with a rigid lens.[41] This value is similar to the 75% of keratoconic patients wearing rigid lenses in the CLEK pilot study[129] and is similar to other reports.[70,130]

A rigid contact lens will neutralize much of the distortion/optical aberrations of the anterior corneal surface and the subsequent VA can be increased several lines on the acuity chart.[131] However, even if VA chart vision is "normal" with rigid contact lens correction, most likely there is some decrement in vision performance. Contrast threshold measurements have shown a vision loss at low-spatial frequencies (0.25 c/deg), which is not improved by contact lens fitting.[132] Therefore, although rigid contact lenses can provide a significant improvement in VA for keratoconic patients, there may still be residual loss of visual function.

Lens-to-Cornea Fitting Relationships

Three common rigid lens-to-cornea fitting relationships have been used in keratoconus. These include apical bearing, apical clearance, and three-point touch.

Apical Bearing: One previously practiced philosophy for fitting keratoconus has been to fit a large diameter, flat base curve lens in an effort to supposedly slow down or halt progression of the condition. It was theorized to result in improved vision versus other fitting relationships. The resulting fluorescein pattern shows excessive central bearing accompanied by midperipheral and peripheral pooling (Fig. 19.7).

This method is now controversial and rarely used today as—although it has been reported that a flatter base curve radius (BCR) design can result in a reduction in higher-order

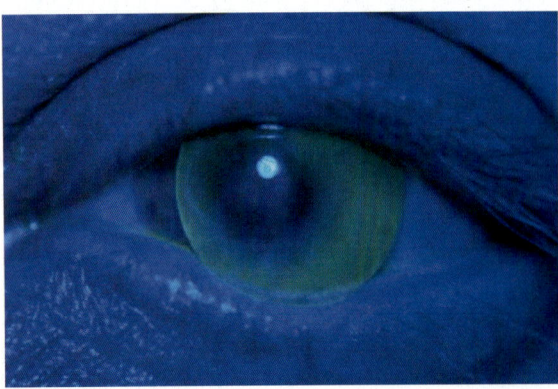

FIGURE 19.7 An apical bearing fitting relationship in keratoconus.

aberrations[133]—it is believed that excessive pressure of the lens on a region of the cornea that is thin and fragile could encourage distortion and apical scarring.[134–136] It is possible that this fitting relationship could also encourage swirl staining, commonly observed over the apex of the cone in keratoconus. Korb et al.[134] compared corneal integrity with an apical bearing fitting relationship with a large-diameter, flat-BCR lens versus an apical clearance fitting relationship achieved with a small-diameter, steep-fitting lens. Seven keratoconic patients exhibiting an absence of corneal scarring were fitted randomly such that one eye had the apical clearance design and the other eye had the apical bearing design. At the end of 1 year, four of the seven eyes in the apical bearing design exhibited scarring; none of the eyes with the apical clearance design had scarring.

Apical Clearance: In an attempt to contour the cornea with a small, steep lens design with total avoidance of bearing, some practitioners have recommended an apical clearance lens design.[134,135,137] This form of fitting relationship should result in minimum lens-induced apical corneal compromise. Essentially, this is accomplished with a small-diameter, steep-base curve lens, which results in an apical clearance fluorescein pattern (Fig. 19.8).

In the CLEK study, the feasibility of this fitting philosophy was assessed using post-fitting frequency of slit-lamp findings such as: (a) moderate epithelial punctate staining; (b) moderate central corneal erosion; (c) corneal edema; (d) contact lens imprint; and (e) the development of central corneal scarring.[137] Investigators fitted 30 eyes with an apical clearance lens design using the CLEK diagnostic fitting set (described below). All lenses had an 8.6 mm overall diameter (OAD) with a 6.5 mm optical zone. An initial diagnostic lens was selected with a BCR equal to the steep keratometry value. After evaluation with fluorescein, lens changes would be made until the First Definite Apical Clearance Lens (FDACL), or the flattest lens that did not demonstrate central bearing, was obtained. Then all 30 eyes were assigned to wear steep-fitting lenses, defined as lenses with BCRs 0.2 mm steeper than the FDACL lens for a 12-month period. The results found that the average wearing time increased from a baseline of 10.5 to 13.7 hours/day at 12 months. In addition, there was not a decrement in VA as compared to the baseline values. Only one eye out of 22 completing the study developed scarring. Nevertheless, if this philosophy is to be utilized, the fluorescein pattern should be monitored to ensure that peripheral seal-off or adherence of lens-to-cornea do not occur.

Three-Point Touch: An especially popular lens-to-cornea fitting philosophy for fitting keratoconic patients is three-point touch. The goal, through diagnostic fitting, is to achieve mild or "feather" touch of the lens over the apex of the cone accompanied by, at minimum, two other areas of touch approximately 180 degree from the apex at the corneal midperiphery.[79] This "feather touch" bearing of the apex and midperiphery creates a bulls-eye appearance upon fluorescein evaluation. Four zones are created: slight apical touch, paracentral clearance,

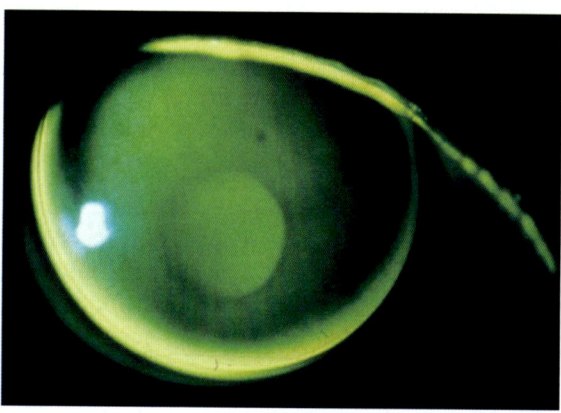

FIGURE 19.8 An apical clearance fitting relationship.

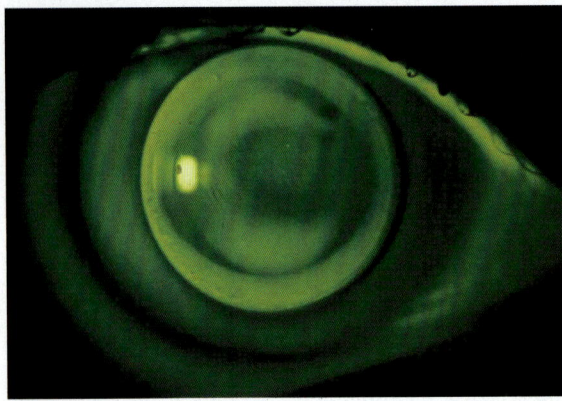

FIGURE 19.9 A three-point-touch fitting relationship.

midperipheral bearing, and peripheral clearance (Fig. 19.9). In this design, the weight of the lens is distributed across a healthy cornea and not focused on one specific area. It is theorized that mild apical bearing will provide some amount of regularity to the anterior corneal surface in that region and possibly improved VA as compared to the apical clearance method. For this fitting relationship to be successful, it should have as little movement as possible that still allows some tear flow under the lens. In addition, it is important to monitor these patients to ensure apical bearing does not become excessive, possibly resulting in the aforementioned corneal complications occurring from apical bearing.

Corneal Topography and GP Lens Fitting

The ability to measure the curvature of the front surface of the cornea is important in fitting the keratoconic patient, both in deciding upon what design to use and also to predict the fitting relationship of that design on the eye.[109] The fitting process is likely to be more efficient and ultimately successful if the cone location and both shape and irregularity of the cornea is considered. For example, a small centrally located "nipple cone" can often successfully be fit with any one of the small-diameter lens designs (to be discussed), whereas larger oval, globus, or decentered cones are often best managed with larger-diameter GP lenses, piggyback combinations, or hybrid designs. Some topographers have the capability of producing an elevation map of the cornea, which can be beneficial in predicting areas of potential bearing or excessive clearance of a GP lens. Many topographers have contact lens software—some with keratoconus-specific designs—such that you can create a simulated fluorescein pattern. The design parameters can then be manipulated to optimize the pattern and a diagnostic lens can be applied that most closely approximates the design to be ordered. Although diagnostic fitting has always been the standard for fitting irregular corneas, this technology does allow for efficient and successful fitting of GP lenses designed empirically. In fact, a study that evaluated virtual fitting of keratoconus comparing topography-predicted fluorescein patterns to actual patterns, there was parity in the great majority of eyes (i.e., 74%, but increased to 95% if a good-quality ring reflection from the placido disk was obtained).[138]

GP Lens Designs

Many GP lens designs have been developed specifically for keratoconus. Available designs for keratoconus can be found at the following site: www.gpli.info/labs/.[139] Typically, these consist of small-diameter, steep-BCR lenses with either spherical or aspheric peripheral curves. These range from conventional designs such as the Soper Cone and McGuire lenses to more recently introduced designs such as the Rose K/Rose K2, ComfortKone, Dyna Z Cone, CLEK, and the I-Kone, as well as intralimbal designs such as the Dyna Intra-Limbal (DIL) and RoseK2 IC. The theory behind these designs as well as the authors' design will be discussed here; for detailed parameter presentation and selection, please refer to the manufacturer's fitting guides.

Small-Diameter Lens Designs: There are a number of different designs that can be fit to the keratoconic patient including small-diameter, intralimbal, and scleral GP designs, custom soft lenses, piggyback combination designs, and hybrids. Small-diameter lenses typically have an OAD in the 8.0 to 9.8 mm range and, until the past decade, comprised the lens of choice for keratoconic patients. Today, they are still commonly used, particularly in patients who have a relatively well-centered and small-cone apex. For GP keratoconic designs, laboratories typically have "loaner" diagnostic fitting sets that can be used when fitting these patients. The laboratories and their keratoconic designs can be found at www.gpli.info. There are a number of small-diameter designs and the following represent a few such designs.

Author's Design and Fitting Philosophy: One of the authors (Bennett) uses an approach that incorporates many of the principles used by other practitioners. The goal is to achieve a three-point touch fluorescein pattern with a spherical GP diagnostic lens and then design the lens to be consistent with the stage of the condition.

The Fitting Process. As mentioned, the use of a diagnostic fitting set is important when fitting a keratoconic patient with GP lenses. The first author's diagnostic fitting set is provided in Table 19.6.

When fitting a keratoconic patient, the application of a topical anesthetic is very beneficial. Keratoconic patients tend to be quite sensitive to initial lens application. Topical anesthetic application will minimize initial lens awareness and reduce chair time. The latter is particularly

TABLE 19.6 Keratoconus Diagnostic Lens Fitting Set (BENNETT)

LENS	OAD/OZD	BCR	SCR/W	ICR/W	PCR/W	POWER (D)
1	9.0/7.2	7.3	8.4/.3	10.2/.3	12.3/.3	−3.00
2	9.0/7.2	7.2	8.3/.3	9.9/.3	12.2/.3	−3.00
3	9.0/7.2	7.1	8.1/.3	9.7/.3	12.1/.3	−3.00
4	8.8/7.0	7.0	8.0/.3	9.6/.3	12.0/.3	−4.00
5	8.8/7.0	6.9	7.9/.3	9.5/.3	11.9/.3	−4.00
6	8.8/7.0	6.8	7.8/.3	9.4/.3	11.8/.3	−5.00
7	8.6/6.8	6.7	7.7/.3	9.3/.3	11.7/.3	−5.00
8	8.6/6.8	6.6	7.6/.3	9.2/.3	11.6/.3	−6.00
9	8.6/6.8	6.5	7.5/.3	9.1/.3	11.5/.3	−6.00
10	8.4/6.6	6.4	7.3/.3	9.0/.3	11.4/.3	−7.00
11	8.4/6.6	6.3	7.2/.3	8.8/.3	11.3/.3	−7.00
12	8.4/6.6	6.2	7.1/.3	8.7/.3	11.2/.3	−8.00
13	8.2/6.4	6.1	6.9/.3	8.5/.3	11.1/.3	−8.00
14	8.2/6.4	6.0	6.8/.3	8.4/.3	11.0/.3	−9.00
15	8.2/6.4	5.9	6.7/.3	8.3/.3	10.9/.3	−9.00

BCR, base curve radius; ICR/W, intermediate curve radius/width; OAD, overall diameter; OZD, optical zone diameter; PCR/W, peripheral curve radius/width; SCR/W, secondary curve radius/width.

important as several lenses may need to be attempted prior to obtaining an acceptable fitting relationship.[140]

The initial lens should have a BCR equal to the steep keratometry reading as the CLEK study has found this to approximate, on the average, the FDACL.[141] The fluorescein pattern should not be viewed immediately after instillation as a false pattern of apical clearance may exist when, in fact, after several blinks, bearing is present. Slit-lamp evaluation with both cobalt blue illumination and the use of a Wratten or Tiffen filter will dictate what change in BCR will be indicated. Often a slight apical clearance fitting relationship will be present. The base curve can then be flattened in 0.50 to 1.00 D steps until apical bearing is first observed. At this time, a three-point touch or "bulls-eye" fitting relationship should be present. Careful evaluation of the peripheral fluorescein pattern is also important to ensure peripheral seal-off is absent. An alignment fluorescein pattern is not expected with this or other keratoconic designs; however, good centration is imperative. If the lens decenters inferiorly due to a corneal apex that is greatly displaced in that direction, either a larger diameter can be attempted in an effort to provide better centration or one of the other keratoconic designs discussed in this chapter may be necessary. A Burton Lamp is also of great value for evaluating fluorescein patterns in keratoconus as the greater field of view allows the practitioner the ability to more easily detect if a three-point touch relationship has been achieved.

Lens Design. Once three-point touch has been obtained, it is important to design the lens to be consistent with the changes in corneal topography. Generally, the optical zone diameter (OZD) should be decreased in size as the BCR steepens to maintain a well-centered lens as the area of the tear meniscus is decreased and bubble formation minimized.[142] In this philosophy, the OZD is typically equal to the BCR in millimeters. For example, if the BCR is 7.00 mm, the OZD will, likewise, be 7.00 mm. Obviously, the OZD can vary depending upon such factors as pupil size, fissure size, and lens position.

Multiple peripheral curves—typically 3 to 4—are necessary to correspond with the rapidly flattening midperipheral and peripheral cornea. The peripheral curve should generally be flatter and wider than conventional designs to provide greater edge clearance and prevent peripheral seal-off and lens-to-cornea adherence.

As almost all lenses ordered will be in minus—if not high minus power—the center thickness should be 0.02 to 0.03 mm thicker than conventional designs to minimize flexure. Lenses with powers >−5.00 D should also be ordered with a plus lenticular or similar peripheral design to minimize edge thickness.

Lens Material. While lens design is the key factor in keratoconus, material selection is also important. Although very low-Dk (i.e., <25) materials are still in use today because of their ability to correct corneal astigmatism while often providing excellent wettability, it is important to select a material that will not further compromise the cornea via hypoxia.[143] With the fact that keratoconic lens designs are almost always of minus power and, therefore, thin in design, a fluoro-silicone/acrylate lens material with a minimum Dk value of 30 is often successful by providing satisfactory oxygen transmissibility (Dk/t) while also providing sufficient rigidity to minimize the effects of flexure. High- and hyper-Dk materials have been found to be successful[144] and are certainly beneficial in minimizing any contact lens-induced complications in an already compromised cornea; however, then one must watch for flexure, notably in thin lens designs. However, it must also be considered that keratoconic patients often will not (or cannot) wear spectacles; therefore, contact lens overwear is certainly possible. Extended wear is contraindicated in keratoconus because of the possibility of further compromising an already compromised cornea.

Soper and McGuire Designs: These are intended to fit over the apex of the keratoconic cornea and, therefore, they are steeper and smaller than conventional GP designs. For historical purposes, two classic designs will be outlined here, which were predominantly used in the 1980s, but are still available and successful today: the Soper design and the McGuire design.

The **Soper Cone** design is fit in an apical clearance manner in which support and bearing are directed off the apex of the cornea and onto the paracentral cornea.[145] This lens design is most effective for small cones, but is also successful for cones with their central apex displaced slightly inferior to the visual axis.[146] The Soper Cone is a bicurve lens design. The two curves on the posterior surface consist of a steep central curve to vault the corneal apex and a flatter peripheral curve to align with the more normal peripheral cornea.[145] The secondary curve of the Soper lens is typically 7.5 mm or 45 D, which is one of the limitations of this design.[146] The constant BCR along with the large diameter of this lens results in an increased sagittal depth and, therefore, a steeper lens. A well-fit Soper Cone lens will vault the central cornea and exhibit slight touch around the periphery.

A representative Soper Cone diagnostic fitting set, available from many CLMA-member laboratories, is given in Table 19.7. The OAD and OZDs are selected depending upon the degree of keratoconus. In mild keratoconus, a 7.4/6.0 mm lens is used; in moderate keratoconus, an 8.5/7.0 mm lens is used, and in advanced keratoconus a 9.5/8.0 mm lens is selected. If the initial lens shows excessive apical clearance and central air bubbles, increasingly flatter lenses with less sagittal depth should be used until a small central air bubble just appears. If the initial lens exhibits apical touch, an increasingly steeper BCR lens with greater sagittal depth may be applied until apical touch disappears or small bubbles appear.

Another classic and historical keratoconic lens design still available today from many laboratories is the **McGuire lens**. This is another apical clearance or alignment-fitting relationship design. This lens design has a steep central curvature with four progressively flatter peripheral curve radii (PCRs).[79,145] The PCRs are flatter than the BCRs by 3, 9, 17, and 27 D. The three inner curves are 0.3 mm wide and the peripheral curve is 0.4 mm wide. It is available in three OADs/OZDs depending upon whether the patient has a nipple cone (8.1/5.5 mm), oval cone (8.6/6.0 mm), or globus cone (9.1/6.5 mm) (Table 19.8). Fitting the McGuire lens is similar to the Soper lens. An advantage of the McGuire design is that it allows adequate edge clearance and movement in comparison to the Soper lens design.[102]

Other, more contemporary, small-diameter corneal lens designs include the Rose K and Rose K2 lens (Blanchard Contact Lenses, Manchester, NH), Comfort Zone design (ABBA Optical, Stone Mountain, GA), the Dyna Z Cone design (Lens Dynamics, Golden, Colorado), and the CLEK design (Conforma, Norfolk, VA). These designs are multicurve designs; that is, the PCRs are spherical and continue to flatten from the base curve through to the final peripheral

TABLE 19.7 Soper Keratoconus Diagnostic Lens Set

BCR/SCR (D)	BCR/SCR (mm)	POWER (D)	OAD (mm)	OZD (mm)	CT (mm)	SAGITTAL DEPTH (mm)
48.00/43.00	7.03/7.85	−4.50	7.50	6.0	0.10	.68
52.00/45.00	6.49/7.50	−8.50	7.50	6.0	0.10	.73
56.00/45.00	6.03/7.50	−12.50	7.50	6.0	0.10	.80
60.00/45.00	5.62/7.50	−16.50	7.50	6.0	0.10	.87
52.00/45.00	6.49/7.50	−8.50	8.50	7.0	0.10	1.00
56.00/45.00	6.03/7.50	−12.50	8.50	7.0	0.10	1.12
60.00/45.00	5.62/7.50	−16.50	8.50	7.0	0.10	1.22
52.00/45.00	5.62/7.50	−8.50	9.50	8.0	0.10	1.37
56.00/45.00	6.03/7.50	−12.50	9.50	8.0	0.10	1.52
60.00/45.00	5.62/7.50	−16.50	9.50	8.0	0.10	1.67

BCR, base curve radius; SCR, secondary curve radius; OAD, overall diameter; OZD, optical zone diameter; CT, center thickness.

TABLE 19.8 Mcguire Cone Trial Sets

BCR (D/mm)	POWER (D)	OAD (mm)	OZD (mm)	PCR/W (mm)
A. NIPPLE CONE				
50.00/6.75	−8.00	8.6	6.0	7.25/.3 8.28/.3 9.75/.3 11.75/.4
51.00/6.62	−9.00	8.6	6.0	7.10/.3 8.10/.3 9.60/.3 11.60/.4
52.00/6.49	−10.00	8.6	6.0	7.00/.3 8.00/.3 9.50/.3 11.50/.4
53.00/6.37	−11.00	8.6	6.0	6.85/.3 7.85/.3 9.35/.3 11.35/.4
54.00/6.24	−12.00	8.6	6.0	6.75/.3 7.75/.3 9.25/.3 11.25/.4
55.00/6.14	−13.00	8.6	6.0	6.65/.3 7.65/.3 9.15/.3 11.15/.4
B. OVAL CONE				
50.00/6.75	−8.00	9.1	6.5	7.25/.3 8.28/.3 9.75/.3 11.75/.4
51.00/6.62	−8.00	9.1	6.5	7.10/.3 8.10/.3 9.60/.3 11.60/.4
52.00/6.49	−10.00	9.1	6.5	7.00/.3 8.00/.3 9.50/.3 11.50/.4
53.00/6.37	−10.00	9.1	6.5	6.85/.3 7.85/.3 9.35/.3 11.35/.4
54.00/6.24	−12.00	9.1	6.5	6.75/.3 7.75/.3 9.25/.3 11.25/.4
55.00/6.14	−12.00	9.1	6.5	6.65/.3 7.65/.3 9.15/.3 11.15/.4
56.00/6.03	−14.00	9.1	6.5	6.50/.3 7.50/.3 9.00/.3 11.00/.4
57.00/5.92	−14.00	9.1	6.5	6.40/.3 7.40/.3 8.90/.3 10.90/.4
58.00/5.82	−16.00	9.1	6.5	6.30/.3 7.30/.3 8.80/.3 10.80/.4
59.00/5.72	−16.00	9.1	6.5	6.20/.3 7.20/.3 8.70/.3 10.70/.4
60.00/5.63	−18.00	9.1	6.5	6.10/.3 7.10/.3 8.60/.3 10.60/.4
C. GLOBUS CONE				
50.00/6.75	−8.00	9.6	7.0	7.25/.3 8.28/.3 9.75/.3 11.75/.4
51.00/6.62	−9.00	9.6	7.0	7.10/.3 8.10/.3 9.60/.3 11.60/.4
52.00/6.49	−10.00	9.6	7.0	7.00/.3 8.00/.3 9.50/.3 11.50/.4
53.00/6.37	−11.00	9.6	7.0	6.85/.3 7.85/.3 9.35/.3 11.35/.4
54.00/6.24	−12.00	9.6	7.0	6.75/.3 7.75/.3 9.25/.3 11.25/.4
55.00/6.14	−13.00	9.6	7.0	6.65/.3 7.65/.3 9.15/.3 11.15/.4

BCR, base curve radius; OAD, overall diameter; OZD, optical zone diameter; PCR/W, peripheral curve radii/width.

curve. These designs differ from the above two designs in that their peripheral curve systems are not immediately accessible to the practitioner, and may be proprietary. Usually the designs are available with a peripheral geometry labeled as standard, flat, or steep. The best place to start in fitting these designs is to attempt the standard peripheral curve system in moderately advanced keratoconus, a steep peripheral system for use with advanced disease, and a flat peripheral system in moderate or early keratoconus.

Rose K and Rose K2 Designs (Blanchard): This popular design utilizes a smaller than average OZD to minimize midperipheral lens impingement as well as pooling or bubbles at the base of the cone.[147] The optical zone ranges from 4.0 for a 5.10 mm BCR to a 6.5 mm OZD for a 7.6 mm BCR. The peripheral lens design consists of a series of five to six computer-controlled spherical radii that clear the midperipheral and peripheral cornea. The curves are blended into a continuum for an aspheric-like periphery. The Rose K2 lens minimizes these aberrations by applying very small changes to the curves on both the front and back of the lens in an attempt to bring the light passing through the lens within the pupil zone to a single point.

TABLE 19.9 Rose K Diagnostic Fitting Set[a]

BCR (D/mm)	POWER (D)	OAD (mm)	PERIPHERAL CURVES	CT (mm)
5.10	−20.75	8.7	Std.	0.10
5.20	−22.00	8.7	Std.	0.11
5.30	−20.75	8.7	Std.	0.12
5.40	−20.75	8.7	Std.	0.10
5.50	−19.25	8.7	Std.	0.11
5.60	−18.50	8.7	Std.	0.11
5.70	−17.25	8.7	Std.	0.12
5.80	−16.00	8.7	Std.	0.13
5.90	−15.00	8.7	Std.	0.10
6.00	−14.25	8.7	Std.	0.13
6.10	−13.00	8.7	Std.	0.14
6.20	−12.00	8.7	Std.	0.14
6.30	−11.00	8.7	Std.	0.14
6.40	−10.12	8.7	Std.	0.14
6.50	−9.00	8.7	Std.	0.15
6.60	−8.00	8.7	Std.	0.16
6.70	−6.87	8.7	Std.	0.17
6.80	−5.87	8.7	Std.	0.18
6.90	−5.00	8.7	Std.	0.19
7.00	−4.12	8.7	Std.	0.19
7.10	−3.00	8.7	Std.	0.20
7.20	−3.00	8.7	Std.	0.19
7.30	−3.00	8.7	Std.	0.20
7.40	−2.00	8.7	Std.	0.20
7.50	−2.00	8.7	Std.	0.19

BCR, base curve radius; OAD, overall diameter; CT, center thickness.
[a]Optical zone diameter varies from 4.0 to 6.8 mm.

As with all other designs, it is important to have their diagnostic fitting set when using this lens. It consists of 26 lenses with BCRs ranging from 5.10 to 7.60, with a standard 8.7 mm OAD and a medium or standard edge lift. This diagnostic set is provided in Table 19.9. It is recommended to start with a base curve equal to the average of the two keratometer readings. A light, feather touch at the apex of the cone is desired. Although 8.7 mm is the standard diameter, any diameter is available and smaller diameters of 8.1 to 8.3 mm tend to be more successful in advanced cases unless a globus cone or an inferior decentered apex exists.

CLEK Design: As part of the CLEK study, a rigid lens diagnostic fitting set was both designed and standardized.[148] This fitting set was developed and tested to simplify the fitting protocol for mild-to-moderate keratoconus patients. The diagnostic lens set and fitting method proposed allows the practitioner an easy-to-follow fitting protocol using an inexpensive diagnostic fitting set.

The parameters for the CLEK diagnostic lenses were standardized and are provided in Table 19.10.

TABLE 19.10 Collaborative Longitudinal Evaluation of Keratoconus Diagnostic Set

BCR (D/mm)	POWER (D)	OAD/OZD (mm)	SCR (mm)
8.00 (42.19)	−3.00	8.6/6.5	9.00
7.90 (42.72)	−3.00	8.6/6.5	9.00
7.80 (43.27)	−4.00	8.6/6.5	9.00
7.70 (43.83)	−4.00	8.6/6.5	9.00
7.60 (44.41)	−4.00	8.6/6.5	8.50
7.50 (45.00)	−4.00	8.6/6.5	8.50
7.40 (45.61)	−6.00	8.6/6.5	8.50
7.30 (46.23)	−5.00	8.6/6.5	8.50
7.20 (46.87)	−5.00	8.6/6.5	8.50
7.10 (47.54)	−7.00	8.6/6.5	8.50
7.00 (48.21)	−6.00	8.6/6.5	8.50
6.90 (48.91)	−6.00	8.6/6.5	8.50
6.80 (49.63)	−8.00	8.6/6.5	8.50
6.70 (50.37)	−7.00	8.6/6.5	8.50
6.60 (51.14)	−6.00	8.6/6.5	8.50
6.50 (51.92)	−8.00	8.6/6.5	8.50
6.40 (52.73)	−8.00	8.6/6.5	8.50
6.30 (53.37)	−7.00	8.6/6.5	8.50
6.20 (54.44)	−9.00	8.6/6.5	8.50
6.10 (55.33)	−8.00	8.6/6.5	8.50
6.00 (56.25)	−7.00	8.6/6.5	8.50
5.90 (57.20)	−9.00	8.6/6.5	8.50
5.80 (58.19)	−8.00	8.6/6.5	8.50
5.70 (59.21)	−7.00	8.6/6.5	8.50
5.60 (60.27)	−9.00	8.6/6.5	8.50
5.50 (61.36)	−8.00	8.6/6.5	8.50
5.40 (62.50)	−8.00	8.6/6.5	8.50
5.30 (63.68)	−8.00	8.6/6.5	8.50
5.20 (64.90)	−8.00	8.6/6.5	8.50
5.10 (66.18)	−8.00	8.6/6.5	8.50
5.00 (67.50)	−10.00	8.6/6.5	8.50

All diagnostic lenses are PMMA with a third curve radius of 11.00 mm and a third curve width of 0.2 mm. The lenses are lightly blended, and the CT is 0.13 mm.
From Edrington TB, Szczotka LB, Barr JT, et al. Rigid contact lens fitting relationships in keratoconus. *Optom Vis Sci.* 1999;76:692–699.

The OAD was established at 8.6 mm and the OZD was set at 6.5 mm. The secondary curve radius was either 8.50 or 9.0 mm and the PCR was 11.00 mm. The contact lens power gradually increased in minus as the base curve became steeper. The diagnostic lenses were fabricated in PMMA material because of its durability, dimensional stability, and low cost. As mentioned previously, a lens fit equal to the steeper keratometry value would represent a good starting point. Based upon the fluorescein pattern, the lens would be changed until first definite apical clearance has been achieved.

I-Kone: The I-Kone design (Valley Contax), developed by Dr. Rob Breece, has a back surface designed to minimize pressure points while the front-surface asphericity reduces aberration-induced problems. The back surface has four conic zones; the central portion vaults the cornea whereas the first and second zones distribute pressure over a larger area to manage corneal ectasia.[149] The peripheral curve system is composed of the third and fourth zones that provide an alignment fit over the nonectatic area of the cornea. As with many of the current designs, the optimum fitting relationship is one that exhibits mild apical touch of slight clearance. The standard 14-lens diagnostic set has a 9.6 mm OAD, although smaller (8.8 mm) and larger (10.4 mm) diameter trial sets are available as well. The BCRs of the diagnostic set range from 44 to 70 D in 2 D steps. The initial diagnostic lens should be selected with a BCR equal to the steeper "K" or "sim K" reading.

Aspheric Lens Designs: Back-surface aspheric lenses have often been used in the fitting of the keratoconic cornea and can provide a better fit and increased success when compared to spherical designs.[150] Many of the designs are progressive aspherics, which gradually flatten from the center of the lens to the periphery to provide better alignment with a highly prolate ectatic cornea. In normal cases, the central cornea has a mean eccentricity (e) of 0.45, with most corneas falling between 0 and 1.0. Aspheric GP lenses designed for non-keratoconic eyes are usually not sufficient except for a mildly keratoconic cornea. However, aspheric back-surface lenses designed to correct presbyopia have eccentricities of approximately 1.0, and these fit well on some keratoconic patients. In aspheric contact lenses, the degree of asphericity or eccentricity increases as the rate of flattening increases.[146] "e-values" of 0.4 to 0.6 are ellipsoidal in shape and fit a mild or nipple cone most effectively, while e-values of >1.0 are paraboloidal and hyperboloidal shaped and fit more advanced or oval-shaped cones.[151]

Examples of aspheric lenses useful for the keratoconic eye include the ABBA-Kone design from ABBA Optical (Stone Mountain, GA), AKS from Art Optical, the Apex Aspheric Cone design (X-Cel Contacts, Duluth, GA), and the Conforma-K design (Conforma Laboratories, Norfolk, VA). These aspheric designs are available in flat, standard, and steep peripheral geometries for use in patients with moderate, moderately advanced, and advanced keratoconus, respectively. Historically, aspheric lenses not specifically intended for keratoconus, which have been successful, including VFL-II and Ellip-See-Con (Conforma, Norfolk, VA).

Finally, there are spherical center/aspheric peripheral designs specifically intended for keratoconus. One such lens is the ComfortKone (Metro Optics, Austin, Texas). The ComfortKone lens is designed with a spherical 4.0 mm OZD that fits the peak of the cone. This lens design incorporates a triaspheric curve in the periphery to maximize overall corneal lens alignment. The aspheric periphery flattens into the aspheric "A" curve. This "A" value is the fitting curve of the lens and depicts the rate of change from the central base curve to the peripheral fitting portion of the lens.[152] The greater the A value, the greater the change from the base curve to the peripheral fitting curve.

Intralimbal Rigid GP Lenses: The advent of high-Dk/t rigid GP lens polymers has allowed us to fit with much larger-diameter designs without the concern of hypoxic complications. In this chapter, large OAD corneal lenses, or intralimbal lenses (because they can fit from limbus to limbus) will be referred to those lenses 10.0 to 12.8 mm in diameter. These designs are typically available with both a conventional periphery and in a reverse geometry design for oblate keratoconic or postsurgical corneas. Examples include DIL design (Lens Dynamics/Firestone), Rose K2 IC (Blanchard), and the G.B.L. lens (ABB Concise Laboratories).

The beauty of an intralimbal lens is that it tends to center better than smaller GP lenses as a result of greater pressure distribution over the midperipheral and peripheral cornea. In addition, in general, these lenses are more comfortable than the smaller designs due to both the centration characteristics and less movement with the blink than the small-diameter designs.[153] Generally these lenses have a large optical zone, which makes the lens forgiving if it decenters in terms of visual function. This is especially important with patients who have large oval, globus, or decentered cones. These designs can be fitted by following three-point touch technique or with minimal apical clearance. However, because of the deep sagittal depth often quickly achieved because of the large chord diameter and steeper base curves, bubbles can easily become trapped in the area surrounding the base of the cone. If this occurs, one has to decrease the sagittal depth by either decreasing the optical zone size or flattening the base curve. Additionally, because of the large optical zone size, the required base curve will likely be flatter than expected to achieve clearance over the conical cornea.

Dyna Intra-Limbal: The DIL is available from Lens Dynamics (Firestone). The standard diameter is 11.2 mm, but this design is available in diameters ranging from 10.0 to 12.0 mm. There are several fitting sets available and two of the standard sets pertaining to conventional periphery and reverse geometry designs are provided in Table 19.11. To select the BCR, it is recommended to use the lens that is 0.2 mm flatter than the mean "K" or sim "K" value. Therefore, if the keratometry readings were 46.00 @ 165; 50.00 @ 069, the mean "K" value would be 48 D (7.04 mm) and the value 0.2 mm flatter would be 7.24 (or rounded off to 7.20 mm). Lens lag of 0.5 to 1.0 mm with the blink is recommended and the fluorescein pattern should exhibit a light feather touch over the apex. These designs are also available in a variable (steep-to-flat) periphery and also in the Quad Sym PC design.

Rose K2 IC: The Rose K2 IC design from Blanchard Contact Lens is available in any diameter from 9.4 to 12.0 mm with a standard diameter of 11.2 mm. It is customarily available in the Boston XO material, although it can be ordered in other materials as well. BCRs of 6.00 to 9.00 mm (in 1 mm steps) are available. The standard 14-lens diagnostic set is provided in Table 19.12. The lenses are available in any one of a series of steep-to-flat edge lifts and if excessive inferior edge lift exists, an Asymmetric Corneal Technology (ACT) design can be used. Wavefront aberration-control aspheric optics are used to enhance vision. The initial BCR is selected to be 3 D flatter than steep "K." A mild apical touch fluorescein pattern is desirable.

G.B.L.: The G.B.L. lens from ABB Concise has a standard 11.2 mm diameter, but can be ordered in any diameter from 10.6 to 11.6 mm. The OZD ranges from 8.2 to 9.2 mm with an 8.8 mm optical zone commonly used with the 11.2 mm OAD. If a keratometer is used, the BCR selected for the initial diagnostic lens should be equal to the mean "K" value. If corneal topography is used, the BCR selected should be equal to 2 to 3 D flatter than steep "sim K."

TABLE 19.11 The Dyna Intra-Limbal Diagnostic Sets

Standard (Elite Series)

DIAMETERS (mm)	NO. LENSES	BCRS (mm)
10.8, 11.2, 11.6, 12.0	14	6.49, 6.62, 6.75, 6.89, 7.03, 7.18, 7.34, 7.50, 7.67, 7.85, 8.04, 8.23, 8.44, 8.65

Reverse Geometry

DIAMETERS (mm)	NO. LENSES	BCRS (mm)
10.8, 11.2, 11.6	18 (A, B, & C)[a]	8.04, 8.23, 8.44, 8.65
	18 (D, E, & F)[a]	8.88, 9.12

BCRs, base curve radii.
[a]Indicates amount of steepening of reverse curve

TABLE 19.12 Rose K2 IC Diagnostic Fitting Set

LENS NO. IN SET	BCR (mm/D)	DIAMETER (mm)	POWER (D)
1	6.50/52	11.2	−11.00
2	6.62/51	11.2	−10.00
3	6.75/50	11.2	−9.00
4	6.89/49	11.2	−8.00
5	7.03/48	11.2	−7.00
6	7.18/47	11.2	−6.00
7	7.34/46	11.2	−5.00
8	7.50/45	11.2	−4.00
9	7.67/44	11.2	−3.00
10	7.85/43	11.2	−2.00
11	8.04/42	11.2	−1.00
12	8.23/41	11.2	−1.00
13	8.44/40	11.2	−1.00
14	8.65/39	11.2	−1.00

Bitoric Lens Applications: Although keratoconic corneas typically have a high level of toricity that, in theory, would benefit from a toric lens, toric back-surface lenses have little application in keratoconus. In a back- or bitoric lens, the toric curvatures and corresponding power corrections are 90 degrees apart. This is often not the case in the irregular astigmatism presented in keratoconus, especially in moderate and advanced cases.[154] If the apex of the cone is decentered, a successful fit is difficult to achieve as well.[4] The corneal toricity error from the central cornea to the apex varies from 0 to 3 D when the apex is decentered by 1 mm and from 0 to about 6 D when the cone is decentered by 2 mm.

If the cone apex is well centered, the astigmatic pattern is relatively symmetrical, and if keratoconus is not advanced, the fitting of a bitoric is possible and has been found to be successful.[6,155,156] However, if the condition continues to progress, other designs will most likely be indicated. Typically, corneal topography is beneficial in determining if the astigmatism is symmetrical and, therefore, a bitoric design is likely to be successful.

Problem Solving

The goal in fitting GPs is not necessarily a certain fluorescein pattern, but rather to allow adequate wearing time with acceptable comfort with best vision while minimizing tissue insult. Complications are often encountered and a simple guide to problem solving is provided in Table 19.13.

As a result of the irregularity and fragility of the cornea, it is important that keratoconic patients are evaluated on a regular basis. Fortunately, these individuals are often receptive to follow-up care as a preventative measure to ensure the condition is successfully managed. When the condition is progressing, patients should be evaluated, at minimum, every 6 months. Once it has stabilized, annual examinations, if not more frequent, should be performed.

It is not uncommon for patients to experience corneal staining, especially at the more fragile apical region of the cone.[157] These mild abrasions or epithelial breaks are not uncommon as a result of the pathogenesis of keratoconus, but can be exacerbated via the mechanical effect of rigid lens wear.[158] Unless this is coalesced, it can simply be monitored. If it coalesces to the point where the patient is symptomatic and an abrasion or severe swirl staining is present,

TABLE 19.13 Keratoconus Problem Solving

PROBLEM	MANAGEMENT
Corneal abrasion/severe swirl staining	D/C CL wear and allow abrasion to heal then clean posterior surface or consider −0.50 D disposable as temporary piggyback; if BCR is too flat, refit with steeper BCR
Paracentral erosion	Most likely due to steep lens with sharp junction; blend pc junctions
Peripheral seal-off	Flatten/widen the peripheral curve
Adherence	Flatten/widen peripheral curve; also can flatten BCR or reduce OZD
Excessive inferior edge lift	Steepen BCR
Poor VA	Select a flatter BCR
Flare	Change to a larger OZD lens
Poor centration	Larger OAD, steeper BCR, or use of a piggyback design
Poor comfort	Ensure edges are thin; +lenticular use if indicated; consider piggyback design; R/O corneal abrasion

lens wear must be discontinued until the staining has been resolved (Fig. 19.10). If necessary, a soft lens can be used as a piggyback under the patient's GP lens during the healing process. The lens can then be cleaned and polished—especially the posterior surface—and an enzyme cleaner added to the care regimen if applicable. If the staining appears to be resulting from an excessively flat lens-to-cornea fitting relationship, a steeper BCR lens should be fit. If a paracentral erosion is present from a steep-fitting lens, the midperiphery can be blended to reduce this problem. If the fitting relationship appears to be acceptable, it would be recommended to return the patients to their previous lens. It is not uncommon for keratoconic patients to overwear their lenses due to the poor vision often achieved with spectacles. If this is compounded by illness, allergies, or any other factor that may result in temporary dryness or hypoxia, significant staining may result.

Other problems may be a result of the lens-to-cornea fitting relationship. If peripheral seal-off is present (Fig. 19.11), the peripheral curve will need to be flatter or wider to increase edge clearance. If adherence is present, either flattening/widening the peripheral curve, selecting a flatter BCR or decreasing the OZD will typically result in lens movement

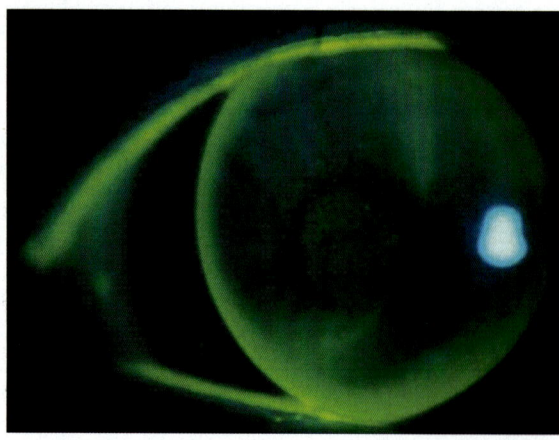

FIGURE 19.10 Central corneal staining. (Courtesy of Craig Norman.)

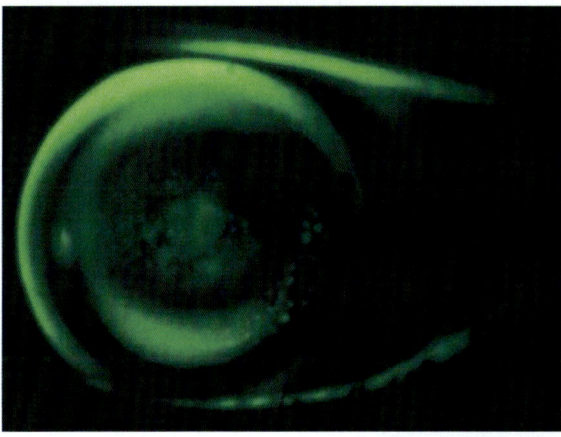

FIGURE 19.11 Minimal edge clearance. (Courtesy of Dr. Larry Davis.)

with the blink. When excessive inferior edge lift is present (Fig. 19.12), the selection of a steeper BCR may reduce this problem. A better modern day design change is to take advantage of new quadrant-specific peripheral curve steepening options available on the newest lathes from multiple laboratories to solve this common problem. Representative designs include the steep–flat option from Lens Dynamics, ACT from Blanchard, and the Quadra-Kone design from TruForm Optics. An example of the benefit of such a design is demonstrated in Figure 19.13A,B, which demonstrates an improved fitting relationship via refitting into a Quadra-Kone design that has different peripheral eccentricities in each meridian.

The Quad Sym (Lens Dynamics/Firestone) is a quadrant-specific design utilizing a technology that was originally successful in Europe. This technology is available for both base curve treatment (BC) or peripheral edge treatment (PC).[159] Computer ray tracing and data analysis has made it possible for software to be developed such that during manufacturing of this design, the front radii cuts can be matched to the various back-surface radii to produce the required power. The Quad Sym BC option allows the lens to have up to four separate BCRs (Fig. 19.14A,B). The Quad Sym PC option allows practitioners to flatten or steepen the edge treatment differently in all four quadrants to match the peripheral cornea. It would be advisable to send a topography map and, if possible, diagnostic lens parameters as well as photographs or video of the fluorescein pattern to the laboratory to assist them in manufacturing this design.

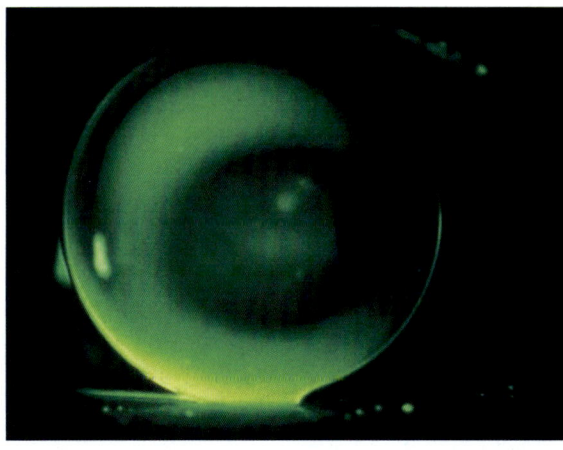

FIGURE 19.12 Excessive edge clearance. (Courtesy of Craig Norman.)

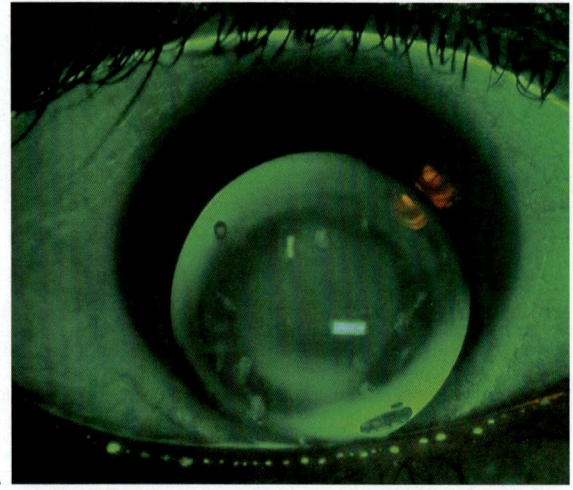

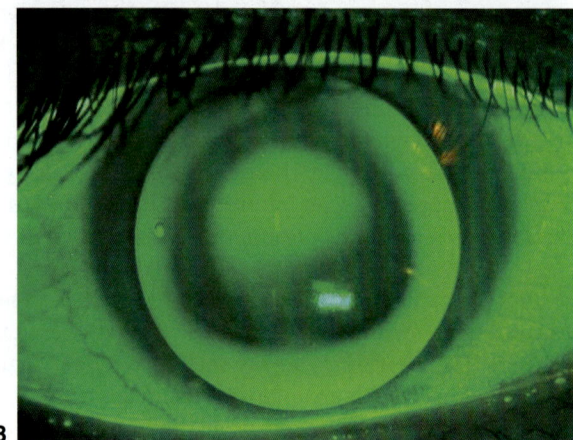

FIGURE 19.13 (A) A decentered gas-permeable lens on a keratoconic cornea with excessive edge lift in some peripheral regions and seal-off in others. **(B)** Same patient with a Quadra-Kone design resulting in a much more uniform peripheral pooling pattern.

Semi-scleral and Scleral Lens Designs

Semi-scleral lens designs have been life changing for a number of irregular cornea patients who were unsuccessful with other designs due to comfort or centration. In the past decade, these designs have literally exploded onto the marketplace and lectures and hands-on workshops provided by the Scleral Lens Education Society (www.sclerallens.org) have been very popular. Success rates of 90% and higher have been reported[160, 162] and, as these designs—if properly fit—vault the cornea, there should be little risk of mechanical abrasion to the cornea when compared to corneal designs. These designs have been found to be successful and result in improved VA when other modalities were unsuccessful and can be considered an essential tool in moderate to advanced keratoconus.[158,160,161]

As is true for the intralimbal designs, semi-scleral designs have become available due to the high-Dk materials allowing us to fit very large lenses without compromise to corneal oxygenation. Semi-scleral lenses are usually, at minimum, 13.8 mm in diameter, and can be manufactured up to about 18.5 mm. They have also been categorized by diameter into corneoscleral, semi-scleral, and mini-scleral.[162] They are differentiated from scleral (haptic) lenses, which range in size from 21 to 28 mm in diameter. Semi-scleral lenses are manufactured in one of a few GP materials that are available in the required material button size. Common materials include Boston XO and XO2, Tyro 97, or Equalens II. Examples include Semi-scleral design

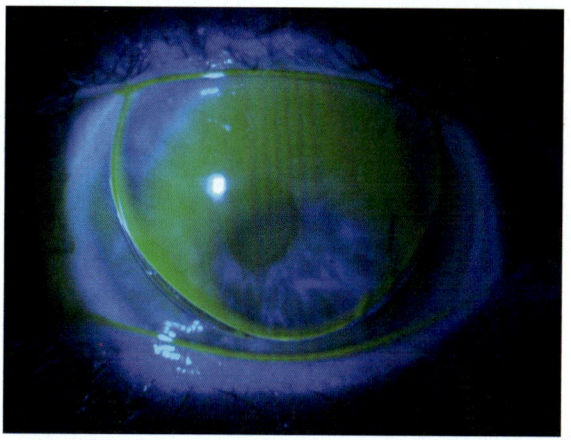
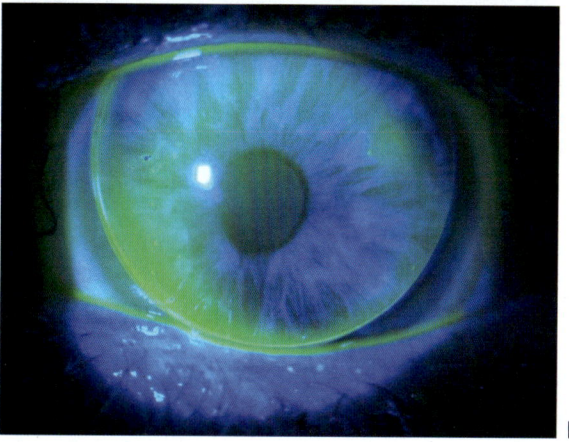

FIGURE 19.14 Quad Sym design shown immediately after dispensing (**A**) and 2 weeks later (**B**). (Reproduced with permission from Bennett ES, Hill S, Grohe RM. Optimizing success with irregular cornea patients, Part 2. *Contact Lens Spectrum.* 2008;23(8).)

(ABBA Optical), the So$_2$Clear Lens (Art Optical/Dakota Sciences), the Jupiter Lens (Essilor), and the msd, One Fit Cone, and Rose K semi-scleral designs (Blanchard).

Perhaps counterintuitive, large semi-scleral lenses are very comfortable when fit well as a result of the large diameters that minimize lens movement and lid interaction. In addition, as the sclera bears the weight of the lens surface, it is unnecessary to achieve a close alignment between cornea and lens, as compared to smaller designs.[163] This has been found to result in good VA in irregular cornea patients due to the larger and flatter OZD.

Some patients may find the excess bulk of the lens to be irritating and the physical size of the lens can discourage patients. Removal of these lenses can also be a problem because of the suction created by the lens–sclera interface. In cases of lens intolerance or discomfort with traditional lenses, however, semi-scleral GP lenses are a very viable option to postpone or prevent surgical intervention. The applications, fitting, care, and problem solving of these designs are described in much detail in Chapter 20.

Scleral lenses made of PMMA materials were historically the first type of contact lenses created. These large lenses are approximately 21 to 28 mm in diameter and the goal in fitting this type of lens is to vault the keratoconic cornea. The major disadvantages of scleral lenses are the time, skill, and expense required to fit them. Only a few centers in the United States are proficient in fitting these lenses. Historically, these lenses were made by creating a negative mold of the patient's eye with dental molding. From this, a PMMA-positive mold was created. The laboratory then lathed the optical zone, back curvatures, and refractive power.

Modern scleral contact lenses are made of high-Dk GP materials that are not thermoplastic and, therefore, they cannot be molded in the manner of PMMA as described above. Preformed

GP scleral lenses are available and can be fitted from an existing fitting set such as the one from Gelflex Laboratories (Donald Ezekial, Perth, Australia) or Innovative Sclerals, Ltd, (Kenneth Pullum, Hertford, UK). In the United States, Dr. Perry Rosenthal who founded the Boston Foundation for Sight (Boston, MA) has established a small network of scleral lens fitters in a few centers nationwide. Nevertheless, fitting true scleral lenses on keratoconic patients is, therefore, reserved for the most advanced patients or in those for whom surgery is contraindicated.

Soft Lenses

Spherical and toric soft lenses have traditionally had little application in keratoconus. Corneal irregularity in keratoconus is best neutralized, and the vision optimum, with a GP lens design with soft lenses having their best application in the mild forms of this condition prior to the onset of significant irregular astigmatism or in combination with a GP lens (i.e., "piggyback").[164] However, the recent introduction of custom lathe-cut soft lens designs, notably in higher-Dk materials, including silicone hydrogel, has resulted in improved designs that are becoming popular as one of the necessary tools for practitioners to have in their management of keratoconus tool box. In addition, aberration-control optics are being implemented into some soft keratoconus designs and appear to be promising in optimizing the quality of vision. The results have been very promising. In one study, 80 eyes were refit into a specialty keratoconic soft lens after experiencing reduced tolerance or poor fitting with other designs. Ninety-one percent resulted in corrected VA of equal to or better than 20/40.[165] Patients with nipple and globus-type cones with a relatively concentric 360-degree peripheral topography appear to be the best candidates, whereas patients with large-diameter, sagging (i.e., inferior) cones may be poor candidates because the inferior steepening of the cornea can result in inferior edge lift.[166] Several designs are commercially available and are shown in Table 19.14.[167]

Representative Soft Lens Designs

KeraSoft (Bausch + Lomb): The KeraSoft lens from Bausch + Lomb and manufactured by Art Optical and other laboratories and has the benefit of being manufactured in the silicone hydrogel Definitive material (Contamac), which has a 74% water content and a Dk of 60.[168–170] This is a recently introduced custom latheable design, which also has a front aspheric or aspheric toric

TABLE 19.14 Soft Contact Lenses for Keratoconus

MANUFACTURER	LENS NAME
ABB Concise	Concise K
	Soft K
Advanced Vision Technologies	Eni-Eye Soft K (hydrogel 67% water)
	Eni-Eye Soft K (Definitive Si-Hy material)
Alden Optical	NovaKone
Bausch + Lomb	Kerasoft IC
Continental SL	Continental Cone
Gelflex USA	Keratoconus Lens
Ocu-Ease	Ocu-Flex K
Orion Vision	Bioperm
SLIC	Solus Soft K Lens
United Contact Lens	UCL-55
X-Cel Contacts	Tricurve Keratoconus
Visionary Optics	Hydrokone

TABLE 19.15 KeraSoft IC ST Fitting Set/Design Information

Standard Fitting Set Parameters (Bausch + Lomb)

BASE CURVE RADIUS (mm)	DIAMETER (mm)	PERIPHERY	POWER
7.80	14.5	STD	Plano
8.00	14.5	STD	Plano
8.20	14.5	STD	Plano
8.40	14.5	STD	Plano
8.60	14.5	STD	Plano
8.80	14.5	STD	Plano
8.20	14.5	FLT2	Plano
8.60	14.5	STD2	Plano

Design Information
BCRs: 7.40 to 9.40 (0.20-mm steps)
Diameter: 14.50 (standard); 14.00, 15.00, and 15.50 mm are available
Periphery options: Standard, STEEP1, STEEP2, STEEP3, STEEP4, FLAT1, FLAT2, FLAT3, FLAT4
Power: sphere: +20.00 to −20.00 D; cylinder: −0.50 to −12.00 D (in 0.25-D steps); axis: 1 to 180 degrees (in 1-degree steps)
Material: Efrofilcon A, 74% water (Definitive material from Contamac); Dk = 60

prism-ballasted design with balanced overall thickness and spherical aberration control. The entire periphery can be steepened or flattened in four gradual steps independent of the overall base curve. In addition, up to two sectors of the periphery can be modified independently of each other. (Sector Management Control or SMC). It is available in up to 12 D of cylinder correction and is replaced on a quarterly basis. The diagnostic fitting set and design parameter information is provided in Table 19.15 and Figure 19.15.

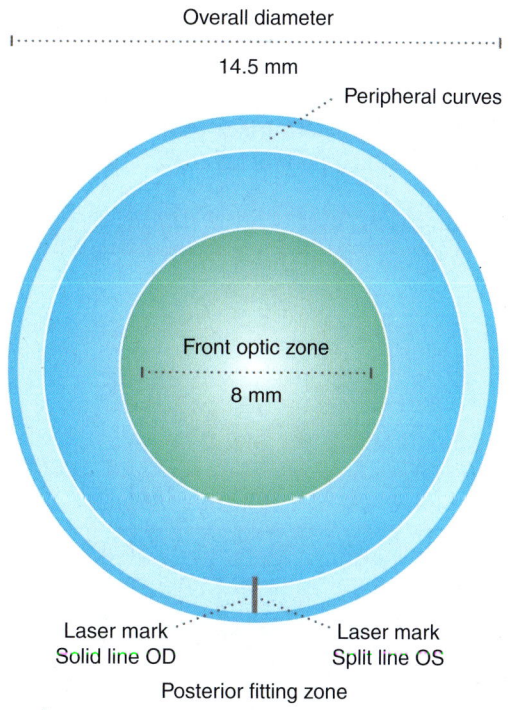

FIGURE 19.15 The KeraSoft lens (Bausch + Lomb).

TABLE 19.16 NovaKone Fitting Set/Design Information

Premium 18-Lens Diagnostic Set (Alden Optical)

BASE CURVE RADIUS (mm)	FITTING CURVE (mm)	SPHERE POWER (D)	I.T. FACTOR
8.6	8.6	−4.00	0, 1, & 2
8.2	8.6	−5.00	0, 1, & 2
7.8	8.4	−6.00	0, 1, & 2
7.4	8.4	−6.00	0, 1, & 2
7.0	8.2	−8.00	0, 1, & 2
6.6	8.2	−9.00	0, 1, & 2

Design Information
BCRs: 5.40 to 8.60 (0.40-mm steps; others available in 0.10-mm steps)
Diameter: 15.0 mm (standard); others available in 0.1-mm steps
Fitting curve: 8.2, 8.4, and 8.6 mm as standard; others available in 0.1-mm steps
Power: sphere: +30.00 to −30.00 D; cylinder: −0.25 to −10.00 D (in 0.25-D steps); axis: 1 to 180 degrees (in 1-degree steps)
Material: Benz G4X, 54% water, Hioxifilcon

NovaKone (Alden Optical): Another recently introduced soft lens for the correction of keratoconus is the NovaKone design. Like KeraSoft, it is replaced on a quarterly basis and corrects a high amount of refractive astigmatism (up to 10 D). It is a unique design in a Benz G4X 54% water content material.[168,169] The base curve is selected equal to the mean keratometry value. Adjacent to the base curve is the fitting curve, which is flatter to align with the peripheral cornea and conjunctiva. This curve can be altered independently of the central base curve. The center thickness can be varied to help mask some of the corneal irregularity in a keratoconus patient. The diagnostic fitting set and design parameter information is provided in Table 19.16 and Figure 19.16.

HydroKone (Visionary Optics): The HydroKone is a custom design, which is available in two different hydrogel materials, a 59% water (Hioxifilcon, Dk = 24), and a 55% water (Methafilcon, Dk = 18). The back surface of the lens consists of a steep central curve, a flatter paracentral curve, and a final peripheral curve. All curves are aspheric and the central curve approximates

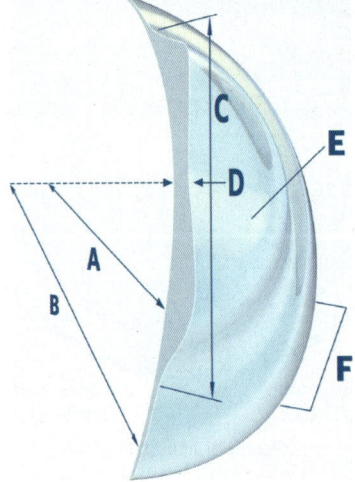

FIGURE 19.16 The NovaKone lens (Alden Optical). *A,* Posterior surface of the lens. *B,* Fitting curve. *C,* Aspheric central optical section of the anterior surface. *D,* Central thickness. *E,* Front-surface cylinder optics. *F,* Dual elliptical stabilizatin.

TABLE 19.17 Hydrokone Fitting Set/Design Information

DIAGNOSTIC SET (VISIONARY OPTICS)

Fitting sets for three different designs:

1. Standard: central steep zone (mild-to-moderate keratoconus)
2. Globus: large sagittal depth (ectasia of most of cornea)
3. Pellucid: reverse geometry (ectasia of large sector of cornea)

Diagnostic lenses: 14.8-mm diameter; 8.6 mm paracentral fitting curve

1. 9-lens diagnostic set: 5.3–8.5 mm BCRs in 0.4-mm steps
2. 6-lens diagnostic set: 6.5–8.5 mm BCRs in 0.4-mm steps

Design Information
BCRs: 4.1 to 9.3 mm
Diameter: 12.0 to 17.0 mm
Power: sphere: +50.00 to −75.00 D (in 0.25-D steps); cylinder: −0.25 to −15.00 D (in 0.25-D steps); axis: 1 to 180degrees (in 1-degree steps)
Material (standard): Hioxifilcon A, 59% water (Dk = 24)
Material: Methafilcon A, 55% water (Dk = 18)

---

hyperbolic aspheres in larger sagittal depths. It is available in almost any conceivable diameter, spherical power, and cylinder power. In addition to a standard design, a globus design, with a larger sagittal depth for a larger cone, and a reverse geometry design for pellucid or inferior apex keratoconus patients are available.[171] The diagnostic fitting set and design parameter information is provided in Table 19.17.

Piggyback Lenses

These designs either consist of a rigid lens fit over top of a soft lens or some form of integration of a rigid lens into a soft lens carrier. It is often a viable option in individuals who either cannot tolerate a rigid lens or a good lens-to-cornea fitting relationship cannot be obtained. The underlying (or adjacent) hydrogel lens improves tolerance and corneal protection while the GP provides optimum vision. The soft lens also offers some amount of protection to the cornea. Two forms of piggyback-type designs will be discussed: (a) Traditional piggyback designs; and (b) Countersunk rigid lens–soft lens carrier.

Traditional piggyback designs: With this combination design, a high-Dk/t soft lens is fitted initially so that both good movement and centration is achieved. A disposable lens, preferably a silicone hydrogel, is recommended. Daily disposable lenses are also popular to avoid additional cleaning steps of soft lenses. The use of a manufacturer who makes custom soft lenses in steeper BCRs, including the KeraSoft design, may be necessary if stock disposable lenses result in edge standoff.

There are two different approaches to fitting the piggyback system.[172] The most common scenario is the GP wearer who loses tolerance to lens wear. In this case, a low minus (i.e., −0.50 D) silicone hydrogel lens is fit underneath the GP. If this is a new fitting, a soft lens can be fit and, if successful, keratometry is then performed over the anterior surface of the soft lens. A hyper-permeable GP lens should be fit with both minimal edge and center thickness to promote good centration and decreased lid sensation.[79,173] This is quite important as the rigid lens is now further away from the cornea as a result of the presence of the soft lens. There are several accepted concepts in the selection of a soft lens power. Some practitioners prefer to fit with negligible power (+ or −0.50 D) and then fit the rigid lens in the same manner as would have been fit without the soft lens in place.[174] This method is especially useful if the patient uses piggyback lenses intermittently for comfort or if the soft lens is expected to be discontinued as the patient's adaptation to the rigid lens improves. A moderate plus power lens (i.e., approximately +6.00 D) has been recommended on patients with an inferior apex and for which the GP lens tends to decenter.[175] This effectively moves the apex of the fitting surface to a centered position. If this method is used, the rigid lens is typically fitted 0.5 to 1.0 D flatter than the steep keratometry value.

The lenses should move independently.[172] That is, the rigid lens and the soft lens neither adhere nor move as one unit. Therefore, the rigid lens should not be fit too steep to encourage lens adherence. If adherence is present, the GP lens periphery should be flattened. If central bubbles are present, the BCR of the GP lens should be flattened; if the bubbles are present peripherally, the BCR should be steepened. The fluorescein pattern of a GP lens can be evaluated on top of the silicone hydrogel lens, because these soft lenses will not readily imbibe the fluorescein molecules. Fluorescein of high molecular weight is required for this purpose when conventional hydrogel lenses are worn.

If the corneal apex is not decentered, the power of a piggyback should be placed in the GP lens as the power is not additive. In fact, the effective power produced by a soft lens will, at average, equal 20% to 25% of the labeled power of the lens.[176,177] For example, a -3.00 D soft lens with a BCR of 7.00 mm will have an effective power of -0.65 D in a piggyback system.[178]

A care system approved for both GP and soft lenses should be used on both systems for ease (i.e., Clear Care, Alcon). However, if needed for wettability, the rigid lens can be cleaned with a compatible rigid lens cleaner and stored in an approved rigid lens storage solution. Most importantly, the rigid lens should be rinsed with soft lens solution (never water) before inserting over the soft lens. Patients should be instructed to insert the soft lenses first, but the rigid lenses are removed first.

Countersunk rigid lens–soft lens carrier

The Flexlens piggyback system: The Flexlens piggyback system (X-Cel Contacts/Walman Optical) was first introduced in the 1970s.[179] It consists of a hydrogel lens with a cutout section in the center for a rigid lens to fit. It is available in a 45% water content hefilcon A or 55% water content methafilcon A. The OAD of the soft lens is 14.5 with a typical cutout diameter of 10.2 mm. A standard thin GP lens design that is 1.0 mm smaller (9.2 mm) is placed within the recessed cutout (Fig. 19.17).[172,180] The main purpose of the Flexlens Piggyback is to assist in the centration of the rigid lens. The biggest drawbacks of this lens include the low-Dk hydrophilic material and nondisposability of the product.

The "Pillow" Lens: The Pillow Lens is manufactured by Fusion Technologies in conjunction with EyeVis Eye and Vision Technologies. Similar to the Flexlens, the GP lens sits within the

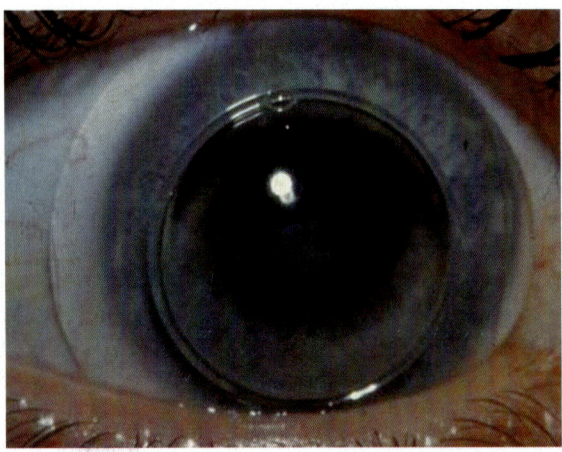

FIGURE 19.17 The Flexlens (X-Cel Contacts/Walman Optical).

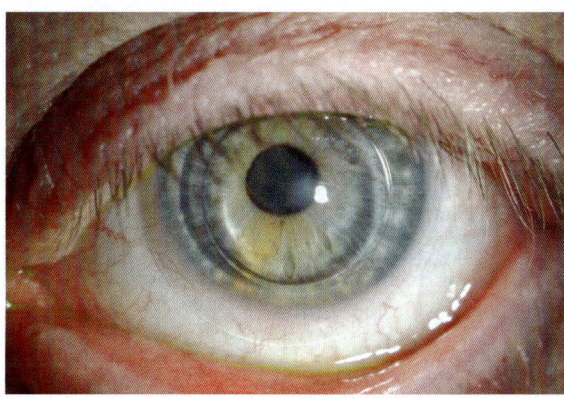

FIGURE 19.18 The Pillow Lens.

recess or "pillow" of a thick customized soft-lens carrier.[172,181,182] This system creates a vision correction modality where the soft recessed pillow positions the lens and the contained GP lens provides the optimal vision correction (Fig. 19.18).

Soft Versus GP Lenses for Aberration Control: The ability of GP lenses to mold and mask the anterior corneal toricity with an irregular cornea, reduce corneal aberrations, often resulting in several Snellen acuity lines improvement in VA, has made this modality the preferable ophthalmic correction.[183–186] However, the impact of GP lenses upon the already highly aberrated keratoconic cornea is highly under debate. The first challenge is that corneal irregularity of the corneal posterior surface, common in keratoconus, cannot be masked by a lens sitting on the front surface, and this may limit a patient's vision potential.[187–189] Secondly, the movement and rotation of the lens can possibly result in an increase in aberrations as the front surface of a GP lens is typically spherical and the movement of a GP lens on an irregular cornea can produce asymmetric refractive surfaces and an increase in coma aberrations.[184,188,190–193] Specifically, it has been found that, in low higher-order aberration (HOA) keratoconic eyes, GP lenses resulted in an increase in HOAs, primarily as a result of increased coma; in high HOA eyes, the HOAs decreased. In both groups, the vertical coma changed directions with GP lens wear.[194] Certainly, the incorporation of front-surface aspheric optics to reduce aberrations can be beneficial; if the lens decenters, coma can be induced, which may eliminate the benefits of aberration control. Overall, it is evident that, due to these factors, the visual performance in GP-wearing eyes in keratoconus is impacted by the limited ability to correct for—and sometimes actually adding to—the already significant presence of HOAs.[195]

The aforementioned results supported the need for providing a custom aberration-correcting soft lens, which is stable on the eye to improve the overall quality of vision.[195,196] Several recent studies have been very promising in the use of custom, typically wavefront-guided, aberration-correcting soft lenses, notably in providing improved visual performance.[197–199] Marsack et al.[199] found that in a small sample of three GP-wearing keratoconic subjects refit into custom wavefront-guided soft lenses, all subjects achieved high-contrast VA equal to or better than what was achieved with their habitual GP lenses. Although not all studies have been this promising when comparing custom soft lenses to GPs,[200] it is evident that custom wavefront-driven soft lenses will represent an important future tool in the contact lens correction of the keratoconic patient.

Hybrid Lenses

Hybrid lenses incorporate a rigid lens center and a soft periphery. One-lens system provides certain benefits over piggyback options such as ease of care, less handling, and perhaps improved comfort as there is no sensation of the rigid lens edge. The previous generations of materials utilized low-Dk materials for both the GP center and the soft lens surround. Problems with these designs included adherence, corneal hypoxia due to the relatively low Dk of both materials, and tearing of the lens at the rigid lens–soft lens junction.[201,202]

The SynergEyes Lens (SynergEyes, Inc.) was long awaited by many practitioners as a way to solve the hypoxic complications of the lower-Dk predecessors. The original SynergEyes lenses introduced to the market incorporates a central 8.2-mm rigid lens center made of Paragon HDS 100 material and a 14.5-mm nonionic 27% water hydrophilic skirt. The benefits of a hyper-Dk GP center and a more durable soft–GP junction resulted in a reduction in both the hypoxia-related and tearing-related problems of previous hybrid designs. There are four types of lenses available, including designs for: typical ametropias (SynergEyes A), keratoconus (SynergEyes keratoconus), multifocals (SynergEyes M), and oblate postsurgical cases (SynergEyes PS).

A fitting set is mandatory to fit these lenses. The SynergEyes K trial set parameters and design information are provided in Table 19.18.

This lens is promoted to be fit with apical clearance to allow for a fluid tear layer beneath the rigid portion to avoid adherence and corneal compromise (Fig. 19.19).[149,172] Multiple skirt radii are available to assist in lens centration and movement. There should be an absence of bubbles centrally and light touch at the rigid lens–soft lens junction. The lens should land evenly on the soft skirt without impingement or edge fluting. Lens movement should be evident with the blink or, at minimum, with the push-up test. The use of OCT can be beneficial to ensure a proper fit.[203] When applying the lens, the bowl of the lens should be completely filled with preservative-free saline solution and a high-molecular-weight fluorescein should also be instilled into the lens bowl. It is recommended to apply the lens to the inferior region of the cornea and push it toward the superior corneas with a single motion.[203] This spreads the

TABLE 19.18 SynergEyes KC Lens Diagnostic Set and Lens Parameters

Diagnostic Fitting Set

ASPHERIC BASE CURVE RADIUS (mm/D)	POWER (D)	FLAT SKIRT (mm)	MEDIUM SKIRT (mm)	STEEP SKIRT (mm)
5.7 (59.00)	−14.00	8.5	8.2	7.9
5.9 (57.00)	−14.00	8.5	8.2	7.9
6.1 (55.50)	−12.00	8.5	8.2	7.9
6.3 (53.50)	−10.00	8.8	8.5	8.2
6.5 (52.00)	−8.00	8.8	8.5	8.2
6.7 (50.50)	−6.00	8.8	8.5	8.2
6.9 (49.00)	−5.00	8.8	8.5	8.2
7.1 (47.50)	−4.00	9.1	8.8	8.5

Lens Parameters
Made-to-Order
Diameter: 14.5 mm
Base curve: 5.7 to 7.1 in 0.2-mm steps
Sphere power: +4.00 to −16.00 D in 0.50-D steps
Skirt curve radius: steep, median, and flat
Custom
Diameter: 14.5 mm
Base curve: 5.7 to 7.1 in 0.2-mm steps
Sphere power: +4.50 to +20.00 D in 0.50-D steps
 −16.50 to −20.00 D in 0.50-D steps
Skirt curve radius: steep, median, and flat

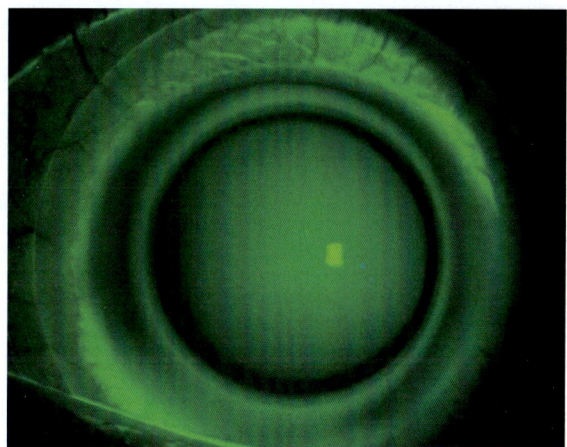

FIGURE 19.19 SynergEyes KC lens. (Courtesy of Dr. Barry Eiden.)

wetting agent to allow coverage of the entire anterior surface, forcing out any air between lens and cornea. The lens should be allowed to sit for 3 to 5 minutes prior to evaluating the lens-to-cornea fitting relationship.[172]

The SynergEyes KC lens is designed for moderate keratoconus with the standard "A" design for early keratoconus. These designs are recommended for central nipple cones or very central prolate corneas.[172] For oval cones and decentered cones, SynergEyes introduced the ClearKone lens in 2009. The ClearKone lens is a reverse geometry design and is fit based upon corneal vault. The center of the lens is alignment fitting whereas the steeper curve of the lens is positioned more peripherally on the GP section of the lens. This design would not be recommended for ectasia that extends beyond the landing zone or for a highly irregular landing pattern as often observed in advanced PMD.[149] Although more suited for postsurgical patients, the SynergEyes PS lens is a viable option in oblate keratoconic corneas.

Recently, SynergEyes introduced their Duette and UltraHealth lenses. These designs have a higher Dk[130] UV-blocking GP center with a low-modulus, higher Dk[84] silicone hydrogel surround. Although the Duette lens is not available in steep BCRs, this design can be a useful option in early keratoconus. The UltraHealth lens is fit on a vault system similar to the Clear Cone design and is targeted for keratoconus patients.

Overall, the SynergEyes designs have been successful when other options are not.[204] However, tight-fitting lens problems can result in patient discontinuation of lens wear, and either short-term edema[158,205] or even lens tightening problems after months of lens wear.[149]

Contact Lens Selection

There are obviously many factors that need to be considered when fitting a keratoconic patient. These include the type of cone and the severity of the condition. Fortunately, there are many tools available to be able to successfully fit almost every keratoconic patient into a specific custom contact lens. One such selection system from the primary author is given in Table 19.19.

ALTERNATIVE METHODS OF MANAGEMENT

Primary Surgical Procedures

Keratoconus represents the most common corneal thinning disorder and, as a group, comprise the second most common indication for corneal transplantation in the United States, totaling nearly 16% of all cases in one study.[110] Anywhere from 10% to 22% of patients diagnosed with keratoconus will require a corneal transplant.[1,4,6,12,115, 206–208] The primary indications for the

TABLE 19.19 Keratoconus Contact Lens Selection	
TYPE OF CONE	RECOMMENDED DESIGNS
Nipple	Small OAD/OZD keratoconic design Custom soft lens design
Oval	Intralimbal GP Small OAD/OZD keratoconic (unless large oval) Custom soft design Hybrid
Globus	Intralimbal GP Mini-Scleral Hybrid or piggyback
Marginal	Same as globus
PROGRESSION	RECOMMENDED DESIGNS
Mild	Small OAD/OZD keratoconic Custom soft design Hybrid
Moderate	Intralimbal GP Small OAD/OZD keratoconic (if nipple cone) Mini-scleral if "1" or "2" decenter/poor comfort
Severe	Intralimbal Mini-scleral (if "1" decenters/poor comfort) Piggyback Hybrid

need for some form of corneal transplant primarily pertain to cases in which a stable contact lens fit was not possible to achieve—or tolerated—or extensive axial corneal scarring was present, which resulted in unacceptable VA and possibly extreme corneal thinning.[41] High risk factors for the eventual need for some form of surgical procedure would appear to be (a) onset at a young age (<20 years of age), (b) >55 D keratometry readings, (c) best-corrected VA less than 20/40, and (d) apical scarring.[4,209] Studies have confirmed, however, that corneal surgery can be delayed or avoided by the application of contact lenses in the large majority of cases.[208,210,211] It is imperative that every attempt should be made to achieve a successful contact lens fit prior to considering a surgical option. This is especially true today as the challenges previously experienced with lens intolerance and poor fitting relationships are minimized with the introduction of semi-scleral, hybrid, and soft lens designs; therefore, the incidence of corneal surgery should decrease in the near future. The primary surgical procedures used today are penetrating keratoplasty (PKP) and deep anterior lamellar keratoplasty (DALK).

Penetrating Keratoplasty (PKP)

When surgery is indicated, a full thickness corneal transplant or PKP is the primary procedure performed. In the CLEK study, 9.8% of patients at baseline had a PKP in one eye; this figure is low as bilateral PKP patients were excluded from the study. During the course of the 8-year study, 12% of those patients who started the study free of PKP in either eye proceeded to a PKP in one or both eyes.[212]

Until recently, PKP has been the surgical procedure performed in the great majority of keratoconus patients requiring surgery. The benefits of PKP are many, including nearly a century of practice with good outcomes. There has been reported as high as 96% success resulting in clear grafts.[112,213–215] This appears to be related, in part, to the integrity of the peripheral cornea in keratoconus. Performing a PKP is not as technically difficult as other surgical procedures;

it can also be performed using a retrobulbar block if the patient is unable to be placed under general anesthesia.[216]

There are also several challenges to PKP that have resulted in DALK and other procedures gaining favor in recent years. The procedure is "open sky" due to the full thickness transplant leaving the remainder of the eye open to the outside world. This increases the risk of two sight-threatening complications: infection and expulsive choroidal hemorrhages during surgery.[216] The fact that free-hand sutures are used to secure the PKP graft to the host cornea often results in a high amount of postoperative astigmatism in the new corneal graft. Studies have found that, although as high as 73% achieve a best-corrected VA of better than 20/40,[215] anywhere from 15% to 31% of PKP patients have postoperative corneal astigmatism >5 D.[217–220] Most PKP patients will require visual correction after surgery, with up to 30% wearing spectacles and 47% contact lenses.[221] After PKP, there is rapid endothelial cell loss over the first 4 years.[222,223]

The use of an excimer laser has recently been used to cut customized donor button edges and corresponding shapes in the recipient bed.[224,225] This eliminates the mechanical trephine currently used and allows for greater healing success as well as a more accurate refraction. However, as with the mechanical procedure, endothelial loss is a concern and the visual recovery may still be slow.[226]

Graft rejection is also probable over time and young graft patients will likely need one or more repeated grafts during their lifetime.[227] It has been found that, within the first 15 years, keratoconus patients will have a greater graft survival rate than the overall survival rate (i.e., 97% vs. overall 90% at 5 years; 92% vs. 82% at 10 years).[228] In a registry study of over 4,800 eyes receiving a corneal graft for keratoconus, the survival rates of first grafts were 89% at 10 years, 49% at 20 years, and 17% at 23 years, and, after 15 years, the survival rates were no better than other causes of PKP surgeries.[227]

Deep Anterior Lamellar Keratoplasty (DALK)

The potential negative outcomes with full thickness transplants have led many surgeons to embrace other procedures, most notably, DALK. The exact procedure tends to vary between surgeons; essentially, the surgery consists of removing all of the corneal tissue anterior to Descemet's membrane and endothelium. A donor corneal graft with both Descemet's membrane and endothelium removed is then placed into the surgically created defect.[216] Often DALK involves using filtered air to separate the underlying Descemet's membrane and endothelium from the corneal stroma, termed the Anwar "big bubble" technique. As keratoconus is a stromal ectasia and not an endothelial dystrophy, the host endothelium does not need to be removed to correct irregular astigmatism. Therefore, the complications potentially resulting from the "open-sky" technique are reduced. DALK also eliminates endothelial rejection and results in less than one-half of the endothelial cell loss that occurs within the first 5 years after surgery.[229–232] Overall, the complication rate has been less with DALK when compared to PKP in most studies,[230–234] although they have been equal in a few other studies.[235,236] In addition, patients in whom a DALK has failed can still undergo a PKP. There is also recent evidence that graft survival is longer with DALK than PKP. In a study of 660 eyes having undergone DALK, 74% as a result of keratoconus, the graft survival rate was 99.3% after 9 years.[237]

However, there are also challenges with DALK. The visual outcomes are typically equal to PKP[230,236,237,238] and may result in reduced VA when compared to PKP.[231] If reduced vision does occur, it could be the result of opacities and light scattering at the host–donor interface.[237] In addition, the procedure itself is technically more difficult to perform. Perforations, although predominantly microperforations, in Descemet's membrane can occur in close to 10% of DALK eyes[229] and some of these eyes will then necessitate PKP surgery.[230]

However, overall, DALK and similar lamellar keratoplasties, can be considered as the first surgical option for patients with keratoconus. This is the result of comparable visual outcomes, better preservation of the integrity of the globe, reduction in intraoperative complications, less endothelial cell loss, and essentially the elimination of endothelial graft rejection.[237] In addition, automated microkeratome-assisted and excimer laser-assisted lamellar keratoplasties are resulting in more refractive accuracy and, therefore, are replacing manual procedures. Outcomes also appear to be improving with the improved techniques to separate Descemet's membrane from the posterior stroma, such as the "small bubble" technique.[239]

Other Procedures

Intrastromal Corneal Ring Segments (Intacs)

Intacs are arclike, PMMA intrastromal corneal ring segments that are surgically inserted into the deep stroma.[240,241] They have been approved by the US Food and Drug Administration (FDA) since 2004 with an expanded range approved by the FDA in 2010. Intacs can be placed manually into the cornea or, more recently, via channels created with the assistance of a femtosecond laser.[242–245] In keratoconus, Intacs are used to flatten the "cone" of the ectatic cornea; therefore, vision is improved.[216] During the surgical procedure, corneal tunnels at approximately 70% of the cornea thickness are created, creating a corneal pocket on each side of the incision. Intacs segments are then inserted into the respective corneal tunnels and the incision sites are then sutured.[240,241] Intacs also come in different sizes and, whereas Intacs are hexagonally shaped, Ferrara rings are triangular, and Bisantis segments are oval. Intacs will typically improve uncorrected and best-corrected VA and often reduce refractive error and flatten keratometry readings by anywhere from 2 to 4 D.[244,246–248]

Good candidates for Intacs include individuals with mild-moderate keratoconus with a steep keratometry reading no higher than the mid-50s, a spherical equivalent refractive error less than 5 D, and a minimum corneal thickness of, at minimum, 450 microns over the region where the Intacs will be inserted.[249–252] In addition, individuals who are contact lens intolerant and not desiring a corneal transplant are often good candidates if they meet the other criteria. It has been found that Intacs is not as beneficial in advanced keratoconus and, in fact, best-corrected VA loss is more likely.[253]

The 5-year results have been positive in terms of the effect on refractive error, vision, and the impact on stabilizing the cornea. However, significant residual refractive error is quite common and other forms of correction (i.e., often GP lenses or secondarily soft lenses or spectacles) are often necessary.[254,255] Also, as many as 10% of Intacs patients may require adjustment surgery.[256] Some possible complications from Intacs include extrusion of the segments, migration of the segments, epithelial defects, infection, halos and glare (in larger pupils), and stromal thinning and corneal melting if the rings are inserted too superficially.[52,253,257,258] It has been found, however, that the use of the femtosecond laser results in less incidence of many of these complications.[244,245,259]

At minimum, it is evident that Intacs is a reversible procedure that likely halts the progression of keratoconus and, in fact, over a 5-year period, 93% of Intacs patients did not experience progression of their keratoconus. Whereas it will not have as significant an effect as a more invasive procedure such as DALK,[260] Intacs may be a therapeutic option to halt this condition and, perhaps, allow some patients to avoid a corneal transplant.

Collagen Cross-Linking (CXL)

Spoerl and colleagues[261–263] introduced a procedure to reduce keratoconus via increasing corneal rigidity through stromal corneal cross-linking. Cross-linking is the addition of molecular bonds to increase the mechanical strength of tissue. Cross-links can be induced enzymatically and in vivo experiments have shown that UV radiation and riboflavin are the most effective and least harmful.[248] Riboflavin, which is vitamin B2, is the primary photosensitizer used in cross-linking; the riboflavin molecule absorbs the UV radiation and causes a cleavage of the oxygen, which splits off and causes the cross-linking in the tissue. Increasing the number of cross-links adds strength to the tissue. CXL increases both the biomechanical rigidity of the collagen lamellae and the collagen fiber diameter; therefore, the progression of the ectasia may be prevented.[52] In other words, the purpose of this procedure is to increase the rigidity of the corneal stroma; therefore, the shape of the cornea is stabilized.[264]

In this procedure, a topical anesthetic is applied and the surgeon removes corneal epithelium over a 7 mm diameter and adds a riboflavin 0.1% applied to the stroma to ensure absorption. Following this procedure, the cornea is exposed to 30 minutes of UV-A radiation, which increases the thickness of the collagen fibrils and results in a more rigid anterior half of the cornea.[73]

Numerous studies have found that CXL appears to stabilize the progression of keratoconus through increased corneal rigidity and often results in both a reduction in myopic refractive error, and flattening of the keratometry readings, typically by an amount equal to 2 to 3 D.[263,265–277] An improvement in corneal shape has been confirmed by a reduction in corneal and wavefront aberrations.[274,275] It has also improved patient's subjective visual functions, including reducing symptoms such as problems with night driving, difficulty reading, diplopia, glare, halos, starbursts, and foreign-body sensation.[278]

The procedure appears to be safe with few reports of complications. As a result of the epithelial removal involved in this procedure, traditional CXL necessitates a minimum corneal thickness of >400 microns.[279] When performed on thin corneas, problems such as posterior corneal elevation[280] and reduction in endothelial cell density[281] have been reported. Mild corneal haze can occur in isolated patients, but is usually gone by 6 months[264,265] and, in one study, a persistent corneal scar occurred in three eyes of treated patients after 1 year.[282] It is also currently believed that intraocular pressure increase may result from this procedure.[283,284] In addition, corneal permeability to topical drugs may be decreased after CXL.[283]

More recently, the procedure has been performed without epithelial debridement.[279,285] To overcome the problem of inability to perform CXL on thin corneas while also making the procedure more comfortable, a transepithelial cross-linking (TE-CXL or "epi-on") procedure has been developed. It has allowed for the treatment of thinner (i.e., 360–400 microns) corneas and may reduce the risk of infection. However, it may also result in a longer procedure as it may take more time to get a sufficient amount of riboflavin into the corneal stroma.[240]

Recently, numerous reports of combining CXL with other procedures have been quite promising in achieving a greater effect. As CXL reinforces stromal collagen and makes the cornea stronger, refractive surgery procedures such as photorefractive keratectomy (PRK) and laser-assisted in situ keratomileusis (LASIK) can be performed in ectatic patients after CXL with little risk postsurgical ectasia.[212] To date, the results have been quite promising.[110,286] CXL has also been successful when performed in combination with Intacs patients.[287,288] It has been found that CXL improves the effect of Intacs and, therefore, appears to act as an enhancement or stabilizing procedure.[287]

However, at this time, there is little CXL activity in the United States. Although Europe had over 300 centers providing CXL, the FDA has only recently approved three clinical trials,[289,290] although 150 centers have applied for the opportunity to initiate studies.[264]

CODING AND REIMBURSEMENT

A common challenge among practitioners who are fitting, refitting, and problem-solving keratoconus patients is the matter of appropriate coding for reimbursement to occur. As keratoconic patients often experience a significant improvement in vision with contact lenses versus spectacles, it is important to emphasize the medical need to third-party plans. Many third-party providers, with the notable exception being Vision Service Plan (VSP), do not customarily recognize keratoconus as a medical condition. The National Keratoconus Foundation (www.nkcf.org) has several useful resources, including an insurance reimbursement form available to send to third-party

TABLE 19.20 Diagnosis Codes for Keratoconus

CODE	CONDITION
370.60	Keratoconus, unspecified
370.61	Keratoconus, stable condition
370.62	Keratoconus, acute hydrops
368.8	Blurred vision
368.15	Monocular diplopia
367.22	Irregular astigmatism
368.13	Photophobia
371.00	Corneal scarring
371.32	Corneal straie
371.10	Fleischer's ring

plans, a brochure on medically necessary contact lens prescribing, and an article on "How to Code" from Dr. Carla Mack.[291]

Much of our understanding on how to bill and code for keratoconus have come from experts such as John Rumpakis,[292] Clarke Newman,[293,294] and Carla Mack.[287] Important diagnosis codes for keratoconus are provided in Table 19.20.

The above-mentioned procedures are often diagnostic of keratoconus and then it can be confirmed with corneal topography (CPT 92025) or pachymetry (CPT 76514). Once the decision to fit the patient into contact lenses is made, a relatively new code, CPT 92072 or "Fitting of contact lens for management of keratoconus, initial fitting" can be used. This code replaces the use of a 9231X code for keratoconus. It is important to note that the 92072 code is just for the initial fit; any subsequent fits/visits should be coded with the appropriate 9921X or 9201X code. This should also be appended with either a RT or LT modifier since it is a unilateral code. It is also very important to always bill for the lens materials separately using the appropriate Level II HCPCS-V-codes such as:

- V2510: Contact Lens, GP, spherical, per lens
- V2531: Contact Lens, GP, scleral, per lens
- V2511: Contact Lens, GP, toric, prism ballast, per lens
- V2520: Contact Lens, hydrophilic, spherical, per lens
- 99070: Contact Lens Supply of material

The fitting fee should not be considered as a global, annual fee to provide unlimited service at no charge. Refitting keratoconic patients is not uncommon and if it is not simply an "incidental revision of the contact lens," then another 9921X or 9201X code is appropriate to bill in addition to the appropriate materials V-code for lens supply. For office visits pertaining to complications, the established patient evaluation and management (9921X) codes can be used, keeping in mind that it is important to use the appropriate diagnostic code for the condition you are monitoring.[292]

RESOURCES

As mentioned before, the National Keratoconus Foundation (www.nkcf.org) has several resources for both patient and practitioner. In addition, the Gas Permeable Lens Institute (GPLI) has a four-part narrated powerpoint series on keratoconus from Dr. Christine Sindt available at www.gpli.info. This includes presentations on etiology and diagnosis, corneal topography, lens designs and fitting, and problem solving. In addition, the GPLI has several other resources, including an online case grand rounds book, a clinical pearls pocket guide, and monthly webinars in which the topic of contact lens management of the irregular cornea is emphasized.

An exceptional resource is your contact lens laboratory consultant. These individuals know their specific designs extremely well and consult on challenging irregular cornea cases every day. In particular, if they can be provided with as much information as possible (diagnostic lens parameters, topography maps, photos, or video), they can assist in both design and troubleshooting and, therefore, will be invaluable in the ultimate success of the keratoconic patient. They can also provide diagnostic sets, including loaner sets, for a given patient.

SUMMARY

Keratoconus is a condition that warrants proper management accompanied by careful monitoring. In most cases, the fitting of contact lenses will delay and often preclude surgical intervention. The most successful option has been the fitting of rigid GP contact lenses. However, other options including spectacles and soft lenses (in early cases) and piggyback, or hybrid, or semi-scleral designs (in advanced cases) should be used when indicated.

CLINICAL CASES

CASE 1

A 16-year-old patient, who is new to your office, presents with symptoms of a slight decrease in vision and a mild ghosting of images. She indicates a desire to simply have her spectacles updated. Your examination reveals the following:
Manifest refraction:

$$OD: -3.75 - 1.75 \times 162 \; 20/25$$
$$OS: -2.00 - 0.75 \times 006 \; 20/20$$

Keratometry:

OD: 44.12 @ 165; 46.00 @ 075 (slight mire distortion)
OS: 43.25 @ 180; 44.25 @ 090 (good mire quality)

Retinoscopy: scissors reflex present OD
Slit-lamp biomicroscopy: Vogt's striae present OD
Videokeratoscopy: localized region of steepening (steepest area equaled 49.00 D) 1 to 2 mm below corneal center

SOLUTION: This patient has keratoconus based on the presence of Vogt's striae, a scissors reflex with retinoscopy, and the 49 D region inferocentrally. In addition, the presence of mild irregular astigmatism in one eye only confirms the pattern of keratoconus, in which one eye progresses before the other eye.

CASE 2

A patient enters your office with symptoms of blurred vision through his spectacle correction. He has been a 20-year rigid lens wearer (10 years PMMA followed by 10 years in a 12-Dk lens material). Your examination reveals the following:
Manifest refraction:

$$OD: -4.75 - 1.25 \times 022 \; 20/25-$$
$$OS: -5.00 - 2.25 \times 162 \; 20/30$$

Keratometry:

OD: 42.12 @ 025; 44.00 @ 118 (slight mire distortion)
OS: 42.25 @ 160; 44.75 @ 071 (slight mire distortion)

Slit-lamp biomicroscopy:
With lenses: superior decentration OU
Without lenses: mild central corneal edema OU
Videokeratoscopy: superior flattening accompanied by inferior steepening with mild distortion OU

SOLUTION: This appears to be CWS. There is an absence of classical slit-lamp signs (i.e., Vogt's striae, Fleischer's ring, scarring), and the patient appears to have complications relating to contact lens-induced hypoxia. It is also likely that the superior fitting relationship is inducing a pseudokeratoconic color map because of superior molding accompanied by inferior steepening. This can be verified by having the patient remove his lenses and rechecking corneal topography a few hours (or days) later. The superior region should steepen, accompanied by inferior flattening.

CASE 3

An 18-year-old patient had been diagnosed with keratoconus 3 years ago. He has been wearing a spectacle correction, but his vision has reached a point where he has decided that contact lenses may be a viable option for him.
Your examination reveals the following:
Manifest refraction:

OD: $-4.75 - 2.50 \times 159$ 20/30$-$
OS: $-4.00 - 1.25 \times 010$ 20/25 $+$ 1

Keratometry (simulated):

OD: 47.12 @ 155; 50.00 @ 039 (mire distortion); apex (paracentral; slightly inferior-temporal)
OS: 45.25 @ 012; 46.75 @ 105 (mire distortion); apex: same as OD

Pupil size: 4 mm (normal room illumination) OU

SOLUTION: This patient would appear to be a good candidate for GP lenses. One method of fitting the patient would be to select a diagnostic lens with a BCR equal to the steep keratometry value. For example, in the right eye in this case that would equal 6.75 mm. Topical anesthetic can be used before lens application. If the fluorescein pattern shows apical clearance, a flatter lens can be used. If apical touch is obtained with a BCR equal to 6.89 mm and the power determined by adding the spherical overrefraction to the diagnostic lens power, the following lens can be ordered:

BCR: 6.89 mm
Secondary curve radius/width (SCR/W): 8.00/0.3 mm
Intermediate curve radius/width (ICR/W): 9.60/0.3 mm
Peripheral curve radius/width (PCR/W): 12.00/0.3 mm
OAD/OZD: 8.8/7.0 mm
Power: -6.50 D
Paragon HDS

CASE 4

A patient was diagnosed with keratoconus 6 years ago and has been wearing rigid GP lenses for the past 4 years. He has observed an increase in lens awareness as well as fluctuating vision over the past 12 months. Your examination reveals the following:
Keratometry:

OD: 46.12 @ 015; 48.00 @ 108 (slight mire distortion)
OS: 50.25 @ 152; 54.75 @ 071 (moderate mire distortion)

Slit-lamp biomicroscopy:
With lenses: inferior decentration with 3 mm of lag with the blink OU
Videokeratoscopy: an inferiorly displaced cone (approximately 2–2.5 mm) is shown OU

SOLUTION: The patient would be a good candidate for one of the keratoconus lens designs recommended for an inferiorly displaced cone. An intralimbal design would be recommended initially. If this design exhibits excessive inferior edge lift, the inferior edge can be "tucked in" via ordering the change recommended by the manufacturer (i.e., "steep-flat," "ACT," "Quadra-Kone," etc.). If this is not successful, a hybrid (i.e., SynergEyes), piggyback, or semi-scleral design can be used.

CASE 5

An advanced keratoconus patient reports to your office with symptoms of gradual left lens awareness for the past 6 months. Your examination reveals the following:
Slit-lamp biomicroscopy:
With lenses: lens adherence is present OS; the fluorescein pattern shows mild apical clearance and peripheral seal-off
Without lenses: central staining is accompanied by an outer compression ring
Lens design: OS: BCR: 7.00 mm; SCR: 8.00/0.4 mm; PCR: 10.00/0.3 mm; OAD/OZD: 9.2/7.8 mm

SOLUTION: The first step in this case would be to apply a flatter peripheral bevel (i.e., 12.00 mm). An additional option that could be helpful would be to decrease the OZD (e.g., from 7.8 to 7.2 or even 7.0 mm). Polishing the back surface of the lens will remove any trapped debris that tends to accumulate and assist in adhering the lens to the cornea.

CASE 6

An advanced keratoconus patient reports to your office with symptoms of intolerance with her GP lenses. Over the past 3 years, she has worn a variety of lens designs, all unsatisfactory from a comfort standpoint. She is very motivated to continue contact lens wear as a result of the vision benefits. Your examination reveals the following:
Slit-lamp biomicroscopy:
With lenses: lenses are decentering inferiorly
Without lenses: mild central staining is present

SOLUTION: This patient would be a good candidate for a piggyback or hybrid (i.e., SynergEyes) lens design. In any case in which comfort and/or lens centration is an ongoing problem, a piggyback or modified piggyback lens system can be used. One of the benefits of the piggyback system is that one can quickly determine whether it will be successful or not (i.e., do both the GP and soft lens fit properly). The selection of a silicone hydrogel lens material in combination with a hyperpermeable GP material is very important. The use of disposable lenses provides the capability of trying a piggyback design on a trial basis. For example, if they are already wearing a high or hyperpermeable Dk GP material, a disposable silicone-hydrogel lens can be worn with their conventional GP lens for a short period of time to see if the patient is more satisfied and comfortable with this lens combination.

CASE 7 (CONTRIBUTED BY LACEY HAINES, OD)

A 31-year-old computer programmer presents with keratoconus OS that has remained fairly stable over the last 4 years. He was not happy with his first attempt at GP lens wear due to discomfort and lens instability while playing sports and he was interested in soft contact lens options. His manifest refraction was OD $-2.25 -0.75 \times 085 = 20/15+$ and OS $-1.50 - 1.75 \times 107 = 20/20-$. Slit-lamp exam revealed mild meibomian gland dysfunction (MGD) OU, inferior Fleischer's ring OS, and mild central striae OS. Pentacam topography showed keratometry values were OD 42.4 @ 115; 42.8 @ 025 and OS 42.7 @ 180; 47.0 @ 090.

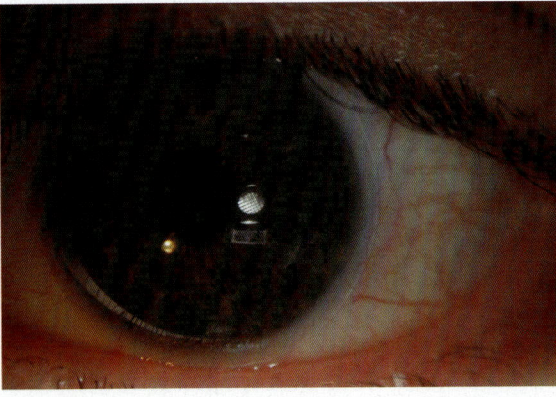

FIGURE 19.20 KeraSoft IC lens.

SOLUTION: He achieved excellent fit, vision, and comfort with a standard toric silicone hydrogel lens in his right eye. The final lens design was Biofinity Toric (CooperVision) 8.7 mm BCR/14.5 mm lens diameter (LD)/−2.00 −0.75 × 080, yielding a centered lens with adequate movement and no rotation, as well as VA of 20/15−. His left eye required more customized lens parameters and the Kerasoft IC lens design (Bausch + Lomb) was employed with the Definitive silicone hydrogel material (Contamac). The final lens design had 8.4 mm BCR/standard periphery/14.5 mm LD/−3.50 −1.25 × 171 = 20/20+ and had good centration and movement with 4 degree clockwise rotation on slit lamp (Fig. 19.20). For management of the mild MGD, a once-daily regimen of warm compresses and lid scrubs along with Blink Contacts artificial tears (Abbott Medical Optics) as needed was recommended.

CASE 8 (CONTRIBUTED BY ALEX NIXON, OD)

A 41-year-old, white female presents for a comprehensive eye exam and contact lens fitting secondary to keratoconus. She was previously wearing small-diameter, GP lenses in both eyes with unknown parameters. She presented wearing glasses because she lost her right lens 3 weeks prior to the visit. She noted longstanding discomfort with contact lenses and symptoms of dryness. She does not use artificial tears due to a previous allergic reaction to an artificial tear.
Manifest Refraction:

OD: −4.25 −5.00 × 063   20/30
OS: −3.00 −5.00 × 118   20/25

SOLUTION: The patient was refit into a larger-diameter, intralimbal GP lens to provide more stable vision and reduce symptoms of discomfort. A diagnostic fitting was performed using the 10.8 mm Dyna-Z Intralimbal fitting set.
Based on her topographies (Fig. 19.21), it appeared as though the right eye would require a lens similar in shape to the left eye. Excessive clearance centrally and adequate edge clearance was found with 10.8 mm, 7.18 BCR lenses in both eyes. Central touch and excessive peripheral clearance was found with 7.50 BCR lenses of the same diameter in both eyes. The lenses were ordered in a smaller OAD (10.4 mm) to reduce the OZD, sagittal depth, and reduce the likelihood of bubble formation. The initial lenses ordered were:

OD: Dyna-Z Intralimbal 10.4 mm OAD/7.25 BCR/STD edge/−4.75 D/Optimum Extra
OS: Dyna-Z Intralimbal 10.4 mm OAD/7.25 BCR/STD edge/−2.50 D/Optimum Extra

DISPENSE 1:

OD: Slight superior and good lateral centration with good lid attachment. There was excessive central clearance with bubble formation supero-centrally. The edge lift was adequate. Vision was correctable to 20/25+2 with a −0.50 D overrefraction.

OS: Slight superior and good lateral centration with good lid attachment. Central pooling was present, but no bubbles formed. There was excessive edge lift present. Vision was correctable to 20/25 with −2.50 D overrefraction. Due to the bubble formation and excessive central clearance, the right lens was ordered 0.05mm flatter and the OAD was again reduced to

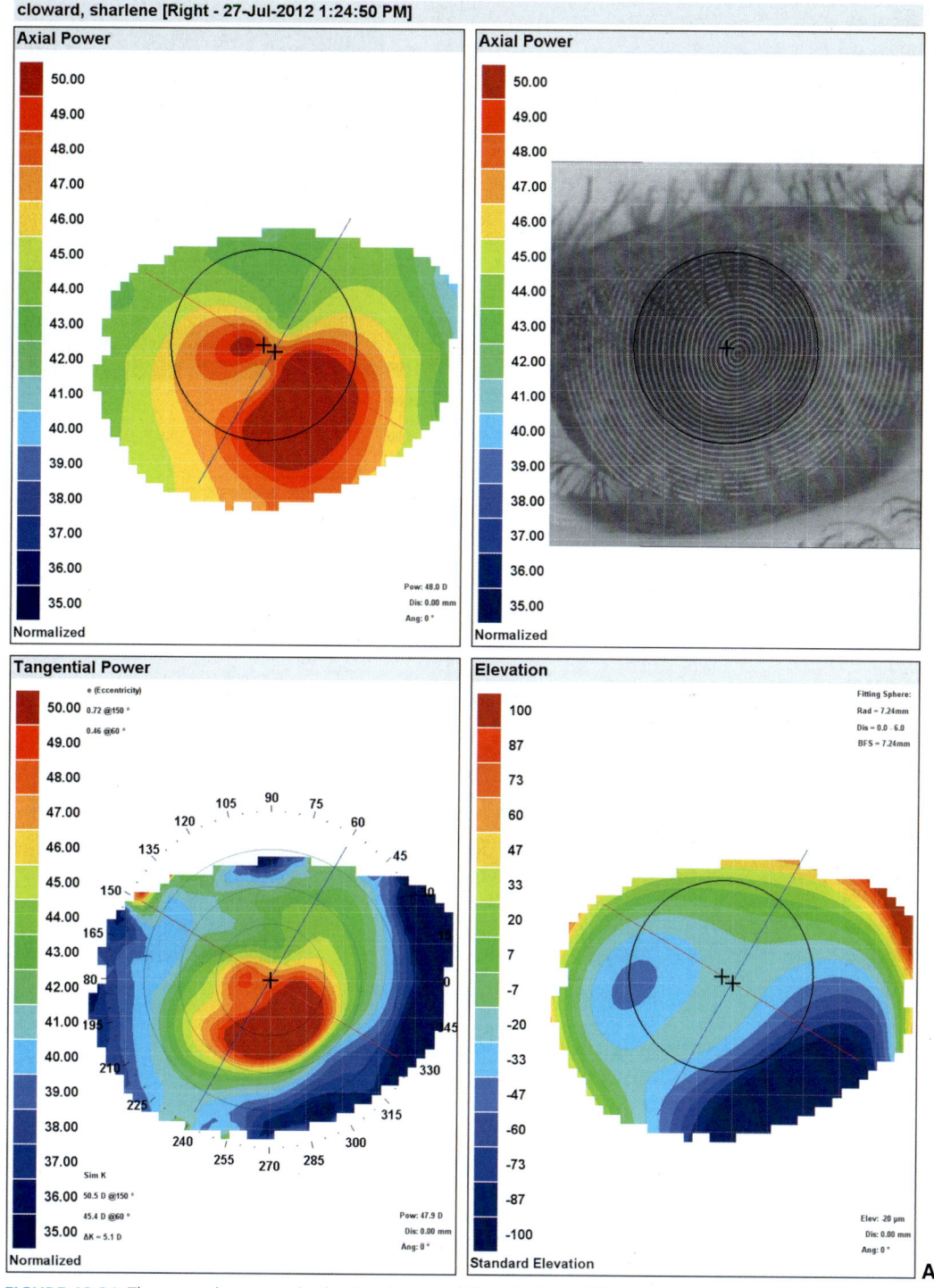

FIGURE 19.21 The corneal topography for the right eye (**A**) and left eye (**B**).

(continued)

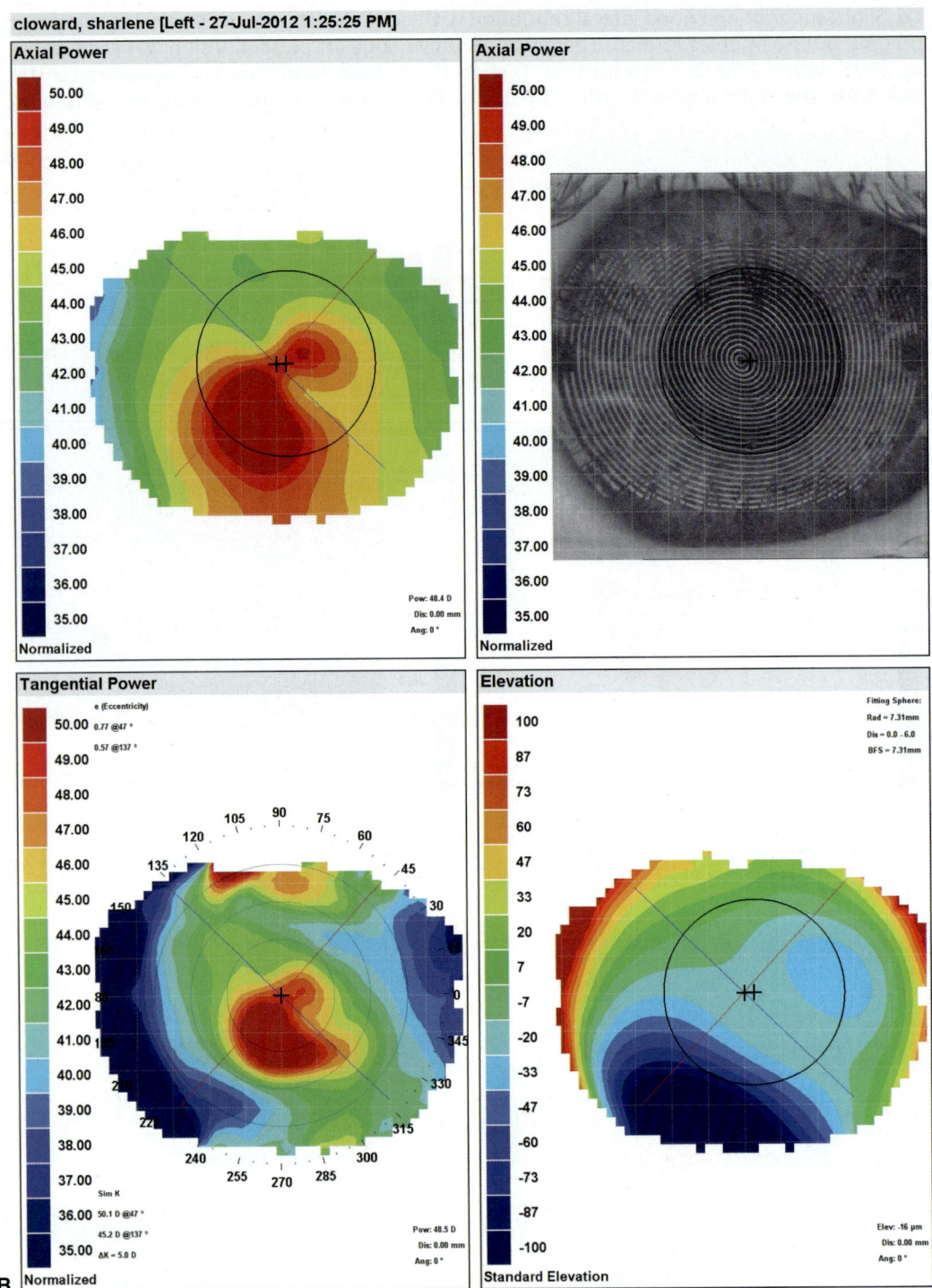

FIGURE 19.21 *(Continued)*

decrease sagittal depth and bubble formation. Since there was no bubble formation OS, this lens was only reduced in diameter and no change was made to the base curve. The peripheral curves were ordered one step steep OS to reduce edge clearance and standard curves were maintained OD.

The following lenses were ordered and the previous lenses dispensed:

OD: Dyna-Z Intralimbal 10.0 mm OAD/7.30 BCR/STD edge/−4.75 D/Optimum Extra
OS: Dyna-Z Intralimbal 10.0 mm OAD/7.25 BCR/1 steep edge/−5.00 D/Optimum Extra

DISPENSE 2:

OD: Slight superior and good lateral centration with good lid attachment. Alignment fit with slight inferior touch. The edge lift was adequate. Vision was correctable to 20/20−2 with a −0.25 D overrefraction (Fig. 19.22A).

OS: Slight superior and good lateral centration with good lid attachment. Alignment fit with slight inferior touch. The edge lift was adequate. Vision was correctable to 20/20 with a −0.50 D overrefraction (Fig. 19.22B).

The lenses were dispensed and there were no further adjustments to the fit or power of either lens. The patient noted improvement in comfort and vision compared to her previous contact lenses. As she was nearing presbyopia, the slight undercorrection provided a near boost in power and reduced her dependence on reading glasses. She was instructed to use Clear Care to clean the lenses and was dispensed samples of Refresh Optive Sensitive to avoid recurrence of the previous preservative toxicity.

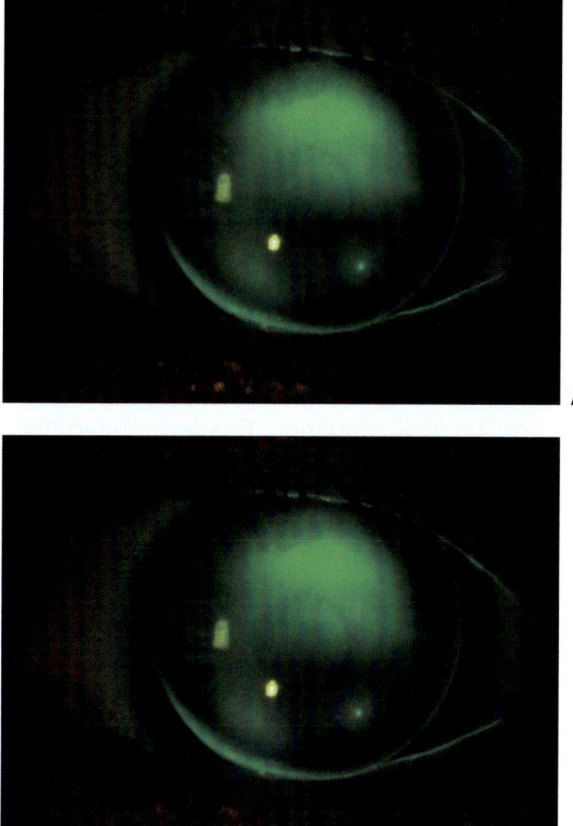

FIGURE 19.22 The fluorescein pattern of the right lens (**A**) and the left lens (**B**).

CLINICAL PROFICIENCY CHECKLIST

- Keratoconus is a progressive, asymmetric disease of the cornea that is characterized by steepening and distortion, apical thinning, and corneal ectasia.
- It is likely to be genetic in origin and often has an association with atopic conditions.
- Early symptoms include gradual blurring, ghost image formation, and distortion of vision.
- Early clinical signs include a scissors reflex with retinoscopy, and increase in irregular astigmatism, lack of parallellism with keratometry mires, and a localized area of steepening as shown with videokeratoscopy.
- Videokeratoscopy is important in the diagnosis and monitoring of keratoconus. The modified Rabinowitz–McDonnell criteria indicates that if the central corneal power is >47.2 D or if the difference between the inferior and superior paracentral regions is >1.4 D, suspect keratoconus. If the central corneal power is >48.7 D and the I–S value is >1.4 D, keratoconus can be diagnosed.
- Classic clinical signs of keratoconus as diagnosed with the slit-lamp biomicroscope are Vogt's straie, Fleischer's ring, and apical scarring.
- Keratoconus can be differentiated from CWS in that it is progressive, it may not be related to contact lens wear, it often progresses to >50 D, the aforementioned slit-lamp signs, and a localized affected region is identified via videokeratoscopy.
- One fitting philosophy utilizes a three-point touch relationship in which a diagnostic lens equal to the steep K reading is selected and, based upon the fluorescein pattern, changes are made to result in minimum apical touch.
- The OZD should decrease as the condition progresses. It is not uncommon for the OZD to approximate the BCR in millimeters unless a globus cone or a decentered apex is present.
- The use of a topical anesthetic during the diagnostic fitting process will be beneficial with keratoconic patients.
- A wide, flat PCR will reduce the risk of peripheral seal-off and adherence. In addition, newer designs have options to reduce edge lift inferiorly (i.e., "Flat-Steep" of ACT) as well as quadrant-specific posterior surfaces.
- A fluoro-silicone/acrylate lens material with a minimum Dk of 30 is recommended.
- A large-diameter (intralimbal) design is recommended when a small lens does not exhibit good centration. This design is recommended in cases of an inferior decentered apex or a large (globus) cone. A semi-scleral lens design can also be beneficial in these cases as well as moderate-severe keratoconus cases in which centration cannot be achieved with other, smaller designs.
- Several soft lens designs for keratoconus have recently been introduced and are indicated, both in early cases and when GP lenses are not well tolerated.
- When comfort or centration are problematic, a piggyback or hybrid lens can be used.
- Full thickness (PKP) and—more recently partial thickness (DALK)—corneal transplantation is highly successful in moderate-severe keratoconus cases in which a stable contact lens fit was not possible (or tolerated) or extensive apical corneal scarring was present.
- Intrastromal corneal ring implants (Intacs) inserted into the stroma have demonstrated promise in improving corrected and uncorrected VA via corneal flattening. It is a reversible procedure that can halt the progression of keratoconus and may allow some individuals to avoid a corneal transplant.
- CXL is a procedure that reduces keratoconus via increasing corneal rigidity. The combination of riboflavin with UV radiation—with or without an abraded corneal epithelium—typically results in a reduction in refractive error and flattening of the keratometry readings.

REFERENCES

1. Rabinowitz YS. Keratoconus. *Surv Ophthalmol*. 1998;42:297–319.
2. Krachmer JH, Feder RS, Belin MW. Keratoconus and related noninflammatory corneal thinning disorders. *Surv Ophthalmol*. 1984;28:293–322.
3. Kok O, Tan GFL, Loon SC. Review: keratoconus in Asia. *Cornea*. 2012;31(5):581–593.
4. Tuft SJ, Moodaley LC, Gregory WM, et al. Prognostic factors for the progression of keratoconus. *Ophthalmology*. 1994;101(3):439–446.
5. Wei RH, Zhao SZ, Lim L, et al. Incidence and characteristics of unilateral keratoconus classified on corneal topography. *J Refract Surg*. 2011;27(10):745–751.
6. Mandell RB. Contemporary management of keratoconus. *Int Cont Lens Clin*. 1997;24:(3&4):43–58.
7. Jimenez JL, Jurado JC, Rodriquez FJ, et al. Keratoconus: age of onset and natural history. *Optom Vis Sci*. 1997;74(3):149–151.
8. Barr JT, Wilson BS, Gordon MO, et al. Estimation of the incidence and factors predictive of corneal scarring in the Collaborative Longitudinal Evaluation of Keratoconus (CLEK) study. *Cornea*. 2006;25:16–25.
9. Kenney MC, Brown DJ, Rajeev B. The elusive causes of keratoconus: a working hypothesis. *CLAO J*. 2000; 26(1):10–13.
10. Kamiya K, Shimizu K, Ohmoto F. Effect of aging on corneal biomechanical parameters using the ocular response analyzer. *J Refract Surg*. 2009;25:888–893.
11. Elsheikh A, Wang D, Brown M, et al. Assessment of corneal biomechanical properties and their variation with age. *Curr Eye Res*. 2007;32:11–19.
12. Kennedy RH, Bourne WM, Dyer JA. A 48 year clinical and epidemiologic study of keratoconus. *Am J Ophthalmol*. 1986;101:267–273.
13. Nielsen K, Hjortal J, Aagaard Nohr E, et al. Incidence and prevalence of keratoconus in Denmark. *Acta Ophthalmol Scand*. July 23, 2007;[Epub ahead of print].
14. Georgiou T, Funnell CL, Cassels-Brown A, et al. Influence of ethnic origin on the incidence of keratoconus and associated atopic disease in Asians and white patients. *Eye*. 2004;18:379–383.
15. Bawazeer AM, Hodge WG, Lorimer B. Atopy and keratoconus: a multivariate analysis. *Br J Ophthalmol*. 2000; 84(8):834-836.
16. Galin MA, Berger R. Atopy and keratoconus. *Am J Ophthalmol*. 1958;45(6):904–906.
17. Harrison RJ, Klouda PT, Easty DL, et al. Association between keratoconus and atopy. *Br J Ophthalmol*. 1989; 73(10):816–822.
18. Al-Hussain H, Zeisberger SM, Huber PR, et al. Brittle cornea syndrome and its delineation from the kyphoscoliotic type of Ehlers-Danlos syndrome (EDS VI): report on 23 patients and review of the literature. *Am J Med Genet A*. 2004;124(1):28–34.
19. Capaccini A, Lampis R, Brogi M. Incidence of mesenchymosic manifestations in keratoconus. *Ann Ottalmol Clin Ocul*. 1963;89(suppl):1118–1122.
20. Gasset AR, Hinson WA, Frias JL. Keratoconus and atopic diseases. *Ann Ophthalmol*. 1978;10(8):991–994.
21. Goodman RM, Gazit E, Katznelson MB, et al. Four new heritable disorders of connective tissue. *Birth Defects Orig Artic Ser*. 1975;11(6):39–51.
22. Greenfield G, Stein R, Romano A, et al. Blue sclerae and keratoconus: key features of a distinct heritable disorder of connective tissue. *Clin Genet*. 1973;4(1):8–16.
23. McMonnies CW. Abnormal rubbing and keratectasia. *Eye Contact Lens*. 2007;33(6, pt 1):265–271.
24. McMonnies CW, Boneham GC. Keratoconus, allergy, itch, eye-rubbing and hand-dominance. *Clin Exp Optom*. 2003;86(6):376–384.
25. Macsai MS, Varley GA, Krachmer JH. Development of keratoconus after contact lens wear. Patient characteristics. *Arch Ophthalmol*. 1990;108(4):534–538.
26. Gasset AR, Houde WL, Garcia-Bengochea M. Hard contact lens wear as an environmental risk in keratoconus. *Am J Ophthalmol*. 1978;85(3):339–341.
27. Phillips CI. Contact lenses and corneal deformation: cause, correlate or co-incidence? *Acta Ophthalmol (Copenh)*. 1990;68(6):661–668.
28. Sommer A. Keratoconus in contact lens wear. *Am J Ophthalmol*. 1978;86(3):442–444.
29. Edwards M, McGhee CN, Dean S. The genetics of keratoconus. *Clin Exp Ophthalmol*. 2001;29(6):345–351.
30. Tuori AJ, Virtanen I, Aine E, et al. The immunohistochemical composition of corneal basement membrane in keratoconus. *Curr Eye Res*. 1997;16(8):792–801.
31. Sawaguchi S, Fukuchi T, Abe H, et al. Three-dimensional scanning electron microscopic study of keratoconus corneas. *Arch Ophthalmol*. 1998;116(1):62–68.
32. Zhou L, Sugar J, Yue BY. Normal lysosomal enzyme staining in skin tissues of patients with keratoconus. *Cornea*. 1996;15:409–413.
33. Rehany U, Lahav M, Shoshan S. Collagenolytic activity in keratoconus. *Ann Ophthalmol*. 1982;14:751.
34. Critchfield JW, Calandra AJ, Nesburn AB, et al. Keratoconus: I. Biochemical studies. *Exp Eye Res*. 1988;46:953–963.
35. Pouliquen Y, Graf B, de KY, et al. Mosphological study of keratoconus. *Arch Ophtalmol Rev Gen Opthalmol*. 1970;30:497–532.

36. Polack FM. Contributions of electron microscopy to the study of corneal pathology. *Surv Ophthalmol*. 1976; 20:375–414.
37. Mathew JH, Goosey JD, Bergmanson JPG. Quantified histopathology of the keratoconic cornea. *Optom Vis Sci*. 2011;88(8):988–997.
38. Gibson IK, Spurr-Michaud SJ, Tisdale AS. Anchoring fibrils form a complex network in human and rabbit cornea. *Invest Ophthalmol Vis Sci*. 1987;28:212–220.
39. Bergmanson JPG. *Clinical Ocular Anatomy and Physiology*. 16th ed. Houston, TX: Texas Eye Research & Technology Center; 2009.
40. Kemp EG, Lewis CJ. Immunoglobin pattern in keratoconus with particular reference to total and specific IgE levels. *Br J Ophthalmol*. 1982;66(11):717–720.
41. Zadnik K, Barr JT, Edrington TB, et al. Baseline findings in the Collaborative Longitudinal Evaluation of Keratoconus (CLEK) study. *Invest Ophthalmol Vis Sci*. 1998;39(13):2537–2546.
42. Ridley F. Eye rubbing and contact lenses. *Br J Ophthalmol*. 1961;45(9):631.
43. Weed KH, MacEwen CJ, Giles T, et al. The Dundee University Scottish Keratoconus study: demographics, corneal signs, associated diseases, and eye rubbing. *Eye (lond)*. 2008;22:534–541.
44. Korb DR, Leahy CD, Greiner JV. Prevalence and characteristics of eye-rubbing for keratoconic and non-keratoconic subjects. *Invest Ophthalmol Vis Sci*. 1991;32:1057. (ARVO abstract)
45. McMonnies C. Is eye rubbing really a contributing factor in keratoconus? Presented at: 2008 Global Keratoconus Congress; January 2008; Las Vegas, NV.
46. Owens H, Gamble G. A profile of keratoconus in New Zealand. *Cornea*. 2003;22(2):122–125.
47. Wang Y, Rabinowitz YS, Rotter JI, et al. Genetic epidemiological study of keratoconus: evidence for major gene determination. *Am J Med Genet*. 2000;93(5):403–409.
48. Tyynismaa H, Sistonen P, Tuupanen S, et al. A locus for autosomal dominant keratoconus: linkage to 16q22.3-q23.1 in Finnish families. *Invest Ophthalmol Vis Sci*. 2002;43(10):3160–3164.
49. Brancali F, Valente VM, Sarkozy A, et al. A locus for automsomal keratoconus maps to human chromosome 3p14-q13. *J Med Genet*. 2004;41(3):188–192.
50. Tang YG, Rabinowitz YS, Taylor KD, et al. Genomewide linkage scan in a multi-generation Caucasian pedigree indentifies a novel locus for keratoconus on chromosome 5q14.3-q21.1. *Genet Med*. 2005;7(6):397–405.
51. Li X, Rabinowitz YS, Tang YG, et al. Two-stage génome-wide linkage scan in keratoconus sib pair families. *Invest Ophthalmol Vis Sci*. 2006;47(9):3791–3795.
52. Yeung KK, Weissman BA. An updated perspective on keratoconus. *Rev Optom*. 2008;145(4):58–66.
53. Pathak D, Nayak B, Singh M, et al. Mitochondrial complex 1 gene analysis in keratoconus. *Mol Vis*. 2011; 17:1514–1525.
54. Li X, Bykhovskaya Y, Haritunians T, et al. A génome-wide association study identifies a potential novel gene locus for keratoconus, one of the commonest causes for corneal transplantation in developed countries. *Hum Mol Genet*. 2012;21(2):421–429.
55. Piccione M, Serra G, Sanfilippo C, et al. A new mutation in EDA gene in X-linked hypohidrotic ectodermal dysplasia associated with keratoconus. *Minerva Pediatr*. 2012;64(1):59–64.
56. Bykhovskaya Y, Li X, Epifantseva I, et al. Variation in the lysyl oxidase (LOX) gene is associated with keratoconus in family-based and case-control studies. *Invest Ophthalmol Vis Sci*. 2012;53(7):4152–4157.
57. Lu Y, Vitart T, Burdon KP, et al. Genome-wide association analyses identify loci associated with central corneal thickness and keratoconus. *Nat Genet*. 2013;4592:155–163.
58. Bykhovskaya Y, Li X, Epifantseva I, et al. Variation in the lysyl oxidase (LOX) gene is associated with keratoconus in family-based and case-control studies. *Invest Ophthalmol Vis Sci*. 2012;53(7):4152–4157.
59. Burdon KP, Macgregor S, Bykhovskaya Y, et al. Association of polymorphisms in the hépatocyte growth factor gene promoter with keratoconus. *Invest Ophthalmol Vis Sci*. 2011;52(11):8514–8519.
60. Li X, Bykhovskaya Y, Haritunians T, et al. A génome-wide association study identifies a potential novel gene locus for keratoconus, one of the commonest causes for corneal transplantation in developed countries. *Hum Mol Genet*. 2012;21(2):421–429.
61. Assiri AA, Yousuf BI, Quantock AJ, et al. Incidence and severity of keratoconus in Asir province, Saudi Arabia. *Br J Ophthalmol*. 2005;89(11):1403–1406.
62. Lee LR, Readshaw G, Hirst LW. Keratoconus: the clinical experience of a Brisbane ophthalmologist. *Ophthalmic Epidemiol*. 1996;3(3):119–125.
63. Rabinowitz YS, Garbus J, McDonnell PJ. Computer-assisted corneal topography in family members of patients with keratoconus. *Arch Ophthalmol*. 1990;108(3):365–371.
64. Rabinowitz YS, Maumenee IH, Lundergan MK, et al. Molecular genetic analysis in autosomal dominant keratoconus. *Cornea*. 1992;11:302–308.
65. Itoi M, Hisae M, Tsuda N, et al. Corneal shape of familial members of keratoconus patients. Presented at: 2011 Annual ARVO Meeting; April 30–May 5, 2011; Fort Lauderdale, FL; A1082–D706.
66. Al-Swailem SA, Al-Assiri AA, Al-Torbak AA. Woodhouse Sakati syndrome associated with bilateral keratoconus. *Br J Ophthalmol*. 2006;90(1):116–117.
67. Shapiro MB, France TD. The ocular features of Down's syndrome. *Am J Ophthalmol*. 1985; 99(6):659–663.

68. Steahly LP. Keratoconus following contact lens wear. *Ann Ophthalmol.* 1978;10:1177–1179.
69. Hartstein J. Keratoconus that developed in patients wearing corneal contact lenses. *Arch Ophthalmol.* 1968;80:345–396.
70. Macsai MS, Varley GA, Krachmer JH. Development of keratoconus after contact lens wear. *Arch Ophthalmol.* 1990;108:435–538.
71. Szczotka L. PMMA lens wear: a probable cause of keratoconus. *Contact Lens Spectrum.* 1999;14(11):10.
72. Kenney MC, Brown DJ. The cascade hypothesis of keratoconus. *Cont Lens Ant Eye.* 2003;26:139–146.
73. van der Worp E. Keratoconus: what do we know? *Contact Lens Spectrum.* 2007;22(10):36–43.
74. Kenney MC. Update on latest studies pertaining to keratoconus. Presented at: 2008 Global Keratoconus Congress; January 2008; Las Vegas, NV.
75. Sugar J, Macsai MS. What causes keratoconus? *Cornea.* 2012;31(6):716–719.
76. Spoerl E, Raiskup-Wolf F, Kuhlisch E, et al. Cigarette smoking is negatively associated with keratoconus. *J Refract Surg.* 2008;24:S737–S740.
77. Sady C, Khosrof S, Nagarah R. Advanced Maillard réaction and cross-linking of corneal collagen in diabètes. *Biochem Biophys Res Commun.* 1995;214:793–797.
78. Kuo IC, Broman A, Pirouzmanesh A, et al. Is there an association between diabètes and keratoconus? *Ophthalmology.* 2006;113:184–190.
79. Bennett ES. Keratoconus. In: Bennett ES, Grohe RM, eds. *Rigid Gas-Permeable Contact Lenses.* New York, NY: Professional Press; 1986;297–344.
80. Wei RH, Khor WB, Lim L, et al. Contact lens characteristics and contrast sensitivity of patients with keratoconus. *Eye Contact Lens: Sci Clin Prac.* 2011;37(5):307–311.
81. Choi JA, Kim MS. Progression of keratoconus by longitudinal assessment with corneal topography. *Invest Ophthalmol Vis Sci.* 2012;53(2):927–935.
82. Chou B, Weissman BA. Making sense of the irregular cornea. *Rev Cornea Contact Lenses.* April 2010.
83. Lim L, Wei RH, Chan WK, et al. Evaluation of higher order ocular aberrations in patients with keratoconus. *J Refract Surg.* 2007;23:825–828.
84. Jafri B, Li X, Yang H, et al. Higher order wavefront aberrations and topography in early and suspected keratoconus. *J Refract Surg.* 2007;23:774–781.
85. Maeda N. Clinical applications of wavefront aberrometry —a review. *Clin Exper Ophthalmol.* 2009;37:118–129.
86. Pantanelli SM, Yoon G, Jeong TM, et al. Aberration characterization of abnormal eyes using the large dynamic range Shack-Hartmann wavefront sensor [E-abstract 2848]. *Invest Ophthalmol Vis Sci.* 2004;45.
87. Alio JL, Shabeyek MH. Corneal higher order aberrations: a method to grade keratoconus. *J Refract Surg.* 2006;22(6):539–545.
88. Atchison DA, Mathur A, Read SA, et al. Peripheral ocular aberrations in mild and moderate keratoconus. *Invest Ophthalmol Vis Sci.* 2012;51(12):6850–6857.
89. Caroline PJ, et al. A new contact lens design for keratoconus: a continuing report. *Contact Lens J.* 1978;12(1):17–20.
90. Perry HD, et al. Round and oval cones in keratoconus. *Am Acad Ophthalmol.* 1980;87(9):905–909.
91. Fiol-Silva Z, Siviglia D. Keratoconus: fitting and managing. *Ophthalmol Clin North Am.* 1989;2(2):291–297.
92. McMahon TT. Topography guided fitting of contact lenses in keratoconus. Presented at: Global Keratoconus Congress; January 2008; Las Vegas, NV.
93. McMahon TT. Collaborative longitudinal evaluation of kertatoconus update. Presented at: Annual Meeting of the American Academy of Optometry; December 2006; Denver, CO.
94. Probst LE. Case 13: LASIK with Forme Fruste Keratoconus. In: Machat JL, Slade SG, Probst LE, eds. *The Art of LASIK.* Thorofare, NJ: SLACK Inc.;1999;504–505.
95. Caroline PJ, Andre MP. Help for screening abnormal corneal topographies. *Contact Lens Spectrum.* 1998; 13(12):56.
96. Klyce SD. Corneal topography in refractive keratectomy. In: Thompson FB, McDonnell PJ, eds. *Color Atlas/Text of Excimer Laser Surgery: the Cornea.* New York, NY: Igaku-Shoin Medical Publishers; 1993;19–36.
97. Wilson SE, Klyce SD, Husseini ZM. Standardized color-coded maps for corneal topography. *Ophthalmology.* 1993;100:1723–1727.
98. Wilson SD, Klyce SD. Screening for cornea topographic abnormalities before refractive surgery. *Ophthalmology.* 1994;101:147–152.
99. Nesburn AB, Bahri S, Berlin M, et al. Computer-assisted corneal topography (CACT) to detect mild keratoconus in candidates for photorefractive keratectomy. *Invest Ophthalmol Vis Sci.* 1995;33/4(suppl):995.
100. Mandell RB, Chiang CS, Yee L. Asymmetric corneal toricity and pseudokeratoconus in videokeratography. *J Am Optom Assoc.* 1996;67(9):540–547.
101. Rabinowitz YS, McDonnell PJ. Computer-assisted corneal topography in keratoconus. *Refract Corneal Surg.* 1989;5:400.
102. Rabinowitz YS, Rasheed K. KISA% index: a quantitative videokeratography algorithm embodying minimal topographic criteria for diagnosing keratoconus. *J Cat Refract Surg.* 1999;25:1327 1135.
103. Li X, Rabinowitz YS, Rasheed K, et al. Longitudinal study of the normal eyes in unilateral keratoconus patients. *Ophthalmology.* 2004;111:440–446.

104. Davis LJ, Barr JT, VanOtteren D. Transient rigid lens induced straie in keratoconus. *Optom Vis Sci.* 1993;70(3):216–219.
105. Zadnik Z, Burger DS. Keratoconus. In: Bennett ES, Weissman BA, eds. *Clinical Contact Lens Practice.* Philadelphia, PA: JB Lippincott; 1995:45-1–45-11.
106. Reinke AR. Keratoconus: a review of research and current fitting techniques. Part 1. *Int Cont Lens Clin.* 1975;2(3):66–80.
107. Barr JT, Schectman KB, Fink BA, et al. Corneal scarring in the Collaborative Longitudinal Evaluation of Keratoconus (CLEK) Study: baseline prevalence and repeatability of detection. *Cornea.* 1999;18(1):34–45.
108. Rizzuti AB. Diagnostic illumination test for keratoconus. *Am J Ophthalmol.* 1970;70:141.
109. DeNaeyer GW, Eiden SB. How technology can help the irregular cornea. *Rev Cornea Contact Lenses.* April 2012.
110. Labiris G, Athanassios G, Sideroudi H, et al. Impact of keratoconus, cross-linking and cross-linking combined with photorefractive keratectomy on self-reported quality of life. *Cornea.* 2012;31(7):734–739.
111. Shovlin JP, DePaolis MD, Kame RT. Contact lens-induced corneal warpage syndrome. *Contact Lens Forum.* 1986;11(8):32–36.
112. Davis LJ. Keratoconus: current understanding of diagnosis and management. *Clin Eye Vis Care.* 1997;9:13–22.
113. Maguire LJ, Klyce SD, McDonald ME, et al. Corneal topography of pellucid marginal degeneration. *Ophthalmology.* 1987;94:519–524.
114. McMahon TT, Szczotka-Flynn L, Barr JT, et al. A new method for grading the severity of keratoconus: the Keratoconus Severity Score (KSS). *Cornea.* 2006;25(7):794–800.
115. Zadnik K, Barr JT, Gordon MO, et al. Biomicroscopic signs and disease severity in keratoconus. Collaborative Longitudinal Evaluation of Keratoconus (CLEK) Study Group. *Cornea.* 1996;15:139–146.
116. Gobbe M, Guillon M. Corneal wavefront aberration measurements to detect keratoconus patients. *Cont Lens Anterior Eye.* 2005;28:57–66.
117. McMahon TT, Edrington TB, Szczotka-Flynn L, et al. Longitudinal changes in corneal curvature in keratoconus. *Cornea.* 2006;25(3):296–305.
118. Feder RS, Kshettry P. Noninflammatory ectatic disorders. In: Krachmer, Mannis MJ, Holland EJ, eds. *Cornea.* 2nd ed. 2005;955.
119. Cooke CA, Cooper C, Dowds E, et al. Keratoconus, myopia, and personality. *Cornea.* 2003;22:239–242.
120. Giedd KK, Mannis MJ, Mitchell GL, et al. Personality in keratoconus in a sample of patients derived from the internet. *Cornea.* 2005;24:301–307
121. Mannis MJ, Morrison TL, Zadnik K, et al. Personality trends in keratoconus. An analysis. *Arch Ophthalmol.* 1987;105:798–800.
122. Vitale S. CLEK study reports on the quality of life. *Am J Ophthalmol.* 2004;138:637–638.
123. Kymes SM, Walline JJ, Zadnik K, et al. Quality of life in keratoconus. *Am J Ophthalmol.* 2004;138:527–535.
124. Kymes S. Walline J, Zadnik K, et al. Changes in the quality of life of people with keratoconus. *Am J Ophthalmol.* 2008;45(4):611–617.
125. Saidel MA, Palk JY, Garcia C, et al. Prevalence of sleep apnea syndrome and high-risk characteristics among keratoconus patients. *Cornea.* 2012;31(6):600–603.
126. Gupta PK, Stinnett SS, Carlson AN. Prevalence of sleep apnea in patients with keratoconus. *Cornea.* 2012; 31(6): 595–599.
127. Ezra DG, Beaconsfield M, Sira M, et al. The associations of floopy eyelid syndrome: a case control study. *Ophthalmology.* 2010;117:831–838.
128. Jinabhal A, Radhakrishnan H, Tromans C, et al. Visual performance and optical quality with soft lenses in keratoconus patients. *Ophthalmic Physio Opt.* 2012;32(2):100–116.
129. Zadnik K, Gordon MO, Barr JT, Edrington TB; the CLEK Study Group. Biomicroscopic signs and disease severity in keratoconus. *Cornea.* 1996;15:139–146.
130. Lass JH, Lembach RG, Park SB, et al. Clinical management of keratoconus: a multicenter analysis. *Ophthalmology.* 1990;97:433–455.
131. Griffiths M, Zahner K, Collins M, et al. Masking of irregular corneal topography with contact lenses. *CLAO J.* 1998;2492:76–81.
132. Carney LG. Contact lens correction of visual loss in keratoconus. *Acta Ophthalmol.* 1982;60(5):795–802.
133. Jinabhal A, Radhakrishnan H, O'Donnell C. Visual acuity and ocular aberrations with different rigid gas permeable lens fittings in keratoconus. *Eye Contact Lens.* 2010;36(4):233–237.
134. Korb DR, Finnemore VM, Herman JP. Apical changes and scarring in keratoconus as related to contact lens fitting techniques. *J Am Optom Assoc.* 1982;53:199–205.
135. Soper JW, Jarrett HA. Results of a systemic approach to fitting keratoconus and corneal transplants. *Contact Lens Med Bull.* 1972;5:50.
136. Ruben M. Treatment of keratoconus. *Aust J Optom.* 1979;62(4):152–157.
137. Gundel RE, Libassi DP, Zadnik K, et al. Feasibility of fitting contact lenses with apical clearance in keratoconus. *Optom Vis Sci.* 1996;73(12):729–732.
138. Sindt CW, Grout TK, Kojima R. Evaluating virtual fitting for keratoconus. *Contact Lens Spectrum.* 2011;26(5):39–43.
139. www.gpli.info. Accessed February 2013.

140. Bennett ES. A common sense approach to fitting keratoconus with RGP lenses. *Optom Today.* 1997;5(3):25–27.
141. Edrington TB, Szczotka LB, Begley CG, et al. Repeatability of two corneal curvature assessments in keratoconus: keratometry and the first definite apical clearance lens. Presented at: Annual Meeting of the American Academy of Optometry; December 1997; San Antonio, Texas.
142. Phan V, Mondino BJ, Weissman BA. Pearls for fitting keratoconus. *Contact Lens Spectrum.* 2012;27(12):43.
143. Weissman B, Chun M, Barnhart L. Corneal abrasion associated with contact lens correction of keratoconus—a retrospective study. *Optom Vis Sci.* 1994;71:677–681.
144. Szczotka-Flynn LB, Patel S. Menicon Z rigid gas permeable lenses for keratoconus and irregular corneas: a retrospective case series. *Eye Contact Lens.* 2008;34(5):254–260.
145. Mannis MJ, Zadnik K. Contact lens fitting in keratoconus. *CLAO J.* 1989;15:282–289.
146. Burger D. Contact lens alternatives for keratoconus: an overview. *Contact Lens Spectrum.* 1993;8:49–55.
147. Caroline PJ, Norman C, Andre M. The latest lens design for keratoconus. *Contact Lens Spectrum.* 1997;12(8):36–41.
148. Edrington TB, Szczotka LB, Barr JT, et al. Rigid contact lens fitting relationships in keratoconus. *Optom Vis Sci.* 1999;76:692–699.
149. Barnett M, Mannis MJ. Contact lenses in the management of keratoconus. *Cornea.* 2011;30(12):1510–1516.
150. Yanai R, Ueda K, Nishida T. Retrospective analysis of vision correction and lens tolerance in keratoconus patients prescribed a contact lens with dual aspherical curves. *Eye Contact Lens.* 2010;36(2):86–89.
151. Henry VA. Irregular Cornea. In: Bennett ES, Henry VA, eds. *Clinical Manual of Contact Lenses.* Philadelphia, PA: JB Lippincott;438–453.
152. Connelly S, Broe D. Comfort for the keratoconus patient: a comparison of lens designs. *Contact Lens Spectrum.* 1999;14(5):42–44.
153. DeNaeyer GW. Managing compromise with large-diameter corneal GPs. *Contact Lens Spectrum.* 2011;26(1):20.
154. Shovlin JP. Bitoric RGPs for keratoconus? *Rev Optom.* 2001;138(1):98.
155. Miller B. Systematic application of toric contact lenses for high astigmatism—aspheric and asymmetric decentered lenses for advanced keratoconus. *Contactologia (German).* 1994;16(1):13–18.
156. Neumann S. Improving the fit and visual acuity by using bitoric keratoconic lenses. Presented at: Global Keratoconus Congress; January 2007; Las Vegas, NV.
157. Weissman B, Chun MW, Barnhart LA. Corneal abrasion associated with contact lens correction of keratoconus—a retrospective study. *Optom Vis Sci.* 1994;71(11):677–681.
158. Vanderhoof SLH, Mathe DS. Troubleshooting keratoconus. *Rev Cornea Contact Lenses.* April 2012.
159. Bennett ES, Hill S, Grohe RM. Optimizing success with irregular cornea patients, Part 2. *Contact Lens Spectrum.* 2008;23(8).
160. Schornack MM, Patel SV. Scleral lenses in the management of keratoconus. *Eye Contact Lens.* 2010;36(1):39–44.
161. Segal O, Barkana Y, Hourovitz D, et al. Scleral contact lenses may help where other modalities fail. *Cornea.* 2003;22:308–310.
162. Sindt CW. Basic scleral lens fitting and design. *Contact Lens Spectrum.* 2008;23(10):32–36.
163. Pullum KW, Buckley RJ. A study of 530 patients referred for rigid gas permeable scleral contact lens assessment. *Cornea.* 1997;16(6):612–622.
164. Zadnik K. Meet the challenge of fitting the irregular cornea. *Rev Optom.* 1994;131(4):77–83.
165. Yamazaki ES, da Silva VC, Morimitsu V, et al. Keratoconus special soft contact lens fitting. *Arq Bras Oftalmol.* 2006;69(4):557–560.
166. Caroline P, Andre M, Kinoshita B, et al. Etiology, diagnosis and management of keratoconus: new thoughts and new understandings. Available at: http://www.pacificu.edu/optometry/ce/courses/15167/etiologypg4.cfm. Accessed Febraurary 2, 2013.
167. Thompson TT. Tyler's quarterly soft contact lens parameter guide. 2012;30(1):19.
168. Brujic M, Miller J. The comfortable side of keratoconus. *Rev Cornea Contact Lenses.* January 2012.
169. Shovlin JP. Softer approach to keratoconus. *Rev Cornea Contact Lenses.* June 2012.
170. Eiden EB, DeNaeyer GW. Keratoconus fitting with specialty soft lenses. *Contact Lens Spectrum.* 2012;27(1):34–37.
171. Andre MP. Soft and hybrid designs for keratoconus. Presented at: 2008 Global Keratoconus Congress; January 2008; Las Vegas, NV.
172. Malooley MM, Faron CA. Contact lens options for irregular corneas. *Contact Lens Spectrum.* 2011;26(5):28–33.
173. Young K, Eghbali F, Weissman BA. Clinical experience with piggyback contact lens systems on keratoconic eyes. *J Am Optom Assoc.* 1995;66(9):539–543.
174. Edrington T, Tran L. Contact lens and surgical management options for keratoconus. *Rev Cornea Contact Lenses.* April 2008.
175. Bennett ES, Grohe RM, Anderson BW, et al. Piggyback applications in modern contact lens practice. *Contact Lens Spectrum.* 2007;22(12):17.
176. Szczotka-Flynn L. Optimizing GP lens designs in the clinical management of irregular astigmatism. Presented at: 2010 Global Specialty Lens Symposium; January 2010; Las Vegas, NV.
177. Brazeau D. Fitting and effective power of soft lenses in piggyback system. Presented at: 2009 Global Specialty Lens Symposium; January 2009; Las Vegas, NV.
178. Woo M, Weissman BA. Effective optics of piggyback soft contact lenses. *Contact Lens Spectrum.* 2011;26(11):50–52.

179. Caroline PJ, Doughman DJ. A new piggyback lens design for correction of irregular astigmatism: a preliminary report. *Contact Lens J*. 1979;13:39–42.
180. Caroline PJ, Andre M. Custom soft contact lenses. *Contact Lens Spectrum*. 1998;13(4).
181. Watanabe R. Keratoconus design options. *Contact Lens Spectrum*. 2011;26(12):23.
182. Davis R, Eiden SB. Constructing a contact lens for multifocal success. *Rev Cornea Contact Lenses*. October 2010.
183. Griffiths M, Zahner K, Collins M, et al. Masking of irregular corneal topography with contact lenses. *CLAO J*. 1998;24:76–81.
184. Atchison DA. Aberrations associated with rigid contact lenses. *J Opt Soc Am A Opt Image Sci Vis*.1995;12:2267–2273.
185. Hong X, Himebaugh N, Thibos LN. On-eye evaluation of optical performance of rigid and soft contact lenses. *Optom Vis Sci*. 2001;78:872–880.
186. Lu F, Mao X, Qu J, et al. Monochromatic wavefront aberrations in the human eye with contact lenses. *Optom Vis Sci*. 2003;80:135–141.
187. DeNaeyer GW. Managing irregular cornea patients. *Contact Lens Spectrum*. 2012;27(4):30.
188. Negishi K, Kumanomido T, Utsumi Y, et al. Effect of higher-order aberrations on visual function in keratoconic eyes with a rigid gas permeable contact lens. *Ophthalmology*. 2007;144(6):924–929.
189. Nakagawa T, Maeda N, Kosaki R, et al. Higher order aberrations due to the posterior corneal surface in patients with keratoconus. *Invest Ophthalmol Vis Sci*. 2009;50(6):2660–2665.
190. Campbell CE. The effect of spherical aberration of contact lens to the wearer. *Am J Optom Physiol Opt*. 1981;58:212–217.
191. Cox I. Theoretical calculation of the longitudinal spherical aberration of rigid and soft contact lenses. *Optom Vis Sci*. 1990;67:277–282.
192. Hammer RM, Holden BA. Spherical aberration of aspheric contact lenses on eye. *Optom Vis Sci*. 1994;71:522–528.
193. Cesnekova T, Skorkovska K, Petrova S, et al. Visual functions and quality of life in patients with keratoconus. *Ceska Slovenska Oftalmologie*. 2011;67(2):51–54.
194. Choi J, Wee WR, Lee JH, et al. Changes of ocular higher order aberration in on- and off-eye of rigid gas permeable contact lenses. *Optom Vis Sci*. 2007;84(1):42–51.
195. Marsack JD, Parker KE, Pesudovs K, et al. Uncorrected wavefront error and visual performance during RGP wear in keratoconus. *Optom Vis Sci*. 2007;84(6):463–470.
196. De Brabender J, Chateau N, Marin G, et al. Simulated optical performance of custom wavefront soft contact lenses for keratoconus. *Optom Vis Sci*. 2003;80:637–643.
197. Marsack JD, Parker KE, Niu Y, et al. On-eye performance of custom wavefront-guided soft contact lenses in a habitual soft lens-wearing keratoconic patient. *J Refract Surg*. 2007;23(9):960–964.
198. Katsoulos C, Karageorgiadis L, Vasileiou N. Customized hydrogel contact lenses for keratoconus incorporating correction for vertical coma aberration. *Ophthalmic Physiol Opt*. 2009;29(3):321–329.
199. Marsack JD, Parker KE, Applegate RA. Performance of wavefront-guided soft lenses in three keratoconus subjects. *Optom Vis Sci*. 2008;85(12):E1172–E1178.
200. Jinabhal A, Neil CW, O'Donnell C, et al. Optical quality for keratoconic eyes with conventional RGP lens and simulated, customized contact lens corrections: a comparison. *Ophthalmol Physiol Opt*. 2012;32(3):200–212.
201. Maguen E, Caroline PJ, Rosmer IR, et al. The use of the SoftPerm lens for the correction of irregular astigmatism. *CLAO J*. 1992;18(3):173–176.
202. Maguen E, Martinez M, Rosner I, et al. The use of Saturn II lenses in keratoconus. *CLAO J*. 1991;17(1):41–43.
203. Davis RL, Eiden SB, Murphy MA. New concepts in combination lenses. *Contact Lens Spectrum*. 2012;27(5):24–27.
204. Abdalla YF, Elsahn AF, Hammerstein KM, et al. SynergEyes lenses for keratoconus. *Cornea*. 2010;29(1):5–8.
205. Fernandez-Velazquez FJ. Severe epithelial edema in Clearkone SynergEyes contact lens wear for keratoconus. *Eye Contact Lens*. 2011;37(6):381–385.
206. Eggink FAGJ, Pinckers AJLG, Van Puyenbroek EP, et al. Keratoconus, a retrospective study. *Contact Lens J*. 1988;16:204.
207. Sayegh FN, Ehlers N, Farah I. Evaluation of penetrating keratoplasty in keratoconus. Nine years follow-up. *Acta Ophthalmol*. 1988;66:400.
208. Smiddy WE, Hamburg TR, Kracher GP, et al. Keratoconus: contact lens or keratoplasty? *Ophthalmology*. 1988;95:487.
209. Crews MJ, Driebe WT, Stern GA. The clinical management of keratoconus: a 6 year retrospective study. *CLAO J*. 1994;20(3):194–197.
210. Kastl PR. A 20-year retrospective study of the use of contact lenses in keratoconus. *CLAO J*. 1987;13:102.
211. Belin MW, Fowler WG, Chambers WA. Keratoconus: evaluation of recent trends in the surgical and nonsurgical correction of keratoconus. *Ophthalmology*. 1988;95:335.
212. Gordon MO, Steger-May K, Szczotka-Flynn L, et al. Baseline factors predictive of incident penetrating keratoplasty in keratoconus. *Am J Ophthalmol*. 2006;142(6):923–930.
213. Boruchoff SA, et al. Comparison of suturing techniques in keratoplasty for keratoconus. *Ann Ophthalmol*. 1975;7:433–436.
214. Martin WRJ, Smith EL. Some points in the surgical technique of keratoplasty. *Am J Ophthalmol*. 1963;55:1199–1208.

215. Pramanik S, Musch DC, Sulphin JE, et al. Extended long-term outcomes of penetrating keratoplasty for keratoconus. *Ophthalmology.* 2006;113(9):1633–1638.
216. Sonsino J, Ewald MD. Corrective options for irregular corneas. *Contact Lens Spectrum.* 2010;25(11):26–29.
217. Frost NA, Wu J, Lai TF, et al. A review of randomized controlled trials of penetrating keratoplasty techniques. *Ophthalmology.* 2006;113:942–949.
218. Troutman RC, Lawless MA. Penetrating keratoplasty for keratoconus. *Cornea.* 1987;6:298–305.
219. Olson RJ, Pingree M, Ridges R, et al. Penetrating keratoplasty for keratoconus: a long-term review of results and complications. *J Catar Refract Surg.* 2000;26:987–991.
220. Javadi MA, Motlagh BF, Jafarinasab MR, et al. Outcomes of penetrating keratoplasty in keratoconus. *Cornea.* 2005;24:941–946.
221. Brierly SC, Izquierdo I, Mannis MJ. Penetrating keratoplasty for keratoconus. *Cornea.* 2000;19(3):329–332.
222. Zadok D, Schwarts S, Marchovich A, et al. Penetrating keratoplasty for keratoconus: long-term results. *Cornea.* 2005;24:959–961.
223. Ing JJ, Ing HH, Nelson LR, et al. Ten year postoperative results of penetrating keratoplasty. *Ophthalmology.* 1998;105:1855–1865.
224. Seitz B, Behrens A, Langenbuchar A, et al. Experimental 193-nm excimer laser trephination with divergent cut angles in penetrating keratoplasty. *Cornea.* 1998;17(4):410–416.
225. Homolka P, Biowski R, Kaminski S, et al. Laser shaping of corneal transplants in vitro: area ablation with small overlapping laser spots produced by a pulsed scanning laser beam using an optimizing ablation algorithm. *Phys Med Biol.* 1999;44(5):1169–1180.
226. Krumeich JH, Daniel J, Knulle A. Live-epikeratophakia for keratoconus. *J Cataract Refract Surg.* 1998;24(4):456–463.
227. Kelly TL, Williams KA, Coster DJ. Australian Corneal Graft Registry. *Arch Ophthalmol.* 2011;129(6):691–697.
228. Thompson RW, Price MO, Bowers PJ, et al. Long-term graft survival after penetrating keratoplasty. *Ophthalmology.* 2003;110:1396–1402.
229. Sarnicola V, Toro P, Sarnicola C, et al. Long-term graft survival in deep anterior lamellar keratoplasty. *Cornea.* 2012;31(6):621–626.
230. Cheng YY, Visser N, Schouten JS, et al. Endothelial cell loss and visual outcome of deep anterior lamellar keratoplasty versus penetrating keratoplasty: a randomized multicenter clinical trial. *Ophthalmology.* 2011;118(2):302–309.
231. Borderie VM, Sandali O, Bullet J, et al. Long-term results of deep anterior lamellar versus penetrating keratoplasty. *Ophthalmology.* 2012;119(2):249–255.
232. Kubaloglu A, Koytak A, Sari ES, et al. Corneal endothelium after deep anterior lamellar keratoplasty and penetrating keratoplasty for keratoconus: a four-year comparative study. *Indian J Ophthalmology.* 2012;60(1):35–40.
233. Hari DC, Mehta JS, Por YM, et al. Comparison of outcomes of lamellar keratoplasty and penetrating keratoplasty in keratoconus. *Am J Ophthalmol.* 2009;148(5):744–751.
234. Kubaloglu A, Sari ES, Unal M, et al. Long-term results of deep anterior lamellar keratoplasty for the treatment of keratoconus. *Am J Ophthalmol.* 2011;151(5):760–767.
235. Bahar I, Kaiserman I, Srinivasan S, et al. Comparison of three different techniques for corneal transplantation for keratoconus. *Am J Ophthalmol.* 2008;146(6):905–912.
236. Cohen AW, Goins KM, Sutphin JE, et al. Penetrating keratoplasty versus deep anterior lamellar keratoplasty for the treatment of keratoconus. *Int Ophthalmol.* 2010;30(6):675–681.
237. Javadi MA, Feizi S, Yazdani S, et al. Deep anterior lamellar keratoplasty versus penetrating keratoplasty for keratoconus: a clinical trial. *Cornea.* 2010;29(4):365–371.
238. Sogutlu SE, Kubaloglu A, Unal M, et al. Penetrating keratoplasty versus deep anterior lamellar keratoplasty: comparison of optical and visual quality outcomes. *Br J Ophthalmol.* 2012;96(8):1063–1067.
239. Parthasarathy A, Por YM, Tan DT. Use of a "small-bubble technique" to increase the success of Anwar's "big-bubble technique" for deep lamellar keratoplasty with complete baring of Descemet's membrane. *Br J Ophthalmol.* 2007;91(10):1369–1373.
240. Barnett M. A dual approach to treating keratoconus. *Rev Cornea Contact Lenses.* April 2011.
241. Colin J, Malet FJ. Intacs for the correction of keratoconus: two-year follow-up. *J Cataract Refract Surg.* 2007;33(1):69–74.
242. Carrasquillo KG, Rand J, Talamo JH. Intacs for keratoconus and post-LASIK ectasia: mechanical versus femtosecond laser-assisted channel creation. *Cornea.* 2007;26(8):956–962.
243. Ertan A, Colin J. Intracorneal rings for keratoconus and keratectasia. *J Cataract Refract Surg.* 2007;33(7):1303–1314.
244. Kubaloglu A, Sari ES, Cinar Y, et al. Intrastromal corneal ring segment implantation for the treatment of keratoconus. *Cornea.* 2011;30(1):11–17.
245. Rabinowitz YS, Li X, Ignacio TS, et al. Intacs inserts using the femtolaser compared to the mechanical spreader in the treatment of keratoconus. *J Refract Surg.* 2006;22(8):764–771.
246. Hamdi IM. Preliminary results of intrastromal corneal ring segment implantation to treat moderate to severe keratoconus. *J Cataract Refract Surg.* 2011;37(6):1125–1132.
247. Gharaibeh AM, Muhsen SM, AbuKhader IB, et al. KeraRing intrastromal corneal ring segments for correction of keratoconus. *Cornea.* 2012;31(2):115–120.

248. Tu KL, Sebastian RT, Owen M. Quantification of the surgically induced refractive effect of intrastromal corneal ring segments in keratoconus with standardized incision site and segment size. *J Cataract Refract Surg.* 2011;37(10):1865–1870.
249. Colin J, Cochener B, Savary G, et al. INTACS inserts for treating keratoconus: one-year results. *Ophthalmology.* 2001;108(8):1409–1414.
250. Levinger S, Pokroy R. Keratoconus managed with intacs: one-year results. *Arch Ophthalmol.* 2005;123(10):1308–1314.
251. Alio JL, Shabayek MH, Belda JI, et al. Analysis of results related to good and bad outcomes of Intacs implantations got keratoconus correction. *J Cataract Refract Surg.* 2006;32(5):756–761.
252. Schanzlin D. Surgical approaches to keratoconus. Presented at: 2008 Global Keratoconus Congress; January 2008; Las Vegas, NV.
253. Kymionis GD, Siganos CS, Tsiklis NS, et al. Long-term follow-up if intacs in Keratoconus. *Am J Ophthalmol.* 2007;143(2):236–244.
254. Tan DT, Por YM. Current treatment options for corneal ectasia. *Curr Opin Ophthalmol.* 2007;18(4):284–289.
255. Pokroy R, Levinger S. Intacs adjustment surgery for keratoconus. *J Cataract Refract Surg.* 2006;32(6):986–992.
256. Ruckhofer J, Twa MD, Schanzlin DJ. Clinical characteristics of lamellar channel deposits after implantation of intacs. *J Cataract Refract Surg.* 2000;26:1473–1479.
257. Kanellopoulos AL, Pe LH, Perry HD, et al. Modified intracorneal ring segment implantations (INTACS) for the management of moderate to advanced keratoconus: efficacy and complications. *Cornea.* 2006;25:29–33.
258. Smiley CA. INTACS® for Keratoconus: advantages and disadvantages. AOA CLCS Newsletter, March 2012.
259. Carrasquillo K, Rand J, Talamo JH. Intacs for keratoconus and post-LASIK ectasia. Mechanical versus femtosecond laser-assisted channel creation. *Cornea.* 2007;26:956–962.
260. Ozerturk Y, Sari ES, Kubaloglu A, et al. Comparison of deep anterior lamellar keratoplasty and intrastromal corneal ring segment implantation in advanced keratoconus. *J Cataract Refract Surg.* 2012;38(2):324–332.
261. Spoerl E. Biomechanical effect of combined riboflavin-ultraviolet A (UVA) treatment for keratoconus. Paper presented at: Global Keratoconus Congress; January 2007; Las Vegas, NV.
262. Spoerl E, Huhle M, Seiler T. Induction of cross-links in corneal tissue. *Exp Eye Res.* 1998;66:97–103.
263. Wollensak G, Spoerl E, Seiler T. Riboflavin/ultraviolet-A-induced collagen crosslinking for the treatment of keratoconus. *Am J Ophthalmol.* 2003;135(5):620–627.
264. Koppen C. Cornea cross-linking update 2013. Presented at: 2013 Global Specialty Lens Symposium; January 2013; Las Vegas, NV.
265. Goldich Y, Marcovich AL, Barkana Y, et al. Clinical and corneal biomechanical changes after collagen cross-linking with riboflavin and UV irradiation in patients with progressive keratoconus: results after 2 years of follow-up. *Cornea.* 2012;31(6):609–614.
266. Vinciguerra P, Albe E, Trazza S, et al. Intraoperative and postoperative effects of corneal collagen cross-linking on progressive keratoconus. *Arch Ophthalmol.* 2009;127:1258–1265.
267. Coporossi A, Baiocchi S, Mazzotta C, et al. Parasurgical therapy for keratoconus by riboflavin-ultraviolet type A rays induced cross-linking of corneal collage: preliminary refractive results in an Italian study. *J Cataract Refract Surg.* 2006;32:837–845.
268. Raiskup-Wolf F, Hoyer A, Spoerl E, et al. Collagen cross-linking with riboflavin and ultraviolet-A light in keratoconus: long-term results. *J Cataract Refract Surg.* 2008;34:796–801.
269. Grewal DS, Brar GS, Jain R, et al. Corneal collagen crosslinking using riboflavin and ultraviolet-A light for keratoconus: one year analysis using Scheimflug imaging. *J Cataract Refract Surg.* 2009;35:425–432.
270. Wittig-Silva C, Whiting M, Lamoureux E, et al. A randomized controlled trial of corneal collagen cross-linking in progressive keratoconus: preliminary results. *J Refract Surg.* 2008;24:S720–S725.
271. FDA trial data positive for corneal collagen crosslinking. Available at: www.modernmedicine.com/modernmedicine/Clinical+News/ASCRS-FDA-trial-data-positive-for-corneal-collagen/ArticleStandard/Article/detail/591528?contextCategoryId=46496&ref=25. Accessed February 2013.
272. O'Brart DP, Chan E, Samaras K, et al. A randomized, prospective study to investigate the efficacy of riboflavin/ultraviolet A (370 nm) corneal collagen cross-linkage to halt the progression of keratoconus. *Br J Ophthalmol.* 2011;95(11):1519–1524.
273. Hersh PS, Greenstein SA, Fry KL. Corneal collagen crosslinking for keratoconus and corneal ectasia: one year results. *J Cataract Refract Surg.* 2011;37(1):201–205.
274. Greenstein SA, Fry KL, Hersh MJ, et al. Higher-order aberrations after corneal crosslinking for keratoconus and corneal ectasia. *J Cataract Refract Surg.* 2012;38(2):292–302.
275. Vinciguerra P, Albe E, Frueh BE, et al. Two-year corneal cross-linking results in patients younger than 18 years with documented progressive keratoconus. *Am J Ophthalmol.* 2012;154(3):520–526.
276. Asri D, Touboul D, Fournie P, et al. Corneal collagen crosslinking in progressive keratoconus: multicenter results from the French National Reference Center for Keratoconus. *J Cataract Refract Surg.* 2011;37(12):2137–2143.
277. Goldich Y, Marcovich AL, Barkana Y, et al. Safety of corneal collagen cross-linking with UV-A and riboflavin in progressive keratoconus. *Cornea.* 2010;29(4):409–411.
278. Brooks NO, Greenstein S, Fry K, et al. Patient subjective visual function after corneal collagen crosslinking for keratoconus and corneal ectasia. *J Cataract Refract Surg.* 2012;38(4):615–619.

279. Filippello M, Stagni E, Buccoliero D, et al. Trans-epithelial cross-linking in keratoconus patients: confocal analysis. *Optom Vis Sci.* 2012;89(10):e1–e7.
280. Kranitz K, Kovacs I, Milhaltz K, et al. Corneal changes in progressive keratoconus after cross-linking assessed by Scheimpflug camera. *J Refract Surg.* 2012;28(9):645–649.
281. Kymionis GD, Portaliou DM, Diakonis VF, et al. Corneal collagen cross-linking with riboflavin and ultraviolet-A irradiation in patients with thin corneas. *Am J Ophthamol.* 2012;153(1):24–28.
282. Koller T, Mrochen M, Seiler T. Complication and failure rates after corneal crosslinking. *J Cataract Refract Surg.* 2009;35:1358–1362.
283. Tschopp M, Stary J, Frueh BE, et al. Impact of corneal cross-linking on drug penetration in an ex vivo porcine eye model. *Cornea.* 2012;31:222–226.
284. Krueger RR, Ramos-Esteban JC. How might corneal elasticity help us understand diabetes and intraocular pressure? *J Refract Surg.* 2007;23(1):85–88.
285. Filippello M, Stagni E, O'Brart D. Trans-epithelial corneal collagen cross-linking: a bilateral, prospective study. *J Cataract Refract Surg.* 2012;38:283–291.
286. Tuwairqi WS, Sinjab MM. Safety and efficacy of simultaneous corneal collagen cross-linking with topography-guided PRK in managing low-grade keratoconus: 1-year follow-up. *J Refract Surg.* 2012;28(5):341–345.
287. Chann CC, Sharma M, Wachler BS. Effect of inferior-segment Intacs with and without C3-R on keratoconus. *J Cataract Refract Surg.* 2007;33(1):75–80.
288. Henriquez MA, Izquierdo L, Bernilla C, et al. Corneal collagen cross-linking before Ferrara intrastromal ring implantation for the treatment of progressive keratoconus. *Cornea.* 2012;31(7):740–745.
289. McPharran R. The link to cross linking: current state of corneal cross linking surgery. AOA CLCS Newsletter, March 2012.
290. Hovakimyan M, Guthoff RF, Stachs O. Collagen cross-linking: current status and future directions. *J Ophthalmol.* 2012;2012: Article ID 406850.
291. Mack CJ. Coding tips for keratoconus from GKC. *Contact Lens Spectrum.* 2007;22(4):46.
292. Rumpakis J. Coding keratoconus—2012. AOA CLCS Newsletter, March 2012.
293. Newman CD. Understanding the new 92071 and 92072 codes. *Contact Lens Spectrum.* 2012;27(2):49.
294. Newman CD. Revisiting coding for medically necessary contact lenses. *Contact Lens Spectrum.* 2009;24(8):47.

Chapter 20

Postsurgical Contact Lens Fitting

Derek J. Louie, Eric Kawulok, Matthew Kauffman, and Arthur Epstein

Prescribing contact lenses for patients following corneal surgery is frequently challenging, but can also be extremely rewarding. Patients presenting for contact lens evaluation following a prior surgical procedure are typically seeking improvement in the postoperative visual result. They may have already seen multiple eye care providers and may be frustrated and impatient after the initial surgery has fallen short of their expectations for visual outcome. Restoring functional vision in these patients while maintaining the gains made by their surgery is potentially life altering. It remains among the greatest thrills that a skilled clinician can experience.

Despite an increased interest in refractive surgical procedures such as photorefractive keratectomy (PRK) and laser-assisted in-situ keratomileusis (LASIK), postoperative contact lens fitting remains a viable and, in many cases, a preferred option. In some situations, contact lenses are still required to restore optimal vision even after refractive procedures have been performed.[1,2]

The postsurgical contact lens design is typically guided by the postsurgical topography of the cornea's anterior surface. It is important that the clinician possesses a good understanding of postsurgical corneal topography and its relation to contact lens fitting to assist in selecting an appropriate lens design. Limbal conjunctiva, bulbar conjunctiva, palpebral fissure anatomy, and patient dexterity should also be considered when discussing and selecting contact lens designs and options.

Increasingly, practitioners are opting for scleral lens options when presented with challenging cases; however, there are multiple situations when a scleral lens is not the most appropriate choice. In cases involving concurrent or previous glaucoma filtering surgery (bleb) or drainage implant (Baerveldt tube shunt or Ahmed valve), a corneal rigid gas-permeable (GP), soft, or hybrid lens may be preferred over a scleral contact lens. Similarly, in cases involving limbal stem-cell transplantation, disrupted bulbar conjunctiva or restrictive palpebral fissure anatomy, a corneal GP lens may be a better initial lens design choice. Lens choice also depends upon practitioner experience and comfort with various possible modalities as well as the availability of specific lens designs in the practitioner's local area.

While each case is always unique, this chapter addresses the most common reasons for postsurgical contact lens fitting. We will explore contact lens options and the rationale for choosing specific designs, including topographic and physiologic needs and limitations. Often, solving a complex case will require clinical creativity and lens designs that deviate from standard, but are increasingly becoming widespread and available locally.

FULL-THICKNESS PENETRATING KERATOPLASTY (PKP)

Full-thickness penetrating keratoplasty (PKP) has long been one of the primary indications for postsurgical contact lens fitting. Post-PKP transplant rates have varied over time. During some periods, high numbers of transplants have reflected complication rates of other surgical procedures such as pseudophakic bullous keratopathy (PBK) following early intraocular lens (IOL) implants.[3] Current indications for corneal transplants include optical correction, tectonic, therapeutic, or cosmetic interventions.

A variety of corneal conditions such as keratoconus, Fuch endothelial dystrophy, previous graft failure, aphakic/PBK, interstitial or herpes keratitis, and corneal stromal dystrophies may benefit from a corneal transplant to help increase visual acuity (VA) or restore globe integrity.[4] A transplant may be performed for tectonic, reparative, or structural purpose. Transplants may also remove actively diseased tissue or unsightly opacities, providing both therapeutic and cosmetic effects.

High degrees of both regular and irregular astigmatism are common following full-thickness PKP. A variety of specific surgical techniques have been devised to reduce postoperative astigmatism and topographic irregularity, which helps the patient better tolerate spectacles or contact lenses. A commonly utilized technique is relaxing incisions (RI). The surgeon creates an arcuate incision along the steep meridian typically adjacent to the host–donor junction. This results in flattening of the steeper meridian, which also effectively steepens the flatter meridian. RI can correct between 4 and 10 D of astigmatism.[5]

Another frequently utilized technique is the compression suture, which may be used independently to steepen the flat meridian or in conjunction with a RI to increase the RIs effect. Compression sutures are placed along the flat meridian. When used in conjunction with RI, compression sutures are typically placed 90 degrees from the RI.[5]

A third technique is the wedge resection, which involves removal of a wedge of corneal tissue at the graft periphery. The remaining edges are then sutured together to produce steepening along that meridian. Graft resections can correct up to 20 D of astigmatism; however, this technique can sometimes induce significant overall myopia and refractive results that may be unstable and often times unpredictable.[6,7]

Intralase-Enabled and Traditional PKP

Corneal transplantation techniques are undergoing a rapid evolution.[4,8] In 2011, 46,196 corneal transplants were performed in the United States.[9] The traditional full-thickness PKP performed with a trephine is becoming increasingly less common, while lamellar keratoplasty is becoming a surgery of choice in patients with corneal disease or opacity that spares the endothelium.[8] However, even when a full-thickness keratoplasty is necessary, techniques and outcomes continue to evolve rapidly.[10] Patients requiring full-thickness keratoplasty benefit from techniques and technology developed for refractive surgery. Femtosecond lasers are currently being used to create both donor button and remove affected host corneal tissue with unprecedented precision. Creating the corneal donor button using the ultraprecise femtosecond laser rather than incisions created by a circular trephine has led to improved wound stability and less corneal astigmatism.[11] Due to increased wound stability, the need for excessive suture tension decreases, reducing distortion from tight or multiple sutures. Healing time and time between suture removal is also decreased.[12] As a result, contact lens fitting can be initiated much sooner for patients who have undergone femtosecond laser-based full-thickness keratoplasty than with previous techniques.

The choice of contact lens design is based largely upon the optical and structural requirements following keratoplasty. A smooth, regular, keratoplasty may yield excellent uncorrected vision or low ametropia easily correctable with spectacles or conventional soft contact lenses. Conversely, a keratoplasty that has several sutures with excessive tension and tissue heaping at the graft–host junction can result in high degrees of irregular astigmatism and a poor visual outcome, with little improvement provided by spectacles or soft contact lenses. The prevalence of irregular astigmatism postkeratoplasty is approximately double that of regular astigmatism.[13,14] Rigid GP lenses offer the best method for correcting induced irregular astigmatism.[15,16]

Running Sutures versus Interrupted Sutures

The donor corneal button may be sutured to the host rim using single or double running sutures, a combination of interrupted and running sutures, or by interrupted sutures alone.[17]

The time interval for suture removal is dependent on the type of sutures utilized, the age of the patient, and underlying disease. If interrupted sutures are used alone, they may be selectively removed as soon as 3 months postoperatively.[18,19] However, if a combination of interrupted and running sutures is used, individual sutures can be removed as soon as 1 month following surgery.[18] In general, the younger and healthier the patient, the sooner after surgery the sutures can be removed. Corneal topography helps best predict which suture or sutures are responsible for induced steepening. Once a suture has been removed, it usually takes 4 to 6 weeks for the change to appear topographically.[18] Postkeratoplasty astigmatism is comparable with the three most common suturing techniques.[20] When fitting a GP lens over running or interrupted sutures, the goal is to have minimal to no interaction between the sutures and the contact lens (Fig. 20.1). If interrupted sutures are in the process of being removed, it is best to delay contact lens fitting until all sutures have been removed.

Timing of Contact Lens Fitting after Surgery

Practitioners can begin fitting patients in contact lenses as soon as the patient's cornea is reasonably stable, regardless if sutures remain or not. However, the decision to initiate fitting should be made in conjunction with the patient's surgeon. Monocular patients are particularly anxious to have functional vision restored. However, the need for visual correction must be balanced by the risk of induced mechanical problems or inflammation. Before proceeding with an initial fitting, it is important to assess the sutures for their potential impact on graft shape. A 2004 study found that the average time from surgery to initial contact lens fitting was 18.2 months.[21] It is important to keep in mind that differences in surgical skill and technique may affect healing rate and extend or reduce the time needed for topographic stability to be achieved. Recent improvements in surgical techniques and lens designs have dramatically decreased the interval between surgery and initial contact lens fitting. In some instances, a contact lens can be fit as soon as the majority of the postsurgical inflammation has subsided, 2 to 3 months after surgery.

Contact lens fitters managing the post-PKP patient must be familiar with graft rejection, which can rapidly lead to graft failure (Fig. 20.2). The role of contact lens wear as a factor in graft failure is controversial; however, rapid treatment with appropriate medications—typically topical steroids—will usually rapidly control rejection episodes.[22,23]

Rigid Gas-Permeable Contact Lens Design

Measurement of corneal shape for the purposes of fitting contact lenses has evolved from keratometry and Placido disk to modern computerized topography instruments that provide detailed topographic images and data. This has dramatically facilitated contact lens fitting and

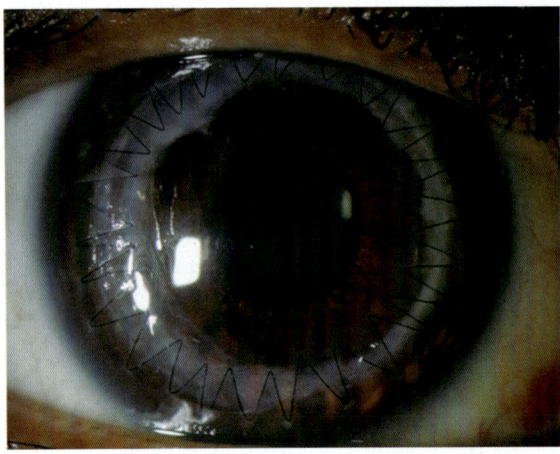

FIGURE 20.1 Intralase-enabled keratoplasty with running suture.

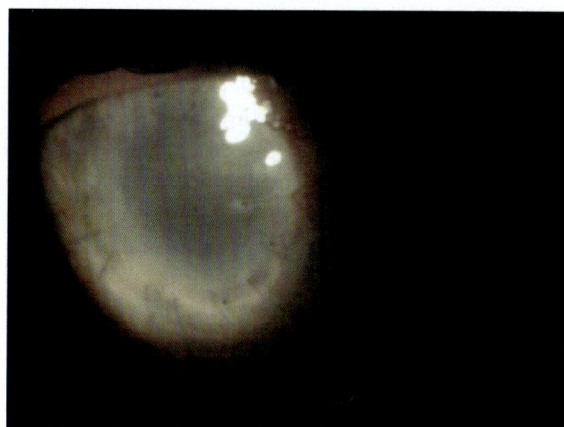

FIGURE 20.2 Corneal graft rejection.

postfitting evaluation of corneal topography. Corneal topography is especially valuable when faced with irregular corneal topography often encountered in complex postsurgical fitting situations.

The lack of availability of computerized corneal topography does not necessarily indicate that successful contact lens fitting cannot be achieved, even in the most complex cases. Evaluation of the fluorescein pattern after trial fitting, using a large-diameter spherical GP lens, reveals underlying topography with reasonable resolution for fitting purposes. An additional benefit is the ability to evaluate potential acuity with good accuracy, even when the fit is unacceptable.

There are two primary philosophies generally applied when fitting contact lenses after corneal surgery or repair. One approach is to fit the lens to approximate the corneal contour, while the second involves masking the underlying corneal contour and vaulting any irregularities. With the former technique, graft shape dictates the GP lens design. The goal in fitting the corneal contour is to provide a centered, stable, comfortable lens that distributes lens weight and bearing forces generated by gravity and lid action as evenly as possible across the transplanted corneal surface. A large-diameter lens (>10.0 mm) with an optical zone diameter (OZD) that spans the size of the graft is required.[24,25] Examples include the Dyna Z intra-Limbal (Lens Dynamics, Kansas City, MO), the GBL lens (ABB Concise, Coral Springs, FL), the Comfort XL (Valley Contax, Springfield, OR), and the Rose K2 IC (Blanchard Contact Lens, Manchester, NH and multiple fabricating laboratories). Masking the corneal contour involves fitting semi-scleral or scleral contact lenses that bridge the majority or entirety of the irregular corneal surface.

Karabatsas et al.[13] classified topographic patterns observed after PKP into several shapes: prolate, oblate, mixed—prolate and oblate—asymmetric, and steep to flat (or tilted). Prolate corneas can simulate normal aspheric topography. The central cornea has a steeper radius, which is surrounded by concentric progressive flattening. Traditional fitting techniques may be used. Prolate corneas are the exception for post-PK corneas. The best contact lens starting point when fitting a prolate-shaped cornea is a traditional keratoconic lens design. Aspheric lenses are also useful in some cases.

Oblate corneas exhibit a flat center with a steeper peripheral topography. This appearance is very common, at least in one meridian. When fitting a contact lens on a cornea with this topography pattern, excessive central clearance may be necessary to achieve proper lens alignment with the peripheral cornea, taking particular caution when assessing the fit over the graft–host junction to avoid excessive bearing and breakdown of underlying tissue. Excessive bearing in any area of the graft–host junction may be heralded by punctate staining, inflammation, focal erosion, scarring, and even graft rejection. Reverse geometry designs are very helpful in fitting this topographic pattern, especially when more conventional designs produce unacceptable central clearance and midperipheral bearing. When designing a reverse geometry lens, it is best to start with an axial topography map.[26] Note both the average central keratometry measurements and the average measurements around the graft–host junction help to select the initial base curve radius (BCR) of the diagnostic lens.[27]

Most GP lens manufacturers offer postsurgical lens designs that incorporate reverse geometry curves. Diagnostic fitting, using one of these designs, will provide an excellent indication of how a lens will perform on the eye. Generally, these lens designs will be between 10.0 and 12.0 mm in overall diameter (OAD), or intralimbal.

Consider modifications to the laboratories' postgraft lens design if there is poor lens–cornea apposition. Excessive central corneal clearance may be controlled by decreasing the optical zone size; however, this may cause significant change in the bearing relationship of the lens periphery on the graft–host junction. If the lens excessively bears over the graft–host junction, an increased reverse curve is likely indicated. A slightly larger OAD (0.5 mm larger) may help to improve centration. To facilitate tear exchange behind the GP lens, attempt the greatest amount of edge lift without causing staining, corneal dehydration, or excessive lens awareness. It is possible that a quadrant-specific peripheral curve system will be needed to accommodate the irregular shape or tilt of a graft.

Modern fabrication techniques have allowed most GP lens manufacturers to produce large-diameter corneal lenses (and scleral lenses) in reverse geometry designs. A reverse geometry lens design refers to any lens that has steeper peripheral curve radii (PCRs) than the central BCR. Generally, a diagnostic lens design should have at least 4 D of difference between central base curve and peripheral curves to effectively reduce excessive clearance over the graft and provide increased clearance over the peripheral areas of the cornea (Fig. 20.3).

Graft tilt likely accounts for some of the challenges presented with postgraft topography. One portion of these grafts will be very steep, while the portion located 180 degrees away is very flat (Fig. 20.4). If a corneal GP lens is utilized, it will tend to center over the steepest portion of the graft. Often this decentration is unavoidable; however, the use of a larger-diameter lens will typically improve centration and reduce glare. Utilizing a quadrant-specific lens design, where the peripheral curves can be varied steeper or flatter per quadrant, can also provide improved centration and comfort, but can be a complex undertaking in some cases. Bitoric lenses are contraindicated in tilted graft corneas. If excessively tilted or proud (Fig. 20.5), where the majority of the graft is elevated away from the host corneal tissue, the application of a corneal GP lens will often result in unacceptable decentration or spontaneous lens ejection. In these cases, a scleral or semi-scleral contact lens will always be a more successful approach.

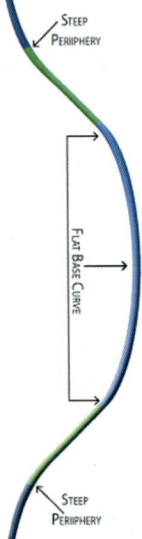

FIGURE 20.3 Reverse geometry contact lens design.

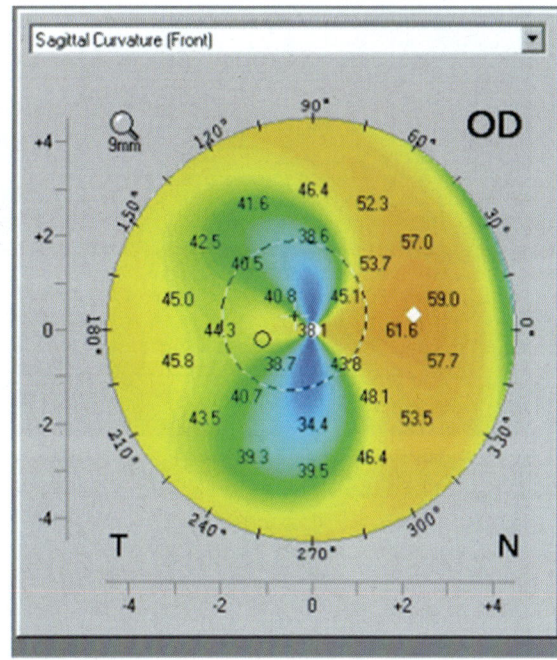

FIGURE 20.4 Corneal topography of a tilted graft.

Post-PKP corneas with mixed astigmatism may have mostly regular astigmatism across the entire topographic map. In these cases, a bitoric lens design can provide good alignment and visual performance.

In general, high oxygen permeable (Dk) and intrinsically wettable lens materials are preferred in fitting postsurgical cases. While lens flexure may be of concern with some high-Dk materials, it is best to start with materials possessing a Dk >90 in patients with already compromised corneas and assess lens flexure with overkeratometry or topography, if flexure is the suspected cause of decreased vision.[28] If lens flexure is causing a loss in best-corrected vision, consider a 0.10 to 0.20 mm increase in central lens thickness.

Soft Contact Lenses

Corneal graft patients may also be prescribed soft lenses, especially when corneal astigmatism is regular. Soft contact lenses can be used as a bandage lens to help heal persistent epithelial defects, epithelial filaments, and extreme height discrepancies at the graft–host junction. It is important to utilize silicone hydrogel materials when fitting soft lenses on a postkeratoplasty

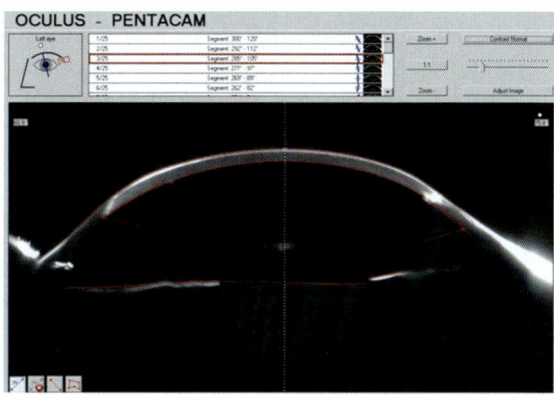

FIGURE 20.5 Scheimpflug image of a proud graft.

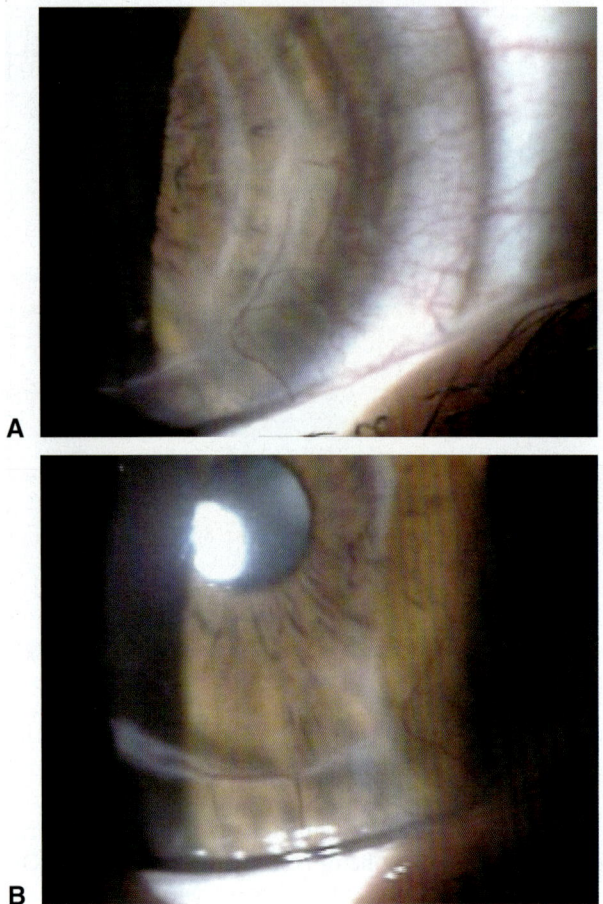

FIGURE 20.6 Neovascularization stopping at the graft interface.

cornea. The use of low-Dk soft lenses is generally inadvisable due to the risk of neovascularization (NV) extending into the graft and subsequent graft rejection.[23] Vascularization of the host cornea occasionally occurs and while it should be avoided, is less problematic than NV that invades the graft (Fig. 20.6). NV into the graft compromises its immune-privileged status.

Silicone hydrogel lenses are a good option for correction of residual ametropia, due to the increased permeability and greater supply of oxygen to the graft. Spherical lenses are primarily used as piggyback lenses, as they rarely correct the majority of postsurgical ametropia. Lenses with a steep base curve are often needed to fit oblate corneal grafts. Custom lenses fabricated from silicone hydrogel materials are available when necessary.

Soft contact lenses can also serve a prosthetic purpose by providing an artificial pupil. Note, however, that prosthetic or custom-painted contact lenses currently are only available in low-Dk hydrogel materials. Special care must be taken and the keratoplasty monitored closely for the development of NV in these cases. Toric silicone hydrogel lenses provide a good option for fitting corneal grafts when the majority of the astigmatism is regular. Stock silicone hydrogel toric lenses or the newer Definitive silicone hydrogel custom toric lens (Contamac US, Grand Junction, CO) (efrofilcon-A 74%, Dk = 60) is appropriate for post-PKP use.

Custom soft contact lenses for postsurgical corneas are available from many lens manufacturers (Table 20.1). These custom lenses, with increased center thickness or reverse geometry peripheral curves, can mask moderate amounts of postsurgical irregularity. A sphero–cylindrical overrefraction to help refine lens parameters, is usually necessary to achieve maximal acuity.

TABLE 20.1 Postsurgical Custom Soft Lens Manufacturers	
LENS MANUFACTURER	WEBSITE
Advanced Vision Technologies	www.avtlens.com
Art Optical	www.artoptical.com
Medlens Innovations/Visionary Optics Inc.	www.visionary-optics.com

Piggyback Contact Lenses

The advantages of a piggyback lens system are improved comfort, reduced mechanical interaction with the graft, and possibly masking of some corneal irregularity by the soft lens, making the GP lens design less complex. Disadvantages include the complexity of applying and caring for two lenses per eye each day, induced distortion, and poorer optics compared to a single lens system, and a possible increased tendency for coatings and deposits on the piggyback lenses. Soft contact lenses can mask some of the corneal irregularity when performing corneal topography or fitting GP lenses on postsurgical corneas. A soft carrier lens also tends to effectively flatten and elevate the corneal apex. This can be controlled somewhat by selection of the carrier. If the postsurgical cornea is excessively steep centrally, a myopic soft lens (−3.00 to −6.00 D) can provide a "flatter" contour and may allow a less complicated GP lens design. Conversely, if the postsurgical cornea is excessively flat, a hyperopic soft lens (+3.00 to +6.00 D) may provide a "steeper" contour to facilitate the piggyback lens. The piggyback lens provides approximately 20% of its original optical power in this system.[29] A silicone hydrogel contact lens along with a moderate-to-high Dk GP lens combination should be selected to allow adequate oxygen availability to the cornea.[30,31] Corneal GP lens designs in a piggyback system should follow fitting guidelines discussed for GP lenses alone. Fitting evaluation of the GP portion of a piggyback lens can be accomplished either using conventional fluorescein or high-molecular-weight fluorescein as conventional fluorescein will be minimally absorbed by most silicone materials. The overall thickness of the piggyback system should be considered when using this type of correction in postsurgical corneas. Practitioners should select the most transmissible materials in both GP and soft lens to maximize oxygen diffusion to the cornea (Fig. 20.7).[30,31]

Hybrid Contact lenses

A hybrid contact lens refers to any lens with a GP lens center and a hydrogel or silicone hydrogel lens fused together. This combination can provide improved comfort and centration over traditional corneal GP lens designs. Early hybrid designs like the Saturn introduced by

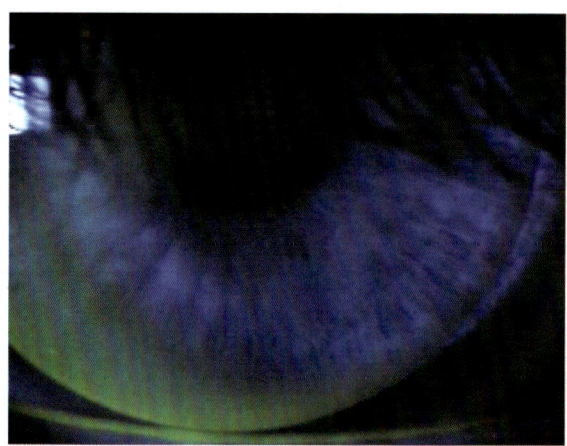

FIGURE 20.7 The piggyback system using the Dyna Intra-Limbal lens GP design.

Precision-Cosmet (Buffalo, NY) in 1984, and later modified and introduced as the SoftPerm lens (Wesley-Jessen), suffered from low Dk of both the GP center and hydrogel surround, and lens tightening, which limited its use. SynergEyes Inc. (Carlsbad, CA) is currently the only contact lens manufacturer to produce hybrid lenses. The company has several lens designs that may provide improved comfort and stability compared to a corneal GP lens.

The selection of a hybrid lens in postkeratoplasty patients rests largely in the topographic appearance of the graft. In patients with moderate amounts of residual, regular, or irregular astigmatism, the Duette or SynergEyes A design may provide an adequate fitting relationship. In steep central grafts or graft with moderate amounts of tilt, the Clearkone or SynergEyes KC design may be useful. In patients with flat central grafts and steep peripheral graft–host junction, the SynergEyes PS or Clearkone design are the lenses of choice.[32]

SynergEyes lens designs use an 8.0 to 9.0 mm GP lens center, a 7.0 to 7.4 mm optical zone with a 14.5 mm OAD. In postsurgical cases, care must be taken to ensure the junction of the hybrid lens does not bear excessively on the graft–host interface. Additionally, the low-Dk skirt of the first-generation SynergEyes lenses should be avoided if possible due to previously mentioned considerations.

The recently introduced SynergEyes UltraHealth may prove useful in postkeratoplasty cases. This reverse geometry lens design incorporates a 130-Dk GP central zone and an 84-Dk silicone hydrogel soft skirt.

LAMELLAR KERATOPLASTY (DALK, DSAEK, DSEK, DMEK)

Deep anterior lamellar keratoplasty (DALK) and endothelial keratoplasty (EK) are the two primary subcategories of lamellar keratoplasty. In addition, there are three subcategories of EK, which include Descemet stripping membrane endothelial keratoplasty (DSEK), Descemet stripping automated membrane endothelial keratoplasty (DSAEK), or Descemet membrane endothelial keratoplasty (DMEK). The goal of most types of lamellar keratoplasty is to remove the diseased portion of the cornea and spare as much patient's healthy, functional tissue as possible.

EK surgery has been rapidly growing in the United States, substantially totaling 44.9% of corneal transplantations in 2010 versus only 4.5% in 2005.[4] The end result of EK is the removal of the poor functioning endothelial cell layer and replacing it with a donor transplant to restore proper corneal function. Once the endothelium is replaced, the anterior corneal curvature often will normalize once excess fluid is removed. Postsurgically, a refractive error shift is usually observed and can either be myopic or hyperopic.[33] In studies by Lee et al.,[33,34] 0.7 to 1.5 D of hyperopia is generally induced after DSAEK postsurgically and is thought to be caused by a reduction in the post corneal radius of curvature of the graft, decreasing the overall effective power of the eye. Once the corneal graft is performed and the cornea clears postsurgically, corneal topography and spectacle refraction will help guide the choice between soft and GP contact lens.

One of the concerns with contact lens wear is stress to the endothelium evidenced by polymegethism and polymorphism of corneal endothelial cells.[35] Practitioners should consider wear time and wear schedule when prescribing contact lenses for patients with an endothelial transplant. A high-Dk lens material, such as a silicone hydrogel, is recommended to allow maximum oxygen transmission. In addition, extended (overnight) wear contact lenses should be avoided to minimize impact on the graft.

The differences between DSEK, DSAEK, and DMEK are related to how the tissue is prepared and the layer of tissue transplanted. DSEK is the manual lamellar dissection of Descemet layer with residual stromal layers. Manual dissection of Descemet layer is imprecise and can lead to a graft with inconsistent thickness. Due to this inconsistency, the use of a microkeratome for dissection has become popular. The microkeratome allows for more consistent graft thickness and can be precut at eye banks, eliminating the need for the surgeon to perform a two-step procedure.[33] DSEK with the use of a microkeratome to prepare the host tissue is coined DSAEK. DMEK is a further refinement of EK in which the stromal portion of the donor is eliminated so that the graft consists only of Descemet's membrane and endothelial cells.[33] Although the handling of the thinner tissue is more challenging, it provides the fastest and best visual recovery of all EK procedures.[33]

In diseases that affect corneal stromal layers, DALK is the lamellar surgery of choice, due to a decreased risk of endothelial rejection. Endothelial rejection is the major cause of transplant failure.[4] Due to the technical difficulty inherent in separating the anterior stromal layers from Descemet's membrane and endothelium, widespread adoption has been limited. Postsurgical mean regular astigmatism between PK and automated lamellar keratolasty (ALK) is approximately 4 to 5 D.[4] As techniques for dissection of the corneal lamellar tissue become more refined and consistent, surgeons may offer this surgical approach more frequently.

Contact lens fitting approaches for DALK are similar to the strategies used in PKP. Surgeon skill, graft quality, and suture tension are all factors that affect overall topography and graft success. Consultation with the surgeons responsible for the new graft is recommended, as they will likely be the referring provider for contact lens fit. Similar to a full-thickness keratoplasty, it can take months for the surgeon to adjust sutures to minimize regular and irregular astigmatism. The course of suture removal is highly dependent on the individual surgeon; presence of sutures, however, is not a contraindication to contact lens fitting. While the presence of sutures may create more challenging corneal topography, a contact lens fit can still be highly successful, without significantly increasing the risk of complications.[36] Sutures may remain indefinitely. Contact lens fitting in these cases should be considered on an individual basis in conjunction with the surgeon, balancing patient need with potential risk to the graft. Fitting becomes generally less complicated when no more sutures are going to be removed.

As indicated in full-thickness keratoplasty, topographic patterns drive the initial diagnostic lens choice. Topography for anterior lamellar keratoplasty will be most influenced by suture tension, suture removal, and healing around the graft–host interface. Commonly, an oblate pattern is observed and a reverse geometry design is indicated. The goal of a reverse curve design is to vault over the sutures and minimize contact with the graft–host interface. Having a flat central base curve and steeper midperipheral curve minimizes excessive central vault. Excessive central pooling can result in dimple veiling and stagnation of tears behind the lens, leading to hazy vision, in some cases within 20 minutes of lens application.

Lid anatomy and contact lens–lid interaction can affect centration and stability of the contact lens. In some cases, an interpalpebral fit may be appropriate due to other surgical obstacles such as a trabeculectomy.

Contact lens OAD should be selected to minimize graft–host interface interaction. Manufacturers' postsurgical contact lens designs generally range between 10 and 12 mm in OAD to help vault the graft–host interface. Vaulting over the graft and irregular sectors improves stability, utilizing the patient's normal peripheral cornea contour. Mini-scleral and scleral contact lenses can be appropriate choices due to their stability and ability to vault significant corneal irregularity; however, in some patients, scleral lenses are contraindicated due to other ocular complications. For more information regarding scleral contact lens fitting techniques and recommendations, refer to Chapter 21.

Contact lens material should also be carefully selected. Due to the larger OAD and decreased movement compared to smaller designs, high-Dk materials should be selected to maximize oxygen diffusion and minimize NV. NV can lead to corneal inflammation and, ultimately, to graft rejection. More wettable materials are also advisable on larger, less mobile lenses as they lead to less deposit buildup.

Care and consideration of lens design should be followed when fitting a postlamellar keratoplasty patient. The overall goals should be to minimize the risk to the transplant as well as provide optimal vision for the patient.

REFRACTIVE SURGERY

Patients who have undergone refractive surgery other than keratoplasty may require contact lenses to improve their VA or manage an operative or postoperative complication. The goal of corneal refractive procedures is to remove or reshape corneal tissue to effect overall corrective refractive change. Although most refractive procedures, especially those performed today, result in acceptable outcomes, complications that are best managed with contact lenses still arise.

Early refractive procedures did not account or compensate for induced higher-order optical aberrations and were therefore more likely to result in postoperative degraded contrast sensitivity, glare, ghosting, and night vision issues, especially in patients with larger pupil sizes.[37,38] Modern excimer treatment generally incorporates wavefront or topographic guidance, which has reduced the incidence of higher-order aberrations and visual problems. Contact lens management of residual higher-order aberrations is difficult, although significant improvement in visual outcomes can be accomplished.

The fitter should be aware that the dissatisfied postrefractive surgery patient seeking care is sometimes extremely challenging to manage. A thorough discussion of the psychological characteristics of the patient who presents with a failed elective refractive procedure is beyond the scope of this text; however, many refractive surgery failure patients suffer from complex psychological as well as refractive issues.[39] As a result, the successful contact lens fitter will need considerable patience and understanding.

Refractive surgeries can be classified based upon structural changes made to the cornea. The categories include surface incisional procedures (radial keratotomy [RK], astigmatic keratotomy [AK]), tissue removal (PRK, ALK, LASIK, laser-assisted sub-epithelial keratomileusis [LASEK]) and tissue addition (Epikeratoplasty, Intacs). Surface incision procedures involve using a diamond blade to make controlled partial thickness incisions into the cornea.

Refractive Corneal Ablation (PRK, ALK, PTK, LASEK, LASIK)

Barraquer first introduced modern corneal reshaping in 1963. Keratomileusis involves removing a section of the cornea with a microkeratome, reshaping it with a specially designed lathe and then resuturing it back onto the corneal surface.[40,41] With the development and clinical refinement of the excimer laser in the late 1980s and early 1990s, newer and more accurate techniques including PRK and LASIK became increasingly popular. Ablative techniques like PRK and LASIK reshape the corneal contour and optics by removing tissue (at a molecular level) and flattening the central cornea.

PRK is typically performed as an outpatient procedure using topical anesthetic. The epithelium is either mechanically removed or flapped back and away from the area to be treated. The excimer laser is then applied to ablate or remove Bowman layer and sufficient stromal tissue to produce the desired refractive effect. In traditional PRK, a bandage lens is placed, which allows the cornea to reepithelize. Complications of PRK and related techniques that are amenable to contact lens correction include under- and overcorrection and corneal irregularity.

LASIK was introduced soon after PRK. It was initially an off-label excimer laser procedure, but because of more rapid healing, shorter recovery time, and increased refractive correction range, it quickly became more popular. The technique entails the use of a microkeratome or, more recently, a femtosecond laser to create a flap consisting of epithelium and anterior stroma. The excimer laser is then applied to the stromal bed to affect the desired refractive change. After treatment, the flap is replaced and seals to the underlying tissue. A bandage contact lens is rarely used. Among the advantages of LASIK is the rapid dramatic improvement in uncorrected vision that is observed.

Early LASIK procedures did not account for the biomechanical consequences of removing excessive amounts of stromal tissue, which resulted in destabilization of the cornea. As a result, some patients, particularly those with higher amounts of treated myopia, subsequently developed postoperative ectasia, a condition mimicking keratoconus. Preoperative measurement and calculation of residual stromal bed depth has reduced the incidence of postoperative ectasia.

The contact lens management of post-LASIK ectasia is complicated by the asymmetric surface irregularity that accompanies the progressive inferior thinning and protrusion seen in this condition. A variety of lens designs are available to fit post-LASIK ectasia patients, including soft, GP, and hybrid lens options. Fitting techniques are similar, but often more challenging than managing keratoconus patients with contact lenses. Decentered treatment zones are another complication of ablative refractive surgery, which may require yet complicate postoperative contact lens management.

Gas-Permeable Lens Design

Central corneal flattening and relative steepening of the surrounding cornea after ablative refractive procedures often complicates GP lens fitting; however, a variety of designs and techniques have been developed to manage these patients. Many fitters prefer to use larger-diameter lenses such as the Dyna Intra-Limbal lenses (Lens Dynamics, Kansas City, MO). Larger reverse geometry designs like the Dyna Intra-Limbal Special Reverse Geometry lens may be necessary due to the perverted topography present in post-LASIK patients (Fig. 20.8). Caution must be exercised to avoid excessive bearing and possible seal-off of the flatter central corneal zone. Many GP fitters prefer to utilize scleral designs that vault over the affected cornea. Scleral lens designs are discussed in Chapter 21.

Soft Lens Designs

Soft contact lenses can be a viable option following ablative refractive surgery for patients primarily requiring refractive correction. Both spherical and astigmatic errors can be successfully managed. Thin, higher-Dk lenses are generally preferred, as they tend to better approximate the reshaped corneal surface. Caution should be observed as some lenses will buckle and be easily dislodged due to the abnormal topography. The lens BCR is typically fit flat, with larger diameter and aspheric designs often being helpful in masking residual irregularity. Caution should be exercised to avoid seal-off of the treated area and lead to hypoxia.

Dry eye is a frequent complaint after ablative refractive surgery and must be managed to insure successful contact lens wear. Preparing and supporting the ocular surface with appropriate adjunctive treatment, including rewetting drops and management of evaporative dry eye, is essential, especially with soft lenses.

In some cases, custom-designed lenses will be necessary. For patients requiring them, hybrid designs are available (SynergEyes PS and UltraHealth, SynergEyes, Inc., Carlsbad, CA).

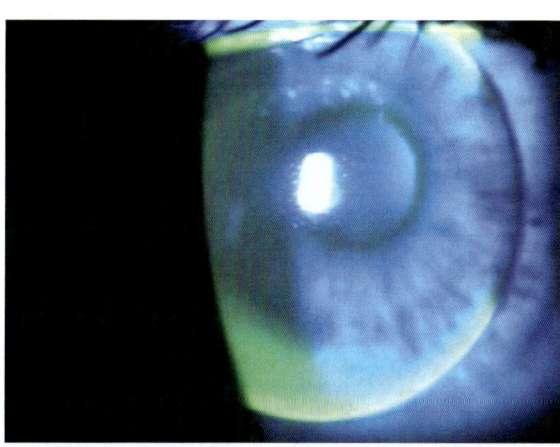

FIGURE 20.8 A good lens-to-cornea fitting relationship of a GP lens in a post-LASIK ectasia patient.

Incisional Refractive Surgery

Incisional refractive surgery includes those patients who have undergone RK, AK, and hexagonal keratotomy. These incisional refractive surgery procedures have been replaced by the more reliable and widely performed modern laser ablative refractive surgical procedures discussed above.

Significant numbers of patients who have undergone RK develop diurnal fluctuations in vision and refractive error.[42,43] These patients may also have significant shifts in corneal curvature.[43,44] Whereas vision with soft contact lens correction can often show diurnal fluctuations similar to changes in spectacle correction, GP contact lenses can mask diurnal visual fluctuations. When hydrogel materials are prescribed in post-RK and -AK cases, corneal NV is associated with lens wear in up to 50% of cases.[45,46]

Similar to postcorneal ablative refractive surgery, the postincisional surgical corneal topography is often oblate. A majority of these patients will require a reverse geometry GP lens design to ensure appropriate clearance over the steeper peripheral cornea.[47]

When selecting a starting BCR of a corneal GP lens, start with a lens 1.00 to 1.50 D steeper than average central keratometry measurements. It is helpful to gather keratometry data in the midperiphery of four quadrants as well. The BCR of the initial diagnostic lens can be equal to the temporal reading or average of four quadrants. Another method of selecting the initial lens BCR is to use the dioptric value 3.5 mm superior to the visual axis on the axial map.[48] On a post-RK cornea, the axial and instantaneous values differ further away from the optical axis. Significant differences occur over the "knee" of the surgical optical zone, where the flat central cornea transitions to a steeper peripheral cornea. To determine the amount of reverse curve necessary, record the axial dioptric change across the transition with topography. Select a lens design that has the secondary curves steeper by an amount greater than or equal to the dioptric transition change. If there are <2 D of astigmatism, the BCR should be 1 D steeper than the flat "K." If more than 2 D of astigmatism are present, the BCR should equal the average "K."

Central vaulting over the RK optical zone is expected (Fig. 20.9). A minus-powered contact lens, determined by overrefraction of the diagnostic contact lens, will help compensate for a plus-powered tear layer. Light touch or pooling will be observed over the inflection point. One may also notice 1 to 2 mm wide bands of midperipheral bearing. It is best to use a larger-diameter lens (i.e., 9.2–10.2 mm), with an optical zone 1 to 4 mm less than the OAD. These lenses will likely exhibit a standard axial edge lift.

The SynergEyes PS, Clearkone, or UltraHealth hybrid lenses may be useful in postincisional refractive surgery cases. These hybrid lens designs can provide stable vision with comfortable, centered GP lens optical properties. However, care should be taken when prescribing low-Dk, high-water-contact lens designs as RK patients are particularly prone to the development of corneal NV along the corneal incisions.

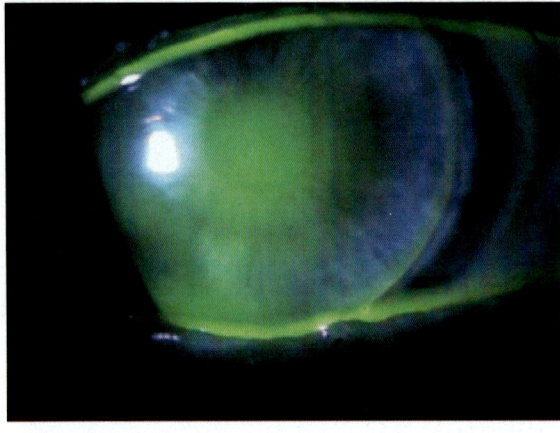

FIGURE 20.9 Postradial keratotomy patient managed with a reverse geometry GP lens design. Central clearance is exhibited with fluorescein.

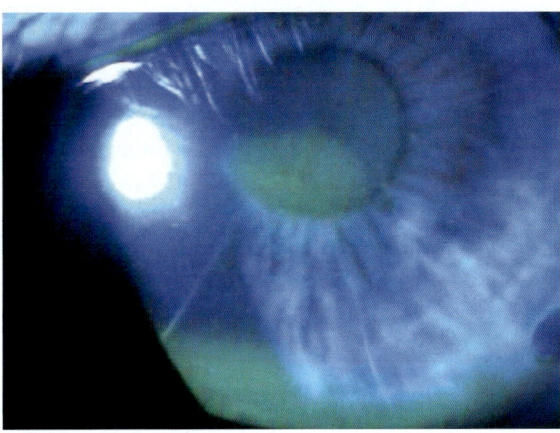

FIGURE 20.10 Postradial keratotomy patient managed with the MacroLens (C & H Contact Lens).

Scleral contact lenses are also becoming more widespread as the lens of choice in postincisional surgical cases. Most lens designs are available with reverse curves and in high-Dk lens materials (Fig. 20.10).

INTRASTROMAL CORNEAL RING SEGMENTS (ICRS) (INTACS)

Intacs, as reviewed in the keratoconus chapter (Chapter 19), are arclike, polymethylmethacrylate (PMMA) ICRS that are surgically inserted into the deep stroma.[49,50] Intacs can be placed manually into the cornea or, more recently, via channels created with the assistance of a femtosecond laser.[51–54] They are used in keratoconus to flatten the cone of the ectatic cornea; therefore, vision is improved.[55] Good candidates for Intacs include individuals with mild-moderate keratoconus with a steep keratometry reading no higher than the mid-50s, a spherical equivalent refractive error <5 D, and a minimum corneal thickness of, at minimum, 450 microns over the region where the Intacs will be inserted.[56–59] At minimum, it is evident that Intacs is a reversible procedure, which likely halts the progression of keratoconus. Whereas it will not have as significant an effect as a more invasive procedure such as DALK,[60] Intacs may be a therapeutic option to halt this condition and, perhaps, allow some patients to avoid a corneal transplant.

Contact Lens Applications

It is evident that Intacs does result in some stabilization of the cornea in keratoconus; however, significant residual refractive error is quite common and other forms of correction (i.e., often GP lenses or, secondarily, soft lenses or spectacles) are often necessary.[61,62]

Typically, GP contact lens fitting can be initiated as soon as 3 months after the segments are implanted.[63,64] In general, post-Intacs corneas remain prolate and can be managed similar to keratoconus (see Chapter 19).[63] As the stabilization of the cornea typically involves flattening of the corneal apex, the fitting can be less complicated than prior to Intacs implantation. Following ICRS implantation, it is best to start with keratoconus-designed corneal GP lenses; however, topographic information should still guide the practitioners lens design selection.[63] A larger-diameter, intralimbal or larger keratoconus design, GP lens can mask remaining irregularity after ICRS implantation. These lens designs center well, and can decrease interaction with the areas of the cornea where the ICRS have been implanted. It is best to begin with a base curve that provides minimal vaulting over the apex of the cornea and avoiding corneal bearing of the lens above the ICRS. Many patients report increased corneal sensitivity if the corneal GP lens rests directly over the ICRS. A large-diameter, (10–12 mm) reverse geometry lens is another useful lens design. Utilize a lens with an optical zone approximately the same as the internal diameter of the ICRS implants (typically 7 mm); the steeper secondary curve can help decrease corneal interaction over the ICRS, while providing improved centration and clearance over the central cornea. A piggyback system, hybrid, semi-scleral, or scleral lens are also good options when fitting corneas with ICRS.

Although typically a GP lens is indicated, soft lenses and, in some cases, spectacles can provide acceptable vision. Intacs patients can be fit into soft lenses—spherical or toric—during the first 3 months, beginning at the end of 7 days.[64] Piggyback lenses have also been quite successful in post-Intacs patients and represented the lenses of choice in over 50% of patients in one study.[65]

POSTOCULAR TRAUMA

Trauma to the anterior segment may be limited to the cornea or more extensive, affecting the posterior structures of iris, crystalline lens, or retina. Contact lenses are useful in the correction of irregular astigmatism created by a corneal scar, glare, high anisometropia, or monocular aphakia, or simply to improve cosmesis. The patient's motivation may be high if contact lenses can dramatically improve best-corrected vision in the affected eye or may be low if the other eye is correctable to 20/20 and the patient is able to suppress the images from the affected eye. In absence of motivation, it is important to educate the patient on the importance of correcting the traumatized eye for multiple reasons: the traumatized eye may become amblyopic if not corrected (depending on patient age), the patient may become strabismic due to loss of sensory stimuli,[66] and the possibility of additional injury or disease affecting the contralateral eye.

Lens Selection

In cases of ocular trauma, the extent of the injury will guide the choice of lens design. Where adequate spectacle correction can be obtained, a soft sphere, soft toric, or custom soft toric may be indicated. In cases where high refractive error and anisometropia, such as monocular aphakia, is the confounding factor, a soft lens may still provide adequate visual correction. This correction may also be combined with a prosthetic lens or custom-painted lens to reduce glare from irregular or loss of pupillary function. Prosthetic and custom-painted lenses are only available in traditional hydrogel materials, not silicone hydrogel or GP materials. Patients must be carefully monitored for formation of corneal neovascular blood vessels.

Corneal lacerations can lead to scarring and localized flattening of the cornea. This flattening can lead to irregular astigmatism and loss of best spectacle correction. In cases with acquired irregular astigmatism due to trauma, a GP or hybrid lens should be considered. Once again, the anterior topographic contours will guide the GP lens design selected. The area of irregularity will be confined to the area of repaired cornea. This may allow a less complicated lens design in postocular trauma contact lens fitting compared to postkeratoplasty. Nevertheless, a larger-diameter GP lens will usually be the lens of choice in postocular trauma cases. Larger diameters can bridge over the irregular portion of the cornea, provide a larger optical zone, and improved comfort with less lens movement (Fig. 20.11). Practitioners should consider 10.0 to 12.0 mm OAD spherical lens designs. Bitoric lens designs are generally not indicated unless there is significant regular astigmatism following trauma. BCR selection should start with the most regular area of the cornea, which will likely be steeper than the area of injury. Excessive clearance over the area of injury is likely, but if centration and comfort are adequate without air bubble formation, then the lens may perform satisfactorily.

Prosthetic Contact Lenses

If ocular trauma patients require improved cosmesis and decreased glare symptoms, a prosthetic contact lens may be indicated. A prosthetic contact lens provides an artificial iris and pupil or may cover an opacified cornea. Prosthetic and custom-painted lenses are only available

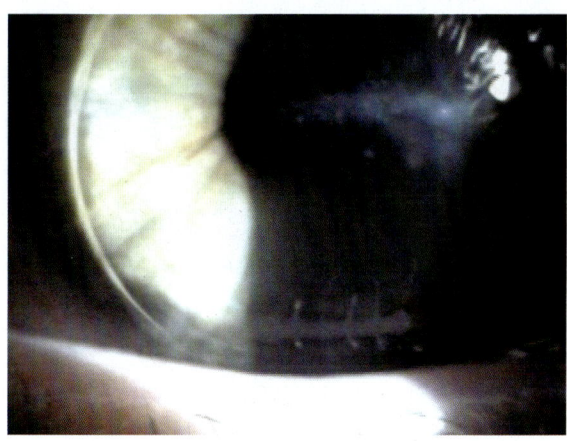

FIGURE 20.11 GP lens over repaired corneal lacerations.

in traditional hydrogel materials, not silicone hydrogel or rigid GP materials. These contact lenses are available in several standard iris tints and with clear or black pupils. Custom-painted prosthetic lenses are also available. First, fit a clear custom soft lens on the injured eye. Once the fit and vision have been optimized with the clear lens, take a digital picture of both the injured and uninjured eye. These hand-painted contact lenses require methafilcon (55% water), ocufilcon (53% water), or hioxifilcon A or B (59%/49% water) lens materials.[67] It is best, when taking a digital image of the eye, to have both wide and close-in images, as well as consistent even lighting across the eye to provide the best image for the artist to match (Table 20.2). Consult with manufacturers for specific guidance when considering custom-painted prosthetic contact lenses.

KERATOPROSTHESIS

KPro type I

The Boston Keratoprosthesis (KPro) is a surgically implantable artificial cornea developed by Claes Dohlman, MD in 1974.[68,69] The KPro is the most common prosthetic corneal device used in the United States.[70] KPro implantation attempts to salvage functional vision in patients with multiple corneal transplant rejections and those with severe ocular surface disease (chemical eye burns, stem-cell deficiencies, Stevens–Johnson syndrome, and ocular cicatricial pemphigoid).[71] Human corneal donor tissue, two PMMA plates, and a locking titanium ring make up the Boston KPro type I. Postoperative management involves chronic treatment with topical corticosteroids, fortified antibiotics (vancomycin), and lifelong therapeutic contact lens use.[72] The new corneal surface is prone to epithelial defects, stromal thinning, tissue melt, and

TABLE 20.2 Custom, Prosthetic Lens Manufacturers

LENS MANUFACTURER	WEBSITE
Alden Optical	www.aldenoptical.com
Adventure in Colors	www.techcolors.com
Cantor Prosthetic Lenses	www.cantor-nissel.co.uk
Crystal Reflections Int'l., Inc.	www.crystalreflectionsintl.com
Custom Color Contacts	www.customcontacts.com
Orion Vision Group/ Marietta Contact Lens Service	www.orionvisiongroup.com www.mariettacontactlens.com
Medcorp International	www.medcorpint.com

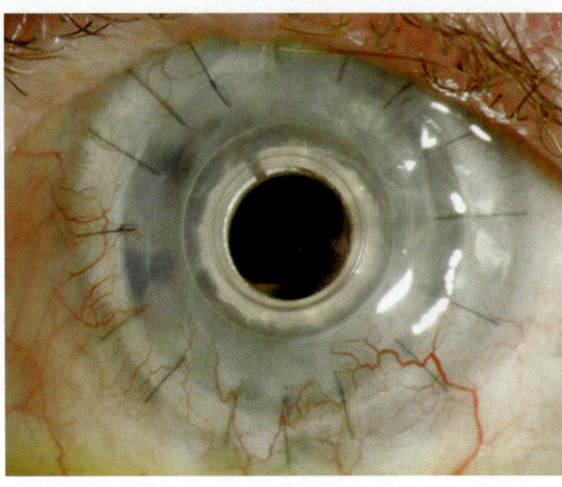

FIGURE 20.12 Boston keratoprosthesis type 1.

necrosis due to desiccation. A 16.0-mm diameter hydrogel soft contact lens with a flat base curve (8.9 mm) is fit over the prosthetic device to decrease surface dehydration.[69] This bandage contact lens also provides protection for exposed sutures and may be tinted to decrease glare as well as correct postoperative refractive error.[73] Some patients rapidly develop lens deposits on this bandage lens, resulting in significantly decreased lens comfort, performance, and vision. In these cases, a hybrid or scleral lens may be required (Fig. 20.12).[74]

CLINICAL CASES

CASE 1 (COURTESY OF JAMIE KUHN, OD)

A 29-year-old male with progressive keratoconus OU underwent PKP OS. The right eye is fit successfully with a limbal GP lens, with BCVA of $20/15^{-2}$. After unsuccessful attempts at correcting his vision with GP contact lenses OS, the patient underwent PKP surgery. He has not been fit with any GP contact lenses since his surgery OS; no spectacle or contact lens correction is worn OS. Uncorrected VA is found to be 20/40 OS. Biomicroscopy reveals a clear corneal graft, without remaining sutures or contraindications to contact lens wear. He wishes to proceed with contact lens correction for his left eye. Keratometry shows significant resultant astigmatism within the 9.0 mm graft OS, with central keratometry values of 48.8 D @ 094 × 41.5 D @ 004. Marked steepening superiorly and inferiorly resembles moderate-to-severe with-the-rule astigmatism (Fig. 20.13).

SOLUTION: The patient is fit with a mini-scleral lens to vault the corneal irregularity. An initial diagnostic lens was chosen from the in-office diagnostic fitting set with the following parameters: 7.40 mm BCR, −2.00 CLP, 15.0 mm OAD. Because of the large irregularity of the cornea corresponding to 7.3 D of corneal astigmatism, true alignment was not observed for the initial lens (Fig. 20.14). As the fitting relationship closely mimics the computerized corneal topography, TruForm Optics notes that a back-surface mini-scleral lens would align well OS.

Because of the large resultant astigmatism, a scleral lens allowing for astigmatic correction was required. Since quadrant-specific technology allows for sectoral peripheral and base curve changes, a new diagnostic lens was ordered to compensate for the large variance in corneal topography utilizing a slit-lamp photo of the lens-fitting relationship in combination with the patient's topography. Several changes for subsequent lenses include an increased central clearance, a toric peripheral curve system, and an increase in peripheral sagittal height resulting in a well-fit lens, with acceptable BCVA at $20/20^{-1}$. The final lens, TruForm Digiform 6.93 mm × 6.36 mm BCR, −11.00 D × −15.25 D CLP, 15.0 mm OAD, showed good

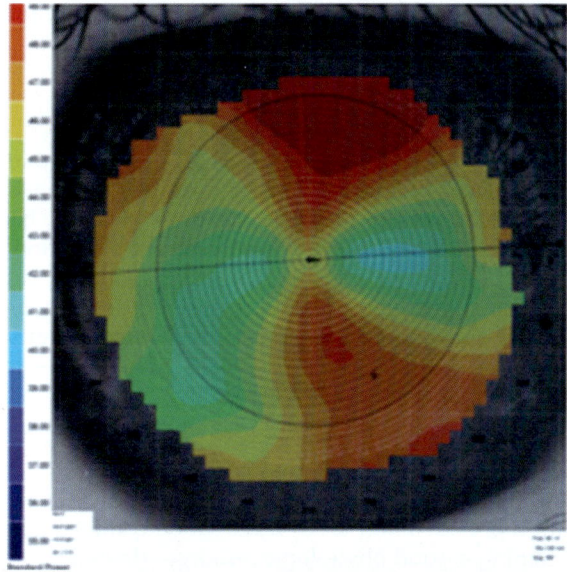

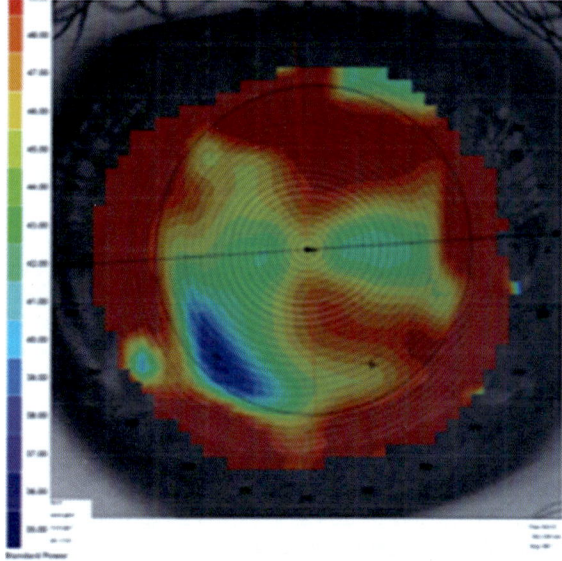

FIGURE 20.13 Computed topography maps OS in Case 1. **(A)** Axial topography: high corneal astigmatism in a near with-the-rule pattern **(B)** Tangential topography showing elevation high corneal surface irregularity.

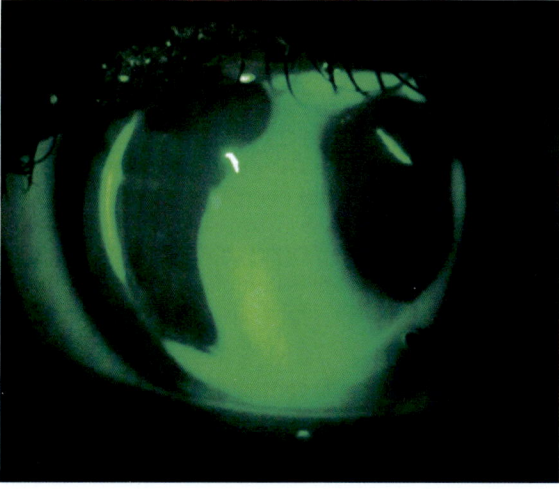

FIGURE 20.14 Bearing in the 180-degree meridian and clearance in the 90-degree meridian can be observed with a diagnostic trial lens in Case 1. A small fenestration can be observed at 4:00 in the periphery.

central corneal vaulting, good limbal vaulting, and good scleral alignment, posing no threat to the graft–host junction and maintaining the health of the graft.

CASE 2

A 53-year-old white male presented with a history of congenital cataract OS, exotropia, and amblyopia OS. He also manifests moderately advanced Fuchs corneal dystrophy OU, and is developing a significant cataract OD. With a best-corrected VA of OD 20/40− and OS CF, his vision is reduced to OD 20/100 with glare source. He elects to undergo cataract extraction, posterior chamber IOL implantation, and PKP OD. Approximately 16 months after surgery his continuous corneal suture is removed, a RI is performed, and wound prolapse ensues, requiring resuturing. Despite a clear corneal transplant and well-positioned IOL, his OD keratometry is 41.50 × 52.00 @ 157 and manifest refraction is OD −5.75 − 5.00×75 = 20/80. As he manifests a highly irregular topography OD, a variety of GP lenses fail due to instability.

SOLUTION: A Ciba Vision Focus Night and Day (lotrafilcon A) 8.6 mm/13.8 mm/−0.25 D Rx contact lens was prescribed as the foundation for a piggyback combination. A Boston XO (Bausch + Lomb) 7.00 mm BCR/9.5 mm OAD/8.1 mm OZD/−9.50 D Rx contact lens was prescribed for visual restoration. This combination provided him VA of 20/20, good comfort, and wearing time of 14 hours daily, while maintaining a good physiologic response. He maintains his lenses with Aquify Multipurpose Solution (Ciba Vision) and Boston Daily Cleaner and Conditioner (Bausch + Lomb).

CASE 3

A 77-year-old male presented with bilateral PKP and IOL implantation. A manifest refraction yields best-corrected VA of OD +2.50 − 3.75 × 116/+2.50 = 20/200 and OS +3.50 − 5.50 × 23/+2.50 = 20/40. As his irregular astigmatism limits VA OD, he is interested in additional surgery or contact lens correction. His surgeon has recommended against additional surgery for the OD, given his irregular astigmatism, secondary glaucoma, and mild background diabetic retinopathy. He does articulate a history of previous GP failure due to frequent-lens dislocation and loss. An initial diagnostic fitting visit confirms keratometry of OD 45.00 × 52.00 @ 90 with grade 4 distortion. Corneal topography reveals irregular astigmatism and PKP "tilt" OD. A number of standard design GP lenses demonstrate variable fluorescein patterns and instability.

SOLUTION: A Dyna Intra-Limbal (Lens Dynamics, Inc.) GP lens was ordered with: 6.50 mm BCR/11.2 mm OAD/−10.00 D Rx. This lens provided exceptional centration, good stability, adequate movement, and a fluorescein pattern of slight apical clearance. Biomicroscopy confirmed an acceptable physiologic response. An overrefraction of OD +1.25 sph/+2.50 = 20/25, and provided reasonable balance with the OS. He uses Optimum Solutions (Lobob) for lens care.

CASE 4

A 69-year-old female has developed PBK OU. She previously underwent a PKP with IOL exchange OD, and is currently having difficulty with her GP lens. The OS is increasingly symptomatic and she is interested in resolving her contact lens problems OD prior to undergoing PK/IOL exchange surgery OS. Best-corrected VA with contact lens and overcorrection is OD 20/40, and with spectacle correction only, OS 20/400. Biomicroscopy demonstrates a nasally displaced and excessively mobile GP, healthy PK, and well-positioned IOL OD. The OS manifests grade 4 bullous keratopathy and an anterior chamber IOL. Her history is complicated by secondary glaucoma OD. Keratometry is OD 46.25 × 47.75 @ 130 with slight distortion. Topography reveals a fairly central, symmetrical, but steep PK OD.

SOLUTION: Given the fairly centered, but steep PK OD, a Rose K contact lens (Blanchard Contact Lens, Inc.) 7.13 mm BCR/9.0 mm OAD/−5.75 D Rx/reduced edge lift profile was ordered. This lens offers slightly superior positioning, moderate fluorescein clearance, and reasonable edge clearance. VA with overrefraction is OD −0.50 − 0.75 × 80/+2.50 = 20/25. The PK remains clear, IOL well positioned, and glaucoma well controlled OD. She has now undergone PK and IOL exchange OS, and is currently corrected with manifest refraction to +1.50 − 2.00 × 55/+2.50 = 20/40. She uses Boston Daily Cleaner and Boston Conditioning Solution (Bausch + Lomb) for lens care.

CASE 5 (PROVIDED ROBERT M. GROHE, OD)[75]

A 56-year-old communications executive presented with distorted vision consisting of halos, spoking, and reduced scotopic vision. He has undergone seven GP refittings in the last 10 years with ongoing GP intolerance. He has had RK performed OU with three enhancements for each eye and bilateral cataracts. He had previously been a 21-year wearer of PMMA lens followed by 3 years of extended soft lens wear and 3 years of daily wear of GP lenses. He has been fitted with four pairs of progressive addition spectacle lenses, all which have failed due to poor vision. He spends 8 to 10 hours per day at a computer.

Keratometry (with −1.00 D extended range):

OD: 33.98 @ 26 × 32.69 @ 112 1+ distortion
OS: 37.62 @ 33 × 37.00 @ 115 Tr distortion

Manifest refraction:

OD: + 2.75 − 1.25 × 115 = 20/40 with monocular diplopia
OS: + 0.75 − 1.00 × 80 = 20/60 with monocular oblique triplopia

Slit lamp:

OD: 8-incision RK with fibrotic recut channels and Tr ASC & 1+ PSC cataracts
OS: 8-incision RK with fibrotic recut channels and 1+ ASC & 1+ PSC cataracts

Corneal topography (Fig. 20.15)

OD: Keratometry = 34.80 × 33.00
Eccentricity = −1.51
Central corneal thickness (CCT) = 426 microns
OS: Keratometry = 37.30 × 36.70
Eccentricity = −1.07
CCT = 453 microns

Diagnostic fitting:
Several different lens designs were attempted including the following:

1. Miniscleral Jupiter 15.0 mm lens (unsuccessful due to intolerance)
2. SynergEyes (unsuccessful due to severe residual monocular diplopia)
3. Piggyback of Ciba Night & Day with Envision 10.2 mm (unsuccessful: similar to #2)

SOLUTION: He was successfully fit into the Rose K2 IC lens OU (Blanchard):

OD: BCR: 9.20 mm (36.62 D)
Power: −0.75 D
OAD: 11.2 mm
PC: standard flat
VA: 20/40 + 2 (trace monocular vertical diplopia)
Lens position: central-to-temporal with 2 mm movement
OS: BCR: 9.25 mm (36.62 D)
Power: −1.00 D
OAD: 11.2 mm
PC: double flat
VA: 20/50 + 1 (1 + monocular vertical diplopia)
Lens position: central with 1 to 2 mm movement (Fig. 20.16)

Prior to the refitting, a long discussion outlined the benefits and lingering compromises we would experience with any contact lens. Given the past history of unsuccessful spectacle and contact lens fittings and the presence of cataracts, it was necessary to reemphasize the need to

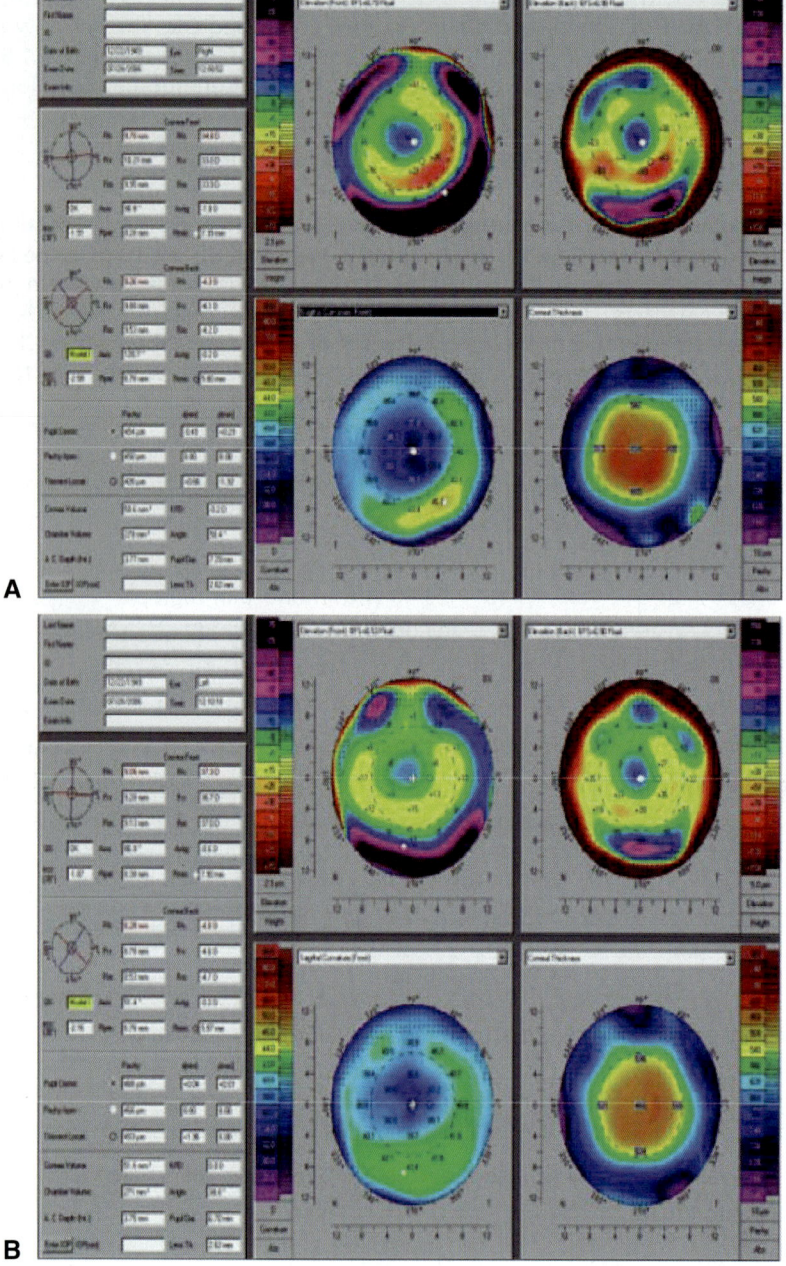

FIGURE 20.15 Case 5 OD topography **(A)** and OS topography **(B)**.

compromise and that no contact lens could provide "perfect" vision. It was also stated that all-day wearing time may be unrealistic given the heavy computer use and antidepressant med, which together would enhance a dry eye-like state. The patient reluctantly agreed.

Success in this case was enhanced by the temporary use of Acular LS dosed:

qid × 1 week
bid × 1 week
qd × 2 weeks
Now: prn

Vision was acceptable and bilaterally resulted in 20/40 − 1 with intermittent but tolerable ghosting and residual diplopia, especially under scotopic lighting. The patient wears his GPs

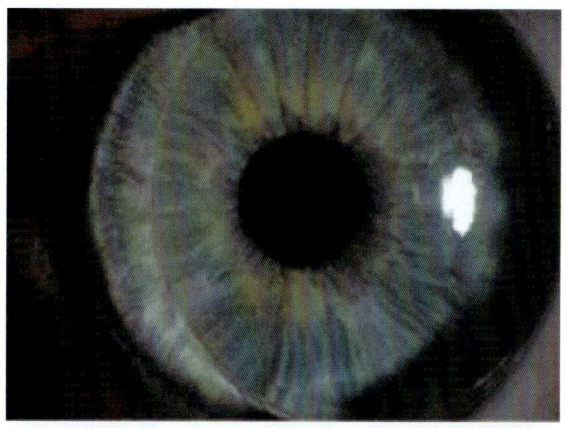
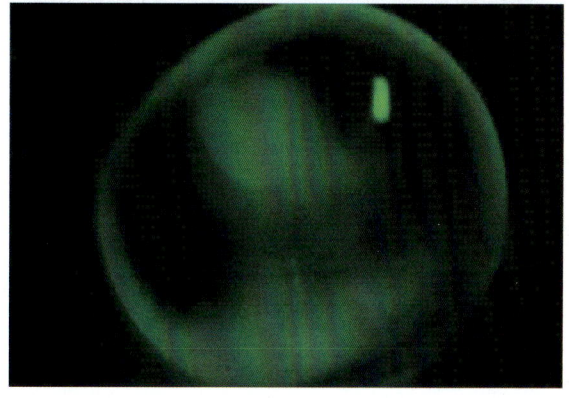

FIGURE 20.16 Lens position for patient in Case 5: with white light **(A)**, with fluorescein application **(B)**.

6 to 12 hours per day, depending on his computer use. He also alternates between two pair of OTC readers (+1.25 or +2.25) for near vision needs.

CASE 6

A 47-year-old female has undergone bilateral LASIK with two enhancements in each eye, resulting in ectasia. Her chief complaint is one of blurry vision and dryness OU. Her spectacle best-corrected VA is OD 20/100 and OS 20/60, with ghosting OU. Biomicroscopy reveals well-healed LASIK with inferior apical thinning OU. Corneal topography confirms keratoectasia with a Pellucid morphology OU. Simulated keratometry is OD 48.00 × 56.00 and OS 42.50 × 49.75. A manifest refraction yields OD +2.00 − 7.50 × 092 = 20/100 and OS +2.00 − 6.50 × 088 = 20/60.

SOLUTION: She achieved excellent vision with a GP contact lens; however, she was intolerant due to her keratoconjunctivitis sicca. She was subsequently fit with a SynergEye KC (SynergEye, Inc.) 6.90 mm BCR, 14.5 mm OAD, −8.50 D OD and SynergEyes A 7.60 mm BCR, 14.5 mm OAD, −3.50 D, 8.6sc OS, yielding an optimal fit and VA of 20/30+ OD and 20/25 OS. We have performed bilateral lower lid punctual occlusion and she uses OptiFree Express (Alcon Labs, Inc.) nightly and Blink Contact Lens lubricating drops (AMO, Inc.) prn.

CASE 7 (COURTESY OF ROBERT MAYNARD, OD)[75]

This 36-year-old male computer sales executive presented in January 2003. He had RK performed OU in 1995 and post-LASIK in 1998 OU.

Visual acuities (with spectacles):

OD: 20/80 − 1

OS: 20/100

Manifest refraction:

OD: −2.00 − 0.75 × 013   20/25 − 1 ghosting & doubling
OS: +3.00 − 5.00 × 098   20/25 − 1 ghosting & doubling

Keratometry:

OD: 41.37 @ 018; 45.37 @ 108
OS: 34.50 @ 109; 43.12 @ 019

SOLUTION:
Initial fit:
Lens parameters:

Power (D)	BCR (mm)	OAD/OZD (mm)	SCR/W (mm)	PCR/W (mm)
OD: −6.50	7.67	11.2/8.8	9.00/.5	11.75/.5
OS: −7.25	7.50	11.2/8.8	9.00/.5	11.75/.5

Overrefraction:

OD: +0.75 DS   20/30
OS: +0.75 DS   20/25

Slit-lamp examination:
OD: The lens is well centered and moved well with the blink. Good fluorescein pooling centrally as well as superior and inferior.
OS: The lens is well centered and moved well with the blink. There was central pooling with slight touch superior-temporal, slight touch nasally, and slight touch inferior-temporal existed.

2-week follow-up visit
Visual acuities (with lenses):

OD: 20/100 (foggy vision)
OS: 20/200 (foggy vision)

Slit-lamp examination:
OD: The lens is centered over the superior limbus with dimple veiling present over the papillary zone; the lens appears to be tilting backward over the superior limbus.
OS: Identical fitting relationship as present OD

Second fit:
Lens parameters:

Power (D)	BCR (mm)	OAD/OZD (mm)	Cap Size (mm)	SCR/W (mm)	PCR/W (mm)
OD: −5.75	7.80	11.2/8.4	8.40	8.80/.7	10.00/.5
OS: −6.75	7.58	11.2/8.4	8.40	8.60/.7	10.00/.5

Overrefraction:

OD: +1.50 DS   20/30
OS: +1.75 DS   20/25 − 2

Slit-lamp examination:
OD: The lens is well centered and exhibits good movement with the blink. A bubble is present at 12:00 superior to the pupil.
OS: Similar fitting relationship as present OD with the additional presence of mild dimple veiling.

Visual acuities:

OD: 20/30 + 2
OS: 20/40 − 1

Overrefraction:

OD: +0.50 DS   20/30 + 2
OS: +1.75 DS   20/25 − 2

Slit-lamp examination:
OD: The lens is well centered with apical clearance and good peripheral edge clearance
OS: Identical fitting relationship as present OD with the exception of mild dimple veiling superiorly

Third fit (new lens OS only):
Lens parameters:

	Power (D)	BCR (mm)	OAD/OZD (mm)	SCR/W (mm)	PCR/W (mm)
OS:	−6.75	7.58	11.2/8.4x9.0 (oval)	8.60/.7	10.00/.5

Overrefraction:

OS: Plano 20/25 − 2 (fluctuates)

Slit-lamp examination:
OS: Good centration and movement although dimple veiling was still present in various regions underneath the lens.

Final fit:
Essentially, the right contact lens was not changed, and continued to provide excellent vision, as well as comfort. The left lens was modified several more times, including fenestrations to reduce the dimple veil problem. The final lens parameters were:

	Power (D)	BCR (mm)	OAD/OZD (mm)	Cap Size (mm)	SCR/W (mm)	PCR/W (mm)
OD:	−5.75	7.80	11.2/8.4	8.20	8.80/.7	10.00/.5
OS:	−6.00	7.50	10.6/6.8x7.8 (oval)	6.80	8.50/.85	10.50/.85

Five fenestrations (OS only)
Overrefraction:

OD: +0.50 DS 20/25 − 2

OS: −0.75 DS 20/20 − 2

Slit-lamp examination:
OD: The lens is decentered slightly superiorly with mild dimple veiling paracentrally at 4:00 and just inside the superior limbus from 11:30 to 12:30.
OS: Similar fitting relationship as present OD with good lid attachment. Fenestrations appear to be successful. There is a minor punctate stain at 4:00, very minor scattered dimple veiling, and some inferior edge standoff. The fluorescein patterns of the lens-to-cornea fitting relationship of both lenses are provided in Figure 20.17.

Overall, he was "delighted" with his vision and comfort. We decided not to correct the prescription on the left eye, since he would not gain that much improvement. We sent him away to return for another complete primary care examination in 3 months. It took 10 months for him to be successfully fit with a lens for his left eye but it was well worth the effort. At the next eye examination visit, his vision was holding steady, the fitting relationship was still good, and he had no complaints; therefore, he was scheduled to return for a routine 6-month contact lens evaluation.

CASE 8

A 33-year-old male became intolerant to contact lens wear, and elected to undergo bilateral LASIK. His preoperative keratometry was OD 43.00 × 45.00 @ 90 and OS 43.25 × 45.00 @ 90. His preoperative manifest refraction was OD −15.25 − 2.75 × 165 = 20/30 and OS −13.50 − 3.00 × 179 = 20/30. He underwent bilateral LASIK, bilateral enhancement, and a flap sweep OD. His final postoperative keratometry is OD 36.25 × 36.75 @ 63 and OS 36.50 × 36.75 @ 82, and his manifest refraction is OD −1.00 DS = 20/25− and OS −0.25 DS = 20/25−. Despite an exceptional outcome, he reports intermittent keratitis sicca symptoms and blurred vision.

SOLUTION: He employs Restasis (Allergen) bid and Refresh (Allergan) artificial tears OU qid. Additionally, he wears a 1-Day Acuvue Moist contact lens (Vistakon): OD 9.0mm BCR/14.2 mm OAD/−1.25 D Rx and OS 9.0 mm BCR/14.2 mm OAD/−0.50 D Rx. These lenses provide VA of OD

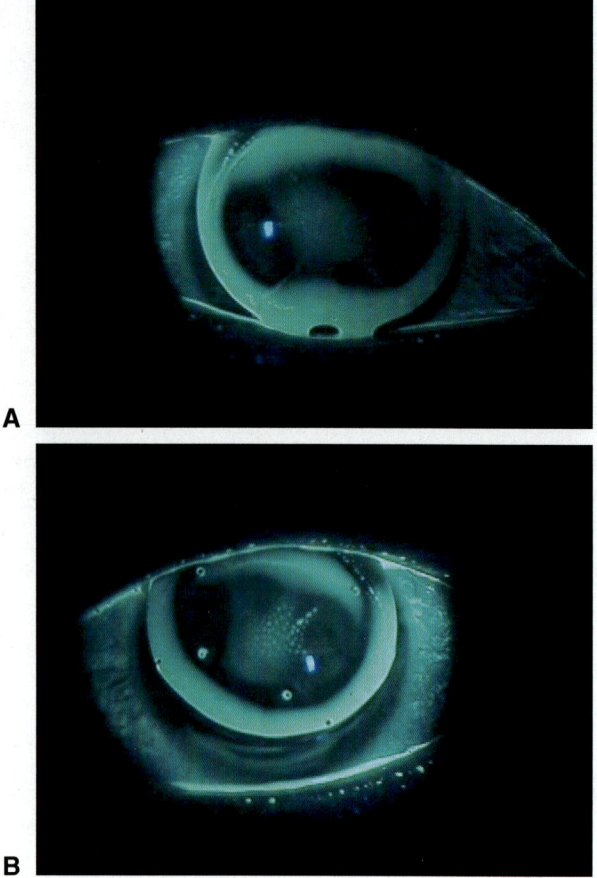

FIGURE 20.17 Fitting relationship of lenses fit in Case 7: right lens **(A)**, left lens **(B)**.

20/25+ and OS 20/25+, good centration and movement, and reasonable comfort. He wears his lenses approximately 4 days each week.

CASE 9 (COURTESY OF MICHAEL WARD)[38]

A 46-year-old male complained of poor VA and decreasing vision from his right eye and desires a contact lens for that eye only. Thirteen months prior to this visit, he had underwent hyperopic LASIK surgery for the right eye as a result of his emerging presbyopia. There was no record of his preoperative prescription. He reported that his vision was good immediately following the surgery. His contact lens history included successful wear of soft lenses prior to the surgery. He stated that he had attempted soft toric and GP lens wear without success during the past 6 months.

VA (without correction):

$$OD: 20/200$$
$$OS: 20/20 - 1$$

Manifest refraction:

$$OD: +3.00 - 3.00 \times 085 \quad 20/80 - 1$$
$$OS: +0.75 - 0.25 \times 138 \quad 20/20$$

Manual keratometry:

OD: 46.7 @ 134; 43.0 @ 044 2+ mire distortion
OS: 43.6 @ 156; 44.2 @ 066 crisp mires

Corneal topography: exhibits keratectasia
Slit-lamp examination:
OD: central and paracentral haze, vertical striae and thinned; nasal-based flap with horseshoe-shaped microkeratome scar noted
OS: cornea clear

Contact lens diagnostic fitting:
Initial diagnostic lens:
Design: Surgical C-4 (reverse geometry postsurgical design from ABBA Optical)
BCR: 40.42 D
Diameter: 10.0 mm

Overrefraction: +2.50 DS 20/25+2

Initial diagnostic lens selection was based on a combination of keratometry readings, topography maps, and fluorescein patterns. This type of lens fitting is similar to fitting keratoconus. It is not recommended in these cases to fit the apex of the ectatic protrusion. The BCR is often fit somewhat flatter than "K," but not as flat as the superior corneal topography. The OAD is slightly larger than normal to increase centration; larger diameters may be beneficial. The fluorescein pattern should show complete tear exchange over the entire corneal surface with each blink.

Contact lens order:
Laboratory: ABBA
Material: Fluoroperm 60
BCR: 41.00 D
OAD/OZD: 10.0/9.0 mm
Power: +2.50 D
Center thickness: 0.23 mm

At the 1-week follow-up visit, the patient's vision was unchanged and he was adjusting well to GP lens wear and enjoying both his vision and depth perception. He was ultimately successful with this design.

CASE 10 (COURTESY OF MATT KAUFFMAN, OD)

A 34-year-old Caucasian female, s/p PKP in her right eye, presented for a contact lens fitting of this eye. She had been suffering with blurry and distorted vision in her right eye ever since her corneal transplant surgery 1 year prior. She has a history of keratoconus in both eyes and underwent corneal crosslinking on her left eye several years previously.
Manifest refraction (s/p PKP OD):

$$OD: -0.50 - 4.25 \times 005: 20/25$$
$$OS: -0.25 - 0.25 \times 090: 20/50$$

Postsurgical corneal topography (Fig. 20.18)
Contact lens fitting OD:

Lens	Power	BCR	OAD	VA	Comments
SynergEyes Duette	Plano	7.50	14.5 mm	20/25	MED skirt; poor comfort; difficulty with I & R
Boston EO Bitoric	−0.25/−3.75	7.76/7.05	9.3	20/20	Excessive movement; poor centration and comfort
Boston EO Bitoric	−0.25/−3.75	7.76/7.05	9.6	20/25^{+2}	Poor comfort, decentered inferiorly
Boston EO Bitoric	+0.75/−2.75	7.94/7.20	9.6	20/30	Decentered inferiorly; excessive inferior pooling

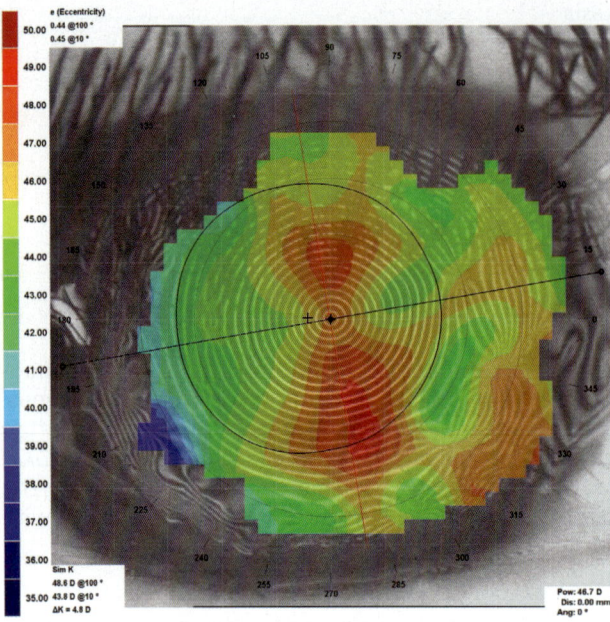

FIGURE 20.18 Postsurgical corneal topography in Case 10.

SOLUTION: The patient was successfully refit into RevitalEyes (Efrofilcon-A Definitive 74% water), a new custom soft silicone hydrogel contact lens manufactured by Metro Optics. The power of the contact lens was $+0.25 -1.00 \times 005$. The patient's VA was $20/25^{-2}$. The lens had a base curve of 8.7 and diameter of 14.5. The lens was rotated 10 degrees nasally, but did not significantly affect her vision (Fig. 20.19). Even though the patient's VA was not as crisp, the patient preferred the custom soft contact lens due to increased comfort and better fit.

CASE 11 (COURTESY OF LACEY HAINES, OD)

A 19-year-old machinist was referred for a GP lens fitting for his left eye only. As treatment for his bilateral but asymmetric keratoconus, he had corneal crosslinking with Intacs performed on his more advanced left eye 4 months prior to his visit and was scheduled to have crosslinking in his right eye once vision was corrected in his left eye. His unaided VA OD was 20/20+ and his manifest refraction OS was $-0.50 -2.00 \times 155 = 20/60+$. Slit-lamp examination of the left eye showed double segment Intacs and central corneal striae. Using anterior segment imaging with Visante OCT (Zeiss Meditec, Germany), the sagittal depth at a 15.8 mm chord for the left eye was calculated to be 4.24 mm (Fig. 20.20).

SOLUTION: Due to the irregularities of the cornea introduced by the Intacs segments, it was decided to use a semi-scleral design to vault over the cornea entirely. Using the MSD 15.8 mm GP lens (Blanchard Contact Lens, Inc.), the initial diagnostic lens was chosen by adding 0.35 mm

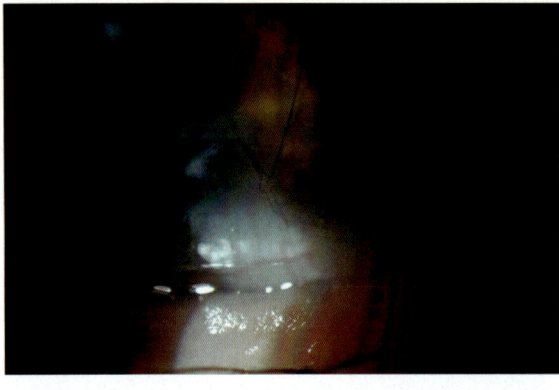

FIGURE 20.19 RevitalEyes soft contact lens shown with three laser etchings for fitting purposes.

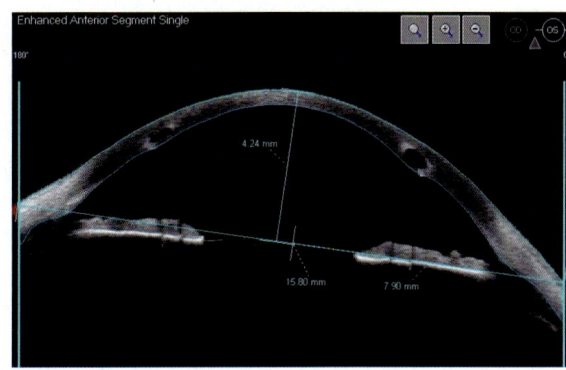

FIGURE 20.20 Anterior segment OCT of the left eye for the patient in Case 11. The calipers show the sagittal depth of the eye at a 15.8 mm chord.

to the measured sagittal depth of the left eye. Since the sagittal depth measured was 4.24 mm, the initial 15.8 mm diagnostic lens had a sagittal depth of 4.60 mm with a standard limbal zone clearance and standard edge clearance. Evaluation of the lens fit showed good centration, complete corneal and limbal clearance with scleral alignment, and a spherical overrefraction of −2.50 D provided a VA of 20/25− (Fig. 20.21). This lens was ordered in Boston XO material. At both the delivery and 2-week follow-up appointments, the lens showed good clearance of the cornea and limbus with scleral alignment and provided 20/20− VA with no overrefraction.

CASE 12 (COURTESY OF ANDREA SEWELL, OD)

History: 21-year-old Hispanic female with keratoconus OD > OS. Previous GP wearer, but was intolerant to the lenses. Intacs was performed OD 1 year prior to visit. She presented for a contact lens fit for OD only.

Objective:
VA's (unaided)

OD: 20/200

OS: 20/25+

SOLUTION: We initially attempted to fit the patient with a scleral lens, but she was intolerant to any rigid lens in the eye. We then successfully fit the patient in the Bausch + Lomb Kerasoft IC lens. She was very satisfied with the comfort and the vision. The lens was well centered, had 5 degrees of nasal rotation, and moved 1.5 mm with the blink.

VA's cc: 20/40+
Final parameters: Kerasoft IC
BCR: 8.2 D
Periphery: Standard
Diameter: 14.5
Power: −3.50 −4.25 × 016

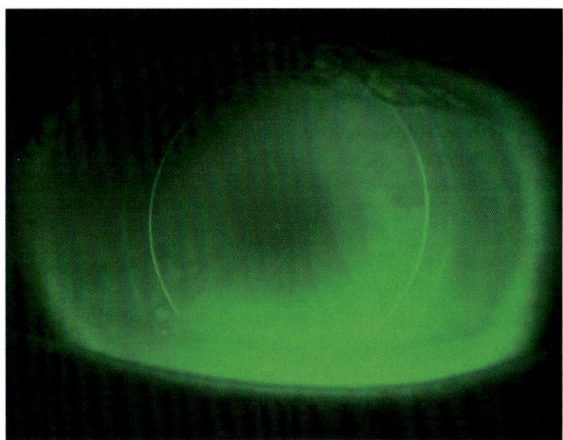

FIGURE 20.21 MSD lens with good corneal and limbal clearance on an eye with corneal cross-linking and double segment Intacs for patient in Case 11.

CLINICAL PROFICIENCY CHECKLIST

- Corneal topography is important in the contact lens management of the postsurgical cornea as it often helps in determining the specific type of lens to be fit.
- Increasingly, scleral lenses are the lens of choice in all forms of postsurgical cases.
- For full-thickness keratoplasty, irregular astigmatism is approximately twice that of regular astigmatism; therefore, rigid GP lenses are the best option for correction.
- After a PKP, a GP lens can be fit as soon as the majority of the postinflammation has subsided, which can be as soon as 2 to 3 months after surgery.
- Intralimbal designs with OADs larger than 10 mm are most often the lens of choice in all forms of corneal transplants. If the cornea is prolate, conventional GP designs are often successful; if the corneas are oblate, a reverse geometry design is indicated; if mixed astigmatism is present, a bitoric design can be successful; if a graft tilt is present, a quadrant-specific design is recommended.
- High-Dk GP lens materials are recommended in postsurgical cases.
- In some postsurgical cases, custom soft lenses can be successful. These lenses have increased center thickness or reverse geometry peripheral curves to provide some assistance in masking corneal irregularity.
- Piggyback designs can be successful in some postsurgical cases in which GP lenses alone do not center or are not well tolerated. A silicone hydrogel lens material should be used in combination with a high-DK GP material. The power should be placed in the GP lens as only approximately 20% of the soft lens power comes through in a piggyback optical system.
- Contact lens fitting approaches in DALK are similar to PKP. Once again, corneal topography will help dictate lens design selection.
- In postrefractive surgery cases, two potential outcomes necessitating GP use are present; one is postsurgical ectasia requiring a keratoconic design or—more likely—an oblate shape necessitating a reverse geometry design. Scleral and hybrid designs are also options in these cases.
- Fitting post-Intacs patients can occur typically 3 months after the procedure and keratoconic GP designs are often successful with soft lenses and piggyback designs presenting additional options.
- Posttrauma patients often have corneal flattening in the region of trauma. Therefore, an intralimbal GP design can be used. If improved cosmesis and decreased glare symptoms are indicated, a prosthetic contact lens is indicated.

REFERENCES

1. Kovoor TA, Mohamed E, Cavanagh HD, et al. Outcomes of LASIK and PRK in previous penetrating corneal transplant recipients. *Eye Contact Lens*. 2009;35(5):242–245.
2. Huang PY, Huang PT, Astle WF, et al. Laser-assisted subepithelial keratectomy and photorefractive keratectomy for post-penetrating keratoplasty myopia and astigmatism in adults. *J Cataract Refract Surg*. 2011;37(2):335–340.
3. Ghosheh FR, Cremona FA, Rapuano CJ, et al. Trends in penetrating keratoplasty in the United States 1980–2005. *Int Ophthalmol*. 2008;28(3):147–153.
4. Tan DT, Dart JK, Holland EJ, et al. Corneal transplantation. *Lancet*. 2012;379(9827):1749–1761.
5. Fronterre A, Portesani GP. Relaxing incisions for postkeratoplasty astigmatism. *Cornea*. 1991;10(4):305–311.
6. Ghanem RC, Azar DT. Femtosecond-laser arcuate wedge-shaped resection to correct high residual astigmatism after penetrating keratoplasty. *J Cataract Refract Surg*. 2006;32(9):1415–1419.
7. Ezra DG, Hay-Smith G, Mearza A, et al. Corneal wedge excision in the treatment of high astigmatism after penetrating keratoplasty. *Cornea*. 2007;26(7):819–825.
8. Reinhart WJ, Musch DC, Jacobs DS, et al. Deep anterior lamellar keratoplasty as an alternative to penetrating keratoplasty a report by the american academy of ophthalmology. *Ophthalmology*. 2011;118(1):209–218.

9. How prevelant is cornea tranplanation? [http://www.restoresight.org/about-us/frequently-asked-questions/]
10. Gaster RN, Dumitrascu O, Rabinowitz YS. Penetrating keratoplasty using femtosecond laser-enabled keratoplasty with zig-zag incisions versus a mechanical trephine in patients with keratoconus. *Br J Ophthalmol.* 2012;96(9):1195–1199.
11. Farid M, Pirouzian A, Steinert RF. Femtosecond laser keratoplasty. *Int Ophthalmol Clin.* 2013,53(1):55–64.
12. Farid M, Steinert RF. Femtosecond laser-assisted corneal surgery. *Curr Opin Ophthalmol.* 2010;21(4):288–292.
13. Karabatsas CH, Cook SD, Sparrow JM. Proposed classification for topographic patterns seen after penetrating keratoplasty. *Br J Ophthalmol.* 1999;83(4):403–409.
14. Brierly SC, Izquierdo L Jr, Mannis MJ. Penetrating keratoplasty for keratoconus. *Cornea.* 2000;19(3):329–332.
15. Alio JL, Belda JI, Artola A, et al. Contact lens fitting to correct irregular astigmatism after corneal refractive surgery. *J Cataract Refract Surg.* 2002;28(10):1750–1757.
16. Jupiter DG, Katz HR. Management of irregular astigmatism with rigid gas permeable contact lenses. *CLAO J.* 2000;26(1):14–17.
17. Lee RM, Lam FC, Georgiou T, et al. Suturing techniques and postoperative management in penetrating keratoplasty in the United Kingdom. *Clin Ophthalmol.* 2012;6:1335–1340.
18. Fares U, Sarhan AR, Dua HS. Management of post-keratoplasty astigmatism. *J Cataract Refract Surg.* 2012;38(11):2029–2039.
19. Sarhan AR, Fares U, Al-Aqaba MA, et al. Rapid suture management of post-keratoplasty astigmatism. *Eye (Lond).* 2010;24(4):540–546.
20. Javadi MA, Naderi M, Zare M, et al. Comparison of the effect of three suturing techniques on postkeratoplasty astigmatism in keratoconus. *Cornea.* 2006;25(9):1029–1033.
21. Wietharn BE, Driebe WT Jr. Fitting contact lenses for visual rehabilitation after penetrating keratoplasty. *Eye Contact Lens.* 2004;30(1):31–33.
22. Genvert GI, Cohen EJ, Arentsen JJ, et al. Fitting gas-permeable contact lenses after penetrating keratoplasty. *Am J Ophthalmol.* 1985;99(5):511–514.
23. Mackman G, Polack FM, Sidrys L. Fluorescein angiography of soft contact lens induced vascularization in penetrating keratoplasty. *Ophthalmic Surg.* 1985;16(3):157–161.
24. Szczotka LB, Lindsay RG. Contact lens fitting following corneal graft surgery. *Clin Exp Optom.* 2003;86(4):244–249.
25. Szczotka-Flynn LB. Fitting contact lenses after a corneal transplant. *Contact Lens Spectrum.* 2011;26(9):16–17.
26. Lin JC, Cohen EJ, Rapuano CJ, et al. RK4 (reverse-geometry) contact lens fitting after penetrating keratoplasty. *Eye Contact Lens.* 2003;29(1):44–47.
27. Lim L, Siow KL, Sakamoto R, et al. Reverse geometry contact lens wear after photorefractive keratectomy, radial keratotomy, or penetrating keratoplasty. *Cornea.* 2000;19(3):320–324.
28. Jaynes J, Edrington TB. Managing scleral lens flexure. *Contact Lens Spectrum.* 2012;27(12):12.
29. Woo M, Weissman B. Effective optics of piggyback soft contact lenses. *Contact Lens Spectrum.* 2011;26(11):50.
30. Weissman BA, Ye P. Calculated tear oxygen tension under contact lenses offering resistance in series: piggyback and scleral lenses. *Cont Lens Anterior Eye.* 2006;29(5):231–237.
31. Lopez-Alemany A, Gonzalez-Meijome JM, Almeida JB, et al. Oxygen transmissibility of piggyback systems with conventional soft and silicone hydrogel contact lenses. *Cornea.* 2006;25(2):214–219.
32. Nau AC. A comparison of synergeyes versus traditional rigid gas permeable lens designs for patients with irregular corneas. *Eye Contact Lens.* 2008;34(4):198–200.
33. Anshu A, Price MO, Tan DT, et al. Endothelial keratoplasty: a revolution in evolution. *Surv Ophthalmol.* 2012;57(3):236–252.
34. Lee WB, Jacobs DS, Musch DC, et al. Descemet's stripping endothelial keratoplasty: safety and outcomes: a report by the American Academy of Ophthalmology. *Ophthalmology.* 2009;116(9):1818–1830.
35. Esgin H, Erda N. Corneal endothelial polymegethism and pleomorphism induced by daily-wear rigid gas-permeable contact lenses. *CLAO J.* 2002;28(1):40–43.
36. DePaolis M, Shovlin J, DeKinder JO, et al. Postsurgical contact lens fitting. In Bennett ES, Henry VA. *Clinical Manual of Contact Lenses.* 3rd ed. Philadelphia, PA: Wolters Kluwer/Lippincott Williams & Wilkins, 2009:508–541.
37. Pasquali T, Krueger R. Topography-guided laser refractive surgery. *Curr Opin Ophthalmol.* 2012;23(4):264–268.
38. Hammond SD Jr, Puri AK, Ambati BK. Quality of vision and patient satisfaction after LASIK. *Curr Opin Ophthalmol.* 2004;15(4):328–332.
39. Morse JS, Schallhorn SC, Hettinger K, et al. Role of depressive symptoms in patient satisfaction with visual quality after laser in situ keratomileusis. *J Cataract Refract Surg.* 2009;35(2):341–346.
40. Barraquer JI. Keratomileusis. *Int Surg.* 1967;48(2):103–117.
41. Reinstein DZ, Archer TJ, Gobbe M. The history of LASIK. *J Refract Surg.* 2012;28(4):291–298.
42. Bourque LB, Cosand BB, Drews C, et al. Reported satisfaction, fluctuation of vision, and glare among patients one year after surgery in the Prospective Evaluation of Radial Keratotomy (PERK) Study. *Arch Ophthalmol.* 1986;104(3):356–363.
43. Schanzlin DJ, Santos VR, Waring GO III, et al. Diurnal change in refraction, corneal curvature, visual acuity, and intraocular pressure after radial keratotomy in the PERK Study. *Ophthalmology.* 1986;93(2):167–175.
44. Kwitko S, Gritz DC, Garbus JJ, et al. Diurnal variation of corneal topography after radial keratotomy. *Arch Ophthalmol.* 1992;110(3):351–356.

45. Szczotka LB, Aronsky M. Contact lenses after LASIK. *J Am Optom Assoc.* 1998;69(12):775–784.
46. Waring GO III, Lynn MJ, Nizam A, et al. Results of the Prospective Evaluation of Radial Keratotomy (PERK) Study five years after surgery. The Perk Study Group. *Ophthalmology.* 1991;98(8):1164–1176.
47. Yeung KK, Olson MD, Weissman BA. Complexity of contact lens fitting after refractive surgery. *Am J Ophthalmol.* 2002;133(5):607–612.
48. McDonnell PJ, Garbus JJ, Caroline P, et al. Computerized analysis of corneal topography as an aid in fitting contact lenses after radial keratotomy. *Ophthalmic Surg.* 1992;23(1):55–59.
49. Cohen AW, Goins KM, Sutphin JE, et al. Penetrating keratoplasty versus deep anterior lamellar keratoplasty for the treatment of keratoconus. *Int Ophthalmol.* 2010;30(6):675–681.
50. Javadi MA, Feizi S, Yazdani S, et al. Deep anterior lamellar keratoplasty versus penetrating keratoplasty for keratoconus: a clinical trial. *Cornea.* 2010;29(4):365–371.
51. Sogutlu SE, Kubaloglu A, Unal M, et al. Penetrating keratoplasty versus deep anterior lamellar keratoplasty: comparison of optical and visual quality outcomes. *Br J Ophthalmol.* 2012;96(8):1063–1067.
52. Parthasarathy A, Por YM, Tan DT. Use of a "small-bubble technique" to increase the success of Anwar's "big-bubble technique" for deep lamellar keratoplasty with complete baring of Descemet's membrane. *Br J Ophthalmol.* 2007;91(10):1369–1373.
53. Barnett M. A dual approach to treating keratoconus. *Rev Cornea Contact Lenses.* April 2011.
54. Colin J, Malet FJ. Intacs for the correction of keratoconus: two-year follow-up. *J Cataract Refract Surg.* 2007; 33(1):69–74.
55. Gordon MO, Steger-May K, Szczotka-Flynn L, et al. Baseline factors predictive of incident penetrating keratoplasty in keratoconus. *Am J Ophthalmol.* 2006;142(6):923–930.
56. Rabinowitz YS, Li X, Ignacio TS, et al. Intacs inserts using the femtolaser compared to the mechanical spreader in the treatment of keratoconus. *J Refract Surg.* 2006;22(8):764–771.
57. Hamdi IM. Preliminary results of intrastromal corneal ring segment implantation to treat moderate to severe keratoconus. *J Cataract Refract Surg.* 2011;37(6):1125–1132.
58. Gharaibeh AM, Muhsen SM, AbuKhader IB, et al. KeraRing intrastromal corneal ring segments for correction of keratoconus. *Cornea.* 2012;31(2):115–120.
59. Tu KL, Sebastian RT, Owen M. Quantification of the surgically induced refractive effect of intrastromal corneal ring segments in keratoconus with standardized incision site and segment size. *J Cataract Refract Surg.* 2011; 37(10):1865–1870.
60. Ruckhofer J, Twa MD, Schanzlin DJ. Clinical characteristics of lamellar channel deposits after implantation of intacs. *J Cataract Refract Surg.* 2000;26:1473–1479.
61. Levinger S, Pokroy R. Keratoconus managed with intacs: one-year results. *Arch Ophthalmol.* 2005;123(10): 1308–1314.
62. Alio JL, Shabayek MH, Belda JI, et al. Analysis of results related to good and bad outcomes of Intacs implantations got keratoconus correction. *J Cataract Refract Surg.* 2006;32(5):756–761.
63. Edrington T, Tran L. Contact lens and surgical management options for keratoconus. *Rev Cornea Contact Lenses.* April 2008;28–32.
64. McCandless K. When to refer keratoconus patients for intacs corneal implants. Presented at: 2008 Global Keratoconus Congress; January 2008; Las Vegas, NV.
65. Russell B. Contact lens management after intracorneal ring segment implantation. Presented at: 2008 Global Keratoconus Congress; January 2008; Las Vegas, NV.
66. Khan AO. Persistent diplopia following secondary intraocular lens placement in patients with sensory strabismus from uncorrected monocular aphakia. *Br J Ophthalmol.* 2008;92(1):51–53.
67. Sanders SM. Prosthetic lens patient management. *Contact Lens Spectrum.* 2008;23(12):25–28.
68. Khan B, Dudenhoefer EJ, Dohlman CH. Keratoprosthesis: an update. *Curr Opin Ophthalmol.* 2001;12(4):282–287.
69. Klufas MA, Colby KA. The boston keratoprosthesis. *Int Ophthalmol Clin.* 2010;50(3):161–175.
70. Zerbe BL, Belin MW, Ciolino JB. Results from the multicenter Boston Type 1 Keratoprosthesis Study. *Ophthalmology.* 2006;113(10):1779 e1–1779 e7.
71. Yaghouti F, Nouri M, Abad JC, et al. Keratoprosthesis: preoperative prognostic categories. *Cornea.* 2001;20(1): 19–23.
72. Greiner MA Li JY, Mannis MJ. Longer-term vision outcomes and complications with the Boston Type 1 keratoprosthesis at the University of California, Davis. *Ophthalmology.* 2011;118:1543–1550.
73. Harissi-Dagher M, Beyer J, Dohlman CH. The role of soft contact lenses as an adjunct to the Boston keratoprosthesis. *Int Ophthalmol Clin.* 2008;48(2):43–51.
74. Beyer J, Todani A, Dohlman C. Prevention of visually debilitating deposits on soft contact lenses in keratoprosthesis patients. *Cornea.* 2011;30(12):1419–1422.
75. GP contact lens case grand rounds troubleshooting guide. www.gpli.info. Accessed February 2013.

Chapter 21

Scleral Lenses

Gregory W. DeNaeyer, Jason Jedlicka, and Muriel M. Schornack

HISTORY

The evolution of contact lenses from their conceptual stage to modern lens designs has brought us full circle when it comes to lens diameter. The late 1800s brought the first mention in the medical literature of scleral lenses that were fabricated for use with patients.[1] Adolf Fick and his blown glass vesicle were mentioned in 1888. In the same year, Eugene Kalt used glass lenses for the correction of vision for a patient with keratoconus. August Muller, who happened to be very nearsighted, attempted to correct his own vision with ground glass lenses in 1889 that were fabricated by Karl Otto Himmler in Berlin.[2] Most descriptions of how these scleral lenses were designed indicate the concept of a fluid reservoir under the lens. Glass was clearly hard to reproduce and oxygen impermeable, making widespread use impractical, but the concept of a scleral lens had been introduced.

The early 20th century resulted in the development of a plastic material, polymethyl methacrylate (PMMA), which allowed for easier molding as well as lathing. Fabrication of lenses was evolving, and lenses could be made with increasing precision. However, because of the lack of oxygen permeability (Dk) of PMMA, lenses were manufactured relatively small to avoid hypoxic complications. The corneal lens, made of PMMA, fit to the cornea and became the first lens that was fit on a widespread basis.

The end of the 20th century and early 21st century saw the barriers to large-diameter designs disappear. As lens materials increased in Dk and manufacturing processes improved in precision and reproducibility, the benefits of larger lens design were able to be realized. The first generations of smaller scleral lenses were being manufactured in the 1990s in the form of the Macrolens, while laboratories under the direction of Perry Rosenthal in Boston and Don Ezekiel in Australia were producing full scleral designs. Using gas-permeable (GP) material, as well as fenestrations in some instances, these initial designs were significant advances and set the stage for the current state of the industry.

Historically, scleral lenses were cast using a mold of the eye surface. This was in no way reproducible with precision, nor did it allow for subtle changes in lens design other than what could be accomplished by removing lens material manually. Today's modern computer-driven diamond tooled lathes can reproduce lenses with microscopic precision as well as make subtle alterations in lens design that allow the lenses to be cut to a near perfect match to most ocular surfaces, limited only by the input of the lens fitter and consultant. The new era of scleral lenses is clearly upon us and has no reason to regress.

CLASSIFICATION

While the renaissance of scleral lenses has opened opportunities for contact lens professionals to help more patients with these exceptional devices, it has introduced numerous designs, which has caused some confusion and controversy as how to describe or categorize them. Initial classification of scleral lenses used lens diameter as the determining factor. The smallest of the large-diameter lenses were classified as "corneoscleral" or "semi-scleral," while larger lenses were "mini-scleral" or "full scleral." The problem with this terminology was that there was no scientific basis for this nor was there anything truly descriptive about "semi-scleral" or "mini-scleral," which would indicate intuitively how the lens should be fit.

In 2010, the Scleral Lens Education Society, a think-tank for scleral lenses, suggested terminology based upon how the lenses fit the eye. Lenses that are fit to the cornea are to be described as corneal lenses; lenses that rest both on the cornea and the sclera are designated as corneoscleral lenses, and lenses that rest strictly on the sclera are designated as scleral lenses. Within the scleral genre, the smaller end of the spectrum could be termed mini-sclerals and the larger full scleral. This terminology is described in Table 21.1.

Corneal and corneoscleral lenses are designed to have at least some amount of bearing on the cornea. In areas where corneal lenses or corneoscleral lenses do vault, the tear reservoir is very limited. Scleral lenses are designed to fully vault the cornea and hold a significant liquid reservoir. It is worth noting that you can certainly fit a lens that is just slightly larger than the cornea itself as a fully vaulting lens, but it is quite likely that the lens is not intended to be fit that way and may not function in a desirable manner. It seems logical to have the desired fit in mind prior to beginning the fitting process and select a lens that is designed to achieve that goal. If the desired fit is a lens that fully vaults the cornea and maintains a fluid reservoir behind the lens, then a lens that is designed as a scleral lens (mini- or full) should be employed.

Within this chapter, the majority of the information will revolve around scleral lens design and fitting, management of the scleral lens wearer, and troubleshooting scleral lenses. However, corneoscleral lenses will be included, as they are similar in many ways to scleral lens fitting and management.

INDICATIONS

Scleral lenses have a broad range of indications. Scleral lenses can be fit for the correction of myopia, hyperopia, corneal astigmatism, residual astigmatism, and presbyopia. Additionally, patients with high myopia or hyperopia and aphakia, may benefit from the visual quality of scleral lenses more than those with standard refractive errors.[2] While the prescription of scleral lenses for the correction of refractive error in the absence of any other ocular disease is still somewhat controversial, the use of scleral lenses is only limited by the comfort level of the patient and the contact lens professional.

Beyond their potential for correcting ametropia and presbyopia, scleral lenses are proving themselves invaluable in the care of the patient with ocular disease. The rigid GP optics of scleral lenses corrects both regular and irregular corneal astigmatism. Moreover, the fluid reservoir of a scleral lens is therapeutic in cases of ocular surface disease (OSD).

TABLE 21.1 Gas-Permeable Lens Terminology

TYPE	ALTERNATIVE NAMES	DIAMETER (mm)	BEARING	TEAR RESERVOIR
Corneal		8–12.5	All lens bearing is on the cornea	No tear reservoir
Corneoscleral	Corneal-limbal Semi-scleral Limbal	12.5–15	Lenses share bearing on the cornea and sclera	Limited tear reservoir capacity
(Full) Scleral	Haptic	15–25 Mini-scleral 15–18 Large scleral 18–25	All lens bearing is on the sclera	Somewhat limited tear reservoir capacity Almost unlimited tear reservoir capacity

Irregular corneas degrade visual acuity (VA), induce polyopia, and increase glare and photosensitivity. Conditions that can result in irregular corneas include keratoconus[3,4] with or without intacs,[5] pellucid marginal degeneration,[3] corneal transplant[3] or refractive surgery,[6] trauma, infection, and corneal degenerations and dystrophies. In many instances, irregular corneas can be managed with traditional corneal GP lenses. However, in those cases where they cannot, scleral lenses can be employed, often with success.

Scleral lenses have many advantages for patients with irregular corneas. Glasses for many irregular cornea patients do not provide adequate visual correction because they do not correct for higher-order aberrations induced by irregularity. Soft contact lenses have the same limitations as spectacle lenses. Corneal GP lenses correct for irregular astigmatism, but issues with corneal GP lenses include lens awareness, lens instability, dryness, and possible corneal scarring from a poorly fit lens. Scleral lenses create very little awareness and are stable because they semiseal to the sclera. Scleral lenses minimize the possibility of causing corneal scarring on the irregular corneal patient because they fully vault the cornea. While scleral lenses are not perfect and certainly have their own potential problems, their advantages for many patients with corneal irregularity are numerous and can be life-changing.

Beyond the irregular cornea, scleral lenses can be utilized to treat OSD that leaves the patient chronically uncomfortable or in pain.[7] Patients with dryness, foreign-body sensation, light sensitivity, and other chronic symptoms secondary to OSD can be successfully managed with scleral contact lenses because the liquid reservoir continuously bathes the anterior ocular surface.[7] The list of conditions that can be managed with scleral lenses includes keratoconjunctivitis sicca,[8] anterior basement membrane dystrophy, recurrent epithelial erosions, and persistent epithelial defects,[9] keratopathies secondary to graft versus host disease,[7,8] superior limbic keratoconjunctivitis (SLK),[10] limbal stem cell deficiency (LSCD),[11] Stevens–Johnson syndrome,[10] ocular cicatricial pemphigoid (OCP),[10,12] and many other corneal dystrophies and degenerations.[4,9] Patients with neurotrophic corneal conditions that lead to break down of the epithelium are also candidates for scleral lens therapy.[9] It has been demonstrated that scleral lenses can be used on an overnight or extended wear basis.[9,13]

Scleral lenses have been shown to improve lid posture for correction of ptosis and blepharospasm.[14,15] The size of the lens as well as the vault and front-surface curves can be used to "push-up" the lids or to provide a protective covering to the eye that allows lids to relax. This area of use has not been fully developed, but the possibility of designing a lens specifically for improving lid posture certainly exists. The application of scleral lenses for the treatment of all these conditions for both the correction of vision, as well as the reduction of pain and healing of the ocular surface, can be applied to pediatric patients as well as adults.[16]

Corneoscleral lenses can be used in many of the same instances as scleral lenses, but caution should be exercised in using them on fragile corneas due to their minimal vault or even light corneal touch. Corneoscleras can be used in cases of refractive error, keratoconus with intact epithelium, corneal grafts, irregular astigmatism, and postrefractive surgery. Scleral lenses that fully vault the cornea will often be more successful at managing OSD, as compared to corneoscleral lenses.

DESIGN

Scleral lenses are typically created in one of two fashions, preformed or impression technique. The vast majority of currently fabricated lenses are preformed, utilizing diagnostic lenses. It is important for clarity of discussion that some lenses are made up entirely of curves of various radii and width, while others use splines, which are zones of (theoretically) infinite curve radii with varying angles of incidence upon the eye. Because the change in curvature of the sclera is typically quite gradual, splines are more commonly introduced in the outer aspects of the lens.

Scleral lenses can range from 15 to 24 mm in diameter, and due to their size, will be comprised of numerous curves or splines that are dependent upon design and individual patient needs. In general, the regions of a scleral lens can be separated into three zones: optical zone, transition zone, and the landing or haptic zone (Fig. 21.1).

The Optical Zone

The optical zone is the central region of the lens, and can be comprised of a single base curve or as many as three curves in some designs. The optical zone serves as the vision correction portion of the lens, as well as helps to determine the uniformity of vault across the central portion of the cornea. Adjusting the curves of the optical zone can increase or decrease vault in the center or midperiphery of the lens, as well as impact the needed power of the lens for optimal vision.

The posterior optical zone curve(s) may be spherical or aspheric. Many designs will employ a spherical central base curve with one or two aspheric ancillary optic zone curves outside of the central zone to aid in fit and to help bridge into the transition zone. When the central base curve is aspheric, it is typically utilized to improve the fit in highly aspheric corneas such as in moderate-to-advanced nipple keratoconus. Changing the curves of the optical zone of the lens may (Fig. 21.2) or may not (Fig. 21.3) affect the sagittal depth of the lens, depending on what else is simultaneously done with the lens design. The front-surface optical zone curves can also be spherical or aspheric. Aspheric front-surface curves are used to improve vision through the reduction of spherical aberrations, although the lens must be centered to gain this benefit.[17]

Toricity can be added to the front-surface optic zone to correct for residual astigmatism (Fig. 21.4). In these cases, the scleral lens has to be ballasted to provide an accurate and stable toric correction. Back-surface toricity in a fully vaulting scleral lens is almost never needed due to the fact that the lens does not touch the corneal surface.

Wavefront correction for higher-order aberrations in scleral lenses is being developed. Using wavefront aberrometry to measure higher-order aberrations through a scleral lens in vivo, it is possible to generate an anterior lens surface with wavefront optics for higher-order aberrations. This technology may allow improved VA for patients who use scleral lenses for irregular cornea conditions such as keratoconus (Fig. 21.5).

The Transitional Zone

The second region of a scleral lens is designated as the transition zone. Alternative terms include the midperipheral zone or the limbal zone. The transition zone may consist of as few as two curves or splines, though in many cases three or even four curves or splines are used in this part of the lens. How this region is designed is very dependent upon the specific lens manufacturer. The curves can be spherical, aspheric, or again, connected splines. The curves can progressively flatten, or there can be a reverse geometry effect, putting a steeper curve or two in the transition zone of the lens.

The transition zone should work in harmony with the optic zone curves to allow for the desired amount of corneal vault under the lens surface. If a lens has significantly more central vault than limbal, it may be useful to flatten the optical zone. However, to compensate, the transition zone will need to be adjusted, otherwise the net effect is only to reduce the central vault, not to increase the midperipheral vault. The opposite of this is also true. Figure 21.3 demonstrates in a simplified fashion how the transition zone and optical zone junction can be moved up and down harmoniously to improve the midperipheral fit. How you alter the lens fit by changes to the optical zone curves and transition zone curves depends upon the shape of the ocular surface you are trying to fit.

In the end, the specific details of the curves or splines of the transition zone are less important than whether they accomplish their goal, which is to transition the lens from the optical zone to the haptic without touching the ocular surface in the process. Having sufficient clearance in this region is important to avoid mechanically injuring the limbal-based corneal stem

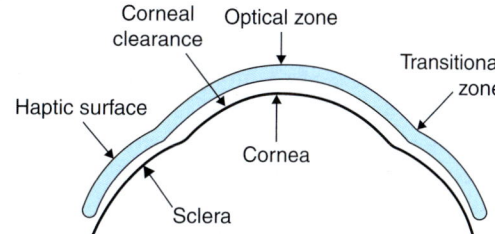

FIGURE 21.1 The zones of a scleral lens and optical transitional and haptic landing zones.

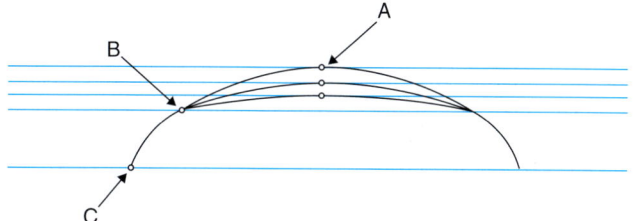

FIGURE 21.2 Changing the optical zone curves of a lens while not altering the transitional zone will affect the sagittal depth of the lens.

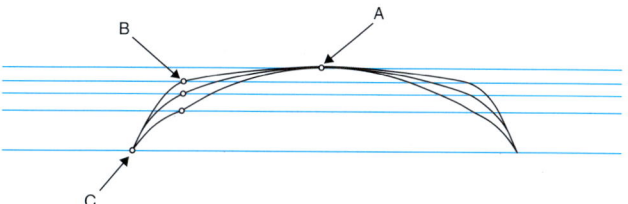

FIGURE 21.3 Changing the curves of the optical zone will not change the sagittal depth of the lens if the transitional zone curves are adjusted as well.

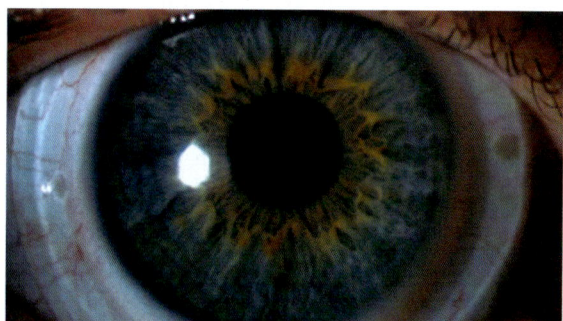

FIGURE 21.4 Front-toric scleral lens with markings evident. (Courtesy of Brooke Messer OD.)

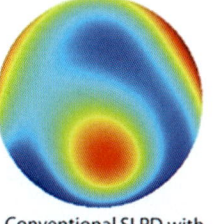
Conventional SLPD with spherical optics

Customized SLPD with wavefront-guided optics

FIGURE 21.5 Spherical versus wavefront-guided optics.

cells. A greater volume of tears in this region will minimize the risk of lens adherence and allow for a better tear pumping mechanism and the avoidance of tight lens symptoms.

Fenestrations are 1 mm holes placed in corneoscleral or scleral lenses to serve a variety of purposes, but their location is almost always in the transition zone. The original purpose for fenestrations was to allow oxygen to reach the cornea in the era of low-Dk materials. Indeed, one type of scleral lens design, the air-ventilated scleral lens, relies upon fenestrations not only for Dk, but also for a proper fit. Fenestrations are most often used to aid in the removal of a tight-fitting corneoscleral or mini-scleral lens. Unfortunately, fenestrations can induce unwanted bubbles into the fluid reservoir, which negates their overall utility.

The Haptic or Landing Zone

The final region of a scleral lens is known as the lens haptic or landing zone. This is the section of the lens that comes into contact with the ocular surface, and is often the region that is most crucial to success of the fit. The lens haptic is often made up of multiple curves or splines, but can also be made up as a tangential section, where the lens is essentially straight.

New technology that allows imaging of the ocular surface has helped us to understand the variability of scleral shape. Daniel Meier, a Swiss eye care practitioner, described five different types of limbal profiles, some having gradual changes in curve across the limbus, while others have a sharp transition. Additionally, scleras can be concave, convex, or tangential at the limbal region.[18]

The landing zone should be as closely aligned to the shape of the sclera to distribute the bearing of the lens over as broad an area as possible. A diagnostic fitting lens is often necessary to evaluate what series of curves or what tangent angle is optimal for an individual eye. It often requires allowing the lens to settle for 20 to 30 minutes to detect a tight-fitting landing zone. Even then a problematic fit may only be evident upon follow-up when a patient has had hours to wear a lens and let it fully settle.

Although the sclera has been described as nonrotationally symmetric, many scleras will exhibit a with-the-rule fitting relationship when using back-surface spherical scleral lens. In these cases, the scleral haptic will exhibit compression in the horizontal meridian and possibly edge lift in the vertical meridian. This fitting relationship can cause lens flexure resulting in residual astigmatism. The use of back-surface toric curves or splines in the landing zone is necessary to improve the fit in this situation. Toric back-surface sclerals demonstrate remarkable rotational stability and recovery.[19]

Quadrant back-surface designs can be utilized in cases of severe scleral irregularity. These lenses can be manufactured with different curves in each of the four quadrants of a lens (Fig. 21.6). Not all manufacturers have the capability of creating quadrant-specific lens designs,

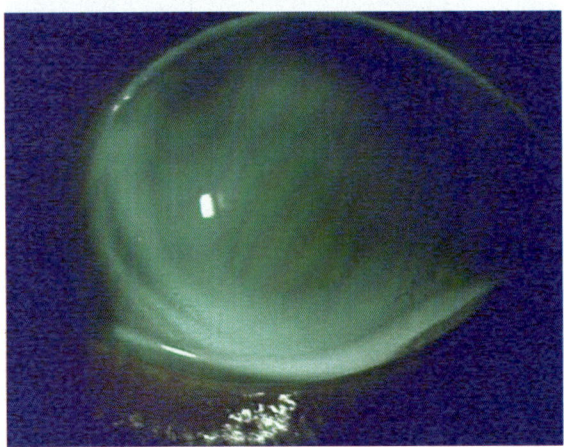

FIGURE 21.6 Quadrant-specific scleral lens. Note etchings on lens surface indicating lens zones.

so in cases where they are needed, it may require use of a specific laboratory. Optical coherence tomography (OCT) imaging of the ocular surface can be very useful in aiding in the creation of a quadrant-specific design.

Reverse Geometry Designs

Standard scleral lens designs incorporate a base curve and a series of curves or splines beyond that which flatten progressively to the edge. This is often successful for prolate corneas. In some instances, the shape of an eye will require a different profile. Most often, eyes that have had previous myopic refractive surgery or corneal transplant will exhibit an oblate cornea where the midperiphery is relatively steeper than the central cornea. These types of eyes will often be better fit with a reverse geometry lens design. A reverse geometry design has a secondary curve(s), which is steeper than the base curve. Typically, the lens will then progressively flatten from the steeper second curve(s) to the edge of the lens. When fitting a cornea with a known oblate profile, it is often advisable to immediately begin the fitting process with a reverse geometry lens design.

Multifocals

Scleral lenses have many positive attributes. Their stability of fit, rigid optics, and fluid reservoir, which can provide better comfort for those with dry eyes, makes scleral lenses an excellent choice for the presbyopic population. Many manufacturers offer scleral lenses with multifocal optics, which can be incorporated on the front or back surface (Fig. 21.7). Scleral lenses do not translate, so all designs utilize simultaneous vision. Therefore, patients should be educated about realistic visual expectations. Additionally, these lenses may not be successful for patients who have significant corneal scarring.

Lens centration is a critical aspect when fitting multifocal scleral lenses. A lens which rides low, which many sclerals lenses are apt to do, is not acceptable with a multifocal. The amount and zone size of the add power are dependent upon the characteristics of the individual patient, as with any multifocal lens. The lenses can be fit as any base scleral lens design and the multifocal surface can be added at the time of fabrication, so a diagnostic fitting set is needed. Laboratories that manufacture multifocal scleral lenses will have a nomogram for choosing add and zone size based upon the information provided by the practitioner about the individual being fit.

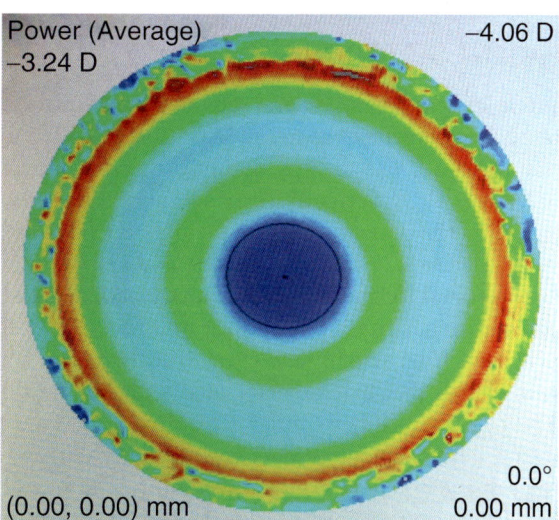

FIGURE 21.7 Power map of multifocal scleral lens.

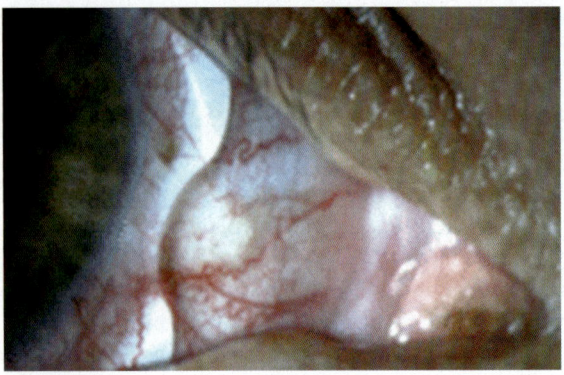

FIGURE 21.8 Scleral lens notched to accommodate pinguecula.

Edge Modifications

Landmarks such as a pinguecula or filtering bleb can interfere with the ability to fit and wear a scleral lens. To accommodate these landmarks, "notching" the edge of a scleral lens can allow the lens to fit bypass these obstacles (Fig. 21.8). Not all lens manufacturers will offer notching, so it is useful to know if that option is available prior to getting too far along in the fitting process. To notch a lens, accurate measurement of the size and location of the landmark is helpful to the laboratory consultant to ensure optimal placement and size. Diagnostic fitting with a scleral lens that has a precut notch can also improve fitting accuracy.

Center Thickness/Lens Materials

Unlike corneal lenses, where lens thickness can be vital to comfort and adaptation, lens thickness with scleral lenses has much less impact on the comfort or fit of the lens. However, thickness does play a role in scleral lenses in other regards. One role of center thickness is reducing lens flexure. Additionally, manufacturing a scleral lens too thin can increase the risk of the lens fitting too tight. For both of these reasons, scleral lenses are often manufactured much thicker than corneal lenses. While many corneal lenses are cut <0.2 mm thick, most sclerals have center thicknesses between 0.3 and 0.5 mm. Despite the thickness of these lenses, corneal swelling can all but be avoided by using hyper-Dk lens materials. Pullum published findings in 1997, which indicated that a lens with a center thickness of 0.6 mm made of a 115-Dk material would cause <3% corneal swelling in 3 hours of wear time.[20]

PATIENT SELECTION

While indications for scleral lens use have been relatively well-established,[4,21-24] there is currently less agreement as to the ideal time at which to introduce this mode of therapy. The position of scleral lens therapy within the patient's overall treatment may depend upon a number of factors. The severity of the ocular condition, outcomes of previous attempted interventions, and even the patient's general mental and physical condition can influence the eye care provider's decision to initiate scleral lens therapy.

In general, scleral lenses are not considered first-line treatment for simple refractive error, corneal irregularity, or OSD. Research has yet to define the risks of various complications that may arise from scleral lens wear. Until we have a clearer understanding of these risks, along with factors that may be associated with a higher likelihood of complications, it may be prudent to exhaust other contact lens options for correction of refractive error before considering scleral lenses. Many patients with primary corneal ectasia or postsurgical corneal irregularity can achieve excellent vision and comfort with one of the many specialty soft, corneal GP, or hybrid lenses on the market today. However, if these primary modalities fail, scleral lenses can be an alternative for visual correction before consideration of surgical intervention. Patients with OSD may wish to consider intervention that is less costly and/or time-consuming (lubricant drops, topical medications, punctal occlusion, moisture chamber goggles) prior to initiating scleral lens therapy.

Case History

The condition for which scleral lenses are being prescribed should be fully evaluated. The time of onset of symptoms and the clinical course of the condition since onset should be investigated. Encourage the patient to articulate the level of severity of current symptoms, ways in which those symptoms impact daily life, and hopes or goals for scleral lens therapy. This information is useful when deciding upon a particular scleral lens design, and helps to establish individualized fitting goals for the patient.

During the initial interview, identify forms of intervention that the patient may have tried prior to scleral lenses. Patients with primary corneal ectasia, postsurgical irregularity, or posttraumatic corneal distortion will generally have already tried at least one form of optical correction prior to considering scleral lenses. The discussion of previous modes of correction should include a description of spectacles or contact lenses that the patient has worn, along with the patient's assessment of vision and comfort with each form of visual correction. An understanding of the patient's experience with other forms of refractive correction gives insight into the patient's visual demands and expectations. Scleral lenses are rarely used as first-line therapy for OSD. By the time they are referred for scleral lens evaluation, most patients with surface disorders have been treated with some combination of lubricant drops, topical steroids, topical cyclosporine, autologous serum drops, punctal occlusion, oral medication, or surgical intervention. Some of these patients may also have used physical barrier devices such as goggles or moisture chamber glasses. Initial discussion with the patient should identify the types of intervention previously attempted, as well as the patient's assessment of the success or failure of each intervention.

In addition to information specific to the patient's current ocular condition, any history of past ocular disease or ocular surgery should be noted. Cataracts, macular disorders, glaucoma, and other forms of optic neuropathy may limit visual potential with scleral lenses. Discussion of these limits prior to scleral lens fitting can help the patient develop reasonable expectations for vision with scleral lenses. Previous corneal surgery such as refractive surgery or keratoplasty can affect the fit of a scleral lens. Lid procedures can change the tension or position of the lids, which may affect lens application and lens positioning on the eye. Procedures that alter scleral contour (i.e., glaucoma filtering surgeries or scleral buckles) can significantly affect the fit of scleral lenses.

Ocular Evaluation

Position of the eye within the orbit can affect lens application and removal. Patients with deeply set eyes may have difficulty controlling lid position when applying scleral lenses. The use of a bulbed plunger may be necessary for these patients, and they may also find it easier to handle a lens with a smaller diameter. Conversely, a relatively proptotic globe may require a larger lens to improve lens stability and provide protection to the entire exposed ocular surface.

Lid position, tension/tone, and structure can affect the position of a scleral lens on the eye. Heavy or unusually taut upper lids may decenter a scleral lens inferiorly, particularly if the lower lid rests below the limbus or lacks tone. Unusually, taut lids can also increase the degree of posterior lens "settling" after application, and may present lens application challenges. The relative position and tension of the lids is easily assessed during slit-lamp evaluation, as is the patient's tolerance of lid manipulation. Vertical fissure height should also be noted prior to initial lens selection. The position of the superior and inferior flange of a scleral lens beyond the lid margins reduces lens sensation and improves lens stability. The relatively large diameter of full scleral lenses virtually assures that this fitting relationship will be achieved in almost all eyes. However, mini-scleral designs may not extend beyond lid margins if the vertical fissure height is considerably greater than average.

The quality of the tear film and the quantity of tears present on the surface of the eye can affect the success of scleral lens wear. If significant meibomian gland dysfunction (MGD) is present, treatment prior to the initiation of lens wear is advised to avoid excessive lipid deposition on the surface of the scleral lens, which may negatively impact both vision and comfort. Decreased tear breakup time (TBUT) in the absence of MGD or general aqueous deficiency do not require resolution prior to scleral lens fitting. However, patients who show signs of tear-film deficiency may need to use lubricant drops during lens wear to maintain surface wetting of the device.

Characteristics of conjunctival tissue can significantly impact the fitting of scleral lenses. Excessively loose conjunctival tissue can be pulled into the postlens reservoir, and can actually "hood" or cover the limbus. Although difficult to assess prior to lens application, the relative elasticity and thickness of the conjunctiva significantly affects scleral lens fitting. Conjunctival tissue that is thick or relatively elastic may allow for more posterior settling of the device during wear, while corneal vault may be better maintained on an eye with thinner or less "spongy" conjunctiva. The presence of pronounced pinguecula, and the position of the pinguecula relative to the limbus should also be noted. Mild pinguecula generally require no special consideration when fitting scleral lenses, but adjustments to lens or haptic diameter, modifications to flange shape, or notched lenses may be required to accommodate some pinguecula.

As most of the conditions that may necessitate scleral lens wear affect corneal tissue, careful evaluation of the cornea is of paramount importance. If epitheliopathy is present, a greater degree of clearance between the cornea and the posterior lens surface may be desirable. Any opacity or neovascularization present prior to the initiation of scleral lens wear should be accurately documented. Corneal neovascularization may indicate relative intolerance for hypoxia, so its presence would indicate caution when fitting scleral lenses. Beyond slit-lamp evaluation of corneal tissue, a cross-sectional view of the cornea can provide considerable insight into overall corneal contour. Not only will an optic cross section allow for assessment of the degree of corneal irregularity, but this view also gives the scleral lens fitter an idea of the depth of the cornea from limbus to apex. The depth of the cornea could be argued to be the most important measurement to be considered when fitting scleral lenses.

PATIENT EDUCATION

Although awareness of scleral lenses has increased dramatically during the past several years, misperceptions about the devices are still common. A discussion of expectations for scleral lens wear will help to avoid misunderstandings and disappointments as the fitting process proceeds.

Patients with severe OSD may think that scleral lenses will replace some or all of their current therapy. However, in most cases, scleral lenses are additive therapy. While scleral lenses may allow these patients to use lubricant drops less frequently, it is unlikely that the devices alone will provide adequate comfort or ocular surface protection. Upon completion of the fitting process, the patient's condition can be reassessed, and therapy can be adjusted accordingly.

Patients may not be able to achieve optimal VA at all distances with scleral lenses alone. While toric and multifocal lens designs exist, some patients will still need spectacle correction over their scleral lenses in order to obtain the clearest possible vision. The patient should be informed that a separate pair of glasses may be necessary for use with scleral lenses to maximize vision at various distances. Moisture chamber glasses may be prescribed for use with scleral lenses in cases of severe OSD.

The size of a scleral lens may be intimidating for some patients, particularly those who have not previously worn contact lenses. A video demonstrating application/removal technique is available online through the Scleral Lens Education Society (http://www.sclerallens.org/

how-use-scleral-lenses). Training in application and removal of a diagnostic lens can be useful for both patient and eye care provider. The patients can gain confidence in their ability to handle the device before committing to the purchase of a lens. Lens design can be altered based upon the patient's ability or inability to successfully apply the diagnostic lens.

Patients who have not worn contact lenses previously may not fully understand the fitting process or how scleral lenses work. Patients that are educated on why they need a specialty contact lens are more likely to start the fitting process. Explaining the need for multiple visits and lenses in order to achieve optimal vision and fit prior to the initiation of scleral lens fitting helps to establish the expectation that the first lens ordered may not be ideal. Patients who understand that scleral lens fitting is a process rather than an event will be less likely to become discouraged if the initial lens is not ideal.

Scleral lenses can be considerably more expensive than other contact lenses, and insurance coverage is not assured. A frank discussion on billing and payment expectations, either before or at the initial evaluation, may prevent misunderstandings, as the fitting process proceeds.

EQUIPMENT

Instruments that have traditionally been used in contact lens fitting may be of limited utility in scleral lens fitting because scleral lens fitting is based upon vault rather than alignment. Manual keratometry estimates the curvature of a very small area of the central cornea. Central corneal contour may not correlate strongly with the depth of the cornea and is of little value in a scleral lens fit.

Corneal topography provides information on the contour of a larger area of the cornea than does manual keratometry. It may be advisable to obtain baseline data on corneal topography prior to scleral lens wear, particularly in patients with corneal ectasia. Manufacturers' guidelines for fitting scleral lenses refer to various topographic indices when describing methods for initial diagnostic lens selection. However, topographic indices have been found to lack predictive value when compared to base curve of appropriately fit scleral lenses.[25] Furthermore, accurate topographic data may be difficult to obtain on highly irregular or extremely dry corneal surfaces. While topography may be useful in following a patient for changes in corneal contour over time, it is not essential for initial diagnostic lens selection.

Anterior segment OCT has the ability to map anterior ocular contour across a 16 mm meridian. With slight modifications to image acquisition techniques, even larger areas have been scanned.[18] With anterior segment OCT, the relationship of the haptic of a scleral lens and the sclera can be observed. The peripheral edges of full scleral lenses still lie just beyond the range of a standard anterior segment OCT. However, the ability to precisely measure the depth of the postlens fluid reservoir beneath either a mini-scleral or full scleral lens can be clinically useful. During the fitting process, images from an anterior segment OCT aid in communication between the eye care provider and the manufacturer when alterations in lens design are needed. If available, anterior segment OCT could also be performed prior to lens fitting, and then be repeated periodically after the initiation of lens wear to monitor for any changes in corneal, conjunctival, or scleral contour.

Anterior segment photography can accurately document the condition of the cornea and conjunctiva before scleral lens wear is initiated, and can be repeated to document any changes that may occur in these tissues. As was the case with anterior segment OCT, digital images of a scleral lens on the eye can allow the eye care provider to show the lens manufacturer any aspect of a suboptimal fit. The ability to precisely communicate with the laboratory should facilitate a more streamlined fitting process.

In cases in which decreased endothelial cell density may compromise the patient's ability to wear lenses successfully, prelens assessment of endothelial cell density with either confocal or specular microscopy is advisable. If these instruments are not available, corneal thickness can be measured prior to and immediately after removal of a diagnostic lens. A significant increase in corneal thickness after 4 to 6 hours of lens wear could be an indication that the patient may not be able to wear the lens successfully.

DIAGNOSTIC LENS FITTING

A well-fit scleral lens bears on the sclera and completely vaults the corneal surface while maintaining a semisealed fit without lens movement. Current limitations in scleral imaging technology make empirical fitting of scleral lenses next to impossible. Diagnostic lenses are generally used as a starting point in scleral lens fitting, and adjustments to standard lens designs can be made if customized lenses are necessary. While each lens design has unique characteristics, the principles of fitting scleral lenses are applicable to all of these designs.

The amount of vault and distribution of space over various areas of the cornea can be assessed with the use of diagnostic lenses. Generous vault beneath the lens can create an optical thick lens system. In such cases, prediction of lens power may be less predictable than with corneal or corneoscleral lenses. Overrefraction performed over a diagnostic lens is likely to yield more accurate refractive results than predictions based upon keratometry readings and lens base curve. Use of diagnostic lenses during the fitting process allows the fitter to assess the alignment of the haptic to the conjunctival tissue overlying the scleral. Areas of vascular compression or impingement will be visible within an hour of lens application. If conjunctival abnormalities are present, diagnostic fitting will show the effect that these irregularities have on lens fit.

The use of diagnostic lenses also allows the patient to experience the sensation of the lens on the eye. Many patients are surprised at the relative comfort of scleral lenses compared to smaller lens designs, but patients frequently note a "thick" or "bulky" sensation with initial lens wear. In most patients, this sensation abates relatively quickly. However, some patients remain quite bothered by this feeling. For such patients, mini-scleral lenses with limited corneal vault may be a more comfortable option than full scleral lenses. Patients may also be able to identify areas of mild conjunctival compression within a relatively short time after application of the diagnostic lens, even before compression becomes obvious upon slit-lamp evaluation. Some patients with severe dry-eye symptoms have very little clinical evidence of dry-eye syndrome. Placement of diagnostic lenses allows these patients to subjectively determine whether or not scleral lenses will provide sufficient relief of symptoms. Finally, diagnostic lens application and removal may relieve some patient anxiety about handling the devices.

Lens Selection and Evaluation

Initial lens selection is guided by manufacturer's guidelines. However, most guidelines are based, at least in part, upon keratometry values or topographic indices. As mentioned earlier, these numbers are not strongly predictive of scleral lens fit. An experienced scleral lens fitter may be able to select an initial diagnostic lens simply based upon the contour of the cornea and sclera as viewed from the lateral side.

Although individual techniques for applying scleral lenses may vary, all require proper positioning of the patient so as not to lose saline. The patient must be in a face-down position. This is easily accomplished in a typical examination chair; the patient is instructed to lean forward from the waist and tuck the chin toward the chest. The fitter places the diagnostic lens either on a bulbed plunger or on a tripod consisting of the thumb, index, and middle fingers. The bowl of the lens is filled with saline, and the lens is applied to the surface of the eye.

A lid fissure that is narrow or restricted does not necessarily preclude the use of a full scleral lens, but may require a slightly different application technique. In such cases, it may be helpful to retract the upper lid sufficiently to create space between the lid and the globe. The superior flange of the lens can be maneuvered into that space, and the lower lid can then be retracted to provide enough space to complete lens application.

Some patients are not able to achieve a fully face-down position. Others may have lid or orbital abnormalities that necessitate more elaborate maneuvering in lens application. For these patients, the bowl of the lens can be filled with off-label use of Celluvisc. The higher viscosity of Celluvisc helps prevent spillage and subsequent bubble entrapment.

If desired, sodium fluorescein can be placed in the bowl of the lens prior to initial application. However, dye in excess fluid may discolor skin or clothing. Some scleral lens fitters prefer to initially evaluate lens fit without fluorescein. If the lens is initially applied with clear saline, observing the rate of transfer of a drop of fluorescein added to the lower fornix into the postlens fluid reservoir allows for an estimation of the rate of tear exchange. Immediately after lens placement, slit-lamp examination can reveal any entrapped bubbles. Small, mobile bubbles that do not approach the visual axis are generally of no significance. However, if a large stationary bubble is present, the lens will need to be removed and reapplied. Repeated bubble entrapment beneath a lens during application despite appropriate application technique may be an indication that the lens is too steep.

Once a bubble-free application has been achieved, the fitting relationship between the cornea and the lens can be observed. While the lens may continue to settle back for some time after application, immediate assessment of the fit will identify a lens that is too shallow. The lens should not touch any portion of the cornea. If central touch is observed, the lens should be removed, and a steeper (or deeper) lens should be applied. The total area of corneal contact provides a clue as to the amount of additional depth needed; a small amount (>2 mm) of touch will probably be eliminated with a relatively slight increase in depth, while a larger amount of touch (<2 mm) would suggest that a more significant change in lens depth will be necessary in order to achieve adequate clearance.

Selecting an initial diagnostic lens that completely vaults the cornea will facilitate an efficient fitting process (Fig. 21.9). If the depth of the postlens fluid reservoir is obviously excessive, a shallower lens can be applied immediately. The amount of vault can be estimated by turning the slit beam to a 45 degree angle and comparing the amount of reservoir with the known thickness of the scleral lens or cornea (Fig. 21.10). If anterior segment OCT is available, an exact measurement of corneal clearance can be obtained. The haptic of a scleral lens rests on the spongy conjunctiva. As the lens settles into this tissue, it can lose up to 150 microns of vault, so a slightly more than the desired central clearance should be observed immediately after application. The amount of clearance desired can be dependent upon the condition being treated with scleral lenses. Treatment of severe OSD may require a more generous fluid reservoir than visual correction of irregular astigmatism. As a general rule, 250 to 500 microns of initial clearance are considered adequate with full scleral lenses. Slightly less clearance is achieved with mini-scleral lenses.

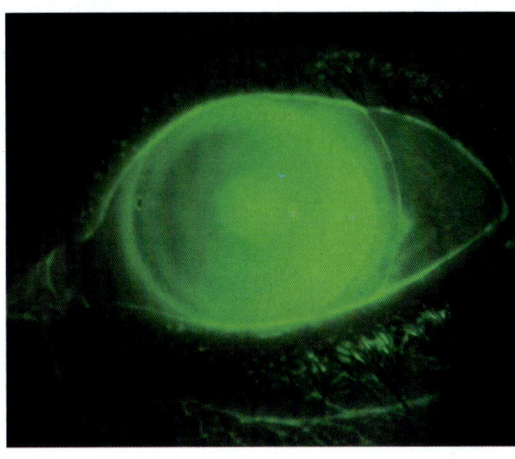

FIGURE 21.9 Scleral lens fully vaulting the cornea.

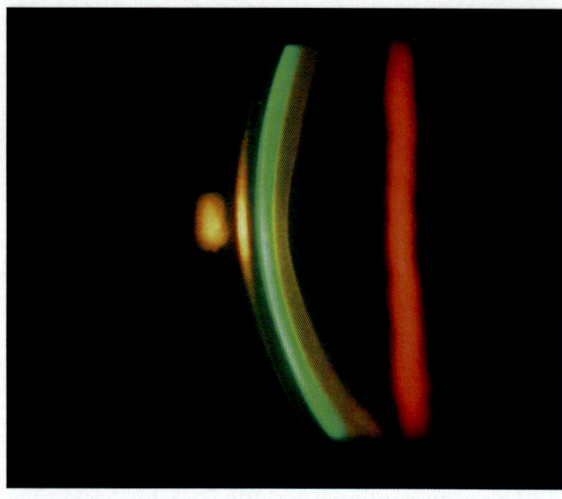

FIGURE 21.10 Cross section with fluorescein highlighting the fluid reservoir.

Once a lens with adequate central clearance has been identified, limbal clearance should be evaluated. In order to avoid mechanical stress on limbal stem cells, scleral lenses should completely clear the limbus. Ideally, the haptic should begin contacting conjunctival tissue between 0.5 and 1.0 mm beyond the limbus. If insufficient limbal clearance is noted with the initial diagnostic lens, a lens of larger diameter may be necessary in order to achieve adequate limbal vault. As changes in lens diameter can significantly impact total sagittal depth, it is important to determine the optimal lens diameter at the onset of the fitting process. If it is not possible to use a larger lens, standard lens designs parameters can be customized to provide additional limbal clearance.

The lens haptic or landing zone is the final area to be evaluated. The haptic should rest evenly upon the conjunctival tissue that overlies the sclera (Fig. 21.11). The lens edge should neither lift off the surface of the conjunctiva nor compress conjunctival vasculature. Once again, standard lens design parameters may need to be customized in order to achieve this fitting relationship.

Once an acceptable preliminary lens fit has been determined, attention can be turned to the optical performance of the lens. Potential VA with scleral lenses in patients with no significant ocular surface irregularity should be similar to what can be achieved with habitual spectacle or contact lens correction. Patients with significant anterior corneal irregularity can expect VA

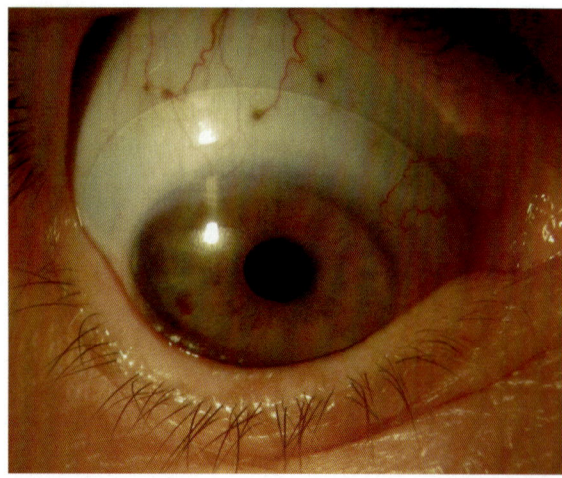

FIGURE 21.11 Scleral lens demonstrating an ideal haptic fit.

that is similar to that which they can achieve through smaller-GP lens designs. In some cases of severe corneal ectasia, corneal lenses that have significant areas of bearing may actually compress corneal tissue. It is possible that this compression reduces the effect of mid-or posterior stromal irregularities. When bearing is relieved, these patients may note a minimal reduction in VA with a scleral lens compared to a flat-fitting corneal GP.

Overrefraction can be performed while waiting for the lens to settle. Lens increments should be large enough to be visually significant for the patient's visual potential. If predicted VA can be achieved with spherical lenses alone, determination of scleral lens power is straightforward; vertex adjusted overrefractive power is simply added to the power of the diagnostic lens. Sphero–cylindrical overrefraction may be necessary if expected VA is not achieved. Several scleral lens manufacturers offer toric refractive correction in scleral lenses. Before ordering a toric power, however, first check to see if unwanted lens flexure is inducing astigmatism by performing keratometry or topography over the diagnostic scleral lens. If significant toricity is noted, the lens can be ordered with increased flange or center thickness to reduce flexure, or an alternate design could be considered.

Final evaluation of the diagnostic lens fit can be completed after the lens has been on the eye for at least 20 to 30 minutes. At that time, corneal clearance should be reassessed. Posterior pressure from the lids, coupled with some degree of conjunctival compression, may reduce overall corneal clearance compared to the evaluation immediately after lens application. Even after lens settling, the lenses should completely and measurably clear the cornea. The amount of clearance is somewhat dependent upon lens design (mini-scleral vs. full scleral) and may be altered based upon the condition to be treated, but no less than 100 to 200 microns of clearance should be observed at this time. Clearance can be considerably higher than this in full scleral designs. Relatively even corneal clearance is ideal, but it is possible to observe differences in the amount of vault over different areas of the cornea in highly irregular corneas (postkeratoplasty, severe ectasia). Complete limbal clearance should also be observed.

The relationship between the lens haptic and the conjunctiva should now be reevaluated. The ideal relationship between the haptic and the conjunctiva consists of even bearing beneath the entire haptic, with minimal disruption of conjunctival vasculature. If the lens has settled back considerably, areas of relative vessel compression or congestion may have developed. Assessment of the location and severity of any vessel blanching is necessary to design a comfortable, well-fit lens.

Consider a toric back-surface haptic if compression is noted along one axis and frank edge lift is observed along the meridian 90 degrees away. Some studies have suggested that haptic toricity can provide improved comfort for a majority of scleral lens patients.[19] If the areas of compression or edge lift are less regular, a quadrant-specific design may be necessary to provide adequate haptic alignment. Lens seal-off results from circumferential compression and will make the lens unwearable secondary to discomfort. Uniform flattening of the peripheral curves will loosen the fit.

The edge of the lens should approximate the contour of the conjunctiva without impingement or edge lift. Impingement of tissue will result in fluorescein staining upon lens removal. Long-term or chronic impingement can result in conjunctival hypertrophy.

In order to assess tear exchange beneath the lens, a drop of fluorescein can be instilled with the lens on the eye. Migration of fluorescein into the postlens fluid reservoir can then be observed. Rapid migration of fluorescein beneath the lens demonstrates minimally obstructed replenishment of newly oxygenated tears into the postlens reservoir. While this level of tear exchange may be preferable, it is not necessary in order to achieve successful scleral lens wear. However, periodic removal of the scleral lenses during the course of the day, followed by reapplication with fresh saline may be advisable in patients with minimal tear exchange, to allow for removal of potentially toxic corneal metabolic waste products and replenishment of freshly oxygenated fluid into the postlens reservoir.

During the 20- to 30-minute adaptation period, the surface of the lens can attract lipid deposits. Areas of the lens surface may become relatively hydrophobic. Patients who experience this phenomenon during initial lens evaluation may require more aggressive therapy for MGD. These patients may need to use lubricant drops over the lenses frequently in order to maintain lens surface clarity, and may benefit from more aggressive cleaning regimens.

Dispensing

Dispensing a scleral lens is a critical step in the fitting process. Allow plenty of time for this appointment, especially if the patient is new to scleral lenses. The first step is to apply the scleral lens to the patient to evaluate fit and vision. The lens should already have been verified and disinfected prior to the patient's appointment time. Fill the lens completely full with saline solution and dip a fluorescein strip into the bowl. Apply the lens to the patient's eye(s) using the same procedure that was used during the diagnostic lens fitting. Next, inspect the lens to make sure it is positioned correctly and check to see if there are any bubbles. If the lens is positioned off center, has a bubble larger than 2 mm, or a central bubble, then remove the lens and reapply with fresh saline and fluorescein. Once you have successfully applied the lens, check the patient's VA, which should be close to the patients known vision potential. It is a good idea to proceed with a sphero–cylindrical overrefraction to check the accuracy of the prescription strength. Next prepare the patient to evaluate the lens with a slit-lamp biomicroscope. Observe the lens with a diffuse cobalt light and Wratten filter. Ideally the lens will be without bubbles or areas of corneal touch. Now observe the vault of the lens with white light using an optical cross section. Compare the liquid reservoir—highlighted with fluorescein—with the known thickness of the scleral lens or cornea. Lastly, use a diffuse white light to observe the fitting relationship of the scleral lens haptic with the sclera. Photographing the lens can help with troubleshooting the lens fit or to track fitting relationship changes over time. Two fitting requirements have to be met in order to start wearing a scleral lens. First, the lens has to provide the patient with adequate VA that meets their visual demand. This includes VA that meets the State standards for driving if the patient operates a motor vehicle. Secondly, the scleral lens has to fit adequately enough that it will not induce secondary anterior surface complications. If the patient has expected VA and the lens is adequately fitting, then you can proceed to show the patient how to manage lens wear and give them care instruction. If the patient's vision or fit is unacceptable, the lens will have to be returned and another lens ordered with adjustments to address its deficiencies. It is important to remember that the lens fit can change during the adaptive period and so it is preferable to wait to make fine-tune adjustment until the patient has had sometime to wear the lens.

Application and Removal Training

The relatively larger size of scleral contact lenses increases the difficulty of application and removal. Additionally, application is further complicated by the fact that the patient has to apply a lens that is filled with a fluid reservoir. Therefore, sufficient time should be allotted for training. If the person is elderly or disabled, make sure to involve the caretaker because they will most likely be helping the patient at home. First, have the patients wash and dry their hands. Then set them up at table in front of a portable mirror. For lens removal, most patients find it easiest to use a lens plunger. Instruct the patients to wet the plunger with saline and to use their free hand to widen their lid aperture. While looking in the mirror, the patient should apply the plunger head to the lens haptic and then lift the lens out. A well-fit scleral lens is semisealed to the eye with significant negative pressure, which will cause the lens to pull on the eye if the plunger is positioned at the lens center. An alternate approach to scleral lens removal is to use the lids. The patients use their upper lid to hold the lens in place while using the margin of the lower lid to break the semiseal between the lens and the sclera. At this point, the patient can grab the contact lens and lift it out.

Once the patients have successfully removed the contact lens, they can be trained on scleral lens application. First, have the patient fill the scleral lens to the contact lens rim with sterile nonpreserved saline solution. Scleral lenses are difficult to balance because of their size and weight after being filled with saline. Most patients will have to support the scleral lens with a large plunger or by making a tripod between their thumb, index, and middle fingers. The patient should hold the scleral lens in the hand opposite of the eye that the lens will be applied. Instruct the patients to use their free hand to widen their lid aperture using their thumb and index finger. At this point, they need to lean over so that their face is parallel to the contact lens table. To help visualize and center the lens, the patients may use a mirror that has been laid flat or they may simply use the lens plunger as a target. Advise the patient to push the lens on center. Once the lens is in position, the patients should let their lids wrap around the lens and pull the plunger or their fingers away. For application, it is preferred the lens simply rests on the plunger without suction. Large plungers are available that have the end of the bulb open to prevent suction. If the patient has a caretaker, he or she may want to participate and help the patient guide the lens because some patients with disability will have difficulty aligning the lens with center of their eye.

Dalsey adaptives (www.dalseyadaptives.com) manufactures a stand that holds a plunger that will support a scleral lens. The patients can hold their lids using both hands and then lower their eye onto the scleral lens. The plunger has a light in the center that the patients can fixate and help guide their eye onto the center of the lens.

Keep in mind that the patients may not be completely successful during the first training session. However, as long as they are able to successfully remove the lens, then they can take it home and practice application. A second training session can be scheduled at a follow-up appointment to reinstruct or troubleshoot.

Contact Lens Solutions

Modern scleral lenses are manufactured using GP materials. Therefore these lenses can be cleaned and disinfected using approved GP care products. Hydrogen peroxide care systems may also be prescribed and are advantageous because there is no risk of residual preservatives getting trapped underneath the lens, which can cause toxicity or hypersensitivity. Larger cases can be purchased from the The Dry Eye Shop (http://www.dryeyeshop.com/prose-case-p277.aspx) for full scleral lenses that do not properly fit in the standard baskets that come with hydrogen peroxide care systems. Extra strength cleaners may also be prescribed for patients who are more prone to lens deposits.

Scleral lenses have to be filled with solution prior to application. Nonpreserved saline solution is preferred in order to avoid hypersensitivity or toxic reactions. Single-use vials of 0.9% sodium chloride can be prescribed off-label in order to eliminate the contamination risk of bottled nonpreserved saline that is used over multiple days. Patients may use contact lens approved rewetting drops as needed.

Safety and Risk

Educate patients concerning the safety and risks of contact lens wear. Written instructions should be reviewed. The patients should sign the documentation that acknowledges their understanding and adherence to the prescribed guidelines. Send the patients home with a small kit that contains all of their starter solutions and accessories. Give them a folder that has detailed instructions reviewing lens handling, contact lens care, and safety and risks. A comprehensive video reviewing scleral lens handling and care can be viewed at the Scleral Lens Education Society website (http://www.sclerallens.org/how-use-scleral-lenses).

TROUBLESHOOTING COMPLICATIONS

Various complications can arise during the scleral lens fitting process that can lead to failure and eventual dropout. Most complications can be successfully remedied if they are properly identified and addressed.

CORNEAL TOUCH

Ideally, a scleral lens vaults the cornea without areas of touch or bearing. There are cases where the best-fitting diagnostic lens of a specific design exhibits residual areas of corneal touch, which can cause the patient discomfort and eventually lead to epithelial breakdown. For instance, this could occur with a keratoconus patient who has a severely steep kone. If the steepest diagnostic lens has insufficient vault, then switch to a design with more sagittal depth. Usually, this means using a larger overall diameter by 3 mm or more. Not only will increase in size give more sagittal depth, but it will also give this relatively steeper lens more area of scleral landing. Midperipheral lens touch is often observed with patients who have oblate corneas, which occurs after myopic refractive surgery and 47% of the time after penetrating keratoplasty.[26] For these patients, use reverse geometry designs to create midperipheral lift for complete corneal clearance.

Persistent areas of touch can be monitored and left uncorrected as long as it does not induce any negative signs or symptoms. If uncorrectable areas of touch cause symptomatic epitheliopathy, then consider piggybacking the scleral lens on a soft bandage lens to improve comfort and prevent epithelial erosion. Start with a bandage soft silicone hydrogel diagnostic lens to maximize Dk. Daily disposables are preferred because they are convenient when using a two-lens system.

Lens Compression and Seal-Off

A well-fit scleral contact lens semiseals to the eye, which means there is no lens translation with blinking or eye movement. Ideally, the haptic portion of the scleral lens should rest evenly on the scleral conjunctiva. Tear exchange occurs secondary to a pumping action that results from lens flexure as the upper lid blinks over its surface. Patients who have more scleral shape asymmetry may exhibit mild intermittent blanching secondary to haptic bearing, especially if a spherical back-surface design is being fit. This scenario may be perfectly acceptable as long as the patient is comfortable and the lens is exhibiting fluid exchange. However, if the scleral lens haptic is fitting too tight, then the lens may move from a semiseal to a complete seal fit. In this case, the haptic will induce a circumferential ring of sclera conjunctival blanching and fluid exchange will cease (Fig. 21.12). The paralimbal area underneath the lens will become red and congested. Metabolic and cellular debris may build up in the reservoir, leading to corneal toxicity. The patient will subjectively complain of irritation and redness. The lens will also be very difficult to remove, secondary to an increase in negative pressure. Late onset seal-off can occur if the lens induces increasing conjunctival congestion, which can cause the lens to gradually fit

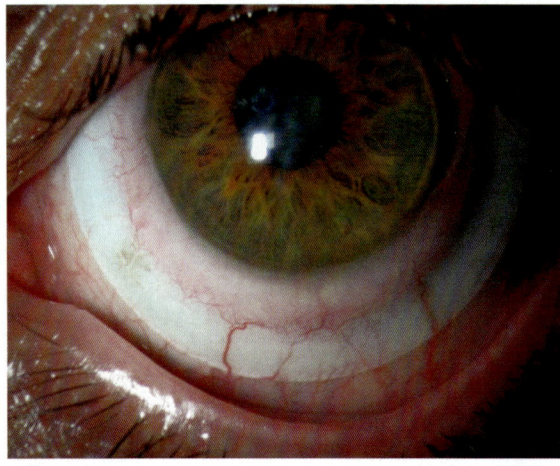

FIGURE 21.12 Scleral lens with circumferential blanching and limbal congestion secondary to seal-off.

tighter. If the scleral lens is compressive and sealing off, then the peripheral curves of the lens haptic need to be flattened in order to loosen the fit and return the lens to a semisealed state. The peripheral curves that correspond to the paralimbal area are the peripheral curves of the lens that need to be flattened to successfully loosen the fit. If the peripheral curves that correspond to the conjunctival blanching are flattened without flattening the paralimbal curves, the scleral lens seal-off will worsen on the eye secondary to the hinge effect. Basically, the edge of the lens is lifted up and the junction between the blanching and the paralimbal area acts like a hinge digging into the sclera, causing the lens to fit tighter. Flattening the peripheral curves will decrease the overall sagittal depth of the lens. Compensate for this by steepening the base curve to maintain corneal vault.

Uneven Haptic Bearing

The majority of scleral designs incorporate spherical back-surface haptic peripheral curves. However, the sclera is not spherical, but rather nonrotationally symmetric.[27] This quadrant asymmetry of the sclera increases with increasing distance from the limbus. Frequently, back-surface spherical haptic lens designs are able to adequately distribute the bearing of the lens to achieve an acceptable fit. The spongy scleral conjunctiva helps to dampen differences between the lens and the eye. Some successfully fit scleral lenses may exhibit relatively small areas of sectorial blanching without affecting lens comfort or performance. Patients who have more severe asymmetrical scleral anatomy will demonstrate an unacceptable fitting relationship—the lens will demonstrate areas of intermittent blanching and edge lift—which will negatively affect comfort and performance (Fig. 21.13). In particular, edge lift of the lens haptic will induce bubbles and excessive debris. If the fit of a spherical back-surface haptic design lens is unacceptable, then you will need to consider a toric or quadrant-specific back-surface haptic design to achieve a successful fit. Toric back-surface haptic designs can be fit with diagnostic lenses. Toric and quadrant-specific haptic back surfaces can be designed with the laboratory consultant using photographs or optical coherence imagery of the scleral lens fit.

Scleral Obstacles

Patients may have scleral conjunctival obstacles that have the potential to negatively affect the fit of a scleral contact lens. The most common scleral obstacles are pinqueculas. The majority of pinqueculas are shallow enough that the scleral lens haptic is able to evenly rest on top of them without negatively affecting the fit. However, more significantly elevated pinqueculas may affect the comfort or fit of the scleral lens. The second most common scleral obstacles are

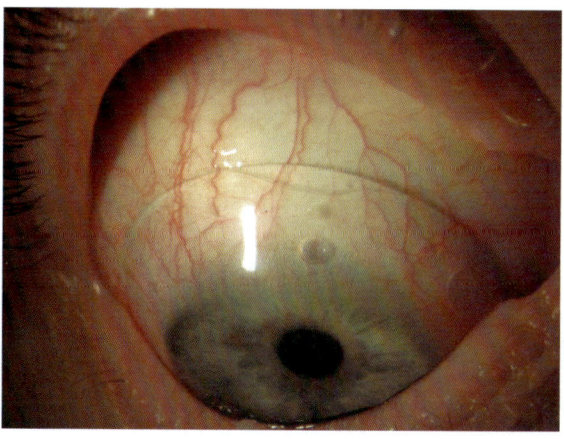

FIGURE 21.13 Edge lift of a scleral lens.

conjunctival blebs that are encountered with glaucoma patients who have had a trabeculectomy. Depending on the location of the obstacle, the haptic edge of the lens may bump into it, causing irritation or negatively affect the fit because the rigid nature of the haptic is unable to drape over the obstacle. In these cases, a notch that is beveled into the scleral lens will allow the lens haptic to bypass the obstacle. A diagnostic lens with a precut notch can be used for measurement or a lens consultant can help design the lens based upon measurement and photographs. The overall lens diameter should be kept relatively small, usually no bigger than 15 mm, because larger-diameter scleral lenses will require deeper notches that may induce bubble formation. The notch should be wide enough to bypass the obstacle and prevent negative lens-to-obstacle interaction. The lens should be placed on the eye like a puzzle piece so that the notch corresponds with the obstacle. For patients with conjunctival blebs, monitor the lens fit and the health of the bleb to detect any lens-induced tissue disruption that could lead to a bleb leak or blebitis.

Conjunctival Hooding

The negative pressure underneath a scleral contact lens can cause conjunctival tissue to be pulled into the scleral zone (Fig. 21.14). This is more likely to occur if the patient has a conjunctiva that is excessive and loose. Conjunctival hooding that is confined to only one quadrant does not usually result in any negative consequences. Larger areas of hooding, especially if it is completely circumferential, may induce scleral lens seal-off. Problematic hooding is difficult to remedy and the patient may be better off switching to an alternate lens modality. If scleral lenses are the patient's only option, then consider having the patient undergo a conjunctival resection.

Lens Flexure

The relatively large overall diameter of scleral lenses leaves them prone to flexure as they rest on the sclera and vault over the cornea. Flexure is more likely to occur if the scleral haptic is not evenly resting on the scleral surface. Lens flexure induces astigmatism, which will degrade the patient's VA. If a sphero–cylindrical overrefraction yields astigmatic error, first determine if the astigmatism is caused by lens flexure or is lenticular astigmatism. This can be accomplished by performing keratometry or topography over the lens. If the scleral lens that the patient is wearing has a spherical front surface, then the resultant reading of this measurement should be spherical. However, if the measurement is astigmatic, then the lens is flexing. The simplest way to prevent flexure is to increase the center or flange thickness. Another strategy to reduce flexure is to use back-surface toric haptic or quadrant-specific peripheral curves to improve the lens-to-eye fitting relationship.

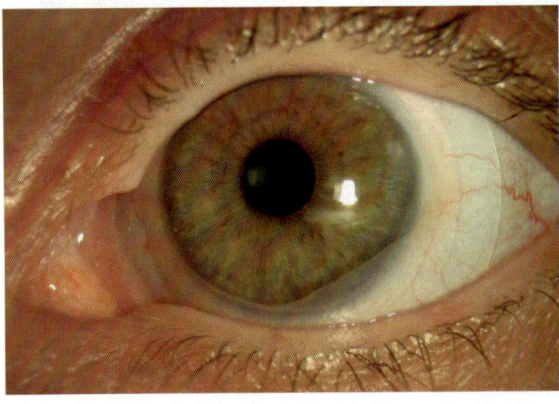

FIGURE 21.14 Loose conjunctiva in the corneal zone.

Reservoir Debris

The accumulation of debris underneath a scleral contact lens is a common complication of scleral lens wear. Reservoir debris consists of one or more of the following: mucus, epithelial cells, or makeup.[28] Patients with OSD are more likely to experience significant debris, especially mucus. Significant debris accumulation may cause a patient's vision to be cloudy, but does not affect lens comfort. Reservoir debris can be viewed with a slit lamp using an optical cross section (Fig. 21.15). If debris accumulation is noted, but the patient is asymptomatic, then no course of action is necessary. However, there are a number of measures that can be taken to reduce the amount of accumulated debris if the patient is visually symptomatic. Instruct the patients that they may have to take their lens out to rinse and refill it one or more times during the day to maintain clear vision. Educating the patients in advance of this potential side effect is important because they might feel dissatisfied if this is an unexpected occurrence. Visser et al.[29] reported that up to 49% of scleral lens patients needed to take one or more of these breaks during the course of a day. The percent of patients increases to 67% for those patients who have keratitis sicca. If the patients are having difficulty with the number of breaks that they need to take over the course of the day, there are several strategies that may reduce the frequency of cloudy vision. First, consider reducing the vault because less fluid reservoir will mean less debris that the patient has to look through. Refitting the patient into a relatively smaller-diameter scleral design that has less fluid reservoir is another option. Having the patients fill their lens with a more viscous solution, such off-label use of Celluvisc, may increase the time for the debris to get behind the lens. Refitting the patient into a toric back-surface haptic or quadrant-specific back-surface haptic design can reduce the gaps between the lens and the sclera so that larger particles can pass through. Patients can be prescribed off-label ophthalmic prepared 10% Mucomyst (acetylcysteine, Bristol-Myers Squibb and generics) two times per day if they are accumulating significant mucus.[27]

Bubbles

Ideally, a scleral lens should hold a uniform liquid reservoir. Air bubbles commonly occur if the patient either inadequately fills the lens bowl with saline prior to application or if some of the saline spills out while the patient is attempting application. Bubbles can also be induced secondary to lens fenestrations. If bubbles are small (>2 mm) and outside of the visual axis, then no corrective actions are necessary. Larger bubbles (<2 mm) will actually prevent the lens from forming a semiseal, which will make wearing the lens uncomfortable. Any bubbles that

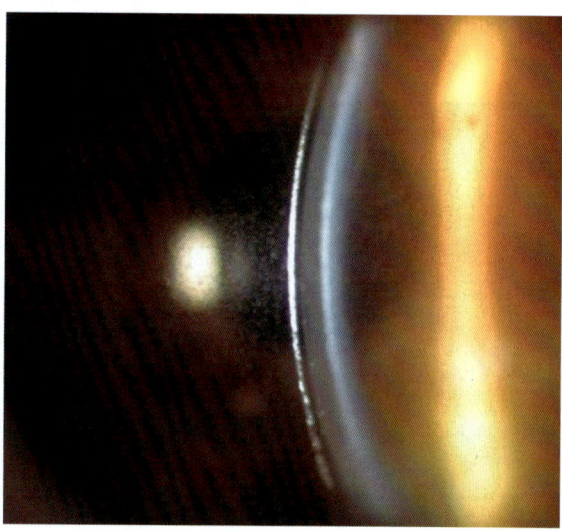

FIGURE 21.15 Reservoir debris viewed with an optical cross section.

are located in the central visual axis will significantly disrupt VA. Persistent bubbles can lead to epithelial desiccation. The only way to remedy a situation in which bubbles are affecting lens fit or VA is to remove and reapply the lens. Have the patients try filling the lens with off-label use of Celluvisc if they consistently lose saline when attempting application. The thicker viscosity of Celluvisc makes it more difficult to spill out. Consider refitting the patient with a nonfenestrated scleral design if a fenestrated design is producing bubbles that are proving to be problematic.

Solution Toxicity/Hypersensitivity

Patients wearing contact lenses can develop problems with lens-related solutions. It is critical that patients use nonpreserved saline solution to fill their scleral lens preapplication. Extended exposure to preservatives trapped underneath the lens can lead to significant epithelial toxicity. Bottled nonpreserved saline may contain buffers that can be toxic for certain patients. Therefore, prescribing off-label individual vials of 0.9% sodium chloride saline solution for preapplication lens filling is the safest alternative because it is preservative and buffer free. Also, the single-use vials reduce the risk of contamination that is inherent with using bottled nonpreserved saline over multiple days. Patients can also develop allergic reactions to cleaning and soaking solutions. Be aware that some of these hypersensitivities take time to develop. A patient may do well with a particular solution for months before sensitizing to it. Patients who develop a hypersensitivity to a solution will start to complain of irritation and redness with scleral lens wear. If an allergic reaction is suspected, then switch the patient to an approved hydrogen peroxide system to eliminate exposure to possible antigens.

Nonwetting

Like any contact lens, scleral lenses require a smooth and even prelens tear film for optimal optics. Scleral lenses that have a nonwettable surface (Fig. 21.16) will result in unacceptable vision. The type of material, laboratory error, and a patient's physiological chemistry can all contribute to poor scleral lens wetting. The best way to improve the wettability of a scleral contact lens is to have it plasma treated by the manufacturer. Occasionally, plasma treatment will need to be repeated 6 to 12 months after lens wear if there is a decrease in the wettability of the lens. This is often the case if the patient has severe OSD.

Lens Deposits

The accumulation of lens deposits can negatively affect vision and the comfort of a scleral contact lens. Depending on individual patient physiology, some patients are prone to significant lens deposition during the normal life of a GP scleral lens. For patients prone to deposits,

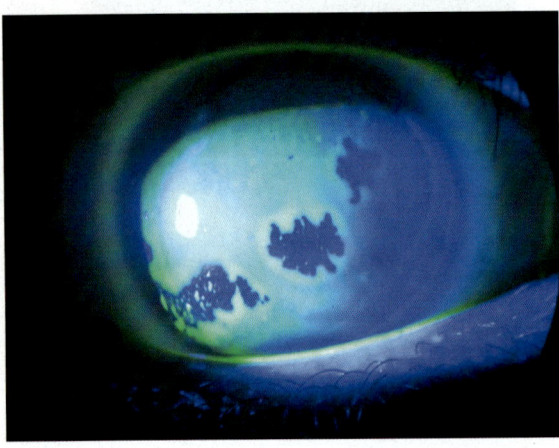

FIGURE 21.16 Nonwetting scleral lens.

prescribe an extra strength cleaner that they periodically use to keep their lens clean, such as Optimum Extra Strength RGP Cleaner (Lobob). For heavy depositors, you should recommend Progent (Menicon) one to two times per month to keep lenses free of deposits.

CONCLUSION

The use of scleral lenses in the management of corneal irregularity and OSD has expanded exponentially during the past decade. The unique fitting characteristics of the lenses eliminate the need to attempt to balance a corneal GP lens on a highly irregular corneal surface. The lack of corneal contact and continuous hydration provided by the postlens fluid reservoir is therapeutic for patients with severe OSD. Some reports have suggested that the ocular surface protection offered by scleral lenses may actually allow for resolution of some corneal conditions[11,30] such as LSCD. Additional applications for scleral lenses may yet be developed, including the possibility of using the lenses to maintain high concentrations of ocular medication at the surface of the eye.[31]

Despite the obvious clinical benefits of scleral lens therapy, we must recognize that we know very little of the potential risks of scleral lens wear. Wearing scleral lenses may create some mechanical challenges for the anterior segment. Long-term effects of conjunctival compression or impingement are possible. Interactions between lenses and irregularities in scleral tissue (such as the presence of tube shunts) deserve further study. The risks of potentially sight-threatening complications of scleral lens wear, namely, microbial keratitis, have yet to be defined. As the use of the devices becomes more widespread, clinical study of these and other issues should help to improve our understanding of the effects of scleral devices on ocular structures.

Regardless of these uncertainties, scleral lenses certainly represent a significant advance in our ability to manage corneal irregularity and severe OSD. Increasing awareness of the potential benefits of the devices, among both patients and eye care providers, will continue to drive demand for this therapy. Eye care providers should identify appropriate candidates for scleral lens wear, fit lenses according to established guidelines, and maintain careful follow-up to maximize visual and ocular benefits while minimizing risks of adverse events.

CLINICAL CASES

CASE 1

A 36-year-old male was referred for a contact lens fitting. He had a history of Marfan syndrome, which led to subluxed lenses in both eyes. The right eye lens was subluxed to an extent that he was functionally aphakic. He subsequently developed keratoconus in the right eye and was having difficulty tolerating his current corneal GP lens. His entering VA with his current lenses was 20/40 OD. Examination of the right eye revealed a subluxed lens. The right cornea had significant vertical striae and mild corneal staining. The right lens was apically touching the cornea, causing secondary erosions. Corneal topography confirmed keratoconus OD (Fig. 21.17).

SOLUTION: The patient was concerned about the progression of the keratoconus, and the idea of wearing a scleral lens that full vaulted the corneal surface was appealing. A scleral lens would also presumably provide better comfort and avoid the recurrent erosion issues. The patient was refit with the following: OD: MSD 4.20 Sag/+10.50/15.8 mm/standard curves/Boston XO.

This lens was dispensed and worn for a few weeks. He returned for a recheck reporting reasonable comfort and vision, but significant redness temporally and decreased comfort as the day progressed. His VA measured 20/40 OD. The fit of the lens demonstrated significant compression on the temporal conjunctiva with 3+ injection just outside of the landing zone. At the same time, the inferior region of the lens was fairly loose. Overrefraction demonstrated

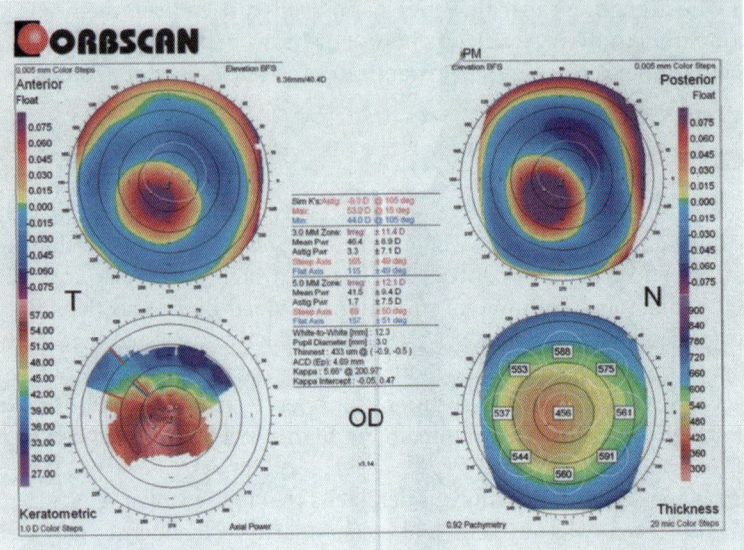

FIGURE 21.17 Orbscan confirming keratoconus with this patient.

uncorrected astigmatism, indicative of lens flexure. After reviewing other options, he was refit: OD: Jupiter 7.34 BC/+8.25/17.5 mm/reverse geometry design/3 D of toricity in the landing zone/Boston XO.

The new lens was dispensed and reevaluated 2 weeks later. The patient reported that his right eye was less red with the new lens and comfort was improved. The VA was 20/30−1. The temporal conjunctiva was minimally injected, with no significant compression. The inferior quadrant was still marginally loose, although tolerable. This lens was reordered with 5 D of landing zone toricity and dispensed. The patient is successfully wearing this lens.

CASE 2

A 62-year-old Caucasian female presented for scleral lens fitting for keratoconus. She had a significant atopic history, which had resulted in lid margin irregularity in both eyes (Fig. 21.18). Her atopic status, along with significant dry-eye disease, had made it impossible for her to wear contact lenses. Her best-corrected VA with spectacles was 20/200 OD and 20/40 OS.

Slit-lamp examination showed thickening of the lid margins, minimal conjunctival injection, and mild corneal scarring (OD > OS) (Fig. 21.19). Topography confirmed keratoconus of both eyes (Fig. 21.20). Cataracts were noted in both eyes upon dilated examination.

SOLUTION: The patient was initially fit with 18.2 mm Jupiter scleral lenses, through which she was able to achieve 20/70 OD and 20/30 OS. She was satisfied with VA, and she was able to wear the lenses comfortably for up to 14 hours daily.

One year later, she presented for follow-up evaluation. VA in the right eye had improved to 20/50, but had decreased to 20/50 OS. Slit-lamp examination showed decreased stromal opacity in the right eye compared to the initial visit (Fig. 21.21). In the left eye, progression

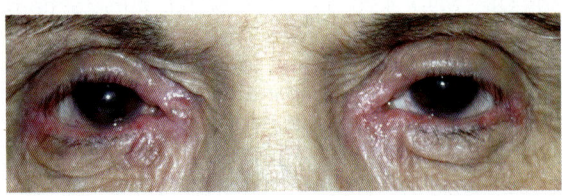

FIGURE 21.18 Lid margin irregularity resulting from patient's atopic history.

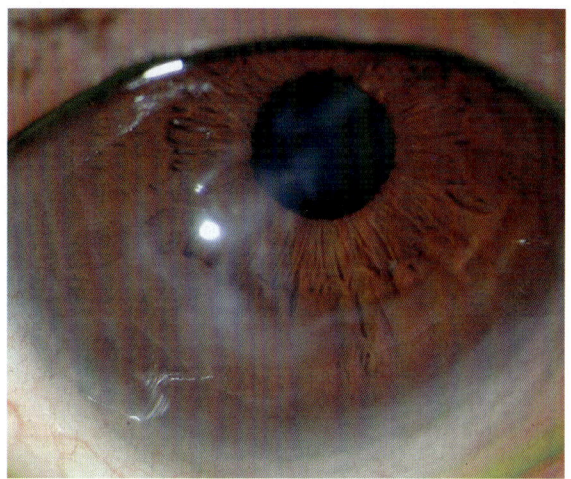

FIGURE 21.19 Corneal scarring resulting from keratoconus.

of the cataract was noted. She chose to pursue cataract surgery for her left eye. Following surgery, we refit her left eye with a new scleral lens, which gave her 20/30 vision.

Patients with keratoconus may have concurrent atopic disease, which can decrease their ability to tolerate corneal GP lenses. Scleral lenses offer a more comfortable alternative for these patients. Protection of the ocular surface with scleral lenses may actually facilitate some

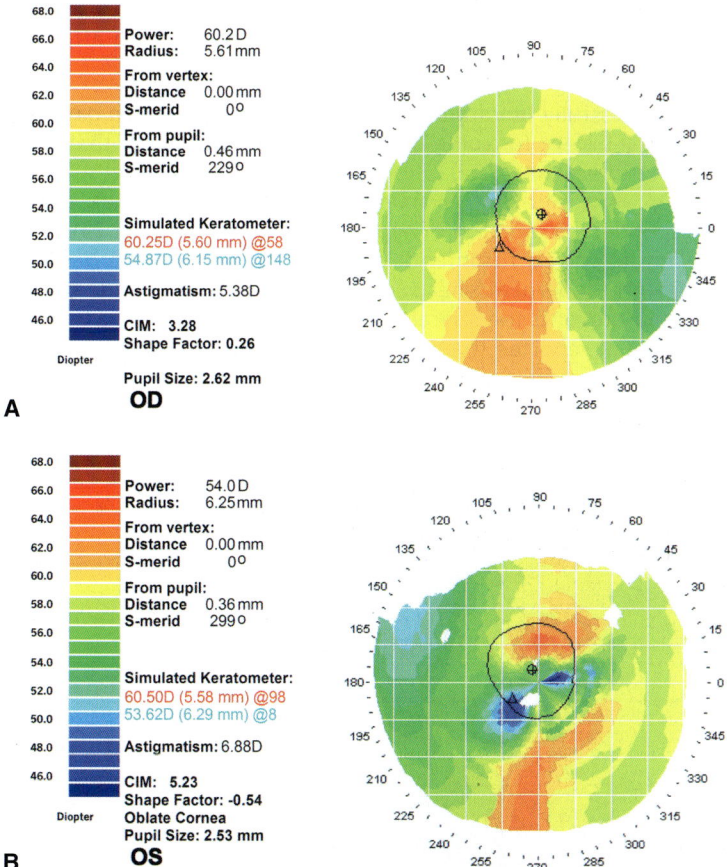

FIGURE 21.20 (A) Keratoconic topography map OD. (B) Keratoconic topography map OS.

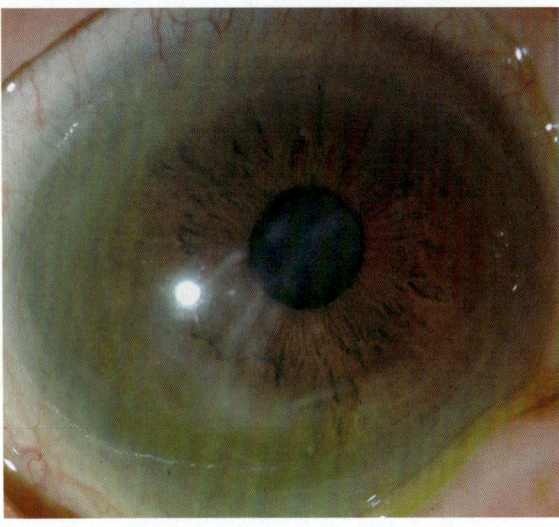

FIGURE 21.21 Reduction in stromal opacification 1 year after scleral lens fitting.

stromal remodeling. In this case, the stromal opacity of the right eye appeared to become less dense over the course of the patient's first year of scleral lens wear.

CASE 3

A 51-year-old patient developed corneal ectasia of her right eye after Laser-Assisted in Situ Keratomileusis (LASIK) surgery. She reported for specialty lens fitting after having failed in soft and hybrid contact lenses.

SOLUTION: She was successfully fit with a full Jupiter scleral lens, which gave her 20/40 vision. Overall, the lens fit well except for some mild superior corneal touch that was attributed to the lens dropping inferiorly (Fig. 21.22). The patient complained of lens-related irritation at subsequent follow-up visits. Slit-lamp examination of her right cornea showed some mild keratitis that corresponded to the area of superior lens touch (Fig. 21.23). As it can be difficult to modify the lens to correct for inferior decentration, the patient was fit with a silicone hydrogel lens to be worn underneath her scleral lens. The soft lens underneath of the scleral acts like a cushion and prevents the scleral lens from disrupting the epithelium. At the next follow-up visit, the patient reported that she had significantly improved comfort with the piggyback system. She was prescribed a daily disposable modality to simplify care regimen and maximize comfort with the soft lens.

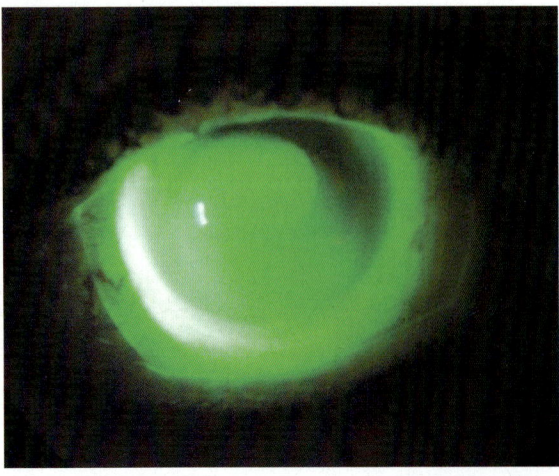

FIGURE 21.22 Scleral lens decenters slightly inferiorly resulting in mild superior-central touch.

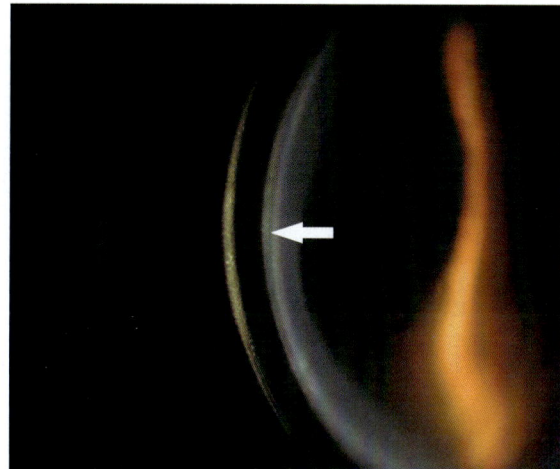

FIGURE 21.23 Arrow points to soft lens between the scleral lens and the cornea.

CASE 4

A 30-year-old male presented for a contact lens fitting. His ocular history was significant for keratoconus, and having had a corneal transplant OS in 2006 and OD in 2009. He typically had worn contact lenses, but over time they had become uncomfortable to wear and he had switched to using glasses.

His uncorrected vision was 20/100 OD and 20/200 OS. With his glasses, his vision was 20/40 OD and 20/30 OS. An updated refraction of +1.75 − 7.00 × 80 improved his right eye vision to 20/20, while the left eye corrected to 20/30 with +1.75 − 5.50 × 075. Examination revealed a thin and clear corneal graft in each eye. Orbscans indicated a high degree of regular against-the-rule astigmatism (Fig. 21.24).

SOLUTION: The patient was fit in SoClear corneoscleral lens OU. Parameters were:

OD: 7.34 BC/−1.87/14.5 mm diameter/standard periphery/Boston XO2 (Fig. 21.25A)

OS: 7.38 BC/−1.75/14.5 mm diameter/standard periphery/Boston XO2 (Fig. 21.25B)

The VA with the lenses was 20/20 OD and 20/25 OS. The fit was generally acceptable in both eyes and the patient reported good comfort. After monitoring the patient for 3 months, he was released to routine follow-up.

CASE 5

An 82-year-old patient developed corneal irregularity after a penetrating keratoplasty of her left eye. The patient was also being managed for glaucoma and previously had trabeculectomy surgery in her left eye for improved intraocular pressure (IOP) control. The trabeculectomy resulted in a superiorly located conjunctival bleb adjacent to the limbus. She was also being monitored for early dry macular degeneration. Her best-corrected spectacle acuity of her left eye was +6.50 − 8.00 × 120 20/300. Corneal topography was attempted, but her irregularity was so severe that a map was unobtainable. The patient was sent for a specialty lens evaluation for her left eye to see if she could achieve improved VA. A corneal GP design was considered but ruled out because of the potential interaction between the lens and the conjunctival bleb.

SOLUTION: Instead the patient was diagnostically fit with a mini-scleral lens that incorporated a beveled notch that would bypass the bleb. The lens parameters were as follows: BCR 47 D, Diameter 15 mm, Plano power, and 4-mm wide by 2-mm deep notch. The lens-to-cornea fitting relationship was assessed and an overrefraction was performed. The diagnostic lens had excessive vault, and the notch slightly impinged the edge of the conjunctival bleb and was deeper than needed. A lens was ordered with the following parameters: BCR 44 D, Diameter 15 mm,

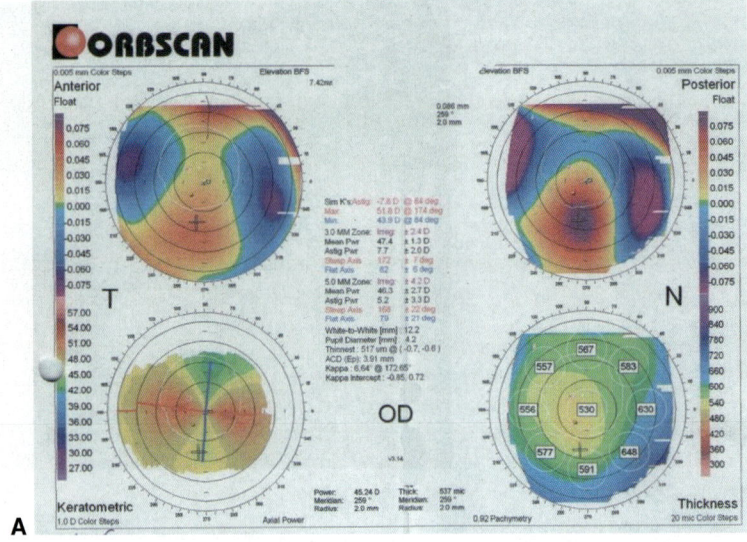

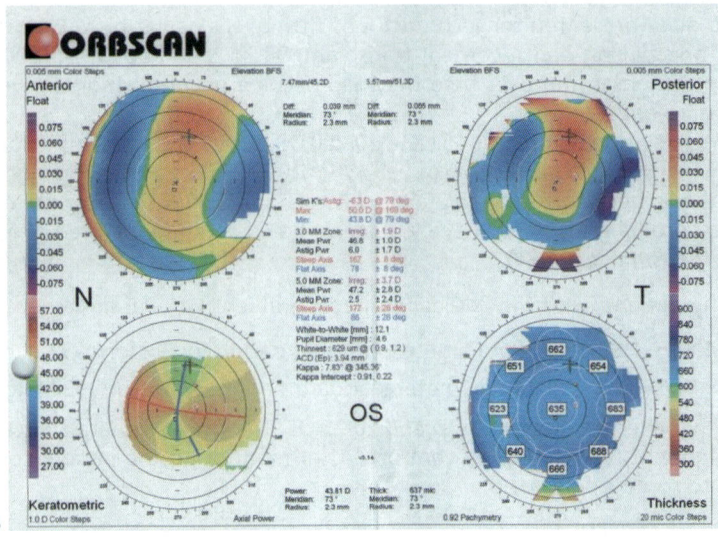

FIGURE 21.24 **(A)** Orbscan OD. **(B)** Orbscan OS.

Power +3.50 D, and the manufacturer was asked to widen the width of the notch and reduce its depth. At the dispensing visit, the patient was able to see 20/50 with the lens, which bypassed the bleb without impingement (Fig. 21.26). The patient was trained to put the lens in like a puzzle piece with the notch toward the conjunctival bleb. She had some difficulty with saline loss during application, which resulted in bubbles underneath the lens. The patient was switched from filling the lens with saline to off-label use of Celluvisc. The increased viscosity of the Celluvisc resulted in her spilling less solution during application so that she was able to apply the lens successfully without significant bubbles in the reservoir. A final overrefraction was plano. Subsequent follow-up visits have not shown evidence of lens-related mechanical injury to the conjunctival bleb.

CASE 6

A 78-year-old male presented for an evaluation with a history of radial keratotomy (RK) OU in 1987, with subsequent photorefractive keratectomy (PRK) and astigmatic keratectomy (AK) in the right eye in 2003, LASIK OU in 2007, cataract and intraocular lens implant surgery OU in

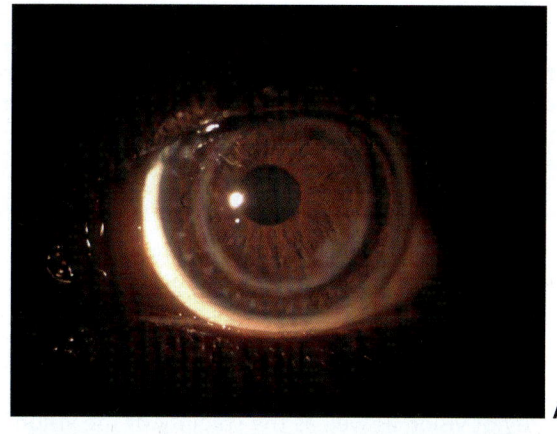

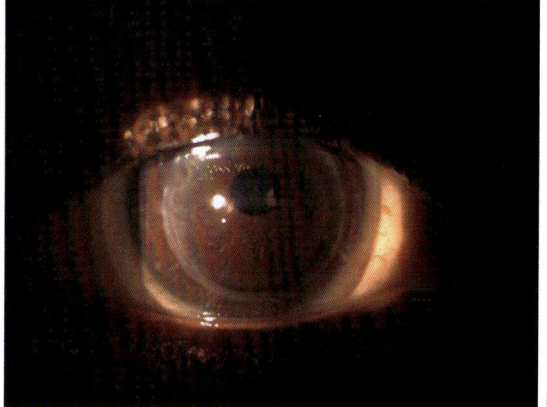

FIGURE 21.25 (A) Corneoscleral lens OD. **(B)** Corneoscleral lens OS.

2008, and corneal cross-linking OU in 2009. He commented that his vision early in the morning was good, but by late morning his vision would deteriorate and stay blurry the remainder of the day. He had no ocular symptoms other than his vision, and had worn contact lenses many years ago, prior to having RK.

His entering acuity without correction was 20/60 OD and 20/40 OS at 4:15 pm. He did note that he felt that his vision was blurry, as was typical of the afternoon, and that he recalled his

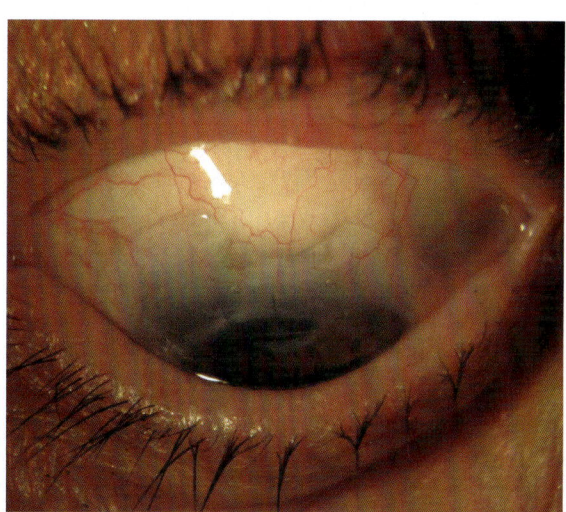

FIGURE 21.26 Scleral lens with beveled notch bypassing the patient's conjunctival bleb.

vision being measured at 20/25 at early morning appointments in the recent past. His pupils were small in each eye, measuring 2 mm. All other entrance testing was normal. A refraction of +0.50 − 2.50 × 180 improved his vision in the right eye to 20/25, while the left eye had no measured refractive error. Slit-lamp examination revealed RK and AK scars on each eye. Intraocular inplants were clear and well-centered OU. Orbscans were performed on each eye, demonstrating a typical postsurgical oblate pattern (Fig. 21.27).

SOLUTION: A scleral lens fitting was undertaken, with final parameters of:

OD: MSD 18.0 mm, 4.60 Sag, increased vault, −7.00 D, standard edge

OS: MSD 18.0 mm, 4.40 Sag, increased vault, −5.00 D, standard edge (Fig. 21.28).

His VA with each eye individually was 20/20 OD and was 20/15 OS. The patient was thrilled with the vision and comfort of the lenses, and was very adept at application and removal. He wears the lenses daily from late morning until late evening. He is extremely happy with the clarity of vision as well as the stability of the vision from morning to evening.

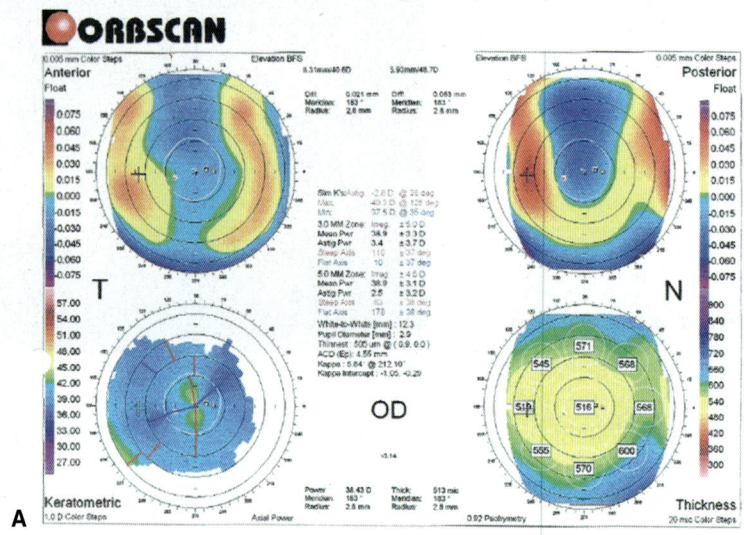

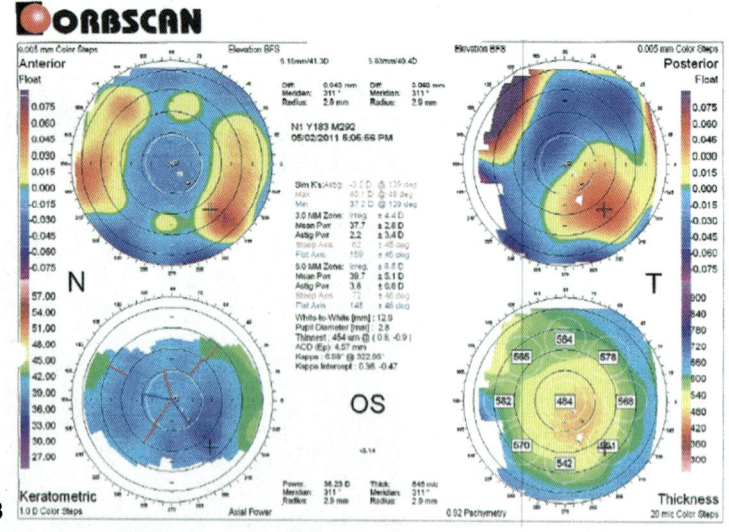

FIGURE 21.27 (A) Orbscan OD. (B) Orbscan OS.

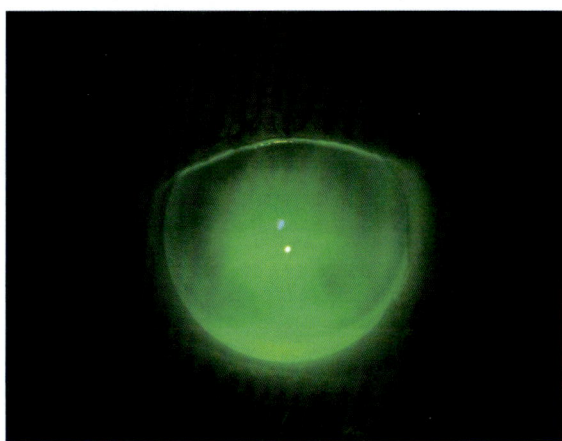

FIGURE 21.28 Fluorescein pattern of scleral contact lens.

CASE 7

A 37-year-old male was referred for a contact lens fitting by his corneal specialist. He had seen several eye care providers for symptoms of photophobia, blurry vision, and chronic irritation. The corneal specialist had diagnosed him with a corneal degeneration, although at this time the specific diagnosis was undetermined. Prior to any surgical intervention, it was recommended that he consider scleral lenses.

At examination, his uncorrected VA was 20/60 OD and OS. Refraction did not improve his vision. Slit-lamp examination revealed 2+ conjunctival injection and 2 to 3+ whorl-like corneal staining (Fig. 21.29). The palpebral conjunctiva were 2+ injected OU, but all other internal and external findings were unremarkable.

SOLUTION: Due to the patient's sensitivity and tight apertures, a relatively smaller scleral lens diameter was chosen. The patient was fit in Jupiter scleral lenses OU, parameters:

OD: 46.00 BCR/−1.75 D/15.6 mm diameter/standard peripheral curves/Boston XO

OS: 46.00 BCR/−2.00 D/15.6 mm diameter/standard peripheral curves/Boston XO

The lens fit provided full corneal vaulting and good centration (Fig. 21.30). The VA with the lenses was 20/20 in each eye. The patient still reported a degree of photosensitivity, but the feeling of irritation was alleviated and he was generally pleased with the comfort and thrilled with his vision. He continues to wear the lenses full time.

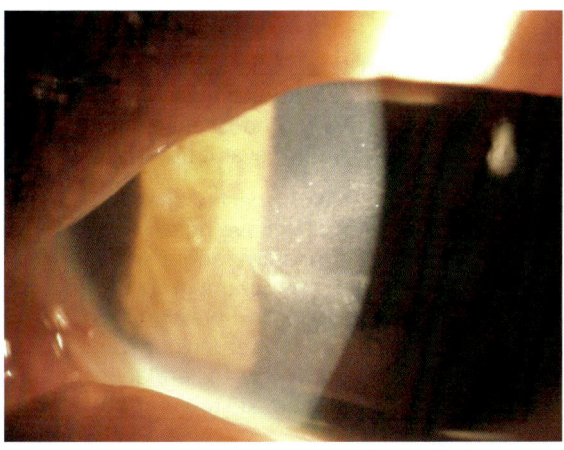

FIGURE 21.29 Corneal stain.

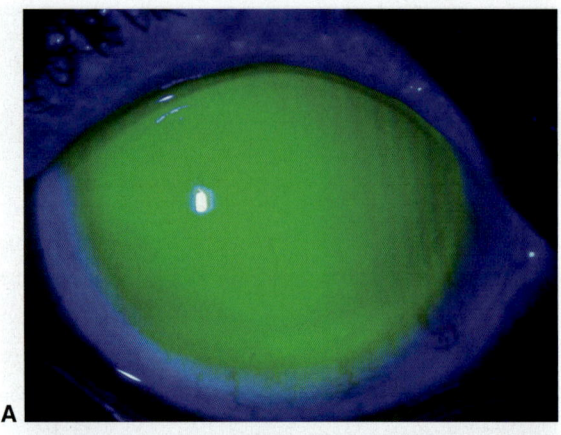

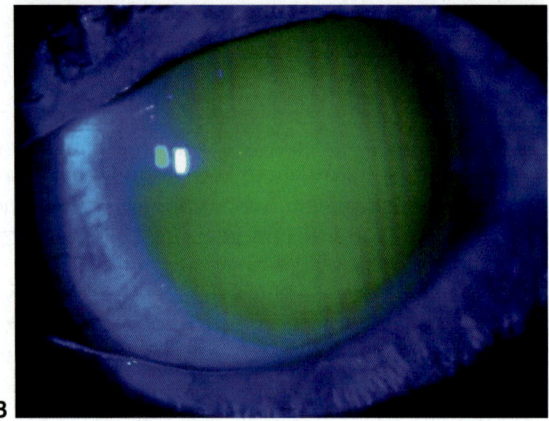

FIGURE 21.30 **(A)** Scleral lens OD. **(B)** Scleral lens OS.

CASE 8

A 56-year-old Caucasian male was referred to our corneal service for management of a nonhealing epithelial defect of his left eye. He had suffered from recurrent iritis in the left eye for approximately 20 years. Long-term steroid use may have contributed to cataract development and elevated IOP in that eye. He had undergone cataract extraction, without intraocular lens implantation, 2 years prior to his appointment. Following cataract surgery, he wore an aphakic soft lens for 1 year until a corneal ulcer of indeterminate etiology forced him to discontinue contact lens wear. He was left with a dense corneal scar and a persistent epithelial defect. His local eye care provider had attempted to treat the defect with a hydrogel bandage lens without success.

His VA at presentation was 1/200 in the left eye. Slit-lamp evaluation revealed a 1.2 × 3.4 mm inferior epithelial defect with mild underlying stromal infiltrate (Fig. 21.31). Diffuse central scarring was also present. Endothelial pigmentation without active keratic precipitates (KP) was noted. Anterior chamber evaluation showed trace cell with no flare.

SOLUTION: A corneal specialist suspected that the epithelial defect was neurotrophic in nature, and that the condition may have been related to HSV keratouveitis. He recommended aggressive therapy, punctal occlusion, aggressive lubrication, scleral lens wear, lateral tarsorrhaphy, and possible amniotic membrane graft or conjunctival flap. Punctal plugs were placed at the initial visit, and a scleral lens fit was initiated.

He was fit with an 18.2 mm Jupiter lens of standard design and +9.75 D, which gave him 20/150. Within 1 month of initiation of scleral lens therapy, the epithelial defect had resolved completely (Fig. 21.32). VA remained stable at 20/150 throughout the patient's follow-up at our clinic.

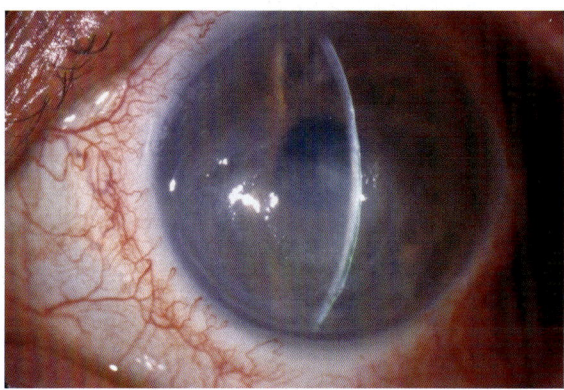

FIGURE 21.31 Persistent epithelial defect.

CASE 9

A 36-year-old Asian male presented for evaluation of eye irritation, redness, photophobia, and blurred vision of approximately 1-year duration. Symptoms had waxed and waned during that time, but his overall eye condition seemed to be worsening. Prior to the onset of his symptoms, he had worn hydrogel lenses for the correction of high myopia. He had been treated with lubricant drops, topical steroids, topical cyclosporine, punctal occlusion, and oral doxycycline without improvement in his symptoms.

At the time of presentation, his VA with glasses was 20/200 OD and 20/70 OS. Moderate–severe conjunctival injection was noted in both eyes. Whorl-like, layered corneal epithelial opacities were present in both eyes (Fig. 21.33). The patient was diagnosed with LSCD OU.

SOLUTION: He was fit with custom 18.2 mm Jupiter lenses. Within days of initiation of scleral lens wear, conjunctival injection and corneal irregularity had improved markedly. As his chemosis resolved, the scleral lens fit was adjusted to provide improved haptic alignment. Two weeks after beginning scleral lens therapy, his vision had improved to 20/40 OD and 20/25 OS (Fig. 21.34).

Nine months after scleral lens fitting, the patient reported that his eyes had remained comfortable with daily lens wear. VA with his scleral lenses was 20/25 OD and 20/20 OS. No active epitheliopathy was noted, but corneal scarring remained (Fig. 21.35). He stated that he wished to discontinue scleral lens wear, and return to spectacles. With the understanding that he would return for further evaluation immediately if symptoms recurred, he was allowed to suspend scleral lens therapy. The patient was given an updated spectacle prescription.

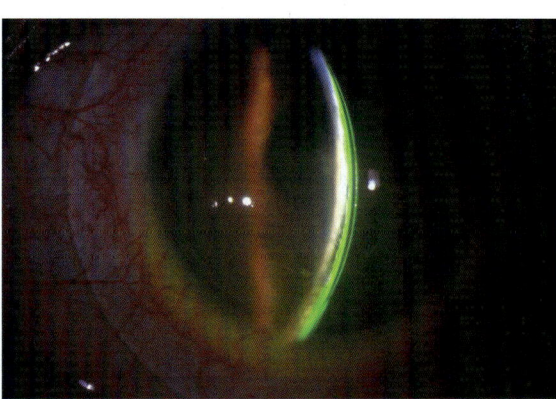

FIGURE 21.32 Resolution of defect.

642 Section IV • Challenging Cases

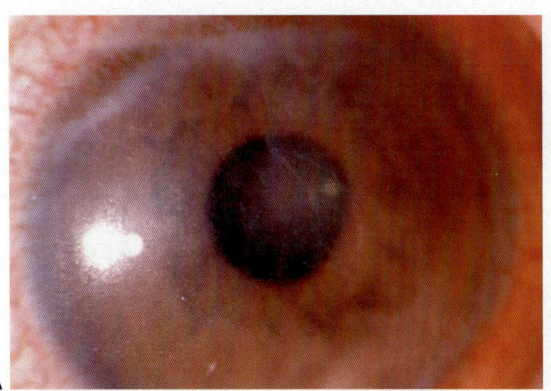

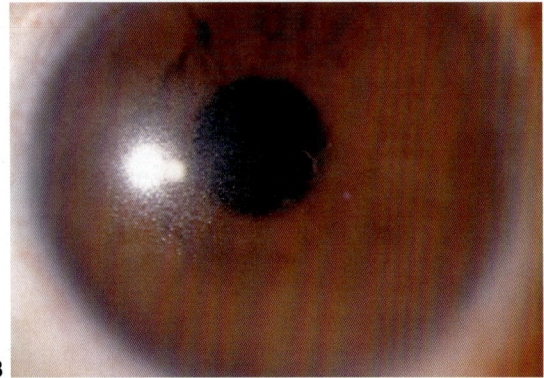

FIGURE 21.33 (A) Corneal epithelial opacities OD. **(B)** Corneal epithelial opacities OS.

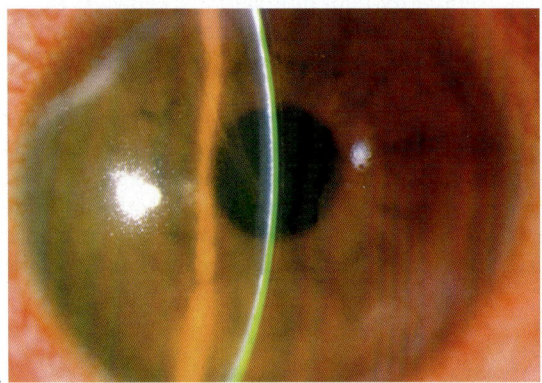

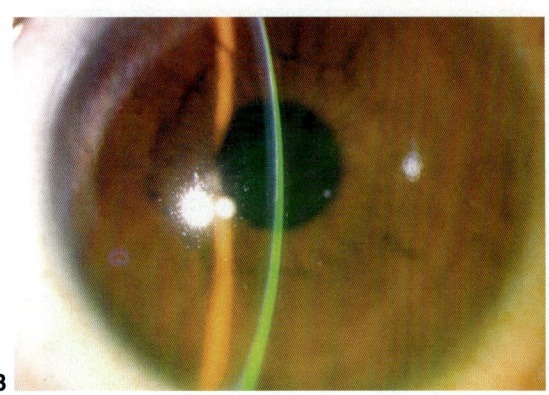

FIGURE 21.34 (A) Scleral lens OD. **(B)** Scleral lens OS.

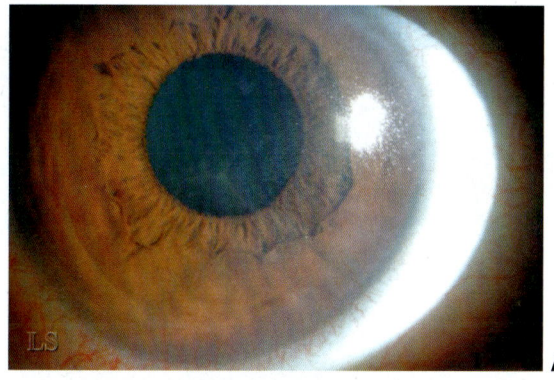
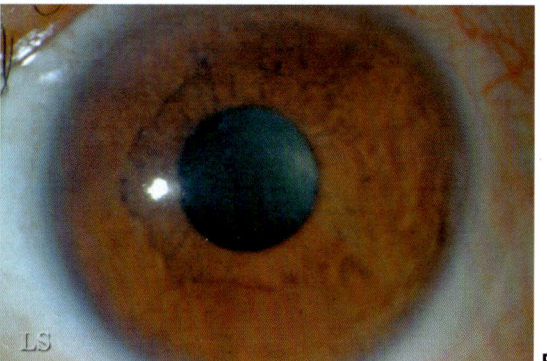

FIGURE 21.35 **(A)** Corneal scarring OD. **(B)** Corneal scarring OS.

At an 18-month follow-up visit, he noted mild irritation in both eyes. Examination revealed very mild peripheral epitheliopathy. He resumed scleral lens wear for a period of 3 to 4 weeks, during which time his symptoms and clinical appearance normalized. He once again discontinued scleral lens wear upon resolution of his symptoms.

LSCD may actually represent dysfunction, rather than destruction of the limbal stem cells. Temporary protection of the limbal area may allow for recovery of limbal stem cell function.

CASE 10

A 35-year-old Caucasian male was evaluated for severe OSD associated with chronic graft versus host disease. He had undergone stem cell transplantation for acute lymphoblastic leukemia 2 years earlier. Within 3 to 4 months of the transplant, he noted ocular dryness and irritation. Those symptoms had worsened considerably since onset. Traditional management (nonpreserved lubricant drops q 15 minutes, topical cyclosporine, topical steroids, punctal occlusion, moisture chamber glasses) had not provided any significant relief.

VA at his initial examination was 20/20 in each eye without correction. Slit-lamp evaluation showed moderate–severe punctate epitheliopathy over the entire cornea, significant lissamine green staining of exposed cornea and bulbar conjunctiva, and mild filamentary keratitis in both eyes.

SOLUTION: He was fit with custom 19.6 mm Jupiter lenses (Fig. 21.36). The scleral lenses provided some conjunctival protection in addition to complete corneal coverage. VA remained 20/20 with the lenses. The patient continued to use nonpreserved lubricant drops over the lenses regularly and occasionally wore moisture chamber goggles in addition to the lenses if he was in a particularly dry, windy, or dusty environment. The addition of scleral lenses to his management strategy for severe dry-eye disease allowed him to resume many of the activities that he had abandoned at the onset of his symptoms.

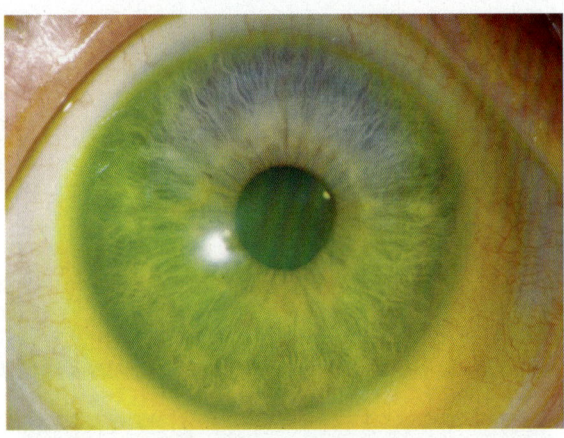

FIGURE 21.36 Scleral contact lens OD.

He continued to wear scleral lenses full time for approximately 4 years. During that time, advances in systemic management of his chronic graft-versus-host disease (cGVHD) improved his overall health. He discovered that he no longer needed the lenses to maintain adequate ocular comfort in anything but the driest environments.

Scleral lens therapy for OSD is frequently additive to a patient's current therapy; patients may still need to continue with other forms of intervention in order to maintain adequate comfort. Scleral lenses allow for healing of the ocular surface in patients with severe dry-eye syndrome, but may not be necessary on a full-time basis once surface integrity has been restored. Advances in systemic treatment for conditions that cause OSD may provide significant relief for dry-eye patients.

CASE 11

A 59-year-old female with a history of dry eyes and ocular allergies had been referred for specialty contact lens fitting. Her history was significant for "hard lens" use many years ago and a "facelift" 3 years prior to her visit. She was using lubricating eye drops as needed and had been started on Restasis at her previous examination. She reported wearing her eyeglasses for driving, but otherwise did not use corrective lenses much, as she could not see at near very well with them.

Her entering VA without correction was 20/70 OD and 20/150 OS. Her near vision without correction was 20/40 OD and 20/30 OS. Keratometry was 43.00/45.50 OU. Her refraction was $+1.50 - 2.75 \times 120$ 20/25 and $-2.50 - 2.50 \times 045$ 20/20. Slit-lamp examination revealed corneal staining in both eyes (Fig. 21.37). The patient was assessed to have myopia, astigmatism, presbyopia, and dry eye with secondary keratitis.

SOLUTION: The patient was fit in the following lenses to manage her refractive error, presbyopia, and dry eye. She was fit with: OD: Digiform Scleral Lens (Truform) N Series 7.65 BCR/ -1.62 D/15.0 mm diameter/standard peripheral curves/$+2.25$ D add/2.0 mm near add zone/ Boston XO.

OS: Digiform Scleral Lens (Truform) N Series 7.65 BCR/-3.00 D/15.0 mm diameter/standard peripheral curves/$+2.25$ D add/2.0 mm near add zone/Boston XO (Fig. 21.38). The lenses were dispensed and she reported good comfort and vision. Her distance VA was 20/20 OD and 20/20 OS. Her near vision was 20/25 in each eye. The patient was thrilled at the improvement in her distance vision versus no correction, while maintaining her ability to read. She managed to apply and remove the lenses successfully. At follow-up, she reported being able to wear the lenses most of the day with good vision and comfort. Her corneal staining, while not resolved completely, was improved versus her prefitting condition. She was happy with the results and was scheduled for follow-up in 6 months.

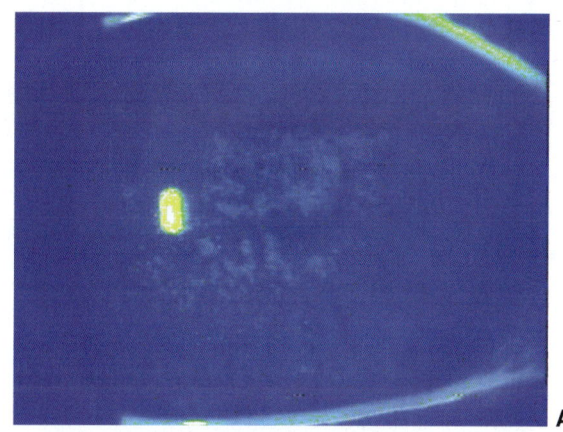
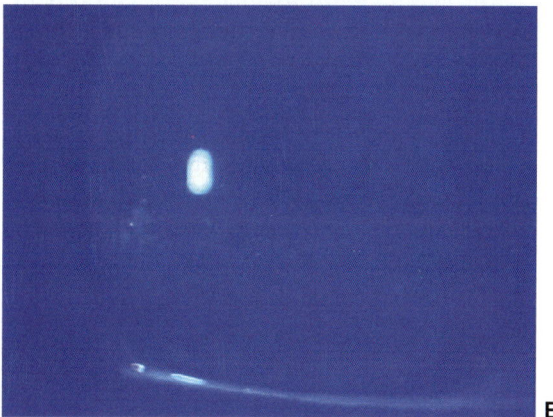

FIGURE 21.37 (A) Corneal stain OD. **(B)** Corneal stain OS.

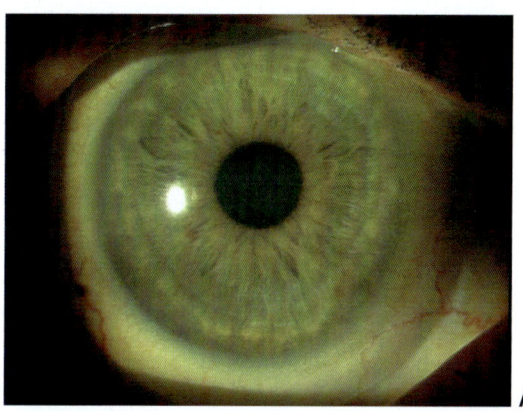
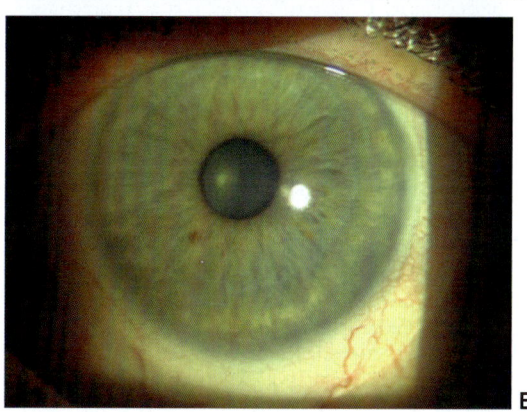

FIGURE 21.38 (A) Multifocal scleral lens OD. **(B)** Multifocal scleral lens OS.

CLINICAL PROFICIENCY CHECKLIST

- Candidates for scleral contact lenses include patients who have corneal irregularity, OSD, or high refractive error.
- Diagnostic lenses are necessary for accurate assessment of fit and determination of lens power.
- Corneal topography is useful for choosing lens diameter and design.
- Assess the diagnostic lenses from the inside out; corneal, limbal, and haptic zones.
- After allowing the lens to settle, the best diagnostic lens should vault the cornea between 100 and 300 microns.
- The lens haptic of the diagnostic lens should rest evenly on the sclera conjunctiva without excessive blanching or edge lift.
- Photographs of the best diagnostic lens are helpful for laboratory consultation and evaluation.
- The appointment for scleral lens dispense should include extra time for training the patient on techniques for application and removal.
- Prescribe single-use vials of 0.9% sodium chloride for preapplication lens filling to avoid allergic or toxic reactions to preserved solutions.
- Periodically monitor the patient for lens deposits, fit changes, and secondary lens-related complications.

REFERENCES

1. Key JE. Development of contact lenses and their worldwide use. *Eye Contact Lens.* 2007;33(6, pt 2):343–345.
2. Pearson RM. Karl Otto Himmler, manufacturer of the first contact lens. *Cont Lens Anterior Eye.* 2007;30(1):11–16.
3. Pullum KW, Buckley RJ. A study of 530 patients referred for rigid gas permeable scleral contact lens assessment. *Cornea.* 1997;16(6):612–622.
4. Cotter JM, Rosenthal P. Scleral contact lenses. *J Am Optom Assoc.* 1998;69(1):33–40.
5. Dalton K, Sorbara L. Fitting an MSD (mini scleral design) rigid contact lens in advanced keratoconus with INTACS. *Cont Lens Anterior Eye.* 2011;34(6):274–281.
6. Steele C, Davidson J. Contact lens fitting post laser-in situ keratomileusis (LASIK). *Cont Lens Anterior Eye.* 2007;30(2):84–93.
7. Jacobs DS, Rosenthal P. Boston scleral lens prosthetic device treatment of severe dry eye in chronic graft-versus-host disease. *Cornea.* 2007;26(10):1195–1199.
8. Schornack MM, Baratz KH, Patel SV, et al. Jupiter scleral lenses in the management of chronic graft versus host disease. *Eye Contact Lens.* 2008;34(6):302–305.
9. Rosenthal P, Cotter J, Baum J. Treatment of persistent corneal epithelial defects with extended wear of a fluid-ventilated gas-permeable scleral contact lens. *Am J Ophthalmol.* 2000;130(1):33–41.
10. Romero-Rangel T, Stavrou P, Cotter J, et al. Gas-permeable scleral contact lens therapy in ocular surface disease. *Am J Ophthalmol.* 2000;130(1):25–32.
11. Schornack MM. Limbal stem cell disease: management with scleral lenses. *Clin Exp Optom.* 2011;94(6):592–594.
12. Schornack MM. Ocular cicatricial pemphigoid: the role of scleral lenses in disease management. *Cornea.* 2009;28(10):1170–1172.
13. Tappin MJ, Pullum K, Buckley RJ. Scleral contact lenses for overnight wear in the management of ocular surface disorders. *Eye (Lond).* 2001;(15, pt 2):168–172.
14. Shah-Desai SD, Aslam SD, Pullum K, et al. Scleral contact lens usage in patients with complex blepharoptosis. *Ophthal Plast Reconstr Surg.* 2011;27(2):95–98.
15. Salam A, Singh AJ, Innes JR, et al. A novel temporary treatment remedy for blepharospasm. *Eye.* 2004;18:324–325.
16. Rathi VM, Mandathara PS, Vaddavalli PK, et al. Fluid filled scleral contact lens in pediatric patients: challenges and outcomes. *Cont Lens Anterior Eye.* 2012;35(4):189–192.
17. Hussoin T, Carrasquillo K, Johns L, et al. The effect of scleral lens optical asphericity on vision in patients with corneal ectasia. Presented at: 26th Biennial Cornea Research Conference; October 2009; Boston, MA.
18. van der Worp E, Graf T, Caroline P. Exploring beyond the corneal borders. *Contact Lens Spectrum.* 2010;25(6):26–31.
19. Visser ES, Visser R, Van Lier HJ. Advantages of toric scleral lenses. *Optom Vis Sci.* 2006;83(4):233–236.

20. Pullum K, Stapleton FJ. Scleral lens induced corneal swelling: what is the effect of varying Dk and lens thickness? *CLAO J.* 1997;23(4):259–263.
21. Schein OD, Rosenthal P, Ducharme C. A gas-permeable scleral contact lens for visual rehabilitation. *Am J Ophthalmol.* 1990;109(3):318–322.
22. Rosenthal P, Croteau A. Fluid-ventilated, gas-permeable scleral contact lens is an effective option for managing severe ocular surface disease and many corneal disorders that would otherwise require penetrating keratoplasty. *Eye Contact Lens.* 2005;31(3):130–134.
23. Pullum KW, Whiting MA, Buckley R. Scleral contact lenses: the expanding role. *Cornea.* 2005;24(3):269–277.
24. Jacobs DS. Update on scleral lenses. *Curr Opin Ophthalmol.* 2008;19(4):298–301.
25. Schornack MM, Patel SV. Relationship between corneal topographic indices and scleral lens base curve. *Eye Contact Lens.* 2010;36(6):330–333.
26. Ibrahim O, Bogan S, Waring GO. Patterns of corneal topography after penetrating keratoplasty. *Eur J Ophthalmol.* 1996;6(1):1–5.
27. van der Worp E. A guide to scleral lens fitting [monograph online]. Scleral Lens Education Society; 2010. Available from: http://commons.pacificu.edu/mono/4/
28. DeNaeyer GW. Decreasing the impact of scleral lens debris. *Contact Lens Spectrum.* 2011;26(3):18.
29. Visser ES, Visser R, van Lier HJ, et al. Modern scleral lenses: part II, patient satisfaction. *Eye Contact Lens.* 2007;33(1):21–25.
30. Cressey A, Jacobs DS, Carrasquillo KG. Management of vascularized limbal keratitis with prosthetic replacement of the ocular surface system. *Eye Contact Lens.* 2012;38(2):137–140.
31. Keating AM, Jacobs DS. Anti-VEGF treatment of corneal neovascularization. *Ocul Surf.* 2011;9(4):227–237.

Chapter 22

Orthokeratology

Marjorie Rah, John Mark Jackson, Beth Kinoshita, Matthew Lampa, Edward S. Bennett, and Cary M. Herzberg

Orthokeratology (OK) is a temporary correction of myopia and astigmatism using specially designed, typically rigid gas-permeable (GP) contact lenses to flatten the central cornea (or in the case of hyperopia, steepen the central cornea). The effect is similar to that from myopic refractive surgery: by flattening the central cornea, the refractive power of the eye is reduced, which makes the refractive error less myopic. This procedure has also been known by a variety of terms, such as orthofocus, corneal reshaping, precision corneal molding, controlled keratoreformation, corneal refractive therapy, and vision shaping treatment, among others. With the recent advancements in designs, instrumentation, and overnight applications, OK is increasing in popularity—especially with young people—and represents 28% of all contact lenses prescribed to minors internationally.[1] Contact lens wear and young people will be addressed in greater detail in Chapter 19.

ORTHOKERATOLOGY TECHNIQUES

Early Orthokeratology Techniques

Early concept of OK has its origins from the days of polymethylmethacrylate (PMMA) corneal contact lenses. Because this lens material did not allow oxygen to pass through, clinicians often made their lenses flatter than the central cornea to allow more tear exchange under the lens, thereby increasing the available oxygen to the cornea. Clinicians observed that this caused a flattening of the central corneal tissue and, usually, "spectacle blur" was the result. Patients noted that their vision was blurred when looking through their habitual glasses for a period of time directly following removal of their contact lenses. Some patients with low myopia reported they saw quite well without any correction at all for some time after lens removal.

The first literature reports of this effect were published in the 1950s.[2–4] In 1962, George Jessen[5] published a paper on what he called "orthofocus." This was the first report of a deliberate attempt to mold the cornea to reduce myopia. Jessen later called the technique "orthokeratology." Jessen's method was to use a standard PMMA lens that was flatter than the cornea by the amount of refractive error. If successful, this would flatten the central cornea enough to eliminate the myopic refractive error. The lens itself had plano power, as the posterior lacrimal lens created by the flat-fitting contact lens provided all the visual correction. Unfortunately, lenses fitted this flat were unstable and very uncomfortable and likely would decenter, creating unpredictable topographical changes and sometimes induce irregular astigmatism.

Although there were other techniques advocated in the early years of OK, the technique of Grant and May was the most utilized by clinicians.[6] Their method was to use a series of gradually flatter large-diameter lenses, starting at about 0.12 to 0.50 D flatter than the flat keratometric value. As the cornea flattened, subsequent flatter lenses were used until the myopia was reduced to the desired level. This process could take many months.

Proponents of OK published many reports of success, but controlled studies using conventional lens designs were not published until the mid-1970s and early 1980s.[7–12] These studies varied in their design and results, but they all reached very similar conclusions: they found that (a) in general, OK was as safe as standard contact lens fits with the PMMA material; (b) reduction in myopia was about 1.00 D on average, although significantly higher amounts were reported; (c) flat-fitting lenses may cause induced with-the-rule and irregular astigmatism; (d) no patient characteristics were found that allowed for prediction of success; (e) improvement in unaided visual acuity (VA) did not necessarily match the amount of corneal flattening or the amount of myopia reduced; and (f) the changes were not permanent and required wear of the lenses for some portion of each day to maintain the effect. After these studies were published, OK was mostly rejected by the eye care community.[13–15] Interest in the procedure did not evaporate completely, and only a few proponents continued to advocate and refine the fitting techniques over the following years.

Modern Orthokeratology

Recent Advances

A major advance in lens design and lens lathing capabilities resulted in a resurgence of interest in OK by practitioners. In contrast to early OK using conventional rigid lens designs, the modern procedure uses an entirely different lens design known as reverse geometry (RG). Conventional rigid lenses have a steeper central base curve radius (BCR) and flatten from center to periphery. When these lenses are fit flat for OK, there is nothing to prevent the lens from decentering as there is no peripheral area of lens-to-cornea alignment. In contrast, RG lenses are designed with a flatter central BCR and a steeper secondary curve radius (reverse curve) to connect with a flatter peripheral curve radius (alignment curve). This allows for alignment with the peripheral cornea and enhanced centration and stability of the lens, even with a very flat central BCR. On average, RG lens designs produce much faster results and can treat greater amounts of myopia.

Although the first use of RG lenses was reported in 1972,[16] manufacturing technology at the time made them difficult to produce. Improvements in the RG design and the introduction of computer-driven lathes in the early 1990s led to more sophisticated designs.[17,18] The improvement in treatment with the new designs was remarkable enough to lead to the term *accelerated orthokeratology* to denote the use of these lenses and to differentiate it from the original OK procedures where multiple successively flatter BCR lenses were required. Results were achieved within weeks rather than months, as with the old procedure. There are now numerous contact lens laboratories that manufacture RG lenses and clinicians now have far more lens options for OK (see section on lens designs).

The use of corneal topography also differentiates modern practice from old. Corneal topography is essential for OK treatment and management because of the much greater area of the cornea measured versus a keratometer. Topography allows for more accurate prediction of treatment success, improved lens design selection, and better monitoring of posttreatment effects. Although some RG OK lenses could be fit without the use of a corneal topographer, it would be very difficult to monitor progress of treatment and for problem solving when the treatment is not optimal.

Another contribution to the resurgence of OK is the advancement in rigid lens materials, specifically the increase in oxygen permeability (Dk), allowing for overnight wear of the modality. The use of the OK lens in the closed-eye state has added to the comfort and convenience of this procedure. The lens is applied before bedtime and removed in the morning. When optimal results are achieved, the patient has stable and good vision during all waking hours. Overnight wear of any contact lens can increase the risk of complications, and patients must be monitored carefully for any signs of problems related to lens wear.

Recent research supports the clinical observations that RG lenses lead to faster results and higher potential corrections than standard lens designs, particularly with overnight wear.[19–23]

In general, these studies show an average treatment of about −2.50 D, with corrections of up to about −4.00 D possible with refractive stabilization occurring, on average, after only 10 days of initiating treatment.[24] In addition, it has been found that significant central corneal flattening and improvement in unaided VA can occur after just 10 minutes of lens wear.[25]

Mechanism

There are numerous theories to account for the mechanism and outcomes of OK. It is apparent, however, that OK-induced changes in anterior corneal topography are achieved through central corneal thinning and midperipheral thickening.[26,27] Studies of structural changes in the cornea that result from RG lens wear showed that the epithelial changes were the largest contributor to the central flattening and midperipheral steepening of the cornea.[26] Some studies suggest stromal thickening may also play a role, but is most likely not the primary reason for topographic changes, especially initially, in the cornea.[28,29] The theories behind how corneal shape changes occur involve fluid forces of the tear film, lid pressure in the closed-eye environment, and surface tension of the tear film at the lens edge.[30] The forces act by both compression and tension at different sites across the corneal surface. The stress created by these forces moves the corneal epithelium. The epithelial layers in the midperiphery are decreased in height and widen laterally, and the movement of corneal epithelium is consistent with the conservation of corneal power, whereby corneal power is able to be redistributed, but not created or destroyed.[30] Cellular volume and surface area are also maintained throughout treatment.[31]

BENEFITS OF ORTHOKERATOLOGY

There are many benefits to overnight orthokeratology (OOK), foremost among them pertaining to the improvement in unaided VA and little to no reliance on spectacles for qualified candidates. This is especially important for young people, especially athletes. It has been found that OK results in a high level of patient satisfaction,[32] results in increased quality of life versus spectacle wear,[33] and is favored versus soft lens wearers as it pertains to concerns about their vision.[34] In addition, when compared to aided vision with disposable soft lenses, unaided high and low contrast VA, via OK, was found to be equivalent.[35] For qualified individuals who either are not eligible—or have no desire—for invasive refractive surgery, OK represents a viable alternative.

However, what is most significant, and has enormous future implications as discussed in Chapter 19, is the effect of OK on eye growth. Several studies have concluded that OOK significantly slows down or retards axial length growth,[33,36,37] which has very important quality-of-life implications.

PATIENT EXPECTATIONS AND SELECTION

OOK is not for every patient. It is important that the practitioner carefully screens potential candidates for this procedure. Although it is not possible to predict success completely, selecting patients carefully and establishing realistic goals will help to eliminate frustration for both the patient and the practitioner. Establishing a realistic goal is important for the success of the procedure. Because the lenses are worn overnight, it is especially important to select patients with no contraindications to overnight contact lens wear. The patient must understand that OOK does not change the cornea permanently and that if treatment is discontinued, myopia will return; however, some patients may be able to wear their OK lenses >7 nights per week, whereas others may achieve functional unaided vision for only a few hours after lens removal.

The current United States Food and Drug Administration (FDA) approvals for OOK are provided in Table 22.1. Although the approvals are for patients with up to −5.00 to −6.00 D of myopia and up to −1.50 to −1.75 D of astigmatism at any axis orientation, the most success will be achieved by initially selecting patients with the lower baseline levels of myopia and low with-the-rule astigmatism.

TABLE 22.1 FDA Approval Criteria for CRT and VST
FDA approval for CRT
Up to −6.00 D of myopia
Up to −1.75 D of astigmatism
No age limitations
FDA approval for VST
−1.00 to −5.00 D of myopia
Up to −1.50 D of astigmatism
No age limitations

Two very important factors in myopia reduction are the prefitting corneal curvature and the asphericity of the cornea. The normal corneal curvature gradually becomes flatter from the center to the periphery and can be described as a prolate ellipsoidal surface. The rate of flattening from center to periphery is known as the corneal eccentricity (denoted by an e-value). Spherical surfaces have an e-value equal to zero, while e-values of elliptical surfaces are <1 but >0. The average eccentricity of the normal cornea is approximately e = 0.50. Corneal eccentricity is typically measured using corneal topography.

Efforts have been made to correlate corneal eccentricity to refractive changes or to use baseline corneal eccentricity values as a predictor of success with OOK. The studies have produced mixed results; some found no correlation between eccentricity and refractive changes,[38] whereas others found good correlation between change in apical corneal power and corneal eccentricity[19] or that shape factor (a measure of corneal shape similar to eccentricity) can be a good indicator of refractive changes.[39]

Good and Poor Candidates

The best candidates for OK are individuals with low myopic refractive errors and low-to-moderate with-the-rule astigmatism. A new contact lens wearer or a soft lens wearer would be preferable to an existing GP wearer, although the latter can be successful if they are willing to discontinue contact lens wear until refractive and corneal stabilization has occurred. This process often takes a minimum of 2 weeks.[40] As the region of the central cornea that is being treated is typically only 5 to 6 mm, individuals with large pupil diameters are not good candidates due to the potential for glare resulting from viewing through the periphery of the treatment area. Individuals exhibiting against-the-rule astigmatism, irregular astigmatism, or a decentered corneal apex are not good candidates due, in large part, to the importance of achieving a well-centered lens-to-cornea fitting relationship. Any patient for whom corneal topography would not be possible (i.e., often individuals with deep-set eyes), would not represent a good candidate for OK.[41]

Individuals who are reluctant to pursue the process due to such factors as satisfaction with their current refractive correction, inability to make follow-up visits, or reluctance with the cost would not be good candidates. The fees for OK are typically competitive with refractive surgery. The actual fee varies from as little as $750 to $2,500, depending upon such factors as the patient's refractive status, and the experience of the fitter.[42] The average fees tend to range from $1,100 to $1400.[43] A list of good, borderline, and poor candidates is provided in Table 22.2.

Screening

OK can represent a very effective practice-building modality. However, it must be promoted ethically (see Table 22.3),[44] although word of mouth via satisfied patients (and parents) is

TABLE 22.2 Good, Borderline, and Poor Candidates for Orthokeratology

GOOD	BORDERLINE	POOR
≤3.50 D myopia	3.75–4.50 D myopia	>4.50 D myopia
<1.50 D WTR cyl	1.50–2.00 D WTR cyl	>2 D WTR cyl
New CL wearer	Current GP wearer	Irregular/ATR cyl
Young, progressive myope	Low "e" value (unless <2 D myope)	High myope with low "e" value
Occupational need for better unaided VA		Loose lids and/or deep-set eyes
Small pupil size	Medium pupil size with moderate myopia	Large (>5 mm room illumination; ≥7 mm dim illumination)
Motivated		Unmotivated for CL wear
Realistic expectations		Unrealistic expectations
History of compliance		Poor history of compliance
Good eye health (no history of dry eyes, anterior segment Dx)		Poor response to overnight trial
Recreational/athletic benefits		Cost or visit schedule is problematic

From Rinehart JM, Bennett ES. Orthokeratology. In: Bennett ES, Hom MM, eds. *Manual of Gas Permeable Contact Lenses*. 2nd ed. St. Louis, MO: Elsevier Science;2004:424–483.

TABLE 22.3 Guidelines for Advertising and Promoting Orthokeratology

- The main responsibility of the Federal Trade Commission (FTC) is to protect consumers from unfair and deceptive acts and practices in advertising and promotion. The main responsibility of the FDA is to promote public health.
- In an FDA Public Health Notification: Illegal Promotion of Contact Lenses dated September 25, 1998, the FDA states, "A licensed practitioner may individually design and prescribe an RGP OK design for a particular patient within the scope of his/her patient. However, eye care practitioners who promote OK in their practice should avoid making exaggerated and unsupported claims of safety or effectiveness."
- The practitioner who is advertising OK is responsible for all statements, regardless of who creates the advertisement. All information must be accurate and must not deceive the patient.
- Claims of safety and efficacy must be supported by competent and reliable scientific evidence. Advertising that claims a specific result, by the individual practitioner, must be documented unambiguously. If the promotion claims a specific result using a particular technique, it is necessary that the orthokeratologist is using the exactly same protocol.
- As a general rule, advertisements using testimonials should be avoided. Far too many variables exist from patient to patient for any testimonial to be considered a typical result.
- Claims of permanence must be avoided. It is important that there be a prominent mention of the need for retainer lens wear.
- The best advertisement of OK is honest, unambiguous, and without deception. One can apply the common person standard: the average person will understand the advertisement and not be misled in any fashion by the content.

OK, orthokeratology.
From Rinehart J. Guidelines for advertising and promoting orthokeratology. *Contacto*. 1999;40(1):7–13.

effective and can result in numerous potential candidates contacting the office. Good candidates can often be identified without the need to see them in-office or, at minimum, via a brief in-office evaluation. Individuals who contact the office—whether or not they express an overt interest in OK—can be informed of this option by the receptionist. If interested, a brief telephone screening can be performed, which could ultimately save them time and money if deemed unqualified. The staff member can inquire about their current mode of correction (if GP lenses, they will need to discontinue lens wear), refractive status, mention about the need for retainer wear, as well as costs and visit schedule. In addition, as presbyopic OK is not as widely prescribed, this could recommend a contraindication in many offices.

An in-office screening should consist of a manifest refraction (cycloplegic, if a young person), a slit-lamp evaluation to rule out anterior segment pathology, and corneal topography to rule out corneal distortion or a decentered apex.

FITTING ORTHOKERATOLOGY LENSES

General Guidelines

Modern OK practice uses RG lenses almost exclusively. The focus of this section will be a description of basic techniques applicable to most RG lens designs.

To flatten the central cornea and reduce myopia, the BCR of a RG lens is made flatter than the central corneal curvature. Exactly how flat is dependent on the lens design, but most manufacturers recommend the selection of a BCR flatter than the cornea by the amount of treatment desired. This technique is sometimes called the Jessen method as this was how George Jessen chose the BCR for his standard lens "orthofocus" procedure.[5] For example, if the patient's spherical refractive error is −3.00 DS, the BCR is made 3.00 D flatter than the flat keratometric reading. Most OK lens design manufacturers will recommend selecting a BCR about 0.50 to 0.75 D flatter than this value to slightly overcorrect the eye to a low amount of pseudohyperopia. This permits for a slight regression of the effect during the day so that the eye is close to plano by bedtime, allowing clear vision for all waking hours. While the RG contact lens is on eye, a minus tear lens created by the flat-fitting contact lens provides all the visual correction needed by the eye, and the contact lens power is close to plano. It should be noted that Mountford[45] argues that selecting the BCR in this manner has no scientific basis (see below).

To aid in centration with such a flat central BCR, the adjacent reverse curve steepens back toward the peripheral cornea. As the contact lens approaches the cornea, it then flattens into an alignment curve. The alignment curve allows the contact lens to stabilize on the peripheral cornea, which "steers" the lens to center. The contact lens must center over the pupil to prevent inducement of irregular astigmatism and provide an acceptable treatment area.

The designs of the reverse and alignment curves vary with each manufacturer, but they all work on the same principles. Some use more than one curve in the reverse and alignment areas, leading to so-called four-and five-zone lenses. Clinically, there is little difference in treatment outcome between lens designs.[23] In effect, the reverse and alignment curves control the overall sagittal depth of the lens to position the BCR close to the cornea without touching it, at least theoretically, while allowing the lens to center. It is thought that the dark central fluorescein pattern of an ideal OK fit is due to the very thin central tear film layer rather than apical touch. The human eye can observe approximately ≥20 μm (microns) of sodium fluorescein. Anything less than approximately 20 μm will be observed as apical touch, although not physically interacting with the cornea.

While the BCR is important, the sagittal depth is more so. A lens with too little sagittal depth (shallow) will decenter, typically superiorly, and a lens with excessive sagittal depth will provide little or no treatment. Typically, when altering an RG lens, the BCR should be left alone and alterations to the reverse curve or alignment curve should be changed, as they have a greater effect on sagittal depth. The BCR acts to achieve the desired central corneal shape change to correct for the appropriate refractive error.

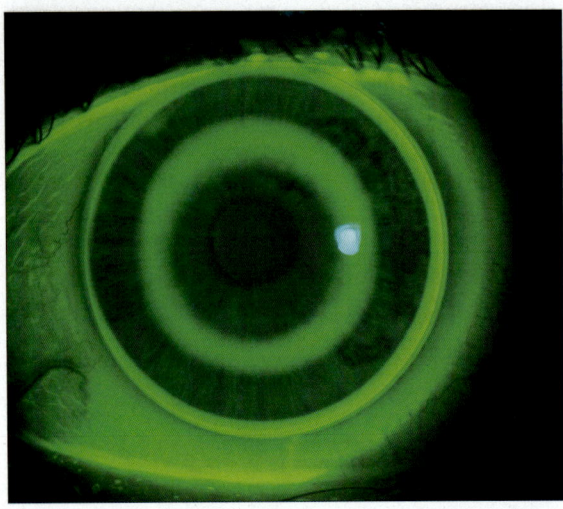

FIGURE 22.1 Reverse geometry lens with ideal "bull's eye" fluorescein pattern.

Most RG lenses have an overall diameter (OAD) in the 10- to 11-mm range. This helps with centration but is also necessary to accommodate the reverse curve and alignment curve zones of the lens. As most OK lenses are worn during sleep, high-Dk materials are used to maximize the oxygen available to the cornea. It has also been found that high-Dk materials optimize the clinical effect versus lower-Dk materials.[46]

A well-fitting RG lens will display a classic "bull's eye" appearance of the fluorescein pattern, where there is about 4 to 5 mm of central thinning of fluorescein, a ring of fluorescein about 1 mm wide in the midperiphery, alignment in the periphery, and a narrow ring of edge clearance (Fig. 22.1). Once an initial lens is chosen based on appearance, postwear topographic changes are used as a useful guide regarding whether the lens parameters are correct to obtain the desired treatment centration and amount. The appearance of the lens in open-eye conditions may not correlate to how the lens performs with the lid closed during sleep.

Mountford[45] has written perhaps the most comprehensive mechanical description of how RG lenses achieve their effect. The tear reservoir that is formed under the reverse curve sets up a dramatic difference in tear film thickness between the center of the cornea and the edge of the optical zone of the lens. The tear film is much greater midperipherally than centrally. This creates a pressure gradient in the tear film. In effect, negative pressure is created near the edge of the optical zone that remodels the corneal epithelium. Mountford terms this the *squeeze-film force*. This force, combined with lid pressure, creates the topographic shape change of OK: central flattening and midperipheral steepening of the cornea.

Mountford also argues that, in order for OK to be successful, there must actually be a very thin layer of tears at the corneal apex; the fluid force model provides little to no reshaping force if the lens touches the cornea centrally. A lens that touches centrally would also lose centration as it would interact with the apex of the cornea. The amount of central clearance is usually on the order of 10 μm. Since fluorescein in the tear film is not visible at tear film thicknesses <20 μm, RG lenses will show an absence of fluorescein centrally, incorrectly but conventionally interpreted as "touch" of the cornea. Also, within the tear reservoir under the reverse curve, small differences in tear film thickness, not discernible by observing the brightness of the fluorescein, make large differences in shaping forces. These observations have led Mountford and others to conclude that the fluorescein pattern of the lens is not a good indication of whether a lens will provide adequate treatment. An overnight trial and evaluation of postwear topography is a much better method to assess the performance of the contact lens. Nevertheless, fluorescein evaluation is helpful to evaluate lens centration and in making parameter changes in some lens designs.

Evaluation of postwear topography involves making a comparison of the pre- and postwear patterns. Most topography systems will produce a difference or subtractive map to show changes from one map to the next. Generally, all visits are compared to the baseline topography map, prewear. The desired difference map pattern will show a circular area of central flattening well centered over the patient's pupil, with a surrounding circular area of midperipheral steepening (Fig. 22.2). This is similar to the appearance of a postrefractive surgery map, with the normally prolate corneal shape changed to an oblate shape. This result indicates that the lens has centered well during closed-eye conditions and is providing adequate central flattening. It is useful to compare the axial, tangential, and refractive maps when evaluating treatment centration and size. Each of these displays information on overview of treatment, position of treatment, and quality of treatment, respectively. By moving the cursor of the topographer over the center of the treatment area on the difference map, an estimate of the amount of refractive change can be assessed.

Patterns other than central flattening indicate that the lens fit is not optimal. A lens that has too little sagittal depth will tend to decenter superiorly, creating a flattened area on the topography map that is superior to the pupil, with an arc-shaped area of steepening below it (Fig. 22.3). This may still result in the correction of the patient's myopia, but the treatment is suboptimal because this combination of treated/untreated area along the visual axis may cause halos or diplopia. The fix for this is to increase the sagittal depth of the contact lens by altering the reverse curve(s), alignment curve(s), or both. The exact fix will depend on the lens design being used, and practitioners should refer to the fitting guide provided by the manufacturer.

A lens with excessive sagittal depth will tend to center well or may decenter slightly inferiorly. The classic topography pattern for a deep lens shows a central island, an area of central steepening (steeper than the baseline corneal curvature in that area) surrounded by an area of flattening, surrounded again by a ring of midperipheral steepening (Fig. 22.4). The patient may show no change in refraction or even an increase in myopia because of the central steepening. A slightly inferiorly decentered pattern may also mean the sagittal depth was too deep. To correct this would be to decrease the sagittal depth of the lens, again using the manufacturer's guidelines to do so. Other variations of topography patterns are possible, but the patterns presented here are the most common.

There are three basic techniques in fitting OK lenses: (a) Inventory fitting technique; (b) Topography fitting technique; and (c) Laboratory fitting technique. The inventory fitting technique is based on the practitioner having access to a full range of OK lens parameters so that adjustments to fit may be made at the initial visit. An example of this technique is the

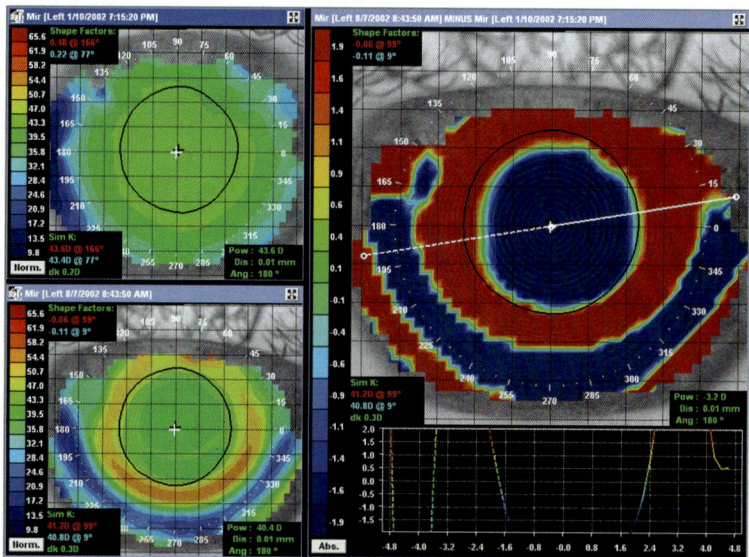

FIGURE 22.2 Well-centered treatment following reverse geometry lens wear. (Courtesy of Randy Kojma.)

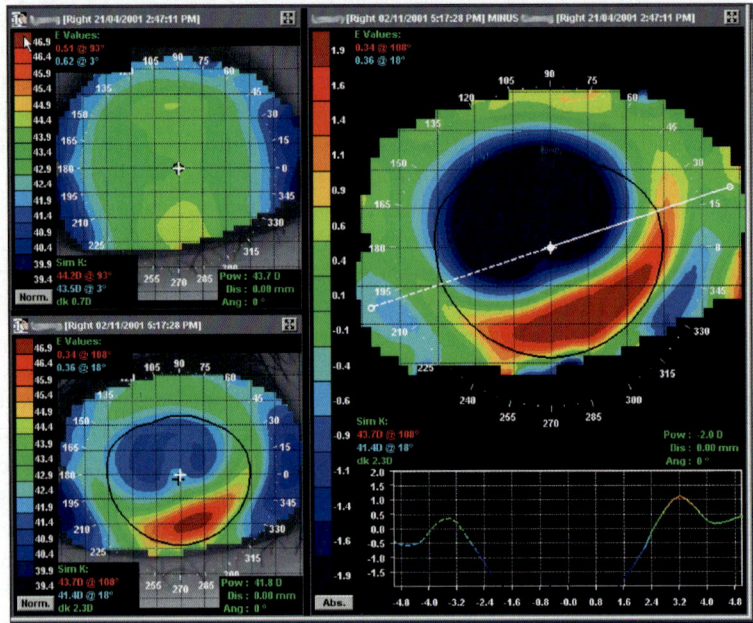

FIGURE 22.3 Superior decentration pattern following wear of shallow sagittal depth reverse geometry lens. (Courtesy of Randy Kojima.)

Paragon corneal refractive therapy (CRT) lens by Paragon Vision Sciences. Each technique aims to achieve the "bull's eye" fluorescein pattern, but differs in how this is achieved. The topography fitting technique is dependent on the topographer to determine the initial lens by inputting information determined by the topographer and the manifest refraction. An example of this is the BE Retainer by Bausch + Lomb. The third technique is where the practitioner calls the manufacturer to specify the patient's keratometric values and manifest refraction. The laboratory then inputs the information into a lens design program to design the initial lens.

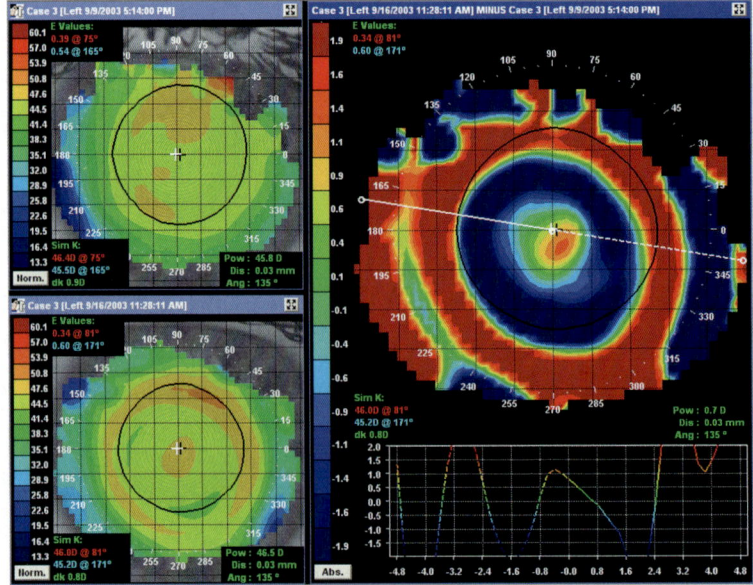

FIGURE 22.4 Central island following wear of deep sagittal depth reverse geometry lens. (Courtesy of Randy Kojima.)

Lens Designs

Corneal Refractive Therapy

The CRT system (Paragon Vision Sciences, Mesa, AZ) was the first lens design FDA approved for overnight treatment. The fitting process uses a slide-rule-type guide to choose the initial lens and fluorescein analysis to refine the lens parameters.

The clinician locates the patient's flat keratometric reading and spherical refractive error on the guide and a set of lens parameters is specified for the first lens. This lens is fitted and evaluated. A good lens fit will center well, have 4 to 5 mm of central alignment (approximately 5–10 microns of fluorescein), and have edge clearance that is about 0.5-mm wide. The lens parameters are changed until an appropriate pattern is found.

The zones of the CRT lens are the treatment zone (BCR), the return zone (reverse curve), and the landing zone (alignment curve). Although this terminology is unique to the CRT lens design, the fitting process is not more complicated.[47] The BCR is chosen by the Jessen method described above with a 0.50 D regression factor. The CRT return zone uses a unique sigmoidal (S-shaped) curve. As it is not a simple spherical curve, the return zone is specified by its sagittal depth. Typical return zone depth (RZD) values are 500, 525, and 550 μm, although others are available in 25-μm steps. A lens with too little sagittal depth will tend to decenter superiorly, indicating the need to increase to the next deeper RZD (such as from 500 to 525 μm). Conversely, a lens that centers well but has <4 mm of central fluorescein thinning indicates the sagittal depth is too deep and the RZD should be decreased one step.

The landing zone is an angle rather than a curvature. Typical landing zone angle (LZA) values are 32, 33, and 34 degrees, available in 1-degree steps. Increasing the LZA will decrease edge clearance, and decreasing it will increase edge clearance by approximately 12 μm. For example, if the lens displays an edge clearance that is wider than 0.5 mm, the LZA should be increased by 1 degree (such as from 33 to 34 degrees) and have an increase in sagittal depth by approximately 12 μm. The standard OAD is 10.5 mm.

Practitioners have the choice of using a 110-lens fitting set or ordering lenses based on the slide-rule guide. The fitting set is valuable because the practitioner can make immediate changes in parameters to achieve an acceptable fit. Lenses can also be dispensed out of this inventory without having to wait for an ordered lens to arrive. For practitioners new to CRT, it may be more economical to order empirical lenses under warranty for the first few patients. The SureFit program allows the practitioner to receive the lens recommended via the slide-rule guide as well as two lens designs that bracket the recommended lens. Conversely, having the set on-hand makes the first fits easier to evaluate because of the access to the different parameters. It is also possible to order the empirical first lens and then Paragon Vision sends two additional lenses that are the most likely options if the initial lens does not provide the optimal fitting relationship.

A new advancement in the CRT lens is the Dual-Axis design, whereby the RZD and the LZA can be changed in two different meridians based on the differences in peripheral corneal elevation, most often seen in corneas with limbus-to-limbus astigmatism. This lens design aids in centration and treatment effect by maintaining a more constant sagittal height and a more uniform central treatment zone (Fig. 22.5).

Vision Shaping Treatment

The following lens designs all have FDA clearance for overnight wear under the Bausch + Lomb vision shaping treatment approval.

BE Lens: The BE Retainer system (Precision Technology Services) uses corneal topography data to design the lens. Fluorescein analysis is not used. The BE system is a lens-design software package and a 24-lens trial set. The patient's topography data and refractive error are entered into the software to design the lens. Necessary topography data include the corneal apical radius,

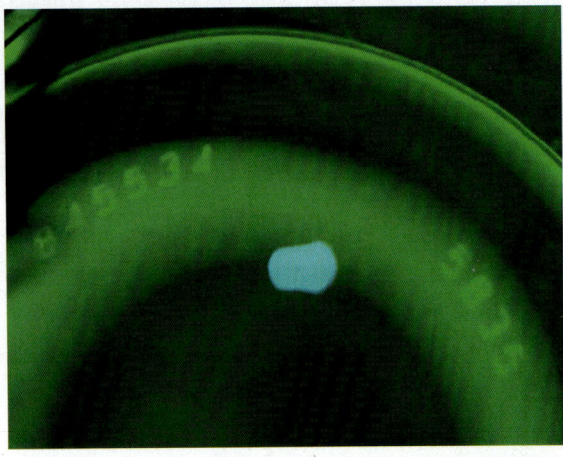

FIGURE 22.5 Dual-axis fluorescein pattern. (From Herzberg CM. An update on orthokeratology. *Contact Lens Spectrum*. 2010;25(3):22.)

sagittal height, and corneal diameter. The Medmont topographer is recommended for the BE system, in part because it generates a value for sagittal height, but other topographers can be used. The software also provides a predicted value for maximum possible treatment for the patient's eye; this is useful to determine whether the patient is a good candidate.

The software calculates lens parameters to provide an ideal tear film profile under the lens to obtain the necessary corneal change. This tear film shape provides what is referred to as the *squeeze-film force*, as discussed in the general fitting section. The BE system does not use the Jessen method of base curve calculation, unlike most other designs. Instead, the lens periphery is calculated to provide good lens centration, the alignment curve is chosen to provide the proper tear film thickness in this area, and the BCR is chosen to provide the correct apical tear film thickness. The lens periphery is flat rather than curved, and is designated by its cone angle.

A problem with using topography for lens design is that the corneal data may be incorrect. The trial lens set is used to overcome this problem. The software selects the trial lens that is closest in sagittal depth to the "ideal" lens based on topography. If the topographer calculated the corneal height correctly, wearing the trial lens overnight should result in the typical well-centered bull's eye of central flattening, although the amount of treatment will likely not be ideal. If this pattern is produced, the "custom" lens can be ordered for the patient. If not, then the topographer miscalculated the corneal sagittal depth. Depending on the type of pattern produced, the software adjusts the lens parameters and a new trial lens is selected. The process is repeated until a well-centered bull's eye is achieved. At this point, the custom lens can be ordered and should give predictable results.

Contex OK E-System: The Contex OK E-System is a RG lens design that utilizes the corneal eccentricity as a key fitting factor in lens design. The lens is composed of a back optical zone, a steeper reverse zone, one or more alignment curves, and a peripheral curve, which provides edge clearance and tear exchange. Each lens has a designated design code specific to the shape of the cornea and the refraction information of the eye. For example, the design code 44.00/−4.00 (0.5 e) refers to a lens design for a cornea with a flat keratometry reading of 44.00 D, a targeted myopia reduction of 4 D, and a corneal eccentricity of 0.5. The BCR, OAD, and lens power are also specified on the lens packaging. The typical OAD of a Contex OK E-System lens is 10.6 mm with an optical zone diameter of 6.0 mm. When fitting a patient in the OK E-System lens design, the initial lens can be selected one of three ways:

1. By providing the laboratory with central keratometry readings and the manifest refraction
2. By providing the laboratory with central keratometry readings, the manifest refraction, and corneal topography maps
3. By trial fitting with an inventory fitting set

When a diagnostic fitting set is not used and information is provided to the laboratory for selection of an initial lens, the laboratory uses the average corneal eccentricity, or 0.5, to select the initial lens design. When corneal topography maps are available, the corneal eccentricity value from the map is used for the initial lens design. Fitting from the fitting set is the recommended method.

When troubleshooting the OK E-System design, the corneal eccentricity value is altered to loosen or tighten the lens fit. For instance, if the lens design code is 44.00/−4.00 (0.5 e) and the lens is too tight, changing to a lens with a design code of 44.00/−4.00 (0.55 e) will loosen the fit while maintaining the same targeted myopia reduction. When adjusting the eccentricity value to alter the fit of the lens, an adjustment of at least 0.05 e (equal to approximately 10 μm) is recommended. If an increase in myopia reduction is needed, the targeted myopia reduction in the design code should be changed. For example, if the patient in this example is undercorrected by 0.50 D, but the topography map and lens fit are ideal, a new lens with a design code of 44.00/−4.50 (0.5 e) should be selected. A troubleshooting computer program and troubleshooting forms are available as an aid in clinical practice.

DreamLens: The DreamLens is also a RG design with a back optical zone, a steep reverse curve, one or more alignment curves, and a peripheral curve for edge clearance and tear exchange. The DreamLens is fitted using the proprietary DreamLens Software program. The program extracts the data from the corneal topography maps and combines the information with the spectacle prescription and the corneal diameter to design the initial lens for the eye. The corneal diameter is used to determine the OAD of the lens (10.0, 10.5, or 10.9 mm).

When troubleshooting a DreamLens fit, if the lens is centering inferior or superior to the pupil, changes in the alignment zone(s) are necessary to provide better lens centration. Changes of at least 0.50 D are recommended. Laboratory consultation is available as an aid in clinical practice.

Euclid Systems Corporation: Emerald Design: The Emerald lens is a RG lens with four zones: the back optic zone, the reverse curve, the alignment curve, and the peripheral curve. When fitting the Emerald lens, the parameters for the initial lens are determined by providing the patient's refraction, keratometry measurements, and horizontal visible iris diameter to Euclid Systems. The laboratory will then use computer calculations to design the initial lens to best fit the patient. The standard lens diameters are 10.2, 10.6, and 11.0 mm and are selected based on the horizontal visible iris diameter. A diameter of 10.6 mm is typically recommended for the initial lens. The initial alignment curve is typically designed as equal to the flat keratometry measurement. The BCR is calculated based on the flat keratometry reading and the targeted myopia reduction (Jessen method described above) plus an additional 0.75 D. Once the alignment curve and base curve are determined, the reverse curve is calculated by Euclid.

Comment on Lens Designs

This is not an exhaustive list of lens designs for OK. Rather, it is meant to give an overview of the different philosophies of the lens designers. A comprehensive list is provided in Table 22.4. Note that some lens designs require decision-making on the part of the practitioner, and some are very proprietary and the laboratory generates the lens design calculations. The decision about which brand to try is up to the practitioner. As mentioned, all the designs can be successfully used and temporarily correct myopia. How easy it is for the practitioner to do so will vary with the brands. It is probably more important for the practitioner to select a method and learn as much as possible about it than to select the "right" brand.

It should also be noted that FDA approval for all these lenses requires that practitioners be certified to fit and order the lenses. This is to ensure that clinicians understand the unique fitting characteristics of RG lenses, the underlying concepts of treatment and follow-up care, and troubleshooting that inevitably has to occur.

TABLE 22.4 Currently Available Orthokeratology Lens Designs

Corneal Refractive Therapy Designs (Paragon Vision Sciences)
CRT (Paragon Vision Sciences)
Z-CRT (Menicon)
FARGO Lens (GP Specialists)
Vision Shaping Treatment (Bausch + Lomb)
BE Retainer (Precision Technology Services)
Contex OK E-System (Contex)
DreamLens (DreamLens)
Emerald (Euclid Systems)
CKR (Eye Care Associates)
MiracLens (MiracLens)
NIghtMove (Advanced Corneal Engineering)
Orthofocus (Progressive Vision Technologies)
Super Bridge and E-Lens (E & E Optics)
VIPOK II (E & E Optics)
WAVE (Custom Craft Lens Service, Metro Optics, and X-Cel Contacts)

DISPENSING

An impressive outcome of several OK studies has been the first-fit success rate with reports of 80.5% and 95%.[48,49] Once the initial lenses have been dispensed, they are evaluated similar to spherical GP lenses. An evaluation of the lens-to-cornea fitting relationship, VA, and instruction on care and handling is to be performed. If the vision and fitting relationship is acceptable, the patient should be scheduled for a follow-up visit for the following morning.

Lens insertion is similar to conventional GP designs. However, the fact that these are larger lenses that exhibit little movement with the blink makes mastering removal more challenging. Simply using one finger at the lateral canthus to eject the lens is typically not successful. Both the upper- and lower-lid margins must be pressed against the eye and pulled laterally to result in the pressure necessary to eject the lens. In addition, it would be recommended to wait, at minimum, 30 minutes after awakening to remove the lenses and to also apply rewetting drops and gently nudge the lower lid against the edge to break any adherence seal prior to removal. The lenses should then be cleaned upon removal in the palm of the hand. The lens should be inserted on the eye 15 to 20 minutes prior to going to bed.

Patients should be educated about what to expect during the adaptation phase. It is not uncommon for the patients to experience some initial awareness the first few evenings of lens wear. However, as a result of the larger OAD and the lesser amount of movement with the blink, the amount of initial awareness and the length of adaptation is much less than with conventional GP lens designs. Patients should also be advised that it is not uncommon to experience some glare around lights and mild ghosting of images, which typically goes away by the end of the treatment phase.

FOLLOW-UP CARE

Follow-Up Visits

It is typically recommended that the first follow-up visit occur on the morning following the first night of lens wear. Although not always possible, it is recommended that the patients

TABLE 22.5 Recommended Testing Procedures for Follow-Up Visits

- Entrance visual acuity
- Unaided visual acuity
- Refraction
- Slit-lamp examination
- Corneal topography
- Lens fit evaluation
- Overrefraction

ideally be examined within a few hours of lens removal or even wear the lenses into their appointment. If, after the first-day visit, a well-centered treatment zone is noted by corneal topography, it is recommended that patients be evaluated again at 1 week, 1 month, 3 months, and 6 months following lens dispensing to monitor the treatment effect. Lens wear is not typically necessary prior to these visits. The basic testing procedures to be conducted at each visit are provided in Table 22.5. If corneal topography is not conclusive (i.e., definite, centered bull's eye) on day 1, a 3-day trial is recommended before a decision is made to continue with these lenses or to change the lens design.

The testing procedures are similar for each follow-up visit. Unaided VA is recorded to monitor the vision and success of the treatment. Biomicroscopy is performed to monitor the ocular health. In addition to these basic procedures, corneal topography is critical for assessing the progress of treatment. If the patient's vision is unacceptable or slit-lamp signs are noted, corneal topography can be helpful in determining the cause. As mentioned previously, lenses with too little or excessive sagittal depth produce characteristic topography patterns, which can be used in addition to evaluating the lens fit on the eye to improve success. Lastly, an overrefraction will determine whether the BCR is appropriate. If minus power is detected in the overrefraction, the BCR should be flattened to fully correct the patient's distance refractive error.

Daily disposable lenses can be provided to the patient to wear during the treatment phase. As regression appears to occur at a greater rate initially than after the treatment period, the patient can be overcorrected initially. For example, if they refract −1.75 DS at the 24-hour visit, they can be provided with two pairs of −2.00 D lenses, two pairs of −1.50 D lenses, two pairs of −1.00 D lenses, and a pair of −0.50 D lenses to wear prior to the 1-week visit. Once the treatment goal (often +0.50 to +0.75 D refractive error) has been achieved, they can initiate retainer wear. As the average amount of myopic regression is 0.50 to 0.75 D per day, some patients may, in fact, wear their lenses every night for retainer purposes.[50] However, patients with a low myopic refractive error may wear their lenses as little as 1 night per week and all patients learn to wear their lenses overnight whenever they begin to experience blur at near.

Complications

As with any contact lens modality, complications are of concern with OK. The quality of vision, as determined via an increase in higher-order aberrations, and a reduction in contrast sensitivity is not uncommon, although it tends to decrease as a problem during the treatment phase[51–53] unless the lens is decentered.[54]

Of greater importance, however, is there have been several reports of microbial keratitis (MK) associated with OOK.[55–57] The majority of reported cases were from Asian countries, predominantly China, Taiwan, and Hong Kong. Most of the cases were children between the ages of 9 and 15 years or young adults between the ages of 16 and 25 years. When interpreting these statistics, it is important to keep in mind that they do not necessarily indicate that patients in Asian countries or patients in the age ranges mentioned are more susceptible to infections. It could simply reflect the populations most likely to be fitted with OOK lenses. Overall, however, it does not appear that the risk of MK is any higher than any other contact lens modalities.[58]

The causative agent is also important in determining the appropriate treatment. In the cases mentioned above, *Pseudomonas aeruginosa* was the offending agent in most of the cases. The second most often noted was *Acanthamoeba*. Because there is a wide range of possible microorganisms that can be present, it is important to obtain a corneal culture before initiation of treatment.

Education of patients regarding hygiene, proper cleaning techniques, and appropriate wearing times helps to reduce the risks of complications. In particular, given the number of cases of *Acanthamoeba* keratitis, patients should be firmly instructed to avoid any tap water coming in contact with the lenses and lens case.[59] In addition, lens cases should be replaced every month. The importance of cleaning the lenses upon removal should be emphasized, as well as OK lenses retain more bacteria adherent to the surface than alignment-fitted GP lenses.[60] Regular follow-up appointments that include similar education are also essential.

CURRENT AND FUTURE USES OF ORTHOKERATOLOGY

Hyperopic Correction

Newer OK designs allow for the treatment and correction of hyperopia, although currently not approved by the FDA, making their use an off-label indication. For the correction of hyperopia topographically, the central cornea steepens and the midperipheral cornea flattens. The corneal compression that occurs in the paracentral region may be the primary mechanism behind the hyperopic OK clinical effect.[49] Histologically, the central corneal epithelium thickens and the midperipheral epithelium thins.[30] The reduction of hyperopia through corneal steepening with the use of OK has undergone less intensive clinical investigation compared to myopic OK.

To steepen the central cornea, ideally the posterior surface of the lens should embody three key elements (Fig. 22.6):

1. A central zone of apical clearance.
2. A contact zone 2 to 3 mm from the geometric center.
3. A relief zone in the midperiphery.[61]

The central zone of clearance allows for tissue molding and corneal steepening. This central zone of steepening is often tightly collected and dynamically flattens over the pupil[62] (Fig. 22.7).

The posterior optical zone responsible for treatment in hyperopic OK can range from 5 to 8 mm in diameter and incorporate a spherical or aspheric radius.[63] The resultant corneal treatment zone diameter with these lenses requires further study to explore the benefits of each design for the treatment of hyperopia.

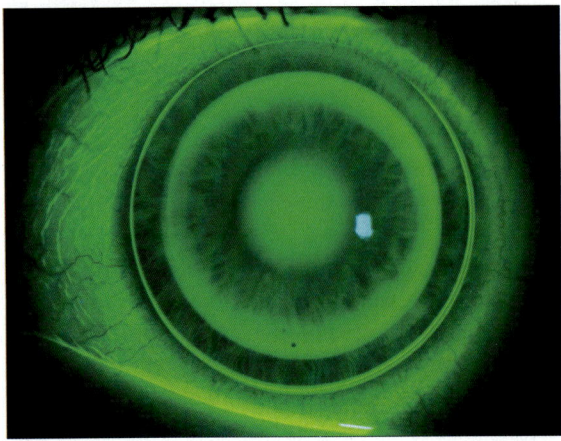

FIGURE 22.6 Hyperopic orthokeratology lens with central apical clearance.

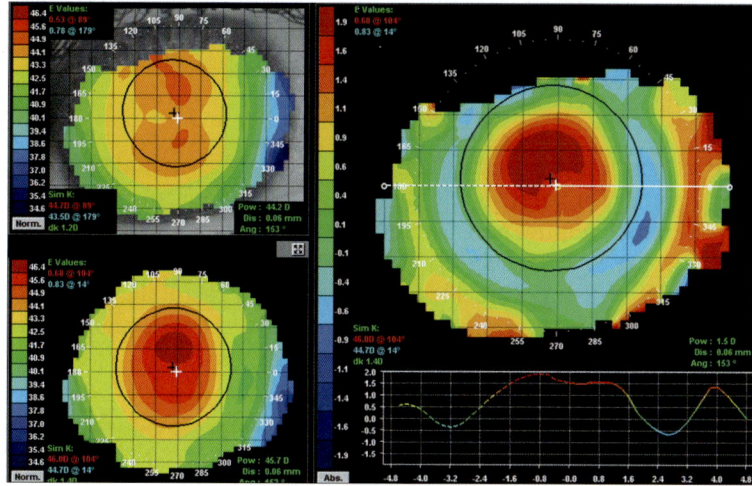

FIGURE 22.7 Topography of a postwear hyperopic orthokeratology difference/subtractive axial display.

The contact or plateau zone 2 to 3 mm from the lens center results in epithelial thinning and in combination with the relief zone or return zone in the midperiphery aids in lens centering and tear circulation.[62,64] The cornea steepens beneath the relief zone, maintaining constancy of corneal power. The ideal fluorescein pattern shows an area of central pooling without evidence of bubbles, juxta-central tear thinning, pooling in the midperiphery, a band of peripheral alignment, and adequate edge lift/clearance. After an adequate fitting relationship is determined, the lenses are dispensed to the patient for overnight wear.

Overnight hyperopic OK results in central corneal steepening with midperipheral flattening with decrease in hyperopic refractive error. Treatment of hyperopia with OK lenses can provide satisfactory vision.

Soft Contact Lenses

An OK-like topographical pattern has been reported to occur with everted high-minus soft contact lenses.[65] This has led to ongoing research utilizing silicone hydrogel soft contact lenses for OK. Two such designs have been investigated by Phillips[66] and Holden.[67] Phillips[66] slowed myopic progression in young people via a dual-focus soft lens that produced myopic peripheral retinal defocus with a simultaneous clear central retinal image. Progression of myopia was also lessened via a silicone hydrogel lens design, which corrected central vision, but reduced relative peripheral hyperopia in young people.[67]

Corneoscleral Lens Designs

Success with semi-scleral lens designs for OK has been reported.[68] The molding effect of such large lenses as well as the initial comfort makes this an option with great future potential.

RESOURCES

There are several resources available to assist interested students, residents, and practitioners in becoming proficient in fitting OK lens designs and successfully incorporating this modality within the practice. As both Bausch + Lomb and Paragon Vision Sciences require certification to fit their designs, this can be achieved online by going to their respective websites (i.e., www.bausch.com; www.paragoncrt.com). Organizations such as the Orthokeratology Academy of America (OAA; www.okglobal.org) and the GP Lens Institute (www.gpli.info) have programs and resources pertaining to OK. The OAA has an annual symposium that includes a fundamentals program for new fitters. The GP Lens Institute has a narrated powerpoint, online cases, and several annual webinars on OK.

SUMMARY

A major advance in lens design, specifically the availability of custom-designed RG GP lenses, resulted in a resurgence of interest in OK. The advanced manufacturing techniques, in combination with corneal topography, have improved the success of OK and brought it back into the mainstream of optometric practice. Higher amounts of myopia can be treated with the newer lens designs and materials available. Further research is still necessary to answer questions regarding topics such as the mechanism of action and the possibility of slowing myopia progression; however, OK is a viable option for many patients.

CLINICAL CASES

CASE 1

A 24-year-old male presented for a contact lens fitting. His chief concern was that he was never being able to wear soft contact lenses successfully due to persistent lens awareness. A pretreatment manifest refraction of OD −2.00 − 0.50 × 160 and OS −2.75 DS with best-corrected VA OD 20/15 and OS 20/15 was obtained. Baseline simulated keratometry readings were OD 42.25/41.25 @ 161 and OS 41.50/41.00 @ 006 with clear and regular mires OU. Baseline topography can be seen in Figure 22.8A.

SOLUTION: Different contact lens options were discussed with the patient including OK. The patient was fitted with Paragon CRT lenses initially selected with the slide rule. The initial parameters were OD 8.7-mm BCR, 525 RZD, 32-degree LZA and OS 8.9-mm BCR, 525 RZD, 32-degree LZA. Both lenses were centered with an appropriate "bull's eye" pattern and plano overrefraction with VA 20/15 in each eye. The patient was taught application and removal and lens care techniques and was instructed to wear lenses overnight and to return to clinic at 7 am the next morning. The patient returned to clinic for his 1-day follow up wearing the OK lenses. VA was 20/15 in each eye. Upon slit-lamp examination, the lenses appeared to be centered well with good movement on blink. After lens removal, corneal topography was taken and revealed well-centered treatment zones in each eye. Unaided VA was 20/30 OD and 20/40 OS.

The patient was instructed to continue wearing the lenses nightly and to return to clinic in 1 week. Entering VA unaided was 20/20+ in each eye and corneal topography continued to

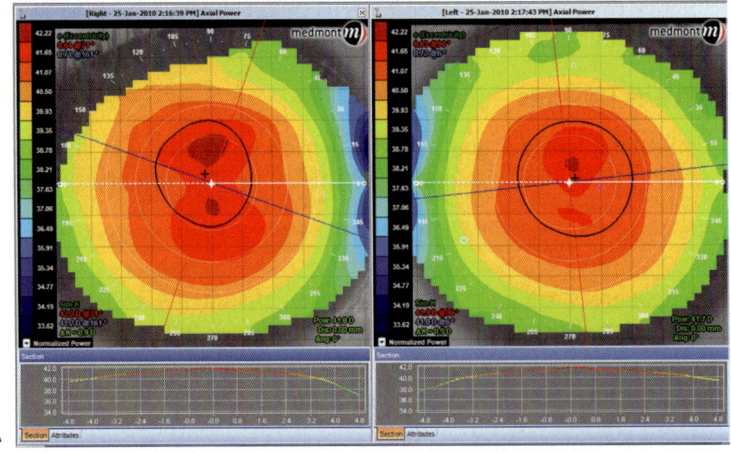

FIGURE 22.8 (A) Baseline topography for Case 1. Difference/subtractive axial topographical map for Case 1 right eye **(B)** and left eye **(C)**.

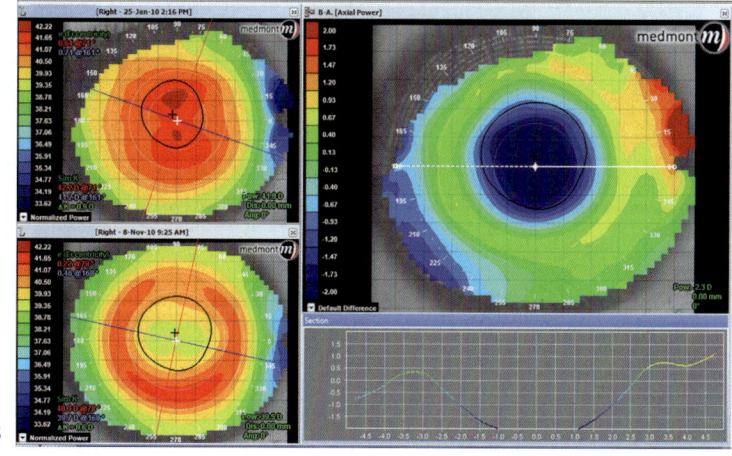

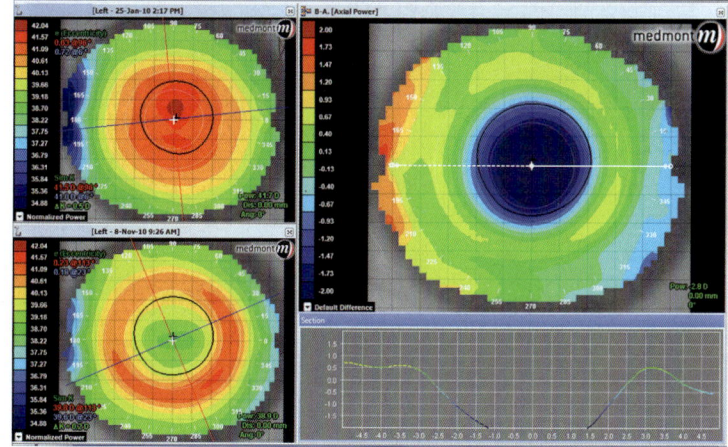

FIGURE 22.8 (Continued)

show well-centered treatment zones in each eye with central corneal flattening corresponding to the patient's pretreatment manifest refractive error.

The patient was again instructed to continue wearing the lenses nightly and return to clinic in 1 month where he reported good visual quality during all waking hours and acceptable comfort while wearing the lenses. Corneal topography was repeated and images are shown in Figure 22.8B,C.

CASE 2

An 11-year-old girl presented for an annual contact lens examination. She had traditionally worn soft contact lenses and her parents were interested in pursuing OK. A pretreatment manifest refraction of OD −2.00 DS and OS −2.50 DS with best-corrected VA OD 20/15 and OS 20/15 was obtained. Baseline simulated keratometry readings were OD 46.37/46.00 @ 170 and OS 46.62/46.25 @ 006 with clear and regular mires OU. Baseline topography can be seen in Figure 22.9A.

SOLUTION: The patient was fitted with Paragon CRT lenses initially selected with the slide rule. The initial parameters were OD 7.8-mm BCR, 550 RZD, 34-degree LZA and OS 7.8-mm BCR, 550 RZD, 34-degree LZA. Both lenses were centered with an appropriate "bull's eye" pattern and plano overrefraction with VA 20/15 in each eye. The patient was taught application and removal and lens care techniques and was instructed to wear lenses overnight and to return to clinic the next morning. The patient returned to clinic for her 1-day follow-up wearing the OK

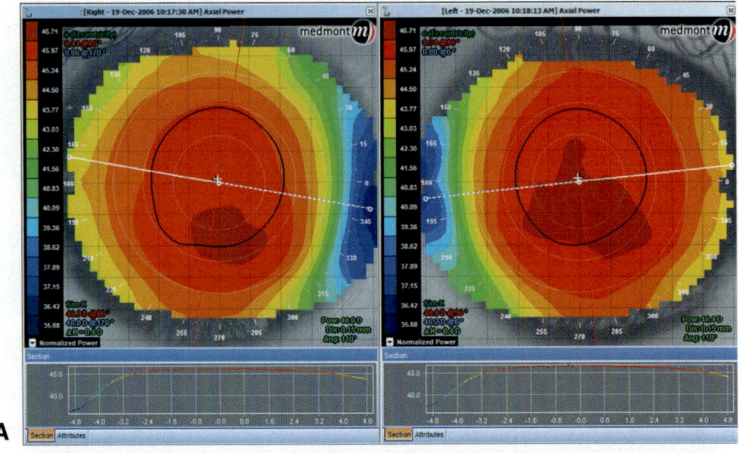

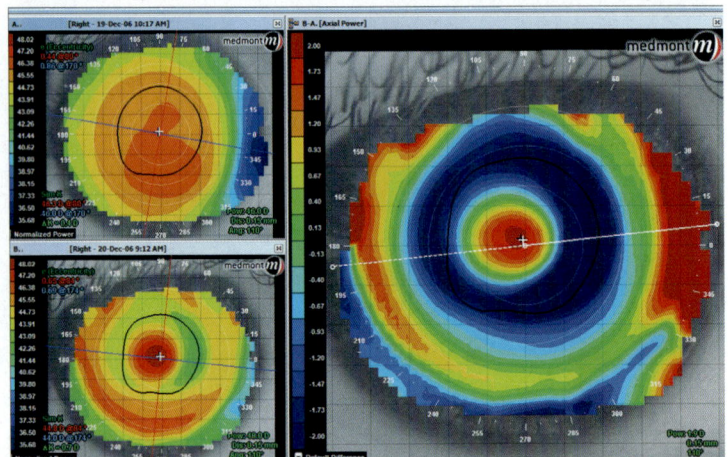

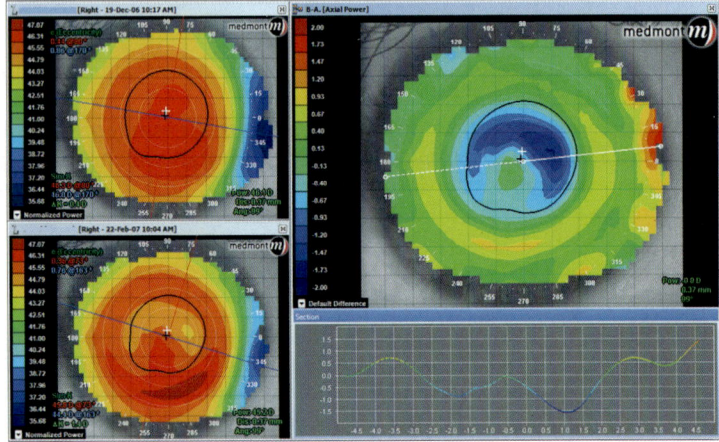

FIGURE 22.9 **(A)** Baseline topography for Case 2. **(B)** Difference/subtractive axial topographical map for Case 2 in the right eye. Note the prominent central island. **(C)** Difference/subtractive axial topographical map for Case 2 in the right eye at the first-day follow-up of the next fitting. The central area of nontreatment is not considered a central island because it is below the baseline axial curvature. **(D)** Difference/subtractive axial topographical map for Case 2 in the right eye at the second-day follow-up. Note the progressive improvement of treatment area.

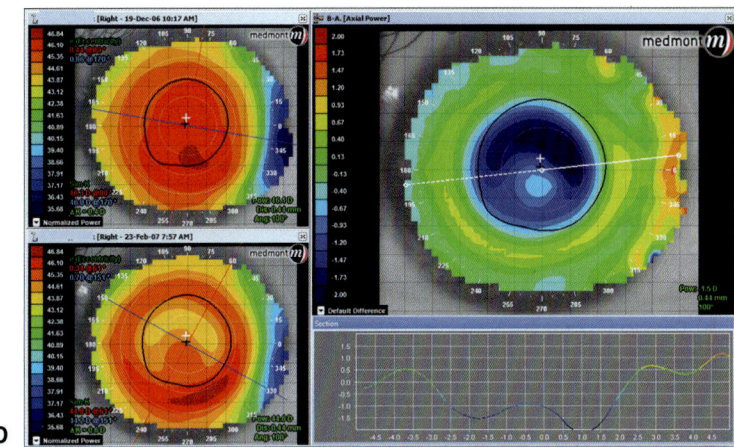

FIGURE 22.9 (Continued)

lenses. VA was 20/15 in each eye. Upon slit-lamp examination, the lenses appeared to be centered well with good movement on blink. After lens removal, corneal topography was taken and revealed a prominent central island OU surrounded by flattening (Fig. 22.9B). Unaided VA was OD 20/100 and OS 20/100.

The patient discontinued lens wear and returned 2 months later due to her busy school schedule. At her return visit, the corneal topography had returned to baseline. The patient was refit into a lens with less sagittal depth by 50 microns OU. Lens parameters were OD 7.8-mm BCR, 500 RZD, 34-degree LZA and OS 7.8 mm BCR, 500 RZD, 34-degree LZA. Lenses maintained centration with a plano overrefraction OU.

At her 1-day follow-up, the treatment zone was well centered with an area that did not exhibit flattening. This was not considered a central island because there was no increase in curvature when compared to the baseline topography (Fig. 22.9C). VA was OD 20/40 and OS 20/25. She was seen the following day and her vision had improved OD to 20/20 and OS 20/20 uncorrected with a noted overall flattening effect in both eyes (Fig. 22.9D). The patient and parents were pleased with the results and continue regular follow-up examinations.

CLINICAL PROFICIENCY CHECKLIST

- OK is a temporary correction of myopia and astigmatism using specially designed rigid contact lenses to flatten the central cornea.
- Modern OK utilizes RG GP contact lenses, which have a secondary curve radius steeper than the BCR. This has resulted in greater refractive error reduction in a shorter period of time compared to earlier designs.
- Corneal topography is much more useful than keratometry in evaluating the corneal changes because it enables the practitioner to measure a much greater area of the cornea.
- The FDA-approved treatment range is up to −5.00 or −6.00 D of myopia and up to −1.50 or −1.75 D of astigmatism, depending on the lens design.
- A well-fitting RG lens will display a classic "bull's eye" appearance fluorescein pattern, where there is about 4 to 5 mm of central absence of fluorescein ("touch"), a ring of fluorescein about 1 mm wide in the midperiphery, alignment in the periphery, and a narrow ring of edge clearance.
- The performance of the lens on-eye after wearing overnight is more important than the fluorescein appearance of the lens, and must be assessed with a corneal topography difference map.

REFERENCES

1. Efron N, Morgan PB, Woods C. Survey of contact lens prescribing to infants, children, and teenagers. *Optom Vis Sci*. 2011;88(4):461–468.
2. Morrison RJ. Contact lenses and the progression of myopia. *J Am Optom Assoc*. 1957;28:711–713.
3. Bier N. Myopia controlled by contact lenses. *Optician*. 1958;135:427.
4. Carlson JJ. Basic factors in checking the progression of myopia. *Opt J Rev Optom*. 1958;95(19):37–42.
5. Jessen GN. Orthofocus techniques. *Contacto*. 1962;6(7):200–204.
6. Grant SC, May CH. Orthokeratology control of refractive errors through contact lenses. *J Am Optom Assoc*. 1971;42:345–359.
7. Kerns R. Research in orthokeratology. Part I: introduction and background. *J Am Optom Assoc*. 1976;47:1047–1051.
8. Kerns R. Research in orthokeratology. Part III: results and conclusions. *J Am Optom Assoc*. 1976;47(8):1505–1515.
9. Binder PS, May CH, Grant SC. An evaluation of orthokeratology. *Ophthalmology*. 1980;87(8):729–744.
10. Polse KA, Brand RJ, Schwalbe JS, et al. The Berkeley orthokeratology study. Part II: efficacy and duration. *Am J Optom Physiol Opt*. 1983;60(3):187–198.
11. Polse KA, Brand RJ, Keener RJ, et al. The Berkeley orthokeratology study. Part III: safety. *Am J Optom Physiol Opt*. 1983;60(4):321–328.
12. Coon LJ. Orthokeratology, part II: evaluating the Tabb method. *J Am Optom Assoc*. 1984;55(6):409–418.
13. Polse KA. Orthokeratology as a clinical procedure (editorial). *Am J Optom Physiol Opt*. 1977;54(6):345–346.
14. Eger MJ. Orthokeratology fact or fiction (editorial). *J Am Optom Assoc*. 1975;46(7):682–683.
15. Safir A. Orthokeratology, II. A risky and unpredictable "treatment" for a benign condition. *Surv Ophthalmol*. 1980;24(5):291–302.
16. Fontana AA. Orthokeratology using the one piece bifocal. *Contacto*. 1972;16(6):45–47.
17. Wlodyga RG, Bryla C. Corneal molding: the easy way. *Contact Lens Spectrum*. 1989;4(8):58–65.
18. Harris HD, Stoyan N. A new approach to orthokeratology. *Contact Lens Spectrum*. 1992;7(4):37–39.
19. Mountford J. An analysis of the changes in corneal shape and refractive error induced by accelerated orthokeratology. *Int Cont Lens Clin*. 1997;24:128–143.
20. Lui WO, Edwards MH. Orthokeratology in low myopia. Part I: efficacy and predictability. *Cont Lens Anterior Eye*. 2000;23(3):77–89.
21. Nichols JJ, Marsich MM, Nguyen M, et al. Overnight orthokeratology. *Optom Vis Sci*. 2000;77:252–259.
22. Rah MJ, Jackson JM, Jones LA, et al. Overnight orthokeratology: preliminary results from the Lenses and Overnight Orthokeratology (LOOK) study. *Optom Vis Sci*. 2002;79:598–605.
23. Tahhan N, Du Toit R, Papas E, et al. Comparison of reverse-geometry lens designs for overnight orthokeratology. *Optom Vis Sci*. 2003;80:796–804.
24. Swarbrick HA, Alharbi A. Overnight orthokeratology induces central corneal thinning. *Invest Ophthalmol Vis Sci*. 2001;42(suppl):S597.
25. Sridharan R, Swarbrick HA. Corneal response to short-term orthokeratology lens wear. *Optom Vis Sci*. 2003;80(3):200–206.
26. Swarbrick HA, Wong G, O'Leary DJ. Corneal response to orthokeratology. *Optom Vis Sci*. 1998;75:791–799.
27. Swarbrick HA. Orthokeratology review and update. *Clin Exp Optom*. 2006;89:124–143.
28. Alharbi A, La Hood D, Swarbrick HA. Overnight orthokeratology lens wear can inhibit the central stromal edema response. *Invest Ophthalmol Vis Sci*. 2005;46:2334–2340.
29. Alharbi A, Swarbrick HA. The effects of overnight orthokeratology lens wear on corneal thickness. *Invest Ophthalmol Vis Sci*. 2003;44:2518–2523.
30. Caroline, et al. Morphologic changes in cat epithelium following overnight lens wear with the paragon CRT lens for corneal reshaping. Paper presented at: American Academy of Optometry Meeting; December 2003; Dallas, TX.
31. Choo JD, Caroline PJ, Harlin DD. How does the cornea change under corneal reshaping contact lenses? *Eye Contact Lens*. 2004;30:211–213.
32. Hiraoka T, Okamoto C, Ishii Y, et al. Patient satisfaction and clinical outcomes after overnight orthokeratology. *Optom Vis Sci*. 2009;86(7):875–882.
33. Santodomingo-Rubido J, Collar CV, et al. Myopia control with orthokeratology lenses in Spain. (RCOS): refractive and biometric changes [E-abstract 110918]. *Optom Vis Sci*. 2011;88.
34. Queiros A, Villa-Collar C, Gutierrez AR, et al. Quality of life of myopic subjects with different methods of visual correction using the NEI RQL-42 questionnaire. *Eye Contact Lens: Sci Clin Prac*. 2012;38(2):116–121.
35. Ritchey ER. The comparison of overnight lens modalities (COLM) study. Presented at the Annual Meeting of the American Academy of Optometry, Dallas, TX, December, 2003.
36. Walline JJ, Jones LA, Sinnott LT. CRAYON study corneal reshaping and myopia progression. *Br J Ophthalmol*. 2009;93:1181–1185.
37. Cho P, Cheung SW, Edwards M. The longitudinal orthokeratology research in children (LORIC) in Hong Kong: a pilot study on refractive changes and myopia control. *Curr Eye Res*. 2005;30(1):71–80.
38. Joe JJ, Marsden HJ, Edrington TB. The relationship between corneal eccentricity and improvement in visual acuity with orthokeratology. *J Am Optom Assoc*. 1996;67(2):87–97.

39. El Hage SG, Leach NE, Colliac JP, et al. Controlled kerato-reformation (CKR): an alternative to refractive surgery. Presented at: American Academy of Optometry; 1995; New Orleans, LA.
40. Subramaniam SV, Bennett ES, Lakshminarayanan V, et al. Gas Permeable (GP) versus non-GP lens wearers: accuracy of orthokeratology in myopia reduction. *Optom Vis Sci*. 2007;84(5):417–421.
41. Mountford JA. Advanced orthokeratology. Part 2: patient selection and trial lens fitting. *Optician*. 2002;224(5867): 26–37.
42. Rinehart JM, Bennett ES. Orthokeratology. In: Bennett ES, Hom MM, eds. *Manual of Gas Permeable Contact Lenses*. 2nd ed. St. Louis, MO: Elsevier Science; 2004:424–483.
43. Cannella A. A guide to overnight orthokeratology. Rochester, NY: Polymer Technology Corporation; 2002.
44. Rinehart J. Guidelines for advertising and promoting orthokeratology. *Contacto*. 1999;40(10):7–13.
45. Mountford J. Design variables and fitting philosophies of reverse geometry lenses. In: Mountford J, Ruston D, Dave T, eds. *Orthokeratology—Principles and Practice*. London: Butterworth-Heinemann; 2004.
46. Lum E, Swarbrick HA. Lens Dk/t influences the clinical response in overnight orthokeratology. *Optom Vis Sci*. 2011;88(4):469–475.
47. McCampbell K, Bennett ES. Corneal reshaping with the CRT lens made easy. *Contact Lens Spectrum*. 2004(19):30–37.
48. Eiden SB, Davis RL, Bennett ES, et al. The SMART study: background, rationale, and baseline results. *Contact Lens Spectrum*. 2009;24(10):24.
49. Gifford P, Au V, Hon B, et al. Mechanism for corneal reshaping in hyperopic orthokeratology. *Optom Vis Sci*. 2009; 86(4):e306–e311.
50. Mountford JA. Retention and regression of orthokeratology over time. *Int Cont Lens Clin*. 1998;25:59–64.
51. Hiraoka T, Okamoto C, Ishii Y, et al. Time courses of changes in ocular higher-order aberrations and contrast sensitivity after overnight orthokeratology. *Invest Ophthalmol Vis Sci*. 2008;49(10):4314–4320.
52. Kobayashi Y, Yanai R, Chikamoto N, et al. Reversibility of effects of orthokeratology on visual acuity, refractive error, corneal topography, and contrast sensitivity. *Eye Contact Lens: Sci Clin Prac*. 2008;34(4):224–228.
53. Stillitano I, Schor P, Lipener C, et al. Long-term follow-up of orthokeratology corneal reshaping using wavefront aberrometry and contrast sensitivity. *Eye Cont Lens: Sci Clin Prac*. 2008;34(3):140–145.
54. Hiraoka T, Mihashi T, Okamoto C, et al. Influence of induced decentered orthokeratology lens on ocular higher-order wavefront aberrations and contrast sensitivity function. *J Catar Refract Surg*. 2009;35(11):1918–1926.
55. Watt K, Swarbrick HA. Microbial keratitis in overnight orthokeratology: review of the first 50 cases. *Eye Contact Lens*. 2005;31(5):201–208.
56. Watt KG, Boneham GC, Swarbrick HA. Microbial keratitis in orthokeratology: the Australian experience. *Clin Exp Optom*. 2007;90(3):188–189.
57. Kim EC, Kim MS. Bilateral acanthamoeba keratitis after orthokeratology. *Cornea*. 2009;28(3):348–350.
58. Bullimore MA, Jones LA, Sinnott LT. The risk of microbial keratitis with overnight corneal reshaping lenses [E-abstract 90583]. *Optom Vis Sci*. 2009;86.
59. Walline JJ, Holden BA, Bullimore MA, et al. The current state of corneal reshaping. *Eye Contact Lens*. 2005;31(5): 209–214.
60. Choo JD, Holden BA, Papas EB, et al. Adhesion of *Pseudomonas* aeruginosa to orthokeratology and alignment lenses. *Optom Vis Sci*. 2009;86(2):93–97.
61. Caroline PJ. Steepening corneal curvature through overnight ortho-k. *Contact Lens Spectrum*. 2006;21(11):56.
62. Geimer TK. OrthoTool 2000 Lens Design Software; 2001.
63. Lu F. *Biomechanical alteration of corneal morphology after corneal refractive therapy* [master's thesis]. Waterloo, Ontario, Canada: University of Waterloo; 2006.
64. Tung, H.T. Dual geometric lenses for hyperopia Ortho-K. *Contact Lens Spectrum*. 2004;19(10):38–40.
65. Caroline PJ, Andre M. Topographical changes after everted silicone hydrogel wear. *Contact Lens Spectrum*. 2005; 20(6):56.
66. Phillips JR, Anstice NS. *Myopic retinal defocus with a simultaneous clear retinal image slows childhood myopia progression*. Fort Lauderdale, FL: ARVO; 2010.
67. Holden BA, Sankaridurg P, de la Jara PL, et al. *Reduction in the rate of progress of myopia with a contact lens designed to reduce relative peripheral hyperopia*. Fort Lauderdale, FL: ARVO; 2010.
68. Herzberg CM. An update on orthokeratology. *Contact Lens Spectrum*. 2010;25(3):22.

Chapter 23

Management of Contact Lens-Associated or Lens-Induced Pathology

Ron Melton and Randall Thomas

INTRODUCTION

Many contact lens wearers experience years of successful wear with no complications associated with or induced by contact lens wear. However, contact lens wearers can experience ocular complications that are related to the type of lens, the wearing schedule, the solutions they are using or not using, self-inoculation of bacteria from handling of the lens, the case or expired solutions, deposits on the lens, hypoxia from the lens, a foreign body trapped by the lens or something totally nonrelated to the contact lens wear, such as lid disease, dry eyes, or nonrelated anterior segment disease. This chapter will address ophthalmic medicines that can help restore afflicted tissues to normal.

ANTIBIOTICS

Antibiotics can be overused with the contact lens patient. As red eyes are more likely to be inflammatory than infectious, prescribing an antibiotic only because the practitioner is unsure of the diagnosis of the red eye, does not justify its use. The most common symptom/clinical sign to warrant antibiotic use is an acute mucopurulent discharge. If this is not present or there is not a threat to the cornea, topical antibiotic use is usually of no clinical value. Typically, the patient is suffering from an inflammatory condition, not an infection. Proper treatment with a steroid results in improvement. The most common contact lens-associated complications that require the use of antibiotics are infectious keratitis (corneal ulcers), corneal abrasion, bacterial conjunctivitis, blepharitis, and hordeola. Bacterial infections do indeed occur, so the following information will examine how best to treat them.

The four preferred ophthalmic medicines to treat *Staphylococcus aureus* and *Staphylococcus epidermidis* (the two most common ocular pathogens) are gentamicin, trimethoprim with polymyxin B, besifloxacin, and vancomycin. These four drugs have been found to be effective and have the least resistance.[1-4] The first two, gentamicin and trimethoprim with polymyxin B, are generically available. Vancomycin eyedrops have to be compounded and besifloxacin is a chlorofluoroquinolone. It is important to note that fluoroquinolones are not the preferred drugs of choice. This has been known to be the case for several years now. In the management of *Pseudomonas* infections, excellent drugs to use are the fluoroquinolones, besifloxacin, the aminoglycosides, and polymyxin B.

Bacitracin and Polymyxin B

From 1943 to 2012, bacitracin was, and continues to be, highly bactericidal against gram-positive bacteria. It achieves this by destroying the cell wall of the bacteria. Bacitracin is available only in ointment form. It is most effective in treating moderate-to-advanced staphylococcal blepharitis in combination with aggressive lid hygiene. The recommended treatment regimen for bacitracin would be to prescribe it for a period of 1 to 2 weeks to be used on the lid margins at bedtime.

The combination of adding polymyxin B, a potent gram-negative bactericidal agent, to bacitracin, results in a very good broad-spectrum antibiotic. This was originally known as Polysporin ophthalmic ointment and is now available as a generic. This combination drug is beneficial in treating staphylococcal blepharitis when used at bedtime for 2 weeks in combination with lid hygiene (i.e., lid scrubs before applying the ointment). Polysporin ointment use at bedtime, in combination with an antibiotic drop during the day, is especially good for severe eye infections. Bacitracin and polymyxin B remain excellent chemotherapeutic agents, despite being available on the market for a long while.

Trimethoprim with Polymyxin B

Trimethoprim with polymyxin B is marketed generically and also as Polytrim (Allergan). Trimethoprim is bacteriostatic by interfering with folic acid production. It is active against common gram-positive and gram-negative organisms with the exception of *Pseudomonas*, which is why it is combined with polymyxin B. It is available as a 10 mL solution and is effective for bacterial conjunctivitis, as adverse effects are rare. When treating a bacterial conjunctivitis, it is recommended that one drop be instilled every 2 hours (q2h) for 2 days, then four times a day (qid) for 5 more days. Trimethoprim is still a drug-of-choice for treating methicillin-resistant *staphylococcus aureus* (MRSA) species.[3] It has been shown by the Ocular Tracking Resistance in U.S. Today (TRUST) study to be more effective than fluoroquinolones in treating *staphylococcal species*.[5] It is interesting to note that the combination of trimethoprim and sulfamethoxazole in oral medicine (known previously as brand names Bactrim and Septra) is the drug-of-choice for the treatment of systemic MRSA infections.[6]

Aminoglycosides

Gentamicin, tobramycin, and neomycin are aminoglycosides that are bactericidal by inhibiting protein synthesis. Gentamicin and tobramycin are effective against gram-negative and gram-positive organisms, although they are most effective against gram-negative organisms, including *Pseudomonas*. Neomycin is not effective against *Pseudomonas*. Although they are all highly effective antibiotics, occasionally their use can result in a type 4 delayed hypersensitivity reaction. The symptoms of this reaction are conjunctival injection, edema of the lid, and superficial punctate keratitis (SPK). Typically any reaction occurs after use of longer than 1 to 2 weeks. Neomycin is most likely to cause this reaction and thus has acquired an undesirable reputation. However, neomycin is an excellent drug and is widely available in numerous combination products. It is the key ingredient in Neosporin, a superb broad-spectrum antibiotic that contains neomycin, bacitracin, and polymyxin B. Neosporin is available in solution and ointment forms. It is rarely used as an ophthalmic drug because of the potential for hypersensitivity reactions.

Tobramycin and gentamicin have been highly used with patients to fight bacterial infections alone or in combination drugs. Both are available in 0.3% solution or ointment forms by many manufacturers. The majority of pathogenic staphylococcal species are now "methicillin-resistant."[4] Studies have shown that aminoglycosides outperform the fluoroquinolones. The drug-of-choice for MRSA infections is gentamicin.[1-2,7]

Macrolides

Macrolides are bacteriostatic by inhibiting bacterial protein synthesis. There are three macrolide drugs erythromycin, azithromycin, and clarithromycin. Erythromycin is available as an ophthalmic ointment, whereas azithromycin is available as a topical eyedrop.

Erythromycin has been overused resulting in resistance. Due to its limited effectiveness and only being available as an ointment, it is not highly used. However, because it is nontoxic, it can be used as a gentle nocturnal lubricant and antibacterial cover for minimally compromised epithelial tissues.

Azithromycin is a relatively broad-spectrum antibiotic. Data from TRUST shows that it is not as effective as many other commonly used antibiotics, including the fluoroquinolones.[8] Orally, azithromycin is known as Zithromax, which comes as Z-Pak or Tri-Pak. Azithromycin has DuraSite as its vehicle, as does besifloxacin. DuraSite is a gel forming drop that extends the contact time of the drug on the eye.[9] The bottle should be tapped or shaken so that the thick solution is forced into the tip of the bottle. The patients should be instructed to hold their eye open for about 5 to 10 seconds after instillation to allow the drop to spread slightly on the ocular surface to enhance absorption. An advantage of topical ophthalmic azithromycin is its long-lasting clinical effectiveness, and thus its enhanced dosing schedule. AzaSite's recommended dosing schedule is one drop every 12 hours for 2 days, then just one drop daily for 5 more days. A total of nine drops will treat bacterial conjunctivitis. This patient-friendly dosing schedule is especially beneficial in children who may fight instillation of eye drops.

Sodium Sulfacetamide

Sulfa drugs are bacteriostatic, meaning they interfere with bacterial replication, in this case by inhibiting folic acid production. Sulfa drugs are broad spectrum; however, many *staphylococcal* and *Pseudomonas* species are resistant to them.[10] Sodium sulfacetamide is available as a 10% solution or ointment and is marketed by numerous companies. Sulfa drugs are rarely used in eye care at present due to the resistance, possible allergic reactions, and the fact that copious amounts of purulent discharge tend to negate the drug's mechanisms.

Fluoroquinolones

Due to aggressive marketing, fluoroquinolones were the predominant drug used and overused for bacterial infections systemically and topically. The dual mechanism of action was thought to make resistance rare; however, overprescribing and overuse has resulted in resistance becoming a major problem. Fluroroquinolones work by inhibiting DNA synthesis.[11] While these drugs still work well for conjunctivitis, practitioners should be cautious to use them in the treatment of microbial keratitis without culture and sensitivities. Table 23.1 provides the dosing frequency.

Chlorofluoroquinolones

Besifloxacin, marketed as Besivance (Bausch + Lomb), is a 0.6% ophthalmic suspension and the only drug in this category. Two studies, the TRUST study and more recently, the ARMOR (Antibiotic Resistance Management in Ocular micRorganisms) study, have guided prescribing.[4]

TABLE 23.1 Dosing Frequency for Antibiotics

CONDITION	TREATMENT
Bacterial conjunctivitis	Every 2 hr until controlled and then four times a day for 4–6 d.
Bacterial keratitis	Besifloxacin, generic Polytrim, or Gentamicin every 15 min for the first 3–6 hr, then hourly until bedtime. Use Polysporin ointment at night until controlled, then discontinue the ointment. Follow the patient daily and modify the therapy based on the clinical response.
Sterile infiltrate with or without epithelial defect	Combination drug (i.e., Zylet, TobraDexST, Maxitrol) every 2 hr for 2 d, then 4 times a day for 4 d, evaluate clinical response.

The research from this newer study demonstrates the antimicrobial abilities of besifloxacin, a bihalogenated quinolone. This study demonstrated that besifloxacin has the effectiveness at a level equal to vancomycin (the gold standard of gram-positive medicines).[12]

Besifloxacin eyedrops have a very thick consistency, as they use the DuraSite vehicle mentioned previously. It is necessary to allow the medicine to spread out on the surface of the eye prior to blinking, about 5 to 10 seconds, in order to prevent the blink from pushing the drop out of the eye.

In summary, based on updated information regarding MRSA bacteria, the four known antibiotics that demonstrate effective activity are gentamicin, trimethoprim, besifloxacin, and vancomycin. At this time, the authors use predominantly gentamicin, tobramycin, trimethoprim with polymyxin B, and besifloxacin for bacterial infections. There are many other products available on the market that may or may not be highly effective. Table 23.2 provides a summary of antibiotics discussed in this section. Ocular conditions and the recommended antibiotic therapy are provided in Table 23.3.

Combination Corticosteroid–Antibiotic Preparations

There are several corticosteroid–antibiotic combination drugs. These can be found in Table 23.2. These combination drugs can be useful when there is a bacterial infection or epithelial disruption combined with inflammation, such as rosacea, vascularized limbal keratitis (VLK), contact lens-induced acute red eye (CLARE), phlyctenular keratoconjunctivitis, noninfectious keratitis, herpes zoster with ocular involvement, peripheral inflammatory epithelial defects, and staphylococcal blepharitis.[13,14] Most red-eye reactions have an inflammatory component. The authors use the following rule of thumb to determine whether to use a steroid alone or a combination drug: use a steroid for a keratitis or conjunctivitis with an intact epithelium, but in those cases of keratitis or conjunctivitis where there is significant corneal epithelial compromise, use a combination drug. The three most commonly used combination drugs by the authors are Maxitrol (Alcon), Zylet (Bausch + Lomb), and TobraDex ST (Alcon). Combination drugs should never be tapered below qid as this creates subtherapeutic levels of the antibiotic, which may cause antibiotic resistance. The section in this chapter pertaining to corticosteroids should be reviewed for a more complete understanding of this class of drugs.

ALLERGY MEDICATIONS

The incidence of allergies is on the rise; therefore, practitioners must be prepared to effectively treat ocular allergies.[15] Unfortunately, patients sometimes resort to over-the-counter drops that "get the red out" without seeing an eye doctor. The key symptom of ocular allergy is itching. However, if there is also a complaint of a "burning" sensation, clinical evaluation should make sure that other forms of ocular disease, such as dry eyes or solution sensitivity, are not the cause. Patients manifesting dry eyes may experience itching and burning; therefore, tear film dysfunction should be ruled out initially. If the patient is using a preserved contact lens care regimen, changing to a nonpreserved system (i.e., hydrogen peroxide) to determine if that eliminates the symptoms, should be attempted. Other helpful tips would include removing the offending source, frequent hand washing, use of cold compresses, refrigerating drops, and discouraging eye rubbing, which causes degranulation of mast cells, thus perpetuating the allergic cycle. Hair washing at night, prior to sleeping, has been found to help prevent irritants (pollution, dirt, etc.) from being released onto the pillow, decreasing ocular allergies.[15]

Allergies should not be confused with the dry-eye patient, who may present with symptoms of dry, scratchy, itchy, burning, and gritty feeling. Even though itching is one of the symptoms, it is likely resulting from ocular surface tear film dysfunction (i.e., dryness). This form of itching is best managed by treating the underlying dry eye.

TABLE 23.2 Topical Antibiotics and Antibiotic Combinations

GENERIC NAME	BRAND NAME	MANUFACTURER	FORM	SIZE
Sodium sulfacetamide	N/A	Generic	Sol.	15 mL
Bacitracin		Fera	Ung.	3.5 g
Bacitracin/polymyxin B	Polysporin	Monarch/generic	Ung.	3.5 g
Bacitracin/polymyxin B/neomycin	Neosporin	Monarch/generic	Sol./ung.	10 mL/3.5 g
Trimethoprim/polymyxin B	Polytrim	Allergan/generic	Sol.	10 mL
Erythromycin 0.5%	Ilotycin	Fera	Ung.	3.5 g
Azithromycin 1%	AzaSite	Merck	Sol.	2.5 mL
Gentamicin 0.3%	Garamycin	Fera/generic	Sol./ung.	5 mL/3.5 g
Tobramycin 0.3%	Tobrex	Alcon/generic	Sol./ung.	5 mL/3.5 g
Ciprofloxacin 0.3%	Ciloxan	Alcon/generic	Sol./ung.	5 mL/10 mL/3.5 g
Ofloxacin 0.3%	Ocuflox	Allergan/generic	Sol.	5 mL/10 mL
Levofloxacin 0.5%	Quixin	Vistakon Pharm.	Sol.	5 mL
Moxifloxacin 0.5%	Vigamox	Alcon	Sol.	3 mL
Gatifloxacin 0.5%	Zymaxid	Allergan	Sol.	2.5 mL
Besifloxacin 0.6%	Besivance	Bausch + Lomb	Susp.	5 mL
Levofloxacin 1.5%	Iquix	Vistakon Pharm.	Sol.	5 mL
Moxifloxacin 0.5%	Moxeza	Alcon	Sol.	3 mL
Antibiotic/Steroid Combination				
Sodium sulfacetamide 10%/Prednisolone acetate 2%	Blephamide	Allergan/generic	Susp./ung.	5 mL/10 mL/3.5 g
Neomycin/Polymyxin B/hydrocortisone 1%	Cortisporin	Monarch/generic	Susp.	7.5 mL
Neomycin/polymyxin B/dexamethasone	Maxitrol	Alcon/generic	Susp./ung.	5 mL/3.5 g
Neomycin/prednisolone acetate 1%	Poly-Pred	Allergan/generic	Susp.	5 mL/10 mL
Gentamicin/prednisolone 1%	Pred-G	Allergan	Susp./ung.	10 mL/3.5 g
Tobramycin/Dexamethasone 0.1%	TobraDex	Alcon/generic	Susp./ung.	5 mL/3.5 g
Tobramycin/Dexamethasone 0.05%	TobraDex ST	Alcon	Susp.	5 mL/10 mL
Tobramycin/loteprednol 0.5%	Zylet	Bausch + Lomb	Susp.	5 mL/10mL/

TABLE 23.3 Ocular Conditions and Recommended Treatments

OCULAR CONDITION	ANTIBIOTIC
Staphylococcal blepharitis	Bacitracin/Polysporin/TobraDex ointments, or Zylet
Acute eyelid infection	Oral antibiotic
Bacterial conjunctivitis	Aminoglycoside, Besifloxacin, or Polytrim
Corneal abrasion	Fluoroquinolone or aminoglycoside drops with ointment at night, NSAID for pain, and a cycloplegic agent
VLK, CLARE	Antibiotic/steroid combination such as Zylet or TobraDex
Corneal ulcer	Besifloxacin or aminoglycoside drops with Polysporin ointment at night

When itching is the primary symptom and there are minimal signs of allergy (i.e., chemosis, conjunctival injection, or eyelid edema), an antihistamine/mast cell stabilizer is an excellent drug-of-choice. There are six antihistamine/mast cell stabilizers, which are effective in suppressing ocular itching. They are epinastine (Elestat-Allergan), azelastine (Optivar-MedPointe), olopatadine (Patanol & Pataday-Alcon), bepotastine (Bepreve-Bausch + Lomb), alcaftadine (Lastacaft-Allergan), and ketotifen. Ketotifen is available over the counter as Zaditor (Novartis), Alaway (Bausch + Lomb), and Refresh Eye Itch Relief (Allergan). Zaditor and Refresh Eye Itch Relief are available in 5 mL bottles and Alaway is available in a 10 mL bottle, which may be beneficial to the patient in quantity and cost. With the exception of Pataday and Lastacaft, which are once-a-day (qd) dosage, the other medications are used twice a day (bid) morning and night. After the first 2 weeks, many patients can decrease to a maintenance dose of once a day. In addition, cold compresses can be used to decrease ocular inflammation (allergies are an expression of inflammation). Warm compresses may aid ocular infections.

Mast cell stabilizers (i.e., pemirolast [Alamast], nedocromil [Alocril], or cromolyn sodium—generic) used alone have been found to have little clinical use, according to Mark Abelson, MD, a renowned ocular allergist at Harvard University. Based on this expert opinion, the authors no longer prescribe these pure mast cell stabilizers.

For contact lens wearers, antihistamine/mast cell stabilizers can be used a few minutes before insertion and again after contact lens removal. If necessary, the drop can be instilled on top of the contact lens. For those contact lens wearers who experience seasonal ocular allergies, use of loteprednol with an antihistamine/mast cell stabilizer morning and evening, before and after contact lens wear, then decreasing the loteprednol to evening use only, will aid the patient in surviving the allergy season. The various topical allergy drops are listed in Table 23.4.

Giant Papillary Conjunctivitis (GPC)

There are various methods of treating GPC (see discussion in Chapter 13). The authors use an initial approach of lens discontinuation for a week or two while using 0.5% loteprednol qid (or loteprednol ointment qhs). After a week or two, conservative wearing schedules may be resumed. Using loteprednol suspension bid (prior to insertion and after removal) or loteprednol ointment qhs for another 2 weeks may be done as needed. While an increase in intraocular pressure (IOP) is rare, always check the IOP at the 2- and 4-week follow-up visits. If possible, fit the patient into a daily disposable lens.

Contact Dermatitis

Contact dermatitis may be caused by an environmental irritant or an allergic response. In either case, removal of the irritant and use of cold compresses and a topical steroid cream (such as 0.1% triamcinolone) applied around the lids (but not in the eye) can be very helpful. In most

TABLE 23.4 Topical Allergy Drops

GENERIC NAME	BRAND NAME	DRUG CLASS	MANUFACTURER	SIZE (mL)
Acute Care Products				
Ketorolac tromethamine 0.4%	Acular LS	NSAID	Allergan, generic	5, 10
Ketotifen fumarate 0.025%	Alaway (OTC)	AH/MCS	Bausch + Lomb	10
	Claritin Eye (OTC)		Schering-Plough	5
	Refresh (OTC)		Allergan	5
	Zaditor (OTC)		Alcon	5
Loteprednol etabonate 0.2%	Alrex	C	Bausch + Lomb	5, 10
Loteprednol etabonate 0.5%	Lotemax	C	Bausch + Lomb	2.5, 5, 10, 15
Bepotastine besilate 1.5%	Bepreve	AH	Bausch + Lomb	10
Epinastine HCl 0.05%	Elestat	AH/MCS	Allergan	5
Emedastine difumarate 0.05%	Emadine	AH	Alcon	5
Alcaftadine 0.25%	Lastacaft	AH	Allergan	3
Azelastine HCl 0.05%	Optivar	AH/MCS	Meda, generic	6
Olopatadine HCl 0.2%	Pataday	AH/MCS	Alcon	2.5
Olopatadine HCl 0.1%	Patanol	AH/MCS	Alcon	5
Chronic Care Products				
Pemirolast potassium 0.1%	Alamast	MCS	Vistakon	10
Nedocromil sodium 2%	Alocril	MCS	Allergan	5
Lodoxamide tromethamine 0.1%	Alomide	MCS	Alcon	10
Cromolyn sodium 4%	Crolom	MCS	Bausch + Lomb	10
	Opticrom		Allergan	10

OTC, over the counter; AH, antihistamine; C, corticosteroid; MCS, mast cell stabilizer.

cases, simply removing the irritant and applying cold compresses will be therapy enough. Moderate-to-severe cases, however, may require the addition of the steroid cream (i.e., 0.1% triamcinolone) or oral prednisone. The allergic response with the recommended medications is provided in Table 23.5.

TABLE 23.5 Summary Table for Allergy Treatments

ALLERGY RESPONSE	MEDICATION
Allergic conjunctivitis (itching only)	Antihistamine/mast cell stabilizer combination
Allergy with associated inflammation	Alrex, FML, or Lotemax
GPC	Loteprednol 0.5% (Lotemax)

CORTICOSTEROIDS

General Information

The inflammatory response is the result of infectious, allergic, or traumatic factors, which cause the tissue to release an array of inflammatory mediators. Adverse effects of the inflammatory response may be mitigated by use of topical or oral corticosteroids. To better understand how anti-inflammatory agents are effective, it is useful to understand what occurs during the inflammatory process. When infections, allergy, or trauma affect the tissue, phospholipids are released from the cell membrane. These phospholipids convert to arachidonic acid. Arachidonic acid is converted to prostaglandins or leukotrienes via one or two enzymes: either cyclooxygenase or lipoxygenase. Corticosteroids work early in the inflammatory process by prohibiting phospholipids conversion to arachidonic acid. Nonsteroidal anti-inflammatory drugs (NSAIDs) exhibit their effect further down in the pathway to inhibit cyclooxygenase, which converts arachidonic acid to prostaglandins. NSAIDs do not affect production of leukotrienes as mediated by lipoxygenase, thus limiting their use in treating inflammatory processes.[11,14,16]

Corticosteroids' ability to suppress inflammation is based on their potency and bioavailability. The most commonly used ophthalmic corticosteroids are loteprednol, prednisolone, dexamethasone, fluorometholones, and rimexolone. An important factor in treatment with corticosteroids is the frequency of instillation, which varies with the nature and severity of the condition. High doses of topical steroids for brief periods of time (typically several days) are usually safe and effective. The treatment regimen should be customized for each case depending on the severity. A summary table of corticosteroid medications is found in Table 23.6.

The treatment regimen for ketone-based corticosteroids most always concludes with an interval of tapering. There are two reasons for the need to taper the patient off this medication. First, the body produces natural steroids. When synthetic steroids are given, the body slows down production of the natural steroids. By tapering the synthetic steroid, the body is given the opportunity to produce the appropriate amount of natural steroids again, without leaving the body momentarily with low levels of natural steroids. The second reason for tapering steroids is that a rebound effect can otherwise occur. The inflammatory process in the body is being inhibited by the synthetic steroids and abruptly discontinuing them may allow the inflammation to rebound. Once the inflammation is controlled, the steroid should be reduced by one-half for a few days, then perhaps by half again for a few more days. Such a tapering schedule will vary considerably from patient to patient.[17] The mechanism of action of the ester-based corticosteroids does not require tapering.

TABLE 23.6 Topical Corticosteroid Drugs

GENERIC NAME	BRAND NAME	MANUFACTURER	FORM	SIZE
Loteprednol etabonate 0.2%	Alrex	Bausch + Lomb, generic	Susp.	5 mL, 10 mL
Loteprednol etabonate 0.5%	Lotemax	Bausch + Lomb, generic	Susp./ung.	2.5 mL, 5 mL, 10 mL, 15 mL/3.5 g
Difluprednate	Durezol	Alcon	Emul.	5 mL
Prednisolone	Pred Forte	Allergan, generic	Susp.	5 mL, 10 mL, 15 mL
Dexamethasone	Maxidex	Alcon, generic	Susp.	5 mL
Fluorometholone	FML	Allergan, generic	Susp./ung.	5 mL, 10 mL/3.5 g
Rimexolone	Vexol	Alcon, generic	Susp.	5 mL, 10 mL

Regarding traumatic corneal abrasions, most reepithelialization should occur prior to steroid use in most cases. This is not the case when stromal inflammation is inhibiting reepithelialization, or when the corneal epithelium is compromised by something other than an infectious agent (i.e., a welder flash). In these cases, an antibiotic/steroid combination or a steroid in combination with a separate antibiotic may be prescribed.

Side effects from steroid use are less likely to occur with topical than with systemic steroids, but may include posterior subcapsular cataracts, increased IOP, retardation of corneal wound healing, mydriasis, and ptosis.[11] Generally, these side effects are rare and only occur after long-term use of a systemic or ocular steroid. If a patient uses a steroid for more than 2 weeks, it becomes important to monitor IOP. Loteprednol is less likely to increase IOP than are other ophthalmic steroids. Concomitant use of a beta-blocker or brimonidine can be used for pressures above 30 mm Hg. The indications and contraindications for steroid use are given in Table 23.7.

TABLE 23.7 Indications and Contraindications for Corticosteroid Use

Indications
Iritis
Episcleritis
Chemical trauma
Uveitic glaucoma
Glaucomatocyclitic crisis
Ocular trauma
Postoperative care
Phlyctenulosis
Corneal microcystic edema
Corneal infiltrates
Ultraviolet keratitis (UV)
Stromal keratitis
Epidemic keratoconjunctivitis (EKC)
Peripheral corneal erosions
Thygeson SPK
Vernal conjunctivitis
Inflammatory blepharitis
Eczemoid blepharitis
Angular blepharitis
Contact blepharodermatitis
Uveitis
Herpes zoster with ocular involvement
Allergic conjunctivitis
Rosacea
VLK
Contraindications
Herpes simplex infectious epithelial keratitis
Acute bacterial infections
Significant epithelial compromise
Fungal infections

Loteprednol

Loteprednol is available in an ophthalmic suspension in two concentrations: 0.5% (Lotemax) and 0.2% (Alrex). Loteprednol differs from other corticosteroids in that it is ester-based as opposed to ketone-based. This is important, as the ester-based corticosteroid has an excellent anti-inflammatory effect, while minimizing the potential for adverse side effects. This occurs as the tissue esterases break down the ester, reducing its residence time in the tissues. The body does not have enzymes to break down ketones; therefore, ketone-based corticosteroids are more likely to cause side effects, especially with long-term use.

Alrex is approved for treating allergic conjunctivitis. If clinical signs accompany the symptoms of itching (i.e., conjunctival injection or chemosis), Alrex is also beneficial in preventing the inflammatory response. Typical dosage is every 2 hours for 2 days, followed by qid and bid or qd for several more days or weeks.

Lotemax is very popular due to its clinical effectiveness and safety profile. It is useful in treating ocular inflammation with little to no increase in IOP. Although the treatment regimen depends on the ocular condition, a typical treatment regimen would be one drop every 1 to 2 hours for a few days until control of the condition is achieved, then taper the drop to qid for a few days, then bid for a few days, then use of the drop is discontinued. As a suspension drop, the patient should be instructed verbally and via written prescription to shake the bottle prior to use.

Prednisolone

Of all topical ophthalmic corticosteroids, prednisone has the greatest anti-inflammatory efficacy. It is available as Pred Forte (Allergan) and in generic forms in 1% concentration, and as Pred Mild (Allergan) in a 0.12% concentration. The 1% concentration is by far the more clinically useful form. Pred Forte has been demonstrated to be the most effective topical corticosteroid in the management of uveitis and corneal inflammation.[18] It can be used for severe ocular inflammation, such as iritis, episcleritis, and chemical and thermal burns of the cornea. The treatment regimen is similar to loteprednol, depending on the severity of the ocular condition.

Dexamethasone

Dexamethasone is available in suspension (0.1%) manufactured by Alcon as Maxidex, and a solution (0.1%) manufactured by Merck as Decadron. Both of these products are available generically. Dexamethasone is not as effective as prednisone and has an increased risk of elevating IOP; therefore, it is not frequently used.

Fluorometholones

Fluorometholones exhibit good anti-inflammatory properties, in addition to being less likely to increase IOP. They are available in two forms: alcohol and acetate. An example of fluorometholone alcohol is FML (Allergan). It is available in 0.1% and 0.25% suspensions and 0.1% ointment. FML suspension is available generically, and is a good choice when long-term therapy (>3–4 weeks) is necessary as it has a reduced risk for elevating IOP. Of note, the 0.25% concentration is no more effective that the 0.1% formulation, and therefore is rarely used. Individuals exhibiting a chronic iridocyclitis or a long-term ocular allergy would likely benefit from use of fluorometholone or loteprednol.

Fluorometholone acetate is available in a 0.1% concentration generically and as Flarex (Alcon). Flarex is an ophthalmic suspension and therefore needs to be shaken before use. The acetate formulation is slightly more effective than the alcohol form. Fluorometholone acetate, like the alcohol form, has the benefit of a reduced tendency to increase IOP.

Rimexolone

Rimexolone is available as Vexol 1% suspension (Alcon). It has an efficacy almost, but not quite, as high as prednisolone acetate 1% and, like fluorometholones, has a reduced risk of increasing IOP. Rimexolone is also used in the treatment of anterior uveitis.

TABLE 23.8 Corticosteroid Use for Ocular Conditions

CONDITION	CORTICOSTEROID
Allergic conjunctivitis	Loteprednol 0.2%, fluorometholone 0.1%
Episcleritis/iritis	Difluprednate 0.05%, loteprednol 0.5%
Uveitis/corneal inflammation	Difluprednate 0.05%, loteprednol 0.5%
Chemical/thermal burns	Difluprednate 0.05%, loteprednol 0.5%
CLARE	Loteprednol 0.5%, fluorometholone 0.1%
Chronic iridocyclitis	Loteprednol 0.5%
Postoperative inflammation	Any potent steroid
CLARE/VLK/staphylococcal blepharitis	An antibiotic/steroid combination

Eye doctors have not utilized corticosteroids as often as indicated, most likely due to a fear of the potential side effects. However, when an accurate diagnosis is made of ocular inflammation and the drugs are used as intended for short periods of time, these agents are extremely successful in treating inflammation. Steroids should not be used in herpes simplex keratitis, acute bacterial or fungal infections, or when the epithelium is compromised, as they may exacerbate the condition and retard healing. Steroids are very beneficial in reducing inflammation, and the results of inflammation: scarring and neovascularization. The most important factors to consider when using steroids include accurate diagnosis, selecting the appropriate steroid based on the severity of the condition, and the aggressiveness of treatment (i.e., every 1–2 hours until the condition is controlled), and the anticipated longevity of treatment. Tapering the drug and monitoring IOP is wise if the drug is used for more than 2 weeks. Ocular conditions treated with corticosteroids can be found in Table 23.8.

NONSTEROIDAL ANTI-INFLAMMATORY DRUGS (NSAIDS)

The use of topical NSAIDs for contact lens-related complications is rare. Systemic NSAIDs do have an anti-inflammatory effect, but topical NSAIDs provide only minimal direct anti-inflammatory effect, thus limiting their use in primary eye care. As discussed in the previous section, NSAIDs only inhibit cyclooxygenase, one of two enzymes that convert arachidonic acid to inflammatory mediators. The other enzyme, lipoxygenase, which converts arachidonic acid to leukotrienes, is not affected by NSAIDs. Therefore, a patient with corneal inflammation and NSAID use may have some reduction in pain, but may also develop corneal infiltrates. The infiltrates are the result of the leukocytes that, in turn, are the result of the lack of inhibition of leukotrienes.

Topical NSAIDs are primarily used to ameliorate ocular surface pain. Ocular treatment options with topical NSAIDs can be found in Table 23.9.

TABLE 23.9 Uses of Topical Nonsteroidal Anti-Inflammatory Drugs

Corneal abrasions
Postoperative care (i.e., penetrating keratoplasty, cataract surgery)
Treatment for inflamed pterygia or pinguecula (after controlled with a corticosteroid)
Post foreign-body removal
Post laser surgery
Allergic conjunctivitis (ketorolac, etc.)
CME

TABLE 23.10 Topical Nonsteroidal Anti-Inflammatory Drugs

GENERIC NAME	BRAND NAME	MANUFACTURER	SIZE
Ketorolac tromethamine 0.4%	Acular LS	Allergan	5 mL
Ketorolac tromethamine 0.45%	Acuvail	Allergan	Unit-dose
Bromfenac 0.09%	Bromday	Bausch + Lomb	1.7 mL
Diclofenac sodium 1%	Voltaren	Novartis	5 mL
Nepafenac 0.1%	Nevanac	Alcon	3 mL

There are several topical NSAIDs, which include Voltaren (Novartis), Acular LS (Allergan), Bromday (Bausch + Lomb), and Nevanac (Alcon). The generic name of Voltaren is diclofenac sodium 0.1% and Acular LS is ketorolac tromethamine 0.4%. Both of these NSAIDs are prescribed qid and have similar responses. Bromday is bromfenac and is used once daily. Nevanac is nepafenac, and is used tid. It is important that the patient not increase the frequency of administration over the U.S. Food and Drug Administration (FDA)-recommended daily dosage for each drug and, except in the setting of cystoid macular edema (CME), these drugs should not be used for more than 1 week because of the rare complication of corneal melting. Topical NSAIDs may need to be used for a month to treat CME. A summary table of topical NSAIDs can be found in Table 23.10.

ANTIVIRAL MEDICATIONS

Contact lens wear does not cause viral infections, but contact lens wearers can still contract viral infections. The three primary viral diseases that eye doctors encounter are herpes simplex virus (HSV), herpes zoster (varicella zoster) disease, and adenoviral infections (i.e., epidemic keratoconjunctivitis [EKC] and pharyngoconjuctival fever [PCF]). The clinical sign of HSV is dendritiform or geographic epithelial keratitis. HSV is best treated with ganciclovir (Zirgan-Bausch + Lomb) 0.15% ophthalmic gel used five times a day for 4 to 5 days, then three times a day (tid) for 4 to 5 more days. This unique medicine comes in a 5 g tube, and represents the state-of-the-art therapeutic intervention for the HSV. As an "infected-cell specific" medicine, it causes little or no epithelial toxicity.

Prior to the advent of ganciclovir, Viroptic (trifluridine 0.1%) ophthalmic solution by Monarch Pharmaceuticals and its generics were commonly used in the treatment of HSV, and are still available. The treatment regimen for this drug is one drop in the affected eye every 2 hours while awake for 4 to 5 days, then qid for 4 to 5 days. Oral acyclovir in the dosage of 400 mg taken five times a day for 1 week is another effective treatment. Other oral antivirals that may be used are valacyclovir, prescribed 500 mg tid for 1 week, or famciclovir, prescribed 250 mg tid for 1 week. In addition, it is recommended that the patient use a lipid-based artificial tear every 2 to 4 hours. HSV tends to recur episodically, and recurrence rates vary widely.

As few cases of HSV occur as stromal immune keratitis or herpetic uveitis, the epithelial form must be treated with antiviral drugs, but these other immune-related forms benefit from treatment with a potent corticosteroid. The recommended treatment would be to use one of these corticosteroids along with ganciclovir tid or oral acyclovir 400 mg 3 to 4 times a day. This antiviral cover should be used until the steroid drops are decreased to bid, which usually takes about 1 month. It usually takes another month or two before the steroid can be tapered to once a day or every other day, depending on the patient's response.

Herpes zoster most commonly affects the trunk, but the second most common location is the trigeminal nerve, specifically the first (or ophthalmic division) with vesicles appearing on the head or face. When there is ocular involvement with herpes zoster, patients may present to eye doctors or be referred to eye doctors by their primary care physician. Herpes zoster is caused by the latent expression of the varicella zoster virus in persons who have had chickenpox. Treatment of herpes zoster is 800 mg of acyclovir orally five times a day for 1 week. Valacyclovir 1,000 mg, or famciclovir 500 mg tid for 1 week can also be used. All of these oral antivirals are generically available. When the eye is involved (this occurs in about 50% of the ophthalmic division cases), it is expressed predominantly as either iritis, or keratitis, or both.[19] In these cases, aggressive use of a corticosteroid is standard–of-care.

Oral antiviral drugs are activated by viral thymidine kinase phosphorylation, which makes them biologically active. This characteristic makes them potent, but safe. Maximum effect occurs when the virus is treated during the first 3 days of symptoms, but these medications are still helpful up to a week postinfection. Patients with poor kidney function should be treated in conjunction with their nephrologist or primary care physician, to calculate the proper dosage.

PCF is found primarily in children. Besides cool compresses, artificial tears, occasionally vasoconstrictors, and perhaps Alrex qid for 4 to 6 days, these children do not need more aggressive treatment. EKC is found primarily in adults and is much more virulent. Symptoms of EKC include acute red eye, watery discharge, clear cornea, petechial hemorrhages on bulbar conjunctiva, palpable ipsilateral lymphadenopathy and, if left untreated, subepithelial infiltrates and pseudomembranes. One eye is typically affected first, with the second eye exhibiting clinical signs about 2 to 3 days later. There is an excellent therapy that, at this time, is an off-label application. The use of Betadine 5% Sterile Ophthalmic Prep Solution (Alcon), which is povidone-iodine, reduces the probability of spreading the virus by its excellent virucidal action, thus decreasing the length of the condition. The authors recommend the following use of Betadine for EKC:

- Rule out allergy to iodine
- Anesthetize the eye with proparacaine; Betadine stings
- Instill a drop of an NSAID as Betadine can cause corneal stippling
- Instill 2 to 3 drops of Betadine 5% Ophthalmic Prep Solution, have the patient close his/her eyes, and roll the eyes around to ensure contact with all ocular surfaces
- While the eye is closed, use a swab moistened with Betadine to wipe across the lid margins to eliminate the virus in that region
- After 60 to 90 seconds, gently lavage the eye with sterile saline irrigation solution. The eye will still be inflamed from the adenovirus. Prescribe a potent steroid qid for 4 to 5 days to reduce inflammation and provide patient comfort
- Instill another drop of an NSAID in the office to maximize patient comfort

This recommended procedure will reduce the time period of EKC, maintain corneal clarity, and decrease the risk of subepithelial infiltrates and pseudomembranes by reducing the ocular residence time of the virus. If the virus has already been present in the eye for 5 to 6 days, the acute infectious phase has passed. Since EKC usually resolves in 7 to 8 days, the authors do not use Betadine therapy for such patients. In these cases, the use of loteprednol qid for a few days will aid in providing comfort to the patient.

Two studies and much anecdotal evidence show that topical ganciclovir (Zirgan) can impact adenoviral replication and help truncate the course of the disease. Studies show that ganciclovir 0.15% gel (Zirgan) can be quite effective for EKC. The first study found that ocular discomfort was alleviated in 1 week and must be prescribed as soon as possible.[20] The second study showed resolution of EKC within 7.7 days.[21] As can be seen from these two studies, Zirgan significantly shortens the clinical course of such adenoviral infections. Currently, the authors are using the Betadine treatment for severe cases of EKC, and Zirgan for mild-to-moderate cases. Both courses of action are most effective when therapy can be initiated early in the infectious

TABLE 23.11 Antiviral Drugs

GENERIC NAME	BRAND NAME	MANUFACTURER	ADMINISTRATION
Ganciclovir	Zirgan	Bausch + Lomb	Topical
Trifluridine 0.1%	Generic	Generic	Topical
Acyclovir	Generic	Generic	Oral
Valacyclovir	Generic	Generic	Oral
Famciclovir	Generic	Generic	Oral
Povidone-iodine	Betadine 5% Ophthalmic Prep Solution	Alcon	Topical

phase. We use the same dosage of Zirgan as would be used in treating HSV infections. A listing of antiviral drugs is provided in Table 23.11.

DRY EYES

Management

A large percentage of the population experiences "dry" eyes and many contact lens "dropouts" attribute their discontinuation of lens wear to "dry" eyes.[22] There are many causes of dry-eye symptoms. Some of these symptoms have been discussed in other chapters, such as solution sensitivity (Chapter 12) and contact lens troubleshooting (Chapters 8 and 13). If the contact lens wearer complains of dry eyes, a thorough evaluation of the precorneal tear film should be performed (Chapter 1). Contact lens wearers should be carefully monitored if they have a less than 10 second tear breakup time (TBUT). Infrequent (<12 blinks per minute) and incomplete blinks may also contribute to dryness symptoms. Express the central meibomian glands for 15 seconds to assess their function. Observation of the lacrimal lake height/volume should be noted as well.

Many times a solution sensitivity mimics dry-eye symptoms; therefore, altering the solution to preferably a nonpreserved solution, such as a hydrogen peroxide system, or using daily disposable lenses with no solution should be beneficial. In gas-permeable (GP) wearers, using a different care regimen, or using daily cleaner and weekly enzyme, can result in more comfortable lens wear. Plasma coating GP lenses may increase the lens comfort and decrease the dryness symptoms.[23-25] Another alternative for soft lens wearers is to use one of the commercially available soft lenses that have claimed to be more comfortable for patients with dry eyes, such as Proclear (CooperVision), Extreme H_2O (Hydrogel Vision Corp.), Dailies Aquacomfort Plus (Alcon), 1 Day Acuvue Moist (Vistakon), and silicone hydrogel materials. Frequent use of a nonpreserved contact lens rewetting drop will hydrate and rinse the lens in the eye. Initiating lid scrubs, warm compresses, and lid massage for 2 weeks prior to lens wear can increase the TBUT. More severe cases of blepharitis or meibomian gland dysfunction (MGD) may require a topical antibiotic/steroid combination, such as Zylet, or oral doxycycline 50 mg qd for 3 to 4 months. If these alternatives do not help and dysfunctional tear film has been diagnosed, rewetting drops, lipid-based artificial tears, punctal plugs, anti-inflammatory therapy, and nutritional supplements, such as 2,000 mg daily of fish oil, may be beneficial.

Severe dry eyes are contraindicated for contact lens wear; however, therapy prior to instituting contact lens wear or concurrent therapy may improve the success of the dry-eye patient. This is especially important in patients who exhibit keratoconus, who need contact lenses to meet their visual needs, but suffer from a dysfunctional tear film. In treating dry-eye patients, the practitioner and the patient need to be flexible to determine what will be most successful

TABLE 23.12 Options to Improve Dryness Symptoms

CONDITION	THERAPY
Mild dry eyes	Lipid-based artificial tears Loteprednol 0.2% bid for 2 mo Omega-3 fatty acid supplementation
Moderate dry eyes	Lipid-based artificial tears and gel at bedtime Loteprednol 0.5% qid for 3 wk, then bid for 3 wk Punctal plugs Omega-3 fatty acid supplementation
Severe dry eyes	Lipid-based artificial tear Loteprednol 0.5% qid for 4 wk, then bid for 4 wk, then pulse-dose prn qid for 1 wk Oral doxycycline 50 mg/d for 2 mo Omega-3 fatty acid supplementation Punctal plugs (after the above measures have been in effect for 1–2 mo) Lacrisert inserts LipiFlow procedure Moisture shields

for each patient. Sometimes combining various therapies may increase success and sometimes a new therapy may replace an old one. For example, a particular lens type with a specific lens care regimen (or solution) used in conjunction with punctal plugs and rewetting drops may be most successful for one patient, while another patient may be able to eliminate rewetting drops after insertion of punctal plugs. Trial and error combined with patience is required to determine what will be most effective for each patient. After utilizing contact lens materials, solutions, and rewetting drops alone without success, some other options to improve dryness symptoms are given in Table 23.12. Each of these therapeutic options may be successful alone, but some patients may require use of two or more therapies concurrently for the relief of symptoms. For the contact lens wearers, it is hoped that the therapies used would improve their likelihood of successful lens wear.

Artificial Tears

When recommending artificial tears, the practitioner must decide on viscosity (low, medium, or high), preservatives (preserved, nonpreserved, or transiently preserved), container (bottled or unit dosage), and preparation (solution, emulsion, gel, or ointment). Probably, the most important factor is the patient usage. Patients tend to be negligent about frequency of instillation of artificial tears. Instilling the drops as directed is the first hurdle in combating dry-eye symptoms. Use of artificial tears every 4 hours is recommended. Use of a gel-type artificial tear, just prior to contact lens instillation with rewetting drops during lens wear, has been found to be beneficial.[26] Realizing that most "dry eye" results from lipid-layer dysfunction, the initial use of a lipid-based artificial tear is recommended.

Punctal Plugs

Punctal occlusion is underutilized. Possible reasons for this underutilization include the cost, the lack of effectiveness of trial occlusion with collagen plugs, and loss of plugs. If punctal occlusion is indicated, it is best to directly proceed with "permanent" silicone plugs. Punctal plugs may be beneficial for patients with moderate tear film volume and those with markedly reduced tear film volume if they use artificial tears concurrently. Infrequent use of artificial tears with punctal occlusion and a small lacrimal lake results in a stagnant tear film, which may increase symptoms of dryness and increase inflammatory agents. Lotemax qid for 2 weeks, followed by bid for 2 weeks and artificial tears should be used prior to punctal occlusion. To prevent loss of the punctal plug, it is suggested that the largest plug size that can be placed in the puncta be used. Punctal gauges aid in determination of the optimal size. The doctor may administer a trial by occluding only the inferior punctum of the more symptomatic eye or by occluding both the lower punctum at the same time.

Anti-inflammatory Therapy

Inflammation results from tear film hyperosmolarity as a result of tear film evaporation. In order to suppress inflammation, a steroid should be used. Some people may be helped with topical cyclosporine-A; however, a short course of a potent topical corticosteroid (qid for 2 weeks, then bid for 2–4 more weeks) rapidly suppresses the inflammatory component and helps patients feel better.

Lipid-based artificial tears are useful for dry eyes, because it is lipid insufficiency that causes most cases of ocular surface inflammatory disease. Systane Balance (Alcon), FreshKote (Focus Laboratories), or Refresh Optive Advanced (Allergan) are all lipid-based artificial tears that can be used to treat the patient. Patients should be encouraged to use the drops as frequently as they would like during the day. When using two different eyedrops, patients should wait 15 minutes between drops.

When using corticosteroid suppression to treat ocular surface inflammatory disease, patients often will aggressively follow the treatment regimen only to lose enthusiasm and lessen their treatment with artificial tears or fish oil supplements. This results in the recurrence of inflammation. At this point, a pulse-dose steroid use (i.e., qid for 1 week) can bring symptoms back under control. Based on patient observation, the authors have found that one 5 mL bottle of the steroid should be all that is needed for a full year. Patients should be encouraged to keep the treatment regimen going to see full benefits.

Management of Meibomian Gland Dysfunction (MGD)

Initially, aggressive treatment with lid scrubs, lid massage, and warm compresses (2–4 times a day) may improve the appearance of the lid margins and the function of the meibomian glands. However, patient compliance is a limiting factor, just as in artificial tear use. If bacterial blepharitis is observed, use of an antibiotic/steroid in conjunction with lid scrubs, warm compresses, and lid massage aid in improving this condition.[27] The use of oral doxycycline has been found to be beneficial in treating MGD.[28] The authors recommend using 50 mg qd for 3 to 4 months. Side effects in adults are uncommon, but may include vaginal yeast infections and photosensitivity. The tetracyclines are contraindicated in pregnant women, nursing mothers, and children under the age of 8 years.

MGD can be improved by encouraging the patients to increase essential fatty acids in their diet. This can be derived from supplements of flaxseed, fish, or krill oil. The authors encourage their patients to take 2,000 mg of fish oil every day. The patient will find that there is less disruption to the digestive system if the fish oil is taken with a meal. Meibomian glands build up the tear's lipid layer. There are many possible reasons why the meibomian glands fail to function optimally, including western diet, ambient air, hormonal imbalance, keratinization of the linings of the gland, or glandular obstruction. If the meibomian glands are not producing adequate amounts of lipids for the tears, supplementing with a lipid-based artificial tear should be helpful.

Two recommendations for patients who have trouble swallowing fish oil capsules are Coromega Orange Squeeze (www.coromega.com) or Nordic Naturals (www.nordicnaturals.com). These supplements can be purchased from online Internet sources (i.e., Amazon.com).

The LipiFlow technology (Tearscience, Inc.) developed by Donald Korb, O.D. and his research team is a device used to treat MGD. The device applies heat to the inside of the upper- and lower-lid margins, while applying pressure on the outside of the upper and lower lids. The massaging action expresses the glandular contents. The entire process takes about 12 minutes and has been shown to give relief for several months from dry-eye symptoms. A deficient lipid layer of the tears causes evaporation which, in turn, causes the tear film to become hyperosmotic. The tear hyperosmolarity effects the inflammation of the ocular surface. This device may benefit patients that remain symptomatic after other medical treatment has been attempted.[29]

In summary, the authors recommend the following steps for treatment of dry eye:

- Use of a steroid qid for 2 weeks and then bid for a month
- Use of a lipid-based artificial tear as frequently as needed
- Taken daily with a meal, 2,000 mg of fish oil by mouth
- If needed after 2 to 4 weeks of steroid treatment, punctal plugs
- If the patient becomes symptomatic, repulse the steroid qid for a week (this might be necessary once or twice throughout the year)

TREATMENT OF FUNGAL INFECTIONS

Fungal infections are rare, but are usually encountered more commonly in hot, humid climates. *Candida*, *Aspergillus* and *Curvularia* are the fungi that can commonly cause infections in the United States.[30] *Fusarium* is the most common cause of fungal keratitis in the United States and *Aspergillus* is the most common cause in the world.[17] Fungi cause ocular damage by the presence of the organism, an infiltrative inflammatory response, and secondary damage is caused by the fungal toxins and enzymes. Risk factors for infection include trauma, extended wear of contact lenses, poor care and hygiene of contact lenses, and diabetes. Presenting symptoms and clinical signs include foreign-body sensation, decreased vision, tearing, redness, stromal infiltration with feathery borders and a dry, whitish-gray, slightly elevated lesion on the cornea. The overlying epithelium may or may not be intact and often satellite lesions, immune rights, and hypopyon may be observed.[31] Laboratory testing of corneal scraping is cytologically diagnostic; however, deeper more invasive biopsy may be required to obtain tissue samples. Due to the deep stromal infection, treatment may be difficult; therefore, partial debridement of the cornea may be necessary to enhance drug penetration. Several weeks of topical therapy is required to achieve clinical success.

The drug-of-choice is natamycin, manufactured by Alcon as Natacyn 5%, which is effective against a variety of fungi. Another drug is amphotericin B, which must be compounded by a pharmacist into an eyedrop formulation. Initially, one drop of natamycin should be used every 15 minutes for a few hours. In treating fungal infections, both natamycin and amphotericin B are typically used, alternating one drop every 30 minutes and a few times during the night until the epithelial defect has reduced in size. Typically, the eye would be cyclopleged during this treatment. Concurrent use of an oral antifungal like ketoconazole or voriconazole is rarely used. When the defect is decreased in size, drop administration can be decreased to alternating every hour. If the eye continues to improve after 2 weeks, amphotericin B can be discontinued as it tends to cause ocular irritation. Natamycin can be used every hour or two for another 10 to 14 days and then decreased to one drop every 4 hours until vision is improved and the lesion appears inactive. At this time, the patient should continue to be observed weekly. Treatment with natamycin will typically take 4 to 8 weeks. In severe cases, a conjunctival flap, penetrating keratoplasty, or corneal graft may be required. Corticosteroids should not be used in these patients unless, after several weeks of antifungal treatment, a corticosteroid is needed to quiet the eye and minimize scarring.

ACANTHAMOEBA KERATITIS

Acanthamoeba is a water-borne protozoa that exists as a cyst or in a trophozoite form. The cyst form is more difficult to eliminate. Fortunately, with increased knowledge and better patient education, this form of infection is rare.[32,33] Thorough contact lens care, proper solution use, not using tap water on contact lenses, and not swimming in contact lenses, especially in fresh water lakes, etc., are the best ways to prevent *acanthamoeba* keratitis. Clinical signs and symptoms of this type of infection include a variably injected eye with pain, photophobia, and tearing. Generally, the symptoms will be more severe than the clinical signs. As the infection increases, epithelial lesions that may appear dendritic and a stromal ring or partial ring of infiltrates may be observed. Left untreated or misdiagnosed, this infection can lead to corneal perforation. As in most conditions, early diagnosis will enable the best results. Tissue biopsy can be helpful in diagnosing *acanthamoeba*. When making a differential diagnosis with herpes simplex, *acanthamoeba* generally has severe pain and few associated clinical signs; generally, herpes simplex will have more clinical signs and less discomfort.[34] Treatment of *acanthamoeba* consists of medications, including antifungals (fluconazole or clotrimazole), cationic antiseptics (polyhexamethylene biguanide or chlorhexidine), diamides (propamidine), and aminoglycosides (neomycin or paromomycin). A combination of two to three of the above medications is generally most effective and treatment should continue for 3 to 4 months after all clinical signs have resolved. Successful treatment with cationic antiseptics and diamide, given every hour for 2 to 4 days, reducing to every 2 hours for 3 to 4 days and then maintained on a maintenance dose of polyhexamethylene biguanide or chlorhexidine for 3 to 4 months, has shown effectiveness.[35] Epithelial debridement will sometimes improve the success of the treatment process. Another treatment regimen is to use a combination of polyhexamethylene biguanide or chlorhexidine, propamidine, and neomycin solution after debridement of the epithelium. The use of antibiotics prophylactically may be used in conjunction with these regimens.[36]

CLINICAL CASES

CASE 1

A rigid GP patient presents with discomfort in his right eye for the last few weeks. Visual acuity is 20/20 OU. Upon slit-lamp examination, there is grade 2 staining at the 3 o'clock and 9 o'clock positions OU, with increased staining on the right eye in the temporal area and a slightly elevated white lesion. The eyes are more injected in the temporal quadrant OU. Evaluation of the lens fit shows the lenses fit intrapalpebral and the lenses come to rest next to the arch of the lesion. The diagnosis is VLK.

SOLUTION: Lens wear is discontinued. An antibiotic/steroid combination drug (e.g., Zylet) is prescribed to be used qid for 1 week, and then tapered to bid. The patient is to return for follow-up in 3 to 4 days. When it is determined that the patient can resume lens wear, the patient should be refitted in a lens that exhibits a tucked-under-the-upper-lid position and provides better tear exchange. The patient is instructed to use a contact lens rewetting drop or a lipid-based artificial tear to aid in lubricating the cornea.

CASE 2

A patient presents for a routine eye examination and contact lenses. She complains of itchy eyes in addition to decreased contact lens comfort toward the end of the day. She has a history of seasonal allergies and is taking Allegra every day. The patient is currently wearing soft contact lenses that are replaced quarterly. Visual acuities are OD 20/30 and OS 20/25. Slit-lamp examination shows grade 3 papillae on the superior tarsal plates, mild injection, and deposits on the contact lenses. The diagnosis is GPC.

SOLUTION: The patient is refit into a daily disposable contact lens and is started on loteprednol 0.5% qid for 2 weeks, or Lotemax ophthalmic ointment qhs for 2 weeks. The patient should return for follow-up in 2 weeks. If an improvement is not observed, contact lens wear should be discontinued until symptoms have subsided.

CASE 3

A patient complains of an irritated, watery, and red left eye since awakening this morning. The patient reports sleeping in her hydrogel contact lenses the prior evening and had removed them upon awakening. Aided visual acuities are OD 20/20 and OS 20/30. Upon slit-lamp examination, four small infiltrates are present in the peripheral cornea OS. Diffuse SPK that stains lightly with fluorescein is also present OU. The bulbar conjunctiva is grade 1+ injected OD and grade 2 injected OS. The diagnosis is CLARE.

SOLUTION: Discontinue contact lens wear until the condition fully resolves. Start the patient on an antibiotic/steroid combination drug (i.e., Zylet or TobraDex) qid OS, and a preservative-free artificial tear qid OU. The patient should follow up in 2 or 3 days, or sooner if there is any worsening of symptoms. After symptom resolution is achieved, the patient should be refitted into contact lenses of silicone hydrogel material, and given a daily wear regimen.

CASE 4

A low-Dk soft contact lens wearer presents complaining of a irritated, red right eye that has existed for 2 days. The patient acknowledges sleeping in his contact lenses 3 to 4 days per week. Entering visual acuities are OD 20/25 and OS 20/20. Slit-lamp examination reveals three midperipheral subepithelial infiltrates located inferiorly on the right cornea. The bulbar conjunctiva is diffusely injected grade 1+. There is grade 1 fluorescein staining of the epithelium over the infiltrates and the anterior chamber is deep and quiet. The diagnosis is infiltrative keratitis.

SOLUTION: Discontinue contact lens wear until the condition resolves. Start an antibiotic/steroid combination (i.e., Zylet or TobraDex), q2h OD for 2 days, the qid day for 4 days. A lipid-based artificial tear may be used every 2 to 3 hours as palliative therapy. Follow up in 2 to 3 days. When the condition is under control, refit the patient into a contact lens of silicone hydrogel material and monitor as needed.

CASE 5

A keratoconic patient complains of discomfort and dryness when wearing his contact lenses. As the patient's visual acuity through spectacles is reduced as compared to contact lens wear, he is highly motivated to continue in his contact lenses. The diagnosis is dry eyes.

SOLUTION: The patient experiences better comfort with a piggyback design contact lens, and frequent use of a lipid-based artificial tear diminishes symptoms of dryness. Punctal plugs are somewhat helpful. The patient is advised to take omega-3 fatty acid supplements. He finds that the supplements and lubricating drops, in conjunction with the piggyback design contact lenses, lengthen his wearing time and increase his contact lens comfort.

CLINICAL PROFICIENCY CHECKLIST

- Never taper antibiotics below recommended dosage.
- Not knowing the diagnosis is not justification for prescribing an antibiotic.
- Bacterial eye infections in adults are uncommon events, whereas inflammatory conjunctivitis or keratoconjunctivitis is common.
- Evidence or history of mucopurulent discharge should be present to diagnose infection.
- Monotherapy with corticosteroids is only contraindicated in herpes simplex keratitis, acute bacterial infection, and fungal infections.

- For bacterial conjunctivitis or prophylaxis, select an aminoglycoside, besifloxacin, or generic Polytrim. When treating an infectious keratitis, use besifloxacin, an aminoglycoside, or fortified antibiotics.
- Prescribe a dosing frequency commensurate with the nature of the clinical presentation. The more severe the condition, the more frequent the dosage should be.
- Regarding steroid use, always gain good control of the inflammatory condition before beginning the tapering process. The longer it takes to gain control, the longer the tapering process should be.
- Any disease process observed at or near the limbus is almost always inflammatory in nature.
- Many inflamed eyes require an antibiotic/steroid combination as opposed to an antibiotic or steroid alone.
- Risk factors for ulcerative keratitis are overnight contact lens wear, poor tear film function, uncontrolled staphylococcal blepharitis, smoking, swimming with contact lenses, respiratory infection, and being under the age of 22 years.
- Perform a therapeutic trial with loteprednol qid for 2 to 4 weeks for symptomatic dry eye. Pulse-dose qid for 1 week once or twice a year as needed for symptomatic breakthrough episodes.
- Drugs such as bacitracin, polymyxin B, the aminoglycosides, and besifloxacin are not used orally; therefore, resistance is exceedingly rare. These drugs remain excellent choices for topical ophthalmic use.

REFERENCES

1. Ta CN, Chang RT, Singh K, et al. Antibiotic resistance patterns of ocular bacterial flora: a prospective study of patients undergoing anterior segment surgery. *Ophthalmology.* 2003;110(10):1946–1951.
2. Deramo VA, Lai JC, Winokur J, et al. Visual outcome and bacterial sensitivity after methicillin-resistant staphylococcus aureus-associated acute endophthalmitis. *Am J Ophthalmol.* 2008;145(3):413–417.
3. Asbell PA, Colby KA, Deng S, et al. Ocular TRUST: nationwide antimicrobial susceptibility patterns in ocular isolates. *Am J Ophthalmol.* 2008;145(6):951–958.
4. Haas W, Pillar CM, Torres M, et al. Monitoring antibiotic resistance in ocular microorganisms: results from the Antibiotic Resistance Monitoring in Ocular micRorganisms (ARMOR) 2009 surveillance study. *Am J Ophthalmol.* 2011;152(4):567–574.
5. McDowell PJ, Sahm DF. Longitudinal nationwide surveillance of antimicrobial susceptibility in ocular isolates (Ocular TRUST 2). Presented at: Annual Meeting of the American Academy of Ophthalmology; November 10–13, 2007; New Orleans, LA. Poster P0052.
6. Diaz E, Fernandez IM, Jimenez L, et al. Is methicillin-resistant staphylococcus aureus pneumonia epidemiology and sensitivity changing? *Am J Med Sci.* 2012;343(3):196–198.
7. Alabiad CR, Miller D, Schiffman JC, et al. Antimicrobial resistance profiles of ocular and nasal flora in patients undergoing intravitreal injections. *Am J Ophthalmol.* 2011;152(6):999–1004.
8. Karlowsky JA, Thornsberry C, Jones ME, et al. TRUST surveillance program. Factors associated with relative rates of antimicrobial resistance among streptococcus pneumonia in the United States: results from the TRUST Surveillance Program (1998–2002). *Clin Infect Dis.* 2003;15;36(8):963–970.
9. http://www.insitevision.com/durasite. Accessed August 20, 2012.
10. Sulfacetamide Sodium Ophthalmic Ointment USP 10% [package insert]. Melville, NY: Fougera; 1998.
11. Dewart MR, Elliott LJ. Management of Contact Lens-Associated or Lens-Induced Pathology. In: Bennett ES, Henry VA, eds. *Clinical Manual of Contact Lenses.* 2nd ed. Philadelphia, PA: Lippincott Williams & Wilkins; 2000;582–610.
12. Haas W, Deane J, Morris TW, et al. Antibiotic Resistance Profile of Ocular Pathogens—an Update from the ARMOR 2011 Surveillance Study. Presented at: Annual Meeting of Association for Research in Vision and Ophthalmology; May 10, 2012; Fort Lauderdale, FL. Poster 6195/D1055.
13. Epstein AB, Quinn CJ. Diseases of the conjunctiva. In: Bartlett JD, Jaanus SD, eds. *Clinical Ocular Pharmacology.* Boston: Butterworth Heinemann; 2001;545–601.
14. Melton R, Thomas R. 2012 Clinical guide to ophthalmic drugs. *Rev Optom.* 2012;149(suppl 6) 1A–48A.
15. Lanier B. Allergy-on the rise and in the news. *Refractive Eyecare.* 2006;10(2):1,32–34.

16. Silbert JA. Inflammatory responses in contact lens wear. In: Silbert JA, ed. *Anterior Segment Complications of Contact Lens Wear*. 2nd ed. Boston: Butterworth Heinemann; 2000;109–131.
17. Krupin T, Mandell AI, Podos SM, et al. Topical corticosteroid therapy and pituitary adrenal function. *Arch Ophthalmol*. 1976;94(6):919–920.
18. Leibowitz HM, Kuferman A. Anti-inflammatory medications. *Int Ophthalmol Clin*. 1980;20(3):117–134.
19. Pavan-Langston D. Herpes zoster ophthalmicus. *Neurology*. 1995;45(12)(suppl 8):S50–S51. Review.
20. Verin PH, Mortemousque B, Barach D. Ganciclovir 0.15% gel, a new treatment in epidemic keratoconjunctivitis (EKC). *Ophthalmic Res*. 1997;29(suppl 1):12–27.
21. Tabbara KF, Goldschmidt PL, Nobrega R. Ganciclovir effects in adenoviral keratoconjunctivitis. Presented at: Annual Meeting of Association for Research in Vision and Ophthalmology; 2001; Fort Lauderdale, FL. Poster 3111-B253.
22. Begley C, Chalmers R, Mitchell L, et al. Characterization of ocular surface symptoms from optometric practices in North America. *Cornea*. 2001;20:610–618.
23. Schafer J. Plasma treatment for GP contact lenses. *Contact Lens Spectrum*. 2006;21(11):19.
24. Bennett ES. To plasma treat of not to plasma treat? *Rev Cornea Contact Lenses*. November 2006;9.
25. Rakow PL. Plasma treatments improve GP comfort. *Vision Care Product News*. October. 2006;76–78.
26. DeKinder JO. Maximizing soft lens comfort. *Contact Lenses Today*. April 2007.
27. Caroline PJ, Andre MP, Kame RT. Dermatologic complications of the lids and adnexa. In: Silbert JA, ed. *Anterior Segment Complications of Contact Lens Wear*. 2nd ed. Boston: Butterworth Heinemann; 2000:171–196.
28. Driver PJ, Lemp MA. Meibomian gland dysfunction. *Surv Ophthalmol*. 1996;40(5):343–367.
29. http://www.tearscience.com/physician/breakthroughtechnology/dry-eye-treatment-science/. Accessed August 20, 2012.
30. Ward MA. Mycotic keratitis and lens care. *Contact Lens Spectrum*. 2006;21(7):27.
31. Schornack MM. Clinical management of fungal keratitis. *AOA News*. April 24, 2006:17–18.
32. Joslin CE, Tu EY, McMahon TT, et al. Epidemiological characteristics of a Chicago-area Acanthamoeba Keratitis outbreak. *Am J Ophthalmol*. 2006;142(2):212–217.
33. Gutman C. Acanthamoeba keratitis increasing at alarming rate. *Ophthalmol Times*. January 1, 2006.
34. Townsend W. Beyond the branches: a closer look at ocular herpes, part 1. *Contact Lens Spectrum*. 2004;19(1):45.
35. Miller W. Acanthamoeba Keratitis. *Contact Lens Spectrum*. 2003;18(3):51.
36. Lingel N, Casser L. Diseases of the cornea. In: Bartlett JD, Jaanus SD, eds. *Clinical Ocular Pharmacology*. 4th ed. Boston: Butterworth Heinemann; 2001:603–672.

Chapter 24

Contact Lens Practice Management

Nicky Lai, Carmen Castellano, Barry Eiden, Jason Jedlicka, Clarke Newman, Thomas Quinn, and Glenda Secor

A good understanding of contact lens design, lens material, and fitting technique is essential to the practice of contact lenses. Another important aspect of contact lenses is the management and administration of the contact lens practice. Knowing how to successfully integrate and incorporate contact lens fitting within the examination flow will maximize practitioner time as well as provide a good contact lens experience for the patient. With successful patient education, effective contact lens care and compliance will improve. Integrating the following ideas into the contact lens practice will increase success and patient satisfaction.

THE PATIENT ENCOUNTER

Patients select a particular practice for a variety of reasons. It may be for the convenience of the practice location to work or home. The provider may be listed on the patient's vision or major medical insurance plan. Patients may have been impressed by media marketing efforts of the practice in the community. Patients may also choose a practice based on a word-of-mouth recommendation of a trusted friend or by referral of another health care provider. Of all the variety of ways to bring patients into your practice, this latter example appears to be the most important. Word-of-mouth recommendations and referrals usually involve a positive previous experience that was provided; therefore, it is important to match that expectation and continue that opinion. Doing so can also help expand that network of satisfied patients.

One of the first impressions a patient has with the practice is the interaction with the initial phone call to the appointment staff. The appointment staff should present themselves as a patient advocate to help navigate the patient through the office. This staff person should be able to triage the appointment by listening to patients' needs and scheduling an appropriate appointment time. An example of something the appointment staff member may say is: "I understand that you are having issues with your contact lenses that we would like to address in your exam. I think the best time for your appointment would be 2 o'clock as this would allow the doctor to best address your concerns. Would this be convenient for you?"

The goal of specifying appointment times for the patient is to maximize the efficiency and flow of the office. Having a staggered schedule of comprehensive examinations and follow-up checks allows the practitioner time to move from one patient to the next to provide expertise without significant wait times for the patient or practitioner.

The next service that the appointment staff member can provide is information to locate the office and expectations of the encounter. These expectations should include arrival time, the type of paper work that may need to be completed, the possibility of pupil dilation to monitor ocular health, special testing that may need to be performed, and costs of the examination and professional fees. The patients should be reminded to bring current contact lens prescriptions, current spectacles, and to wear their contact lenses into the examination such that the practitioner can evaluate the contact lenses. A range of professional fees can be presented at this time, but should not be specifically quoted until the patient has been evaluated. An example of appointment staff script is: "During your examination, the doctor will determine your visual needs and present you with the best option for your vision and eye health. Professional fees will be discussed with you before any services are performed." This would be an appropriate time to clarify insurance coverage and address those issues. The appointment staff may ask the patient to speak to the insurance staff at a later time if the patient has more specific questions on insurance coverage. The insurance staff can better explain details of coverage plan as well as provide information on the difference between vision plans and major medical plans.

Upon arrival on the day of the appointment, the check-in staff should verify personal and insurance information. The technician or intake staff should start working with the patient to obtain pretesting examination data. This should include contact lens histories, lens wear and replacement schedule, cleaning systems and regimen, including specific solutions used, any eye medication either prescribed or over the counter, and any specific complaints with the contact lenses. Depending on the level of staff training, the contact lenses can be evaluated and an overrefraction can be performed before the practitioner enters the examination room. During the examination, the staff or technician can help as a scribe for the doctor in documenting examination findings. After the examination is complete, a staff member should be present as the practitioner reviews the examination findings and recommendations as well as general fees associated with the services. At this time, the staff member can discuss exact fees and costs with the patient. If a new contact lens is to be fit, the staff can obtain the diagnostic lenses from the practitioner and apply the lenses on the patient's eye. While the new lenses are settling, this would be a good time for the technician to review contact lens wear and care as well as the expectations of contact lens wear. When the practitioner returns to perform the final evaluation, the patients will have already been educated on their contact lenses and the doctor can review and reinforce the information.

After the examination is complete, the technician or staff can escort the patient to the optical dispensing area for spectacle selection or contact lens orders.

The check-out staff member can then complete billing and payments as well as schedule follow-up visits, or make preappointments for the next annual examination.

Of course, any of the tasks may be performed by many of the staff members as well as the same staff member and can be performed by the doctor given the personnel resources available to each practice. The issues that may arise from the patient encounter will be discussed in greater detail.

STAFF EDUCATION

In order for this type of examination flow to work, the technician or staff must be well trained. The staff should be able to answer patient questions and make recommendations regarding general contact lens product information, care regimens, and basic ocular health in line with the practitioner's preferences and practice. The well-trained technician is the "right hand" of the doctor and acts as the bridge between the patient and doctor. In a practice with multiple doctors, it may be helpful for each doctor to have a dedicated staff member or team that works closely with that doctor as opposed to questions or phone calls fielded by any of the staff members.

In any office, the level of training and experience of a new staff member can range from years of experience as a certified optometric technician to a complete novice. A variety of resources can help with basic contact lens education. Many contact lens manufacturers provide training resources for optometric staff specific to contact lens materials and designs, as well as general practice management. Manufacturer representatives can also provide valuable information on products used in the office. Any information that is provided to the doctor on pharmaceuticals, care systems, or contact lens materials should be shared with the staff. The American Optometric Association has a paraoptometric center that provides reference to educational materials, textbooks, handouts, and continuing education for Paraoptometric certification (http://www.aoa.org/). Staff should also be encouraged to attend local, state, or national organization conferences.

In order to encourage communication in the office, regularly scheduled meetings with key staff leaders as well as all staff members to promote education of staff should be conducted. The meetings should address updates in contact lens materials and designs, contact lens-related care products, patient care and management issues, as well as other areas of discussion. This helps to insure that everyone in the practice is on the same page and has the information to provide in the best interest of the patient.

Billing and Fees

Third-party insurances can improve access to eye care and bring new patients into a practice. Established patients may also come to the practice on a more regular basis for routine care because these benefits are available to them. These benefits are sometimes balanced out by increased administrative burden, decreased reimbursement for services, and limited coverage for materials. Patients may also have expectations that their insurance plan covers all services and costs. Learning to work with third-party insurance is a reality of today's contact lens practice.

Optometry is unique in the ability to bill a third party for vision-related services as well as medical and surgical services. With the widespread use of third-party insurances, it is important to clarify to the patients the services that fall into each category. Vision insurance often covers routine vision examinations for refractive errors and preventative care. Major medical insurance may cover treatment and monitoring of ocular disease with a nonrefractive diagnosis. Contact lenses also fall into two similar categories: contact lenses to manage refractive errors and medically necessary contact lenses to manage and treat an ocular disease or medical condition.

It is important to educate the patient that cosmetic contact lenses for the correction of refractive error is often considered a noncovered service and there are out-of-pocket costs associated with wearing contact lenses. These costs include professional fees, cost of contact lens materials, and cost of care systems. Some third-party vision insurance may provide discounts on professional fees and include an allowance for contact lens materials.

Unfortunately, medical insurance plans differ greatly from one patient's plan to the next, and most do not cover contact lenses, even in cases of medical necessity such as irregular astigmatism or keratoconus. There are a few strategies to help with receiving reimbursement for these cases. Initial examinations with diagnosis and treatment of the medical condition can be billed under the appropriate evaluation and management medical level visit according to the examination elements performed. Medically indicated procedures can also be performed and billed with the appropriate diagnosis, including corneal topography, specular microscopy, anterior segment imaging, and anterior segment photography. Several procedure codes are available to use that fall under contact lens fitting for the treatment of ocular disease and keratoconus (Table 24.1). As these codes can change over time, it is important to check with the insurance providers as to which codes are covered services. Follow-up and monitoring of ocular health associated with the ocular condition can also be billed with the appropriate evaluation and management level. A good resource for contact lens coding and billing are the archive articles in Contact Lens Spectrum (http://www.clspectrum.com/).

One additional option once a diagnosis and treatment plan is established is to submit a letter of prior authorization to the major medical insurance to seek coverage or reimbursement for the condition. An example of a letter to seek coverage for keratoconus can be found at the National Keratoconus Foundation website under the Resources page (www.NKCF.org). Of course, it should be explained to the patients that they are responsible for any charges or

TABLE 24.1 Examples of CPT Codes Useful in Contact Lens Billing

PROCEDURE	2012 CPT CODE
	CODE
Corneal topography	92025
Specular endothelial cell microscopy	92286
Anterior segment scanning imaging (OCT)	92132
Anterior segment photo	92285
Fitting of contact lens for treatment of ocular surface disease	92071
Fitting of contact lens for management of keratoconus, initial fitting	92072
Contact lens material	V2510
Prescription and fitting of contact lens with medical supervision	92310
Supplies and material over and above those usually included with office visits	99070
Corneal lens for aphakia one eye/both eyes	92311/92312
Corneoscleral lens	92313

costs that are not covered by their insurance plan, but billing the medical insurance correctly can reduce some of those costs. It may be more efficient for the patient to pay for services and materials up front and seek reimbursement from their third-party carrier.

Contact lens services are services performed in addition to the comprehensive examination, and as such additional fees should be assessed accordingly. The implementation of the Fairness to Contact Lens Consumer Act (FCLCA) by the Federal Trade Commission in 2003 has changed the way contact lens practitioners gain profitability in a practice (http://business.ftc.gov/documents/bus62-contact-lens-rule-guide-prescribers-and-sellers). The FCLCA states that the contact lens prescriber must provide the patient with a copy of the contact lens prescription after the fitting is complete and all fees are paid. This rule also requires that the contact lens seller verifies the details of the contact lens prescription with the prescriber through direct communication. The prescriber has 8 business hours to respond to the validity and accuracy of the prescription request. If the prescriber does not respond to the request within the 8-hour time period, the prescription is considered "passively" verified and the seller can fill the prescription request. The intent of this rule is to protect the contact lens consumer. Although this rule may appear to favor the third-party contact lens seller, it can actually have a positive impact on the practitioner.

In a traditional optometric practice, a proportion of the profit is derived from material sales from spectacles and contact lens supplies. With the increase in consumer access to contact lens materials through outside sources, practitioners should change their focus from material sales to a focus on providing services to the patient. The contact lens practitioner should market his or her expertise in prescribing contact lenses that provide the best ocular health, wearing comfort, and visual performance to the patient. Contact lens material pricing should cover the cost of the material itself as well as costs associated with the time spent administrating the processing and order of the lenses by staff members. With a competitive contact lens pricing established in the practice compared to other sources, the discussion of material costs can become secondary to the clinical decision of lens choices and further emphasis can be placed on the care that the practitioner provides.

Expertise in the prescribing of contact lenses and the aftercare should be impressed on the patient as a value and professional fees should be assessed accordingly. The fees assessed should reflect the chair time costs within the practice. It is important to know the time spent with each patient encounter within a typical day of the practice. This includes doctor time as well as staff and technician time for each comprehensive examination, follow-up visit, and ophthalmic materials provided. This information can help determine the amount of the professional fees associated with the time it takes for each contact lens fit.

One method of establishing a fee schedule is with a global contact lens professional fee, which covers all contact lens-related services within an established time period. This fee can vary depending on the complexity of the lens fit and the potential time required to finalize the lens fit. With a brand new contact lens wearer, the time required to train and educate the patient on lens application and removal as well as lens care habits should be considered. For a more complex refractive need, such as contact lenses for astigmatism and presbyopia, more follow-up visits may be expected as there are more factors to consider and, as such, a higher fee would be justified. With a global fee, the patients will not hesitate to return to the office for follow-up visits and checks because they will not be assessed additional fees while within the time frame. This can help establish open communication with the patient so that they do not feel penalized to return for follow-up visits to troubleshoot any problems, which will lead to happier and healthier contact lens wear.

The reasoning for the fees should be explained clearly and honestly to the patients along with any policies associated with them. This can include refunds, time periods limits, and additional costs as well as what visits are covered. Typically, a contact lens professional fee does not cover costs associated with treatment and diagnosis of medical conditions even if they are related to contact lens wear. With any professional fee, there should be written policies in place to address specific issues including services (Fig. 24.1). A list of those issues is included in Table 24.2.

Another method of determining the contact lens professional fee schedule is to charge for each additional contact lens visit after the initial evaluation and fit. This allows the practitioner to easily cover any chair time costs associated with care of the contact lens patient without the patient paying a large global fee for services he or she may not need.

In addition to professional fees for contact lens evaluations, a practice can implement a service agreement as coverage for additional services or office visits relating to contact lens wear. These service agreements usually include discounts on the purchase of contact lens supplies as well as discounts on spectacles. These service agreements usually include unlimited office visits, laboratory services, lens polishing, and a certain supply of lenses for a given amount of time, usually 1 year. The benefits of the service agreement can defray the cost of the service agreement when services are used and materials are purchased. A service agreement helps to create patient loyalty to a practice, establish continuity of care, and acts as a safety net for contact lens wearers in need of further services that may not be included by other fees.

PRACTICE PROMOTION AND INCREASING PROFITABILITY

There is a perception by some in the eye care community that prescribing contact lenses is not profitable, and they are only provided because the patient requests them. This may be related to traditional modes of practice where emphasis is placed on sale of spectacle and ophthalmic materials. As discussed, an emphasis on eye care and patient services can shift profitability away from material sales to professional service fees. Effective use of third-party plans and service agreements can also help optimize profitability in a contact lens practice.

In order for a contact lens practice to sustain, the needs of established patients need to be met so that patients continue to return for care and services. In order for the contact lens practice to grow, it will need to attract new patients to seek care and services. There are many methods to promote the contact lens practice. Keep in mind that promotion means not only attracting new patients, but also reaffirming to established patients that they have made the right choice in choosing this practice.

Practice promotion can be achieved via a variety of methods. Media advertising can help potential patients become aware of the practice and seek out more information either with a

> **CORNEA AND CONTACT LENS INSTITUTE**
> **CONTACT LENS FITTING AGREEMENT**
>
> Congratulations on the decision to wear contact lenses. Contact lenses can provide many benefits to your life, but proper fitting, care, and use is vital to optimize your experience with your lenses.
>
> To be fitted with lenses involves various steps, including determining the best lens options for you as an individual, ensuring proper fit and maximum vision, teaching you to handle your lenses properly if necessary, and following your for signs of problems related to lens wear. Most of these steps are NOT part of a general eye exam, and therefore the fitting and follow-up of someone wearing contact lenses is not included in the fee for a comprehensive eye examination.
>
> After or as a part of your eye examination, the following extra tests may be done: corneal mapping to determine the curve and size of your corneas, evaluation of lens fit, measurement of vision through lenses and overrefraction to determine proper prescription, and instruction on inserting, removing, and caring for your lenses. In addition, a certain number of follow-up visits are included to allow for later evaluation and modification if needed.
>
> Payment for the professional fees associated with contact lens wear is always required whether you decide to keep your lenses or not. Disposable contact lenses are only purchased after a trial period has been completed and you are satisfied with your lenses. Custom lenses, including custom soft and rigid lenses and any special lens design must be paid for before the lenses can be taken from the office. If the lenses do not work and are returned, a refund can be given minus any cost for restocking if returned in original packaging, in good condition, and within the warranty period of the lenses, typically 60–90 days.
>
> The cost of lenses and fitting can be submitted to your vision insurance if you wish. If you do want these costs submitted, please let us know that you wish us to do so. Once submitted, you are responsible for any balance not covered by your insurance. Contact lenses cannot be submitted to medical insurance unless they are being used for the treatment of an approved medical condition.
>
> The cost of various types of contact lens fittings are listed below. Please make sure you are notified of the cost of your fitting before signing this agreement if you wish. The cost of your lenses may vary depending upon which lenses you are fitted in. Please ask for an estimate of your annual lens cost prior to signing this if you wish.
>
> It is our desire to provide you the best possible contact lens experience and at a great value compared with other offices. Please let us know if you have any questions about any of this agreement.

FIGURE 24.1 Example of contact lens fitting agreement.

phone call or through the practice website. Established patients who are exposed to the media advertisement can feel connected to the practice and may be reminded to return for services. When a patient calls the practice, there may be occasions when they are put on hold on the phone. This is an opportunity to utilize "On-hold" messages to communicate new products

TABLE 24.2 Issues to Address in Written Fee Policy

—Length of time of service
—Amount of fee patient is responsible for
—Types of services covered and not covered
—Materials prescribed or provided with fee
—Replacement of lost or damaged contact lens
—Refund of exchange of contact lenses
—Refund of professional fees

and services or to educate patients on ocular conditions and treatments. Brochures, newsletters, or e-mail blasts can highlight the doctors' expertise and introduce services in the practice that patients were not aware of. Practices can hold an open house or fitting workshops to introduce new contact lens designs or materials.

In order for a contact lens practice to stand out, the doctors need to be willing and able to fit those challenging-to-fit patients. Some patients are told over and over that they are not good candidates for contact lenses, not because contact lenses for their refractive needs are not available, but because the practitioner does not have the expertise and confidence to fit the patient. These patients may be aware of the complexity of their visual needs or refractive error and are often willing to pay for these services, especially if you can provide contact lenses that other practices may not be able to. A strong specialty contact lens practice can provide these complex patients with contact lenses that may not be available from another provider. These lenses come in a variety of soft and gas-permeable (GP) lens materials to manage ametropia, astigmatism, presbyopia, aphakia, or irregular and postsurgical corneas. Most often, specialty contact lenses are custom lenses, which are made and created to exact specifications for that patient and must be purchased from the practitioner. Fitting specialty lenses is a way for a successful contact lens practitioner to assess higher professional fees for these complex fits and retain contact lens material purchases through custom-made specialty lenses that are designed by the practitioner. These satisfied patients are more likely to recommend the expertise of the practitioner to others, increasing the word-of-mouth referrals to the practice.

Electronic health records (EHR) are becoming a reality in the eye care practices. The initial time and costs associated with converting to electronic health records is significant, and the benefits of EHR may take many years to be realized. Converting from paper records to EHR requires training and support of all staff members and doctors, as well as additional equipment costs and changes to physical infrastructure of the practice. All this can be overwhelming to staff, doctors, and patients. So it is important to keep in mind the ultimate benefits of EHR. EHR can facilitate access to medical records and information, thereby saving staff time. It can provide feedback on medical coding and billing, which can increase reimbursement. It can help the practice monitor patient flow, material inventory, and prescription capture rates. All this information can help the practice seek new strategies to increase profitability and aid in the growth of the practice.

DIAGNOSTIC LENSES, STORAGE AND INVENTORY

There are advantages to different modes of contact lens fitting, either by empirical or diagnostic. One strategy of contact lens fitting is to fit the lenses empirically. The comprehensive examination is performed and all the data is gathered concerning patient visual needs, ocular health and physiology, and refractive status. The addition of topography data, information about lid aperture position and pupil size can help to attain a more successful empirical lens design. With that information, the appropriate diagnostic lens, either a soft or GP modality, is ordered and the patient returns for the dispensing. From a practice standpoint, this can reduce administrative time of keeping diagnostic lenses in stock, which takes up valuable office space. From a patient perspective, it reflects the practitioner's time and expertise in ordering a specific lens. At the dispensing visit, the patient will always have the correct lens for them, instead of the closest lens parameter that is in stock. This is especially true for astigmatic lenses or specialty lenses where visual needs may exceed availability of that in a diagnostic lens set.

Another strategy is to have a stock of diagnostic lenses available that you can use diagnostically or dispense at the fitting visit. For this purpose, it would be helpful to have options of a few different lenses in each category to make this as efficient as possible. Keep in mind these diagnostic soft contact lens sets require office space and staff attention to keep stocked in order to be effective. When patients present for a contact lens examination and fitting, there is some expectations of being able to experience the contact lens the day of the visit. It is helpful to have access to diagnostic contact lenses for a few reasons. Having the particular lens can be helpful in evaluating the fit of the lens on the patient's eye and how it interacts with the physiology of the eye. The patient is able to experience the initial comfort and vision correction the lens has to offer. Often small changes in lens parameters can have a large effect on patient's experience, such as that with astigmatic or multifocal lenses where a change in axis or power can dramatically improve the visual performance.

Most specialty GP lenses require a diagnostic lens set for fitting, including lenses for presbyopia correction, irregular corneas, or hybrid-type lenses. It may be difficult to order these lenses empirically, so it is important to have these diagnostic lens fit sets available. Even when using a diagnostic lens set for fitting, sometimes the practitioner may experience some challenges with lens designs. This is an opportunity for the practitioner to utilize laboratory consultation. Each lens laboratory provides consultation on the fit and design of the specialty lens. The laboratory consultants are often the people who directly manufacture the lens and therefore have insight and advice on possible parameter changes that can enhance the fit of the lens. A list of suggested soft and GP diagnostic lenses is available in Table 24.3.

These diagnostic lenses must be stored in a safe manner for reuse. GP contact lenses can be disinfected using a contact lens-approved hydrogen peroxide system and stored dry in the appropriate case. Some GP lens materials are recommended by the manufacturer for storage in solution, which need to be replaced every 30 days or as recommended by the solution. GP lenses can be cleaned and conditioned with a compatible GP lens solution prior to insertion for diagnostic fitting. Most diagnostic soft contact lenses are available in disposable blister packs and are not reused. Specialty soft contact lenses that are reused can be disinfected in a hydrogen peroxide system as well and stored in a multipurpose disinfecting solution with replacement of this solution every 30 days or as recommended by the manufacturer.

Whether they are designed empirically or by diagnostic fitting, GP lenses that are ordered are custom made specifically for that patient and are dispensed to the patient as their lens supply. Some specialty soft lenses are dispensed this way as well. When fitting a frequent-replacement lens, a lens supply needs to be ordered after the diagnostic fitting is finalized. The annual lens supply can be ordered through a distributor or directly through the manufacturer and often shipping is included when the year supply is ordered. If the patient does choose to order less than a 1-year supply, the practice should have a system to send reminders for patients to order more contact lenses to complete the annual supply. Patients with access to an annual supply may be more compliant with lens replacement as they do not feel the need to prolong lens wear because they have depleted their supply of lenses.

Even with the trend of ordering lens supplies and shipping them to patient, some practices may choose to keep an inventory of contact lenses to improve capture of contact lens material purchases. If the practice is able to offer the patients their annual supply of contact lenses at the day of their office visit, this can save the patient time in ordering lenses and waiting for

TABLE 24.3 Diagnostic Lens Sets

DIAGNOSTIC LENS SETS	
Soft Spherical	2 sets of silicone hydrogel and 1 set of hydrogel
Soft Toric	2 sets with different stabilization designs
Soft Multifocal	2 sets with different add power designs
GP Spherical	2 sets with different overall diameters
GP Bitoric	1 SPE set with 2 D difference in base curves
GP Multifocal	1 set of aspheric design and 1 set of translating design
Irregular Cornea	1 corneal lens set, 1 large-diameter corneal lens set, 1 scleral lens set, 1 hybrid lens set

the supply to come in. Having access to that supply of lenses immediately can encourage the purchase of the annual supply at one time. Keeping an inventory of contact lenses requires storage space and staff to maintain the stock. Staff time is dedicated to ordering lenses to replace the stock instead of placing orders to ship to patients. If the 1-year supply is encouraged and dispensed, there should not be any more time necessary other than processing the shipping order, or sometimes multiple times per year if patients order only a 3- or 6-month supply. This can actually help productivity and increase patient compliance. It is also possible to maintain a stock of spherical GP lenses with common base curve radii in a standard diameter in a range of powers that can be beneficial in diagnostic fitting as well as to dispense to the patient as necessary.

PATIENT EDUCATION

A successful contact lens practice relies on successful contact lens patients. The patient's success depends on the doctors' expertise as well as on the patient's ability to comply with recommendations from the doctor. Patient education is key to this equation. There are numerous other opportunities to provide patient education through various points of contact with the patient. During the initial phone call, an office can utilize the on-hold message to share information on new products or services and to educate on common eye conditions and treatments. Informational pamphlets throughout the reception area can also relay the same messages in written form.

Patients are presented with much information throughout the examination, from their refractive and eye health conditions, to various fees and costs, to different contact lens and spectacle recommendations. That is why it is important to provide some of the information in writing so that patients can review it at a later time.

Certain information presented needs to be understood immediately so that patients can make decisions on their care and treatment. When discussing fees and contact lens options, this is a good place to have written material that patients can refer to while they are being educated (Fig. 24.2). A detailed version of the same information should be provided to the patient to take home so that they can process the information on their own.

When educating patients on treatment plans or pertaining to their contact lens care regimen, written materials can be a helpful reference for the patient to follow along so that they can both hear and read the information to better understand what is explained and ultimately improve compliance with recommendations (Fig. 24.3). The Association of Optometric Contact Lens Educators provides an easy-to-follow handout for patients called "Healthy Soft CL Habits," which is a useful guide for contact lens care (http://www.aocle.org/healthyHabits.html).

Patient education is the key to compliance with contact lens wear. Even with the best-trained staff and technicians, the patients rely heavily on the recommendation of the doctor. After all, that is why the patient selects a particular practice. There are a number of key factors that the doctor must communicate to the patient. First, the doctors' recommendations on contact lens wear modality and options. Patients receive a wide variety of information on contact lenses, ranging from media advertisement to hearsay from a friend. It is the doctors' responsibility to filter that information and guide the patient toward the correct decision in their contact lens options. The doctor should explain that the reason for their recommendation is based on the examination findings and the patient's visual needs. The patient should be presented with risk and benefits of contact lens wear and the options available. The doctor should set up realistic expectations of contact lens visual performance and limitations. The doctors should also explain fee structures with both short-term and long-term costs of contact lens wear. All of this information can and should be repeated by a staff member to impress upon the patients the importance of these issues. The more the patients are informed and educated on issues with contact lens wear, the more likely they will be compliant to the doctors' recommendations.

SOFT MULTIFOCAL CONTACT LENSES

Cost

Professional services	$XXX.XX
(Includes fitting, dispensing, follow-up care for up to 90 days)	
Materials	
Right eye	$XXX.XX
Left eye	$XXX.XX
Tax	$ XX.XX
Total*	$XXX.XX

Refund Policy

If you do not successfully adapt to your lenses:
1. You will be fit into a different type of lens, returning the original lens or.
2. The contact lenses may be returned within the first 90 days for refund of all material fees.
3. The service fee is nonrefundable.

Eight Great Reasons to Buy a 1-Year Supply[†]

1. Free shipping
2. Healthier, more comfortable lens wear due to improved compliance with lens replacement
3. Complimentary diagnostic lenses, if ripped/lost lenses result in running out before annual exam
4. Unused lenses can be returned if prescription changes
5. 30% discount on complete pair of prescription glasses same day of contact lens order
6. 20% discount on complete pair of prescription glasses up to 1 year after contact lens order
7. Money-back rebates on all eligible brands
8. Buy now, pay later! interest-free financing allows you to spread payment over 1 year

*This total does not include exam fees or contact lens check fee.
[†]Restrictions apply. See an associate for details.

FIGURE 24.2 Example of fee schedule.

PRACTITIONER RESOURCES

The contact lens practitioner's skills and expertise is the primary factor in a successful contact lens practice. It is the responsibility of the doctor to stay informed of new advances in contact lens technology in order to offer the best option to patients. The doctor also needs to stay informed on clinical research by reading professional journals and attending local and national educational meeting. The Annual Meeting of the American Academy of Optometry and American Optometric Association's Optometry's Meeting both have excellent continuing education programs on the latest in clinical research and patient care topics. Publications such as Contact Lens Spectrum (http://www.clspectrum.com/) and Review of Cornea and Contact Lenses (http://www.reviewofcontactlenses.com/) are good resources for contact lens practitioners. Internet websites may provide more up-to-date information than printed material because of

> **Hot Compress Application Technique**
>
> - Moisten two clean cotton cloths.
> - Place one cloth in the microwave. Heat for 20 seconds. (Microwaves vary. Test the first cloth on arm to make sure it is not too hot. If too hot, decrease heating time and retest.)
> - Apply cloth to affected area for 2 minutes.
> - Begin heating second cloth when first cloth has been applied to affected area for 1.5 minutes.
> - Switch cloths and repeat so heat is applied for at least 10 minutes.
>
> **Lid Scrub Technique**
>
> - Use OCuSOFT Lid Scrub Formula (Foaming Eyelid Cleanser)
> - First wash and clean hands.
> - Pump desired amount of OCuSOFT Lid Scrub Foam onto a clean, lint-free washcloth, or fingertip. (People with long fingernails should use caution if using fingertip application.)
> - Close the eye and gently cleanse lids using lateral side to side strokes.
> - Rinse thoroughly with warm water. Avoid touching the eye directly.
> - Perform twice a day for the first 2 weeks, then taper to once a day. If problems recur, return to twice a day cleaning.

FIGURE 24.3 Examples of patient education materials.

the dynamic nature of the Internet. Trusted websites like Contact Lens Update (http://www.contactlensupdate.com/) and the Gas-Permeable Lens Institute (http://www.gpli.info/) can provide useful information as well. These websites contain interactive learning tools to help seasoned and novice practitioners increase their expertise in contact lens practice.

SUMMARY

A successful contact lens fit relies on the skill and expertise of the doctor, but a successful contact lens practice also relies on a number of other factors discussed in this chapter. Integration of a well-trained staff can provide value to the overall care of the contact lens patient. Utilizing some of the ideas discussed in this chapter in billing and fee schedules can help the contact lens practice be profitable. The contact lens practitioner can set the practice apart from others by providing specialty contact lens fits to those more complex patients. The results can be more satisfied patients and increased word-of-mouth referrals to grow the practice. When the practice embraces the advantages of providing contact lenses to patients, it can be rewarding both financially and personally to everyone involved.

Appendices

APPENDIX 1 KERATOMETER DIOPTER CONVERSION TO MILLIMETERS

CURVATURE (D)	CONVEX RADIUS (mm)	CURVATURE (D)	CONVEX RADIUS (mm)	CURVATURE (D)	CONVEX RADIUS (mm)
38.00	8.88	45.00	7.50	52.00	6.49
38.25	8.82	45.25	7.46	52.25	6.46
38.50	8.77	45.50	7.42	52.50	6.43
38.75	8.71	45.75	7.38	52.75	6.40
39.00	8.65	46.00	7.34	53.00	6.37
39.25	8.60	46.25	7.30	53.25	6.34
39.50	8.55	46.50	7.26	53.50	6.31
39.75	8.49	46.75	7.22	53.75	6.28
40.00	8.44	47.00	7.18	54.00	6.25
40.25	8.39	47.25	7.14	54.25	6.22
40.50	8.33	47.50	7.11	54.50	6.19
40.75	8.28	47.75	7.07	54.75	6.16
41.00	8.23	48.00	7.03	55.00	6.14
41.25	8.18	48.25	7.00	55.25	6.11
41.50	8.13	48.50	6.96	55.50	6.08
41.75	8.08	48.75	6.92	55.75	6.05
42.00	8.04	49.00	6.89	56.00	6.03
42.25	7.99	49.25	6.85	56.25	6.00
42.50	7.94	49.50	6.82	56.50	5.97
42.75	7.90	49.75	6.78	56.75	5.95
43.00	7.85	50.00	6.75	57.00	5.92
43.25	7.80	50.25	6.72	57.25	5.90
43.50	7.76	50.50	6.68	57.50	5.87
43.75	7.72	50.75	6.65	57.75	5.84
44.00	7.67	51.00	6.62	58.00	5.82
44.25	7.63	51.25	6.59	58.25	5.79
44.50	7.58	51.55	6.55	58.50	5.77
44.75	7.54	51.75	6.52	58.75	5.75

APPENDIX 1 (Continued) KERATOMETER DIOPTER CONVERSION TO MILLIMETERS

CURVATURE (D)	CONVEX RADIUS (mm)	CURVATURE (D)	CONVEX RADIUS (mm)	CURVATURE (D)	CONVEX RADIUS (mm)
59.00	5.72	61.50	5.49	66.00	5.11
59.25	5.70	61.75	5.47	66.50	5.08
59.50	6.67	62.00	5.44	67.00	5.04
59.75	6.65	62.50	5.40	67.50	5.00
60.00	5.63	63.00	5.36	68.00	4.96
60.25	5.60	63.50	5.31	68.50	4.93
60.50	5.58	64.00	5.27	69.00	4.89
60.75	5.56	64.50	5.23	69.50	4.86
61.00	5.53	65.00	5.19	70.00	4.82
61.25	5.51	65.50	5.15	70.50	4.79

APPENDIX 2 EFFECTIVE SPECTACLE LENS POWER AT THE CORNEAL PLANE (12-mm VERTEX DISTANCE)

SPECTACLE LENS POWER	EFFECTIVE POWER	SPECTACLE LENS POWER	EFFECTIVE POWER
Minus Lenses (D)			
−4.00	−3.82	−9.25	−8.33
−4.25	−4.05	−9.50	−8.53
−4.50	−4.27	−9.75	−8.73
−4.75	−4.49	−10.00	−8.93
−5.00	−4.72	−10.25	−9.13
−5.25	−4.94	−10.50	−9.33
−5.50	−5.16	−10.75	−9.52
−5.75	−5.38	−11.00	−9.72
−6.00	−5.60	−11.25	−9.91
−6.25	−5.82	−11.50	−10.11
−6.50	−6.03	−11.75	−10.30
−6.75	−6.25	−12.00	−10.49
−7.00	−6.46	−12.25	−10.69
−7.25	−6.67	−12.50	−10.87
−7.50	−6.88	−12.75	−11.06
−7.75	−7.09	−13.00	−11.25
−8.00	−7.30	−13.25	−11.43
−8.25	−7.51	−13.50	−11.62
−8.50	−7.71	−13.75	−11.80
−8.75	−7.92	−14.00	−11.99
−9.00	−8.13	−14.25	−12.17

Continues

APPENDIX 2 (Continued) EFFECTIVE SPECTACLE LENS POWER AT THE CORNEAL PLANE (12-mm VERTEX DISTANCE)

SPECTACLE LENS POWER	EFFECTIVE POWER	SPECTACLE LENS POWER	EFFECTIVE POWER
−14.50	−12.38	−16.50	−13.78
−14.75	−12.54	−16.75	−13.95
−15.00	−12.72	−17.00	−14.12
−15.25	−12.90	−17.25	−14.30
−15.50	−13.07	−17.50	−14.47
−15.75	−13.25	−17.75	−14.64
−16.00	−13.43	−18.00	−14.80
−16.25	−13.61		

Plus Lenses (D)

SPECTACLE LENS POWER	EFFECTIVE POWER	SPECTACLE LENS POWER	EFFECTIVE POWER
+4.00	+4.20	+11.25	+13.01
+4.25	+4.48	+11.50	+13.30
+4.50	+4.76	+11.75	+13.68
+4.75	+5.04	+12.00	+14.02
+5.00	+5.32	+12.25	+14.37
+5.25	+5.60	+12.50	+14.71
+5.50	+5.89	+12.75	+15.06
+5.75	+6.18	+13.00	+15.41
+6.00	+6.47	+13.25	+15.76
+6.25	+6.76	+13.50	+16.11
+6.50	+7.05	+13.75	+16.47
+6.75	+7.35	+14.00	+16.83
+7.00	+7.64	+14.25	+17.20
+7.25	+7.94	+14.50	+17.56
+7.50	+8.24	+14.75	+17.93
+7.75	+8.55	+15.00	+18.30
+8.00	+8.85	+15.25	+18.67
+8.25	+9.16	+15.50	+19.05
+8.50	+9.52	+15.75	+19.43
+8.75	+9.83	+16.00	+19.81
+9.00	+10.09	+16.25	+20.02
+9.25	+10.41	+16.50	+20.59
+9.50	+10.73	+16.75	+20.97
+9.75	+11.05	+17.00	+21.37
+10.00	+11.36	+17.50	+22.16
+10.50	+12.02	+17.75	+22.57
+10.75	+12.35	+18.00	+22.97
+11.00	+12.68		

APPENDIX 3 EXTENDED KERATOMETER RANGE WITH +1.25 D LENS

ACTUAL DRUM VALUE READING (D)	EXTENDED VALUE (D)	ACTUAL DRUM VALUE READING (D)	EXTENDED VALUE (D)
43.00	50.13	47.62	55.53
43.12	50.28	47.75	55.67
43.25	50.42	47.87	55.82
43.37	50.57	48.00	55.96
43.50	50.72	48.12	56.11
43.62	50.86	48.25	56.25
43.75	51.01	48.37	56.40
43.87	51.15	48.50	56.55
44.00	51.30	48.62	56.69
44.12	51.44	48.75	56.84
44.25	51.59	48.87	56.98
44.37	51.74	49.00	57.13
44.50	51.88	49.12	57.27
44.62	52.03	49.25	57.42
44.75	52.17	49.37	57.57
44.87	52.32	49.50	57.71
45.00	52.46	49.62	57.86
45.12	52.61	49.75	58.00
45.25	52.76	49.87	58.15
45.37	52.90	50.00	58.30
45.50	53.05	50.12	58.44
45.62	53.19	50.25	58.59
45.75	53.34	50.37	58.73
45.87	53.49	50.50	58.88
46.00	53.63	50.62	59.02
46.12	53.78	50.75	59.17
46.25	53.92	50.87	59.31
46.37	54.07	51.00	59.46
46.50	54.21	51.12	59.61
46.62	54.36	51.25	59.75
46.75	54.51	51.37	59.90
46.87	54.65	51.50	60.04
47.00	54.80	51.62	60.19
47.12	54.94	51.75	60.33
47.25	55.09	51.87	60.48
47.37	55.23	52.00	60.63
47.50	55.38		

APPENDIX 4 EXTENDED RANGE WITH −1.00D LENS

ACTUAL DRUM VALUE READING (D)	EXTENDED VALUE (D)	ACTUAL DRUM VALUE READING (D)	EXTENDED VALUE (D)
36.00	30.87	39.12	33.55
36.12	30.98	39.25	33.66
36.25	31.09	39.37	33.77
36.37	31.20	39.50	33.88
36.50	31.30	39.62	33.98
36.62	31.41	39.75	34.09
36.75	31.51	39.87	34.20
36.87	31.62	40.00	34.30
37.00	31.73	40.12	34.41
37.12	31.84	40.25	34.52
37.25	31.95	40.37	34.63
37.37	32.05	40.50	34.73
37.50	32.16	40.62	34.84
37.62	32.27	40.75	34.95
37.75	32.37	40.87	35.05
37.87	32.48	41.00	35.16
38.00	32.59	41.12	35.27
38.12	32.70	41.25	35.38
38.25	32.80	41.37	35.48
38.37	32.91	41.50	35.59
38.50	33.02	41.62	35.70
38.62	33.13	41.75	35.81
38.75	33.23	41.87	35.91
38.87	33.34	42.00	36.02
39.00	33.45		

INDEX

Page numbers followed by *f* denote figures; those followed by *t* denote tables.

Aberrations, optical, 38–39, 39*t*
Abrasions, corneal, 450
Abrasive surfactants, 159–160
Absolute scale, 68–69
Acanthamoeba, 90, 177, 288, 289, 291, 293, 662, 686–687
    minimizing risk of, 179*t*
Accelerated orthokeratology, 649
Accelerated stability, 371
Accommodation, 9
Accommodative demand, 38, 43
Acidosis, 444
Acrylate gas-permeable lenses, 96–97
Acular, 506*t*, 681
Acuvue Oasys for Presbyopia (Vistakon), 406
Adaptation
    overnight contact lens wear and, 453–454
    patient education, 173–174
    symptoms, 173*t*
Addition
    of minus power, 243–244
    of plus power, 244–245
Adjunct therapy, 22
Adolescent and Child Health Initiative to Encourage Vision Empowerment (ACHIEVE) study, 497–498
AEC. *See* Axial edge clearance
AEL. *See* Axial edge lift
Age
    gas-permeable lenses and, 103
    silicone hydrogel lenses and, 274
Air Optix Aqua Multifocal lenses, 402, 403*t*
Alamast, 506*t*, 675
Alaway, 506*t*, 675
Alcon, 256, 275, 292, 443
Alignment fluorescein patterns, 121*f*
Allergy medications, 506, 673–676
    drops, 676*t*
    summary table of, 676*t*
Alocril, 675
Alomide, 506*t*
Alrex, 506*t*, 679
Anatomic measurements, 4–6
    blink rate, 6
    corneal diameter, 4*f*
    horizontal visible iris diameter, 4
    lid position, 5

lid tension, 6, 124–125
palpebral aperture height, 5, 5*f*, 124
pupil diameter, 4–5, 5*f*, 68, 124
Anesthetics, topical, 113–114
Aniseikonia, 37
Anisometropia, 37
Anterior CN bevel, 130, 131*f*
Anti-inflammatory therapy, 685
Antibiotics, 670–673
    topical, 674*t*
Antiviral medications, 681–683
Aphakia, 473–478
    anatomic considerations and, 481–482
    care regimen, 487–488
    complications of, 478
    contact lens fitting and, 482–483
    effective power, 494
    fitting principles, 474
    gas permeable lenses and, 474–476
    hydrogel lenses and, 476–477
    lens handling and care, 483
    lens materials and, 474–476
    lens parameters in, 482
    lens-to-cornea fitting relationship, 483
    lenticular trial lens set, 476*t*
    magnification and, 495
    minus carrier, 475*f*
    optical considerations, 494–495
    parent education, 487–488
    patient selection, 473–474
    pediatric lenses, 481*t*
    pediatric patients, 478–488
    potential problems, 487
    silicone hydrogel lenses and, 274, 476–477
    single-cut, 476*t*
    vertex power, 494–495
    wearing schedules, 487–488
Apical bearing, 121, 532–533
Apical clearance, 121, 139*t*, 533, 537
Artificial tears, 684
Aspergillus, 686
Aspheric design, 147–148, 354
Aspheric lenses, 81, 355*f*
    for keratoconus, 541–542
Aspheric multifocals, 413–416
Aspheric optical zone, 148
Aspheric periphery, 148

Asthenopia, 424
Astigmatism
　addition, 40
　amount of, 367
　axes, 75
　central, 82f
　contact lens correction of, 43
　corneal, 81–83
　corneal topography of, 134f
　gas-permeable lenses and, 92, 344–366
　high, 354–366
　irregular, 366
　peripheral, 82f
　refractive, 367
　residual and high, 39
　soft lenses and, 315
　types of, 368
　uncorrected refractive, 315
Asymmetric Corneal Technology (ACT) design, 542
Asymmetry, 75
Atopic relationship, 519
Autokeratometer, 7
Axial edge clearance (AEC), 136f
Axial edge lift (AEL), 135, 136f
　maintaining, 137t
Axial map, 140
Axis location, 372–373
Azithromycin, 671–672

Bacitracin, 670–671
Back surface designs
　high eccentricity, 415
　low eccentricity, 414–415
Back surface toric lenses, 355–358
Back toricity, 371, 378
Back vertex power (BVP), 30–31, 39, 42
Bacteria biofilm formation, 176f
Base curve radius, 125–127
　determining, 141, 188f
　diagram of, 188f
　selection, 134–135, 135t
　of silicone hydrogel lenses, 276–277
　verification of, 187–189
Bausch and Lomb's PureVision material, 441–443
BE Retainer system, 657–658
Benzalkonium chloride, 158
Benzyl alcohol, 159
Besifloxacin, 670, 672, 673
BiExpert, 416–417
Bifocal contact lenses
　aging changes, 396–397
　candidates, 399t, 417t
　comprehensive preliminary evaluation, 396–398
　diagnostic lenses, 410–411
　educational resources, 422
　fitting, 409–411, 417–418
　follow-up care, 412–413
　hybrid designs, 421
　irregular cornea designs, 420
　lens design, 402–408
　patient consultation, 398–400
　patient selection, 396–400, 401

　patient success, 399t
　performing tests, 397–398
　practice promotion, 396
　preliminary testing for, 409–410
　problem solving, 412–413
　scleral designs, 421
　soft, 401–413, 510
　translating, 407–408, 416–422, 421f
Billing and fees, 693–695
Binocular vision
　and perception, 35–39, 40–41
　status, 8–9
Biofinity, 257f
Biomicroscope, 120–121, 418
Biotrue, 275, 291, 292
Bitoric design, 358–366
Bitoric lens, 358–366
　applications, 543
　center thickness of, 365
　educational resources, 366t
　fitting methods, 358–359
　keratoconus and, 543
　Mandell-Moore guide, 360
　peripheral curve design of, 365
　spherical power effect, 361–365
Blanket technique, 485f
Blending
　guidelines, 236t
　peripheral curves, 233–236
Blepharitis, 9
Blink rate, 6
Blur
　at distance, 424
　at intermediate distance, 424
　at near, 424–425
　persistent, 425
　slight, 425
Boston Keratoprosthesis (KPro), 593, 594f
Bubbles, 629–630
Bulbar conjunctiva, 10
Bulbar conjunctival disruptions, 449
Bull's eye effect, 235f
Burning sensation, 319–320
Burton lamp, 120

Candida, 686
Care regimen, 157–161
　aphakia, 487–488
　patient education, 168–170
　soaking, 157–159
　wetting, 157–159
Care systems, 21
"Cascade Hypothesis," 520
Cast molding, 264
CCC. *See* Central corneal clouding
CDC. *See* Centers for Disease Control
　　and Prevention
Center edge, 191
Center of gravity, 133
Center thickness, 128–129, 137, 138t
　of bitoric lenses, 365
　gas-permeable lenses, 129t

gauge, 192f
  of silicone hydrogel lenses, 278–279
  verification of, 191
Centers for Disease Control and Prevention (CDC), 117, 177
Central astigmatism, 82
Central corneal clouding (CCC), 217–218
Chemical disinfection, 287–289
Children, insertion for, 486f
Chlorhexidine, 158
Chronic hypoxia, 447
CLARE. *See* Contact lens acute red eye
Clarithromycin, 671
Cleaning, 159–161
  daily, 161t
  patient education, 168
  solutions, 159–161
CLEK. *See* Collaborative Longitudinal Evaluation of Keratoconus
CLEPA. *See* Contact Lens Edge Profile Analyzer
CLMA. *See* Contact Lens Manufacturers Association
Collaborative Longitudinal Evaluation of Ethnicity and Refractive Error (CLEERE) study, 506
Collaborative Longitudinal Evaluation of Keratoconus (CLEK), 91
  design, 539–540
Collagen cross-linking (CXL), 558–559
Collimator angle, 58
Color vision defects, 3
Comfort, 19
  corneal topography and, 83–84
  optimizing, 112–114
  overnight contact lens wear and, 453–454
  reduced, 210–211
Compliance, 175–177
  common rules for, 300t
  nomogram, 178f
  silicone hydrogel lenses and, 275
  soft lenses and, 298–301
  test, example of, 506t
Computational method, 359
Concave surface, 241
  polishing, 243f
Concentric alternating designs, 418
Cone tool, 237
Cone types, 523t
Confusion, 179–180
Conjunctiva, 9–10
  tarsal, 10
Conjunctival hooding, 628
Constant axial edge lift, 136–137
Contact dermatitis, 675–676
Contact lens(es). *See also specific types*
  ability to taking care of, 500
  adjunct therapy, 22
  age factor, 499
  applications, 591–592
  benefits of, to young people, 497–498
  bifocal soft lenses, 510
  borderline dry-eye patients and, 20–22
  care and compliance instructions, 503–504
  care systems, 21
  children and, 497
  comfort of, 19
  contact lenses and myopia control, 508–510
  corneal topography and, 76–84
  decision-making process, 501–502
  decorative, 501
  diameters of, 55f
  discussion with parents, 501
  examination, 501
  fitting, based on corneal topography, 79
  flexure of, 33–34
  follow-up visits, 505
  gas-permeable lenses, fitting, 502–503
  handling, 503
  history of, 2–4
  initial comfort, 112–114
  interest and motivation, 499–500
  keratoconus and, 532–555
  maturity, 500
  and myopia control, 508–510
  myopia development, 505–507
  myths regarding, 19–20
  non-prescription to young people, 498–499
  noncontact lens methods, 507–508
  optical aberrations, 38–39, 39t
  patient education and follow-up care, 503
  patient selection, 499–501
  personal hygiene habits, 500
  preexisting medical conditions, 501
  prescription requirements, 500–501
  prismatic effects of, 37–38, 38t
  reasons for wearing, 2–3
  soft lenses, fitting, 502
  spectacles v., 18–19
  in sports, 20t
  sports, 500
  wearing schedule, 22
Contact lens acute red eye (CLARE), 451
Contact Lens Edge Profile Analyzer (CLEPA), 130, 130f
Contact Lens Manufacturers Association (CLMA), 113, 232
Contact lens optics
  clinical guidelines from, 42–44
  formulae for, 39–41
Contact lens papillary conjunctivitis (CLPC), 450–451. *See also* Giant papillary conjunctivitis (GPC)
Contact lens peripheral ulcer (CLPU), 438f, 451
Contact lens practice management, 691
  billing and fees, 693–695
  diagnostic lenses, storage and inventory, 697–699
  patient education, 699
  patient encounter, 691–692
  practice promotion and increasing profitability, 695–697
  practitioner resources, 700–701
  staff education, 692
Contact Lenses in Pediatrics (CLIP) study, 498
Contex OK E-System, 658–659
Continuous wear. *See* Extended wear
Convergence, 9
Convex surface, 240–241

CooperVision, 256, 273, 406, 443
Cornea, 11
    abrasions of, 450
    astigmatism, 81–83
    chronic changes in, 446
    curvature of, 124
    disruption, 78f
    erosions of, 450
    flattening, 80
    gas-permeable lenses and, 77, 91
    irregularity of, 73–76, 91
    oxygen requirements, 436
    postsurgical, 91
    reflections in, 55f
    scarring of, 526f
    shape of, 79–81
Corneal and corneoscleral lenses, 610
Corneal astigmatism, 368
Corneal desiccation, 211
    edge clearance and, 212
    lens centration and, 212
    lens material and, 212
    management, 214f
    tear film stability and, 213
Corneal edema
    clinical evaluation of, 326–327
    epithelial, 327–328
    management, 328
    signs and symptoms of, 326t
Corneal graft rejection, 581f
Corneal lacerations, 592
Corneal refractive therapy (CRT) lens, 651t, 656, 657
Corneal staining, 447
Corneal swelling, 327
Corneal topographer, 7
Corneal topography, 6–8, 60, 138–142, 398, 583f, 619
    of astigmatism, 134f
    comfort and, 83–84
    contact lens fitting based on, 79
    in contact lens practice, 76–84
    contour, 6
    evaluation of, 6–8
    final analysis, 8
    of gas-permeable lenses, 101, 103, 534
    history of, 54–58
    hydrogel lenses and, 77–79
    introduction to, 54
    irregularity of cornea in, 73–76
    in keratoconus, 521–524
    keratoscopy and, 59–64
    maps, 67–73
        absolute scale, 68–69
        curve, 67
        relative scale in, 68–69
        sagittal scale in, 69–70
        tangential scale in, 69–70
    measuring procedure, 65–67
Corneal touch, 626
    bubbles, 629–630
    conjunctival hooding, 628
    lens compression and seal-off, 626–627
    lens deposits, 630–631

    lens flexure, 628
    nonwetting, 630, 630f
    reservoir debris, 629
    scleral obstacles, 627–628
    solution toxicity/hypersensitivity, 630
    uneven haptic bearing, 627
Corneal vascularization
    abnormal, 331–332
    appearance, 332
    initiating factors, 332
    management, 332–333
    normal, 331–332
    stages, 332
    treatment, 332–333
Corneal warpage syndrome (CWS), 218–219, 527–528, 528t
Corneal zone, loose conjunctiva in, 628f
Corneoscleral lens designs, 502, 610, 663
Corticosteroid–antibiotic preparations, 673
Corticosteroids, 673, 677–680
    contraindications for, 678t
    for ocular conditions, 680t
    topical, 678t
Cosmetic wear
    of gas-permeable lenses, 93
    patient education on, 172
    of soft lenses, 304
Countersunk rigid lens-soft lens carrier, 552–553
CPE. *See* Cylinder power effect
CRA (calculated residual astigmatism), 8
Crolom/Opticrom, 506t
Curvularia, 686
Custom soft contact lenses, 584
CWS. *See* Corneal warpage syndrome
Cyclopleging nonaphakes, 502
Cylinder power effect (CPE), 363

Dailies Total 1, 273
Daily cleansers, 161t
Dalsey adaptives, 625
Decentration
    inferior, 206–207
    lateral, 207
    reduced vision and, 205–207
    superior, 207
Decision-making process, 501–502
Decorative contact lenses, 501
Deep anterior lamellar keratoplasty (DALK), 557–558, 586, 587
Defective lenses, 316
Delefilcon A, 254
Deposited lens, 323
Deposits
    silicone hydrogel lenses and, 273
    soft lenses and, 294–295, 314–315
Descemet membrane endothelial keratoplasty (DMEK), 586
Descemet stripping automated membrane endothelial keratoplasty (DSAEK), 586
Descemet stripping membrane endothelial keratoplasty (DSEK), 586–587

Desiccation, corneal, 211–213, 214f
Design
    aspheric, 147–148, 354
    back surface, 414–415
    bifocal lenses, 401–407
    bitoric, 354
    CLEK, 539–540
    concentric alternating, 418
    custom, 146–147
    edge thickness, 137
    and fitting resources, 148–149
    front surface aspheric, 415–416
    lens, 147
    McGuire, 537
    modification of, 245
    multifocal lenses, 401–407
    peripheral curve, 365
    plus lens, 132t
    plus lenticular, 131f
    pseudoaspheric, 148
    segmented translating, 418
    semi-scleral and scleral lens, 546–548
    Soper Cone, 537
    standard, 146–147
Dexamethasone, 679
Diagnostic fitting, 115. *See also specific types*
    empirical fitting v., 115t
    inventories, 116–119
Diagnostic lens fitting, 620
    application and removal training, 624–625
    contact lens solutions, 625
    dispensing, 624
    lens selection and evaluation, 620–624
    safety and risk, 625
Diagnostic lens formula, 40
Diagnostic lenses
    procedures, 373
    storage of, 117, 697–699
Difference maps, 70, 79f
Dimple veiling, 206f
Discomfort, 112
    burning, 319–320
    on insertion, 317–318
    during lens wear, 319
    after removal, 319
    soft lenses and, 317–320
    sudden, 319
Disinfection solutions, 158t
    for silicone hydrogel lenses, 292
    for soft lenses, 287–293
Dispensing visit, 162–175
    patient education, 163–175
    procedures, 162
Disposability
    of gas-permeable lenses, 93
    of presbyopic contact lenses, 401t, 404t
    of silicone hydrogel lenses, 279
Disposable lenses, 372
DreamLens, 659
Dry eye, 589
Dry-eye questionnaire, 17

Dry Eye Shop, 625
Dryness, 211–217, 683–686
    anti-inflammatory therapy, 685
    artificial tears and, 684
    borderline, 20–22
    environmental factors, 322
    improving, 684t
    management, 683–684
    meibomian gland dysfunction and, 685–686
    punctal plugs for, 684–685
    silicone hydrogel lenses and, 273–274
    soft lenses and, 321–322
    spots, 13f
Dual-axis fluorescein pattern, 658f
Duette lens, 103, 292, 555, 586
Duffens modification unit, 230f
Dumbbell-shaped fluorescein patterns, 123f
Durability, of gas-permeable lenses, 90
Dyna Intra-Limbal (DIL), 542, 542t
Dynamic stabilization, 370–371

Eccentric lenticulation soft lenses, 371
ECFs. *See* Edematous corneal formations
Edema, 11
    corneal, 326–328
    epithelial, 327–328
Edematous corneal formations (ECFs), 218
Edge clearance
    corneal desiccation and, 212
    excessive, 545f
    high, 213f
    minimal, 545f
Edge lift, 127
    constant axial, 136–137
Edge polishing, 237–240, 239f
Edge shaping, 237–240
Edge thickness, 129–132
    design, 137
EDTA. *See* Ethylenediamine tetraacetate
EGDMA. *See* Ethylene glycol dimethacrylate
EKC. *See* Epidemic keratoconjunctivitis
Electronic health records (EHR), 697
Elestat, 506t, 675
Elevation maps, 70–73, 140, 141f
Emadine, 506t
Emerald lens, 659
Emergencies, overnight contact lens wear, 455
Empirical fitting, 114–115
    diagnostic fitting v., 115t
Endothelial keratoplasty (EK), 586
Endothelial polymegethism, 445
Endothelium, 11
Entropion, 9
Environmental limitations, 93
Enzymatic cleaners, 296
Enzymes, 160
Epidemic keratoconjunctivitis (EKC), 681
Epithelial edema, 327–328
Epithelial microcysts, 445
Epithelial staining, 11
Erosions, corneal, 450
Erythromycin, 671–672

Ethylene glycol dimethacrylate (EGDMA), 253
Ethylenediamine tetraacetate (EDTA), 158
Evaluation, 114–149
   case history, 203
   process, 203–204
   of silicone hydrogel lenses, 279–282
   visits, 280t
Excessive edge clearance, 545f
Extended wear (EW), 211, 288, 328, 435–436, 439, 536
External observation, 9
Extraction of soft lenses, 263
Eye-Dock, 148
Eye switching, 425
Eyelid. *See* Lid

Fairness to Contact Lens Consumer Act (FCLCA), 694
False fluorescein patterns, 123
Fatigue and flare, 425
Final contact lens power (FCLP), 35, 40
Finger polishing, 237
Finishing, 263
First Purkinje image, 55
Fitting, 114–149. *See also* Diagnostic fitting
   aphakia and, 474
   axis location and orientation, 372–373
   bifocal lenses, 409–411, 417–418
   bitoric lens, 358–359
   computational method, 359
   considerations, 148
   form, 146t
   guides, 411t
   interpalpebral, 132–138, 138t
   inventory, 93
   lens selection and, 372
   lens-to-cornea relationships, 483, 532–534, 544
   lid-attachment, 124–132
   methods, 114–115
   monovision, 422
   multifocal lenses, 409–411
   nomograms, 132f
   optical cross method, 360
   philosophies, 123–146
   principles, 372–379
   Rose K diagnostic, 539t
Flare, fatigue and, 425
Flat lens, 323
Flat sponge, 239–240, 239f
Flattening, 233–236
Fleischer's ring, 525f
Flexlens Multifocal (X-Cel Contacts), 405, 552f
Flexlens piggyback system, 552
Flexural resistance, 95
Flexure, 205
   of contact lenses, 33–34, 40
Fluorescein, 419f
   application, 119–123
   description, 119
   evaluation, 119–123
   methods of observation, 119–123
   patterns
      alignment, 121f
      apical clearance, 122f
      dumbbell-shaped, 123f
      evaluation of, 121–123
      false, 123
Fluoro-silicone lens materials, 97–100
Fluorometholones, 679
Fluoroquinolones, 670, 672
Focus Dailies Progressive lenses, 403
Foggy vision, 324
Folds, 444–445
Follow-up care
   bifocal lenses, 412–413
   multifocal lenses, 412–413
   patient education on, 455–456
Foreign-body particles, 171
Free-standing bowl modification unit, 230f
Front curve radius, 189–190
Front surface aspheric designs, 415–416
Front surface toric gas-permeable lenses, 348–354
Front toricity, 378
Front vertex power (FVP), 31, 39, 42
Full-thickness penetrating keratoplasty (PKP), 578
   hybrid contact lenses, 585–586
   intralase-enabled and traditional PKP, 579
   piggyback contact lenses, 585, 585f
   rigid gas-permeable contact lens design, 580–583
   running sutures v. interrupted sutures, 579–580
   soft contact lenses, 583–584
   timing of contact lens fitting after surgery, 580
Fungal infections, 686
Fusarium, 288, 686

Ganciclovir (Zirgan), 682
Gas-permeable lenses, 19
   advantages of, 19t
   age and, 103
   applications of, 90–92
   aspheric multifocal, 413–416
   astigmatism and, 92, 344–366
   base curve selection criteria and, 126t
   benefits, 89–90
   bifocals, 413–422
   center thickness, 129t
   cornea and, 91
   corneal changes in, 77
   corneal topography of, 101, 103
   cosmetic wear of, 93
   custom design, 129t
   designs, 149t, 534–535, 589
   diameter selection, 133t
   disposability, 93
   durability of, 90
   environmental limitations of, 93
   evaluation process, 203–204
   fitting, 502–503, 534
   fitting inventory, 93
   flexural resistance of, 95
   fluoro-silicone, 97–100
   front surface scratches on, 242f
   front surface toric, 348–354
   hardness of, 96
   high-DK, 116t

high-riding, 528
initial comfort, 93
intralimbal rigid, 541–545
inventory lens set, 118t
for keratoconus, 534–543
limitations of, 92–93
low-DK, 116t
material properties of, 93–96
material selection, 101–103
material types and composition, 96–101
modification procedures, 246t
multifocals, 413–422
myopia reduction and, 90–91
occupation and, 103
ocular health and, 89–90
oxygen permeability of, 93–94
palpebral aperture size of, 93
patient instruction manual, 175t
patient retention and, 90
plasma treatment, 100–101
presbyopia and, 91
problem solving, 216–217t
profitability of, 90
progress evaluation procedures, 204t
proper insertion of, 164f
quality of vision and, 89
refits, 103, 217–220
refractive error of, 101
rules for designing, from corneal topography, 139
selection, 21
silicone, 96–97
soft lens refits, 92
soft lenses v., 21, 219–220
specific gravity of, 96
spherical, 347
stability of, 90
surface wettability of, 94–95
ultraviolet blockers, 100
verification of radius, 187–190
G.B.L. lens, 542
Gentamicin, 670, 671
Giant papillary conjunctivitis (GPC), 10f, 333–336, 675
    signs, 333–335
    stages of, 334t
    symptoms, 333–335
    treatment, 335–336
Glyceryl methacrylate (GMA), 253
GP Eye Care Professional Locator, 149
GP Lens Institute (GPLI), 123, 148, 174
GPC. See Giant papillary conjunctivitis
GPLI toric and spherical lens calculator, 360
Guesstimates, 349

Handling, 163–168
    of silicone hydrogel lenses, 273
Haptic lenses, 546
Haptic/landing zone, 614–615
Hardness
    of gas-permeable lenses, 96
    of soft lenses, 255
Hazy vision, 324
Headaches, 425

Headband frames, 479f
Height contours, 62f
Height maps, 61
HEMA. See Hydroxyethyl methacrylate
Herpes simplex (HSV), 681
High astigmatism, 354–366
    correcting, 362f
High eccentricity back surface designs, 415
High refractive index, 101
High riding gas-permeable lens, 528
Higher-order aberration (HOA) keratoconic eyes, 553
History
    contact lens, 2–4
    of corneal topography, 54–58
    evaluation process and, 203
    medical, 3–4
    ocular, 3
    of overnight contact lens wear, 435–436
    soft lenses, 367
Horizontal visible iris diameter, 4, 277f
HSV. See Herpes simplex
Hybrid contact lenses, 585–586
Hybrid designs, 421
Hybrid lens disinfection and care, 292
Hybrid lenses, 553–555
Hydration, 257–258, 263
Hydrogel lenses, 77–79. See also Silicone hydrogel lenses
    aphakia and, 476–477
    applications, 366–379
    common conventional, 439t
    complications associated with, 451–453
    corneal disruption under, 78f
    high minus silicone, 79f
    for overnight contact lens wear, 439
    silicone, 260t
Hydrogen peroxide, 289–292
    warnings on, 290f
Hydrokone fitting set/design information, 496t
Hydroxyethyl methacrylate (HEMA), 252–253
Hygiene, 303–304
Hypergel material, 273
Hyperopic correction, 662–663
Hyperopic orthokeratology lens, 662
Hypersensitivity, 630
Hypoxia, 444

I-Kone, 541
IK. See Infiltrative keratitis
In-office disinfection, 293
Incisional refractive surgery, 590–591
Incorrect prescriptions, 315
Infants
    insertion, 484f
    speculum on, 484f
Infiltrates, 11
Infiltrative keratitis (IK), 451–452
Inflammatory complications, 452
Informed consent, 453
Initial comfort, 93
Initial presentation, 112–113
Initial vision, 114

Injection, 329–331
    factors resulting in, 329t
    generalized, 329–331
    lens-related, 329–330
    not relating to contact lens wear, 331
    sectorial, 331
Insertion, 301f
    in children, 486f
    discomfort on, 317–318
    infant, 484f
    by patient, 163–164
    patient education, 163–164, 301, 303
    by practitioner, 164
    proper, 164f
    of soft lenses, 301, 303
    toddler, 484
Interference phenomena evaluation, 13
Internal astigmatism, 368
Interpalpebral fitting, 132–138
    parameters of, 138t
Intralase-enabled keratoplasty, 580f
Intralimbal rigid gas permeable lenses, 541–542
Intrastromal corneal ring segments (ICRS) (Intacs), 558, 591
    contact lens applications, 591–592
Inventories, 116–119
Inversion, 317
Inverted lens, 323
Ionic charge, 257
Irregular cornea designs, 420

Jackson Cross Cylinder (JCC), 521
Jelly bumps, 295, 295f

KeraSoft lens, 548–549
Keratoconus
    aspheric lenses, 541–542
    bitoric lens applications, 543
    "Cascade Hypothesis," 520
    characteristics of, 518
    classification, 529–531, 529t
    clinical signs, 527t
    coding and reimbursement, 559–560
    collagen cross-linking (CXL), 558–559
    color map in, 522f
    contact lenses, 520, 532–555
    corneal topography and GP lens fitting, 534
    deep anterior lamellar keratoplasty (DALK), 557–558
    diagnosis of, 521–527
    diagnosis codes for, 560t
    diagnostic lens fitting set, 535t
    differential diagnosis, 527–528
    Dyna Intra-Limbal (DIL), 542, 542t
    epidemiology of, 518
    etiology, 519–520
    gas-permeable lenses in, 534–543
    G.B.L. lens, 542
    heredity, 519–520
    histologic changes, 519
    lens selection, 556t
    lens-to-cornea fitting relationships, 532–534
    management, 555–559
    ophthalmoscopy, 526
    patient consultation, 531
    penetrating keratoplasty (PKP), 556–557
    Pillow Lens, 552–553, 553f
    primary surgical procedures, 555–558
    problem solving, 543, 544t
    progression of, 529–531
    protective associations, 520
    Quad Sym, 545
    reimbursement, 559–560
    rigid lens fitting, 532–545
    Rose K2 IC design, 542, 543t
    scleral lenses, 547
    semi-scleral lens, 546
    severity score, 530t
    soft lenses and, 548–552
    spectacle management in, 531–532
    surgical management of, 555–559
    symptoms of, 521
    tomography applications, 526
    topography map of, 65f
    videokeratography, 522–524
Keratoglobus, 528
Keratometer, 6–7
Keratometer diopter conversion, to millimeters, 702–703
Keratometry, 55, 58–59
    in keratoconus, 521–522
    principle of, 56f
Keratoprosthesis, 593
    KPro type I, 593–594
Keratoscopy, 59–64
Ketotifen, 675
KPro type I, 593–594

Laboratory consultants, 149
Lacrimal lens power (LLP), 34–35
    example, 35
    formulae, 40
Lamellar keratoplasty, 586–587
LARS (left add, right subtract) principle, 350, 350f
Laser-assisted in situ keratomileusis (LASIK), 559, 588–589
Lathe cutting, 262–263
Lens(es). *See specific types*
Lens attachment devices, 231
Lens centration, 615. *See also* Decentration
    corneal desiccation and, 212
Lens compression and seal-off, 626–627
Lens crack, 198f
Lens edge
    inspection of, 191–194
    palm test for quality of, 192f
    soft, 196
    view of, 193f
Lens fitting relationship, 330
Lens inversion, 317
Lens modulus values, 255
Lens mount, 188f
Lens movement, 323
Lens power
    of silicone hydrogel lenses, 277–278
    of soft lenses, 196
    verification of, 190–191, 196

Lens-related injection, 329–330
Lens removal
    procedure after, 204
    procedure before, 203–204
Lens-to-cornea relationships, 483, 532–534, 544
Lensometer, 191*f*
Lenticular aphakia trial lens set, 476*t*
Lid
    anatomy, 368–369
    attachment fitting, 124–132
    configuration, 368–369
    contour, 420*f*
    position, 5
    retraction, 163
        improper, 166*f*
        proper, 163*f*
    tear prism on margins of, 67*f*
    tension, 6, 124–125
Lid wiper epitheliopathy (LWE), 16
Light filament, 189*f*
Limbal hyperemia, 445
Limbal vasculature, 11
Limbal vessel engorgement, 281–282
Linear dimensions, 194–196
LipiFlow technology, 685
Lissamine green, 16
Lotemax, 679
Loteprednol, 678, 679
Low eccentricity back surface designs, 414–415
Lubrication, 161*t*
    for soft lenses, 296–297, 297*t*

MAA. *See* Methacrylic acid
Maastricht Shape Topographer (MST), 61, 62*f*
Magnification, 495
Mandell-Moore bitoric lens guide, 360
Mandell-Moore fit factor, 355*t*
Maps
    corneal topography, 67–73
        absolute scale in, 68–69
        curve, 67
        relative scale in, 68–69
        sagittal scale in, 69–70
        tangential scale in, 69–70
    difference, 70, 78
    elevation, 70–73
McGuire lens design, 537
    trial sets, 538*t*
Measurements
    anatomic, 4–6
    in corneal topography, 65–67
Medical history, 3–4
Medications
    allergy, 673–676, 676*t*
    antiviral, 681–683
Medmont topographer, 658
Meibomian gland dysfunction (MGD), 9, 618, 683, 685–686
Menicon Inc., 158*t*, 160, 161*t*, 209, 241, 256, 289, 443
Menicon Progent Intensive Protein Remover, 161
Menicon Z, 97, 161, 212, 440
Meniscus, 12*f*

Methacrylic acid (MAA), 253
Methyl methacrylate (MMA), 253
Methylcellulose derivatives, 159
Microbial keratitis (MK), 452–453, 501, 661
Microcysts, 328
    epithelial, 445
Minimal edge clearance, 545*f*
Minus lens design parameters, 132*t*
Minus Power, 243–244
Mires, 58
MK. *See* Microbial keratitis
MMA. *See* Methyl methacrylate
Modification
    "do's" and "don'ts," 247*t*
    equipment, 231–232
    of high-oxygen permeability lens, 245–247
    procedures, 233–245, 246*t*
    proficiency at, 247
    reasons for, 229–230
    of special designs, 245
    unit, 230
Modified monovision, 411–412
Modulus of elasticity, 255
Monomers, 253*t*
Monovision, 411–412, 422–426
    disadvantages, 423
    fitting considerations, 423–424
    lens selection, 423–424
    overview, 422–423
    patient selection, 423
    problem solving, 424–426
Motivation, evaluation of, 18
Movement, lens, 323
MST. *See* Maastricht Shape Topographer
Mucin balls, 448–449
Mucoprotein film, 209*f*
Multifocal contact lenses
    diagnostic lenses, 410–411
    educational resources, 422
    fitting, 409–411
    follow-up care, 412
    lens design, 401–407
    patient selection, 401
    preliminary testing for, 409–410
    problem solving, 412
    scleral lenses, 615
    soft, 401–413, 401*t*
    soft toric, 408–409
    translating, 407–408
Myopia, 20
    development, 505–507
    gas-permeable lenses and, 90–91
    progression, 507*t*
Myopia control, contact lenses and, 508
Myopic shift, 447
Myths, 19–20

N-vinyl pyrrolidone (NVP), 253
National Keratoconus Foundation, 559
Naturalens inventory, 119*f*
Near Vision chart, 410*f*
Neomycin, 671

Neosporin, 671
Neovascularization, 379, 446
  overnight contact lens wear and, 447f
Nesofilcon A, 257
Newman's GP Toric Guide, 361
Nipple cone, 523f
Nomograms
  compliance, 178f
  fitting, 132f
Nonabrasive surfactants, 159
Noncontact lens methods, 507–508
Noninvasive tear breakup time (NIBUT), 8, 13
Nonpolishing alternatives, 241
Nonsteroidal anti-inflammatory drugs (NSAIDs), 114, 680–681, 680t
Nonwetting scleral lens, 630, 630f
NSAIDs. See Nonsteroidal anti-inflammatory drugs
NVP. See N-vinyl pyrrolidone

Observation, 9
Occupation
  gas-permeable lenses and, 103
  silicone hydrogel lenses and, 275
  soft lenses and, 369
OCT. See Optical coherent tomography
Ocular disease, 274
Ocular examination, 281–282
Ocular health, 89–90
Ocular history, 3
Ocular surface disease (OSD), 610–611
1-day Acuvue TruEye, 273
1-2-3 principle, 357f
Opacities, 11
Ophthalmometry, 55
Ophthalmoscopy, 526
Opti-Free PureMoist, 275, 291, 292
Optical aberrations, of contact lenses, 38–39, 39t
Optical coherent tomography (OCT), 58, 63–64, 526
  front segment, 64f
Optical considerations, in contact lens practice, 30
Optical cross method, 360
Optical zone, 612
Optical zone diameter (OZD), 124–125, 125f, 135
  peripheral curve radii and, 135
  verification of, 194
Optimum Extra Strength Cleaner (Lobob), 209
Optivar, 506t, 675
Optometry, 693
Ordering the lenses, 145–146
Orinda Longitudinal Study of Myopia (OLSM), 505
Orthokeratology, 509, 648
  BE Retainer system, 657–658
  benefits of, 650
  candidates, good and poor, 651
  complications, 661–662
  Contex OK E-System, 658–659
  corneal refractive therapy, 657
  corneoscleral lens designs, 663
  current and future uses of, 662
  dispensing, 660
  DreamLens, 659
  early techniques, 648–649
  Emerald lens, 659
  fitting orthokeratology lenses, 653
  follow-up visits, 660–661
  general guidelines, 653–656
  good, borderline, and poor candidates for, 652t
  guidelines for advertising and promoting, 652t
  hyperopic correction, 662–663
  lens designs, 657, 659
  mechanism, 650
  modern, 649
  patient expectations and selection, 650
  recent advances, 649–650
  resources, 663–664
  screening, 651–653
  soft contact lenses, 663
  vision shaping treatment, 657
Orthokeratology-like patterns, 79
OrthoTool, 139
Osmolarity, of tear film, 16–17
Overall lens diameter (OAD), 133–134
  demonstration of, 195f
  determining, 140
  methods to determining, 194f
  silicone hydrogel lenses, 277
  verification of, 194
Overnight contact lens wear
  adaptation to, 453–454
  comfort and, 453–454
  emergencies, 455
  history of, 435–436
  hydrogel materials for, 439
  material selection for, 439–443
  neovascularization and, 447f
  patient education for, 453–456
  patient selection for, 437–439
  rewetting and, 455
  rigid lenses for, 440
  silicone elastomers, 439–440
  silicone hydrogel lenses, 441, 444t
  soft lens, 444–453
  suitable candidates for, 437–438
  unsuitable candidates for, 438–439
  wearing schedule for, 454–455
Overnight orthokeratology (OOK), 498, 650
Overrefraction, 162, 623
Oxidative disinfection, 289–292, 292t
Oxidative Stress Pathway, 520
Oxygen permeability
  of gas-permeable lenses, 93–94
  of soft lenses, 258–259, 258f
Oxygen transmissibility, 436
OZD. See Optical zone diameter

Pain, 112
Palpebral aperture height, 5, 124
  measurement of, 5f
Palpebral aperture size, 93
PAPB. See Polyaminopropyl biguanide
Papoose board, 485f
Parameter changes, 133t
Part-time wearers, 275

Pataday, 506t, 675
Patanol, 506t, 675
Patient agreement, 453
Patient education, 163–175
    adaptation, 173–174
    care regimen, 168–170
    checklist, 299t
    cleaning, 168
    compliance, 175–177
    contact lens practice, 699
    cosmetics, 172
    emergencies, 455
    follow-up care, 455–456, 503–505
    foreign-body particles, 171
    handling, 163–168
    insertion, 163–164, 301, 303
    lens case, 170–171
    lid retraction, 163
    medication use and GP wear, 172
    methods, 174–175
    overnight contact lens wear, 453–456
    placement, 164
    positioning, 163
    removal, 164–166, 301, 303
    rewetting, 455
    scleral lenses, 618–619
    scratches, 171
    soft lenses and, 297–305
    solution confusion, 179–180
    swimming, 173
    tap water, 177–179
    wearing schedule, 454–455
Patient retention, of gas-permeable lenses, 90
Pattern evaluation, 121–123
PCF. *See* Pharyngoconjunctival fever
PCR. *See* Peripheral curve radius
Pediatric Refractive Error Profile, 498
Pellucid marginal degeneration (PMD), 72, 76, 528
Penetrating keratoplasty (PKP), 556–557
Periballast, 353–354
    soft lenses, 371
Peripheral astigmatism, 82f
Peripheral curve(s)
    blending, 233–236
    design, 365
    flattening, 233–236
    light blend of, 197f
    medium blend of, 197f
    widths, 127–128, 196
Peripheral curve radius (PCR), 127–128, 135, 355
    verification of, 190
Pharyngoconjunctival fever (PCF), 681
Phenol red thread test, 14–15, 15f
Photodiagnosis, 526f
Photokeratoscopy, 7, 59
Photophobia
    causes of, 321
    soft lenses and, 320–321
    treatment of, 321
Photorefractive keratectomy (PRK), 559, 588
Piggyback lenses, 551–552, 585, 585f
Pillow Lens, 552–553, 553f

Placido disks, 55–58, 56f
    of irregular cornea, 57f
    photographic image of, 57f
Plasma treatment, 161
    gas-permeable lenses, 100–101
Plus lens design, 132t
Plus lenticular design, 131f
Plus power, 244–245
PMD. *See* Pellucid marginal degeneration
PMMA lenses. *See* Polymethylmethacrylate
Polishing
    compounds, 233
    concave surface, 243f
    edge, 237–240, 239f
    soft lenses, 263
Polyaminopropyl biguanide (PAPB), 158–159
Polymegethism, 218
Polymethylmethacrylate (PMMA) lenses, 77, 233, 440, 547, 609, 648
    refitting, 217–219
Polymyxin B, 670–671
Polyquaternium-1, 159
Polyvinyl alcohol (PVA), 159, 253
Positioning lenses, 163
Postocular trauma, 592
    lens selection, 592
    prosthetic contact lenses, 592–593
Postsurgical contact lens fitting, 578
    contact lens applications, 591–592
    full-thickness penetrating keratoplasty (PKP), 578
    gas-permeable lens design, 589
    hybrid contact lenses, 585–586
    incisional refractive surgery, 590–591
    intralase-enabled and traditional PKP, 579
    intrastromal corneal ring segments (ICRS) (Intacs), 591
    keratoprosthesis, 593
    KPro type I, 593–594
    lamellar keratoplasty, 586–587
    lens selection, 592
    piggyback contact lenses, 585, 585f
    postocular trauma, 592
    prosthetic contact lenses, 592–593
    refractive corneal ablation, 588
    rigid gas-permeable contact lens design, 580–583
    running sutures v. interrupted sutures, 579–580
    soft contact lenses, 583–584
    soft lens designs, 589
    timing of contact lens fitting after surgery, 580
Power change, 210
Power determination, 142–146
Prednisolone, 679
Prentice's rule, 37, 41
Presbyopia, 91
Presbyopic contact lens, 397t
    correction, 424–426
    disposable, 401t, 404t
Prescription
    incorrect, 315
    requirements, 500–501
Preservatives, 157–159
Primary surgical procedures, 555–558

Prism, 37
    verification of, 191
Prism ballast, 349, 352, 418
    for soft lens, 370
    trial lens set, 353t
Prism thickness formula, 41
Prismatic correction, 9
Prismatic effects
    accommodative demand, 38
    of contact lenses, 37–38, 38t
    of lens correction, 38f
Proclear and Biofinity Multifocals, 406
Proclear EP, 406
Proclear 1 day Multifocal lens, 404
    power selection for, 405t
Profitability, of gas-permeable lenses, 90
Progent protein remover, 160
Projection topography, 61–63
Prosthetic contact lenses, 592–593
Protein remover, 160
Pseudoaspheric design, 148
Pseudomonas, 158, 170f, 321, 501, 671
Pseudomonas aeruginosa, 90, 452, 662
Punctal plugs, 684–685
Pupil diameter, 4–5, 68, 124
    measurement of, 5f
PureVision Multi-Focal lens, 402–403
PureVision 2 (PV2), 403
PVA. *See* Polyvinyl alcohol

Quad Sym, 545, 547f
Quattro lens, 403
    power selection, 404t

Radius tools, 234f
Radiuscope, 188f, 189f
Reading glasses, 422
Recentration, 167–168
Reduced comfort, 210–211
Reduced vision, 204–210
    decentration and, 205–207
    flexure and, 205
    power change and, 210
    soft lenses and, 314–317
    warpage and, 205
Refits
    gas-permeable lenses, 103, 217–220
    PMMA lenses, 217–219
    procedures, 220
    of silicone hydrogel lenses, 275
    soft lenses, 219–220
    strategy, 219
Reflection topography, 60–61
Refraction, 8, 398
Refractive astigmatism, 367–368
Refractive corneal ablation, 588
    gas-permeable lens design, 589
    soft lens designs, 589
Refractive correction, 30–35, 39–40
Refractive error
    of gas-permeable lenses, 101
    silicone hydrogel lenses, 272

Refractive index, 256
Refractive information, 6–8
Refractive power, 124
    clinical measurement of, 31
    with vertex distance, 31–33
Refractive surgery, 588
    gas-permeable lens design, 589
    incisional refractive surgery, 590–591
    refractive corneal ablation, 588
    soft lens designs, 589
Relative scale, 68–69
Relative spectacle magnification (RSM), 37
Relubricating drops, 161
Removal, 165f
    discomfort after, 319
    patient education, 164–166, 301, 303
    by practitioner, 166–167
    of soft lenses, 301, 303
Replacement schedules, 264–266
Repowering, 241, 243–245
Reservoir debris, 629
Residual astigmatism, 39, 344–354
    actual, 344–346
    calculated, 344–346
    correcting, 347–354, 362f
    spherical gas-permeable lenses for, 347
    spherical soft lenses for, 347–348
Retinoscopic reflex, 378
Reverse geometry designs, 615
Revitalens, 275, 288, 291
Rewetting, 161
    overnight contact lens wear and, 455
    for soft lenses, 296–297
Rigid gas-permeable contact lens
        design, 580–583
Rigid lens form 1040, 44f
Rigid lenses, 34
    common materials for, 441t
    fitting, 532
    front and back vertex powers for, 32t
    modification of, 229–230
    OAD of, 124
    for overnight contact lens wear, 440
    and soft lenses, 552
Rimexolone, 679–680
Ring jam, 67
Rose bengal, 15
Rose K diagnostic fitting set, 539t
Rose K2 IC design, 542, 543t
Rounded sponge pad, 245f

Sagittal scale, 69–70
Sagittal topography, 59f
SAI (surface asymmetry index) value, 75
Saline, 293–294
Scale
    absolute, 68–69
    relative, 68–69
    sagittal, 69–70
    tangential, 69–70
Scars, corneal, 11, 438f
Scheimpflug correction system, 61, 63f

Scheimpflug imaging, 526
Scheiner disk, 58
Schirmer tear test, 14, 14*f*
Scleral Lens Education Society, 610
Scleral lenses, 547, 609
    application and removal training, 624–625
    bubbles, 629–630
    case history, 617
    center thickness/lens materials, 616
    with circumferential blanching, 626*f*
    classification, 609–610
    conjunctival hooding, 628
    contact lens solutions, 625
    corneal touch, 626
    demonstrating ideal haptic fit, 622*f*
    design, 421, 611
    diagnostic lens fitting, 620
    dispensing, 624
    edge lift of, 627*f*
    edge modifications, 616
    equipment, 619–620
    haptic/landing zone, 614–615
    indications, 610–611
    lens compression and seal-off, 626–627
    lens deposits, 630–631
    lens flexure, 628
    lens selection and evaluation, 620–624
    with limbal congestion, 626*f*
    multifocals, 615
    nonwetting, 630, 630*f*
    ocular evaluation, 617–618
    optical zone, 612
    patient education, 618–619
    patient selection, 616
    reservoir debris, 629
    reverse geometry designs, 615
    safety and risk, 625
    scleral obstacles, 627–628
    solution toxicity/hypersensitivity, 630
    transitional zone, 612–614
    troubleshooting complications, 625
    uneven haptic bearing, 627
Scleral obstacles, 627–628
SCR. *See* Secondary curve radius
Scratches, patient education, 171
SEALs. *See* Superior epithelial arcuate lesions
Secondary curve radius (SCR), 127, 355
Sectorial injection, 331
Segmented, translating designs, 418–419
Semi-scleral lens designs, 546–548
Shack–Hartmann analyses, 403
Silicone elastomers, 439–440
Silicone hydrogel lenses, 96–97, 260*t*, 584
    advantages of, 272*t*
    age and, 274
    aphakia and, 274, 476–477
    applications, 366–379
    base curve radius, 276–277
    bulbar conjunctival disruptions, 449–450
    center thickness, 278–279
    compliance, 275
    complications associated with, 448

    contraindications, 270–271
    deposit-prone patients and, 273
    disadvantages of, 272*t*
    disinfection of, 292
    dry eye and, 273–274
    fitting, 275–279
    handling issues, 273
    indications, 270–271
    lens diameter, 277
    lens selection, 275–279
    materials, 442*t*
    occupation and, 275
    ocular disease and, 274
    ocular examination and, 281–282
    overnight contact lens wear of, 441, 444*t*
    part-time wearers, 275
    patient selection, 270–271
    power of, 277–278
    progress evaluation, 279–282
    refits, 275
    refractive error, 272
    superior epithelial arcuate lesions (SEALs) and, 449
    therapeutic use, 274
    tinted, 279
Siloxane, 257*f*
Single aspheric curve posterior surface, 148
Single-vision contact lenses, 422
Sjögren's syndrome, 3
Slit-lamp beam rotation, 349
Slit-lamp biomicroscopy, 162
    in keratoconus, 524–525
Slit-lamp evaluation, 9–11, 63*f*
Soaking, wetting and, 157–159
Sodium fluorescein, 621
Sodium sulfacetamide, 672
Soflens Multi-Focal lens, 402
Soft lenses, 19, 548. *See also* Hydrogel lenses
    advantages of, 19*t*
    applications, 366–379
    astigmatism and, 315
    bifocal, 401–413
    cast molding, 264
    classification of, 259, 261
    clinical signs, 324–336
    cosmetic wear of, 304
    defective, 316
    deposits, 294–295, 314–315
    designs, 589
    diameter of, 196
    discomfort, 317–320
    disinfection of, 287–293
    dryness and, 321–322
    eccentric lenticulation, 371
    edge inspection of, 196
    enzymatic cleaners for, 296
    extraction of, 263
    fitting, 502
    fitting pearls with, 413*t*
    foggy vision, 324
    full-thickness penetrating keratoplasty and, 583–584
    gas-permeable lenses v., 21, 219–220
    hardness of, 255

Soft lenses (*continued*)
  hazy vision, 324
  history and, 367
  hydration of, 257–258, 263
  HydroKone, 550–551
  incorrect prescriptions and, 315
  insertion of, 301, 303
  inversion, 317
  ionic charge, 257
  KeraSoft lens, 548–549
  keratoconus and, 548–552
  lathing, 263
  lens movement of, 323
  lubricants for, 296–297, 297t
  material properties of, 252–261
  modulus of elasticity of, 255
  multifocal, 401–413
  NovaKone design, 550
  occupation and, 369
  orthokeratology and, 663
  oxygen permeability of, 258–259, 260t
  patient education, 297–305
  periballasting, 371
  photophobia and, 320–321
  physiologic problems, 378–379
  polishing, 263
  power of, 196
  prism ballasting for, 370
  problem solving, 313–339
  reduced vision and, 314–317
  refitting, 219–220
  refractive index of, 256
  removal of, 301, 303
  replacement schedule, 264–266
  rewetting, 296–297, 297t
  saline, 293–294
  selection of, 21
  spherical, 347–348
  spin casting, 263–264
  staining, 325–326
  sterilization of, 263
  stiffness of, 255
  surface inspection of, 196
  surfactant cleaners for, 295–296
  symptoms, 314–324
  tensile strength of, 255
  terminology, 313–314
  tinting, 263
  toric, 348, 354–355, 376
  toric lens rotation and, 316
  toric multifocal, 369t
  truncation, 370
  verification of, 196
  wear, 271t
  wearing schedules for, 264
  wet cell power, 196, 199f
  wettability of, 256–257
Solution toxicity, 630
Solutions, combination, 158t
Solvents, 160–161
Soper Cone design, 537
  diagnostic lens set, 537t
Specific gravity (SG), 96
Spectacle lens power, at corneal plane, 704–705
Spectacle magnification (SM), 35–37
  clinical implications of, 36–37
  formulae, 40
  relative spectacle magnification (RSM), 37
Spectacles, 317, 497
  contact lenses v., 18–19
  in keratoconus, 531–532
  management, 531–532
Speculum, 484f
Spherical lenses
  calculator, GPLI toric and, 360
  gas-permeable, 347, 354
  soft, 347–348
  verification of, 190–191
Spherical optical zone, 148
Spherical power effect, 359f
  bitoric diagnostic lenses, 361–365
Sphero–cylindrical OR, 373
Spin casting, 263–264
SPK. *See* Superficial punctate keratitis
Sponge tool, 238
Sports, contact lens in, 20t, 500
Squeeze-film force, 658
SRAX index, 75
Stability
  accelerated, 371
  dynamic, 370–371
  of gas-permeable lenses, 90
  techniques for, 370–371
Staff education, 692
  billing and fees, 693–695
Staining, 81
  corneal, 447
  patterns, 325f
  soft lenses, 325–326
Staphylococcus aureus, 670
Staphylococcus epidermidis, 670
Sterilization, 263
Stiffness, 255
Stinging sensation, 319–320
Storage solutions, 158t
Striae, 444–445
  Vogt's striae, 524, 525f
Suction cups, 231f
Sulfa drugs, 672
Superficial punctate keratitis (SPK), 378
Superior epithelial arcuate lesions (SEALs), 379
  silicone hydrogel lenses and, 449
Surface polishing, 240–241
Surface quality
  of soft lenses, 196
  verification of, 196
Surface wettability, 94–95
Surfactants
  abrasive, 159–160
  cleaners, 295–296
  nonabrasive, 159
  soaking solutions, 160

Swimming, 173
SynergEyes lens, 292, 421, 554–555, 586

Tangent streak, 418f, 419f
Tangential map, 140
Tangential scale, 69–70
Tap water, 177–179
Tarsal conjunctiva, 10
Tear breakup time (TBUT), 12–13, 322, 618
Tear film evaluation, 11–18, 398
Tear film stability, 213
Tear layer power, 142–143
Tear lens calculations, 144f
Tear meniscus evaluation, 12
Tear osmolarity, 16–17
Tear prism, 67f
TearLab Osmolarity System, 17
Tensile strength, 255
Tetracurve, 127
Thermal disinfection, 292–293
Thickness. *See* Center thickness; Edge thickness
Thimerosal, 158
3 and 9 o'clock staining management, 81
Three-point touch, 533–534
Tight lens syndrome, 328
Tinting
    silicone hydrogel lenses, 279
    of soft lenses, 263
Tobramycin, 671
Toddlers, insertion, 484
Tomography applications, 526
Topical anesthetics, 113–114
Topical antibiotics, 674t
Topography. *See specific types*
Toric lenses, 191
    back surface, 355–358
    physiologic problems, 378
    rotation, 316
    soft, 348, 354–355, 369t
    soft lenses and, 316
    verification of, 190, 191
Toricity
    back, 371, 378
    front, 378
Transitional zone, 612–614
Translating
    absence of, 421f
    bifocal lenses, 407–408, 416–422, 420f
    multifocal lenses, 407–408
Transparency, 254–255
Trial frame, 349, 350f
Trichiasis, 9
Trimethoprim, 670, 671
Triton Translating Bifocal lens, 407

Truncation
    prism ballast and, 352–353
    for soft lens, 370

Ultraviolet blockers, 100
Uneven haptic bearing, 627

Vancomycin eyedrops, 670
Vascularized limbal keratitis, 213, 215f
Vertex distance, 31–33, 39, 42, 144–145
Vertex powers, 494–495
Vertical meridian, 73–74
    asymmetry in, 75f
Videokeratograph, 7–8, 59
    in keratoconus, 522–524
Vision, binocular, 35–39
Vision quality, 89
    foggy, 324
    hazy, 324
    reduced, 204–210, 314–317
Vision Service Plan (VSP), 559
Vision shaping treatment, 657
    BE Retainer system, 657–658
    Contex OK E-System, 658–659
    DreamLens, 659
    Emerald lens, 659
Vision therapy, 3
Visions Ultra Thin lenses, 115
Vistakon, 443
Visual acuity, 162, 317
Visual response, 376–378
Vogt's striae, 524, 525f

Warped lenses, 190
    reduced vision and, 205
    verification of, 190
Water, tap, 177–179
Watermelon seed principle, 370
WAVE system, 139
Wearing schedules
    aphakia and, 487
    overnight contact lens wear, 454–455
    for soft lenses, 264
Wettability, 256–257
Wetting, 157–159
    agents, 159
    poor surface, 207–210
    preservatives in, 157–159
    solutions, 161t

X-Cel Contacts, 115

Zaditor, 506t, 675